Table of Contents

**Information
on IMIA**

Review Section

**Research and
Education Section**

3605296010

Yearbook

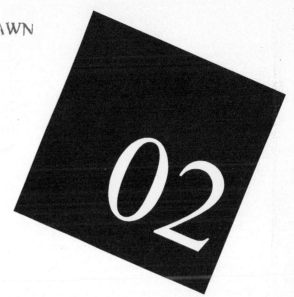

02

of
Medical Informatics

Medical Imaging Informatics

Editors:
  Reinhold Haux
  Casimir Kulikowski

Managing Editors:
  Elske Ammenwerth
  Andreas Bohne
  Klaus Ganser
  Petra Knaup
  Christoph Maier
  André Michel
  Reiner Singer
  Astrid C. Wolff

Regional Editors:
  Arie Hasman
  Sedick Isaacs
  Jochen Moehr
  Charles Safran
  Chun Por Wong

Advisory Board:
  Marion Ball
  Jan H. van Bemmel
  Alexa T. McCray

Guest Editors:
  Stephen Chu
  Gregory F. Cooper
  Jens Dørup
  Ralf Hofestädt
  Sedick Isaacs
  Michio Kimura
  Pablo Laguna

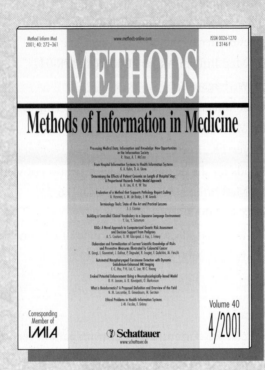

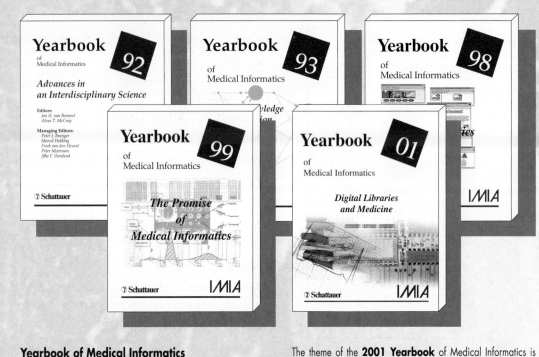

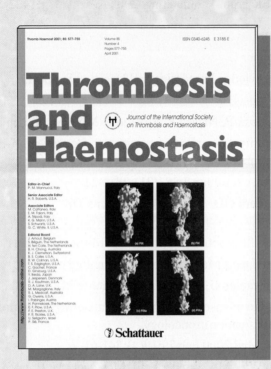

Section 7:
Bioinformatics

Faculty of Informatics and Communication
Central Queensland University

Central Queensland University's Faculty of Informatics and Communication is the only faculty of its kind in Australia. It aims to bring together in a creative and innovative way a range of disciplines which are concerned with the Information Age, such as
- information technology,
- human and computer-mediated communication,
- information systems,
- multimedia, and
- mathematics.

As a faculty our goals are to maximise opportunities for courses that meet student and employer needs, to create new synergies between discipline areas which stimulate and support teaching and research, and to seek partnerships with industry and the wider community in order to contribute to social and economic development.

The faculty offers a Bachelor of Nursing Informatics (Post registration), Bachelor of Nursing Informatics (Honours), a Graduate Diploma and Masters degree in Health Informatics with a choice of specialisations, nursing, management or e-health, Masters by research and Doctorate by research. All programs are offered by distance education using various combinations of print based and on line teaching methods. The University's information literacy program has been a focus for numerous teaching and learning research grants and recognised as a flagship program internationally, as well as within Australia. CQU has an excellent infrastructure supporting students engaged in flexible (distance) learning. Students can choose to locate in any of our 14 campuses ranging from Queensland regional centres, large Australian cities and international locations. Around 60% of the Faculty's students are from overseas.

Contact course advisor k.bloxsom@cqu.edu.au or

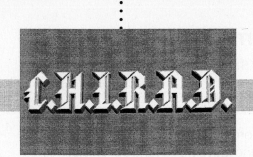

C.H.I.R.A.D.

Centre for Health Information Research and Development, King Alfred's College, Winchester, UK

A new **MSc in Health Informatics** has been designed by experts from CHIRAD at King Alfred's College Winchester that enables students to:-

- Distinguish their competencies from others working in the domain; give yourself the edge
- Position themselves to manage complex projects and develop sound organisational strategies involving ICTs
- Effectively harness ICTs to contribute to clinical practice and health management appropriately
- Engage in productive dialogue and critical review, setting user demands in context and technology in its place
- Keep pace with the rapid development of ICTs, changing clinical demands and organisational environments and be able to assess their impact on your own workplace situation
- Recognise the human and organisational issues raised by ICTs and how they can be resolved
- Play a significant role in the release and realisation of predicted benefits from ICT use in the health domain
- Operate effectively with the support of the world-wide evidence base in health and informatics themes
- Empower themselves with generic skills in research methodologies, evaluation, critical analysis and effective dissemination of messages

It will have a mix of taught and independent study supported by a Virtual Learning Environment on the Internet.

Taught Modules will include:
- Health Informatics in Clinical Practice
- Developments in Informatics
- Strategic Management
- Human and Organisational Issues
- Research Methods

Taught by a team of world-renowned Health Informatic experts who will help you to make a difference to patient care through the application of informatics concepts. www.chirad.org/

**For more details contact
Professor Graham Wright**

**G.Wright@wkac.ac.uk
Telephone - fax 01962 827373**

Department of Medical Informatics
University of Heidelberg

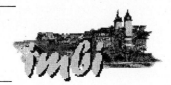

Research

Information infrastructures for health care are investigated with special emphasis on fully electronic medical records, authentication and digital signature, records shared among institutions and professions.

Medical documentation research concentrates on registries, quality assurance of records, ontology-based electronic data capture (EDC) for multi-center clinical trials, and usage of speech recognition for note taking.

Knowledge based decision support spans from basic decision theoretic investigation to implementing guidelines in clinical pathways.

Projects are normally run in close cooperation with clinical partners. In several cases they include health technology assessment activities. The conjoint Department of Medical Biometry becomes involved whenever experimental investigations of new methods are aimed at.

Education

Education covers the full from graduate, post-graduate and Ph.D. academic curricula to vocational classes for radiology and laboratory assistants. In cooperation with the University of Applied Sciences Heilbronn, the department is responsible for the only German Master's (Diploma) program in Medical Informatics and a post-graduate program for physicians on Information Management in Medicine. The Akademie Medizinische Informatik (akadeMIe) offers several courses for IT career development in the health care sector. Online courses have just been started.

Professional organizations and international contacts

International education and career development is supported through a cooperation with other leading curricula in Amsterdam, NL, Minneapolis, MN, and Salt Lake City, UT which constitute the IΦE (International Partnership in Health Informatics Education). Besides serving in several national organizations such as GMDS (German Society for Medical Informatics, Biometry and Epidemiology) or GI (Association for Informatics), the department edits the Methods of Information in Medicine and the IMIA Yearbook of Medical Informatics.

Contact: Thomas Wetter, University of Heidelberg, Department of Medical Informatics, Im Neuenheimer Feld 400, D-69120 Heidelberg, Germany, Thomas_Wetter@med.uni-heidelberg.de

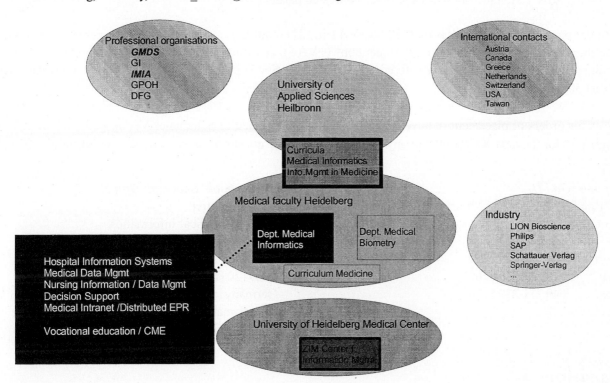

Impressum

The Yearbook of Medical Informatics gives an overview of the latest outstanding research contributions in the field of Health and Medical Informatics.

The Yearbook includes original reviews, reports on research and educational programmes in Health and Medical Informatics, information about IMIA activities and member societies as well as original papers which have been selected as best papers of the recent year. These papers are selected based on an international review process, taking into account their significance, their quality, their originality, and their clarity and organization. The Yearbook of Medical Informatics 2002 covers papers which appeared in refereed journals between April 2000 and March 2001.

Suggestions for high-quality papers for the Yearbook of Medical Informatics 2003 are welcome. They must have been published between April 2001 and March 2002. Suggestions should be sent to the Editorial Office before May 1, 2002.

The publication of the IMIA Yearbook of Medical Informatics is a joint project of the International Medical Informatics Association (IMIA) and F.K. Schattauer Verlagsgesellschaft mbH, Stuttgart – New York. The copyright on the Yearbook remains vested in IMIA and Schattauer. The Yearbook is published annually in March and is thereafter delivered to IMIA's Member Societies and other interested parties.

The regular price of the Yearbook is EUR 30,00 +VAT in EU countries and US$ 30 elsewhere per copy including surface shipping, the student price is EUR 10 per copy (+VAT). Discounts are given if the Yearbook is ordered in larger quantities. The Yearbook will be offered to IMIA Member Societies for a special price if ordered in quantities of at least 50 copies.

Requests for orders of placement of advertisements should be directed to Schattauer Verlagsgesellschaft before September 1st for the next Yearbook. For any other suggestions or questions, please contact the Editorial Office.

Schattauer GmbH
Verlag für Medizin und Naturwissenschaften
P.O. Box 104543
D-70040 Stuttgart
Germany
Tel: +49 711 229 870
Fax: +49 711 229 8750

IMIA Yearbook Editorial Office
Martina Hutter
Dept. of Medical Informatics
University of Heidelberg
Im Neuenheimer Feld 400
D-69120 Heidelberg
Germany
E-mail: martina_hutter@med.uni-heidelberg.de
Homepage: http://www.yearbook.uni-hd.de

ISBN 3-7945-2193-5
ISSN 0943-4747

Nicholas Ayache

INRIA - The French National Institute for
Research in Computer Science and Control
Sophia-Antipolis, France

Preface

From Digital Anatomy to Virtual Scalpels and Image Guided Therapy

Medical imaging informatics will bring about a revolution in medicine in the 21st century, introducing a collection of powerful new tools designed to better assist clinical diagnosis and to model, simulate, and guide patient's therapy more efficiently. A new discipline is emerging in computer science, closely related to others such as computer vision, computer graphics, artificial intelligence and robotics.

How could a plausible scenario of tomorrow's hospital room look? First, all imaging modalities will be interconnected to fuse the available anatomical and functional data of a patient and exploit them in a coherent manner. The images involved will not only be radiographs, computed tomographies, magnetic resonance, nuclear medicine, or ultrasound images, but also video, endoscopic, confocal, microscopic, histological, or molecular images. This information will be processed in 3-D, as most imaging modalities are volumetric, but also in 4-D whenever temporal sequences are available, either to detect subtle changes or to quantify a dynamic motion (typically for cardiac analysis). The physician will, therefore, be provided with new sets of quantitative measurements to assess a more accurate and objective diagnosis. At this stage, digital image processing will often play the same role as the microscope during the 17th century, allowing visualization of details or changes which otherwise, would have remained invisible, by a direct visualization of the original images(*).

When a therapy has been decided upon, pre-operative diagnostic images will serve to optimally prepare a therapy. Mostly interactive, the software tools will enhance the capacities of the physicians, offering the possibility to experiment various approaches before selecting the best one. Virtual reality display and force feed-back (haptic) devices will provide realistic training for therapy, allowing the surgeon to practice on virtual but highly realistic models and scalpels. Once the actual treatment has to be delivered, image-guided therapy procedures will rely on various types of intra-operative images. Augmented reality tools will enhance the perceptual capacities of the physician by fusing the intra-operative images with pre-operative images and models, including, for instance, high resolution digital atlases.

High speed networks will permit the transmission of images and gestures to remote sites, where medical robots will enhance, or replace, the physicians' gestures, often with help of real-time processing of intra-operative images.

This will allow, for instance, compensation of a moving organ (e.g. the beating heart), offering the possibility for surgeons to operate on a quasi-still image while a robot adds the required computed motion to his gestures. Finally, post-operative images will be automatically compared to pre-operative images, in order to better assess the efficiency of the therapy. This will also be useful to objectively measure the efficiency of a drug treatment and, thus, better control the design of new medication and therapeutic protocols.

Is this scenario a dream? Certainly not. We know that parts of this scenario are already operational in a few leading medical centers. Also, research on these topics is more active than ever across the globe, in all areas of medical image processing and analysis, including the acquisition, reconstruction, enhancement, compression, storage, transmission, visualization and understanding of medical images. The major methodological research topics that have emerged include segmentation, registration and fusion, dynamic analysis from temporal sequences, modeling of anatomy and physiology from anatomical or functional images, content-based indexing, statistical analysis of shapes and signals, surgery simulation and image-guided medical robotics. These topics often involve interdisciplinary methodologies. For instance, to create a digital model whose behavior mimics the actual body of a given patient as well as possible, surgery simulation requires geometric anatomical modeling with various modalities of medical imaging, bio-mechanical modeling of soft tissues, and the physiological modeling of organs and vessels.

A leading selection of articles in this Yearbook describe the state of the art developments of some of the most advanced research centers in medical informatics, and suggest some contours of this upcoming revolution.

(*) Citation from Gilles Kahn, Scientific Director of INRIA.

References

1. Bankman I, editor. Handbook of Medical Imaging – Processing and Analysis, Academic Press; 2000.
2. CAS: Int. Journal of Computer Aided Surgery, Wiley, http://www3.interscience. wiley.com/cgi-bin/jtoc?ID=56867
3. Duncan J, Ayache N. Medical Image Analysis: Progress over two decades and the challenges ahead. IEEE Transactions on Pattern Analysis and Machine Intelligence 2000;22(1):85-106.
4. Grimson E, Kikinis R, Jolesz F, Black P, Image Guided Surgery, Scientific American, June 1999.
5. Marescaux J, Clement JM, Tassetti V, Koehl C, Cotin S, Russier Y, et al. Virtual Reality Applied to Hepatic Surgery Simulation: The Next Revolution. Ann Surg 1998 Nov;228(5):627-34.
6. MedIA: Int. Journal on Medical Image Analysis, Elsevier. http://www.elsevier.nl/ locate/media
7. Medinfo'01: 10th World Congress on Health and Medical Informatics; http:// www.medinfo2001.org/
1. MICCAI'01: 4th Int. Conf. on Medical Image Computing and Computer-Assisted Intervention Conference, Utrecht, Holland, Oct. 2001; http://miccai.isi.uu.nl/
8. Robb RA. Biomedical Imaging, Visualization and Analysis. New York, NY: John Wiley and Sons, Inc.; 1999.
6. Taylor RH, Lavallee S, Burdea G, Mosges R, editors. Computer-Integrated Surgery. Cambridge, Massachusetts: MIT Press; 1996.
8. TMI: IEEE Transactions on Medical Imaging, http://ieeexplore.ieee.org/lpdocs/ epic03/RecentIssues.htm?punumber=42

Address of the author:
Nicholas Ayache
Research Director, Epidaure Project,
Medical Imaging and Robotics
INRIA Sophia Antipolis
2004 Route des Lucioles
F-06902 Sophia-Antipolis, France
E-mail: nicholas.ayache@sophia.inria.fr
URL: http://www.inria.fr/personnel/ Nicholas.Ayache

Casimir A. Kulikowski[1]
Reinhold Haux[2]

Editors

[1] Department of Computer Science
Rutgers - The State University of New Jersey
New Brunswick, New Jersey, USA
[2] Department of Medical Informatics
University of Heidelberg
Heidelberg, Germany
and
University for Health Informatics and Technology Tyrol
Innsbruck, Austria

Editorial

Medical Imaging Informatics

The 2002 Yearbook of Medical Informatics takes as its theme the topic of Medical Imaging Informatics. The visual nature of so much critical information in the practice, research, and education of medicine and health care would suggest that computer-based imaging and its related fields of graphics and visualization should be central to the practice of medical informatics. Yet, historically, this has not usually been the case. The need for technological sub-specialization on the part of imaging researchers and the frequently opposite tendency towards generality of information systems studied and developed by informatics researchers may have contributed to an increasing separation between the fields in the period from the 1970's to the 1990's.

A trend towards re-convergence, however, began in the early 1990's as important new image database, mapping, registration, and segmentation issues arose in the context of neuro-imaging with the Human Brain Project [1,2], and multimodal, whole body imaging with the Visible Human Project [3,4]. There was early recognition of the need for computer-based knowledge representations, not only of anatomy at the tissue level, but also at the multiple underlying biological levels (cellular, molecular, atomic) leading to the definition of structural informatics [5], and the development of a Foundational Model of Anatomy [6]. Meanwhile, knowledge representations for integrating multimodal image interpretations [7], methods for modeling elastically deformable anatomical objects [8], integrated segmentation and visualization systems [9], knowledge-based methods [10], and model-driven systems for surgery and education [11] have been gradually helping renew connections between imaging and mainstream informatics work. Encouraging further productive collaborations between researchers in imaging and informatics was one of our motivations in the choice of Medical Imaging Informatics as the theme for this Yearbook.

The Yearbook of Medical Informatics is distributed through IMIA's Member and Corresponding Member Societies worldwide. For the 2002 Yearbook we expect that over 7,000 copies will reach the memberships of 45 Member and 8 Corresponding member societies. The Yearbook's editors are grateful for the contributions of distinguished researchers in medical informatics who have prepared five invited review papers, six research and education papers, and six synopses of papers included in the different disciplinary fields covered. In addition we owe a debt of gratitude to the 49 reviewers who assisted in the selection of papers from the recent refereed literature.

The present Yearbook includes papers selected from the literature for the period April 2000 to March 2001. The criteria for selection include topic significance, representativeness and coverage of research in a given subfield, subject to appropriately high levels of quality in presentation and results. A more detailed description of these quality criteria can be downloaded from http://www.Yearbook.uni-hd.de/ quality_criteria.pdf. The referees score and rank the papers, and the final selection is made by the editors with the advice of editorial board members from each of the specialty areas. We expect to publish a description of the quality criteria used in selection in the medical informatics literature in the coming year to help provide more general insight on this process [12].

This year's preface to the Yearbook „From Digital Anatomy to Virtual Scapels and Image Guided Therapy" has been prepared by Nicholas Ayache, Research Director for the Epidaure Project, Medical Imaging and Robotics of INRIA (The French National Institute for Research in Computer Science and Control), Sophia Antipolis, France.

Imaging Informatics and Medical/Health Care Informatics: The Opportunities and Constraints of Interdisciplinarity

Medical informatics researchers have contributed to the development of medical imaging methods and systems since the inception of this field

approximately 40 years ago. Starting in the mid-1970's rapid progress in computer-based imaging research and practice came from the increasingly specialized, highly mathematical, bio-physical, and engineering models of different imaging modalities (CT, MRI, digital angiography, ultrasound, nuclear medicine imaging, etc.). Various specialties such as radiology, cardiology, and nuclear medicine distinguished themselves by concentrating their efforts on the technologies most effective for their own diagnostic and therapeutic goals. Hospital or enterprise-wide storage and retrieval of large numbers of patient image studies led to the development of PACS systems, but, technological, organizational, and economic constraints tended to divorce them from novel imaging research, and they frequently became just another part of the IT infrastructure for hospitals and clinics. Meanwhile, professional societies and conferences devoted exclusively to biomedical imaging and its subdisciplines proliferated. The number of researchers in the mainstream of medical informatics who remained professionally active in medical imaging began to shrink, and this trend continued until recently.

The combination of more advanced and user-friendly medical image data bases, coupled with improved 2D and 3D reconstruction, visualization and navigation algorithms, is making medical imaging results more accessible to physicians at the point of care. Starting in the early 1990's the Visible Human Project produced a widely available reference set of multimodal images of the whole body. Its wide dissemination has led to much anatomically-detailed education software, but more importantly, it has raised important informatics issues of knowledge representation, modeling, and information retrieval for dealing with large-scale repositories of such multimodal digital image sets. The Human Brain

Project initiated at around the same time led to a very large number of projects in brain data mapping, registration and segmentation, all of which made clear the new informatics, biometrics, and computational imaging challenges inherent in integrating massive visual datasets of subject-specific data which needed to be abstracted and summarized into atlases and retrievable maps of the brain. Possibly as result, there has been a re-awakened interest of medical informatics researchers in imaging problems, and the development of what can be identified as a medical imaging informatics subspecialty [13]. This is centered around the problems of image data representation and abstraction, where ontologies for describing the underlying medical knowledge needed to interpret images are now being developed in computationally explicit form [14]. This will not only assist in standardization and interoperability, but will be crucial in making image data more usable for data mining, decision support, and visual modeling and simulation.

Fundamental issues in imaging that are well-known to medical informatics researchers include: standards for image information exchange, communication protocols, underlying computer data and knowledge representations, coding, nomenclature and vocabulary for including imaging information in the electronic medical record, relation to computerized guidelines for health care, information compression, efficient indexing of image databases, security and confidentiality of imaging records, etc.

There are also many informatics challenges that require deeper scientific, technical, and medical expertise as imaging information becomes more integrated and pervasive to the practice of medicine. These include:
· the development of better human-computer interaction models for

health care that rely not only on the increasing power of graphics and visualization but also on good psychophysical and cognitive science studies, given the multiresolution nature of many medical imaging studies, and how this affects perception and interpretation of data;

· developing better techniques for automatic segmentation and registration of medical images in 3D as well as 2D;

· data abstraction, summarization, and graphical (iconic) representation involved in atlas construction;

· representation of biological variability across repositories of bioimaging data to interpret imaging data across populations, and the linking of phenotype to genotype data;

· improving ways of integrating results from automatic image segmentation with expertly derived manual segmentations and annotations - and methods for evaluating the outcomes;

· developing annotation languages for extracting key patient findings found within the massive quantity and great level of detail inherent in medical imaging data;

· creating underlying computer-based representations of knowledge (ontologies, atlases, etc.) to help formalize such communication, while also preserving the flexibility needed for capturing novelty and enabling discovery;

· embedding advanced imaging systems in more general health care delivery software and evaluating their results within health care environments with effective feedback for learning how to modify and update the imaging methods in different clinical contexts.

As researchers in medical imaging informatics begin to address these and other topics, we hope that the 2002 IMIA Yearbook's theme will stimulate greater interaction among imaging and informatics researchers in the development of working systems for the practice of health care, and the improvement of education.

Review Sections

As is customary, the 2002 Yearbook includes a number of original review articles, which focus primarily on this year's theme. An article by Michael Ackerman on "Visible Human Project: From Data to Knowledge" updates the status of this seminal project for the field. "Imaging Informatics and the Human Brain Project: The Role of Structure" by Jim Brinkley and Cornelius Rosse, provides a comprehensive review of how imaging informatics approaches were essential for the Human Brain Project and the development of structural informatics, and have led to the development of a computer-based foundational model of anatomical structure. Wieslaw Nowinski gives a systematic review of the application of different modeling methods for enhancing neuroimaging results. Two papers address other important topics to medical informatics: Bonnie Kaplan and Nicola T Shaw use evaluation processes to review how people, organizations, and social issues impact medical informatics concerns; and Gunnar Klein reviews advances in standards-setting activities in the field.

Education and Research in Medical Informatics

The Yearbook provides an opportunity for highlighting an international selection of current education, training, and research programs in Medical Informatics. This year Russ B. Altman describes the program in Biomedical Computation at Stanford University which increasingly introduces biomolecular as well as clinical applications of informatics. Marius Fieschi,

D. Fieschi, J. Gouvernet, M. Joubert, and G. Soula provide an overview of Research and Development in Health Informatics at the Faculty of Medicine of Marseille, while György Kozman of Veszprem University describes how education in medical informatics is based on an information technology curriculum at his university. Yu-Chuan Li presents the Evolving Biomedical Informatics Program at Taipei Medical University, and Wendy McPhee writes about Education Downunder from the Centre of Medical Informatics at Monash University. Finally Edward H. Shortliffe describes the changes in the program in Bio-Medical Informatics at Columbia University, where he has recently assumed the chairmanship.

Challenges in Medical Informatics

In this section, three papers can be found dealing with the future of Medical Informatics. Incoming IMIA President KC Lun (Singapore) describes important future tasks of IMIA. Mark Musen (Stanford) reports on the outcomes of an IMIA satellite conference on this topic. Finally, the result of a panel discussion on the future impact of information and communication technology on health care, addressed by clinicians, researchers and industrial representatives, is presented.

Guest Editors

After the selection of papers to be included in the Yearbook had been accomplished, guest editors were asked to write Synopses reviewing the papers in the different sections. The section on Health and Clinical Management was edited by Steven Chu of the University of Auckland; that on Patient Records by Michio Kimura of Hamamatsu University, that on Health Information Systems by Sedick Isaacs of South Africa, the section on Signal Processing by Pablo Laguna of Zaragoza University, and that on Knowledge Processing and Decision Support by Greg Cooper of the University of Pittsburgh. Computer-supported education had as guest editor Jens Dørup of Aarhus University, and the section on Bioinformatics was edited by Ralf Hofestädt of the University of Bielefeld.

IMIA

The Yearbook contains detailed information about IMIA, its Member Societies, Working Groups, and Special Interest Groups. Preparation of the general pages describing IMIA activities received considerable assistance from Steve Huesing, the Executive Director. The section on IMIA Working Groups and Special Interest Groups was greatly aided by contributions from Nancy Lorenzi.

For the first time in this Yearbook, a more detailed report on the activities of IMIA regions is included with the help of Regional Editors. We would like to thank Arie Hasman (for EFMI), Sedick Isaacs (for Helina), Jochen Moehr and Charles Safran (for the North American IMIA Member Societies), and Chun Por Wong (for APAMI) for their support.

The IMIA representatives from the individual countries provided the material for their own national societies.

The 2003 IMIA Yearbook

The theme of the 2003 Yearbook will be on the Informatics Foundations of the Quality of Healthcare. With the increasing automation of health care systems, the more widespread introduction of electronic patient records, and the application of evidence-based

medicine guidelines for care, as well as the world-wide concerns for controlling costs in health care systems, there has been growing research on the impact of informatics systems on the quality of health care, and its implications for patients and health care practitioners.

The 2003 Yearbook will continue its coverage of all topics in medical informatics, including the one newly added this year, that of bioinformatics, which, due to its long-term implications for the development of molecular medicine and its methodological connections to medical informatics, will now become a permanent section of the Yearbook.

Advisory Board

The Editors wish to thank the members of the Advisory Board for their invaluable contributions to the planning of this Yearbook. They are: Marion Ball, Vice-President of Health-link, Inc. of Baltimore, MD, Jan H. van Bemmel, Rector of Erasmus University Rotterdam, The Netherlands, and Alexa McCray, Director of the Lister Hill Center of the National Library of Medicine, NIH, USA (Figure 1). Their

experience has been essential in helping chart a course of excellence and world-wide coverage for the Yearbook during this period of rapid change in medical informatics.

Acknowledgements

The editors gratefully acknowledge the contributions of the Referees and Guest Editors. They would also like to thank the writers of the professionally critical Review Papers and the contributors to the Education and Research Section.

They are most appreciative of the considerable skill, time, and effort devoted by the Managing Editors, especially the Executive Managing Editor Elske Ammenwerth, and by the Section Managing Editors, Andreas Bohne, Klaus Ganser, Petra Knaup, Christoph Maier, Andre Michel, Reiner Singer, and Astrid Wolff. A considerable amount of the organizational support was carried out by the staff at the Department of Medical Informatics at the University of Heidelberg, where we most especially thank the Editorial Assistant, Martina Hutter, without whose untiring efforts the Yearbook would not have been completed.

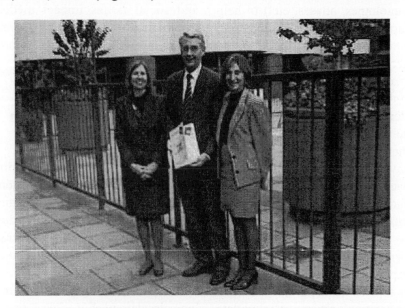

Fig.1. IMIA Yearbook Advisory Board Members (Alexa T. McCray, Jan H. van Bemmel, Marion J. Ball)

The referees who contributed to the selection of articles in the 2002 Yearbook of Medical Informatics are:

A. Abu-Hanna The Netherlands
H. Åhlfeldt, Sweden
R. Beuscart, France
A. Bolz, Germany
T. Bürkle, Germany
J.J. Cimino, USA
H. Dickhaus, Germany
J. Dørup, Denmark
M. Egmont-Petersen, The
    Netherlands
U. Engelmann, Germany
K.-H. Englmeier, Germany
G. Eysenbach, Germany
M. Fischer, Germany
D. Gamberger, Croatia
G. Gell, Austria
W.T.F. Goossen, The Netherlands
A.M. Grant, Canada
J. Grimson, Ireland
L. Hanmer, South Africa
E. Hovenga, Australia
H.K. Huang, USA
R. Jané Campos, Spain
M. Kaus, Germany
G. Kozmann, Hungary
T. Lehmann, Germany
N. Maglaveras, Greece
V. Maojo, Spain
F. Martin Sánchez, Spain
W. McPhee, Australia
A. Merzweiler, Germany
J. Möhr, Canada
P. Molholt, USA
P.W. Moorman, The Netherlands

J. Murphy, United Kingdom
C. Nøhr, Denmark
N. Oliveri, Argentina/USA
C. Quantin, France
C. Safran, USA
G. Schiff, USA
B. Seroussi, France
Y. Shahar, Israel
M. Stefanelli, Italy
I.M. Symonds, New Zealand
M. van Gils, Finland
R. Walton, United Kingdom
A. Winter, Germany
W. Wolf, Germany
T. Yoo, Korea
J. Zvárová, Czech Republic

References

1. Toga AW. Three Dimensional Neuroimaging, Raven Press, NY, 1990.
2. Koslow SH, Huerta MF, editors. Neuroinformatics: an overview of the Human Brain Project. Mahwah, New Jersey: Lawrence Erlbaum; 1997.
3. National Library of Medicine (U.S.) Board of Regents. Electronic imaging: National Institutes of Health. NIH Publication 1990. p. 90-2197.
4. National Library of Medicine (U.S.). Proceedings of the Third Visible Human Project Conference. Banvard RA, editor. October 5-6, 2000, Bethesda, MD: US Department of Health and Human Services, Public Health Service, National Institutes of Health; 2000.
5. Brinkley JF. Structural informatics and its applications in medicine and biology. Academic Medicine 1991;66(10):589-91.
6. Rosse C, Mejino JL, Modayur BR, Jakobovits RM, Hinshaw KP, Brinkley JF. Motivation and organizational principles for anatomical knowledge representation: the Digital Anatomist symbolic knowledge base. Journal of the American Medical Informatics Association 1998;5(1):17-40.
7. Höhne KH, Pflesser B, Riemer M, Schiemann T, Schubert R, Tiede U. A new representation of knowledge concerning human anatomy and function. Nature Medicine 1995;1(6):506-10.
8. Gee JC, Reivich M, Bajcsy R. Elastically deforming 3D atlas to match anatomical brain images. J Comput Assist Tomogr 1993;17(2):225-36.
9. Robb RA, Hanson DP, The ANALYZE software system for visualization and analysis in surgery simulation. In Lavalle S, Taylor R, Burdea G. Mosges R, editors. Computer Integrated Surgery. MIT Press, Cambridge, MA 1995. p. 175-90.
10. Gong L, Kulikowski CA. Composition of image analysis processes through object-centered hierarchical planning. IEEE Trans Pattern Analysis and Machine Intelligence 1995:997-1009.
11. Kikinis R, Shenton ME, Iosifescu DV, McCarley RW, Saiviroonporn P, Hokama HH, et al. A digital brain atlas for surgical planning, model-driven segmentation, and teaching. IEEE Trans. Visualization and Computer Graphics 1996;2(3):232-41.
12. Ammenwerth E, Wolff AC, Knaup P, Skontzki S, van Bemmel JH, McCray AT, Haux R, Kulikowski CA. Quality criteria for medical informatics research papers, submitted for publication, 2002.
13. Kulikowski CA. Medical imaging informatics: challenges of definition and integration. J Am Med Inform Assoc 1997;4(3):252-3.
14. Mejino JLV, Noy NF, Mussen MA, Brinkley JF, Rosse C. Representation of structural relationships in the foundational model of anatomy. IN: Proc. AMIA Fall Symp, Washington DC, 2001. p. 973.

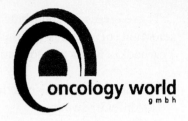

Company Profile

Oncology World offers a new dimension of services in oncology providing complete knowledge management solutions for all executives in the healthcare industries. The company's weapon to fight cancer is based on its unique database-technology, extensive oncological expertise and in-depth technical know-how of its staff.

Technology

Oncology World has built up a highly sophisticated IT-architecture - a worldwide unique combination of a Data Warehouse and an object-oriented Knowledge Base. The Data Warehouse contains terabytes of worldwide cancer-relevant data. By modeling a pre-defined structure in which all the data from the various sources can be integrated, **Oncology World** reorganizes these data in a meta-structure model interlinked by UID (unique identifiers) or merge keys to create an interlinked data platform for further analysis. Business-Intelligence-Tools perform impact analysis and derive new data from the interlinked platform. By creating and deploying data marts – where customer specific scaled-down warehouse concepts are realized - crucial information is delivered. The Knowledge Base system excels in giving direct and fast access to knowledge content and provides valid and high quality retrieval results. It is easy to maintain and up-date since all information is not stored as document, but as information fragment in a defined interchangeable location in the Knowledge Base system.

Portfolio

Oncology World´s portfolio contains strategic, scientific consulting, technical consulting, reports and scientific information (available at www.oncology-world.com) tailored to the individual requirements of today´s healthcare industries. The company´s products and services provide increased dynamics of innovation and empower to make faster, smarter and more confident decisions resulting in an optimised product development process with significantly reduced time-to-market and reduced costs. **Oncology World** is already co-operating with renowned companies in worldwide healthcare industries.

Contact

Oncology World GmbH
Behringstr. 12
D-82152 Planegg
Germany
Phone +49-89-895 44 300
Fax +49-89-895 44 398
info@oncology-world.com
www.oncology-world.com

Information on IMIA

General

The International Medical Informatics Association is an independent organization established under Swiss law in 1989. The organization was established in 1967 as Technical Committee 4 of the International Federation for Information Processing (IFIP). In 1979, it evolved from a Special Interest Group of IFIP to its current status as a fully independent organization. IMIA continues to maintain its relationship with IFIP as an affiliate organization.

The organization also has close ties with the World Health Organization (WHO) as a NGO (Non Government Organization).

The working language of IMIA is English.

Purpose, Goals, Objectives

IMIA plays a major global role in the application of information science and technology in the fields of healthcare and research in medical, health and bio informatics. The basic goals and objectives of the association are to:

- promote informatics in health care and research in health, bio and medical informatics;
- advance and nurture international cooperation;
- to stimulate research, development and routine application;
- move informatics from theory into practice in a full range of health delivery settings, from physician's office to acute and long term care;
- further the dissemination and exchange of knowledge, information and technology;
- promote education and responsible behaviour; and
- represent the medical and health informatics field with the World Health Organization and other international professional and governmental organizations.

In its function as a bridge organization, IMIA's goals are:

- moving theory into practice by linking academic and research informaticians with care givers, consultants, vendors, and vendor-based researchers;
- leading the international medical and health informatics communities throughout the 21st century;
- promoting the cross-fertilization of health informatics information and knowledge across professional and geographical boundaries; and
- serving as the catalyst for ubiquitous worldwide health information infrastructures for patient care and health research.

Membership

IMIA membership consists of National, Institutional and Affiliate Members and Honorary Fellows.

National Members represent individual countries. A member is a society, a group of societies, or an appropriate body, which is representative of the medical, and health informatics activities within that country. Where no representative societies exist, IMIA accommodates involvement through "Corresponding" members within developing countries.

National IMIA members may organize into regional groups. Currently, such regions exist for Latin America and the Caribbean (IMIA LAC), Europe (EFMI), Asia/Pacific (APAMI) and Africa (Helina); an initiative to structure a North American region was started in 2001.

Institutional Members consist of corporate and academic members. Corporate members include vendor, consulting, technology firms as well as national professional organizations. Academic members include universities, medical centres, research centres and like institutions.

Affiliate Members consist of international organizations that share an interest in the broad field of health and medical informatics.

Honorary Fellows are individuals who have earned exceptional merit in furthering the aims and interests of the IMIA; fellowship is conferred for life.

Governance

IMIA is governed by its General Assembly which consists of one representative from each IMIA member, Honorary Fellows, Chairs of IMIA's Working Groups and a representative from IFIP, the World Health Organization, and each of IMIA's Regions. Only National Members have full voting rights. The General Assembly meets annually.

The Board of IMIA, elected by the General Assembly, conducts the association's affairs. The day-to-day operations are

International Medical Informatics Association (Continued)

supported by the association's Executive Director who is also responsible for IMIA's electronic services.

The officers of the Board and IMIA's vice presidents vigorously pursue IMIA's mission to:

- Monitor the range of special interest areas and focus support on new developments.
- Capitalize on the synergies and collective resources of IMIA's constituents.
- Minimize fragmentation between scientific and professional medical informaticians.
- Ensure successful adaptation to changes in the medical informatics marketplace and discipline.
- Raise the profile and awareness of IMIA within and outside of the IMIA organization.
- Encourage cooperation between the scientific and commercial health informatics communities.
- Equitably balance support to emerging and existing IMIA members.
- Establish and maintain cooperation and harmony with organizations that emerge to address medical informatics issues.
- Continue to position IMIA as the gatekeeper for medical informatics issues in the international community

Activities

MEDINFOs

IMIA organizes the internationally acclaimed tri-annual "*World Congress on Medical and Health Informatics*", MEDInfo. MEDInfo 2001, held in London, UK, September 2-5, 2001 at the newly developed Docklands area was hosted by the British Computer Society: Health Informatics Specialist Group. It was a highly successful scientific event.

MedINFO 2004 will be held at the Hilton Hotel in San Francisco, USA on September 7 –11, 2004. Potential participants and exhibitors are encouraged to visit their web site at www.medinfo2004.org. The American Medical Informatics Association (AMIA) hosts MedINFO 2004.

Previous MEDInfos have been held in Stockholm (1974), Toronto (1977), Tokyo (1980), Amsterdam (1983), Washington (1986), Beijing/Singapore (1989), Geneva (1992), Vancouver (1995) and Seoul (1998).

Working and Special Interest Groups

The IMIA family includes a growing number of Working and Special Interest Groups, which consist of individuals who share common interests in a particular focal field. The groups

hold Working Conferences on leading edge and timely health and medical informatics issues.

Current and future activities of the Working and Special Interest Groups are posted on the IMIA Website at www.imia.org

Other Initiatives

In the next few years IMIA will focus on "bridging the knowledge gap" by facilitating and providing support to developing nations. Specific goals include supporting the ongoing development of the African Region, and, on a broader basis, the development of the "Virtual University", an ongoing initiative of IMIA's working Group 1, Health and Medical Informatics Education.

IMIA reached a major milestone in completing a major redevelopment of its web-site www.imia.org. The site now contains profiles on its members, working groups and activities. The site uses a dynamic database to facilitate user-friendly communications for news, announcements, and an events calendar for the public, and access to e-mail communications, minutes, reports and association information for its members.

IMIA is constantly striving to further the services it provides to its members and the informatics community in general. The organization will expand its existing database in the support of the development of a Professional Resource Index, a database that will serve the purpose of providing access to the vast knowledge, skills and expertise of individuals who have participated in IMIA activities. Completion of this project is expected in 2002.

At the fall meeting of 2000, a task force was established by the General Assembly to develop an Ethical Code of Practice for adoption by IMIA. The resulting draft was reviewed by the General Assembly in the 2001 meeting, following detailed consultation with IMIA member countries it is planned that a formal draft will be submitted for approval in the fall of 2002. This work is being conducted under the umbrella of IMIA WG4 on Data Protection in Health Information Systems.

The goal of these initiatives is to provide the health professional and the patient with information when they need it, where they need it, and how they need it.

Progress Report by the President of IMIA

Immediate Past President:
Jan H. van Bemmel
Department of Medical Informatics
Erasmus University Rotterdam
PO Box 1738
NL-3000 DR Rotterdam
The Netherlands
Tel: +31 10 408 1749
Fax: +31 10 408 9447
E-mail: vanbemmel@mi.fgg.eur.nl

This report of the President of IMIA covers the period between the General Assembly meeting in Hannover, Germany, August 2000, and the GA meeting held during MEDINFO 2001 in London, September 2001.

Preparation of the Spring Board meeting 2001

Much effort was invested to organize IMIA's 2001 Spring Board meeting in the Middle East. The President had correspondence with several colleagues, to find out whether a medical/health informatics conference could be organized in the Middle East, at the same time as our Board meeting. Contacts were made with representatives of Ministries in Israel, Egypt and Jordan to find out whether such a combined meeting was feasible. In spite of all positive intentions and favorable answers from the authorities in all three countries, it appeared regretfully not possible to have these events in any of the three countries, because of the emerging political situation in the Middle East. Therefore, after contacting our Spanish colleagues in Barcelona and Madrid, and in agreement with the Board and IMIA's Director, the Spring Board meeting was organized in Madrid on March 30 and 31, 2001. IMIA is very indebted to the very efficient and constructive help of our Spanish member society.

IMIA 2001 Satellite meeting on Challenges in Medical and Health Informatics

The President organized, together with Dr. Mark Musen of Stanford University, an IMIA satellite meeting on *Challenges in Medical and Health Informatics*, at the time of the 2001 Spring Board meeting. This satellite meeting was held in Madrid, preceding the Board meeting. The outcomes of this satellite meeting have been presented at MEDINFO 2001 in London and will be published in issue 1/2002 of *Methods of Information in Medicine*. A summary of the Working Conference can be found in this 2002 Yearbook.

MEDINFO 2001, held in London

Our British colleagues organized a perfect tri-annual world congress MEDINFO. At the location where we had MEDINFO in the Docklands area, only two years earlier a large pit in the ground could be seen; an area covered with concrete, and for the rest a desert. Nevertheless, the Brits had full confidence that at the time of MEDINFO the congress center would be fully operational. And, indeed, the circumstances were ideal, such as the nearby City Airport, closeness to the city of London, a large exhibition area, proximity to the river Thames, etc. Some of the participants from the Continent made the journey to London even by a tall sailing ship (see the picture on next page).

The scientific program, the tutorials and the exhibition were very attractive. Jean Roberts and her Organizing Committee have to be congratulated for the success of MEDINFO 2001. The same thanks are to be conveyed to the Scientific Program Committee, chaired by Arie Hasman and Hiroshi Takeda, for the time and effort they spent to present the state-of-the-art in our profession to the world community of medical and health informatics. The editors as well – Vimla Patel, Reinhold Haux, and Ray Rogers – have accomplished a tremendous task by offering both paper Proceedings and a CD-ROM. Last, I want to pay tribute to the full Organizing Committee of this Congress, chaired by Jean Roberts: Bud Abbott, John Bryant, John Bryden, Sheila Bullas, Glyn and Judy Hayes, Frances Jackson, Brian Layzell, Peter Murray, Mike O'Flynn, Andrew Ogilvie, Joy Reardon, Bernard Richards, Ray Rogers, Nikki Shaw, and Graham Wright.

Other key issues

Many other important issues have been taken care of in close collaboration with the Executive Director and members of IMIA's Board, such as:

1. Strengthening IMIA as professional organization

On this issue much progress has been made, primarily thanks to the activities of IMIA's Executive Director, Steven Huesing. This does not imply that IMIA is already a full-blown professional society. This goal is perhaps still far away, as long as IMIA remains to be an Association of National Societies, and has no individual members. Very valuable first steps were already made at

Progress Report by the President of IMIA (Continued)

the end of Otto Rienhoff's presidency, and were continued and widened during the last three years, such as the realization of IMIA's central database and website and its expanding membership. In collaboration with the Executive Director, a host of new institutional members, both corporate and academic, could be welcomed to IMIA at the past General Assembly meetings.

the 'corporate memory' of IMA and is very valuable for giving advice to IMIA's Board. Therefore, I want to acknowledge the continuing leadership of this group, given by Hans Peterson and Marion Ball, both of them past Presidents of IMIA.

4. Making IMIA better visible to the outside world

During the past years, electronic services of IMIA were taken care of in an excellent

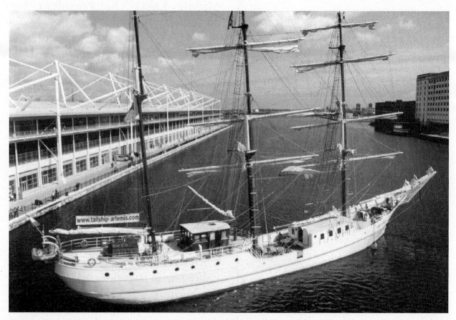

The picture shows how the Institute of Medical Informatics of Erasmus University Rotterdam sailed to MEDINFO 2001.

2. Building bridges to other organizations

The ties with several organizations have been strengthened during the past years. Discussions on collaboration were started and/or continued with the International Federation for Medical and Biological Engineering, the International Federation of Health Record Organizations, the Society for The Internet and Medicine, the International Society of Telemedicine, and WONCA.

3. Tapping the experience of former officers and honorary members

Former IMIA officers and honorary members serve IMIA by reflecting on plans of IMIA's Board, by coming forward with ideas on long-range planning, or by giving advice on a model for accreditation of persons/ institutions by IMIA. This group embodies

way by Thomas Kleinoeder from Göttingen, Germany. This activity has now been taken over by IMIA's Executive Director, Steven Huesing. The new website and the growing corporate and academic membership are living proof that the visibility of IMIA has increased. The Executive Director took the initiative to make an agreement with the journal *Health Informatics* on a regular presentation of IMIA in their periodicals.

At the end of MEDINFO 2001, I transferred the gavel with great gratitude and happiness to the most capable successor I could think of, my friend Dr. K.C. Lun from Singapore. In closing, I would like to thank all my friends and colleagues in IMIA for their continuous support and friendship. I wish IMIA a great future with lots of creative and bright ideas.

National and Corresponding Members

National Members

Argentina	Asociacion Argentina de Informatica Medica
Australia	Health Informatics Society of Australia
Austria	Österreichische Computergesellschaft
Belgium	Belgian Society for Medical Informatics
Bosnia & Herzegovina	Society for Medical Informatics
Brazil	Brasilian Society of Health Informatics
Canada	COACH: Canada's Health Informatics Association
China	China Medical Informatics Association
Croatia	Croation Society for Medical Informatics
Cuba	Cuban Medical Informatics Association
Czech Republic	Czech Society for Biomedical Engineering and Medical Informatics
Denmark	Danish Society for Medical Informatics
Finland	The Finnish Society for Medical Informatics
France	Association pour les Applications de l'Informatique à la Médecine
Georgia	Georgian Association of Medical Informatics and Biomedical Engineering (Observer Status)
Germany	Deutsche Gesellschaft für Medizinische Informatik, Biometrie und Epidemiologie
Hong Kong	Hong Kong Society for Medical Informatics
Hungary	Biomedical Section of John von Neumann Society
Ireland	Healthcare Informatics Society of Ireland
Israel	Israel Society for Medical Informatics
Italy	Italian Medical Informatics Society
Japan	Japan Association for Medical Informatics
Kazakstan	Kazakstan MedPharmInfo Association
Korea	The Korean Society of Medical Informatics
Mexico	Assucion Mexicana de Informatica Medica (Observer Status)
Netherlands	Society for Medical and Biological Information Processing
New Zealand	New Zealand Health Informatics Foundation
Nigeria	The Nigerian Health Informatics Society
Norway	The Norwegian Society for Medical Informatics
Peru	Peruvian Health Informatics Association (Observer Status)
Philippines	Philippine Medical Informatics Society, Inc.
Poland	Polish Society of Medical Informatics
Romania	Romanian Society for Medical Informatics
Singapore	Association ofInformatics in Medicine
Slovakia	Slovak Society for Biomedical Engineering and Medical Informatics
Slovenia	Slovenian Society for Medical Informatics
South Africa	South African Health Informatics Association
Spain	Sociedad Española de Informatica de la Salud (SEIS)
Sweden	Swedish Society for Medical Information Processing
Switzerland	Swiss Society for Medical Informatics
Turkey	Turkish Medical Informatics Association
Ukraine	The Ukrainian Association for Computer Medicine (Observer Status)
United Kingdom	British Computer Society: Health Informatics Specialist Groups
Uruguay	Sociedad Uruguaya de Informatica en la Salud
USA	American Medical Informatics Association

Corresponding Members

Armenia (Provisional Status), Chile, Egypt, Iran, Malaysia, Saudi Arabia (Provisional Status), Syria (Provisional Status), Tanzania

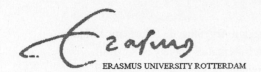

ERASMUS UNIVERSITY ROTTERDAM

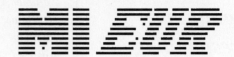

Department of Medical Informatics at the Erasmus University Rotterdam, The Netherlands

Medical Informatics is an interdisciplinary research group at the Medical School of the Erasmus University Rotterdam in the Netherlands. The group creates and validates knowledge and data models that are used in biomedicine. In as far as these models have signals or images of specific organs as their input, signal analysis and image processing are also part of our research. Our research staff and students study new methods for acquiring, representing, processing, and managing knowledge and data within health care and the biomedical sciences.

Our research clusters on two main themes: structuring medical data, with the electronic patient record as an important application area, and structuring of medical knowledge, with decision support as main focus.

Information about our department can be found at

http://www.eur.nl/fgg/mi/

The Department of Medical Informatics forms, together with the Departments Epidemiology, Health Services Research, and Public Health, the Netherlands Institute for Health Sciences (NIHES). NIHES offers a variety of educational programs including MSc, MPH, DSc, and PhD degree programs (see www.nihes.nl for more information).

Surface address:
Department of Medical Informatics
School of Medicine, Erasmus University Rotterdam
PO Box 1738
3000 DR Rotterdam
The Netherlands
tel: +31 10 408 7050
fax: +31 10 408 9447

Institutional Members

CORPORATE MEMBERS

American Health Information Management Association (AHIMA)
Chicago, IL - USA
Cerner Corporation
Kansas City, MO - USA
Covansys (Formerly Complete Business Solutions, Inc.)
Farmington Hills, MI - USA
DynCorp
Reston, VA - USA
Healthcare Informatics, McGraw-Hill Healthcare Information Group
Minneapolis, MN - USA
Healthcare Information & Management Systems Society (HIMSS)
Chicago, IL - USA
HISCOM - Health Information Solutions
Leiden - The Netherlands
Oncology World GmbH
Planegg bei Muenchen – Germany
Schattauer GmbH
Stuttgart - Germany
Siemens Medical Solutions
Erlangen - Germany
TILAK Tiroler Landeskrankeanstalten GmbH
Innsbruck - Austria
Wolters Kluwer International Healthcare Publishing
Philadelphia, PA - USA

ACADEMIC MEMBERS

Academic Medical Center (AMC) (Provisional)
Amsterdam, the Netherlands
Central Queensland University
Rockhampton, NSW, Australia
Centre for Health Informatics Research and Development
Winchester, UK
Erasmus University Rotterdam
Rotterdam, The Netherlands
Fundacion de Informatica Medica
Buenos Aires, Argentina
Institute of Healthcare Informatics (Provisional)
Dublin, Ireland
Monash University
Victoria, Australia
National Cancer Institute
Bethesda, MD, USA
Stanford University
Stanford, CA, USA
Tasmanian University Department of Rural Health
Launceston, Tasmania, Australia
University of Heidelberg
Heidelberg, Germany
University of Sydney (Provisional)
Sydney, Australia
University of Victoria, School of Health Information Science
Victoria, BC, Canada
University of Waterloo
Waterloo, ON, Canada
University of Wollongong
Wollongong, Australia

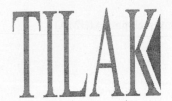

TILAK (Tiroler Landeskrankenanstalten) is a publicly owned holding company responsible for 5 hospitals, one health care education institution (AZW), several IT-solution providers and consulting firms based in Tyrol, Austria. The **TILAK** hospitals hold 2,100 beds and employ a staff of 5,500 persons, including 1,000 physicians.

By far the largest and most important organization of **TILAK** is the Innsbruck University Hospital, one of three university teaching hospitals in Austria. As a center of excellence for patient care, Innsbruck University Hospital covers all medical disciplines and comprises some 40 medical departments.

The **TILAK**-Hospitals utilize highly sophisticated IT-solutions, such as MEDAS (patient administration and billing), Cerner HNA Millennium (Clinical Information System), SAP (Human Resources, Controlling, Material Management, Datawarehouse) and comprehensive, hospital wide PACS- and Image Management solutions. For further information please consult our Internet homepage www.tilak.at, or contact Dr. Georg Lechleitner (georg.lechleitner@tilak.or.at).

The IT solution providers amongst **TILAK**'s affiliated companies are "ITH" (for hospital information systems), "icoserve" (for PACS and image management) and "AT solution partner" (for SAP solutions in healthcare). These companies are part of the newly founded Competence Center for Health Informatics.

University for Health Informatics and Technology Tyrol

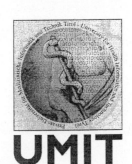

UMIT

In 2000, TILAK also initiated the founding of a new academic school for health informatics, the **Private Universität für Medizinische Informatik und Technik Tirol / University for Health Informatics and Technology Tyrol** (UMIT). UMIT was accredited by the Austrian Government in October 2001.

The University aims to reach a top international position in Medical Informatics in research and education.

Its headquarters are in Innsbruck. University instruction began in the academic year 2001/2002 with two educational programs. They lead to a B.Sc. (3 years) and a M.Sc. (1.5 – 2 years) degree in Medical Informatics. In parallel, Ph.D. students work in research projects. From the very beginning, an international integration of the programs is planned. For further information please visit www.umit.at.

UMIT's Mission Statement

The **University for Health Informatics and Technology Tyrol** sets for itself the following goals:
- To explore opportunities and practical applications of information and communication technologies, so as to contribute to high-quality, efficient health care that does justice to the individual and to society, and to contribute to progress in medical and health sciences research.
- To respect the freedom of science and its teachings in a community of students and teachers, who engage in open scholarly inquiry following principles of good scientific practice, always striving towards the highest quality in research and education.
- To promote the development and intellectual growth of the students, so that upon graduation they are well prepared for professional and related social responsibilities.
- To seek cooperation with other universities and research institutions, in particular with the LEOPOLD-FRANZENS-University of Innsbruck, and with health care institutions and other health related enterprises.

Publications

MEDINFO Proceedings

Anderson J, Forsythe JM, editors. MEDINFO 74. Amsterdam: North-Holland; 1974

Shires DB, Wolf H, editors. MEDINFO 77. Amsterdam: North-Holland ; 1977.

Lindberg DAB, Kaihara S, editors. MEDINFO 80. Amsterdam: North-Holland; 1980.

Van Bemmel JH, Ball MJ, Wigertz O, editors. MEDINFO 83. Amsterdam: North-Holland; 1983.

Salamon R, Blum BI, Jørgensen M, editors. MEDINFO 86. Amsterdam: North-Holland; 1986.

Barber B, Cao D, Qin D, Wagner G, editors. MEDINFO 89. Amsterdam: North-Holland; 1989.

Lun KC, Degoulet P, Piemme TE, Rienhoff O, editors. MEDINFO 92. Amsterdam: North-Holland; 1992.

Greenes RA, Peterson HE, Protti DJ, editors. MEDINFO 95. Amsterdam: North-Holland; 1995.

Cesnik B, McCray AT, Scherrer J-R, editors. MEDINFO 98. Amsterdam: IOS Press; 1998.

Patel V, Rogers R, Haux R, editors. MEDINFO 01. Amsterdam: IOS Press; 2001

Yearbooks of Medical Informatics

Van Bemmel JH, McCray AT, editors. 1992 Yearbook of Medical Informatics: Advances in an Interdisciplinary Science. Stuttgart: Schattauer; 1992.

Van Bemmel JH, McCray AT, editors. 1993 Yearbook of Medical Informatics: Sharing Knowledge and Information. Stuttgart: Schattauer; 1993.

Van Bemmel JH, McCray AT, editors. 1994 Yearbook of Medical Informatics: Advanced Communications in Health Care. Stuttgart: Schattauer; 1994.

Van Bemmel JH, McCray AT, editors. 1995 Yearbook of Medical Informatics: The Computer-based Patient Record. Stuttgart: Schattauer; 1995.

Van Bemmel JH, McCray AT, editors. 1996 Yearbook of Medical Informatics: The Integration of Information for Patient Care. Stuttgart: Schattauer; 1996.

Van Bemmel JH, McCray AT, editors. 1997 Yearbook of Medical Informatics: Computing and Collaborative Care. Stuttgart: Schattauer; 1997.

Van Bemmel JH, McCray AT, editors.1998 Yearbook of Medical Informatics: Health Informatics and the Internet. Stuttgart: Schattauer; 1998.

Van Bemmel JH, McCray AT, editors. 1999 Yearbook of Medical Informatics: The Promise of Medical Informatics. Stuttgart: Schattauer; 1999.

Van Bemmel JH, McCray AT, editors. 2000 Yearbook of Medical Informatics: Patient-centered Systems. Stuttgart: Schattauer; 2000.

Haux R, Kulikowski C, editors. 2001 Yearbook of Medical Informatics: Digital Libraries and Medicine. Stuttgart: Schattauer; 2001

Conference Proceedings

Peterson HE, Isaksson AI. Communication networks in health care. Amsterdam: North Holland; 1982 ISBN0444865136

Scholes M, Bryant Y, Barber B. *The Use of Computers in Nursing.* London, UK; 1982. ISBN-0-444-866-825

Cote RA, Protti DJ, Scherrer JR. Role of informatics in health data coding and classification systems. Amsterdam: North Holland; 1985 ISBN0444876820

Hannah KJ, Guillemin EJ, Conklin DN. *Nursing Uses of Computers and Science,* Calgary, Canada. Amsterdam: Elsevier North Holland; 1985. ISBN-0-444-87904-8

Van Bemmel JH, Gremy F, Zvarova J. Medical decision making: diagnostic strategies and expert systems. Amsterdam: North Holland; 1985 ISBN0444878408

Harris EK, Yasaka T. Maintaining a healthy state within the individual. Amsterdam: North Holland; 1986 ISBN 0444702709

Peterson HE, Gerdin-Jelger U, editors. *Preparing Nurses for Using Information Systems* (Working conference) 1986 Stockholm, Sweden. N.Y.: National League for Nursing; 1987. ISBN-0-88737-416-6

Willems JL, Van Bemmel JH, Michel J. Progress in computer/assisted function analysis. Amsterdam: North Holland; 1987 ISBN0444703845

Daley N. and Hannah KJ. *Proceedings of the Third International Symposium on Nursing Use of Computers and Information Science.* 1988 Dublin, Ireland. St. Louis: Mosby; 1988. ISBN-0-8016-3258-8

Bakker AR, Ball MJ, Scherrer JR, Willems JL, editors. *Towards new hospital information systems.* Amsterdam: North-Holland; 1988.

Hayes GM, Robinson N, editors. *Primary Care Computing.* Amsterdam: Elsevier Science Publ (North Holland); 1990.

Ozbolt JG, Vandewal D, Hannah KJ. *Decision Support Systems in Nursing.* (Working conference) 1988 Dublin, Ireland. St. Louis Mosby; 1990. ISBN-0-8016-3236-6

Hovenga EJS, Hannah KJ, McCormick KA, Ronald JS. *Nursing Informatics '91.* Melbourne, Australia, Berlin: Springer-Verlag; 1991. ISBN-3-540-53869-0 / ISBN-0-387-53869-0

Marr PB, Axford RL, Newbold SK. *Health Care Information Technology; Implications for Change.* (Post conference) Melbourne, Australia, 1991. Berlin: Springer-Verlag; 1991. ISBN-3-540-54124-1 / ISBN-0-387-54124-1

Turley J. P and Newbold S. K . *Nursing Informatics '91: Preconference Proceedings*

Publications (Continued)

(Preconference) Melbourne, Australia 1991. Berlin: Springer-Verlag; 1991.

Van Bemmel JH, Zvárová J, editors. *Knowledge, Information and Medical Education.* Amsterdam: Elsevier Science Publ (North-Holland); 1991.

Timmers T, Blum B, editors. *Software Engineering in Medical Informatics.* Amsterdam: Elsevier Science Publ (North-Holland); 1991.

Duisterhout JS, Salamon R, Hasman A, editors. *Telematics in Medicine.* Amsterdam: Elsevier Science Publ (North-Holland); 1991.

Bakker AR, Ehlers CT, Bryant JR, Hammond WE, editors. *Hospital Information Systems:Scope-Design-Architecture.* Amsterdam: Elsevier Science Publ (North-Holland); 1992.

Williams BT, Collen MF, Schmidt RM, editors. *Special Issue on International Health Evaluation* (IHEA/IMIA). Meth Inform Med 1993;32:187-264.

Haux R, Leven FJ, Moehr JR, Protti D, editors. *Special issue on Health and Medical Informatics Education.* Heidelberg/Heilbronn, Germany. Methods Inf Med 1993;34/3.

Mandil SH, Moidu K, Korpela M, Byass P, Forster D, editors. *Health Informatics in Africa - HELINA '93.* Amsterdam: Elsevier Science Publ (North Holland); 1993.

Van Gennip EMSJ, Bakker A. *Challenges and opportunities for technology assessment in medical informatics - Case Study: PACS.* Med Inform 1993;18:209-18

Ball MJ, Silva JS, Douglas JV, Degoulet P, Kaihara S, editors. *The Health Care Professional Workstation.* Special Issue of Int J Biomed Comput 1994;34:1-415.

Barber B, Bakker AR, Bengtsson S, editors. *Caring for Health Information: Safety, Security and Secrecy.* Amsterdam: Elsevier Science Publ (North-Holland); 1994.

Grobe SJ, Pluyter-Wenting ESP. *An International Overview for Nursing in a Technological Era.* (San Antonio, Texas, USA, 1994). Amsterdam: Elsevier North-Holland; 1994.

Henry S, Holzemer W, Tallberg M, Grobe SJ. *The Infrastracture for Quality Assessment and Improvement in Nursing.* 1994 Austin, Texas, USA (postconference). 1995.

Bakken HS. Holzemar W, Tallberg M, Grobe SJ. *The Infrastructure for Quality Assessment and Improvement in Nursing.* (Austin, Texas, USA, 1994 - Post-conference) 1995.

Van Bemmel JH, Rosenfalck A, Saranummi N, eds. Special Issue on *Biosignal Interpretation.* Proceedings of a IMIA/IFMBE Working Conference. Methods Inf Med 1994;33:1-160.

Bakker AR, Barber B, Tervo-Pellikka R, Treacher A, editors. (IMIA WG4). *Communicating Health Information in an Insecure World :* (Proceedings of the Helsinki Working Conference 1995). Amsterdam: Elsevier Publishing Co; 1995. 43:1, 2:1-s (also Special Issue of the Int J Biomed Comput, Vol. 43).

McCray AT, Scherrer J-R, Safran C, Chute CG, editors. *Concepts, Knowledge, and Language in Healthcare Information Systems.* Methods Inf Med 1995;34: 1-231.

Hammond WE, Bakker AR, Ball MJ, editors. *Information Systems with fading Boundaries.* Special issue of Int J Biomed Comput 1995;39:1-192.

PAHO and Koop Foundation Meeting: *Telecommunications in Health and Healthcare for Latin America and the Caribbean,* November 12-15, 1996, Washington DC, USA.

1st Argentine Symposium of Nursing Informatics, December 4-6, 1996, Buenos Aires, Argentina.

Gerdin U, Tallberg M, Wainwright P. *Nursing Informatics: the impact of nursing knowledge on health care informatics.* Stockholm, Sweden 1997. Amsterdam: IOS Press; 1997.

Van Bemmel JH, Saranummi N, Yana K, Sato S, editors. *Biosignal Interpretation.* Proceedings of an IMIA/IFMBE Working Conference. Methods Inf Med 1997;36:235-375.

Haux R, Swinkels W, Ball MJ, Knaup P, Lun KC, editors : Special Issue on *Health and Medical Informatics Education : Transformation of Healthcare through innovative use of Information Technology.* Int J Med Inf 1997;44.

Bakker AR, Barber B, Ishikawa K, Yamamoto K, editors. *Common Security Solutions for Communicationg Patient Data.* Int J Med Inf. Special Issue; 1998;49.

Chute CG, Baud RH, Cimino JJ, Patel WL, Rector AL, editors. *Special Issue on Coding and Language Processing.* Methods Inf Med 1998;37.

Ehnfors M, Grobe SJ, Tallberg M. *Nursing Informatics: Combining Clinical Practice Guidelines and Patient Preferences Using Health Informatics* (postconference). Stockholm: SPRI 1998.

Kay S, editor. Special Issue on *Health Informatics: Challenges to Progress.* Methods Inf Med 1999;38.

Talmon JL, Lorenzi N, van Gennip EMSJ, Nykänen P, editors. *Organisational issues and technology assessment in health informatics.* Int J Med Inform 1999, Vol. 56.

Van der Lei J, Moorman PW, Musen M. Special Issue on *Electronic Patient Records in Medical Practice.* Methods Inf Med 1999;38.

Bakker AR, Barber B, Moehr J, editors. *Security of the Distributed Electronic Patient Record* (EPR). Int J Med Inf. Special Issue; 2000;60.

Oliveri N, Sandor T, Lazaro C, Wiese B, Porta C, editors. Informedica 2000: 1st Ibero-American Virtual Congress of Medical Informatics. Proceedings of the Congress. CD Rom Spanish and English Edition. Fundación de Informática Médica. Argentina. 2000.

Saba V, Carr R. Sermeus W, Rocha P. *One Step Beyond: The Evolution of Technology and Nursing.* Auckland, New Zealand: Adis International; 2000. ISBN 0-86471-081-X.

Addresses of IMIA Member Societies

Argentina

Argentine Association of Medical Informatics
Asociación Argentina de Informática Médica (AAIM)
http://www.aaim.org.ar

National Office:
Guido 1948 1° B
Buenos Aires CP 1119, Argentina
Tel: +54 11 4807 5923
Fax: +54 11 4807 5982

President:
Carlos Hugo Leonzio
Fundacion Favaloro
Health Informatics
Tel: +54 11 4378 1200 Int 4438
Fax: +54 11 4378 1311
E-mail: hleonzio@fibertel.com.ar
          leonzio@hugo.net.ar

IMIA Representative:
Dr. Nora Oliveri
Fundacion de Informatica Medica
Iberoamerican Projects
Tel: +54 11 4807 5923
Fax: +54 11 4807 5982
norao@mifound.org

Treasurer:
Tonas A. Sandor
Tel: +54 11 4309 5479
Fax: +54 11 4309 5400
E-mail: tsandor@boldt.com.ar

Australia

Health Informatics Society of Australia Ltd. (HISA)
http://www.hisa.org.au

HISA Executive Director:
Ms. Joan Edgecumbe
Health Informatics Society of Australia
413 Lygon Street
Brunswick East 3057
Australia
Tel: +61 3 9388 0555
Fax: +61 3 9388 2086
E-mail: hisa@hisa.org.au

President:
Paul Cohen
IT Relationship Manager
Medibank Private
E-mail: Paul_Cohen@
          medibank.com.au

Secretary:
Ms. Robyn Cook
South Eastern Sydney Area
Health Service, ISD
E-Mail: CookR@
          sesahs.nsw.gov.au

IMIA Representative:
Prof. Jeffrey Soar
University of Wollongong
School of Information Technology
and Computer Science
Tel: +61 2 4221 5321
Fax: +61 2 4221 4170
E-mail: jeffrey@uow.edu.au

Treasurer:
Steve Tipper
University of South New Wales
Centre for Health Informatics
E-mail: s.tipper@unsw.edu.au

Austria

Austrian Computer Society
Working Group Medical Informatics
Österreichische Computergesellschaft
Arbeitskreis Medizinische Informatik
http://www.kfunigraz.ac.at/imiwww/ak/

President and IMIA Representative:
Prof. Dr. Günther Gell
Graz University
Institute of Medical Informatics,
Statistics and Documentation
Engelgasse 13
A–8010 Graz, Austria
Tel: +43 316 385 3201
Fax: +43 316 385 3590
E-mail: guenther.gell@uni-graz.at

Secretary/Treasurer:
Dr. Andreas Holzinger
Graz University
Institute of Medical Informatics,
Statistics and Documentation
Engelgasse 13
A-8010 Graz, Austria
Tel: +43 316 385 3883
Fax: +43 316 385 3590
E-mail: andreas.holzinger@
          kfunigraz.ac.at

Belgium

Belgian Medical Informatics Association
http://www.bmia.be

President:
Dr. Etienne De Clercq
Ecole de Santé Publique - SESA
Université Catholique de
Louvain
Clos Chapelle aux Champs, 30.41
1200 Brussels
Tel: +32 2 764 3262
Fax: +32 2 764 3031
E-mail: declercq@sesa.ucl.ac.be

IMIA Representative:
Prof. F.H. Roger France
Université Catholique de
Louvain
Centre for Medical Informatics
Tel: +32 2 764 4711
Fax: +32 2 764 4717
E-mail: roger@infm.ucl.ac.be

Secretary:
Dr. P. Piette
E-mail: p.piette@hopiteaux-
          gilly.be

Bosnia and Herzegovina

Society for Medical Informatics of Bosnia and
Herzegowina

President and IMIA Representative:
Prof. Dr. Izet Masic
Medical Faculty
Center for Medical Informatics

Mose Pijade 6, 71000 Sarajevo
Tel/Fax: +387 71 444 714
E-mail: imasic@utic.net.ba

Brazil

Brazilian Society of Health Informatics
Sociedade Brasileira de Informática em Saúde - SBIS
http://www.sbis.org.br

SBIS Office Address:
Rua Trisão de Campos276
São Paulo SP - Brazil

President and IMIA Representative:
Dr. Lincoln de Assis Moura Jr.
Tel: +55 11 5056 0458
Fax: +55 11 9182 7495
E-mail: lamoura@uol.com.br

Secretary/Treasurer:
Ms. Fabiane Bizinella Nardon
Heart Institute - University of Sao
Paulo Medical School Hospital
Research and Development Group
Tel: +55 11 3069 5547
Fax: +55 11 3069 5311
E-mail: fabiane.nardon@
        incor.usp.br

Canada

COACH, Canada's Health Informatics Association
http://www.coachorg.com

Secretariat:
Andrew Parr (executive director)
1304 - 2 Carlton Street
Toronto, Ontario M5B 1J3
Tel: +1 416 979 5551
Fax: +1 461 979 1144
E-mail: info@coachorg.com

President:
Brendan Seaton
CareLink Incorporated
Tel: +1 416 321 9857
Fax: +1 506 459 3001
E-mail: brendan.seaton@
        carelink.ca

Secretary/Treasurer:
Dr. Don Newsham
Sierra Systems Consulting
Tel: +1 780 424 0852
Fax: +1 780 426 0281
E-mail: donnewsham@
        sierrasystems.com

IMIA Representative:
Prof. Jochen Moehr
University of Victoria
School of Health Information
Science
Tel: +1 250 721 8581
Fax: +1 250 472 4751
E-mail: jmoehr@uvic.ca

Executive Director:
Andrew D. Parr
Tel: +1 416 979 5551
Fax: +1 416 979 1144
E-mail: info@coachorg.com

China

China Medical Informatics Association (CMIA)
China Medical Informatics Association of Chinese
Institut of Electronics
http://www.cmia.net

CMIA Office Address:
17 Zhengjue Jiadao
Xinjiekou, Xicheng District
Beijing 100035
P.R. China

President:
Prof. Debing Wang
Peking University
Tel: +86 10 6275 7072
Fax: +86 10 6275 1207
E-mail: wdb@pku.edu.cn

Secretary/Treasurer:
Mr. Ying I. Liang
China Medical Informatics
Association
Tel: +86 10 6615 3078
E-mail: medinfo@cmia.net

IMIA Representative:
Dr. Ling Zhu
Golden Medicine Commodities
Network Co., Ltd.
Tel: +86 10 6489 0022 ext.166
Fax: +86 10 6492 4861
E-mail: lzhu_md@yahoo.com

Croatia

Croatian Society for Medical Informatics (CSMI)
Hrvatsko drustvo za medicinsku informatiku
http://www.snz.hr/wnew/csmi.html

President:
Prof. Dr. Gjuro Dezelic
Medical School, University of
Zagreb
Department of Medical Statistics,
Epidemiology and Medical
Informatics
Tel: +385 1 468 4440
Fax: +385 1 468 4441

IMIA Representative:
Prof. Dr. Josipa Kern
Andrija Stampar School of
Public Health
Medical School
University of Zagreb
Tel: +385 1 468 4440
Fax: +385 1 468 4441
E-mail: jkern@snz.hr

Croatia

Croatian Society for Medical Informatics (CSMI)
Hrvatsko drustvo za medicinsku informatiku
(Continued)

Secretary:
Ms. Mira Hercigonja-Szekeres
Polimedika, Ltd.
Tel: +385 1 663 6500
E-mail: mira.hercigonja-
        szekeres1@zg.tel.hr

Cuba

Cuban Society of Medical Informatics
Sociedad Cubana de Informática Médica
http://www.cedisap.sld.cu

Office Address:
CEDISAP
Calle 23 No. 177 entre N y O,
Vedado, Plaza
Ciudad de la Habana, Cuba

President:
Prof. Dr Esperanza O'Farrill
Center of Cybernetics Applied
to Medicine (CECAM)
Tel: +537 21 1354
E-mail: espe@cecam.sld.cu

IMIA Representative:
Prof. Dr. Emilio Morales
Medical Faculty Finlay-
Albarran
Tel: +537 28 2571
E-mail: emorales@
        infomed.sld.cu

Secretary/Treasurer:
Ms. Maria Vidal
Ministry of Public Health
Centro de Desarollo Informatico
de Salud Publica
Tel: +537 55 3325
Fax: +537 55 2222
E-mail: swmedic@infomed.sld.cu

Czech Republic

Czech Society of Biomedical Engineering
and Medical Informatics
Ceska spolecnost biomedicinskeho inzenyrstvi a
lekarske
http://www.cls.cz/

President:
Dr. Jaromir Cmíral
Institute of Aviation Medicine
Generála Piky 1
160 60 Prague 6
Czech Republic
Tel: +420 2 2020 8120
Fax: +420 2 2431 1934
E-mail: ulz@telecom.cz

Secretary/Treasurer:
Jiri Holcik
Inst Biomedical Engineering
FEI VUT Bro
Purkynova 118
61200 Brno
Tel: +420 5 4114 9546
Fax: +420 5 4114 9542
E-mail: holcik@
        dbme.fee.vutbr.cz

IMIA Representative:
Prof. Dr. Jana Zvárová
Charles University
EuroMISE Center
Pod vodarenskou vezi 2
182 07 Prague 8
Czech Republic
Tel: +420 2 6605 3097
Fax: +420 2 6897 013
E-mail: zvarova@euromise.cz

Executive Director:
Dr. Alexander Stozicky
Czech Medical Society HJ.E.
Purkyne
Tel: +420 2 2426 6223
Fax: +420 2 2426 6226

Denmark

The Danish Society for Medical Informatics
Dansk Selskab for Medicinsk Informatik
http://www.dsmi.dk

Office Address:
Dansk Selskab for Medicinsk
Informatik
St. Kongensgade 59 A
København K
Denmark

President :
Henrik Lindholm
WM-data eSolutions
Tel: +45 4582 2200
E-mail: henrik@dsa-net.dk

Secretary/Treasurer:
Ms. Lise Therkelsen
Dansk Sygeplejerad
Tel: +45 3315 1555

IMIA Representative:
Dr. Knut E. Bernstein
Danish Centre for Health
Telematics
Heden 18
DK-5000 Odense C
Denmark
Tel: +45 6613 3066
Fax: +45 6613 5066
E-mail: kbern@inet.uni2.dk

Finland

Finnish Social and Health Informatics Association
(FinnSHIA)
Sosiaali-ja terveydenhuollon tietojenkäsittely
-yhdistys ry ry
http://www.oskenet.fi/tty

*President and IMIA
Representative:*
Dr. Mikko Korpela
University of Kuopio
Computing Centre
P.O. Box 1627
FIN-70211 Kuopio
Tel: +358 17 16 2811
Fax: +358 17 282 5566
E-mail: mikko.korpela@uku.fi

Treasurer:
Kauko Hartikainen
Association of Finnish Local and
Regional Authorities
Tel: +358 9 771 2647
Fax: +358 9 771 2291
E-mail: Kauko.Hartikainen@
         Kuntaliitto.fi

Executive Director:
Ms. Ursula Cornér
National Research and
Development Centre for
Welfare and Health
Tel: +358 9 3967 2329
Fax: +358 9 3967 2443
E-mail: Ursula.Corner@stakes.fi

France

Association pour les Applications de l'Informatique à la
Médecine

IMIA Representative:
Prof. Patrice Degoulet
Pompidou University Hospital
Hospital Informatics Department
Tel: +33 1 5609 2030
Fax: +33 1 5609 2052
E-mail: patrice.degoulet@
         egp.ap-hop-paris.fr

Georgia

Georgian Association of Medical Informatics and
Biomedical Engineering (GAMIBE)

*President and IMIA
Representative:*
Prof. Gaioz S. Vasadze
51 Iv. Javakhishvili str.
380002 Tbilisi, Georgia
Tel: +995 32 953 418
Fax: +995 32 960 300
E-mail: aiha@nilc.org.ge

Germany

German Association for Medical Informatics, Biometry
and Epidemiology
Deutsche Gesellschaft für Medizinische Informatik,
Biometrie und Epidemiologie (GMDS) e.V.

GMDS-Geschäftsstelle
Schedestrasse 9
D-53113 Bonn, Germany
http://www.gmds.de

Berufsverband Medizinischer Informatiker (BVMI)
P.O. Box 101308
D-69003 Heidelberg, Germany
http://www.bvmi.de

President:
Prof. Dr. Rüdiger Klar
University Hospital Freiburg
Medical Informatics
Stefan-Meier-Str. 26
D-79104 Freiburg
Germany
Tel: +49 761 203 6701
Fax: +49 761 203 6711
E-mail: klar@
         mi.ukl.uni-freiburg.de

President BVMI:
Prof. Dr. D.P. Pretschner
TU Braunschweig
Fallersleber-Tor-Wall 22
D-38100 Braunschweig
Tel: +49 531 391 9501
Fax: +49 531 391 9502
E-mail: d.p.pretschner@
         umi.cs.tu-bs.de

IMIA Representative:
Prof. Dr. Herbert Witte
Institute of Medical Statistics
Computer Sciences and
Documentation
Friedrich Schiller University Jena
Jahnstr. 3
D-07740 Jena
Germany
Tel: +49 3641 933 133
Fax: +49 3641 933 200
E-mail: iew@imsid.uni-jena.de

Hong Kong

Hong Kong Society of Medical Informatics
http://www.hksmi.org.hk

President and IMIA Representative:
Dr. Chun Por Wong
Ruttonjee Hospital
266 Queens's Road East
Hong Kong
Tel: +852 2291 1345
Fax: +852 2291 1335
E-mail: cpwong@iohk.com

Secretary/Treasurer:
Anthony Cheung
IT Division, Hospital Authority
147B Argyle Street
Kowloon, Hong Kong
Tel: +852 2300 6538
Fax: +852 2300 5395

Hungary

Biomedical Section of John von Neumann Society for Computing Sciences
http://www.njszt.iif.hu

President and IMIA Representative:
Prof. Dr. Attila Naszlady
National Inst. of Pulmonology
Cardiopulmonary Department
Budapest
Hungary
Tel: +36 1 200 2573
Fax: +36 1 200 2573
E-mail: irgalmas@elender.hu

Ireland

Healthcare Informatics Society of Ireland
Cumann Riomheolais Sláinte
http://www.mater.ie/hisi/hisi.htm

Office Address:
58 Eccles Street
Dublin 7
Republic of Ireland

President:
Prof. Jane Grimson
Trinity College, Dublin
Center for Health Informatics
Tel: +353 1 608 1780
Fax: +353 1 608 2512
E-mail: jane.grimson@tcd.ie

Executive Director:
Gerard Hurl
Institute of Healthcare Informatics
Mater Misericordiae Hospital
Tel: +353 1 830 7958
Fax: 830 7728*IMIA*

Representative:
Diarmuid UaConaill
Biochemistry Laboratory
Mater Misericordiae Hospital
Eccles Street, Dublin 7
Ireland
Tel: +353 1 803 2423
Fax: +353 1 803 4781
E-mail: duaconaill@mater.ie

Secretary:
Ms. Ann Sheridan
Eastern Regional Health Authority
Tel: +353 1 4065 600
Fax: +353 1 4065 611
E-mail: ann.sheridan@erha.ie

Israel

The Israeli Association for Medical Informatics

Office Address:
P.O. Box 50006
Tel Aviv, Israel

President and IMIA Representative:
Dr. Batami Sadan
MDG Medical Inc.
Tel: +972 3 6340 404
Fax: +972 3 6340 411
E-mail: sadanba@netvision.net.il

Secretary/Treasurer:
Ms. Dorit Shaul
ILA/The Israeli Association for Medical Informatics
Tel: +972 3 5140 503
Fax: +972 3 5140 077
E-mail: ILA@kenes.com

Italy

Italian Society for Medical Informatics (AIIM)

Office address:
c/o MGA
Viale Mazzini
Rome, Italy

President and IMIA Representative:
Prof. Angelo A.S. Serio
Università di Roma "La Sapienza"
Facoltà die Medicina
Tel: +39 6 3542 0351
Fax: +39 6 3973 0351
E-mail: angelo.serio@tiscalinet.it

Japan

Japan Association for Medical Informatics
http://plaza.umin.ac.jp/~jami/jamiM.html

President:
Dr. Michitoshi Inoue
President
Osaka National Hospital,
Japan
Tel: +81 6 6946 3500
Fax: +81 6 6946 8031
E-mail: inoue@onh.go.jp

Secretary:
Kiyomu Ishikawa
Professor
Hiroshima University
c/o MEDIS-DC
E-Mail: kiyomu@
        hiroshima-u.ac.jp

IMIA Representative:
Prof. Ken Toyoda
Asahi Arthur Andersen Limited
Healthcare Group
Tel: +81 3 3266 7241
Fax: +81 3 3266 8370
E-mail: ken.toyoda@
        jp.arthurandersen.com

Kazakstan

Medical Pharmaceutical Information Association
(MedPharmInfo)
http://www.med.kz

Office address:
47 Mynbaev Street
Almaty
Republic of Kazakstan 480008

President :
Dr. Arsen Abdrakhmanov
Tel: +7 3272 4534 04
Fax: +7 3272 4575 78
E-mail: arsen@med.kz

Executive Director:
Dr. Aliya Kusherova
MedPharmInfo Association
Tel: +7 3272 4790 54
Fax: +7 3272 4575 78
E-mail: aliya@ean.kz

IMIA Representative:
Prof. Azat Abdrakmanov
Tel: +7 3272 4575 78
Fax: +7 3272 4575 78
E-mail: azat@med.kz

Korea

The Korean Society of Medical Informatics (KOSMI)
http://www.kosmi.org

President:
Prof. Hank-Ik Cho
Seoul National University
College of Medicine
Tel: +82 2 760 2542
E-mail: hanik@snu.ac.kr

Secretary/Treasurer:
Prof. Hyeoun-Ae Park
Seoul National University
College of Nursing
Tel: +82 2 740 8827
Fax: +82 2 765 4103
        +82 11 786 3284
E-mail: hapark@plaza.snu.ac.kr

IMIA Representative:
Prof. Taiwoo Yoo
Seoul National Univ Hospital
Department of Family Medicine
Tel: +82 2 760 3329
Fax: +82 2 766 3328
E-mail: tyoo@mydoctor.snu.ac.kr

Mexico

Mexican Medical Informatics Association
Assucion Mexicana de Informatica Medica (AMIM)

IMIA Representative:
Dr. Cesar Colina Ramirez
Universidad Nacional Autonoma
de Mexico
Facultad de Medicina
Tel: +52 623 24 85
Fax: +52 623 24 80
E-mail: ccolina@
        drbaz.fmed.unam.mx

The Netherlands

Society for Healthcare Informatics
Vereniging voor informatieverwerking in de zorg
(VMBI)
http://www.vmbi.nl

President and IMIA
Representative:
Prof. Dr. Arie Hasman
Dept of Medical Informatics
Maastricht University
PO Box 616
6200 MD Maastricht
The Netherlands
Tel: +31 43 388 2242
Fax: +31 43 388 4170
E-mail: hasman@mi.unimaas.nl

Treasurer:
Gijs G. Andrea
Inview BV
Tel: +31 35 692 2848
Fax: +31 35 692 2849
E-mail: G.Andrea@InView.nl

New Zealand

Health Informatics New Zealand

Office Address:
PO Box 62-578
Kalmia Street PO Boxes
Auckland, New Zealand

President:
Ms. Ann C. Browett
Mercy Hospital and Health
Services
Tel: +64 9 623 5700
Fax: +64 9 623 5701
E-mail: annb@mercy.co.nz

Secretary/Treasurer:
Ms. Anne Andrews
Waitemata Health Ltd.
Tel: +64 9 489 9134
E-mail: andrewsp@whl.co.nz

IMIA Representative:
Ian H. Symonds
Wellington Pathology Ltd.
Tel: +64 4 801 5111
Fax: +64 4 801 5432
E-mail: ihs@welpath.co.nz

Norway

Norwegian Society for Medical Informatics
Forum for Databehandling i Helsesektoren (FDH)
http://www.fdh.no

President:
Prof. Margarethe J. Lorensen
University of Oslo
Institute of Nursing Science
E-mail: m.j.lorensen@
           sykepleievit.uio.no

IMIA Representative:
Ms. Irma Iversen
Pasientombudet for Akershus
Fylkeskommune
Tel: +47 221 70491
Fax: +47 221 75270
E-mail:irma.iversen@po.ah.no

Peru

Peruvian Health Informatics Association
Asociacion Peruano de Informatica en Salud (APIS)
http://www.apisnet.org

President and IMIA
Representative:
Dr. Crisogono Rubio Nieto
Telefonica Data Peru S.A.A.
Tel: +51 1 210 4592
Fax: +51 1 422 0591
E-mail: crubio@tp.com.pe

Secretary/Treasurer:
Dr. Jorge Ballon Echegaray
Unversidad Nacional San Agustin
Facultad de Medicina
Tel: +51 1 447 0472
E-mail: francis@LaRed.net.pe

Philippines

Philippine Medical Informatics Society, Inc.
http://www.pmis.org

Secretariat:
Dr. Alex C. Yu
Philippine Medical Informatics Society, Inc.
University of the Philippines
College of Medicine Class of 2000
547 Pedro Gil Street
Ermita, Manila, Philippines 1000
Tel: +63 2 526 0371
Fax: +63 2 526 0371
E-mail: alexcyu@eudoramail.com

President:
Dr. Herman D. Tolentino,
University of the Philippines
College of Medicine
Medical Informatics Unit
Tel: +63 2 526 4254
Fax: +63 2 874 6992 0918
           +63 2 874 9040 294
E-mail: hermant@
           i-manila.com.ph

IMIA Representative:
Dr. Alvin B. Marcelo
University of the Philippines
Department of Surgery
Division of Trauma
Tel: +1 301 435 3278
Fax: +1 603 452 3657
E-mail: amarcelo@cm.upm.edu.ph

Poland

Polish Society of Medical Informatics

President and IMIA Representative:
Prof. Dr. Edward Kacki
Institute of Computer Science
Technical University of Lódz
Ul. Sterlinga 16/18
90-217 Lódz, Poland
Tel: +48 42 329 757
Fax: +48 42 303 414
E-mail: ekacki@ics.p.lodz.pl

Romania

Romanian Society of Medical Informatics
Societatea Romana de Informatica Medicala
http://medinfo.umft.ro/rsmi/

Office Address:
Spl. T.Vladimirescu 14
Timisoara
Romania

President and IMIA Representative:
Prof.dr. George I. Mihalas
Univ. Medicine and Pharmacy
Dept. Medical Informatics
P-ta Eftimie Murgu 2
RO-1900 Timisoara
Romania
Tel: +40 56 19028
Fax: +40 56 190 28
E-mail: mihalas@medinfo.umft.ro

Secretary:
Ms. Mariana Bazavan
Center for Health Computing
Statistics and Medical
Documentation
Tel: +40 1 314 0890
Fax: +40 1 311 2998
E-mail: mbazavan@yahoo.com

Singapore

Association for Informatics in Medicine, Singapore
(AIMS)
http://www.aims.org.sg

Office Address:
Medical Informatics Program
Clinical Research Ctr, Blk MD 11
10 Medical Drive
National University of Singapore
Singapore

President and IMIA Representative:
Prof. Kwok-Chan Lun
Nanyang Technological University
School of Biological Sciences
Tel: +65 790 3726
Fax: +65 896 8874
E-mail: kclun@ntu.edu.sg

Treasurer:
Ms. Swee Wah Chew-Goh
National University of Singapore
Computer Centre
Tel: +65 874 2480
Fax: +65 778 0198
E-mail: ccegohsw@nus.edu.sg

Slovak Republic

Slovak Society for Biomedical Engineering
and Medical Informatics
http://www.fmed.uniba.sk/~biofyzika/engin.html

President:
Prof. Peter Kneppo
Slovak Institute of Metrology
Tel: +421 7 654 262 08
Fax: +421 7 654 295 92
E-mail: pkneppo@smu.gov.sk

IMIA Representative:
Dr. Mikuláš Popper
Comenius University
Faculty of Mathematics,
Physics and Informatics
Tel: +421 2 6542 7469
E-mail: popper@fmph.uniba.sk

Secretary:
Dr. Milan Tyšler
Slovak Academy of Science
Institute of Measurement
Sciences
Tel: +421 7 5477 5950
Fax: +421 7 5477 5943
E-mail: umertyssl@savba.sk

Slovenia

Slovenian Medical Informatics Society (SMIS)

President and IMIA Representative:
Dr. Marjan Premik
Medical Faculty
Institute for Social Medicine
Zaloska 4
SI-1105 Ljubljana, Slovenia
Tel/Fax: +386 61 131 4210
E-mail: premik@
ibmi.mf.uni-lj.si

South Africa

South African Health Informatics Association

President:
Dr. Sedick S. Isaacs
Groote Schuur Hospital/
University of Capetown
Tel: +27 21 404 2058
Fax: +27 21 404 2070
E-mail: seisaacs@
pawc.wcape.gov.za

IMIA Representative:
John D. Tresling
Meditech SA
Tel: +27 11 805 1631
Fax: +27 11 805 1430
E-mail: jdt@pc.meditech.co.za

Secretary/Treasurer:
Ms. Lyn A. Hanmer
Medical Research Council
Tel: +27 21 938 0343
Fax: +27 21 938 0315
E-mail: lyn.hanmer@mrc.ac.za

Spain

Spanish Society of Health Informatics
Sociedad Española de Informática de la Salud (SEIS)
http://www.seis.es

Office Address:
CEFIC (SEIS Secretary)
C/Olimpo, 33 1° C
28043 Madrid, Spain

President:
Prof. Luciano Saez-Ayerra
Institute of Health "Carlos III"
Dept. of Health Informatics
Tel: +34 91 387 7835
Fax: +34 91 387 7790
+34 62 937 1639
E-mail: lsaez@isciii.es

Secretary:
Dr.Salvador Arribas
Hospital Universitario La Paz
Tel: +34 91 350 2600 ext. 1156
E-mail: sarribas@hulp.insalud.es

IMIA Representative:
Dr. Fernando J. Martin-Sanchez
Institute of Health "Carlos III"
Public Health Bioinformatics
Tel: +34 91 509 7027
Fax: +34 91 509 7917
E-mail: fmartin@isciii.es

Sweden

Swedish Society for Medical Information Processing
Svensk Förenig för Medicinsk Databearbetning
http://www.sfmi.org

President and IMIA Representative:
Hans Adolfsson
Tel: +46 855 670 155
Fax: +46 855 670 155
E-mail: hans.adolfsson@
telia.com

Secretary/Treasurer:
Claes Schonqvist
Uppsala County Council
Tel: +46 18 611 6055
Fax: +46 18 611 6299
E-mail: claes.schonqvist@
it.ck.lul.se

Switzerland

Swiss Society for Medical Informatics (SSMI)
Schweizerische GEsllschaft für Medizinische Informatik
Société Suisse d'Informatique Médicale
http://www.sgmi-ssim.ch/

SSMI Secretariat:
SGMI / SSIM
PO Box 229, Daelhoelzliweg 3
Bern 6, Switzerland

President:
Dr. Judith Wagner
H+ die Spitäler der Schweiz
Spitalinformatik und -statistik
Zähringerstraße 33
CH-3012 Bern
Switzerland
Tel: +43 41 31 306 6130
Fax: +43 41 31 306 6110
E-mail: judith.wagner@hplus.ch

IMIA Representative:
Prof. Dr. Antoine Geissbuhler
Geneva University Hospital
Division of Medical Informatics
Switzerland
Tel: +43 41 22 372 6201
Fax: +4341 22 372 6255
E-mail: antoine.geissbuhler@
hcuge.ch

Switzerland

Swiss Society for Medical Informatics (SSMI)
Schweizerische GEsllschaft für Medizinische Informatik
Société Suisse d'Informatique Médicale
(Continued)

Executive Director:
Ms. Anita Eymann
Sekretariat SGMI c/o VSAO
Tel: +43 31 436 4499
Fax: +43 31 436 4498
E-mail: admin@sgmi.ssim.ch

Secretary:
Dr. Ruedi Tschudi
Spital Thurgau AG
Tel: +43 41 716 864 550
Fax: +43 41 716 864 549
E-mail: ruedi.tschudi@kttg.ch

Turkey

Turkish Medical Informatics Association (TURKMIA)
TIP BILISIMI DERNEGI
http://www.turkmia.org

President:
Mehmet T. Kitapci
Gazi University School of
Medicine
Tel: +90 312 214 1000/6161
Fax: +90 312 215 6456
E-mail: mkitapci@yahoo.com

IMIA Representative:
Erdal Musoglu
NAMSA, HQ
Tel: +90 352 3063 6702
Fax: +90 352 3063 6653
E-mail: erdal_musoglu@
          yahoo.com

Secretary:
Dr. Tamer Calikoglu
Oncology Hospital
Tel: +90 312 435 5343
Fax: +90 312 435 4006
E-mail: tamer@pleksus.net.tr

Ukraine

The Ukraine Association for "Computer Medicine"
(UACM)
http://www.uacm.cit-ua.net

IMIA Representative:
Prof. Oleg Yu. Mayorov, Ph.D.,
M.D., Dr.Sc.
Kharkiv Medical Academy
National Institute of Children
and Adolescents
Tel: +380 572 118 032
Fax: +380 572 118 025
E-mail: mayorov@
          uacm.kharkov.ua

United Kingdom

British Computer Society Health Informatics Specialist
Group
http://www.bcs.org.uk/siggroup/siglist.htm

President:
Dr. John S. Bryden
Bryden Consulting Ltd.
Tel: +44 141 427 2959
E-mail: jsbry@healthinfo.win-
          uk.net

Secretary/Treasurer:
John Bryant
University of Surrey
Tel: +44 1483 876700 ext.2972
Fax: +44 1483 259 395
E-mail: j.bryant@surrey.ac.uk

IMIA Representative:
Peter Murray
E-mail: peter@
          lemmus.demon.co.uk

Uruguay

Uruguayan Society of Medical Informatics
Sociedad Uruguaya de Informática en la Salud
http://www.suis.org.uy

IMIA Representative:
Dr. Alvaro Margolis
Tel: +598 2 401 4701
Fax: +598 2 402 6170
E-mail: margolis@mednet.org.uy

USA

American Medical Informatics Association (AMIA)

http://www.amia.org

AMIA Office:
4915 St. Elmo Avenue, Suite 401
Bethesda, MD 20814 USA

President:
Dr. Patricia Flatley Brennan,
University of Wisconsin -
Madison School of Nursing
1513 University Avenue
Madison, WI 53706, USA
Tel: +1 608 263 5251
Fax: +1 608 263 5252
E-mail: pbrennan@engr.wisc.edu

Executive Director:
Dennis J. Reynolds
American Medical Informatics
Association
Tel: +1 301 657 1291
Fax: +1 301 657 1296
E-mail: dennis@mail.amia.org

IMIA Representative:
Marion J. Ball
Healthlink, Inc.
Tel: +1 410 433 1889
Fax: +1 410 433 6314
E-mail: marionball@earthlink.net

Treasurer:
Dr. Nancy M. Lorenzi
Vanderbilt University Medical
Center
Informatics Center
Tel: +1 615 936 1423
Fax: +1 615 936 1427
E-mail: nancy.lorenzi@
          mcmail.vanderbilt.edu

EFMI (IMIA Europe)

European Federation for Medical Informatics
http://www.hiscom.nl/efmi

President:
Dr. Rolf Engelbrecht
MEDIS - Institut
GSF-National Research Center
for Environment and Health
Ingolstädter Landstr. 1
D-85764 Oberschleißheim
Germany
Tel: +49 89 3187 4138
Fax: +49 89 3187 3008
E-mail: engel@gsf.de

Vice President:
Dr. Assa Reichert
SAREL House, Hgavish St, Ind.
Zone south Netanya POB 8466
Netanya, Israel
Tel: +972 9 892 2005
Fax: +972 9 892 2111
E-mail: reichert@sarel.co.il

Vice President IMIA:
Prof. Dr. Attila Naszlady
National Inst. of Pulmonology
Cardiopulmonary Department
Sahegyi ut 18, H-1124 Budapest
Hungary
Tel: +36 1 200 2573
Fax: +36 1 200 2573
E-mail: irgalmas@elender.hu

Secretary:
Dr. Robert Baud
Hospital of Geneva
Div. Informatique Médicale
Rue du Crest
CH-1211 Geneva 14
Switzerland
Tel: +41 22 372 6203
Fax: +41 22 372 6255
E-mail: robert.baud@
          dim.hcuge.ch

Treasurer:
Dr. Camilla Glaso Skifjeld
Universitets Klinikken
Montebello
Norske Radiumhospital
N-0310 Oslo
Norway
Tel: +47 22 935 656
Fax: +47 22 732 944
E-mail: c.g.skifeld@labmed.uio.no

Executive Officer:
Dr. Peter McNair
Department of Clinical
Biochemistry
Hvidovre Hospital
Kettegaard alle 30
DK-2650 Copenhagen-Hvidovre
Denmark
Tel: +45 36 32 2345
Fax: +45 31 75 0977
E-mail: peter.mcnair@
          dadlnet.dk

Information Officer:
Dr. Jacob Hofdijk
HISCOM
Schipholweg 97
NL-2316 XA Leiden
Netherlands
Tel: +31 71 525 6708
Fax: +31 71 521 6675
E-mail: Jacob@hiscom.nl

Publication Officer:
Prof. Dr. Arie Hasman
University Maastricht
Dept. of Medical Informatics
P.O. Box 616
NL-6200 MD Maastricht
The Netherlands
Tel.:   +31 43 3882 240
Fax: +31 43 367 1052
E-mail: hasman@mi.unimaas.nl

IMIA-LAC (Latin America)

Federation of Health Societies in Latin America

President and IMIA Representative:
Dr. Lincoln de Assis Moura Jr.
Saude24Hs
Sao Paulo SP, Brazil
Tel: +55 11 5056 0458
Fax: +55 11 9182 7495
E-mail: lamoura@uol.com.br

APAMI (IMIA Asia Pacific)

Asia Pasific Association for Medical Informatics

IMIA Representative:
Dr. Chun Por Wong
Chief of Integrated Medical Services
Ruttonjee Hospital
Tel: +852 2291 1345
Fax: +852 2291 1335
E-mail: cpwong@iohk.com

Helina (African Region)

IMIA Representative:
Dr. Sedick S. Isaacs
Integrated Business Information Systems
Groote Schuur Hospital/
University of Cape Town
Observatory, Western Cape
Tel: +27 21 404 2058
Fax: +27 21 404 2070
E-mail: seisaacs@
              pawc.wcape.gov.za

Information on IMIA Societies

Argentina

General Information:

The Argentine Association of Medical Informatics (*AAIM*) is an academic institution born as an umbrella organization to fulfill the needs related to the development and application of Medical/Health Informatics overall the country. Some of these needs are the interchange of information and ideas, the development of norms, standards and joint projects, the promotion of international relationship and the diffusion of scientific papers and specific programs. *AAIM* is open to all representative groups that produce developments in the field of Medical/Health Informatics all over the country.

The Main Goals of AAIM are:

- The objectives of *AAIM* are of scientific, bibliographic and educational characters. These objectives are aimed at promoting the development and application of Medical Informatics to improve patient care, use teaching programs in the area of Health Informatics and carry out research and administration projects in the field of health.
- To promote interchange among the different local groups and similar foreign ones.
- To spread and provide knowledge about informatics in the field of health.
- To represent its associates in local and international organizations.

Australia

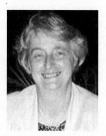

Evelyn Hovenga, IMIA Representative

HISA Mission Statement

HISA is a member-friendly, professional organisation, focussing on healthcare informatics with benefits for practitioners, disciplines and sectors of healthcare in any geographic region of Australia and the world.

Member services are developed with the aim of value-adding knowledge for the individual member and enhancing networking opportunities between members.

HISA Objectives

- A national focus for health informatics in Australia Management and administration of HISA
- National assistance to members and others Publishing through print and electronic media
- Information collection, analysis and distribution
- Research promotion, support and co-ordination

Austria

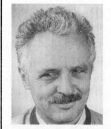

Günther Gell, President

Computers have become more important for medicine. At the edge of the 21st Century, informational technology, computer science, knowledge management and communications engineering are of increasing importance as Interfaces between humans and machines. Improved medical technology has helped doctors to raise the level of health care.

Teaching and learning technology has proved to be equally valuable in the education and training of medical students. We aim to achieve an improved interdisciplinary cooperation between medical and technological personnel.

Topics:
- Information Systems
- Internet - Intranet
- Knowledge Management
- Knowledge Technology
- Multimedia in Medicine
- Telemedicine
- PACS
- Human - Computer - Interaction
- Quality Management
- Standards

Belgium

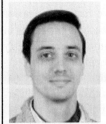

Etienne De Clercq, President

The Belgian Society for Medical Informatics ("MIM") was established in 1974 to promote and develop medical information science and technology in Belgium. It is a national bilingual (French and Dutch) society consisting of about 300 members, all involved or interested in the use of computers and telematics in the health-care environment. The administrative board includes 15 members (physicians, engineers and computers specialists) from academic institutions, hospitals, computers and the software industry.

The MIM is a scientific society. Its major activities focus on improving communication among researchers and developers in the field of medical computing and telematics. It is also the place of choice where problems related to the role of medical informatics in society and its ethical aspects are discussed. International related medical informatics societies:

- The MIM is the Belgian member of EFMI (European Federation for Medical Informatics) and of IMIA (International Medical Informatics Association). As such, the MIM is involved in the setting up of whose congresses, scientific events and publications.
- The MIM cooperates closely with the Dutch (VMBI), French (AIM) and Swiss (SSIM) medical informatics societies to organize annual scientific meetings: the « Medish Informatica Congres » (MIC) and the « Journées Francophones d'Informatique Médicale » (JFIM).

Bosnia and Herzegovina

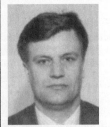

Izet Masic, President

The Society of Medical Informatics of the Republic of Bosnia and Herzegovina (DMI BiH) was founded in 1998, and has now over 80 members. The Society has its statutory bodies- the Administrative Board and Committees. The members of the administrative Board are the President of the Society, two Vice-Presidents, a Secretary, a Treasurer and four additional members. The current president is Prof.Dr. Izet Masic, the founder of the Society. Prof. Masic is also the official representative of the Society in EFMI and IMIA.

The society became an official member of EFMI and IMIA in 1994.

The Society carries out the following activities:

a) Promotion and improvement of informatics within the health-care system, health insurance and bio-medical research,

b) Engagement of experts in the field of medical informatics in B&H on development and establishment of health care information systems

c) Assistance in research, development and professional work in the field of medical informatics in B&H

d) Distribution and development of technical information in the field of medical informatics in B&H

e) Assistance in education of medical informatics experts

f) Exchange of professional experience on national and international level

g) Publishing activities in the field of medical informatics.

The society edits its own professional journal-ACTA INFORMATICA MEDICA, and has organized four scientific and professional symposia during wartime in BIH. In November 1992, the Society has organized the First Symposium of Medical Informatics in BIH about Nomenclatures and classification systems in Bosnia and Herzegovina. Next Symposium was organized in 1993 with the theme:

Health Information Systems in Bosnia and Herzegovina. In 1994 the Society of Medical Informatics prepared new Symposium: Medical informatics according to the War medicine. Several books and monographs in the field of Medical Informatics have been published. Our experts have taken part in various scientific and professional gatherings and symposia at home and aboard on EFMI and IMIA Congresses and workshops during last eight years. They also participate in development and realization of information system health care, at regional as well as national levels. In this way the Society contributes considerably to the improvement of health care in Bosnia and Herzegovina.

The First congress of Medical informatics in B&H that was held in Sarajevo on November 5 & 6, 1999 gave us the opportunity to discuss the experiences in the current state of this science and its practical use in the world and our country. The Congress attracted over 100 participants, who attended seven very attractive sessions.

Brazil

The Brazilian Health Informatics Association - SBIS - aims at improving the quality and reducing the costs of healthcare via the use of Health Informatics techniques, concepts and technologies, by:

- Stimulating educational activities related to Health Informatics;
- Stimulating scientific research and technical development in Health Informatics;
- Organising conferences, symposiums, courses, seminars, and other activities

that lead to experience and knowledge exchange;
- Joining individuals, groups and organizations together;
- Cooperating with sister societies;
- Contributing to the construction of healthcare policies;
- Promoting of Health Informatics as a means to reduce costs and improve the quality of healthcare services;
- Promoting the use of standards for healthcare information.

Canada

COACH, Canada's Health Informatics Association is an organization of more than 700 health executives, physicians, nurses, and allied health professionals, researchers, educators, information technology managers and vendors.

COACH Members form a network of specialists in the Healthcare industry across Canada. This network provides an opportunity for the exchange of information and ideas through personal contact with colleagues, locally and nationally.

COACH's mandate is to promote the understanding and effective use of information technologies in the Canadian Health Care environment through: education, information, communication and networking.

China

The China Medical Informatics Association (CMIA), established in 1980, is an academic organization constituted by physicians, researchers, technologists, and administrators who are researching how to utilize computer science and information science in health care field. CMIA is a National Member in International Medical Informatics Association (IMIA), and is the only representative of China in IMIA. There are more than 5,700 members, 31 professional committees and 22 regional branches in CMIA.

The development of CMIA, also named as China Medical Informatics Association of Chinese Institute of Electronics, has won support from Ministry of Information Industry, Ministry of Health, State Economy and Trade Commission, State Drug Administration, etc. CMIA has built up broad relationship with hospitals, universities, academic institutions and industries.

Medical informatics is developed with a rapid speed in today's China. CMIA's goals and objectives are to advance the understanding and use of information technologies in China health care; to support the development of medicine and pharmacy; to build up the bridges among researchers, scientists, practitioners, suppliers, managers in health care field.

The 3rd China-Papan-Korea Joint Symposium on Medical Informatics is scheduled for Oct. or Nov. 2001 in Japan

Croatia

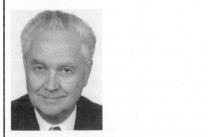

Gjuro Dezelic, President

The Croatian Society for Medical Informatics is a non-profit organization concerned with the scientific field of medical informatics, which comprises the theory and practice of information science and technology within health care and health care science. The basic objectives of the CSMI are as follows:

(1) to advance dissemination of information in the field of MI in Croatia,

(2) to promote high standards in the application of work in this field,
(3) to promote research and development in this field,
(4) to encourage high standards in education in this field,
(5) to advance international cooperation in this field.

Croatia (Continued)

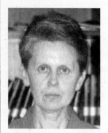

Josipa Kern, IMIA Representative

CSMI organizes professional and scientific meetings. Four national symposiums with international participation were organised so far. Recently, two working groups were established:

WG1 - standardization in medical informatics

WG2 - data protection and data security.

The Society publishes a bulletin with papers of the CSMI members, and relevant information two times a year.

Cuba

The Cuban Society of Medical Informatics groups specialists of different fields working on Medical and Health Informatics throughout the country. Health Research Centers, Medical Sciences Faculties, Specialized Informatics Centers working on Medical and Health Computerized Applications are also involved. The main goal of the Society is to develop and widespread scientific and updated informatic knowledge in all medical and health fields supporting the Health Policy of the National Health System. A major movement towards generalizing Medical Informatics is being developed through the creation in Provincial and Municipal Health Administrative Levels as well as in most Health Institutions of Health Informatics Groups. These groups are in charge of training the current staff of health organizations and institutions on the use of computers and the application of specific Medical and Health Informatics Systems performed. A National Policy on Health Informatics is ongoing with the active support of the Society.

Czech Republic

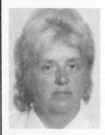

Jana Zvárová, IMIA Representative

The Czech Society of Biomedical Engineering and Medical Informatics is one of the medical societies gathered in the Czech Association of Medical Societies of J.E. Purkyne. Medical Informatics Section of the Czech Society of Biomedical Engineering has been established in 1978. Through this section the activities in the field of medical informatics have been developed. Nowadays the Society is mostly concerned with activities in three sections "Medical Informatics Section" "Clinical Engineering Section" and "Biophysics" section. The Czech Society of Biomedical Engineering is the member of International Medical Informatics Association (IMIA), European Federation for Medical Informatics (EFMI) and International Federation for Medical and Biological Engineering (IFMBE).

The general board of eleven elected society members rules the Society. The president of the Czech Society of Biomedical Engineering and Medical Informatics is J. Cmíral, the Medical Informatics Section is headed by J. Zvárová (IMIA representative and EFMI representative), the Clinical Engineering Section by V. Grošpic and Biophysics Section by Z. Grossman. The Czech Society of Biomedical Engineering and Medical Informatics has issued the journal Physician and Technology, edited by J. Zvárová. The journal is published bimonthly and basic information about the journal can be found at the www address http://lat.euromise.cz/. The Society has structural links with other medical societies J.E. Purkyne http://www.cls.cz/ and co-operates with other Czech scientific societies in this field, mainly Society for Cybernetics and Informatics and Czech Scientific and Technical Society. The Society has close contacts with scientific societies in Hungary, Bulgaria, Poland and Austria.

The main activities of the Czech Society of Biomedical Engineering and Medical Informatics developed in the past together with Slovakia, were seminars, conferences and congresses, namely three international biomedical engineering conferences held in Mariánské Lázne (1983), Bratislava (1987) and Prague (1991, 1997). The Society has co-

Czech Republic (Continued)

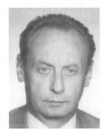

Jaromir Cmíral, President

sponsored the international conference System Science in Health Care in Prague 1992 and has been involved in Biosignal international conferences in Brno each two years. The next conference Biosignal co-sponsored by EURASIP will be held in Brno, June 26th – 28th, 2002 (*http://www.fee.vutbr.cz/UBMI/bs2002.html*).

The medical informatics section of the Society has organized the main activities in the field of medical informatics. Apart from several national seminars held on different topics of medical informatics each year, the conferences on medical informatics were held in Prague 1981 and 1988, and IMIA international working conference took place in Prague in 1985 and 1990. The proceedings of the IMIA working

conferences were published by Elsevier Publishing Company (North Holland) under the titles "Diagnostic Strategies and Expert Systems" and "Knowledge, Information and Medical Education".

In 2001 the activities of the Society concentrated in the following areas. The Society was the main organizer of the international workshop The International HL7 Standard – a Pathway to Better Healthcare (Prague, April 20th 2001), participated in the 25th Workshop on Medical Biophysics (Mozolov, May 30th – June 1st 2001) and is organizing the main organizer of the workshop Telemedicine, October 10th 2001 in Prague. Further the Society participates in the workshop MediForum 2001 organized at the congress MEFA in Brno, November 9th 2001.

Denmark

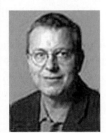

Henrik Lindholm, President

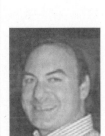

Knut Bernstein, IMIA Representative

The interest in medical informatics, or more appropriate - health care informatics - is increasing in the Danish community. The awareness among health care professionals is growing, the topic is clearly on the political agenda, and the marketplace is expanding.

It is interesting to note, that

- the Government has published its IT strategy - where health care has a very high priority. An agreement has been reached with the Counties (which runs the hospitals) for a strategy and the financing of an expansion of IT use in hospitals.
- the national health care network programme (MedCom) has been made a permanent activity. More than 1,5 million health care messages are sent via the network every month. (www.health-telematics.dk/)
- the Ministry of Health is supporting 10 project regarding the development of Danish electronic patient records. An increasing number of hospitals are starting to use electronic health care records. (www.hep.dk/)
- the National Panel for Standardisation of Medical Informatics has published a popular booklet on standardisation of electronic health care records.
- the use of Internet in health care is increasing. The Danish Medical Association has established a medical Intranet and supplies all Danish doctors with free Internet access. (A public part is on www.dadl.dk)
- the post graduate education in health care informatics is running at Aalborg University for the forth year, graduating Masters of Information Technology.

DSMI has once again supported some of the students with grants. (www.v-chi.dk/)
- the number of members in The Danish Society for Medical Informatics is increasing. (www.dsmi.dk)

The Danish Society for Medical Informatics - Dansk Selskab for Medicinsk Informatik (DSMI) was established in 1966. It is an independent society with an associated status to the Danish Medical Societies. The aim of the society is to compile and disseminate theoretical and practical knowledge in medical informatics, and to stimulate research and the use of medical information systems. The 350 members are physicians, nurses and others who work with theoretical or practical aspects of medical information technologies.

DSMI organises meetings, conferences and courses to pursue the goals of the society. One of the largest efforts for the Society was the organisation of MIE'96 in Copenhagen. More that 1000 participants participated in the high quality scientific programme and the large exhibition.

Other meetings have been successfully organised on electronic patient records, classification and semantics, clinical databases, resource management, the information highway etc.

The Society is represented in various groups, i.e. the Ministry of Health's advisory group and the Danish Standardisation Committee. The Society publishes a newsletter with abstracts of the meetings, papers, book reviews, announcements of international conferences and other relevant information. The DSMI homepage is playing a large role in the communication with the members: www.dsmi.dk.

Finland

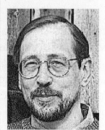

Mikko Korpela, IMIA Representative

The Finnish Social and Health Informatics Association was founded in 1974 and it organised the MIE conference in 1985. After that the association's activities decreased and it became dormant by the mid 1990s.

Since research, education and development projects in health informatics have been increasing strongly in Finland recently, the association was re-vitalised in May 2000. The scope of the association was expanded to social services informatics in June 2001.

The activities of the association focus on international relations, establishing a new membership base, and in building up a web site for information dissemination. The main event of the association is the annual national Social and Health Care Informatics Research Days SoTeTiTe-tutkimuspäivät), the fifth of which will be held in May 2002.

France

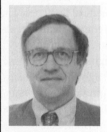

P. Degoulet, IMIA Representative

AIM, the acronym for *the Association pour les Applications de l'Informatique en Médecine* was created in 1968. Since its beginning, the association has been involved in the promotion of computer applications in health care through the organization of scientific meetings, publications and various educational efforts. In the early seventies, AIM was directly involved in the organization of the *Journées d'Informatique Médicale de Toulouse*, which were among the first international meetings devoted to medical informatics. AIM is the official representative of France within the IMIA and EFMI boards and counts approximately 500 affiliate members. AIM currently organizes one or two meetings per year.

Proceedings of major meetings have been published since 1989 in a special series called *Informatique et Santé* and published by Springer-Verlag France.

Recent volumes include:

Volume 7: *Informatisation d l'Unité de Souns du Futur.* J. Demongeot, P. Le Beux, G. Weil, eds, 1994.

Volume 8: *Information Médicale: Aspects Ethiques, Juridiques et de Santé Publique.* L. Dusserre, M Goldbert, R. Salamon, eds, 1996.

Volume 9: *Informatique et Gestion Médicalisée.* F. Kohler, M. Brémond, D. Mayeux, eds, 1997.

Volume 10: Santé et *Réseaux Informatiques.* A. Albert, F. Roger France, P. Degoulet, M. Fieschi, eds, 1998.

Volume 11: *L'informatisation du Cabinet Médical du Futur.* A. Venot, H. Falcoff, eds, 1999.

Additional information is available at the following URL address: http://www.hbroussais.fr/Broussais/InforMed/AIM.html

Georgia

The Georgian Association of Medical Informatics and Biomedical Engineering (GAMIBE) was founded in 1990 on the basic of the former Georgian Division of the All-Union Medical-Technical Society. However, the activities in Georgia in the field of the implementation of mathematical tools and computer techniques in medicine and health care began as early as 1968, when the Department of Medical Cybernetics at the Research Institute of Clinical and Experimental Surgery was organized.

Medical informatics specialists, under the guidance of the above mentioned predecessor of GAMIBE, have developed and implemented a number of projects, particularly information systems for medical statistics, for sanitary-epidemiological surveillance, several hospital and policlinical information systems, medical personnel retrieval systems, various accounting systems, etc. They have conducted research in psychophysiology (together with colleagues from Germany), in modeling processes in the human organism, and other investigations. The Georgian specialists of medical informatics took part in many conferences and congresses in Moscow and other parts of the former Soviet Union.

There are many publications on different issues in the field, mostly in the Georgian or Russian language.

Since 1971, four National Conferences on Medical Informatics and Biomedical Engineering were held. Especially the fourth Conference of 1990 is worth mentioning. At this Conference, which took place in the capital of Georgia, Tbilisi, specialists of many countries took part, particularly the members of the IMIA Board. The IMIA Board Meeting was held during that Conference. The Proceedings of the 4th National Conference were then published in original languages in which they were presented.

After 1991, when Georgia became independent, GAMIBE tried to take active part in the activity of IMIA. Since September 1993, GAMIBE is a national member of IMIA.

Since 1993, the activities of GAMIBE substantially slowed down, mainly because of the critical political and economic situation in the Georgian society as a whole, which is characteristic for a transition period. The year 1998 is expected to be a turning-point. A number of working groups have restarted their activities. Organizing the 5th National Conference on Medical Infor-matics and Biomedical Engineering is envisaged.

Germany

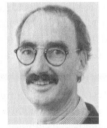

Rüdiger Klar, President

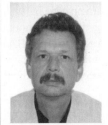

Herbert Witte, IMIA Representative

The GMDS, Deutsche Gesellschaft für Medizinische Informatik, Biometrie und Epidemiologie (German Association for Medical Informatics, Biometry and Epidemiology) is the only scientific organization in this field and as such the official national member within EFMI and IMIA. It closely cooperates with two professional organizations: the Berufsverband Medizinischer Informatiker (BVMI) and the Deutsche Verband Medizinischer Dokumentare (DVMD).

The scientific association GMDS was founded in the Fifties and is with more than 1600 members one of the largest scientific societies in this field in the world.

The basic structure of the GMDS consists of four divisions (medical informatics, medical biometry, epidemiology and medical documentation), with a wide variety of working groups. The management board of the GMDS is led by its president (Prof. Klar, Freiburg, 1999-2001; Prof. Lehmacher, Köln 2001-2003). The full structure of the GMDS and its work is described in www.gmds.de.

The GMDS issues a national scientific journal: Biometrie, Informatik und Epidemiologie in Medizin und Biologie (Gustav Fischer Verlag, Stuttgart, Eugen Ulmer Verlag, Stuttgart). The journal includes a newsletter of the national society.

Besides a spring congress on Hospital Information Systems and some smaller working conferences, the GMDS annually organizes one large national meeting with about 700 to 900 participants. The 2000 GMDS congress was held in Hannover together with MIE 2000. The 2001 congress will be held in Köln (Sept. 16th-20th). All national congresses have been published in proceedings volumes.

As education is a main concern of GMDS it has published a national strategic plan for education in medical informatics as well as for medical biometry.

The GMDS is also actively involved in the definition of the medical curriculum and of the content of CME for physicians and for certified further professional qualification of medical informaticians, biometricians, epidemiologists and medical documentalists.

Hong Kong

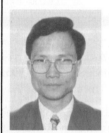

Chun Por Wong, President

The Hong Kong Society of Medical Informatics was founded in April 1987 by a group of medical practitioners with special interests in medical informatics and computing. It expanded rapidly and now encompasses all workers in the health care information technology industry. In 2000, the Society had more than 1000 members.

The specific objectives of the Society are:

1. To promote applications of computers and information technology in medicine, and to maintain knowledge on information science and computer basics for health care workers in Hong Kong.
2. To provide a forum for the exchange of ideas and experience in medical computing among its members.
3. To hold lectures, seminars, exhibitions and conferences on subjects related to medical informatics.

4. To liaise with overseas medical informatics organizations, in order to capture first-hand information on the development of medical informatics.

The most important projects undertaken by the Society were the hosting of the series of five Hong Kong Asia-Pacific Medical Informatics Conferences since 1990. The Society has also acted as the technical organizer in the Medical Informatics Pavilions of various computer exhibitions in Hong Kong.

Hong Kong is now the President of the APAMI for the year 2000-2003. We look forward to a joint effort in Asia Pacific countries to further promote the standing of Medical Informatics in the region to a more prominent level in the global scene, and more importantly, to assist under-developed countries to develop and improve the medical informatics development in their region.

Hungary

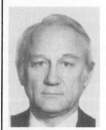

Attila Naszlady, President

The Biomedical Section of the Hungarian John von Neumann Society for Computing Sciences was founded in 1968. A team of the Attila Jozsef University of Science in Szeged, which has biocybernetical interest, and its leader, Laszlo Kalmar, mathematician and academician, had a decisive role in founding this Society. An excellent initiative was launched by organizing Von Neumann Colloqia in Szeged each year. The name "colloqium" is not by chance; it expresses the essential aims of computer science and informatics in a scientific forum, i.e., the discussion of the themes. Vivid discussions, a critical spirit, and a high professional level still have great value today, which concerns not only research, but also the distribution of knowledge and continuing training.

The first colloquium of 1970 dealt with themes which are even of interest today: analysis of amplitude-time dependence curves, capnograms, pneumotachograms, electroencephalograms, correlation analysis of blood-circulation curves, mathematical-statistical analysis of data, computerization of telemetric and nuclear data, and modelling of receptor fields.

In the middle of the 1970s, as a continuation of previous themes, the first computer studies of clinical and hospital information processes, compartmental analysis, image processing, hospital management, decision-support systems, cell automation, and data processing for population screening completed the list of subjects.

Starting in 1980, taking into consideration the wishes of the members of the Society, which increased to 3,400, we decided that the colloquium in each even year should be largely theoretical, related to basic research, and in each following year application oriented.

Soon, software houses, programming groups, and computer companies began to be interested in these themes. Exhibitions were organized during the time of the colloquia. Application-oriented colloquia were organized by Institutes dealing with medical informatics in different cities, usually with international participation. In 1987, we applied for joining the International Medical Informatics Association (IMIA) and its European regional organization, the European Federation for Medical Informatics (EFMI).

Hungary (Continued)

In 1988 we became members of both organizations. Rory O'Moore, the president of EFMI at that time, took part in the colloqium in Szekszard, and reported with great appreciation to the International Society. In 1990, the Biomedical Section of NJSZT had the honor that its president was elected to one of the 6 members of the EFMI Board, as the first one from the previous socialist countries. The Biomedical Section of NJSZT is building connections with other international and home organizations. So, we were happy to welcome the initiative of the International Measurement Confederation (IMEKO) to organize common meetings.

We regularly invite a representative of the Hungarian Health Informatics Society to our Board meetings, and we organized the colloquium of 1991 together with them, the Medical Science Society, and the Hospital Federation. This meeting can be called a jubileum, as this was the 20th during the previous 20 years. The President of our Society, Prof. Attila Naszlady, M.D., was elected to be EFMI Secretary in Jerusalem in 1993. He has been elected as Vice President of EFMI in (Copenhagen) 1996, then President of EFMI in (Porto Karras) 1997. The most important events have been the Computers in Cardiology World Congress in Vienna-Budapest in 1995, and the IFIP World Congress in Vienna-Budapest in 1998.

Ireland

From 1976 to 1996, Healthcare Informatics interests in the Republic of Ireland were represented by the Health Care Specialist Group of the Irish Computer Society. This group represented Ireland at the European Federation for Medical Informatics (EFMI) and the International Medical Informatics Association (IMIA). It hosted the European Medical Informatics conference, MIE 82, and was associated with the IMIA Working Group 8 international symposium on Nursing Informatics held in Dublin in 1988.

In May 1996 the members of the Health Care Specialist Group formed a new society, the Healthcare Informatics Society of Ireland (Cumann Ríomheolais Sláinte), in order to broaden the base of membership and increase the range of services offered. By formal agreement with the Irish Computer Society, the Health Care Specialist Group was disbanded, and its functions, assetts and liabilities transferred to the new Society, which then became affiliated to the Irish Computer Society.

The Healthcare Informatics Society of Ireland was inaugurated formally at its First Annual Conference in the Burlington Hotel, Dublin, on Thursday 10th October 1996. The new society incorporates the Healthcare Informatics section of the Royal Academy of Medicine in Ireland. Thus the Healthcare Informatics Society is in a position to build bridges between computer professionals interested in health care, and health care professionals interested in

computing, while supporting and embracing the new professionals of health care informatics. There are currently some 270 members, drawn from information technology, medicine, nursing, other professions allied to medicine, education, government and industry.

The officers of the Society are:

President: Prof. Jane Grimson, Trinity College, Dublin.

Chair: Mr. Gerard Hurl, Mater Misericordiae Hospital, Dublin.

Secretary: Ms. Ann Sheridan, St. John of God Hospital, Dublin.

Treasurer: Mr. Diarmuid UaConaill, Mater Misericordiae Hospital, Dublin.

The objectives, as set out in the Constitution, are:

1. To develop and disseminate knowledge of the use of informatics in health care.
2. To promote research and education in health care informatics.
3. To participate internationally with bodies of similar interests.

In pursuit of the third objective, the Healthcare Informatics Society of Ireland has been accepted as a member of the European Federation for Medical Informatics, and the International Medical Informatics Association.

For further information, see our website at: http://www.mater.ie/hisi/hisi.htm or http://hisi.ie.eu.org/hisi.htm

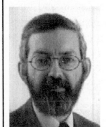

Diarmuid UaConaill, IMIA Representative

Israel

The Israeli Association of Medical Informatics(IAMI) was established in 1983 with the following goals:

- To promote knowledge of Medical Informatics by organizing scientific and professional conferences, seminars courses and exhibitions.

- Advance cooperation among health professionals in the field of Medical Informatics.
- Provide forums for exchange of information and ideas.
- Present the interest of health professionals in goverment committees and other bodies.

Italy

The Italian Association for Medical Informatics (AIIM) was founded on 1997 to promote the applications of informatics in the different areas of medicine.

The objectives of the AIIM are the dissemination and exchange of information on medical informatics, for support patient care, teaching, research and health care administration; to advance international cooperation in medical informatics; to promote medical informatics education and to organize courses for health services personnel.

The AIIM is a Member of the European Federation for Medical Informatics (EFMI) and the International Medical Informatics Association (IMIA).

The Members categories are: (a) Regular members including physicians, nurses, dentists, teachers, researchers, biomedical engineers, health services administrators, other health care professionals who have a strong interest in medical informatics; (b) Honorary members: very important persons in the field of medical informatics; (c) Correspondent members, including representatives of other Organizations and Associations having similar aims (European Society for Medical Decision Making; National Association for Informatics in Neuroscience, Italian Telematics Forum, etc).

The President of AIIM, who has to be a physician, and the national council (10 members), are elected every four years by the membership.

At present, AIIM organize a National Congress every two years, and annually other meetings and workshops on specific top-

ics. The previous AIIM National Congresses have been held in Parma (1997), Catania (1985), Firenze (1988), Como (1989), Cassino (1990), Catania (1991), Genova (1992), Roma (1994), Venezia (1996); furthermore AIIM organized in Rome the Seventh European Congress on Medical Informatics (MIE 1987): about 1,000 participants coming form 32 countries all over the world took part in the Congress.

The proceedings of the national congresses published by AIIM are an important source of information for the knowledge of medical informatics progress in Italy.

At present, the following Working Groups are operating in AIIM:

- Data Protection and Security in Health Information Systems, Bio-Ethics
- Standards in Health Information Systems
- Computerized Medical Records, Cards
- Telemedicine and Health Telematics
- Decision-Support Systems

AIIM cooperates with governmental bodies as an adviser in the field of medical informatics.

Guidelines on Telemedicine and Telematics in Health Care and on Health Cards, were approved during the last national Congress in Venice with the participation of representatives of governmental and military health organizations, health professionals and scientific associations, researchers, telecommunication and information technology companies and industries, national research council, and citizens associations.

Japan

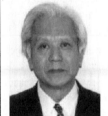

Michitoshi Inoue, President

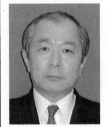

Ken Toyoda, IMIA Representative

Activities of the Japan Association for Medical Informatics (JAMI) are mainly performed through 8commitees and 16 research groups supported by 2,112 members.

The president of JAMI is Dr. Inoue, President of Osaka National Hospital and Professor Emeritus of Osaka University.

Six issues of „Iryo Jouhou Gaku" (Japan Journal of Medical Informatics), the official journal of JAMI, have been published in 2001 (Volume 21). Included are two supplements for „The JAMI Symposium" and „The 21st Joint Conference on Medical Informatics".

The „JAMI Symposium 01" entitled „Medical Informatics in the 21st century" was held at MailParc at Nagoya on June 16. There was a special lecture on the topic „Risk Management to Patient Safety -Data is Key" by Dr. Luke Sato, Vice President of Harvard Risk Management Foundation.

„The 21st Joint Conference on Medical Informatics" was held on November 26-28 at the Waterfront of Tokyo. The chairperson of the organizing committee was Dr. Hiroshi Inada, Professor of Tokyo University. The main theme was „Medicine in the New Century by IT Application". More than 1,800 members participated and about 500 papers were presented. As a special program contribution there were two special lectures, one by Dr. Edward H. Shortliffe, Professor of Columbia

University, on the topic „Networking Health : Prescription for the Internet" and other by Prof. Yusuke Nakamura, Tokyo University, on the topic „Order made medicine based on Genome Information".

The 3rd China-Japan-Korea Joint Symposium on Medical Informatics" (CJKMI'01) was held on November 27 at the same place of „The 21st Joint Conference on Medical Informatics". There were tree keynote lectures, „The Telemedicine in China" by Ms. Yanjie Gao, Deputy Director, Leading Group Office, IT Application, MOH., P.R. China; „Global Standardization and Non-Western Medicine" by Mr. Ken Toyoda, Director, Andersen Japan and „Current Status and Scope of Medical Informatics Education in Korea" by Dr. Hune Cho, Department of Medical Informatics, Kyungpook National University.

The JAMI Symposium 2002, entitled „Evaluation and Management of Medical Information Systems" will be held at Kokuyo Hall in Tokyo on May 31-June 1, 2002.

The 22nd Joint Conference an Medical Informatics will be held in Fukuoka on November, 2002. The chairperson of the organization committee is Prof. Yoshiaki Nose, Kyusyu University.

For more information about JAMI, contact the home page of JAMI (http://jami.umin.ac.jp/) or MEDIS-DC by telefax: 81-3-3505-1996 or by phone: 81-3-3586-6321.

Kazakstan

MedPharmInfo Association (medical - pharmaceutical information) was established in March, 2000 on the basis of The Information Center and Institute of Standardization, Metrology and Certification jointly with an inquiry-information bureau under the private company ZdravTechStandard. Besides mentioned organizations founders of the Association include several non-governmental medical centers, pharmaceutical companies, educational and scientific institutions.

The need for such association was due to an absolute necessity of an operational and professional information for specialists engaged in various healthcare organizations. First and foremost, this provides an opportunity to obtain the full code of laws and standard Acts, regulating public healthcare activity, production and supply of medicines and medical

products etc. In the course of professional activities medical men quite often search for specialized information covering different fields of medical sciences as well as practical issues. Population lacks accessible sources of popular information as to preventive methods, diseases, treatment and so forth. The list of problems can be extended further.

Taking into account the aforesaid grounds, founders of the Association set a goal to create a public organization uniting all the concerned medical and pharmaceutical organizations, scientific institutions, chemists, institutes of higher education and colleges, industrial enterprises etc., which are in need of access to contemporary information technologies. The Association initiated the creation of a large specialized informational center, which already comprises highly qualified specialists

Kazakstan
(Continued)

(doctors, pharmacists, marketing and information experts, computer programmers, electronics engineer etc.).

Modern material and logistic support is being created, new communication and technological solutions are in the process of implementation. This Center is meant for a large-scale information support in the field of healthcare in Kazakhstan, medical achievements and rendering various information to both specialists and vast population strata.

Activities: In the sake of the users large marketing and analytical research of the pharmaceutical market is being conducted in Kazakhstan, wholesale and retail prices for medications and medical equipment are being monitored. The Center has developed unique schemes for gathering and processing of information concerning wholesale and retail pricing in Almaty and other regions of Kazakhstan.

A free of charge round-the-clock phone inquiry office Medicines and Medical Services is successfully working under the jurisdiction of the Association.

Every month more than 70000 citizens use its services by multi-line telephone (3272) 50-50-60. This number is constantly growing.

The Center regularly publishes information bulletins: "Wholesale Prices for Medicines in Almaty, Kokshetau, Karagandy, Petropavlovsk and Shymkent" (twice a month), "Average Retail Process for Medicines in Almaty City" (monthly), and "Cost of Medical Services in Almaty" (at request). The bulletins are being distributed at pharmacists and clinics, in large pharmaceutical companies in Almaty, Astana, Aktyubinsk, Atyrau, Karagandy, Kokshetau, Kostanai, Pavlodar, Petropavlovsk, Semipalatinsk, Taraz, Ust-Kamenogorsk, Shymkent.

The Center's information database has been updated every day. Electronic versions of any information are available at the first request. Analytical data as to the population's requests allow obtaining extra information on the demand for certain medications.

For the first time in Kazakhstan The Center is publishing information materials on diverse healthcare issues in the Internet - on the website http://www.med.kz, which enlarges possibilities of the users to get necessary information such as code of laws and standards Acts on pharmaceutical and medical undertakings in the Republic of Kazakhstan; medical equipment producers and manufacturers; wholesale pharmaceutical companies; pharmacists in Almaty; medicines registered in Kazakhstan, wholesale and retail prices; international conferences and exhibitions, and many other aspects.

Since August 2000 there was launched a project "Telemedicine in Kazakhstan" http://www.tele.med.kz, within which framework the Association started to implement educational projects - monthly seminars Contemporary Internet technologies in the healthcare sphere (for free), and quarterly 3-day computer courses for medical specialists.

The Association is intended to widen up its services in the future for local and foreign organizations. It's planned to establish international co-operation in informational support for the healthcare system.

Conferences: Conferences and meetings are being held on the regular basis. Conference Achievements of Internet Technologies in Healthcare was arranged in Almaty on November 14, 2000 with the participation of local and foreign pharmaceutical companies and medical organizations. In the City of Taraz, on March 21, 2001 conference Prospective of telemedicine application under diagnostics and treatment of Kazakhstan's children was held on the basis of a children's hospital. conference IT in Healthcare took place in Pavlodar on May 25, 2001. The Association is planning the regularly arrange such conferences and seminars with medical workers.

Korea

The Society was established in October 1989 and Prof. Chang–Soon Koh was elected as the first Chairman of the Society. The first Conference of the Society was held in November that year, in which 7 papers were presented. Since then, every year, KOSMI organizes a conference. In 1990, KOSMI was registered for IMIA membership. In 1992, KOSMI was registered by the Ministry of Information and Communication as a corporation aggregate. In 1992, the 6th Conference of the Society was held, in which 21 papers were presented, and many applications were demonstrated, including computerization of medical record systems, and medical order communication systems, an automatic dispensing system for prescription order. The 9th International World Congress on Medical Informatics MEDINFO 98 has been held in Seoul, August 18-22, 1998.

The Netherlands

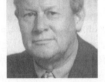

Arie Hasman, President

The goal of the VMBI, the Dutch Society for Health Care Informatics, is to promote research, development, and applications in medicine and health care, and in the biological sciences.

The Society is a meeting place for people in medical informatics in the broadest sense, i.e. physicians, nurses, informaticians, physicists, hospital administrators, and health care managers.

All hospitals in The Netherlands have systems installed to support administration, communication and patiënt care. In primary care, over 85% of GPs, all retail pharmacists, dentists, and the majority of physio-therapists have systems in use. An increasing numberv of systems are interconnected by EDI and networks. Development of computer-based patient records has much attention in R&D institutions. The Dutch professional medical societies play a major role in the promotion of information systems in healthcare. Most universities offer some training in medical informatics as part of the curriculum. This dynamic activity is a very healthy environment for the VMBI.

The activities of the VMBI include monthly meetings (lecturers, demonstrations) in Utrecht, in the center of the country, most of them in the late afternoon / early evening, annual two-day Conferences (called MIC, Medical Informatics Conference), together with the Belgian Society for Medical Informatics MIM, where about 400 people meet around lecturers, workshops and a large exhibition, an which is alternately held in The Netherlands and Belgium. The VMBI publishes a quarterly called I& (Informatie & Zorg, in english: Information & Care).

Over the past years, several IMIA Working Conferences have been organized in The Netherlands on subjects such as Tele-matics in Health Care, Hospital Information Systems, Electronic Patient Records in Medical Practice and Software Engineering in Health Care.

The VMBI developed a strategy to reinforce the relationships with professional medical societies and to increase its membership of practicing physicians. A working group has been established to develop concrete plans to widen the scope of the Society.

New Zealand

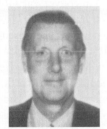

Ian H. Symonds, IMIA Representative

Health Informatics New Zealand is a national group open to anyone interested in Health Informatics We also have international members. Membership can be Individual or Corporate, (which allows unlimited members), Honorary or an affiliate. Health informatics relates to information technology in all areas of health care: clinical practice, administration, research, and education. It is the use of computers, information systems and other technologies which will provide better outcomes for patients who require health interventions.

We exist to :

- To promote and contribute to the growth of knowledge in Health Informatics

- To participate in the development of health information technologies and their use
- To lobby government on related health informatics issues to ensure informed input into decisions which affect health care outcomes in New Zealand
- To network and support those people interested in the use and application Health informatics Network with related national and international health informatics groups

Benefits for our members:

- Regular newsletters
- Bi annual conferences
- Study days/seminars
- Travel/conference funding/grants
- Website

Norway

The Norwegian Society for Medical Informatics - Forum for Databehandling i Helsesektoren (FDH) was established in 1972 as a special interest group of The Norwegian Informatics Society - Den Norske Dataforening (DND). Since 1989 FDH has been an independent society with primary interest in medical informatics and an associated status to DND. FDH has a long-established membership in EFMI and IMIA.

The society has both individual and institutional members. Most of the individual members are health care workers

FDH organizes meetings, seminars and courses to share knowledge and information with the members as well as to promote involvement of medical informatics in the Norwegian health care system.

FDH arranges seminars and meetings regularly on topics like EPR, Data Security, Trusted Third Parties, Legal Issues and Healthcare Legislation, Healthcare Politics.

Poland

(PTIM) was officially established in 1988 in Warsaw. It was constituted according to the Polish law and its statute was accepted by the State Authorities. According to the statute, the objective of PTIM is to improve efficiency in health service, medical education and environment protection, and thus its basic aims are: (1) to construct medical computer systems; (2) to propagate rational use of computer systems in medical diagnosing and therapy, management of health care centres, scientific research in various fields of medicine, academic teaching and professional training; (3) to promote environment protection and environment-friendly behaviour. The Society's activities cover the whole territory of the country. At present, PTIM has four branch offices: in Warsaw, Cracow, Lódz, and Wroclaw.

Prof. Dr. Jerzy Janecki was chosen as the first president of the Society. In accordance with the statute, in 1991 a new Society Board was chosen and Prof.Dr. Edvard Kacki the Main Board president of PTIM.

PTIM organized about 60 seminars and lectures on applications of computer systems to medical fields, and 4 exhibitions of computer equipment and software for hospital use. In the years 1993, 1994 and 1995 members of the Society Board co-organized and lectured at one-year-long postgraduate studies on medical informatics.

PTIM was the main organizer of 7 scientific conferences: (a) two international conferences on "System-Modelling-Control" (Zakopane, 1993 and 1995), with 6 volumes of conference proceedings published by

PTIM in the English language; (b) three Polish conferences on "Computer in Medicine (Lódz, 1989, 1991, 1994) with conference proceedings in 5 volumes; (c) a Polish conference on "Computer Assisted Health Care Facility Management, Medical Diagnosis and Treatment Recording (Wroclaw, 1995) with one volume of conference proceedings in the Polish language. Six conferences mentioned above (a, b, c) were organized by the Lódz Department of PTIM and one by the Wroclaw Department of PTIM.

PTIM is the main organizer of the International Conference on "Computers in Medicine", 2-5 May, 1997 in Zakopane (Poland) and the co-organizer of the International Conference on "System-Modelling Control", 3-6 May 1998 in Zakopane.

PTIM became the Polish national representative of IMIA at the 8th World Congress MedInfo'95 in Vancouver, on July 20th, 1995 and on 21st January, 1997 became a representative at EFMI. The present president of PTIM is the official representative of the Society in IMIA en EFMI. He is a member of the Scientific Council at the Institute of Biocybernetics and of the Biomedical Engineering Committee of the Polish Academy of Science. He is also organizer and chairman of the Medical Informatics Group joining scientists working at the Technical University of Lódz and the Medical University of Lódz.

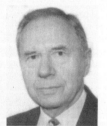

Eduard Kacki, IMIA Representative

Romania

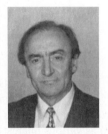

George I. Mihalas, President and
IMIA Representative

The Romanian Society for Medical Informatics, RSMI, is a scientific, professional, non-governmental organisation aimed to promote the activities in the development of medical informatics in Romania and to represent the activities in the country and abroad.

RSMI was founded in 1990 and has now almost 200 members: physicians, computer scientists, engineers, mathematicians and other professionals working in the field of medical informatics. It continues the tradition of a group of specialists who started to work in this field in 1977.

The activities of RSMI concern stimulation and co-ordination of the activities of its members in promoting medical informatics in the country and to support international co-operation in this field, which implies:

- organising scientific and professional conferences, symposia, courses and exhibitions and collaboration in such activities with related organisations;
- publishing scientific, professional and educational publications in the field of medical informatics;
- promoting scientific and professional contacts with similar societies at the international level;
- collaboration with the Romanian Academy and with the Academy of Medical Sciences in medical informatics research;
- collaboration with medical universities in developing education in medical informatics.

RSMI members serve in several professional and scientific committees and also in various expert groups of the Ministry of Health and the Ministry of Education.

During 1999 and 2000 the participation of RSMI members in international events has increased: 14 participants at MIE'99 in Ljubljana and 23 at MIE 2000 in Hanover (with a generous support of EFMI and GDMS). The Romanian Society of Medical Informatics expressed its gratitude to all those who helped the contacts of their members either as sponsorship for participation to meetings and/or direct collaboration in international projects; the society aims to increase its efforts in this line.

Romania was represented as a corresponding member in IMIA since 1986 and RSMI has become a full member in 1994, having now representatives in several active working groups of IMIA. In the same year 1994 RSMI also joined EFMI.

The 23rd National Conference on Medical Informatics, organised by the Romanian Society of Medical Informatics, was held in Iassy 2-4 Nov. 2000, and the 24th Conference will be held in Timisoara, Oct. 2001.

Singapore

The Association for Informatics in Medicine, Singapore (AIMS) was established in 1986 with the following aims:

- promote the growth, development and usage of information science and information technologies as applied to health care and to the education of health professionals in Singapore;
- advance cooperation among health professionals in the field of medical informatics;
- provide a forum for the dissemination, exchange and analysis of information through education and participation of its members;
- offer recommendations to international or governmental agencies and other appropriate bodies concerning the need for, and the structure of eductional programs in the field of medical informatics. Attention will be given to the mechanisms for implementing such educational programs in informatics;
- represent the interests of health professionals in the promotion and pursuit of informatics with international or governmental agencies and other bodies.

AIMS (www.aims.org.sg) currently has about 100 members who are mainly health, medical or IT professionals. AIMS promotes its activities in a variety of ways including organizing local conferences and seminars, the publication of a newsletter and an annual Medical Informatics Lecture. The Association was also instrumental in assisting IMIA to stage MEDINFO 89 Part II in Singapore on short notice.

Nationally, the Association works closely with the governmental IT agencies, health and medical professional associations and the IT and healthcare industries while internationally, the Association is a member of IMIA and actively supports the international organization in its activities. AIMS was instrumental in helping IMIA to establish the Asia Pacific Association of Medical Informatics (APAMI) which was inaugurated in Singapore on November 10, 1994. APAMI (www.apami. org) currently has 13 national members.

Slovak Republic

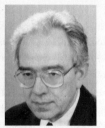

Peter Kneppo, President

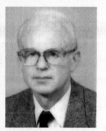

Mikulas Popper,
IMIA Representative

For the year 2001 the following major activities are planned regarding medical informatics:

- Seminar on Developments in Medical Informatics - as an accompanying action of the SLOVMEDICA EXHIBITION (September-October)
- Conference on Hospital Information Systems NIS'2001 (October/ November)
- Seminar on Developments in Bionics (preliminary tittle, the approx. date is to be specified)

The steering board of our Society meets 3-4 times in a year (i.e. approx. quarterly)

Slovenia

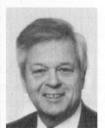

Marjan Premik, President

The Slovenian Society for Medical Informatics (SSMI) was founded at the general meeting of interested professionals on the 10th of October 1988 at the Medical Faculty in Ljubljana as a voluntary and non-governmental association. One of the principal tasks of the Society is to enhance the development of medical informatics, to take care of professional progress of its members, and to present those activities to the people, feeling responsible for them in our society.

The Society has its seat at the Medical Faculty Ljubljana. The Slovenian Society for Medical Informatics is a member of IMIA and EFMI.

In 1994, the Society began to publish its professional journal "Informatica Medica Slovenica", in which scientific and professional articles as well as various interesting reports and items from Slovenia and abroad are published.

The most important project of the Society is now to organise the 15th International Congress of the European Federation of Medical Informatics, MIE 99, which will be held August 22nd-28th, 1999 at the Congress Center Cankarjev dom, Ljubljana, Slovenia. In addition to organize this Congress the Society published in their journal and on a home page on the World Wide Web an internet site: http://www.mie99.org

South Africa

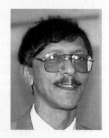

Sedick Isaacs, President

The South African Health Informatics Association (SAHIA) was formed to promote the professional application of Health Informatics in South Africa.

The goals of the organisation include:

- to represent South African Health Informatics nationally and internationally
- to promote and uphold the status of the Health Informatics profession
- to stimulate the advancement of Health Informatics in South Africa, and
- to promote the interests of members.

The focus of SAHIA activities is in the HISA (health informatics for Southern Africa) conferences, which will be held annually from 2000.

Members are involved in a wide range of Health Informatics activities in both the public and private sectors.

Spain

The Spanish Society of Health Informatics is a non-profit scientific society, built up in 1976 and joining today more than five hundred professionals, technicians or health scientists with interest in the promotion of the use of Information and Communications Technologies in the health environment. In this way it arises as a common debate forum for the professional of medicine, informatics, pharmacy, nursery, biology, and all the other Health Sciences, as well as for the students of any related career.

Among the multiple activities and projects developed by our society in the recent years, outstands the National Congress on Health Informatics that, in a biannual basis, has had three editions until date.

In addition to this general congress (INFORSALUD), the society organises more specific congresses targeted to professional sectors (Pharmacy and Informatics, Medical Informatics, Nursery and Informatics, Bioinformatics) or technological aspects (Internet in Health, medical data protection, ...).

Sweden

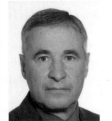

Hans Adolfsson, President

The Swedish Society of Medical Informatics (SFMI) was established in 1967. The number of members is around 500 representing physicians, nurses, dentists and many other health care professions as well as computer sciences.

SFMI is also a section of the Swedish Society of Medicine. This Society has its annual assembly in late autumn each year. During this assembly SFMI arranges a half-day long scientific session and seminar. The aim of the scientific session is to present recent research results in the field and to create a meeting place for members and other persons interested in Medical Informatics.

SFMI has its annual general meeting in May. The meeting is rotated between different

university towns with the intention to present different regional activities within the area of medical informatics in Sweden. In 1999 the meeting was held in Stockholm in cooperation with Spri and Exponova as a Conference and Exhibition. The Conference "IT in Healtcare" was attended by ca 300 visitors. The Conference Program with some international speakers is documented on CD-Rom.

SFMI publishes a newsletter four times a year and has a website http://www.sfmi.org with actual and relevant information about Medical Informatic topics. The Society also gives scholarships to members to promote their participation and presentation of papers at international conferences.

Switzerland

Before February, 1985, the date of the creation of the Swiss Society for Medical Informatics (SSMI), most of the medical activities related to the application of computer sciences, were held within the Swiss Society for Biomedical Engineering where, as expected, most of the professionals were engineers. The SSMI, on the contrary, has been set up and led, since its creation, by a majority of health-care professionals: physicians as well as nurses. Already from its first year the SSMI became a member of the Swiss Federation for Informatics, which regroups all the other Swiss informatics Societies being the Swiss national society and a member of IFIP (which in 1960 had just been created under the auspices of UNESCO). Furthermore, it is worthwhile to highlight that in 1969 the IFIP permanent secretariat was established in Geneva and since 1991 has also been associated with the IMIA secretariat at the same address.

Naturally, the SSMI became an IMIA and EFMI member, within the Swiss IFIP Chapter, and the former place of TC4 (Technical Com-

mittee 4) is held by the IMIA representative delegated by the SSMI. It follows that our IMIA national society is associated with all the other computer science activities handled by the IFIP special interest groups as well as its technical committees.

The SSMI is managed by an executive committee of 11 members, of them 10 are devoted to technical committees or special interest groups following in this respect the IFIP structure:

- General Practice Informatics and Communication Systems.
- Nursing Informatics.
- Medical Education.
- Biostatistics.
- Medical Imaging and Expert Systems.
- Hospital Information Systems.
- Nomenclature Classification and Health Data Coding.
- IMIA/EFMI/EEC (EU-European Union) activities and relationships with the SSMI
- Norms for Medical Informatics.
- Ethics in Data Communication in Health Care Systems.

Turkey

TURKMIA is a nonprofit membership organization, dedicated to guiding development and organisation of health and medical informatics in Turkey.

TURKMIA was founded in 1999 in Ankara. It organized First Medical Informatics Symposium in November 1999.

Aims of TURKMIA include:

- to collect, process and distribute information about the activities related to health and medical informatics of companies, governmental and non-governmental organizations.
- to stimulate all the professionals related to health and medical informatics to reach the contemporary level of knowledge and skills, prepare the background for communication and interaction between the professionals in the field, promote multidisciplinary study.
- to determine the problems related to health and medical informatics domain in Turkey, suggest solutions to these problems, collaborate with other organizations to realize the projects, announce the results of the projects or applications.
- to enhance the knowledge of health care providers and demanders about health and medical informatics, organize meetings and publish materials to shape public opinion.
- to inform, sensitize and stimulate the

decision making and administrating people and organizations about the issues related to medical informatics.

Activities of TURKMIA:

- TURKMIA started SBS 2000 (Health Information Strategies of Turkey in the New Millenium) project in June 2000 by a meeting in Ankara. Preliminary reports of the study groups discussed in the First Congress of Medical Informatics which was held in 28-29th April 2001 in Istanbul. Final reports were collected in a book and in press. This book will be presented to the governmental and civil organizations, healthcare institutions, professional associations, commercial companies and non governmental organizations which are active in the healthcare sector in order to establish the health information vision, goals, strategy and politics of Turkey

- TURKMIA is in collaboration with Turkish Informatics Foundation (Turkiye Bilisim Vakfi) for informatics projects in healthcare domain.
- A study group is founded to prepare guidelines for electronic medical journals in Turkey.
- TURKMIA organizes regular monthly meetings in Istanbul, the largest city of Turkey, to bring together people responsible of and/or interested in hospital information systems.

Ukraine

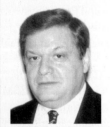

Oleg Mayorov, IMIA Representative

UACM was set up in August 1992 in Kharkiv, where the IVth World Congress of WFUPS (World Federation of Ukrainian Physicians Societies) was taking place.

UACM became a national member of International Medical Informatics Association (IMIA) in September 1993 (Kyoto, Japan).

In May 1994 UACM was adopted as a National Member of European Federation of Medical Informatics (EFMI) at the IVth European Congress on Medical Informatics in Lisbon (Portugal).

It unites 78 scientific research institutes, universities, scientific societies, enterprises and hospitals. Over 900 scientists are individual members of the UACM.

The structure of the UACM has Scientific Council including 68 leading scientist-experts in medical informatics, medicine, radioelectronics from Ukraine, NIS, USA, UK, Canada, France, Japan, Israel and Turkey.

This Council's terms of reference cover:

- elaboration and discussion of complex computerisation programmes in various fields of healthcare;
- analysis and sharing of experience of computer technologies usage according to the situation in Ukraine;
- consideration of foreign proposals dealing with introduction and selling of computer technologies in the field of medicine to Ukraine and making proposals to the Ministry of Healthcare of Ukraine to buy them;

Ukraine
(Continued)

· progressive directions on elaborating and consideration of possible joint projects;
· carrying out expert estimations for receiving state licences.

A Regulation on certification information technologies in Healthcare was worked out with the help of the UACM Scientific Council and was approved by   t h e Ministry of Healthcare and the State Committee for Standards. Committee on certification was set up under the Ministry of Healthcare. Starting from 1998 its work will be based on the Ukrainian Institute of Public Health. All programme products for medical application will be forwarded to this Institute for certification. Since 1998 all medical software used in Healthcare of Ukraine must receive the certificate from the mentioned Committee.

Purposes:

Working out new medical software and biotechnical systems. Carrying out independent expert control and preparing materials to receive certificate.

Putting the best Ukrainian and foreign systems into medical practice.

Organising educational activity to train for new and postgraduate education; patent search; author's rights protection. Contacts with IMIA and EFMI members, foreign scientific societies, universities. Participation in state and foreign programs of Informatization of Healthcare in Ukraine. Organising symposia, forums, exhibitions and competitions.

The UACM experts has worked out the Concept of State Policy of Informatization of the Ukraine Healthcare adopted by the Ministry of Healthcare, agreed with Academy of Medical Sciences (http://www.uacm.cit-ua.net (Ukr. Radiological Journal 1996. №2.p. 115-118). The National Program of Healthcare Informatization to be put into practice has created.

National healthcare network of direct access UkrMedNet is being set up. The Concept of creation of the direct access State National Healthcare Network (UkrMedNet) has been developed by UACM experts (http://www.uacm.cit-ua.net).

The Information Analytical System (its medical part) for emergency situations within Cabinet of Ministers of Ukraine is under development.

The project of the system of medical information exchange in the NIS is worked out.

The UACM is an initiator of the National Program Hospital Information Systems.

The fact that the UACM joins the Internet plays an important role in its development. In 1996 the UACM has created of its own WWW-server in 3 languages: Ukrainian, Russian and English (http://www.uacm.cit-ua.net). The UACM members have the possibility to use data bases and scientific information on medical informatics world-wide and Europe-wide in Ukrainian and Russian (WWW-servers of EFMI, IMIA, WHO, EHTO European Observatory on Telemedicine), UNESCO and different WWW-servers of IMIA/EFMI (WG's and SIGs). The UACM has received an offer and has created affiliate Web-EHTO-UKRAINE server in Ukraine (http://www.ehto-ukr.cit-ua.net).

In 1996 the United Commission on Telemedicine of the Ministry of Healthcare and the Academy of Medical Sciences has been created. The Commission co-operates with the UN International Telecommunication Union (ITU) and European Commission on Telemedecine (DGXIII). In June 1997 the UACM specialists took part in the 1st World Symposium on Telemedecine for developing countries and made a report. The Symposium took part in Lisbon, Portugal, under the patronage of UN and WHO. In July 1998 the UACM specialists took part in the Conference “Telemedecine International Medical Care Networks” in Visby (Sweden) for co-operation and efficient use of resources by building networks within the Baltic Region. In 1998 under the initiative of UACM started the Ukrainian-American project on monitoring of birth defects in Ukraine.

The annual scientific conferences, exhibitions and sales of medical software are carried out with the participation of leading foreign firms and Ukrainian enterprises within the Programme of Health Care Informatization.

Since a 1993 UACM conducts annual International Conference Computer Medicine.

United Kingdom

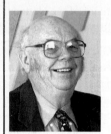

John Bryden, President

HIC is a body formed to co-ordinate the work of the five BCS Special Interest Groups involved in healthcare computing - Nursing, Primary Health Care, London Medical, Northern Medical, and Scotland Medical.

HIC's role is threefold: to assist these groups; to act for BCS in all aspects of health care matters; and to run its own activities, the most important of which is the annual Healthcare Computing Conference. This is held in spring, and attracts over 1200 delegates and 5000 visitors to the associated exhibition. Those interested in further information should contact the appropriate Group.

USA

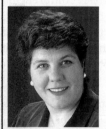

Patricia Flatley Brennan, President

The American Medical Informatics Association (AMIA) was incorporated in the District of Columbia in 1988 following more than a year of discussions among the boards of directors of the American Association for Medical Systems and Informatics, the American College of Medical Informatics, and the Symposium on Computer Applications in Medical Care (SCAMC). It brings together a professional association solely devoted to medical informatics, the organization responsible for the major annual meeting in the field, and the College of recognized leaders who have made major contributions to the field.

The oldest of the three organizations was the Symposium on Computer Applications in Medical Care. The Symposium was first conducted in 1977 as a regional effort in the Washington-Baltimore area. Two years later, SCAMC expanded its horizon, and quickly grew to a meeting attracting more than 2,000 participants. The name of the meeting was eventually changed to the AMIA Annual Symposium. Now over 100 organizations/ companies and 2,000+ attendees participate in the Annual Symposium featuring scientific paper presentations, panel discussions, tutorials, workshops, system demonstrations, posters and commercial product exhibits. The Proceedings of the Annual Symposium reflects the body of work that is accomplished each year in medical informatics in the United States and abroad and is indexed by the National Library of Medicine.

The American Association for Medical Systems and Informatics (AAMSI) was formed in 1981 through a merger of the Society for Computer Medicine and the Society for Advanced Medical Systems.

This union of two organizations with nearly 500 members each resulted in the largest membership society in the country at that time, with a principal interest in the advancement of medical informatics. A tradition was established of a spring meeting held annually on the West Coast, known as the AAMSI Spring Congress.

In response to a perceived need for the recognition of experts and leaders in the medical informatics field, the American College of Medical Informatics was established in 1985. Candidates are proposed by the Fellows and elected by mail ballot. ACMI meets three times each year, which includes an ACMI Symposium and meetings held in conjunction with the AMIA Annual Symposium and the AMIA Spring Congress.

By 1987 it had become clear that the leadership of the three organizations created an interlocking directorate. It appeared to many that the interests of the organizations and of the field would best be served by a merger. Early in 1988 representatives of the three organization began meeting and in November, 1988 they formed the American Medical Informatics Association (AMIA), a society that can speak with one voice to the United States and to the international medical informatics community.

Purpose

The purpose of AMIA is to advance the public interest through charitable, scientific, literary and educational activities and by promoting the development and application of medical informatics in the support of patient care, teaching, research and health care administration.

USA
(Continued)

AMIA contributes to the advancement of medical systems and informatics by:

- Serving as an authoritative body in the field of medical informatics and providing representation with respect to such matters in international forums;
- Fostering liaisons between disciplines involved in health care, computers, information, communications, systems sciences, engineering and technology;
- Promoting training and development of professional and allied health personnel necessary to support medical informatics;
- Planning and conducting scientific, technical, and educational meetings and programs;
- Publishing and distributing educational materials through various media;
- Coordinating medical informatics activities with other national and international organizations to advance the public's interest; and
- Carrying on other activities as are necessary, suitable, and proper for the fulfillment of the Association's charitable, scientific, literary and educational purposes.

These objectives are accomplished through a variety of activities and services that AMIA offers:

- Holding scientific, technical and educational meetings;
- Publishing and disseminating reports, digests, proceedings and other pertinent documents and contributing to the professional literature;
- Publishing a journal, the Journal of the American Medical Informatics Association (JAMIA);
- Sponsoring Working Groups (WGs) and Special Interest Groups (SIGs);
- Providing a communications network via telematics (information systems databases, computer and telecommunications);
- Providing a focus for the development of standards, terminology and coding systems;
- Stimulating, conducting and sponsoring research into the application and evaluation of technical systems as they apply to health care and health sciences;
- Representing the United States in the international arena of medical systems and informatics; and
- Advising and coordinating matters of mutual interest to its members.

In late 1999, the Board of Directors and members of AMIA undertook a strategic planning exercise to re-define the vision, mission and goals of the association. As of the fall of 2000, these are the draft statements.

Vision

The American Medical Informatics Association is the premier organization to advance discovery and innovation in the use of information in health and biomedicine.

Mission

The mission of the American Medical Informatics Association is to improve healthcare through innovation in the use of information by advancing the field, fostering scientific exchange, educating professionals and the public, and influencing decision makers and policy makers.

Goals

I. Be the premier membership and peer communication organization in medical informatics.
II. Promote and integrate medical informatics as a field.
III. Expand and maintain multiple forums for interchange and dissemination of advances in the field.
IV. Promote research, development, and diffusion of medical informatics to solve healthcare problems and improve health quality.
V. Foster cooperation and establish relationships with relevant organizations.
VI. Foster and ensure an effective governance and management foundation to enable the American Medical Informatics Association to achieve all of its goals.

Membership Categories

- Regular Member: Physicians, nurses, dentists, biomedical engineers, educators, medical librarians, researchers and other health care professionals who have a strong interest in medical informatics. Regular members receive JAMIA (both print and on-line versions), Access AMIA, AMIA Alert, AMIA Yearbook & Directory and the IMIA Yearbook of Medical Informatics at no

USA
(Continued)

extra charge. Regular members also receive membership in two working groups as part of their membership fee. Discounts for AMIA Annual Symposium, Spring Congress and Site Visits apply. $240/year

• Institutional Member: Nonprofit organizations, nonprofit associations, non-profit universities, nonprofit hospitals and libraries. All regular member benefits apply for one individual designated as the AMIA contact person. Additional benefits include JAMIA on-line access, conference publications and promotional opportunities offering support and exposure. $375/year

• Corporate Member: For-profit corporations that are supporters of the medical informatics community. Numerous corporate membership benefits apply at the three levels of membership —silver, gold, and platinum. Corporate members have representatives that receive all the benefits of regular members plus additional advertising and sponsorship opportunities. $2,500, $5,000 or $10,000/year

• Retired Member: Retirees at least 60 years of age who have been members of AMA for the past two years or longer. All benefits of regular membership apply. $100/year

• Student Member: Persons currently enrolled full-time in a degree-granting program or in an academic program such as a medical residency or post-doctoral fellowship. A certified letter attesting to the student's full time status at an academic institution is required along with membership application. JAMIA is not included in student membership fees, but students may subscribe at a special rate of $35 for a year's subscription (6 issues) and on-line access. Students are automatic members of the student working group at no additional charge. Special conference discounts apply. $35/year

• Associate Member: Individuals may join one working group or special interest group for one year only. No regular member benefits apply. No journals or conference discounts will be given. $30/year

Member Services

Membership in AMIA provides a means of staying abreast of the rapid changes in medical systems and informatics, and is open to anyone with interest in the field.

AMIA offers a growing array of services designed to meet professional needs:

• Meetings & Conferences: AMIA's meetings and conferences offer the best in panels, tutorials, paper presentations, workshops and exhibits. By joining AMIA, you will receive significant discounts to meetings and conferences. AMIA holds two major meetings each year, the AMIA 2001 Spring Congress being held May 15-17 in Atlanta, Georgia and focused on developing a national agenda for public health informatics and the AMIA 2001 Annual Symposium being held November 3-7, 2001 in Washington, DC. AMIA 2001, A Medical Informatics Odyssey, is expected to draw 2,000+ attendees interested in the multidisciplinary arena of medical informatics.

• Site Visit Program: Members can see medical informaticians at work on internationally acclaimed projects at the finest centers of excellence in medical informatics research and development.

• Working Group Program: AMIA members are encouraged to join and participate in the association's working groups and special interest groups. The working groups conduct programs and activities and produce products to benefit AMIA and the medical informatics community. Working groups are also important in helping members develop personal networks within specific professional or topic areas.

• Continuing Education Credits: By attending the AMIA Annual Symposium and Spring Congress, members may earn valuable continuing medical education credits and nursing contact hours.

• Job Exchange: Members can learn "who's looking" and "what's available" for various positions within the medical informatics field.

• President's Club: AMIA's Member-Get-A-Member Campaign: Any AMIA member can participate in the campaign. Each new member who signs-up for membership and indicates the name of the AMIA member who sponsored his/her membership, will earn the current AMIA member one point toward the campaign. All current AMIA members earning at least one point in the campaign will be invited to the President's Club Reception held at the Annual Symposium

USA
(Continued)

where awards are given. The more points accumulated during the campaign, the more prestigious the award.

- Web Site: AMIA's newly designed web site provides valuable information to members and prospective members about the association and member services. The site also has a resource center which contains information about academic and training programs, conferences and meetings, publications of interest, the health IT marketplace, public policy and news developments and research and grant information. Be sure to visit the site at www.amia.org.

Publications

AMIA members have the opportunity to subscribe at discounted rates to the Journal of Biomedical Informatics (formerly Computers & Biomedical Research) which is a refereed journal that provides researchers and clinicians with up-to-date information about the application of computers to health care.

We also offer the following periodical publications when you join:

- JAMIA: The Journal of the American Medical Informatics Association: AMIA's timely and informative journal is the primary source of information for professionals in medical informatics. All regular, institutional, corporate and retired members receive JAMIA bi-monthly and receive 24 hour on-line access. Students may order JAMIA at a special student member rate (which also includes on-line access).
- Access AMIA and AMIA Alert: Two monthly e-mail alerts letting you know about what's going on at your association's headquarters, new services on the horizon, messages from AMIA's leaders and the latest information about the field.
- AMIA Yearbook & Directory: This valuable networking tool, available exclusively to AMIA members for noncommercial purposes, provides completed address, phone, fax and e-mail information for each AMIA member. It also provides an overview of the current year, and lets you know what's in store for the following year.
- IMIA Yearbook of Medical Informatics: Published by the International Medical Informatics Association, this annual publication includes the best papers in medical informatics from an international arena.

JAMIA

AMIA's own journal is called JAMIA, the Journal of the American Medical Informatics Association. This peer-reviewed specialty journal is the official publication of AMIA and is published by Hanley & Belfus. The content of the regular issues emphasizes the publication of peer-reviewed, original and unsolicited full-length manuscripts dealing with hypotheses and findings that are relevant to medical informatics in all arenas of health care delivery, biomedical education and biomedical research. Also included are brief technical notes, abstracts or full-length papers submitted for presentation at meetings of AMIA, state-of-the-art papers, refereed discussion forums, invited editorials and news and announcements of the association. An occasional regular issue may be dedicated to a collection of invited full-length manuscripts on a single topic. The Proceedings of the AMIA Annual Symposium are published as a supplement to JAMIA. Those who pay full registration to the Annual Symposium receive a CD-ROM copy of the Proceedings. The Proceedings may also be purchased independently of the meeting in either print form or on CD-ROM.

JAMIA is regarded by investigators as the premier vehicle for the archival publication of peer-reviewed papers containing original hypotheses and findings. Submitted material is judged on the originality and quality of work. The journal is reviewed as relevant by the many constituencies that make up AMIA's membership. Each issue contains one or more practical papers addressing the problems facing individuals in the biomedical and health profession who are interested in informatics but do not consider themselves to be researchers. State-of-the-art papers and refereed discussion forums can meet this need while outlining the issues in the field that are controversial or require further investigation.

JAMIA is owned, copyrighted and sponsored by AMIA and is an automatic member benefit to most AMIA members. When subscribing to JAMIA, members also receive access to the on-line version of the journal available at www.jamia.org. Outside subscriptions are also available.

Uruguay

Uruguay is a small country located in the Southern Cone of the Americas, on the River Plate and the Atlantic Ocean, between Argentina and Brazil. Its population is three million, and it was once called the Switzerland of the Americas because of its highly educated people and good standards of life. The capital is Montevideo, which now also hosts the administrative headquarters of the Mercosur, the growing economic market involving Brazil, Argentina, Paraguay and Uruguay.

Health Informatics is not new in Uruguay: (1) The Latin American Perinatal Information System was designed in Montevideo. It was created by the Latin American Perinatology Center, which has its headquarters in Uruguay, and was implemented in the region over ten years ago; (2) The Libraries at the School of Medicine and University Hospital, together with the one at the Cancer Society, have been linked together and provide remote access to information to clinicians, including several CD-ROM databases as well as the *Internet*; (3) The Uruguayan Medical Association has created *Red Médica* (Medical Network) which involves over 700 physicians, and provides its own medical discussion lists, full access to *Internet*, and other services; (4) One of the groups in Uruguay has created and implemented a decision-support system for the management of oral anticoagulation, called *Warfarin*. (5) There is great interest among the private and public health care facilities to implement clinical information systems, as well as to continue improving their financial and administrative systems.

There was a growing interest in health informatics in our country. Therefore, a decision was made to create SUIS on November, 1996. There were 39 professionals during the founding meeting, and the number is over 150 today.

Goals

SUIS is a multidisciplinary society, and some of its current goals are:

- To create a favorable environment for the development of health informatics.
- To promote the inclusion of informatics in the education of health professionals.
- To create multidisciplinary links among professionals.
- To create ties with similar Societies in the Americas and the World.
- To promote the use of standards in health informatics.
- To contribute to regulate the integrity and confidentiality of electronic medical records.
- To disseminate the importance and use of informatics among health professionals.

Governing Board and Members

The Governing Board has been elected for a period of two years, and is composed by professionals with different backgrounds (physicians, computer engineers and medical librarians). The members' background is also diverse.

Activities

Regarding the activities of SUIS for 1997, several have been performed. These are some examples: (1) A three-hour interactive videoconference was done on May with Dr. Brent James at Utah about "Informatics and Quality in Health". (2) A Health Informatics Congress was held on October, with the participation of foreign experts. (3) A health informatics discussion list is already on-line, at <compu_med @chasque.apc.org>. (4) A Web page, at http://www.chasque.apc.org/suis/ (5) Promotion of courses regarding health-oriented computer literacy for health care professionals. In 1998, we are starting a Bulletin called *InfoSuis*, published three times a year, both electronically and on paper. SUIS is also supporting continued efforts to improve health-oriented computer literacy for health care professionals. Finally, through the organization of seminars with national or foreign speakers, the Society tries to increase knowledge and skills in some medical informatics tracks, i.e., *Information Access and Retrieval, Internet Applications in Medicine, Health Information Systems*, and *Computer-Assisted Medical Education*.

EFMI

Regional Editor: Arie Hasman

Structure

The constitutional bodies of EFMI are

- The EFMI-Council, a General Assembly of all members, officers and working group chair persons.
- The Board of officers, treasurer, vice presidents and president
- Working Groups organised by a chairperson (see also the EFMI-homepage, addresses, member societies)

Objectives

The objectives of the European Federation for Medical Informatics (EFMI) founded in 1976 are:

- To advance international co-operation and dissemination of information in Medical Informatics on a European basis;
- To promote high standards in the application of medical informatics;
- To promote research and development in medical informatics;
- To encourage high standards in education in medical informatics;
- To function as the autonomous European Regional Council of IMIA

Activities

All European countries are entitled to be represented in EFMI by a suitable Medical Informatics Society. The term medical informatics is used to include the whole spectrum of Healthcare Informatics and all disciplines concerned with Healthcare and Informatics. The organisation operates with a minimum of bureaucratic overhead and each national society supports the Federation by sending and paying for a representative to participate in the decisions of the Federation's Council. Also, and again to reduce overhead, English has been adopted as the official language, although simultaneous translation is often provided for congresses in non-English speaking countries.

Countries

Currently, 29 countries have joined the Federation, and are named as

Austria, Belgium, Bosnia, Herzegovina, Bulgaria, Croatia, Cyprus, Czech Republic, Denmark, Finland, France, Germany, Georgia, Greece, Hungary, Ireland, Israel, Italy, The Netherlands, Norway, Poland, Portugal, Romania, Slovakia, Slovenia, Spain, Sweden, Switzerland, Ukraine and United Kingdom. Application are open to representative societies in countries within the European Region of WHO. The EFMI council and board normally meets twice a year. Furthermore, it is represented by a Vice President (Europe) at meetings of the Board and the annual General Meetings of the International Medical Informatics Association (IMIA).

Congresses and Publications

So far 16 general congresses (Medical Informatics Europe – MIE) have been organised by EFMI. These have taken place in Cambridge (1978), Berlin (1979), Toulouse (1981), Dublin (1982), Brussels (1984), Helsinki (1985), Rome (1987), Oslo (1988), Glasgow (1990), Vienna (1991), Jerusalem (1993), Lisbon (1994), Copenhagen (1996), Thessaloniki (1997), Ljubljana (1999), and Hannover (2000). In 2001, EFMI started organizing spring conferences. The first conference was held in Buchares in Romania, the next one will be held in Cyprus.

The proceedings of these congresses were usually published by Springer in the series *"Lecture Notes in Medical Informatics"* and by IOS Press in the series *"Studies in Health Technologies and Informatics"*.

A selection of the best papers from the MIE-conferences were published in a special volume of the International Journal of Medical Informatics. The next MIE congress will take place in Budapest 2002.

To date four official journals adopted by the Federation are: *Methods of Information in Medicine, Medical Informatics, and Health Informatics Europe, International Journal of Medical Informatics*.

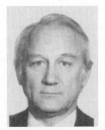

Attila Naszlady, IMIA Representative

EFMI (Continued)

Working Groups

The following EFMI-Working Groups are operating:

Working Group 1

MBDS, Case Mix, Resource Management and Outcomes of Care

Chair:
Prof. F.H. Roger France,
Centre for Medical Informatics
University of Louvain
10 av. Hippocrate, Box 3718
B-1200 Brussels
Tel. +32-2-7644709
Fax: +32-2-7644717
roger@infm.ucl.ac.be

Co-chair/Secretary:
J. Hofdijk
HISCOM, Schipholweg 97
NL-2316 XA LEIDEN, The Netherlands
Fax: +31-71-216675
jacob@bazis.nl

Objectives:
The organisation of special topic conferences, workshops, Teaching sessions in the European Region on MBDS, Case Mix and Severity of cases and their applications to Resource management and outcomes of care.

The communication of up to date experiences and/or references between members, including national uniform data sets, terminology, coding system and patient classification methods for resource management and quality of care.

The dissemination of results about informatics tools and telematics systems in this specific area among EFMI and IMIA affiliated members and participants to their meetings.

Recent activities:
Workshop at the MEDINFO 98 Conference in Seoul

Workshop at MIE 99, Ljubljana, Slovenia

Special Topic Conference 2001 in Collaboration with PCS-E, Patient Classification Systems Europe. "Case Mix: Global Views, Local Actions" Bruges, 10-13 October 2001.

Publications:
Roger France F.H., De Moor G., Hofdijk J., Jenkins L. (Eds.) Diagnosis Related Groups in Europe, Ghent, Goff BVBA, ISBN 90-73045-01-0, 259 p., 1990
Roger France F.H., Noothoven van Goor J.,

Staehr Johansen K. (Eds) Case-Based Telematics Systems towards Equity in Health Care, IOS Press, Amsterdam, ISBN 90-51991-82-7, 207 p., 1994
Roger France F.H., Mertens I., Closon M.C., Hofdijk J. (Eds) Case Mix: Global Views, Local Actions – Evolution in Twenty Countries, IOS Press, Amsterdam, No 86, in press (2001)

Working Group 2

Data Protection and Security in Health Information Systems

Chair:
Francois-André Allaert
apsis@ipac.fr

Working Group 3

Standards in Medical Informatics has been replaced by CEN TC 251 (a European entity covering the scope of Telematics in Healthcare)
Chair:
Gunnar Klein
gunnar.klein@spri.se

Working Group 4

Information Planning and Modelling in Health Care

Chair:
Bryan Manning
bryan.manning@btinternet.com

Objectives:
To develop generic approaches across an ever-widening range of health and linked social care domains

To develop working links to other National and International bodies

Recent activities:
This year were have been focusing on Risk and Security Modelling and presented some of these concepts at a two day Conference "Making Medical Informatics Work" held in Manchester in the Spring. These types of event have proved are an ideal vehicle for disseminating the results of our work more widely at no cost other than the time involved.

Future activities:
Our aim is to set up a Working Conference with a core theme of:

"Joining-up Healthcare Services in the 21st

EFMI (Continued)

Century: Modelling the Best Practice"

Its aim will be to examine how to identify Best Clinical and Health Management Practice through:

- the use of appropriate workflow analysis and modelling techniques to provide in-depth mappings of the range of Service Provision Pathways used in delivering care across the spectrum of patient need
- the use of these Pathways as a "back-bone" upon which to attach clinical/management protocols, guidelines, check-lists, decision support tools [including risk analysis], etc.
- the interactive use of these Pathways for case planning and semi-automatic record generation for transfer in to full multimedia record databases.
- the integration of diagnostic and bio-medical data into these records
- the use of summary data extracts from multimedia record databases to:
- establish resource profiles/parameters for planning/rostering
- support to clinical governance
- monitor service efficacy, effectiveness, efficiency and economy
- the application of domain-based security modelling and other techniques to determine the varying levels of security required both within agencies and between agencies, and similarly between the professionals involved
- the impacts of the use of semi-secure intranets communicating over public networks and the introduction of public key infrastructure [PKI] controls on clinical practice
- the use of Telemedicine and Telecare
- the opportunities and lessons learnt form e-commence in improving and optimising supply chains

Working Group 5

Nursing Informatics in Europe

Chair:
Patrick Weber
CEO Nice Computing
Rte de Fey
CH-1414 Rueyres Switzerland
patrick.weber@nicecomputing,ch
URL: www.nicecomputing.ch/nieurope

Objectives:
To support nurses and nursing organisations in the European countries with information

and contacts and the field of informatics

To offer nurses opportunities to build contact networks within the informatics field. This could be accomplished by arranging sessions, workshops and tutorials in connection with the Medical Informatics European (MIE) conferences or by arranging separate meetings.

To support the education of nurses with respect to informatics and computing.

To support research and developmental work in the field and promote publishing of achieved results.

Recent activities:
Working group meeting in Hanover 2000.

Active presentation at the EFMI spring meeting in Bucharest, spring 2001.

Future activities:
We will have a presentation at the next EFMI spring meeting in 2002 and a workshop at MIE 2002, Budapest.

All information is published at the Website.

Working Group 6

Education and Training in Health Informatics

Chair:
Prof. John Mantas
Health Informatics Laboratory
University of Athens, Greece
Email: jmantas@cc.uoa.gr

Co-chair/Secretary
Prof. Arie Hasman
Dept. of Medical Informatics
University Maastricht, The Netherlands
Email: hasman@mi.unimaas.nl

Objectives:
To organize workshops and possibly tutorials dedicated to the WG topics at each MIE conference, and other events.

To cooperate with IMIA WG 1 regarding Recommendations about Health Informatics Curricula and other subjects involving education and training in health informatics.

To disseminate knowledge about education and training in health informatics by various activities, such as conferences, educational events, publications and electronic means.

To encourage individuals to publish their research and other work in journals.

EFMI (Continued)

To provide a forum for discussion and debate.

Recent activities:
The last activities of the working group were organized in Hannover, 2000 and Bucharest, 2001.

Both in Hannover and Bucharest workshops were held. In Hannover the workshop on organisational issues was organized jointly with the EFMI working group on Human and Organisational issues.

At the MIE special topic conference in Bucharest a workshop was organized in which five speakers from Rumania presented work in the area of Training and Education in Medical Informatics.

Future activities:
At MIE2002 the working group will organise a tutorial and jointly with the EFMI working group on Human and Organisational issues a workshop on organisational issues in health informatics education. Discussions are held with the Cyprus Medical Informatics Association to organise a workshop during their forthcoming local meeting.

Working Group 7

Primary Care Informatics

Chair:
Dr. N.T. Shaw
E-mail: nikki.shaw@dial.pipex.com
Tel: +44 (0) 7976 618879

Objectives:
To organize workshops and tutorials dedicated to WG topics at each MIE conference, and other events and to provide a forum for discussion and debate.

To establish networks of people involved in primary care informatics throughout Europe, and to learn about new developments and their activities.

To represent EFMI at IMIA WG5; to represent EFMI at MEDINFO; to represent EFMI at WONCA Informatics (the group has recently agreed to act as a European arm of WONCA Informatics); to collaborate with AMIA and other National Organisations.

To disseminate knowledge about primary care informatics issues by various activities, such as conferences, educational events, publications and electronic means.

To encourage individuals to publish their research and other work in journals.

Recent activities:
During MIE2000 a workshop, called 'Primary Care and Electronic prescribing - Towards patient-focussed prescribing' was organized.

Members of the group participated in leading and organising a workshop during MEDINFO2001 discussing the need for a global strategy for the use of IT in Primary Care in conjunction with IMIA WG5, WONCA, the Australian GPCG, and AMIA PCI WG.

Members of the group ran a workshop during the British Computer Society's Primary Health Care Specialist Group Annual Conference discussing the potential for international ground level collaboration in primary care informatics focusing on achievability and sustainability.

Future activities:
The working group has offered to support the Cypriot Health Informatics society in running a conference in Spring 2002 in conjunction with the EFMI Council meeting.

Members of the group will participate in leading and organising a workshop during MIE2002 in Budapest.

Publications:
Shaw N.T. (2001) Going Paperless: A Guide To Computerisation In Primary Care, Radcliffe Medical Press.

Working Group 8

Natural Language Understanding

Chair
Robert Baud
Division d'Informatique Médicale
Hôpitaux Universitaires de Genève
CH-1211 GENEVA 14 Switzerland
robert.baud@dim.hcuge.ch

Objectives:
To organize workshops dedicated to the WG topics at each MIE conference, and other events.

To have personal connections with people involved in NLP in the medical domain, and to learn about their current developments and activities.

EFMI (Continued)

To represent EFMI at IMIA WG6; to represent EFMI at AMIA new SIG on NLP. In general, to participate to events of those entities.

To develop a website with information on WG8 topics and links to linguistic resources.

Recent activities:
A full day workshop on NLP was organized during MIE2000 at Hannover.

At MEDINFO2001 a tutorial on the multilingual lexicon was given.

At MEDINFO2001 a workshop was organized on aspects on NLP, ontologies and knowledge representation.

Future activities:
A special interest conference on NLP and knowledge representation will be organized during the next EFMI spring conference in Cyprus.

To develop a section on the EFMI website about WG8.

To be active and to encourage the usage of open source distribution channel as set up by EFMI, regarding NLP topics.

Working Group 9

Human and Organisational issues

Chair:
Jos Aarts
Dept. Of Health Policy and Management
Erasmus University Rotterdam
PO Box 1738, 3000 DR Rotterdam
j.aarts@bmg.eur.nl

Objectives:
To organize workshops and tutorials dedicated to the WG topics at MIE conferences and other events

To establish networks of people involved in human and organisational issues in the healthcare domain, and to learn about new developments and their activities

To disseminate knowledge about human and organisational issues by various activities, such as conferences, educational events, publications.

To encourage individuals to publish their research and other work in journals

Recent activities:
At MIE2000 in Hannover both a tutorial and a workshop (together with the EFMI

working group on Education and Training in Health Informatics) were organised.

Together with IMIA WG13 panel sessions on organisational issues were organised during MEDINFO2001.

The WG chairman delivered a keynote address on the organisational issues surrounding the design, implementation and evaluation of knowledge based systems at the conference Artificial Intelligence in Medicine Europe in Cascais, Portugal.

A working conference on organisational issues, called "Information Technology in Health Care: Sociotechnical Approaches" was organized in Rotterdam after the MEDINFO2001 conference.

Publication of an electronic newsletter together with IMIA WG13 and the AMIA People and Organizational issues WG.

Future activities:
At MIE2002 in Budapest a tutorial and workshop will be organized.

Working Group 10

Health Informatics for Development

Chair:
Prof. Dr. George I. Mihalas
University of Medicine and Pharmacy
P-ta Eftimie Murgu 2
1900 Timisoara, Romania
Tel+Fax: +40-56-190288
mihalas@medinfo.umft.ro

Co-chair/Secretary:
Dr. Marcelo Sosa-Iudicissa
Telemedicine and Information Society Area
Instituto de Salud Carlos III
(National Health Institute)
Gardenia 28, 28109 Alcobendas
Madrid, Spain
Tel: +34 91 387.78.46
Fax: +34 91 387.77.90
Email: Sosa@ISCIII.Es

Objectives:
To promote exchange of information between actors in Europe, developing regions and world-wide, for improved access and use of data and knowledge

To investigate the needs, opportunities and obstacles for health information systems, informatics and telematics in developing regions

---

EFMI (Continued)

To disseminate European and world-wide results and experiences across developing regions and professionals

To facilitate access to European groups and their facilities and outcomes by students, medical practitioners, nurses, health managers and any other person from developing regions interested in learning and working together with partners in Europe and other industrialised countries

To analyse and promote the use of Internet resources and applications to bridge gaps between north and south and between west and east, to act as a clearinghouse of information on resources of all kinds of mutual interest to health informatics and telematics participants in Europe and developing regions.

Recent activities:
Active participation at the workshop organized by IMIA WG9 at MEDINFO'98 in Seoul, Korea.

Workshop organized by the WG at MIE2000, Hannover, Germany, entitled: "Let's face reality: differences between expectations and achievements".

Organizer of the working conference entitled *MIE2001 Special Topic Conference "Healthcare Telematic Support in Transition Countries"*, *Bucharest, June 7-9, 2001*, in co-operation with Romanian Society of Medical Informatics and other EFMI working groups (esp. the EFMI working group on Human and Organisational issues))

Future activities:
Organize a Workshop at MIE2002 in Budapest.

Working Group

Electronic Healthcare Records

Chair:
Dr. Bernd Blobel
Otto-von-Guericke University Magdeburg
Medical Faculty
Institute of Biometry and Medical Informatics
Leipziger Str. 44
D-39120 Magdeburg
bernd.blobel@mrz.uni-magdeburg.de

Objectives:
The working group deals with the issue of electronic health records at different levels.

Such levels concern the case level, organisational level, regional level, national level, and international level. In that context, the Working Group supports:

Studies on specification, implementation, and promotion of standards for EHR,

The modelling of its architecture and its interoperability, as well as education on that topic.

The organisation of workshops dedicated to the WG's topics.

The working group especially deals with the analysis of different EHCR approaches, harmonising tools and methods for specification, presentation, implementation and use for common views, consideration and evaluation of the single model versus the dual model approach,

The EFMI Working Group "Electronic Healthcare Records" strongly co-operates with the EUROREC initiative and its supporting institutions.

Recent activities:
· Organisation of an international workshop on EHCR standards, held in February 2001 in Göttingen, Germany.
· Active participation in TEPR 2000 (San Francisco), TEHRE 2000 (London), TEPR 2001 (Boston) as representative of EFMI Working Group "Electronic Healthcare Record"

Future activities:

· Organisation of a set of workshops for providing insight and understanding of the methodologies developed and applied around the globe. A workshop and a tutorial will be organised at the next EUROREC Conference at Fall 2001 in France.
· Moving the structure-based models to real components specifying structure and functionality.
· Development of a set of UML models for meeting the challenges and requirements.
· Development tools for facilitating EHCR specification and implementation.
· Participation to established EHCR conferences to publish and to promote the EFMI's engagement.
· Contribution to activities within ISO TC 215 for representing EFMI interests.

APAMI

Regional Editor: Chun Por Wong

Regional President's Report - CP Wong

1. **Membership of APAMI**
   To date, medical informatics societies of 13 countries were members of the APAMI (Australia, the People's Republic of China, Hong Kong, Indonesia, Japan, South Korea, Malaysia, New Zealand, Pakistan, the Philippines, Singapore, Taiwan and Thailand). Sri Lanka and Vietnam have been observer members. Bangladesh and India have also shown interests in joining.

   WONCA, APOHN (Asia Pacific Online Health Network), CJK (China-Japan-Korea) and APAN are the organizations working in close linkage to APAMI countries.

2. **AGM of the APAMI**
   The AGM of the APAMI was held in Hong Kong on 29th September 2000. Eleven member societies (Philippines, Japan, Indonesia, Malaysia, Vietnam, Singapore, Korea, PR China, Taiwan, Sri Lanka and Hong Kong) were represented.

   In the AGM the following were resolved:
   a. The Philippine Medical Informatics Society was unanimously agreed to be the official national representative in APAMI.
   b. Korea was voted to be the hosting country for APAMI 2003 Conference, and also the next President-elect of APAMI.
   c. Hong Kong was elected the President (2000-2003), Korea the Vice-President, Philippines the Secretary and Japan the Treasurer.
   d. It was suggested that members' society names rather than country names should be used in the APAMI to avoid conflicts in the Asia region.

3. **APAMI Conference**
   The APAMI Conference 2000 was held in Hong Kong on 28-29th September 2000. A total of 331 participants from 17 countries attended. Thirteen plenary sessions, 71 papers, 13 posters and 5 pre-conference tutorials were presented.

Members' Activities 2000-2001

China (from Dr. Ling Zhu)

1. There are more than 5,700 members, 31 professional committees and 22 regional branches in CMIA.

Hong Kong (from Dr. Chun Por Wong)

1. APAMI Conference and AGM were held in Hong Kong in September 28-29, 2000.
2. A satellite symposium on medical informatics was held successfully in collaboration with the Hospital Authority Convention and International Hospital Federation Conference in May 2001.
3. Significant progress was made in the development and implementation of Hospital Information Systems to all 14 acute hospitals in Hong Kong. All modules will be completed before 2003. Extension of HIS to the remaining 30 health institutions will be planned within 5 years.
4. Funding of HK$ 800 million for a territory-wide health information infrastructure has been ear-marked to cover both government and private sectors health service agencies.

India (from Prof. Saroj K. Mishra)

1. A national society for medical informatics has been formed few years ago. The Indian Society for Telemedicine was launched in 2001 with the first ever national conference on telemedicine held in April 2001 at Lucknow.
2. Many government and corporate hospitals have introduced hospital information systems. The range of applications ranges from few to many modules depending on the size of the hospital. Teleradiology facility is available at few places.
3. Virtual medical university has been launched by one private agency. Video-conferencing facility is available at few places.
4. Ministry of Health, Government of India has digitized the National Library of Medicine located at New Delhi and getting it connected to peripheral medical colleges gradually.
5. Isolated centers in private sector started setting up telemedicine as stand alone facility to provide teleconsultation. Two corporate hospitals have started telecardiology facility.

APAMI (Continued)

Korea (from Prof. Yun Sik Kwak)

1. A successful CJK (China-Japan-Korea) Medical Informatics Meeting was held on 2nd December 2000 at Jeju Island in South Korea with 3 plenary lectures, 65 full paper presentations and over 350 participants from China, Japan, Korea and guests from Australia and Mongolia.
2. Seoul hosted the ISO Technical Committee 215, Health Informatics 5th General Meeting from March 26-30, 2001 with 131 experts from 17 countries attending. Delegates from People's Republic of China attended as observer-member for the first time. More than 10 Draft International Standards were produced.
3. An International Conference on Human-Society-Internet will be held in Seoul from July 4-6, 2001. Speakers from 10 different countries will be invited.
4. Korea inaugurated Health Level 7-Korea in May 2000. Seoul National University Hospital and Kyunpook National University Hospital have started to use HL7 interface to communicate HIS and PACS.

Taiwan (from Prof. Jack Li)

1. Taiwan Association of Medical Informatics (TAMI) is steadily growing into a society of more than 500 members. Since January 2001, more than 12 conferences on topics ranging from security standards to electronic health record were hosted by TAMI. TAMI is also actively involved in the planning of multi-million US dollar knowledge-based healthcare project starting 2002.
2. Hosted by TAMI, we have had one of the most successful annual symposiums in Taiwan last year - MIST 2000. More than 80 papers and posters were presented to an attendance of about 500 people. This year, MIST 2001 will be held in conjunction with Taiwan Bioinformatics Association in a multi-function conference/mall complex near Taipei during 10/26-28. Details will be sent to APAMI once it is available.
3. Taiwan has formally joined HL7 as the 11th international affiliate. HL7 Taiwan has also successfully attracted about 100 initial members starting June this year when it formally materialized as a non-profit organization. Taiwan has formally joined DICOM committee and government liaison was assigned to communicate with all public agencies.
4. TAMI is still actively pursuing to host APAMI of 2006.

Vietnam (from Prof. Nguyen Hoang Phuong)

1. The VJMEDIMAG 2001 - a first Vietnam-Japan Bilateral Symposium on Biomedical Imaging/Medical Informatics and Applications will be held on 24-25 November 2001 in Hanoi. A call for papers has been distributed to member countries.

Helina

Regional Editor: Sedick Isaacs

The First International Working Conference on Health Informatics in Africa, HELINA'93, was held in Ile-Ife, Nigeria, in 19-23 April 1993. In the closing session of HELINA'93, it was proposed that this successful conference should be periodically organised and along the lines of HELINA'93. Helina 96 was held in South Africa, Helina99 took place in Zimbabwe and Helina2002 will be in Cairo Egypt.

The only African Country who thus far is a full member of IMIA is South Africa. Corresponding member countries are Egypt, Tanzania and Nigeria. Countries who are in the process of establishing their national societies are Zambia, Kenya and Zimbabwe.

The African health informatics community also has an electronic bulletin board - HELINA-L@uku.fi. HELINA-L is for news, information and requests for information concerning the informatics (computer and communications) support for health care in Africa. It is not for general health-related or general computer-related information, as there are other lists for such purposes. In order to contain the cost for subscribers in Africa with low-capacity facilities, the maximum length of any message is about 100-200 lines. More voluminous contributions are abstracted and the full text is made available by order from an archive of files. The maximum number of messages is about 5-10 per month, i.e. 1-2 per week in the long run. These limitations are based on a questionnaire among the subscribers in 1996. Editing policy HELINA-L is moderated, i.e. the bulletins distributed through the list will be selected by the list administrators, who reserve the right to select, edit and adapt, if necessary, materials they consider suitable for distribution. Commercial information is not distributed. The HELINA-L is initially operated by the HELINA'93 Overseas Bureau, in coordination with colleagues from IMIA (International Medical Informatics Association) and WHO (World Health Organisation). You are welcome to contribute by sending news, announcements, reports on practical experience of using informatics in a health care setting in Africa, etc. If you wish to distribute some information through the HELINA-L, please send the text to: HELINA-L@uku.fi.

Forthcoming African Event: Helina2002 (the African Regional Health Informatics Conference) in Cairo in October 2002.

Dr. Sedick Isaacs
Department of Information Management
Groote Schuur Hospital
Observatory
7925 South Africa
E-mail: seisaacs@pawc.wcape.gov.za
Tel: +27 21 404 2058
Fax: +27 21 404 2070

IMIA Members in North America

Regional Editors:
Jochen Moehr, Charles Safran

Although there is not an IMIA region in North America, medical informatics activity in North America has been vibrant in 2001. IMIA's national members in this region are Canadian Organization for Advancement of Computers in Health (COACH) with Jochen R. Moehr as its IMIA representative, and the American Medical Informatics Association with Marion Ball as its IMIA representative. In addition we report some activities of Société québécoise de l'informatique biomédicale et de la santé - Quebec Biomedical and Health Informatics Society, The Health Evidence Application and Linkage Network, HEAL*Net,* the Medical Records Institute's TEPR conference and activities, and the American National Standards Association's Healthcare Informatics Standards Board.

United States related Health Informatics Organizations and Activities

AMIA

The American Medical Informatics Association (AMIA) was formed just over a decade ago through the merger of three medical informatics organizations including the Symposium on Computer Applications in Medical Care (SCAMC), the American Association for Medical Systems and Informatics (AAMSI), and the American College of Medical Informatics (ACMI).

Today AMIA has more than 3,200 members including individuals, institutions, and corporations. It is governed by a Board of Directors that include 16 elected and 2 ex-officio members. The business of the Association is conducted through a division of responsibility among the Board, 14 standing and ad hoc committees, 18 Working Groups and Special Interest Groups, and a headquarters office with a staff of 11. AMIA holds two meetings per year – an Annual Symposium in the autumn and a Spring Congress in May – publishes a scholarly journal and several electronic bulletins, engages in public policy initiatives both on its own and in collaboration with other organizations, and carries out a number of other programs.

Highlights of 2001

The last half of year 2000 and the year 2001 marked an extremely active period for AMIA. Following are some of the highlights over that period:

AMIA 2001 Annual Symposium

The 2001 AMIA Annual Symposium celebrated its 25th Anniversary in 2001, having spent the first 14 of those years pre-dating AMIA as the Symposium on Computer Applications in Medical Care (SCAMC). The 2001 Annual Symposium, with the theme *"A Medical Informatics Odyssey: Visions of the Future and Lessons from the Past,"* took place November 3-7 in Washington, DC. The 2001 Symposium was chaired by Suzanne Bakken, RN, DNSc, of Columbia University. The meeting was held in a time of great uncertainty in the U.S., having suffered less than two months before from terrorist incidents in New York, Washington, and Pennsylvania that claimed more than 5,000 lives of Americans and visiting citizens of more than 80 other countries as well, followed weeks later by an outbreak of anthrax in Washington, DC, the location of the meeting, and elsewhere along the U.S. Atlantic Coast.

Despite the enormously adverse conditions, the 2001 Annual Symposium ranked as among the more successful in its esteemed history. Registration through the summer had the 2001 Symposium on target to be among the largest in several years, but the subsequent chilling effect of terrorist threats made itself evident through higher-than-normal cancellations and a slowing of registrations. Nevertheless, registration in the end was nearly 1,600, remarkably only about 8% fewer than had attended the previous year's AMIA Annual Symposium in Los Angeles. In addition to the regular scientific sessions, the 2001 meeting featured a series of unique presentations. Several distinguished AMIA leaders presented special overviews of the development of the field over the past 25 years including the evolution of research, clinical practice, professional education, and the Symposium itself. Case study presentations provided a unique format combing formal presentation, poster, and discussion. In response to the previous weeks' events, there was a special panel on *"The Medical Informatics Response to Bioterrorism, War, and Disaster"* attended by nearly 800 of the registrants and underwritten by three corporate supporters, DynCorp, Eclipsys, and TheraDoc.

<table>
<tr><td>

IMIA Members in North America (Continued)

</td></tr>
</table>

AMIA 2001 Spring Congress

The AMIA 2001 Spring Congress was held in Atlanta, Georgia on May 15-17, 2001. The theme was *"Developing a National Agenda for Public Health Informatics."* The Program Committee was chaired by William A. Yasnoff, MD, PhD, of the Centers for Disease Control. The attendance surpassed 500 for the first time in several years for an AMIA Spring Congress. Major funding was provided by the Robert Wood Johnson Foundation and two U.S. government institutions, the National of Medicine and the Agency for Healthcare Research and Quality. The Congress held the endorsement of several U.S. public health associations, and brought together representatives from both the informatics community and the public health community to discuss ways in which medical informatics could play a role in the improvement of public health care in the U.S. A series of recommendations coming out of the meeting was published in AMIA's journal *JAMIA* and in the public health literature. In addition, all of the plenary presentations were captured on videotape and made available on the Internet for subscription through DigiScript, Inc.

JAMIA – the Journal of the American Medical Informatics Association

AMIA's scholarly journal continued to excel through its rigorous publishing schedule of 6 issues per year. *JAMIA* maintained its prestigious ranking for the third year in a row as having the top citation impact factor among all medical informatics journals indexed by the Institute for Scientific Information (ISI). In addition, the Web-accessible electronic edition of JAMIA saw its first full year after the initial appearance of the online edition in mid-2000. Archives of past years' issues were converted to online in early 2001. At the end of the year, AMIA announced Randolph Miller, MD, as only the second editor of *JAMIA* effective with the 2003 volume, succeeding William Stead, MD, who was founding editor of the journal and is serving as editor-in chief through the 2002 volume.

AMIA Online – AMIA's Web Site and other Online Publications

Bringing JAMIA online represented one of several tangible developments within AMIA in mid-2000 that began moving the association to the forefront of online communications with its members. In October, 2000, AMIA unveiled a new Web site. In addition to information about AMIA as an association, AMIA's Web site now includes extensive sections of news and updates about events within the discipline of medical informatics as well as developments in other realms of activity that promise to have a bearing on the field. These are organized into an online Resource Center, with sections covering News and Developments, Public Policy and Legislation, Research and Grants, the Health Information Technology Marketplace, Academic and Training Programs, Publications of Interest Conferences and Meetings, and a link to a wide range of other relevant Web sites. In addition, AMIA now regularly issues two online communiqués to members – *AMIA Alert* which reports news and developments in academia, industry, government and elsewhere that have a bearing on issues of relevance to medical informatics, and *Access* AMIA which details activities of the association itself that members may find of special interest.

Member Initiatives – Reflecting Trends in Medical Informatics

The role of AMIA, as an association, as a conduit to developments in the field of medical informatics is nowhere so evident as in AMIA's Working Groups structure. There are currently 14 Working Groups and 4 Special Interest Groups in AMIA, each focusing on a leading content area. In 2001, many groups held programs at the AMIA Annual Symposium and carried out other activities throughout the year. As examples of some of the leading efforts of these groups, AMIA's Primary Care Working Group continued to spearhead a multi-organizational National Alliance for Primary Care Informatics, bringing together representatives from a variety of associations to set forth an agenda to develop a primary care infrastructure in the U.S. with information technologies playing a central role. Another AMIA Working Group, Consumer Health Informatics, sponsored an intensive two-day post-conference at the AMIA 2001 Annual Symposium.

Public Policy Initiatives

For the past several years, AMIA has been closely involved in advocating for a measured approach to medical privacy that

IMIA Members in North America (Continued)

both protects citizens and provides opportunities for meaningful use of aggregate data by researchers and in applied settings. These efforts have taken on added significance as the U.S. government has sought to deal with the electronic generation and flow of medical information through changes to the Health Insurance Portability and Accountability Act (HIPAA). Many of AMIA's efforts on medical privacy advocacy have been through its participation in the Coalition on Health Information Policy (CHIP), a four member collaborative including AMIA, the American Health Information Management Association (AHIMA), the Center for Healthcare Information Management (CHIM), and the Health Information Management and Systems Society (HIMSS). In addition to the medical privacy and confidentiality initiative, the AMIA Public Policy and an ad hoc task force developed a strong position statement in late 2001 with recommendations regarding the role of U.S. federal government in facilitating the creation of a national health information infrastructure (NHII).

The AMIA Board

AMIA President Patricia Flatley Brennan, RN, PhD, described in last year's *IMIA Yearbook* the strategic planning process the AMIA Board launched in 2000. The Board continued in 2001 to work at a high level on refining how the association can play a facilitative role in fostering the evolution of the field of medical informatics as a vital discipline in the intersection of health care, information science, and technology. On January 1, 2002, W. Ed Hammond, PhD, assumed the Presidency of AMIA.

Medical Records Institute

The year 2001 has seen a switch from the e-Health activities that dominated the last couple of years. Although some of the industry has not survived, the consumer movement has increased in the United States. The trend is to involve the patient as a partner in health care by providing more information. In leading provider organizations, patients are given access to some of their personal health information (laboratory reports, allergies, appointments, immunization, etc.) on web sites. Some 13 million patients are reported to have personal health records on websites.

However, the key issue in medical informatics concerns the computer interface. An interesting event was the 'Documentation Challenge" at the 17th TEPR conference. Ten companies were demonstrating how to best capture an encounter in their information systems. Close to a thousand people were analyzing information capture methods such as speech recognition, free text and template systems for more than four hours. The annual TEPR conference had 3,800 attendees, 438 speakers and 158 exhibitors exploring best practices of medical informatics.

Two issues dominate the healthcare field in the United States. One is mobile health, i.e., the use of mobile computing devices in applications such as emergency rooms, order entry, and mobile computing in various hospital applications, etc. Still in its infancy, m-Health promises to be a major factor in US health care in the coming years. The second issue is security. The HIPAA legislation will introduce a national approach to privacy and security. Providers are forced to develop their own strategy for security.

In the standards world, ANSI HISB (American National Standards Association's Healthcare Informatics Standards Board) is coordinating the efforts toward electronic signatures and is addressing the future use of XML in health care. HL7 has continued to grow into the world's dominating standard for healthcare communication. Version 3 of HL7 is in its ballot stage. When it will be ready for implementation, it will be a major step toward interoperability in medical informatics.

Canadian Health Informatics Organizations and Activities

COACH

COACH, the Canadian Organization for Advancement of Computers in Health (http://www.coachorg.com/) is an organization of more than 750 health executives, physicians, nurses, and allied health professionals, researchers, educators, information technology managers and vendors.

The mission of COACH is "to promote understanding and effective utilization of information technologies in the Canadian health care environment through:

IMIA Members in North America (Continued)

- Education
- Information
- Communication
- Networking

Members form a network of specialists in the Healthcare industry across Canada. This network provides an opportunity for the exchange of information and ideas through personal contact with colleagues, locally and nationally. COACH provides an educational and professional program, which includes:

- Regional workshops and seminars: Held in major centers across Canada, these COACH sponsored events are topic specific and feature experts that have direct knowledge in the field.
- A National Conference, which brings over 800 members and vendors together to interact on a national level.

COACH's annual Conference is designed to enable members of the Healthcare community to participate on a national level in the exchange of information, developments, ideas and concepts. In recent years, COACH has collaborated with both the Canadian Institute for Health Information (CIHI) and the Canadian Health Record Association (CHRA). Both of these organizations have held their annual meetings in conjunction with COACH.

The formal component of the Conference's three day agenda includes plenary sessions and concurrent sessions which deal with a broad range of topics presented by leading authorities from Canada and abroad. In addition to the General Program, the conference includes Scientific Sessions under the direction of a Scientific Program Committee; papers for this segment of the conference are peer-reviewed.

Vendor exhibits complement the educational component of the Conference. The COACH Conference has emerged as "THE" Canadian venue for firms who provide application software, hardware and services to the Canadian Healthcare information and telecommunications technology market place. Typically, over fifty vendors from Canada, the U.S. and abroad exhibit at the Conference.

The 2001 conference, e-health 2001, in Toronto, Ontario, marked the release of the second edition of the "Guidelines for the Protection of Health Information". This publication is the culmination of more than a year of research and writing efforts of the ten member Security and Privacy Committee. This publication gives health informatics professionals the framework needed to develop and implement security and privacy programs. As technology and information management techniques evolved over time, COACH decided that it needed to update its original guidelines published in 1995 under the authorship of Brendan Seaton, the current President of COACH.

SOQIBS

The SOQIBS - Société québécoise de l'informatique biomédicale et de la santé - Quebec Biomedical and Health Informatics Society (*www.soqibs.org*) has been formed in 2001 to encourage scientific exchange between all persons interested in the role of informatics in relation to the health system. The three health system pillars of research, education and service are seen as equally important with outreach to all interested whether the public or private sectors or the community at large. The attempt is to make a single meeting place for diverse elements and to link positively and reciprocally to different special interest groups nationally and internationally. Furthermore, the society seeks to be a source of expertise for policy development linked to the discipline. In May 2002, the society will host for the first time in North America the 9th French speaking international medical informatics meeting: JFIM, Journées francophones d'informatique médicale. The current President of SOQIBS is Dr. Andrew Grant, Professor at the University of Sherbrooke, Sherbrooke, Quebec.

CHRA

The Canadian Health Record Association (CHRA) (http://www.chra.ca/org/index.html) was founded in 1942 to provide a forum for health record professionals to share their expertise. Its federal charter was obtained in 1949. The Canadian College of Health Record Administrators was federally chartered in 1972 to deal with

IMIA Members in North America (Continued)

the educational standards and professional certification of the health record professional. These bodies operate jointly, under the acronym CHRA in pursuit of CHRA's mission and goals.

The CHRA **mission** is: To contribute to the promotion of wellness and the provision of quality healthcare through excellence in health information management.

Its **goals** are:

- To ensure entry level competency of practice through standards and certification.
- To support continued professional learning.
- To promote the expertise of health record professionals.
- To strengthen the membership through the delivery of relevant and timely services.
- To research, develop and disseminate "theory and practice" of health information management.
- To maintain an effective organization.

The CHRA has 3000 certified members nationwide. CHRA members provide leadership and expertise regarding health record/information systems and management, patient access to health information, confidentiality, record security, record retention, data quality, analysis and utilization.

CIHI

Created by Canada's Health Ministers, the Canadian Institute for Health Information (CIHI, www.cihi.ca) is an independent, national, not-for-profit organization working to improve the health of Canadians and the health care system by providing quality health information.

Committed to safeguarding the privacy and confidentiality of personal health information, CIHI's mandate is to coordinate the development and maintenance of a common approach to health information for Canada. To this end, CIHI is responsible for providing accurate and timely information that is needed to establish sound health policies, manage the Canadian health system effectively and create public awareness of factors affecting good health.

The Institute's mandate is based upon collaborative planning with key stakeholder groups, including all provincial, territorial and federal governments, national health care agencies and service providers.

The Institute's core functions are to:

- identify and promote national health indicators;
- coordinate and promote the development and maintenance of national health information standards;
- develop and manage health databases and registries;
- conduct analysis and special studies and participate in research;
- publish reports and disseminate health information; and
- coordinate and conduct education sessions and conferences.

Among its many initiatives, is *The Partnership for Health Information Standards* (www.cihi.ca/partship/partner1.shtml). Created in 1996, The Partnership is a forum that brings together the public and private sectors to share, connect and map the future of health information standards in Canada. The Partnership organizes two conferences a year (spring and fall) focusing on major Canadian and international health information standards activities.

Among the projects currently underway by CIHI in the area of technical/interoperability standards is the development of an enhanced health data model that has been adopted by ministries of health in British Columbia, Alberta and Ontario. This model will serve to guide users who are involved in the development of health information systems. CIHI has also completed the development of a draft data dictionary, which describes/defines some of the elements currently used in its databases.

CIHI has also worked on a number of PKI-related documents, produced to assist in the establishment of a health PKI within and across jurisdictions. These documents provide a framework and guidelines for the secure electronic communication of health information. A number of demonstration projects are currently underway to ensure the relevance and usefulness of these tools.

IMIA Members in North America (Continued)

Additionally, CIHI is the sponsoring agency for HL7 Canada, the forum for Canadian health information stakeholders to decide how HL7 is adopted and adapted for use in Canada. HL7 Canada is a recognized international affiliate and a voting member of the HL7 International Committee. HL7 Canada is organized to identify and support the unique requirements of its member groups—health information system users, vendors, and administrators.

On the international front, CIHI has been actively involved in standards development activities within the ISO community, including support Canadian leadership on standards for country identifiers, a conceptual health indicators framework and an information architecture framework (data model).

HEALNet

The Health Evidence Application and Linkage Network, HEAL*Net*, is one of 18 federal Networks of Centres of Excellence (NCE) funded through the federal granting councils - the Natural Sciences and Engineering Research Council, the Canadian Institutes of Health Research (formerly the Medical Research Council),

and the Social Sciences and Humanities Research Council - in partnership with Industry Canada, Canadian universities and corporate and public sector partners. HEALNet was funded from 1995 to 2002 and is dedicated to enhancing the use of evidence-based knowledge and technologies to improve health-related decision-making in the health system and in the workplace. HEAL*Net* research focuses on the delivery and promotion of the best available research evidence in the making of health decisions at the individual, administrative, and policy levels.

HEAL*Net* included close to one hundred researchers and a similar amount of graduate students from about 30 universities, research institutions and companies. In the health informatics context HEAL*Net* is important in Canada since it provided a focus for national collaboration of many Canadian researchers in health informatics, working on novel approaches to providing, accessing, assessing, and using research evidence. From the perspective available at the close of the year 2001, it appears that this consolidation of a part of the academic health informatics community may be one of the lasting legacies of HEAL*Net*.

Health Informatics in Computer Science at the University of Waterloo

Computer Science at the University of Waterloo has three major initiatives in Health Informatics (HI):

- **An HI specialization option for M.Sc. and Ph.D. candidates.**
  Our objective is to engage graduate students in research on new concepts and tools that facilitate the development of HI solutions. We currently offer two graduate-level courses: "Frontiers of Computer Science Research in HI", and "Health Natural Language Processing".

- **Research on the Computer Science foundations of HI.**
  The Center for Computer Science Research in HI (CCSRHI) includes faculty and students pursuing research in key areas, including: health natural language processing, clinical workflow automation, clinical utilization management, medical image understanding, health data mining, the economics of health IT, and concepts and methods in HI education. Several major companies serve as industry partners.

- **The Education Program Health Informatics Professionals (EPHIP).**
  This is a synchronous distance education program for practicing professionals in the health field. It offers 7 courses: Introduction to Applied HI, An HI Perspective of the Health System, The Nature of Health Information and Systems, Health Process and Product Innovation, AHI Management and Personal Competencies, Evaluating IT/IM in Health, and Managing the Health Systems Life Cycle. For more information visit: http://ephip.uwaterloo.ca.

Information on our research and graduate education programs can be found at:
http://www.math.uwaterloo.ca/CS_Dept/health_info/index.htm

For Further Information:

Health Informatics
Computer Science
Room 3320 Davis Centre
University of Waterloo
200 University Ave. West
Waterloo, ON Canada
N2L 3G1
Telephone: 519-888-4567 ext 5996
E-mail: healthinfo@logos.math.uwaterloo.ca

Nancy M. Lorenzi,
Guest-editor

Vanderbilt University,
Medical Center,
Nashville, Tennessee, USA

IMIA's Working Groups and Special Interest Groups:

Connecting the World's Medical Informatics Working Groups

While Informatics is not a new discipline, it is still an evolving discipline, and many people are working toward better understanding and developing informatics concepts and tools. There are informatics experts throughout the world with no one part of the world having all the answers - we are developing the informatics answers for the future together today.

Working Groups and the content experts who are in these groups are the future of Medical Informatics. Each group and person deliberates, helps to understand, and moves forward the scientific content area of informatics. As part of creating more dynamic interactions among IMIA's Working Groups and also identifying content areas where working groups are needed, I began to evolve a scientific content map (Table 1). The scientific content map has seven areas: 1) applied technology, 2) information technology infrastructure, 3) data infrastructure related, 4) applications and products, 5) human organizational, 6) education and knowledge and 7 the clinical disciplines that underpin and need information from each other and content from each of the major areas. Each of the major topic areas have specific content topics that working groups are or could work on in the future.

The original IMIA effort led to looking for other health/medical informatics working groups worldwide. The Asian-Pacific group (APAMI), COACH (Canada), the IMIA African Region or the IMIA Latin America Region do not have working groups. Three major informatics organizations have working groups, They are the American Medical Informatics Association, the European Federation of Medical Informatics, and the International Medical Informatics Association. Table 2 illustrates how the world's working groups connect to the scientific content map. The categories focus on infrastructure/technical research, standards and representations, applications and products, education and health related issues. Needing content from these topics are those working groups for developing countries, clinical-based discipline working groups that cross all of the above content areas and the AMIA student working group, that needs to be connected to all of the content areas plus the developing countries and clinical discipline working groups.

On behalf of the IMIA Working Group Chairs we hope that people from all of the working groups in all of the associations mentioned as well as others who are interested will look at this material and determine how the efforts can be integrated or connected. There is much work to do that supporting or being complementary is important for all of us. We hope that by working together we can enhance the area of informatics for the basic and clinical science.

Table 1: Proposed Medical Informatics Scientific Content Map

Applied Technology	Information Technology Infrastructure	Data-Infrastructure Related	Applications and Products	Human-Organizational	Education and Knowledge
• Algorithms • Bioinformatics • Biosignal processing • Boolean logic • Cryptology • Human genome related • Human interfaces • Image Processing • Mathematical models in medicine • Pattern recognition	• Archival-repository systems for medical records- EPR-CPR-EMR • Authentication • Chip cards in health care • Distributed systems • Health professional workstation • Interfaces • Knowledge based systems • Networks • Neural networks • Pen based • Security • Speech recognition • Standards • Systems architecture • Telehealth • User interfaces	• Classification • Coding systems • Concept representation-preservation • Data acquisition-data capture • Data analysis-extraction tools • Data entry • Data policies • Data protection • Database design • Indexing • Syntax • Language representation • Lexicons • Linguistics • Modeling • Nomenclatures • Standards • Terminology-vocabulary • Thesaurus tools	• Biostatistics • Clinical trials • Computer-supported surgery • Decision support • Diagnosis related • Disease mgt. • EPR-CPR-EMR • Epidemiological research Hospital IS • Event-based systems • Evidence based guidelines • Expert systems • Health services research • HIS management • Knowledge-based systems • Laboratory data • Image processing • Operations/Resource management • Outcomes research and measurement • Quality management • Patient identification • Patient monitoring • Minimum Data Sets • Supply chain • Telematics • Telemedicine	• Assessment • Compliance • Cognitive tasks • Collaboration • Communication • Economics of IT • Ethics • Implementation-deployment • Diffusion of IT • Evaluation • Human Factors • Legal issues, implementing national laws • Management • Managing Change • Needs assessment • Organizational redesign processes • Organizational transformation • Planning • Policy Issues • Privacy • Project Management • Security • Strategic plans • Unique identifiers • User-computer interface	• Bibliographic • Cognitive learning • Computer aided instruction • Computer-supported training • Consumer education • Continuing education • Digital Libraries • E-Business • H/MI education • Information management-dissemination • Knowledge bases • Knowledge management • Learning models • Online/distance education

Clinical Disciplines: Anesthesia, Behavioral, Cardio/Thoracic, Cardiovascular, Dentistry, Dermatology, Emergency Medicine, Environmental health, Gastroenterology, Human genetics, Internal Medicine, Neurosurgery, Nursing, Obstetrics & Gynecology, Ophthalmology, Orthopedics, Pathology, Pediatrics, Pharmacy, Primary care, Psychiatry, Radiology, Surgery, Urology

Table 2: World-wide Informatics Association's Working Groups

Infrastructure/Technical/Research	Standards & Representation	Applications & Products	Education and Human Related Issues
• Data Protection and Security (EFMI) -Francois Allaert • Data Protection in Health Information Systems (IMIA) - Ab Bakker • Intelligent Data Analysis and Data Mining (IMIA) - Riccardo Bellazzi, Blaz Zupan • Biomedical Pattern Recognition (IMIA) - Christoph Zywietz • Biomedical Statistics and Information Processing (IMIA) - Jana Zvarova, Leon Bobrowski • Genomics (AMIA) - John McCarthy	• Standards in Health Telematics (EFMI) • Natural Language understanding (EFMI) - Robert Baud • Medical Concept Representation (IMIA) - Christopher G. Chute • Standards in Health Care Informatics (IMIA) - Open • Natural Language Processing (AMIA) - Stephen B. Johnson	• Clinical Information Systems (AMIA) - Richard Gibson • Clinical Trials (AMIA) - Joyce Niland • Computerized Patient Records (IMIA) - Johan van der Lei, Mark Musen • Health Information Systems (IMIA) - Klaus Kuhn, Dario Giuse • MDBS, Case Mix and severity of cases (EFMI) - Francis Roger-France • Telematics in Healthcare (IMIA) - Regis Beuscart • Information Planning and Modelling in Health Care(EFMI - Brian Manning • Internet (AMIA) -Bradford J. Richmond • Telehealth (AMIA)- Luis G. Kun, PhD	• Consumer Health Informatics (IMIA) - Alejandro Jadad, Betty L. Chang, Gunther Eysenbach • Consumer Health Informatics (AMIA) - Betty L. Chang • Education in Health Informatics (EFMI) - Arie Hasman • Education (AMIA) - Paul N. Gorman • Ethical, Legal, and Social Issues (AMIA) - Peter Winkelstein • Health and Medical Informatics Education (IMIA) - Evelyn Hovenga, John Mantas • Human and organisational issues in medical informatics (EFM) - Jos Aarts • Organizational and Social Issues (IMIA) - Bonnie Kaplan • People & Organizational Issues (AMIA) - Cynthia Gadd and Annette L. Valenta • Prevention and Public Health AMIA) - Jeff Luck • Quality Improvement (AMIA) - E. Andrew Balas • Technology Assessment & Quality Development (IMIA) - Jan Talmon

Developing Countries—Need Content From all of the Above Topics	
Health, Informatics and Development (EFMI) - George I. Mihalas	Health Informatics for Development (IMIA) - Nora Oliveri

Clinical Based Discipline Working Groups that Cross all of the Above	
• Anesthesiology/Critical Care and Emergency Medicine (AMIA) - Vasu Brown • Dental Informatics (AMIA) -Heiko Spallek • Dental Informatics (IMIA) - Wook-Sung Yoo, John Eisner • Mental Health (IMIA) - Michael Rigby, Ann Sheridan • Nursing Informatics (AMIA) -Patricia S. Button	• Nursing Informatics in Europe (EFMI) -Patrick Weber • Nursing Informatics (IMIA) - Virginia K. Saba, Heather Strachan • Primary Care Informatics (AMIA) - John A. Zapp • Primary Care Informatics (EFMI) - Nicolas Robinson • Primary Health Care Informatics (IMIA) - Michael Kidd, H.C. Mullins

Student Working Group (AMIA)—Christoph Lehmann

WG 1 - Health and Medical Informatics Education

Chair:
Dr. Evelyn J.S. Hovenga RN
School of Mathematical and Decision
Sciences,
Informatics and Communication,
Central Queensland University,
Blg 18, Room G20,
Rockhampton CQMC 4702, Australia
Tel: +61 749-309-839
Fax: +61 749-309-871
E-mail: e.hovenga@cqu.edu.au

Prof. Dr. John Mantas, co-chair
University of Athens, Dept. of Nursing,
Laboratory of Health Informatics.
PO Box 77313
GR-17510 Athens, Greece
E-mail: jmantas@dn.uoa.gr

Objectives:

· To disseminate and exchange information on Health and Medical Informatics (HMI) programs and courses.
· To promote the IMIA HMI database on programs and courses on HMI education.
· To produce international recommendations on HMI programs and courses.
· To support HMI courses and exchange of students and teachers.
· To advance the knowledge of: (1) how informatics is taught in the education of health care professionals around the world, (2) how in particular health and medical informatics is taught to students of computer science/informatics, and (3) how it is taught within dedicated curricula in health and medical informatics

Recent Activities:

· The Recommendations of the IMIA on Education in Health and Medical Informatics have now been translated into Spanish, Chinese, Italian, Turkish, Czech and Japanese. Anyone undertaking further translations must (1) formally seek permission from our publisher of the recommendations, Schattauer, (2) notify Dr Reinhold Haux (Reinhold_Haux@med.uni-heidelberg.de) and (3) forward the URL to Dr Evelyn Hovenga (e.hovenga@cqu.edu.au) so that a link can be established on the WG1 website.
· IMIA HMI has a new mailing list and anyone with an interest is able to join this list by sending a message to majordomo@cqu.edu.au and subscribe to imia-wg1@cqu.edu.au or to Dr Evelyn Hovenga.
· New webpages are now accessible via the IMIA homepage at http://www.imia.org

Future Activities:

· The Recommendations of the IMIA on Education in Health and Medical Informatics will be reviewed and updated.
· A Global (Virtual) University initiative is being undertaken. A steering committee consisting of Dr John Mantas, Dr. Jim Turley, Dr Umberto Giani, Dr. William Hersh and Dr Yu-Chuan (Jack) Li was established at the last meeting held during Medinfo 2001 in London. A glossary of terms describing the many data elements used to describe various aspects of programs and courses is being complied. Around 20 issues needing exploration from which recommendations can be made have been identified. A number of members are contributing to this effort. It is expected that the results of this work will be published in a textbook. One of the objectives is to meet educational needs of developing countries.
· The next meeting is scheduled to be held mid 2002 in conjunction with another international working conference in the USA.

WG 2 - Consumer Health Informatics

Co-Chairs:
Alejandro (Alex) R. Jadad, MD DPhil
Director, Program in eHealth Innovation
Rose Family Chair in Supportive Care
Senior Scientist, Div. of Clinical Decision
Making and Health Care Research
Professor, Departments of Health
Policy, Management and Evaluation
and Anesthesiology
University Health Network
University of Toronto
Tel   +1 416 340 4800 Ext. 6823
Fax: +1 416 340 3595
E-mail: ajadad@uhnres.utoronto.ca

Betty L. Chang
Professor
School of Nursing, Box 956918
University of California, Los Angeles
Los Angeles, CA 90095-6918, USA
Tel: +1 310 206-3834
Fax: +1 310 206-0914

Gunther Eysenbach, MD
Research Unit for Cybermed. & eHealth
Clinical Social Medicine/Health
Systems Research
Heidelberg University Hospitals
Bergheimer Str. 58
69115 Heidelberg, Germany
Tel: +49 6221 56 88 97
Mobile   +49 172 82 49 086
Tel.:   +49 6221 56 47 42 (secr)
Fax   +49 6221 56 55 84

Objectives:
· To provide a forum to enhance collaboration, share experiences, and promote research in Consumer Health Informatics (CHI).
· To increase communication with other working groups at IMIA and other informatics organizations relevant to CHI.
· To establish itself as a group for funding agencies to consult on issues related to information technology projects in health care.

Recent Activities:
· The working group developed a temporary website, <http://www.jmir.org/imia-chi/> which provides a framework for WG activities. This CHI-WG website will be moved to the IMIA website on a central IMIA-server <http://www.imia.org> when the IMIA infrastructure is in place. We discussed the use of the IMIA site for active discussions, and considered the desirability of creating an active mailing list for the group.
· Members of CHI WG presented a panel to promote international collaboration, and papers on the ascertaining the quality of information on the web, and the outcomes of telehealth advice nursing as part of the Medinfo 2001, September 2-5. Several members of the IMIA WG are taking part as presenters at the forthcoming American Medical Informatics Association (AMIA) conference November 2-7, 2001 as well as participating in the AMIA CHI-WG co-sponsored post-conference on Critical Issues in Consumer Health Informatics to be held in Washington DC on November 7 and 8, 2001.

Future Activities:
· During the coming year, designated members of the IMIA CHI WG will explore the possibility of drafting a project proposal that provides a roadmap of activities of IMIA CHI participants. Examples of questions the roadmap may address are: who is engaged in certain CHI activities? Who has done so in the past? What are some lessons learned from previous projects?
· We plan to increase communication and collaboration by the possible use of the IMIA website for discussion groups. We will also promote an exchange of ideas and experiences with other working groups. The most likely IMIA working groups are: Health and Medical Informatics Education, Data Protection in Health Information Systems, Mental Health Informatics, Health Informatics for Development, Health Information Systems, Organizational and Social Issues, Telematics in Healthcare, and Special Interest Group I - Nursing Informatics. As a beginning, the Chairs or Co-Chairs of several of the Working Groups and the Special Interest Group met with an IMIA WG (2) Consumer Health Informatics during the working group chairs' meeting at Medinfo 2001 to explore future avenues of communication and information exchange.
· The CHI WG will explore ways to increase student travel grants and reduced registration fees in order to encourage student participation. Finally, we plan to explore the potential role of IMIA CHI-WG in interacting with funding agencies on issues related to CHI.

WG 3 - Intelligent Data Analysis and Data Mining

Chair:
Dr. Riccardo Bellazzi
Dipartimento di Informatica e Sistemistica
Università di Pavia
via Ferrata 1
27100 Pavia, Italy
Tel: +390382505511
Fax: +390382505373
E-mail: Riccardo.Bellazzi@unipv.it

Co-Chair:
Dr. Blaz Zupan
Faculty of Computer and Information Sciences
University of Ljubljana
Trzaska 25
SI-1000 Ljubljana, Slovenia
and Department of Human and Molecular Genetics
Baylor College of Medicine,
Houston, Texas, USA
Tel: +38614768402
Fax: +38614264647
E-mail: blaz.zupan@fri.uni-lj.si

Objectives:
· To increase the awareness and acceptance of intelligent data analysis and data mining methods in medical community.
· To foster scientific discussion and disseminate new knowledge on AI-based methods for data analysis and data mining techniques applied to medicine.
· To promote the development of standardized platforms and solutions.
· To provide a forum for presentation of successful intelligent data analysis and data mining implementations in medicine, and for discussion of best practices in introduction of these techniques in medical and health-care information and decision support systems.

Recent Activities:
On occasion of Medinfo 2001, working group members organized IDAMAP 2001 (chair: R. Bellazzi, co-chair: Blaz Zupan), a full-day workshop on the working group topics. Seventeen papers were presented; they are available at the working group web site: http://magix.fri.uni-lj.si/idamap2001. Moreover, a panel for reporting the results of the workshop was organized within the main conference. The results of the workshop were also presented in a workshop within AMIA 2001. Finally, a Special Issue on IDAMAP of *Methods of Information in Medicine* was published in the November-December 2001 issue.

Future Activities:
The working group will focus on specific topics of interest for the scientific community. In particular, the following issues will be explored: the relationships between predictive data mining and evidence based medicine, knowledge-based functional genomics, temporal data abstractions within clinical guidelines and intelligent visualization techniques. The working group Web site will be restructured, in order to offer a list of most relevant publications, technical notes and recent results to the general audience. Finally, the WG will organize IDAMAP 2002 within ECAI 2002.

WG 4 - Data Protection in Health Information Systems

Chair:
Prof. Ab R. Bakker
Atjehweg 10
2202 AP Noordwijk
The Netherlands
Tel: +31713621984
Fax: +31713617500
E-mail: abakker@addabit.demon.nl

Other contact person:
Kees Louwerse (secretary)
LUMC Central Information Processing Department
PO Box 9600, 2300 RC Leiden
The Netherlands

Objectives:
To examine the issues of data protection and security within the health-care environment. The Data Protection in Health Information Systems Working Group addresses state-of-the-art security of distributed electronic patient records (EPR).

Recent Activities:
· Working conference "Security of the Distributed EPR", Victoria Canada June 21-24 2000. Proceedings published as special issue of the International Journal of Medical Informatics, Vol 60 NO.2. CD-ROM with presentations during the conference available through Jochen Moehr (email: jmoehr@uvic.ca).
· As follow-up to the recommendations of this working conference the IMIA AGM asked this working group to develop a draft for an Ethical Code of Practice and a draft for a Security Policy Framework. Two working teams were created to prepare the drafts. Eike Kluge (Canada) is leading the team for the Ethical Code of Practice; Barry Barber (UK) is leading the team for the Security Policy Framework.
· A workshop was organized at Medinfo2001 to discuss a draft of the Ethical Code of Practice
· A panel session was organized at Medinfo2001 to discuss the approach to arrive at a draft for the Security Policy Framework.

Data Protection in Health Information Systems (IMIA WG4) (Continued)

WG 5 - Primary Health Care Informatics

Co-chairs:
Dr. Michael Kidd, Professor and Head
Department of General Practice
The University of Sydney
37A Booth Street
Balmain 2041, Sydney, Australia
Tel: +61 2 9818 1400
Fax: +61 2 9818 1343
E-mail: michael.kidd@
           med.usyd.edu.au

Dr. H. C. "Moon" Mullins, MD
Crozer Keystone Health Systems
PO Box 545
Montrose, AL 36559, USA
Tel: +1 334 928 0905
Fax: +1 334 928 0106
E-mail: hmullins@
           jaguar1.usouthal.edu

Future activities:

1. Updated draft of an Ethical Code of Practice to be sent to the IMIA members in January 2002, asking them for comments within 3 months. Proposal for an Ethical Code of Practice to be offered to the IMIA AGM 2002 (at Taipei) for endorsement.
2. Preparation of a draft Security Policy Framework, time schedule: first draft ready end 2002.
3. Exploration of possibilities to have next working conference in Italy in the year 2003.

Objectives:
· To promote primary care computing by
    · acting as a forum for exchange of ideas between its members,
    · providing information to its members to assist them in progressing primary care computing in their own country, and
    · increasing the understanding of primary care computing issues with a view to publishing the results of these discussions.

Recent Activities:
· Primary Health Care Informatics Working Group 5 met at Medinfo 2001
· A combined meeting with members of the EFMI Working Group 7 (Primary Care), members of the Informatics Working Party of WONCA (The World Organization of Family Doctors), and IMIA Working Group 5 also occurred at the Medinfo conference.
· The Working Group consolidated its work plan for the next three years at the Medinfo meeting.
· There was strong representation of Primary Health Care issues among the papers, workshops, seminars, and panels being presented at Medinfo 2001. Jean Roberts produced an excellent overview of the Primary Health Care topics that were widely circulated.
· After the Medinfo meeting many individuals also attended the annual conference meeting of the British Computer Society Primary Health Care Specialist Group at Downing College, Cambridge, on September 7th & 8th, 2001. This was an excellent opportunity for networking as well as to discover what is happening in primary health care informatics in the UK.

Future Activities
· Seeking continued collaboration with members of the EFMI Working Group 7 (Primary Care), members of the Informatics Working Party of WONCA (The World Organization of Family Doctors), the American Medical Informatics Association's Primary Care Informatics Working Group, and IMIA Primary Health Care Informatics Working Group.
· Development of recruitment plan.
· Development of work plan to deliver our stated objectives
· Collaboration with Journal of Primary Care Informatics
· Website presence through the IMIA web site.
· Sharing outcomes from each nation

WG 6 - Medical Concept Representation

Chair:
Dr. Christopher G. Chute
Department of Health Sciences
Research, Mayo Foundation
Rochester, MN 55905, USA
Tel: +1 507 284 5541
Fax: +1 507 284 1516
E-mail: chute@mayo.edu

Co-chair:
Dr. Werner Ceusters
Director R&D
Language & Computing
Hazenakkerstraat 20a
B-9520 Zonnegem, Belgium
Tel: +32 53 62 95 45
Fax: +32 53 62 95 55
http   www.landc.be
E-mail: werner@landc.be

Objectives

To provide a forum for state of the art dialogue and collaboration on natural language processing and concept representation in healthcare applications. IMIA's Medical Concept Representation Working Group is the international forum for issues related to informatics in the classification and coding of health data. The working group is charged with: 1) reviewing health data nomenclature and classification needs for the world community; 2) evaluating information processing technology in meeting these defined needs; and 3) recommending methods for future classification and nomenclature systems.

Recent Activities:

· This Working Group sponsored a conference on Natural Language and Medical Concept Representation in Jacksonville, Florida in 1997.
· The Proceedings of the working conference were published in *Methods of Information in Medicine* in 1998, issues 4 and 5.
· The Working Group on Medical Concept Representation held its triennial conference on Natural Language Processing and Medical Concept Representation in late 1999, in Phoenix, Arizona, USA. This fifth conference, spanning a 15-year history, provided a forum for presentation and discussion of the state of the art in health terminology issues relevant to informatics research and applications.
· The working group had several papers and meeting at the Medinfo 2001 conference in London.

Future Activities:

· Planning for content and foci are underway for the 6th Triennial meeting, to be held in Europe around January 2003.
· The European Commission is offering possibilities for European research groups to involve US, Japanese, Australian, etc experts, within the 6th Framework Program that begins in 2002

Homepage: http://www.mayo.edu/imia-wg6/

WG 7 - Biomedical Pattern Recognition

Chair:
Christoph Zywietz
Medizinische Hochschule Hannover
Biosignalverarbeitung - 8440 -
Carl-Neuberg-Strasse 1
30625 Hannover, Germany
Tel: +49 511 532 4412
Fax: +49 511 532 4295
E-mail: zywietz.christoph@
          MH-Hannover.de

Objectives:

· To explore the field of biosignal interpretation, model-based biosignal analysis, interpretations and integration, extending existing signal-processing technology for the effective use of biosignals in a practical environment.
· To provide a forum for discussion and collaboration on problems of Biosignal Processing, Biomedical Pattern Recognition and on Quality Assurance in this field. This includes the following topics:
  · Measurement and interpretation of physiological signals
  · Signal-based modeling and simulation in biomedicine
  · Biological control systems, e.g., the human autonomous regulation system
  · Quality assurance and evaluation of physiological analysis systems

Recent Activities:

· Web pages for this working group provide information on the Working Group itself, information on working conferences and workshops (including their proceedings) organized/prepared specifically by this working group, links to the Proceedings publications in the *Methods of Information* as well as information on upcoming events.

Biomedical Pattern Recognition (IMIA WG 7) (Continued)

· The group presented a workshop "Quality Assurance in Biosignal Processing and Evaluation of Physiological Analysis Systems" during Medinfo 2001.

· Christoph Zywietz (Medical School Hannover, Hannover, Germany), Thomas Penzel (Medical Clinic, Philips University, Marburg, Germany), Paul Woolman (Royal Infirmary, Glasgow, United Kingdom) from this working group presented a "Quality Assurance in Biosignal Processing and Evaluation of Physiological Analysis Systems" workshop at Medinfo 2001. The workshop focused on medical devices that have built in computing capabilities for data acquisition, signal or image processing, diagnostic classification and result export (e.g. display, printing, storage and transmission). Performance analysis of such systems requires particular care. Besides general accuracy requirements, psychological and legal implications for patient and physician have to be considered on both the development and the user site. Cybernetics and control engineering have provided the basic methodology for performance analysis of systems: in pure technical systems often mathematically defined functions and signals can be fed into the system and its response and output provide the necessary performance characteristics after adequate mathematical analysis. However, the mathematical tools as well as the still used performance and test specifications within the official system standards very often imply that the systems to be tested are *linear* systems. Implementation of digital processing has introduced many *non-linear* properties into the behavior of devices and device systems. Consequently, many new test procedures (including new test signals) have to be developed for performance analysis and quality assurance. The Workshop discussed examples from three application areas in medical care: Computer assisted ECG analysis, Multi-parameter sleep monitoring, and Monitoring of vital signs in anesthesia and during surgery.

Future Activities:

· This working group will hold the IMIA 4th International Workshop on Biosignal Interpretation (http://www.BSI2002.polimi.it/FirstA.html) (June 24-26, 2002 in Villa Olmo, Como, Italy). http://wwwBSI2002.polimi.it/Committee.html. Program Committee members include: Metin Akay, Dartmouth, Collage Hanover, USA, Sergio Cerutti (Chairman) Polytechnic University of Milan, Bin He, University of Illinois, Chicago, USA, Shunsuke Sato, Osaka University, Japan, Christoph Zywietz, Medizinische Hochschule of Hannover, Germany

· The working group will have a portion of the papers presented published in a special issue of the Methods of Information. Sergio Cerutti and Christoph Zywietz will be the editors.

WG 8 - Mental Health Informatics

Chair:
Michael Rigby
Centre for Health Planning and
Management
Darwin Building, Keele University,
Keele, Staffordshire, ST5 5BG, UK
Tel: +44 1782 583193
Fax: +44 1782 711737
E-mail: hma10@keele.ac.uk

Co-chair:
Ann Sheridan
Assistant Director
Nursing/Midwifery Planning &
Development Unit ERHA
Canal House
Canal Road Dublin 6, Ireland
Tel: +44 406 5600
Fax: +44 406 5611
E-mail: ann.sheridan@erha.ie

Objectives:

This group was established at the IMIA Board meeting in August 2000 with the formal confirmation being received in October 2000. The proposal was triggered by an increasing recognition of the need to consider the special information and informatics needs of this domain, which represents some 10% of all healthcare activity. The domain has special information-handling requirements, and a range of challenges commencing with the longer-term, multi-site nature of much mental health care and the emphasis on qualitative and attitudinal data. At the same time, it is hoped that techniques to assist with these particular needs in health informatics will enrich more biophysical care domains as well.

Recent Activities:

· The chair and co-chair attended the IMIA board meeting in Madrid in 2001.
· The chair and co-chair presented a paper in the 'Patients Rights and New Technology' session at the joint Royal College of Psychiatrists/World Psychiatric Association Meeting in London in 2001.
· An open forum meeting took place at Medinfo in September.
· The HISI (Health Informatics Society of Ireland) approved a proposal to host an inaugural conference with support from the Nuffield Trust in London.
· A meeting was held with the Royal College of Psychiatrists/World Psychiatric Association. The event received interest from a number of delegates from UK, the rest of Europe, and wider afield.
· The inaugural scientific event of the WG, linked to the HISI conference on 14/15 November 2001 in Dublin, has the topic "Critical Success Factors in Mental Health Electronic Patient Record Systems". It now has confirmed key international speakers: Cheryl Plummer (Chief Information Officer, Riverview Hospital, Port Coquitlam, British Columbia, Canada. Organizational, Provincial and National Issues of Mental Health EPRs), Bosse Ivarsson Consultant Psychiatrist (Boras Psychiatric Unit, Western Sweden, Electronic Records–Challenges in Addressing the Clinical Culture), Per Lund (Chief Executive Officer, Skt. Hans Hospital, Copenhagen, Denmark, The Organizational and Managerial Issues of Implementing a Mental Health EPR), and Walter Gulbinat (Executive Secretary, International Consortium for Mental Health Policy and Service formerly Head Scientist, Mental Health Division, WHO.)
· An open forum was held at the Medinfo 2001 and drew representatives from three continents.

Future Activities:

It is planned that as a result of these activities, it should be possible to establish a work program for 2002 onwards, and to widen the organizational base.

WG 9 - Health Informatics for Development

Chair:
Nora Oliveri
Medical Informatics Foundation
801 Brickell Bay Drive,
Box 4, PMBC 134,
Miami, FL, 33131, USA
Tel: +1 786 425-381/+1 305 710-1528
Fax: +1 509 752-5912
E-mail: norao@fim.org.ar

Objectives:
· To find out how health care informatics could improve live conditions in developing regions and implement programs in that direction.
· Organization of forums to exchange of experiences of colleagues working in the field of health informatics.
· Making a list of the needs and resources in medical informatics for each country.
· Organization of educational activities in developing regions, especially through the implementation of professors' exchange.
· Organizing workshops and seminars with international experts participation

General Information
· Information about activities, publications, how to join the WG 9 and links to web sites related are available at www.fim.org.ar/wg9/
· To facilitate communication between members and all professionals interested in IMIA-Health Informatics for Developing Countries goals. Language: English and Spanish. To subscribe, send a message to: IMIA-WG9@pccorreo.com.ar. Subject: Subscribe. Body: name last name e-mail contact data

Recent Activities:
· This Working Group held a day workshop during Medinfo 2001 on Issues for Health Informatics for Developing Countries: Globalization and Development
· During year 2001 this working group collaborated with Informedica 2000's First Iberoamerican Virtual Congress of Medical Informatics. Oct 30, 2000-April 30, 2001. [www.informedica.org] / [www.informedica.org.ar]
· This working group maintains a valuable exchange of ideas and experiences with IMIA's Health and Medical Informatics Education Working Group and the European Federation of Medical Informatics working group on Health Informatics for Development

Future Activities:
· To develop a close collaboration and action program with IMIA-LAC (Latin America), the African Region and APAMI (Asian Pacific Association of Medical Informatics).
· To improve access to information for health care workers
· To support HELINA Conference for the African continent that will take place at the end of March in 2002.

Homepage: http://www.fim.org.ar/wg9/

WG 10 - Health Information Systems

Chair:
Dr. Klaus A. Kuhn
Professor of Medical Informatics
Philipps-University Marburg
Bunsenstr. 3
D-35037 Marburg, Germany
Tel: +49 6421 286 6205
Fax: +49 6421 286 3599
E-mail: kuhn@mailer.uni-marburg.de

Co-chair:
Dr. Dario A. Giuse
Informatics Center
Vanderbilt University Medical Center
Informatics Center,
Eskind Biomedical Library
Nashville, TN, 37232-8340, USA
Tel: +1 615 936 1435
Fax: +1 615 936 1427
E-mail: Dario.Giuse@
             mcmail.vanderbilt.edu

Objectives:
· To provide a forum for collaboration among world members, and to promote systematic development and research in the field of health information systems.
· To identify and assess problems and success factors of health information systems and to provide intensive feedback between the scientific community, healthcare professionals, and the health IT industry. This implies a "horizontal" orientation with close contact to other working groups.

Recent Activities:
· The working group organized a workshop during MEDINFO 2001 on "Challenges in deploying Health Information Systems".
· During its MEDINFO working group meeting, this working group decided to change its name from "Hospital Information Systems/Health Professional Workstations" to "Health Information Systems".

Future Activities:
· A working conference will be held in Heidelberg, Germany, from April 8-10, 2002. The following topics are planned: (1) The basic bottlenecks - WG HIS recommendations revisited, (2) Pathways to open architectures, (3) Socio-technical aspects of HIS, (4) Outcome of HIS implementations/possible metrics, (5) Patient empowerment.
· It is also planned to present real systems in close cooperation with the HIS industry.

WG 11 - Dental Informatics

Chair:
Dr. Wook-Sung Yoo
Computer and Information Sc. Dept.
Gannon University
109 University Square
Erie, PA 16506 USA
Tel: +1 814 871 7692
Fax: +1 814 871 7616
E-mail: yoo@gannon.edu

Co-chair:
Dr. John Eisner
School of Dental Medicine
University of Buffalo
315A Squire Hall
Buffalo, NY 14214, USA
Tel: +1 716 829 2057
Fax: +1 716 833 3517
E-mail: John_Eisner@sdm.buffalo.edu

Objectives:
To bring the small, but rapidly growing, community of dental informaticians around the world into closer contact.

Recent Activities:
· The Dental Informatics working group home page (http://www.ecs.gannon.edu/IMIA) has recently been updated and a new link to "Dental Informatics Literature Survey" site has been added. The purpose of this site is to provide a library of dental informatics related paper abstract to the members. This site includes "abstract entry page", "author information page" and "search engine". The Working Group members have entered published paper abstracts and we expect continuing growth.
· The Third International Conference for Computers in Dental Education was held November 29 - December 1, 2001 at The Westin Riverwalk in San Antonio, Texas USA. This conference is intended to promote the sharing of ideas and experiences on how computer-based technology has and will be implemented to support missions of Dental Academic institutions around the world. The working group chair and co-chair represented IMIA at this meeting.

Future Activities:
The next addition to the home page will be a "News" page identifying current dental informatics activities in countries and posting summaries or links to news items or web-sites related to these activities.

Homepage: http://tasc.sdm.buffalo.edu/imia/

WG 12 - Biomedical Statistics and Information Processing

Chair:

Dr. Jana Zvárová
EuroMISE Center, Charles University
and Academy of Sciences
Pod vodarenskou vezi 2
182 07 Prague 8
The Czech Republic
Tel: +420 2 6605 3097
Fax: +420 2 689 7013

Co-Chair:

Dr. Leon Bobrowski
Institute of Biocybernetics and
Biomedical Engineering,
Polish Academy of Sciences,
Trojdena 3, Warsaw, Poland
Tel: +48 22 659 9143 (Ext 416)
Fax: +48 22 6597030

Objectives:

The working group activity will focus on the development and correct application of statistical methods and tools in biomedicine and health care. It will promote computational statistics, exploratory data analysis including visualization methods, and confirmatory data analysis on the broad scale of biomedical and healthcare applications. Great emphasis will be given to clinical and epidemiology statistics, stochastic genetics, and statistics in pharmacology. Bayesian, as well other approaches, will be considered. Attention will be paid to the use of statistical approaches for data mining and decision support systems.

Recent Activities:

The IMIA General Assembly approved this working group in 2001.

Future Activities:

The WG members have been active in the past in different conferences and workshops connected with statistics in biomedicine and healthcare. Every two years, workshops on Statistics in clinics have been organized at the Institute of Biocybernetics and Biomedical Engineering and the Polish Academy of Sciences. The most recent workshop was held in June 2000. These workshops combine education and research in the field of clinical statistics. The working group seeks to organize sessions at these conferences, as well as in the future MIE, IMIA conferences. It intends to establish closer co-operation in this field with IMIA member countries as well as with international societies and other bodies in the field of biomedical and health statistics, e.g. Biometric Society, International Society for Clinical Biostatistics, and International Society for System Science in Health Care.

WG 13 - Organizational and Social Issues

Chair:

Dr. Bonnie Kaplan, Ph.D.
Center for Medical Informatics
Yale University
School of Medicine
59 Morris Street
Hamden, CT 06517, USA
Tel: +1 203 777 9089
Fax: +1 203 777 9089
E-mail: bonnie.kaplan@yale.edu

Objectives:

· To investigate organizational, social, and individual behavioral issues surrounding the introduction and use of informatics applications.
· To determine strategies for product design and technological change to support health care delivery through information and communication technologies.
· To incorporate organizational change management and human concerns into information technology projects.

Recent Activities:

· Joint panels with AMIA People and Organizational Issues (POI) WG and EFMI WG 9 at the AMIA Fall 2000 Symposium, and the IFIP 8.2 IS 2000 Conference.
· Three sessions at Medinfo 2001 on "New Approaches To Evaluation: Alternatives to The Randomized Controlled Trial," organized by WG13 and AMIA POI WG. These sessions included a workshop on Evaluation in the UK National Health Service, a panel on Qualitative Approaches to Design and Evaluation: Theory and Practice, and a panel on Quantitative Models for Evaluation
· The chair of WG13 served on the Scientific Program Committee for the AMIA Fall Symposium 2001.
· Produce and distribute an on-line newsletter and maintain a listserv.
· Working Group 13 in conjunction with the AMIA People and Organizational Issues WG and EFMI WG 9.
· Endorsed a conference planned by EFMI WG9, IT in Health Care: Sociotechnical Approaches in Rotterdam, September 6-7, 2001.
· Tutorial at Medinfo on "Organizational readiness for clinical information technologies: culture, change management and evaluation," taught by WG chair.

Organizational and Social Issues (IMIA WG 13) (Continued)

- Tutorial at the AMIA Fall Symposium 2001 on "Evaluating the Impact of Health Care Information Systems," taught by James G. Anderson, chair of AMIA Ethical, Legal, and Social Issues WG.
- Submitted papers for a new section on organizational and social issues for the IMIA Yearbook 2002.

Future Activities:
- Bibliography on evaluation and assessment, in collaboration with WG15, EFMI WG9, and the AMIA POI WG.
- The chair of WG13 will serve as a Program Chair for the IFIP 8.2 2004 conference in Manchester, England.
- Submit papers on social and organizational issues for future IMIA yearbooks.
- Participate in IMIA's Technology Assessment and Quality Improvement working group efforts to develop a framework for assessment.
- Provide suggestions for WG1's curriculum guidelines revision.
- Coordinate with the EFMI WG9 and AMIA POI WG on electronic communications and web sites.
- Encourage the formation of sister WGs in other organizations and geographic regions.
- Review criteria for papers to be included in the IMIA Yearbook or published in *Methods of Information in Medicine,* as requested by the editors.

WG 15 - Technology Assessment and Quality Improvement (TAQI)

Chair (2001-2004):
Dr. Jan Talmon
Dept. Medical Informatics
Maastricht University
PO Box 616
6200 MD Maastricht
The Netherlands
Tel: +31 43 388 2243
Fax: +31 43 388 4170
E-mail: talmon@mi.unimaas.nl

Objectives:
- To promote comprehensive assessments of healthcare information technologies.
- To demonstrate the value of assessment methods in healthcare information technologies.
- To promote international cooperation toward developing methodological issues.

Recent Activities:
- The working group organized a MEDINFO 2001 workshop during which time Dr. Jytte Brender from Aalborg University in Denmark presented a framework for assessing the value of assessment studies. This framework, when fully developed, will allow decision makers to assess the quality of assessment studies. Also researchers can utilize the framework for the design of assessment studies.
- The chairman of this working group presented the global design for a repository of resources with respect to Technology Assessment. A prototype implementation is available at the VATAM website (http://www-vatam.unimaas.nl)

Future Activities:
- During the MEDINFO meeting a new modus operandi of TAQI was discussed. Many of those interested in the objectives of the working group have as primary interest other topics covered by one or more of the other IMIA working groups. Therefore, it has been difficult to get active contributions of the members of the working group. In the new model, a core group will further develop the above-mentioned framework as well as the design of the repository. The other members of the working group - can be considered, as "customers" of the developed "products" - will be invited to comment on the results of the core group.
- Further collaboration with other working groups will be established. Specifically Organizational and Social Issues working group has shown interest in the repository.

WG 16 - Standards in Health Care Informatics

Chair:
Open

Objectives:

· To facilitate the exchange of information between different standards bodies of different continents.
· To ensure broad dissemination and create awareness of standards.
· To involve end-users in the standards process.
· To analyze and compare the standards needs and priorities in the different countries.
· To provide feedback from the scientific medical community to the standards developers.

Future Activities:

The IMIA Vice President for Working Groups in conjuction with several people from all parts of the world are investigating how to re-created this working group so that it enhances the world's standards efforts, but does not compete with existing standards organizations. If you have any suggestions, please contact: Nancy.Lorenzi@mcmail.vanderbilt.edu.

WG 17 - Computerized Patient Records

Chair:
Dr. Johan van der Lei
Institute of Medical Informatics
Medical Faculty
Erasmus University
P.O. Box 1738
3000 DR Rotterdam
The Netherlands
Tel: +31 10 408 7050
Fax: +31 10 408 9447
E-mail: vanderlei@mi.fgg.eur.nl

Co-Chair:
Dr. Mark A. Musen
Section of Medical Informatics
Stanford University
School of Medicine
Medical School Office Building
Room X-215, Route 5
Stanford, CA 94305-5479 USA
Tel: +1 650 723 3390
Fax: +1 650 725 7944
E-mail: musen@stanford.edu

Objectives:

· To support studies of the electronic patient record in the clinical environment.
· To study the electronic patient record in relation to evidence-based medicine.
· To stimulate the infrastructure required by an electronic patient record by supporting development and testing of the definition (1) of medical terms, (2) specific data sets, and (3) standards for electronic data exchange.

Recent Activities:

· The working group held its first conference on October 8-10, 1998 in Rotterdam. The Proceedings of this conference appeared in a special issue of *Methods of Information in Medicine* (1999; 38).
· During the MEDINFO 2001, the WG had a workshop discussing the role of academia in the development of electronic patient records. Although an increasing number of vendors have initial versions or partial implementations of electronic patient records on the market, members of the WG believed there was still a significant role for academia.
· The issue of merging with other working groups was raised, but no decisions were made.

Future Activities:

· The working group will schedule its a major meeting at the Medinfo 2004 meeting. In preparing that meeting, collaboration with other WGs will be sought.
· The working group also is considering hosting a workshop that would explore requirements for management of genomic information with electronic patient records.

WG 18 - Telematics in Healthcare

Chair:
Dr. Regis Beuscart
Professor of Medical Informatics
The University of Lille
1, Place de Verdun
59045 Lille, France
Tel: +33 3 2052 6970
Fax: +33 3 2052 1022
E-mail: rbeuscart@chru-lille2.fr

Objectives:
· To explore the rationale and perspective of health telematics.
· To promote the design and development of open architectures and inter-operability tools.
· To promote the analysis, design and development of methodologies and tools to support collaborative work in healthcare information systems.

Recent Activities:
· During 2001, the Working Group debated about recommendations that could be proposed for the development of Telematics in Healthcare (Telemedicine, Professional Networks): Reimbursement of Telemedicine activities, unique ID for Healthcare access, Standards and security, etc.
· A workshop was organised during the Medinfo Congress in London. During this meeting, presentations by leaders of the domain (from USA, Australia, France, Italy, Denmark) allowed a tour d'horizon of the field, drawing the state of the art of the discipline. The workshop included the usages of Telematics for a better management of Healthcare. This workshop demonstrated that Telematics is not only penetrating the activities of the Healthcare professionals but involves more and more patients, patients organizations, and health care providers, giving access to medical information that is not available elsewhere.
· Access to any type of information appears to have become more easy and efficient now that global access to Internet and Websites exist. This is equally the case for Healthcare and Medicine. The number of the sites devoted to Healthcare is continuously growing. Health Telematics presents a striking challenge
· The objective of the workshop was oriented towards sharing experiences of successful or failing medical networks or Health Telematics Projects. The focus was on technical characteristics, but also on human and organizational factors that have to be taken into account to make an experience successful.

Future Activities:
· The next meeting of the Working Group will be in Lille, France in January 2002.

Nursing Informatics (Special Interest Group 1)

Chair:
Dr. Virginia K. Saba
Distinguished Scholar
Georgetown University
2332 South Queen Street
Arlington, VA 22202, USA
Tel: +1 703 521 6132
Fax: +1 703 521 3866
E-mail: vsaba@worldnet.att.net

Objectives:
· To foster collaboration among nurses and others interested in nursing informatics.
· To explore the scope of nursing informatics and its implications for information handling activities.
· To support the development of nursing informatics in member countries.
· To provide informatics conferences and meetings.
· To encourage publication and dissemination of research and development materials.
· To develop recommendations, guidelines, tools, and courses.

General Information
Homepage: http://www.infocom.cqu.edu.au/imia-ni/
NI-SIG Executive Committee consists of
Chairperson: Virginia K. Saba, USA;
Vice-Chairperson & Treasurer: Heather Strachan, UK; and
Secretary, Robyn Carr, NZ.

Nursing Informatics (Special Interest Group 1) (continued)

It currently has 30 official members, including its officers, from 27 IMIA member countries. It has several working groups addressing several nursing informatics activities: They are:

- Concept Representation Models: Virginia Saba, USA
- Reference Terminology Model: Suzanne: Bakken, USA
- International Nursing Minimum Data Set: Connie Delaney, USA
- Research: Heather Strachan, UK
- Management: Robyn Carr, NZ
- Education: Margareta Ehnfors, SW & Diane Skiba, USA
- Standards: Kathleen McCormick, USA
- History: Marianne Tallberg, FN
- Evidenced-Based Practice: Connie Weaver, USA
- Consumer Health: Betty Chang: USA
- Nursing Telematics: Paula Proctor, UK

NI-SIG meets annually - either at its International Conference held every three years, at Medinfo, or at other IMIA and Nursing Informatics-related meetings.

Recent Activities:
- NI-SIG hosted its Annual Meeting at Medinfo in London, UK on 2 September 2001.
- It also conducted workshops during ICN in Copenhagen in June and AMIA in November, 2001
- NI-SIG has been actively involved in the development of a Nursing Informatics Standards within the International Standards Organization (ISO) Technical Committee (TC) 215. It sponsored a New Work Item Proposal (NWIP) # 142 entitled "Integration of a Reference Terminology Model for Nursing" to ISO/TC 215 via the Working Group 3—Concept Representation—US TAG Regional Technical Advisory Group. The Proposal was submitted in November 2000, approved 24 January 2001, followed by the Working Draft submitted on 26 July and reviewed In Copenhagen in June, 2001 and during the London ISO meeting on August, 2001 and plans to submit its Committee Draft on 24 January 2002. This Model is co-sponsored by NI-SIG and the International Council of Nursing (ICN). The Model is being overseen by a Steering Committee, Chaired by Virginia Saba and three other members—Kathleen McCormick, Amy Coenen and Evelyn Hovenga—who are responsible for the coordination and final preparation of the submission of the Drafts. Also, by two other committees established to facilitate the work: Work Item Task Group Chaired by Suzanne Bakken, USA and her Technical Advisory Group, and an Expert Committee consisting of numerous ISO and other national and international experts who review the prepared documents.

Future Activities:
- The Nursing Informatics SIG will meet in Budapest in August, 2002 during Medical Informatics Europe
- Support the development of the "Integration of a Reference Terminology Model for Nursing" to ISO/TC 215, WG3 Group 3—Concept Representation—US TAG Regional Technical Advisory Group.
- Support the activities of the NI-SIG Working Groups.
- Conduct workshops at all IMIA-related conferences and meetings including one at MIE in Budapest, August 2002.
- Assist in the planning of the 8th International Congress Nursing Informatics to be held in Rio de Janeiro, Brazil in June, 2003 Chaired by Heimar Marin.

IFHRO
IMIA Affiliate
Member

The International Federation of Health Records Organizations (IFHRO) supports national associations and health records professionals to implement and improve health records and the systems which support them. IFHRO was established in 1968 as a forum to bring together national organizations committed to improvement in the use of health records in their countries. The founding organizations recognized the need for an international organization to serve as a forum for the exchange of information relating to health records and information technology.

The purposes of IFHRO are to:
· promote the development and use of health records in all countries
· advance the development and use of international health records standards
· provide for the exchange of information on health records education requirements and training programs
· provide opportunities for communication between persons working in the field of health records in all countries

IFHRO is a non-profit organization affiliated with the World Health Organization (WHO) as a non-governmental organization (NGO). The Federation sends representatives to WHO meetings and works closely with WHO on specific projects of particular concern to WHO in the field of health records and information systems. IFHRO also has a partnership with the International Medical Informatics Association (IMIA) which provides opportunities for interested professionals to share information through newsletters and to participate in meetings dedicated to healthcare informatics. The partnership also provides an opportunity for IFHRO and IMIA to work together to promote health informatics and health records throughout the world.

Why health records?

Health records (medical records) are the foundation upon which quality healthcare is based. A well-designed and utilized health record can contribute significantly to the effectiveness and quality of healthcare. The documentation in the health record provides communication and facilitates continuity of care between healthcare professionals throughout the continuum of care, serves as a legal document which is also useful for research, education, epidemiology and planning. Whether paper-based or computerized, it is important that every country has health records that comply with international standards wherever possible.

IFHRO activities include:

· *International Health Records Congress*:
Every three years IFHRO holds the International Health Records Congress which is hosted by one of the national member organizations. This is an opportunity to bring together member countries, other interested countries and individuals in an international forum to participate in educational sessions and networking opportunities.
· *Newsletter*:
The International Health Records Newsletter is published quarterly and provides information about health records activities in member countries as well as interesting and informative articles on the latest health information standards and technology.
· *Educational programs*:
Educational programs and consultations may be provided to countries as needed. Health records educational tools are also available for the training of health records professionals in all areas of health information management.

IFHRO (Continued)

· *International Committees, Task Groups and Projects*

Members have the opportunity to serve on international committees, task groups or projects, which focus on health information and health records.

IFHRO leadership

The leadership of IFHRO is comprised of the Executive Committee, which is made-up of elected officials, these being the President, the President-elect, the Secretary/Treasurer, and four Regional Directors. The Executive Committee reports to the General Assembly, which is made up of the representatives from the national member countries. The member countries are:

Australia
Canada
China
Denmark
France
Germany
Hongkong
India
Indonesia
Ireland
Israel
Jamaica
Japan
Korea
Malaysia
The Netherlands
New Zealand
Nigeria
The Philippines
United Kingdom
United States of America
Venezuela

Regional organization

In order to improve communication and participation of the member countries, IFHRO is organized into 4 regions: Europe, Americas, Africa/Eastern Mediterranean/South-East Asia, and the Western Pacific. Coordination of IFHRO activities in each region is the responsibility of the Regional Directors.

IFHRO Executive Committee

President:
Willem Hogeboom,
The Netherlands
W.Hogeboom@Bigfoot.com

Regional Directors:
Europe:
Lorraine Nicholson,
United Kingdom
l.nicholson@zen.co.uk

Americas:
Jean Clark,
United States
jean.clark@carealliance.com

Africa/Eastern Mediterranean:
Lourdes Palapal,
The Philippines
llpalapal@edsamail.com.ph

Western Pacific
 (Secretary/Treasurer):
Philip Roxborough,
New Zealand
PhilipR@ahsl.co.nz

Review Section

B. Kaplan[1], N.T. Shaw[2]

[1] Yale University School of Medicine
New Haven, CT, USA
Kaplan Associates, Hamden, CT, USA
[2] Lancashire Postgraduate School of
Medicine & Health, UCLAN
Preston, Lancashire, UK

Review

People, Organizational, and Social Issues: Evaluation as an exemplar

Introduction

Many promising applications of information and communication technologies have been applied in health care over the past 50 years. During this time, it also has become apparent that attention to people, organizational, and social issues is required in order to realize the potential benefits of informatics applications [1]. Clinically, the most pressing questions surrounding information and communication technologies are: (1) Are information and communication technologies clinically effective? and, (2) Do information and communication technologies deliver positive outcomes for patients?

A system must be used in order to be effective clinically. It has been estimated that nearly 50% of technically sound systems have foundered on staff revolt, boycott, sabotage, or dissatisfaction [2]. With reports of "surprisingly frequent failures" [3], it is not surprising that informatics experts rank organizational change issues and barriers to use among the most important research priorities in health informatics [4]. Effectiveness depends as much on these concerns as on technical excellence. Organizational culture, professional values, work practices, change management, and effective leadership are crucial.

Barriers to using information and communication technology in health care have been discussed since the 1950s (e.g., [5, 6]). In 1987, Kaplan classified barriers previously identified in the literature into four categories [6]:
1. barriers of insufficiency (i.e., not enough funding, knowledge, or sufficiently advanced technology),
2. barriers inherent in the medical environment (i.e., the fragmentation of health care institutions into separate departments and organizations, and difficulty in organizing and standardizing medical knowledge),
3. barriers pertaining to project management (i.e., difficulties of coordinating teams of clinicians, computer scientists, and professionals from other disciplines); and
4. user resistance (especially what is perceived as resistance by physicians to medical informatics applications). These barriers concern people, organizational, and social issues. For example, concern over user resistance and adoption of clinical applications has been long-standing [6]. In 1980, Dowling studied user sabotage, providing case examples, a classification scheme for types of sabotage, and management recommendations [2]. "Resistance" may be understood as a response to people, organizational, or social issues that need addressing [3, 7, 8, 9].

Much attention has been paid to physician resistance. However, physicians readily adopt some information technologies and applications, but not others. Historically, physicians were faulted for overenthusiasm, rather than resistance, in adopting CT scanning [6]. Now, the same physicians who use electronic mail, the Internet, and personal productivity software are disenchanted with their electronic medical record system [10]. Physicians use technologies they see as being worth the time it takes to use them, ones that facilitate their work flow while not interfering with patient rapport, quality of care, and privacy. They are more favorable to informatics applications that enhance their sense of what it means to be a physician: autonomous architect of patient care, artful and compassionate practitioner of scientific medicine, provider of quality individualized care, and cultivator of good patient rapport [10, 11]. Some researchers further explain differential adoption as related to cultural considerations such as these physician values as compared with the values of others within a health care institution [11, 12, 13]. For example, Kaplan argued that how physicians view a system, and conflicts between developers' goals and physicians' values, affect physicians' adoption and use of informatics applications [11, 14, 15, 16]. Regulatory and economic incentives, as well as strong leadership, also clearly are important, and help explain why nearly all general practitioners in the UK use computers, while fewer than 10% of UK hospital physicians do [17].

More recently, concern about physician resistance to informatics applications has been underlying efforts towards gaining physician adoption of clinical practice guidelines and practices deriving from evidence-based medicine, as embodied in clinical decision support systems [18, 19]. Also, physician order entry, rather than physician resistance *per se*, has been addressed. Few hospitals - 20% in Japan, 32% in the US - have physician order entry, and few physicians use it [3, 20, 21, 22]. As found in early studies of record systems such as COSTAR [23], these rates may be due, at least in part, to physicians' seeing more benefits of such systems to others than to themselves [3, 24, 25, 26, 27]. In a series of studies, Ash *et al.* identified a variety of other issues surrounding house staff concerns pertaining to physician order entry: educational issues, benefits, problems, feelings, implementation strategies, and future of physician order entry [28]; technical and implementation issues, organizational issues, clinical/professional issues, organization of information and knowledge issues, and personal issues of the system [21, 29]; and communication within the institution and management style [30]. They developed a taxonomy of ten high level themes from their study: (1) language and misunderstandings; (2) the importance of context; (3) benefits and tradeoffs; (4) contrasts, conflicts, and contradictions; (5) collaboration and trust; (6) special people; (7) customization and the organization of information; (8) defining the boundaries of physician order entry; (9) the ongoing nature of implementation; and (10) time [30].

Their analysis indicates some of the problems that occur with physician order entry even in institutions where it is used, and suggests recommendations for more successful implementation [27].

As these studies of resistance and of physician order entry indicate, people, organizational, and social issues are important aspects of informatics. Such issues have been addressed directly within the field of medical informatics [1, 31, 32], and also by incorporating insights and research from other disciplines, such as the social sciences [1] and organizational theory [33]. Within the past few years, the International Medical Informatics Association (IMIA), American Medical Informatics Association (AMIA), and European Federation for Medical Informatics (EFMI) established working groups concerning these aspects:

· IMIA Working Group 13: Organizational and Social Issues http://www.imia.org
· AMIA People and Organizational Issues Working Group http://www.amia.org
· EFMI Working Group 9: Human and Organizational Issues of Medical Informatics http://www.efmi.org

These working groups have been building on years of activities and research by organizing conference sessions and publications. One such session resulted in a White Paper in *The Journal of the American Medical Informatics Association* proposing a research agenda for key people and organizational issues. The authors indicate that these concerns are more challenging now because technological and institutional changes in health care contribute to making complex organizational, social, and personal arrangements even more complex [1].

In this paper, we review some streams of activity relating to people, organizational, and social issues.

Because of its long history in medical informatics, we take evaluation (sometimes called "assessment") as our primary focus and draw on it for examples.

Evaluation

Evaluation serves multiple purposes [34, 35, 36]. Such studies are done not only for research, but also to provide information, inform action, and enhance decision making by using the knowledge generated in order to solve problems. Because change is required when introducing information and communication technologies, evaluation has been thought imperative for identifying where such change may need fine tuning or major adjustment, preventing harm, and minimizing disruption, as well as for providing evidence for decision-making and extending knowledge [37]. Thus, evaluation and change management are closely related in that they address similar concerns and involve related theories [3, 8, 34, 38], and because evaluation can inform change and generate management recommendations.

Foundation studies

Evaluation addressing people, social, and organizational issues has accompanied informatics projects in health care at least since the 1960s, resulting in a stream of publications during the 1970s and 1980s. Representative work from this period is collected in [31]. These early papers, many by researchers who have stayed active in the field, report insights that remain relevant.

In the United States, for example, an evaluation of the PROMIS system was published in 1981 [39, 40]. This multi-method study by external evaluators is exemplary both methodologically and for the people, organizational, and social issues insights it produced, including how this new records and clinical guidance system was related to issues concerning professional roles and status; change management; user involvement; and relationships between the medical record, philosophy of health care delivery, and clinical work. Other early evaluations focusing on these kinds of issues include a series of studies at what was then called the Rockland Research Institute in New York [e.g., 41, 42], and another series at Methodist Hospital in Indiana [e.g., 43, 44]. The new hospital information system at El Camino Hospital in California also was extensively evaluated by independent researchers during the 1970s [45]. Originally developed by Lockheed Missiles and Space, it became the popular Technicon, then TDS, and, later, the Eclypsis system.

During the 1970s, analyses began to appear of lessons learned and prescriptions for success [46]. Management issues, user acceptance, and diffusion and adoption of information systems have been discussed in the medical informatics literature at least since the early 1980s [47]. From early on, authors linked diffusion studies, evaluation research, and change management [e.g., 16, 48, 49, 50, 51, 52]. Studies of diffusion of a hospital information system, for example, showed that physicians' professional networks influenced adoption [43, 44], so that these professional networks could be used to encourage system use. Others analyzed medical informatics applications according to innovation characteristics known to affect adoption [51, 53].

Current studies

Evaluation [34, 35, 36] and change management [54, 55] by now have come into their own. The UK's National Health Service, for example, advises that evaluations should include business,

user (i.e., organizational), and technical impact [56]. In a discussion of problems, challenges, and perspectives on the transition from hospital to health information systems, Kuhn and Giuse [3] include a variety of human-computer interaction, socio-technical, and organizational issues, including: the importance of user perspectives on benefits and stresses; adaptation to users' work practices, work flow, and terminology; and "common ground" [57] between physicians' thought processes and knowledge structures embodied in software. They emphasize that organizational and social issues are crucial for successful implementation.

In another recent literature review, Kaplan summarizes evaluation findings in terms of people, organizational, and social issues and the fit of information and communication technologies with various aspects related to these concerns [19]. These include how information and communication technologies fit other contextual issues surrounding their development, implementation, and use. Researchers have addressed work flow [27, 58, 59, 60, 61], clinicians' level of expertise [59], values and professional norms [11, 62], institutional setting [63, 61], communication patterns [64], organizational culture and status relationships [27, 40, 65], cognitive processes [66], congruence with existing organizational business models and strategic partners [67], and compatibility with clinical-patient encounter and consultation patterns [61, 68]. Authors also have addressed (in various combinations) the fit between information technology and how individuals define their work, user characteristics and preferences (e.g., information needs), the clinical operating model under which the system is used, and the organization into which it is introduced [69, 70, 71, 72, 73, 74]. Others have discussed interrelationships among key components of an organization, such as organizational structure, strategy, management,

people's skills, and technology [75]; and compatibility of goals, professional values, and cultures of different groups within an organization, including developers, clinicians, administrators, and patients [11, 12, 13, 29, 75, 76, 77, 78, 79, 80]. Some have discussed difficulties of transferring to another country a system designed for use under a different country's health care system [61]. In addition, there has been work on ways in which informatics applications incorporate values, norms, representations of work and work routines; assumptions about usability and about links between medical knowledge and clinical practice; and how these assumptions influence design [79, 81, 82, 83, 84, 85, 61]. The concept of "fit" thus links evaluation and design [86, 87, 88, 89, 90].

Newer applications of information and communication technologies, such as for telehealthcare, have given rise to a body of research literature reporting results from small-scale demonstration projects and feasibility studies. This literature also discusses a range of problems that relate to evaluation [91, 92, 93, 94, 95, 96, 97, 98, 99, 100, 101, 102, 103, 104]. Among these issues are how technology incorporates new rules and resources that embody new structures for health care [105]. As with previous medical technologies and information systems, as well as newer consumer informatics applications, telehealth technologies may be used in ways that redefine how health care is delivered, or change the relationship and personal distance between practitioner and patient [68, 106, 107, 108, 109]. Imaging technologies, among others, have provoked discussion of how the meaning of clinical findings is negotiated among clinicians, and of the effects of making visible clinical work and procedures that previously had been seen only by those involved [109, 110, 111]. Another new use of technology, telephone keypads which patients/consumers use for input into a voice-response intelligent consultation system [112], like some older applications [29, 61, 70, 113, 114], raises issues of the different meanings information and communication technologies have for different users, even among those who appear to be of the same group. Additionally, telehealth involves ethical questions not traditionally considered in evaluation - such as empowerment, effect on home-care and home-care givers, equity and equality of services, how health care roles change, medicalization of social phenomena, and individuals' relationships both with practitioners and technologies - suggesting that such concerns should be reflected in evaluations of other areas of information technology in health care as well [105, 112]. Lastly, evaluation studies themselves may need to change from a focus on individual technologies, individual institutions, and individual users, to the changing context of patient-centered care and integrated delivery systems, and networked technologies that support them [67].

Current Concerns

As these many studies indicate, system success depends not only on system functionality, but also on organizational and behavioral issues, such as organizational readiness, diffusion of innovation, work flow, change management, and human factors, as well as on clinical context, cognitive factors, and methods of development and dissemination [1, 19, 73, 115, 116 , 117]. Numerous studies support the observations that: "Sociologic, cultural, and financial issues have as much to do with the success or failure of a system as do technological aspects" [118] because "information technologies are "embedded within a complex social and organizational context" [119]. Thus evaluation needs to address not only how well a system works, but also how

well it works with particular users in a particular setting. This focus is needed in order to help answer such key questions as:

· Why are the outcomes that are studied as they are?

· What might be done to affect outcomes?

· What influences whether information and communication technologies will have the desired effects?

· Why do individuals use or not use an informatics application?

· What from one study might be generalizable to other sites or applications?

To help do this, five areas need additional development:

1. Many evaluations focus on practitioners, primarily physicians [19]. While some studies include nurses, administrators, patients, or personal caregivers, more evaluations are needed to address concerns of the many individuals involved in or affected by informatics applications.

2. Attention is needed not only to successes, but also to failures, partial successes, and changes in project definition or outcome. Although, over the years, some researchers have examined failures, removals, or sabotage of systems [e.g., 2, 75, 120, 121, 122, 123, 124, 125, 126, 127], and some high-profile failures have been reported for UK National Health Service projects [128] - the failure of the London Ambulance Service's dispatch system, for example, has been studied extensively [e.g., 129, 130, 131] - or how failures became successes or were otherwise redefined [e.g., 30, 75, 80], publication bias in medical informatics provides little opportunity to learn from studies in which technology interventions resulted in null, negative, or disappointing results [132].

3. Comparative studies, while exceedingly difficult [133], are important for illuminating contextual

issues. Such studies might compare similar groups using the same technology at different sites, different groups using the same technology at one site, or various other combinations. The value of such research is illustrated by comparative studies of an electronic medical record [134], physician order entry [29], pediatric office systems [113], CT scanning [135], and physicians' use of images [111]. Extending such considerations not only across sites, but cross-culturally, remains a challenge [136].

4. Reporting and dissemination mechanisms are needed for work that is not published in traditional research outlets. Insights gained through evaluations of governmental projects world-wide, and experiences in non-western countries need to be disseminated.

5. More work is needed to develop both evaluation methods and theory, and to bring together understanding developed through studies undertaken in different areas of health care as well as studies undertaken by researchers in other disciplines (e.g. information systems, social studies of science, organizational behavior, computer science, and information studies), as discussed in the remainder of this paper.

Evaluation methods and project life cyle

There has been considerable debate about the appropriateness of methods evaluation researchers use. Because what happens when a new technology is introduced is affected by organizational and implementation processes, as well as affecting them, evaluation is inherently political. Some, therefore, resist evaluation for fear of potential disruptiveness of the investigation or its findings [37]. Others may view evaluation results as site specific.

Consequently, some discount either conducting evaluation studies or accepting their results [137]. Efforts have been undertaken to address these concerns while providing a structure for evaluations. For example, The National Health Service in the UK has issued an evaluation framework with the intent to improve the quality of evaluations [56]. In the European Union, the first phase of ATIM, the Accompanying Measure on Assessment of Information Technologies In Medicine, was undertaken as an Accompanying Measure in the Programme for Telematics Systems in Areas of General Interest (DG XIII) in the area of AIM (Advanced Informatics in Medicine). Its goal was to develop consensus on both methods and criteria for assessment [137]. In addition, IMIA WG15: Technology Assessment and Quality Development in Health Informatics, is directly concerned with these issues [37], as are the three sister working groups listed above.

Jones classified evaluation approaches into four models: randomized controlled trials, scientific/quantitative/objectivist, project management, and qualitative/interpretive/subjectivist [128]. Randomized controlled trials and experimental designs dominate [19] and are advocated as the best evaluation approaches [138, 139]. However, they have come under increasing criticism [19, 119, 133, 140, 141, 142, 143, 144, 145]. Other approaches, when used under controlled conditions, also have been criticized for excluding a variety of human, contextual, and cultural factors that affect system acceptance in actual use [19]. Some have called for making it a priority "to develop richer understanding of the effects of [system] benefits in health care and to develop new evaluation methods that help us to understand the process of implementing it" [119].

A school of thought has developed suggesting that neither randomized controlled trials, experimental designs, nor economic impacts are suitable in and of themselves for evaluating informatics applications. Such designs may pinpoint *what* changed, but they make it hard to assess *why* changes occurred. Additionally, these traditional designs prove difficult for following changes as they are developing, or in determining system design and implementation strategies that are well suited to particular institutional setting and societal considerations. Longer-term field studies and more interpretive approaches are better for investigating processes, multiple dimensions of causality, and relationships among system constituents and actors [8, 38, 127, 146].

Evaluation methods and questions depend upon both system development phase and purpose of the evaluation [3, 34, 56, 137, 147, 148]. Evaluation, therefore, should be an on-going process throughout the life of a project, and include a variety of approaches, selected from, for example, randomized controlled trials, experimental designs, simulation, usability testing, cognitive studies, record and playback techniques, network analysis, ethnography, economic and organizational impacts, content analysis, data mining, actor-network theory based approaches, balanced score cards, soft systems and participatory design methodologies, surveys, qualitative methods of data collection and interpretive analyses of it, technology assessment, benchmarking, SWOT (Strengths, Weaknesses, Opportunities, and Threats) analysis, and social interactionism [3, 34, 35, 36, 56, 142, 143, 144, 145].

The need for evaluation to influence system design, development, and implementation also has become apparent. While results of post-hoc or summative assessments are useful for future development, evaluation (or, some argue, technology assessment) that precedes or is concurrent with the processes of systems design, development, and implementation can be a helpful way to incorporate people, social, organizational, ethical, legal, and economic considerations into all phases of a project [8, 38, 137, 149, 150, 151]. Because evaluation is both theoretically based and practically oriented, some authors draw on their research to make project management or system design recommendations [e.g., 2, 27, 55, 65, 75, 79, 152, 153, 154]. Thus, evaluation and other project phases may converge.

Evaluation theory

Most evaluations are based on positivist, rationalist, or rational choice theoretical perspectives [19]. However, many alternatives have been developed, and these efforts continue. Evaluations informed by a variety of theoretical work in both organizational theory and the social and behavioral sciences have been undertaken for some time [1, 19]. Lorenzi [54] gives an overview of organizational theory influences. Earlier examples of work based in the social sciences are in [31, 39, 40, 47] and cited in [1, 46]. More recently, in order to address people, organizational, social, and other contextual issues, Forsythe advanced ethnography [141]; Lau and Hayward discussed the value of action research [153]; Weaver [155] and Ash *et al.* [27] use diffusion of innovation theory, while Schubart and Einbinder also based their study on it and provided a brief review of others who have [156]; and Anderson, Aydin, and Kaplan have been advocating social interactionism based on diffusion of innovation theory in their various publications [e.g., 7, 19, 157]. Among other recent examples are a variety of studies drawing on a constructivist tradition emphasizing organizational, political, social, and cultural concerns: Aarts employs actor-network theory [158], while Whitley and Pouloudi apply concepts connected with it [80]; Berg and colleagues have been advancing a sociological approach that employs sociocultural analyses and sociotechnical design as well as drawing on actor-network theory and situated action/design[159, 160, 161, 162], and others have drawn on this work [163]; Bygholm uses activity theory [164]; Sicotte *et al.* and Kristensen both take a social constructionist approach [60, 122, 165]; while Klecun-Dabrowska and Cornford combine construtionist theories and structuration theory [105]. These efforts are reflected in working group activities. The AMIA People and Organizational Issues Working Group established the Diana Forsythe Award in 2000 to recognize new publications at the intersection of medical informatics and social science; EFMI WG 9 on Human and Organizational Issues held a conference in 2001 that drew on the disciplines of medical informatics, information systems, and social studies of science [166]; and IMIA WG 13 on Organizational and Social Issues, together with these sister working groups, co-sponsored sessions on evaluation alternatives to randomized controlled trials at the AMIA Fall 2000 Symposium and at Medinfo 2001 [142, 143, 144, 145]; and the AMIA People and Organizational Issues Working Group organized panels at the AMIA 2001 Fall Symposium, one on "Situational Implementation: Human Factors in the Diffusion Process," and the other on "Organizational Issues for Design of Medical Informatics Systems" and, together with the AMIA Consumer Health Informatics Working Group, one on "Decreasing Disparities in Access to Health Care for Vulnerable Populations." These efforts are bringing together researchers from different traditions and creating opportunities for findings from evaluation studies of different applications areas to enrich each other. This developing tendency should help counteract the insulation such studies (and researchers) have had from each other, resulting in an impoverished analysis of evaluations and consequent understanding of people, organizational, and social issues that could result from them [19].

Social science influences also are apparent in efforts towards informing design. Using evaluation to influence system design enables building into the system an understanding of users' goals, roles, tasks, and how they think about their work. To do this, situated action and participatory design approaches - often based on Suchman's influential work on situated action [167, 168, 169] - have been undertaken in efforts to link work design and software design, including attempts to model work according to users' views [19]. The underlying principle is that "knowledge can never be decontextualized" because knowledge "is situated in particular social and physical systems" and "emerges in the context of interactions with other people and with the environment" [170]. These themes are apparent in a special issue of *Artificial Intelligence in Medicine* [171]. The authors draw on Scandinavian participatory design approaches [172] and on the writings of Winograd and Flores [173], as well as on Suchman. A stream of work undertaken by Timpka and colleagues promotes action design, a combination of action research, participatory design, and situated action [e.g., 84, 85, 174, 175].

Kaplan argues that each of these theoretical threads is a form of social interactionist theory [19]. She sees in social interactionism an explanation for the concept of "fit" summarized above, and also a theoretical base from which to derive evaluation frameworks, principles, and guidelines [8, 19, 38].

A recent trend in evaluation takes a more post-modern stance and turns reflexively to examine evaluation itself [176]. Instead of seeing evaluation as a neutral technical process of applying specific methods, evaluation results and reports are recognized to be affected by decisions such as: what evaluation is, how it is to be done, which questions are addressed, what methods are selected, and how it relates to other aspects of care delivery (service).

Moreover, the focus of evaluation itself changes throughout a study as various actors adapt, modify and transform themselves, the technology, and the evaluation. Political, professional, and commercial interests play into such processes. In this view, evaluation is seen as a component of extended social and technical networks that grow throughout the life of an intervention. Within these networks, the individuals involved define and negotiate ideas about the appropriateness of particular technologies and models of practice as they deal with contingent and structural factors (e.g., service take-up - the rate at which a new method/delivery route of providing care is accepted by users, and costs); interpersonal relations (e.g., inter- and intra-professional networks, professional-patient interaction); and technical considerations (e.g., how the technology itself functions and is used). In the process, they develop definitions of efficacy and utility that meet their situational demands.

These contingent processes present major challenges for evaluators who are dealing with a technology that is applied and deployed in the real world of health care provision, rather than the laboratory of system developers [177]. A conceptual model that places information and communication technologies and their evaluation in context as products of networks of professional and organizational activities, and of their internal and external processes of negotiation, may help illuminate some of the complex dynamics of evaluation. Producing evidence of efficacy and utility comprises relatively fluid processes, even where the design of evaluation or research projects apparently is structured in a rigid and "objective" way [68, 127, 178]. However, because much existing research in this vein has focused on historical examples like ultrasonography [179], new studies are needed to develop this kind of understanding for contemporary systems [180]. Both organizational and technological complexity are increasing as telecommunications integrated delivery networks support healthcare integration, new organizational forms, and new modes of health care delivery [67]. More work is needed to improve approaches to people, social, and organizational issues in this changing environment.

Evaluation frameworks

A number of authors have suggested frameworks for conducting evaluation studies that draw on different theories, combine methods, and address a variety of concerns. Kaplan's 4Cs framework - focusing on communication, control, care, and context - and her set of evaluation guidelines call for flexible multi-method longitudinal designs of formative and summative evaluations that incorporate a variety of concerns are examples [8, 19, 38]. Shaw identifies six aspects in her CHEATS framework: clinical, human and organizational, educational, administrative, technical, and social [148]. Lauer, Joshi, and Browdy illustrate how an equity implementation model can apply to evaluating user satisfaction [9]. Aarts and Peel discuss stages of implementation and change [181, 182]. Others elaborate or extend Donabedian's well-known structure-process-outcome evaluation model [183, 184] for use in evaluating information systems in health care [e.g., 56, 185, 186]. IMIA WG15 is attempting to create a framework for assessing the validity of a study [187], and Jones is concerned with how to evaluate evaluations [128].

Conclusion

The underlying basis for attention to people, organizational, and social issues is that human and organizational concerns should be taken into account during system design, implementation, and use. International perspectives are converging to a broad and encompassing multi-method approach to evaluation throughout the life of a project, with studies conducted in actual clinical settings so as to allow for complex contextual issues to be addressed through a variety of theoretical lenses [19, 148]. Considerable work has been undertaken concerning appropriate evaluation paradigms. Newer evaluations build on the work of early evaluation researchers to focus on roles of different actors and the connections between them; on contextual, organizational, and social concerns; on meanings attributed to the experiences by the persons involved; and on the processes and interactions among these different aspects of system design, implementation, and use.

Acknowledgements

We are grateful to Cynthia S. Gadd, PhD, of the University of Pittsburgh, USA, and to Tony Cornford, PhD, of the London School of Economics and Political Science, UK for their helpful suggestions and encouragement.

N. Shaw is funded as a National Health Service Executive (North West Region) Research & Development Post-Doctoral Training Fellow. The support of the National Health Service Executive (North West Region) Research & Development Department and Oldham Primary Care Group is therefore gratefully acknowledged.

References

1 Kaplan B, Brennan PF, Dowling AF, Friedman CP, Peel V. Towards an informatics research agenda: key people and organizational issues. J Am Med Inform Assoc 2001 May-June;8(3):234-41.

2 Dowling AF Jr., Do hospital staff interfere with computer system implementation? Health Care Management Review 1980;5:23-32. Reprinted in: Anderson JG, Jay SJ, editors. Use and impact of computers in clinical medicine. New York: Springer;1987:302-17.

3 Kuhn KA, Guise DA. From hospital information systems to health information systems - problems, challenges, perspectives. In: Haux R, Kulikowski C, editors. Yearbook of Medical Informatics. Stuttgart: Schattauer; 2001, p. 63-76.

4 Brender J, Nøhr C, McNair P. Research needs and priorities in health informatics. Int J Med Inform 2000 Sep;58-59:257-89.

5 Ellis NT. Telemedicine and information for health: the impediments to implementation. In: HC'99 Information At The Heart Of Clinical Practice. March 22-24 1999, Harrogate.

6 Kaplan B. The medical computing 'lag': perceptions of barriers to the application of computers to medicine. Int J Technol Assess Health Care. 1987;3(1):123-36.

7 Anderson JG, Aydin CE. Overview: theoretical perspectives and methodologies for the evaluation of health care information systems. In: Anderson JG, Aydin CE, Jay SJ, editors. Evaluating health care information systems: Approaches and applications. Thousand Oaks, Cal.: Sage;1994:5-29.

8 Kaplan B. Organizational evaluation of medical information systems. In: Friedman CP, Wyatt JC. Evaluation methods in medical informatics. NY: Springer;1997:255-80.

9 Lauer TW, Joshi K, Browdy T. Use of the equity implementation model to review clinical systems implementation efforts: a case report. J Am Med Inform Assoc 2000 Jan/Feb;7(1):91-102.

10 Gadd CS, Penrod LE. Assessing physician attitudes regarding use of an outpatient EMR: a longitudinal, multi-practice study. Proc AMIA Symp; 2001; 194-8.

11 Kaplan B. The influence of medical values and practices on medical computer applications. In: Proc, MEDCOMP '82: The First IEEE Computer Society International Conference on Medical Computer Science/Computational Medicine. Silver Spring, Md.: IEEE Computer Society Press, 1982:83-8. Reprinted in: Anderson JG, Jay SJ, eds. Use and impact of computers in clinical medicine. New York: Springer;1987:39-50.

12 Kaplan B. Culture counts: how institutional values affect computer use. MD Computing. 2000 Jan/Feb;17(1):23-6.

13 Friedman CP. Information technology leadership in academic medical centers: a

tale of four cultures. Acad Med 1999;74(7):795-9.

14 Kaplan B. User acceptance of medical computer applications: a diffusion approach. In: Blum BI, editor. Proc, Symp Computer Applications in Medical Care, Silver Spring, Md.: IEEE Computer Society Press, 1982;6:398-402.

15 Kaplan B. The computer as Rorschach: implications for management and user acceptance. In: Dayhoff RE, editor. Proc, Symp Computer Applications in Medical Care. Silver Spring, Md.: IEEE Computer Society Press, 1983;7:664-7.

16 Kaplan B. Barriers to medical computing: history, diagnosis, and therapy for the medical computing 'lag'. In: Ackerman MJ editor. Proc, Symp Computer Applications in Medical Care. Silver Spring, Md.: IEEE Computer Society Press, 1985;9:400-4.

17 Benson, T. Why British GPs use computers and hospital doctors do not. Proc AMIA Symp; 2001; 42-6.

18 Kaplan B. Evaluating informatics applications - clinical decision support systems literature review. Int J Med Inform. 2001;64:15-37.

19 Kaplan B. Evaluating informatics applications - some alternative approaches: theory, social interactionism, and call for methodological pluralism. Int J Med Inform. 2001;64:39-56.

20 Ash JS, Gorman PN, Hersh WR. Physician order entry in U.S. hospitals. Proc AMIA Symp. 1998;235-9.

21 Ash JS, Gorman PN, Lavelle M, Lyman J, Fournier L, Carpenter J, et al. Physician order entry: results of a cross-site case study. Methods Inf Med. Submitted.

22 Haruki Y, Ogushi Y, Okada Y, Kimura M, Kumamoto I, Sekita Y. Status and perspective of hospital information systems in Japan. Methods Inf Med 1999;38(3):200-6.

23 Campbell JR, Givner N, Seelig CB, Greer AL, Patil K, Wigton RS, et al. Computerized medical records and clinic function. MD Computing. 1989;6(5):282-7.

24 Kaplan B. Reducing barriers to physician data entry for computer-based patient records. Tops Health Inform Management 1994 Aug;15(1):24-34.

25 Shu K, Boyle D, Spurr C, Horsky J, Heiman H, O'Connor P, Lepore J, Bates D. Comparison of time spent writing orders on paper with computerized physician order entry. In: Patel V, Rogers R, Haux R, editors. Medinfo 2001. Amsterdam: IOS Press, 2001: 1207-11.

26 Weiner M, Gress T, Thiemann DR, Jenckes M, Reel SL, Mandell SF, Bass EB. Contrasting views of physicians and nurses about an inpatient computer-based

provider order-entry system. J Am Med Inform Assoc 1999 May/June;6(3):234-44.

27 Ash JS, Lyman J, Carpenter J, Fournier L. A diffusion of innovations model of physician order entry. Proc AMIA Symp; 2001; 22-6.

28 Ash JS, Gorman PN, Hersh WR, Poulsen SP. Perceptions of house officers who use physician order entry. Proc AMIA Symp. 1999;471-5.

29 Ash JS, Gorman PN, Lavelle M, Lyman J. Multiple perspectives on physician order entry. Proc AMIA Symp. 2000;27-31.

30 Ash J, Gorman P, Lavelle M, Lyman J, Fournier L. Investigating physician order entry in the field: lessons learned in a multi-centered study. In: Patel V, Rogers R, Haux R, editors. Medinfo 2001. Amsterdam: IOS Press, 2001:1107-11.

31 Anderson JG, Jay SJ, editors. Use and impact of computers in clinical medicine. New York: Springer; 1987.

32 Protti DJ, Haskell AR. Managing information in hospitals; 60% social, 40% technical. Proc IMIA Working Conference on Trends in Hospital Information Systems. North Holland Publishing; 1992; 45-8.

33 Lorenzi NM, Riley RT, Blyth AJC, Southon G, Dixon BJ. Antecedents of the people and organizational aspects of medical informatics: review of the literature. J Am Med Inform Assoc 1997 Mar-Apr;4(2):79-93.

34 Anderson JG, Aydin CE, Jay SJ, editors. Evaluating health care information systems: methods and applications. Thousand Oaks, CA: Sage Publications; 1994.

35 Friedman CP, Wyatt JC. Evaluation methods in medical informatics. New York: Springer; 1997.

36 van Gennip EMS, Talmon J, editors. Assessment and evaluation of information technologies, Studies in Health Technology and Informatics, vol 17. Amsterdam, IOS Press; 1995.

37 Rigby M. Evaluation: 16 powerful reasons why not to do it - and 6 over-riding imperatives. In: Patel V, Rogers R, Haux R, editors. Medinfo 2001. Amsterdam: IOS Press; 2001. p.1198-201.

38 Kaplan B. Addressing organizational issues into the evaluation of medical systems. J Am Med Inform Assoc 1997 March/April;4(2):94-101.

39 Fischer PJ, Stratman WC, Lundsgaarde HP, Steele DJ. User reaction to PROMIS: issues related to acceptability of medical innovations. In: O'Neill JT, editor. Proc Symp Computer Applications in Medical Care Silver Spring: IEEE Computer Society Press, 1980;4:1722-30. Reprinted in: Anderson JG, Jay SJ, editors. Use and impact of computers in clinical medicine.

New York: Springer; 1987;284-301.

40 Lundsgaarde HP, Fischer PJ, Steele DJ. Human problems in computerized medicine. Publications in Anthropology, 13. Lawrence, KS: The University of Kansas; 1981.

41 Siegel C, Alexander MJ, Dlugacz YD, Fischer S. Evaluation of a computerized drug review system: impact, attitudes, and interactions. Comp Biomed Res 1984;17:19-435. Reprinted in: Anderson JG, Jay SJ, editors. Use and impact of computers in clinical medicine. New York: Springer; 1987:238-66.

42 Dlugacz YD, Siegel C, Fischer S. Receptivity toward uses of a new computer application in medicine. In: Blum BI, editor. Proc Symp Computer Applications in Medical Care Silver Spring: IEEE Computer Society Press; 1980;6:384-91.

43 Anderson JG, Jay SL. Computers and clinical judgment: the role of physician networks. Soc Sci Med 1985;20:967-79. Reprinted in: Anderson JG, Jay SJ, editors. Use and impact of computers in clinical medicine. New York: Springer; 1987;161-84.

44 Anderson JG, Jay SL, Schwerr HM, Anderson MM, Kassing D. Physician communication networks and the adoption and utilization of computer applications in medicine. In: Anderson JG, Jay SJ, editors. Use and impact of computers in clinical medicine. New York: Springer; 1987:185-99.

45 Barrett JP, Barnum RA, et al. Evaluation of a medical information system in a community hospital. Battelle Columbus Laboratories (NTIS PB 248 340); Dec. 19, 1975.

46 Kaplan BM. Computers in medicine, 1950-1980: the relationship between history and policy. Doctoral Dissertation, University of Chicago, 1983.

47 Collen MF. A history of medical informatics in the United States: 1950 to 1990. [Bethesda, MD]: American Medical Informatics Association; 1995.

48 Farlee C, Goldstein B. Hospital organization and computer technology: the challenge of change. New Brunswick, NJ: Health Care Systems Research; 1972.

49 Brown B, Harbort B, Kaplan B, Maxwell J. Guidelines for managing the implementation of automated medical systems. In: Heffernan HG, editor. Proc. Symp Computer Applications in Medical Care. Silver Spring: IEEE Computer Society Press; 1981;5:791-6.

50 Brown B, Harbort B, Kaplan B. Management issues in automating medical systems. J Clinical Eng 1983 Jan-Mar;8(1):23-30.

51 Kaplan B. Pre-installation strategies:

setting the social stage for user acceptance. National Report on Computers and Health 1983 Jan;28:special report.

52 Sigurdardottir H, Skov D, Bartholdy C, Wann-Larsen S. Evaluating the usefulness of monitoring change readiness in organisations which plan on implementing health informatics systems. In: IT in Health Care Sociotechnical Approaches. International Conference Proceedings, 6-7 September 2001. Erasmus University Rotterdam, The Netherlands. p. 52.

53 Hanmer JC. Diffusion of medical technologies: comparison with ADP systems in the medical environment. In: O'Neill JT, editor. Proc Symp Computer Applications in Medical Care Silver Spring: IEEE Computer Society Press; 1980;4:1731-6.

54 Lorenzi N, Riley R T. Managing change: an overview. J Am Med Inform Assoc 2000 Mar-Apr;7(2):116-24.

55 Ash J. Managing change: analysis of a hypothetical case. J Am Med Inform Assoc 2000 Mar-Apr;7(2):125-34.

56 Department of Health, NHS Executive. Information Management Group. Project review: objective evaluation. Guidance for NHS managers on evaluating information systems projects. Department of Health, NHS Executive, 1996. IMG D 4042

57 Coiera E. When conversation is better than computation. J Am Med Inform Assoc 2000;7(3):277-86.

58 Kaplan B. Information technology and three studies of clinical work. ACM SIGBIO Newsletter 1995 May;15(2):2-5.

59 Safran C, Jones PC, Rind D, Booker B, Cytryn KN, Patel VL. Electronic communication and collaboration in a health care practice. Artif Intell Med 1998 Feb;12(2):137-51.

60 Sicotte C, Denis JL, Lehoux P. The computer based patient record: a strategic issue in process innovation. J Med Syst 1998 Dec;22(6):431-43.

61 Mitev N, Kerkham S. Organization and implementation issues of patient data management systems in an intensive care unit. J End User Computing 2001 July-Sep; 13(3):20-9.

62 Grémy F, Fessler JM, Bonnin M. Information systems evaluation and subjectivity. Int J Med Inform 1999;56(1-3):13-23.

63 Kaplan B. Development and acceptance of medical information systems: an historical overview. J Health Human Resources Admin 1988 Summer;11(1):9-29.

64 Aydin C. Computerized order entry in a large medical center: evaluating interactions between departments. In: Anderson JG, Aydin CE, Jay SJ, editors. Evaluating health care information systems:

Approaches and applications. Thousand Oaks, Cal.: Sage;1994. p. 260-75.

65 Massaro TA. Introducing physician order entry at a major academic medical center:1. Impact on organizational culture and behavior. Acad Med.1993;68(1):20-5.

66 Patel VL, Allen VG, Arocha JF, Shortliffe EH. Representing clinical guidelines in GLIF: individual and collaborative expertise. J Am Med Inform Assoc 1998 Sep-Oct;5(5):467-83.

67 Harrop VM. Virtual healthcare delivery: defined, modeled, and predictive barriers to implementation identified. Proc AMIA Symp; 2001; 244-8.

68 May CR, Gask L, Atkinson T, Ellis NT, Mair F, Esmail A. Resisting and promoting new technologies in clinical practice: the case of 'telepsychiatry.' Soc Sci Med 2001, 52(12):1889-901.

69 Kaplan B, Duchon D. Combining qualitative and quantitative approaches in information systems research: a case study. Manag Inform Sys Q 1998 December;12(4):571-86.

70 Nordyke RA, Kulikowski CA. An informatics-based chronic disease practice: Case study of a 35-year computer-based longitudinal record system. J Am Med Inform Assoc 1998, Jan./Feb;5(1):88-103.

71 Aarts J, Peel V, Wright G. Organizational issues in health informatics: a model approach. Int J Med Inform 1998 Oct-Dec;52(1-3):235-42.

72 Folz-Murphy N, Partin M, Williams L, Harris CM, Lauer MS. Physician use of an ambulatory medical record system: matching form and function. Proc AMIA Symp. 1998;260-4.

73 Clarke K, O'Moore R, Smeets R, Talmon J, Brender J, McNair P, et al. A methodology for evaluation of knowledge-based systems in medicine. Artif Intell Med 1994 Apr;6(2):107-21.

74 Dixon DR. The behavioral side of information technology. Int J Med Inform 1999 Dec;56(1-3):117-23.

75 Southon G, Sauer C, Dampney K. Lessons from a failed information systems initiative: issues for complex organisations. Int J Med Inform. 1999 Jul;55(1):33-46.

76 Heathfield HA, Wyatt J. Philosophies for the design and development of clinical decision-support systems. Methods Inf Med 1993;32:1-8.

77 Kaplan B. The computer prescription: medical computing, public policy, and views of history. Science, Technology, and Human Values 1995 Winter;20(1):5-38.

78 Demeester, M. Cultural aspects of information technology implementation. Int J Med Inform 1999 Dec;56(1-3):25-41.

79 Forsythe DE. New bottles, old wine: hidden cultural assumptions in a computerized explanation system for migraine sufferers. Med Anthropology Q 1996;10(4):551-74.

80 Whitley EA, Pouloudi A. Studying the translations of NHSnet. J End User Computing 2001 July-Sep; 13(3):31-40.

81 Covvey HD. When is a system only a system? Healthcare Inform Management & Comm Canada 2001;15(1):46-7.

82 Graves W III, Nyce JM. Normative models and situated practice in medicine. Inform Decision Technologies 1992;18:143-9.

83 Nyce JM, Graves W III. The construction of knowledge in neurology: implications for hypermedia system development. Artif Intell Med 1990 Dec;292):315-22.

84 Nyce JM, Timpka T. Work, knowledge and argument in specialist consultations: incorporating tacit knowledge into system design and development. Med Biol Eng Comput.1993 Jan;31(1): HTA16-HTA19.

85 Timpka T, Rauch E, Nyce JM. Towards productive Knowledge-Based Systems in clinical organizations: a methods perspective. Artif Intell Med 1994 Dec;6(6):501-19.

86 Gadd CS, Baskaran P, Lobach DF. Identification of design features to enhance utilization and acceptance of systems for Internet-based decision support at the point of care. Proc AMIA Symp. 1998;91-5.

87 Gamm LD, Barsukiewicz CK, Dansky KH, Vasey JJ, Bisordi JE, Thompson PC. Pre- and post- control model research on end-users' satisfaction with an electronic medical record: preliminary results. Proc AMIA Symp. 1998;225-9.

88 Kaplan B, Morelli R, Goethe J. Preliminary findings from an evaluation of the acceptability of an expert system in psychiatry. Extended Proc AMIA Symp. 1997; (CD-ROM).

89 Karlsson D, Ekdahl C, Wigertz O, Forsum U. A qualitative study of clinicians ways of using a decision-support system. Proc AMIA Symp. 1997:268-72.

90 Moore LA. Reaction of medical personnel to a medical expert system for stroke. In: Anderson JG, Aydin CE, Jay SJ, editors. Evaluating health care information systems: Approaches and applications. Thousand Oaks, Cal.: Sage;1994:226-44.

91 Grigsby J. You got an attitude problem, or what? Telemed Today 1995:32-4.

92 Burghgraeve P, De Maeseneer J. Improved methods for assessing information technology in primary health care and an example from telemedicine. J Telemed Telecare 1995;1:157-64.

93 Wyatt JC. Commentary: telemedicine trials - clinical pull or technology push? BMJ 1996;313:380-1.

94 Perednia DM. Telemedicine system evaluation, transaction models, and multicentred research. J Am Health Inform Manag Assoc 1996;67:1:60-3.

95 Grigsby J, Schlenker R, Kaehny M, Shaughnessy P. Analytic framework for evaluation of telemedicine. Telemed J 1995;1(1):31-9.

96 Grigsby J. Sentenced to life without parole doing outcomes research. Telemed Today.1996:40-1.

97 McIntosh E,Cairns J. A framework for the economic evaluation of telemedicine. J Telemed Telecare 1997;3:132-9.

98 Yellowlees P. Practical evaluation of telemedicine systems in the real world. Tele Med 1997; 36:90-3; also J Telemed Telecare 1998;4 Suppl 1:56-7.

99 Bashshur R. On the definition and evaluation of telemedicine. Telemed J 1995;1(1):19-30.

100 Nykanen P, Chowdhury S, Wigertz O. Evaluation of decision support systems in medicine. Comp Meths Programs Biomed 1991;34:229-38.

101 Filiberti D, Wallace J, Koteeswaran R, Neft D. A telemedicine transaction model. Telemed J 1995;1(3):237-47.

102 DeChant H, Tohme W, Mun S, Hayes W. Health systems evaluation of telemedicine: a staged approach. Telemed J 1996;2(4):303-12.

103 Tohme WG, Hayes WS, Dai H, Komo D. Evaluation of a telemedicine platform for three medical applications Comp Assisted Rad 1996;505-11.

104 Allen D. Telemental health services today. Telemed Today 1994;2(2):1-24.

105 Klecun-Dabrowska E, Cornford T. Evaluating telehealth: the search for an ethical perspective. Cambridge Q Healthcare Ethics 2001;10(2):161-9.

106 Kaplan B, Brennan PF. Consumer informatics supporting patients as co-producers of quality. J Am Med Inform Assoc 2001 Jul-Aug;8(4):309-16.

107 Reiser, SJ. Medicine and the reign of technology. Cambridge: Cambridge University Press; 1978.

108 Bosk C, Frader J. The impact of place of decision-making on medical decisions. In: O'Neill JT, editor. Proc Symp Computer Applications in Medical Care Silver Spring: IEEE Computer Society Press; 1980;4:1326-9.

109 Qavi T, Corley L, Kay S. Nursing staff requirements for telemedicine in the neonatal intensive care unit. J End User Computing 2001 July-Sep; 13(3):5-13.

110 Aanestad M., Edwin B, Mǻarvik R. Image quality as a sociotechnical network. In: IT in Health Care Sociotechnical Approaches. International Conference proceedings, 6-7 September 2001. Erasmus University Rotterdam, The Netherlands, p.16.

111 Kaplan B. Objectification and negotiation in interpreting clinical images: implications for computer-based patient records. Artif Intell Med 1995;7:439-54.

112 Kaplan B, Farzanfar R, Friedman RH. Ethnographic interviews to elicit patients' reactions to an intelligent interactive telephone health behavior advisor system. Proc AMIA Symp. 1999;555-9.

113 Travers DA, Downs SM. Comparing the user acceptance of a computer system in two pediatric offices: a qualitative study. Proc AMIA Symp. 2000;853-7.

114 Kaplan B. Computer Rorschach Test: what do you see when you look at a computer? Physicians & Comput 2001 Jan;18(5):12-3.

115 Nøhr C. The evaluation of expert diagnostic systems - How to assess outcomes and quality parameters? Artif Intell Med 1994 Apr;6(2):123-35.

116 Grémy F, Bonnin M, Evaluation of automatic health information systems. What and how? In: van Gennip EMS, Talmon JL editors. Assessment and evaluation of information technologies, Studies in Health Technology and Informatics, vol 17. Amsterdam: IOS Press;1995. p. 9-20.

117 Jørgensen T. Measuring effects. In: van Gennip EMS, Talmon JL editors. Assessment and evaluation of information technologies, Studies in Health Technology and Informatics, vol 17. Amsterdam: IOS Press; 1995. p. 99-109

118 Miller RA. Medical diagnostic decision support systems - past, present, and future: a threaded bibliography and brief commentary. J Am Med Inform Assoc 1994;1:8-27.

119 Heathfield HA, Buchan IE. Current evaluations of information technology in health care are often inadequate. BMJ October 19 1996;313(7063):1008.

120 Dambro MR, Weiss BD, McClure C, Vuturo AF. An unsuccessful experience with computerized medical records in an academic medical center. J Med Ed 1988;63:617-23.

121 Chessare JB, Torok KE. Implementation of COSTAR in an acaedmic group practice of general pediatrics. MD Computing 1993 Jan-Feb;10(1):23-7.

122 Sicotte C, Denis JL, Lehoux P, Champagne F. The computer-based patient record: challenges towards timeless and spaceless medical practice. J Med Syst 1998 Aug;22(4):237-56.

123 Tonnesen AS, LeMaistre A, Tucker D. Electronic medical record implementation barriers encountered during implementation. In: Proc AMIA Symp 1999:625-66.

124 Balka E. Getting the big picture: The macro-politics of information system development (and failure) in a Canadian hospital. In: IT in Health Care Sociotechnical Approaches. International Conference proceedings, 6-7 September 2001. Erasmus University Rotterdam, The Netherlands. p.17.

125 Jeffcott M. Technology alone will never work: Understanding how organisational issues contribute to user neglect and information systems failure in healthcare IT. In: Health Care Sociotechnical Approaches. International Conference Proceedings, 6-7 September 2001. Erasmus University Rotterdam, The Netherlands. p. 35.

126 Zuiderent T. Changing care and theory: a theoretical joyride as the safest journey. In: IT in Health Care Sociotechnical Approaches. International Conference Proceedings, 6-7 September 2001. Erasmus University Rotterdam, The Netherlands. p. 62.

127 May C, Ellis NT. When protocols fail: technical evaluation, biomedical knowledge, and the social production of 'facts' about a telemedicine clinic. Soc Sci Med 2001 Oct;53(8):989-1002.

128 Jones MR. An interpretive method for the formative evaluation of an electronic patient record system. In: Remenyi D, Brown A, editors. Procs of the 8th European Conference on IT Evaluation. Oxford:17-18 September 2001, p349-56.

129 Beynon-Davies P. The London Ambulance Service's computerised dispatch system: a case study in information system failure. University of Glamorgan Pontyprid, 1993.

130 Beynon-Davies P. Information systems 'failure': the case of the London Ambulance Service's Computer Aided Despatch project. European J Inform Syst 1995;4:171-84.

131 Silva L, Backhouse J. Becoming part of the furniture: the institutionalization of information systems. In: Lee AS, Leibenau J, DeGross JI. Information Systems and Qualitative Research, London: Chapman & Hall; 1997. p. 389-414.

132 Friedman CP, Wyatt JC. Publication bias in medical informatics. J Am Med Inform Assoc 2001 Mar/Apr;8(2):189-91.

133 Heathfield HA, Peel V, Hudson P, Kay S, Mackay L, Marley T, et al. Evaluating large scale health information systems: from practice towards theory. Proc AMIA Symp. 1997;116-20.

134 Penrod LE, Gadd CS. Attitudes of

academic-based and community-based physicians regarding EMR use during outpatient encounters. Proc AMIA Symp; 2001; 528-32.

135 Barley SR. Technology as an occasion for structuring: evidence from observations of CT scanners and the social order of radiology departments. Adm Sci Q 1986;31:78-108.

136 Isaacs S. The power distance between users of information technology and experts and satisfaction with the information system: implications for cross-cultural transfer of IT. In: Patel V, Rogers R, Haux R, editors. Medinfo 2001. Amsterdam: IOS Press; 2001. p. 1155-7.

137 van Gennip EMS, Talmon JL editors. Introduction. In: van Gennip EMS, Talmon JL editors. Assessment and evaluation of information technologies, Studies in Health Technology and Informatics, vol 17. Amsterdam, IOS Press, 1995;1-5.

138 van der Loo, RP. Overview of published assessment and evaluation studies. In: van Gennip EMS, Talmon JL editors. Assessment and evaluation of information technologies, Studies in Health Technology and Informatics, vol 17. Amsterdam: IOS Press; 1995. p. 261-82.

139 Tierney WM, Overhage JM, McDonald CJ. An plea for controlled trials in medical informatics. J Am Med Inform Assoc 1994 July/Aug;1(4):353-5.

140 Heathfield H, Pitty D, Hanka R. Evaluating information technology in health care: barriers and challenges. BMJ 1998 June 27;316(7149):1959-61.

141 Forsythe D, Buchanan B. Broadening our approach to evaluating medical expert systems, In: Clayton PD, editor. Symposium on computer applications in medical care. McGraw-Hill, New York;1991:8-12.

142 Ellis NT, Aarts J, Kaplan B, Leonard K. Alternatives to the controlled trial: new paradigms for evaluation. AMIA Symp. Los Angeles, CA, 2000.

143 Kaplan B, Aarts J, Hebert M, Klecun-Dabrowska E, Lewis D, Vimarlund V. New approaches to evaluation: alternatives to the randomized controlled trial - qualitative approaches to design and evaluation: theory and practice. In: Patel V, Rogers R, Haux R, editors. Medinfo 2001. Amsterdam: IOS Press; 2001. p. 1531.

144 Kaplan B, Atkinson C, Ellis N, Jones M, Klecun-Dabrowska E, Teasdale S, et al. Evaluation in the UK's National Health Service. In: Patel V, Rogers R, Haux R, editors. Medinfo 2001. Amsterdam: IOS Press; 2001. p. 1529.

145 Kaplan B, Anderson JG, Jaffe C, Leonard

K, Zitner D. New approaches to evaluation: alternatives to the randomized controlled trial - quantitative models for evaluation. In: Patel V, Rogers R, Haux R, editors. Medinfo 2001. Amsterdam: IOS Press; 2001. p. 1456.

146 Kaplan B, Maxwell JA. Qualitative research methods for evaluating computer information systems. In: Anderson JG, Aydin CE, Jay SJ, editors. Evaluating health care information systems: approaches and applications. Thousand Oaks, Cal.: Sage;1994. p. 45-68.

147 Talmon J, Enning J, Castãneda G, Eurlings F, Hoyer D, Nykänen P, et al. The VATAM guidelines. Int J Med Inform 1999 Dec;56(1-3):107-15.

148 Shaw NT. CHEATS: A generic evaluation framework for information communication technologies: invited paper. Comp Meths Programs Biomed In press 2001.

149 Gardner RM, Lundsgaarde HP. Assessment of user acceptance of a clinical expert system. J Am Med Inform Assoc 1994 Nov-Dec;1(6):428-38.

150 Saranummi N. Supporting system development with technology assessment. In: van Gennip EMS, Talmon JL eds. Assessment and evaluation of information technologies, Studies in Health Technology and Informatics, vol 17. Amsterdam: IOS Press; 1995. p. 35-44.

151 Faber M. User involvement in design and introduction of a Electronic Patient Record. On the never predicatble interplay between technical objects and social organisations. In: IT in Health Care Sociotechnical Approaches. International Conference Proceedings, 6-7 September 2001. Erasmus University Rotterdam, The Netherlands. p. 27.

152 Kaplan B. Fitting system design to work practice: using observation in evaluating a clinical imaging system. In: Ahuja MK, Galletta DF, Watson HJ, editors. Proc: Americas Conference on Information Systems, Volume IV: Information Systems—Collaboration Systems and Technology, and Organizational Systems and Technology. Pittsburgh: Association for Information Systems; 1995. p. 86-8.

153 Lau F, Hayward R. Building a virtual network in a community health research training program. J Am Med Inform Assoc 2000 Jul/Aug;7(4):361-77.

154 Timpka T, Arborelius E. The GP's dilemmas: a study of knowledge need and use during health care consultations. Meths Inform Med. 1990 Jan;29(1):23-9.

155 Weaver RR. Evaluating the Problem Knowledge Coupler: a case study. In: Anderson JG, Aydin CE, Jay SJ, editors. Evaluating health care information systems: approaches and applica-

tions. Thousand Oaks, Cal.: Sage;1994. p. 203-25.

156 Schubart JR, Einbinder JS. Evaluation of a data warehouse in an academic health sciences center. Int J of Med Inform 2000;60:319-33.

157 Anderson JG, Aydin CE, Kaplan B. An analytical framework for measuring the effectiveness/impacts of computer-based patient record systems. In: Nunamaker JF, Sprague RH Jr., editors. Proc: Twenty-Eighth Hawaii International Conference on Systems Science, Vol IV: information systems – collaboration systems and technology, organizational systems and technology. Los Alamitos, Cal: IEEE Computer Society Press;1995. p. 767-76.

158 Aarts J. On articulation and localization - some sociotechnical issues of design, implementation, and evaluation of knowledge based systems. In: Quaglini S, Barahona P, Andreassen S, editors. Artificial Intelligence in Medicine, Proc of the 8th Conference on Artificial Intelligence in Medicine in Europe, AIME 2001. Berlin: Springer; 2001. p. 16-9.

159 Berg M. Patient care information systems and health care work: a sociotechnical approach. Int J Med Inform 1999 Aug;55(2):87-101.

160 Berg M, Gorman E. The contextual nature of medical information. Int J Med Inform 1999 Dec;56(1-3):51-60.

161 Berg M, Langenberg C, v.d. Berg I, Kwakkernaat J. Considerations for sociotechnical design: experiences with an electronic patient record in a clinical context. Int J Med Inform.1998 Oct/Dec;52(1-3):243-51.

162 Stoop A, Berg M. Health care ICT evaluation: state of the art in a dynamic field. In: IT in Health Care Sociotechnical Approaches. International Conference Proceedings, 6-7 September 2001. Erasmus University Rotterdam, The Netherlands. p. 55.

163 Reddy MC. Sociotechnical requirements for healthcare systems. In: IT in Health Care Sociotechnical Approaches. International Conference Proceedings, 6-7 September 2001. Erasmus University Rotterdam, The Netherlands. p. 49.

164 Bygholm A. Activity thepry as a framework for conducting end-use support. In: IT in Health Care Sociotechnical Approaches. International Conference Proceedings, 6-7 September 2001. Erasmus University Rotterdam, The Netherlands. p. 21.

165 Kristensen M. Assessing a prerequisite for a constructivist approach – change readiness in organisations implementing health informatics systems. In: IT in Health Care Sociotechnical Approaches.

International Conference Proceedings, 6-7 September 2001. Erasmus University Rotterdam, The Netherlands. p. 38.

166 IT in Health Care Sociotechnical Approaches. International Conference Proceedings, 6-7 September 2001. Erasmus University Rotterdam, The Netherlands.

167 Suchman L. Representations of work. Commun ACM 1995;38(9):33-4.

168 Suchman LA. Plans and situated actions: the problem of human-machine communication. Cambridge: Cambridge University Press; 1987.

169 Butler KA, Esposito C, Hebron R. Connecting the design of software to the design of work. Commun of the ACM 1999;42(1):38-46.

170 Musen MA. Architectures for architects. Methods Inf Med 1993;32:12-3.

171 Artificial Intelligence in Medicine. 1995 Oct;7.

172 Greenbaum J, Kyng M. Design at work: cooperative design of computer systems. Hillsdale NJ: Lawrence Erlbaum Associates;1991.

173 Winograd T, Flores F. Understanding computers and cognition: a new foundation for design. Norwood NJ: Ablex;1986.

174 Sjöberg C, Timpka T. Participatory design of information systems in health care. J Am Med Inform Assoc 1998 Mar-Apr;5(2):177-83.

175 Timpka T, Hedblom P, Holmgren J. Action design: using an object-oriented environment for group process development of medical software. In: Timmers T, editor. Software engineering in medical informatics. Amsterdam: Elsevier; 1991. p. 151-65.

176 May CR, Mort M, Mair F, Ellis NT, Gask L. Evaluation of new technologies in health care systems: what's the context? Health Inform J 2000;6(2):67-70.

177 Williams TR, May CR, Mair F, Mort M, Shaw N, Gask L. Normative models of health technology assessment and the social production of evidence about telehealth care. In review 2001.

178 May C, Gask L, Ellis NT, Atkinson T, Mair F, Smith C, et al. Telepsychiatry evaluation in the north west of England: preliminary results. Telemed Telecare 2000;6 (Supplement 1):20-2.

179 Yoxen, E. Seeing with sound: a study of the development of medical images. In: Bijker WE, Hughes T, Pinch T, editors. The social construction of technological systems. Cambridge, Mass: MIT Press; 1987. p. 281-306.

180 May M, Mort M, Williams T, Mair F, Shaw NT. Understanding the evaluation of telemedicine: The play of the social and the technical, and the shifting sands of reliable knowledge. In: IT in Health Care Sociotechnical Approaches. International Conference Proceedings, 6-7 September 2001. Erasmus University Rotterdam, The Netherlands. p. 43.

181 Aarts J, Peel V. Using a descriptive model of change when implementing large-scale clinical information systems to identify priorities for future research. Int J Med Inform 1999 Dec;56(1-3):43-50.

182 Aarts J, Peel V, Wright G. Organizational issues in health informatics: a model approach. Int J Med Inform 1998 Oct-Dec;52(1-3):235-42.

183 Donabedian A. The quality of medical care: methods for assessing and monitoring the quality of care for research and for quality assurance programs. Science 1978;200:856-64.

184 Donabedian A. Explorations in quality assessment and monitoring. Vol I: The definition of quality and approaches to its assessment. Ann Arbor: Health Administration Press; 1980.

185 Hebert M. Telehealth success: evaluation framework development. In: Patel V, Rogers R, Haux R, editors. Medinfo 2001. Amsterdam: IOS Press; 2001. p. 1145-9.

186 Cornford T, Doukidis GI, Forster D. Experience with a structure, process and outcome framework for evaluating an information system. Omega, Int J of Manage Sci 1994;255(5):491-504.

187 Talmon JL. Workshop WG15: technology assessment and quality improvement. In: Patel V, Rogers R, Haux R, editors. Medinfo 2001. Amsterdam: IOS Press; 2001. p. 1540.

Address of the authors:
Bonnie Kaplan, PhD
Yale University School of Medicine
New Haven, CT, USA 06520

Kaplan Associates,
59 Morris Street
Hamden, CT, USA 06517
E-mail: bonnie.kaplan@yale.edu

Nicola T Shaw, PhD
Lancashire Postgraduate
School of Medicine & Health
UCLAN
Preston, Lancashire PR1 2HE
United Kingdom
E-mail: nikki.shaw@dial.pipex.com

G.O. Klein

Centre for Health Telematics
Karolinska Institute
Stockholm, Sweden

Review

Standardization of health informatics - results and challenges

Abstract: A number of standardization initiatives have been in progress for more than ten years in several parts of the world with the aim to facilitate different aspects of the exchange of health information. Important results have been achieved, and in some fields and parts of the world, standards are widely used today. Unfortunately, we are still facing the fact that most healthcare information systems cannot exchange information with all systems for which this would be desired. Either the existing standards are not sufficiently implemented, or the required standards and necessary national implementation guidelines do not yet exist. This causes unacceptable risks to patients, inefficient use of healthcare resources, and sub-optimal development of medical knowledge. This article will review some of the difficulties surrounding standards, as well as highlight the achievements and main global actors, while focusing on the challenges facing the international consensus process.

Introduction

The health sector is still a rather immature user of information technology (IT) compared to other parts of society, especially considering the very strong dependence on information management. While there are many good exceptions where IT is used to provide better quality of care and more efficient use of resources, unfortunately, the over-all picture is different. Many routines still depend on the exchange of paper documents often not available when needed. Most often, information systems excellent in some aspects of the healthcare process are isolated islands, unable to communicate with other systems.

There are several reasons why obstacles may be overcome in the relatively close future.

Healthcare is extremely complex. Even though important international shared scientific background is available, many variations in information exchange requirements exist within the different specialty fields, countries and organizations. The standards that have been developed had to address these diverse requirements and rapidly changing technology. This is paired with a resistance toward change within a large installed basis of different systems owned and operated by different organizations in the network of collaborating healthcare entities.

An increasingly difficult issue for achieving interoperability is the rapid general development of IT with important, radically new software tools, and, not the least, standards from a large number of non-health related organizations. Still, the formal international standards, especially from the collaboration of ISO and IEC in JTC1 (Joint Technical Committee no 1) are very important in providing basic tools for interoperability, both with many lower layer standards, and also for e.g. character encoding (where the gradual introduction of the ISO/IEC 10646 character set, which provides for most international characters, is one important contribution sometimes underestimated by the English language speaking countries). The modern security techniques with public key infrastructures are very much dependent on such basic standards, which are sometimes developed jointly with the ITU (International Telecommunications Union). However, today, we are also seeing the formation of more and more other special bodies targeting the provision of important IT standards. Some examples are the IETF (Internet Engineering Task Force), which not only provides basic Internet standards, but also for many aspects of intranet applications. W3C (the World Wide Web Consortium), which developed HTML, and more recently XML, with many additional techniques, such as XSL and XML schemas, is another important actor. The open group OMG has developed UML (unified modeling language) which is now widely used for healthcare information management and standards. This organization is also behind Corba (Common Object Request Brokering Architecture).

While these inter-sector techniques and standards are very important for interoperability, we also need health specific standards for many issues to achieve interoperability.

In this article some of the achievements of the following organizations will be reviewed: IEEE, which is focusing on device communication; DICOM for imaging; CEN (the European Committee for Standardization) with very diverse objectives; Health Level Seven, based in the US, but with many international affiliates, mainly for messaging; and the relatively recently formed ISO/TC 215 Health Informatics Committee. The reader should be aware of a possible bias by the author, since he has been the chairman of CEN's Health Informatics Committee since 1997, and of the ISO Committee, which he helped establish in 1998. In the latter he leads the working group on security.

Objectives of standardization

Relation between standards and political goals

CEN (Comité Européen de Normalisation), established in 1961, is a federation of official national standards bodies of the twenty European countries. It now has strong links to the political European Union, but is, nevertheless, an independent institution.

Generally, this European collaboration follows two objectives: Their first objective is to facilitate a European market for products and services and to remove the different national standards as barriers to this. This goal has generally been extended to include a global market wherever possible, and CEN is collaborating with the International Standards Organization (ISO) in many areas, now including Health Informatics. However, it is often easier to develop regional technical standards and it has been possible to achieve more precise requirements in Europe than under a global approach. Because of the links to trade policies within the European Union and EFTA, the CEN standards, which have been adopted by a qualified majority (with weighted votes, meaning countries with larger population have more votes than the smaller ones), automatically become valid in all CEN countries, even if a country is actually against a particular standard. This is unlike the situation for ISO, in which each national standards body decides if they want to adapt an international standard in their specific country. Because of this, unfortunately, many examples exist of ISO standards not becoming truly global. Large countries like the USA have often maintained national technical standards in direct conflict with ISO standards. However, in international trade the WTO agreement stresses the importance of the ISO for technical requirements.

The second important objective of the European standardization collaboration is related to the safety of its citizens. In many respective areas, common legislation (national laws following European Union directives) exist, in which the general safety requirements are set out, but to be used in connection with detailed technical specifications which have been developed and maintained by the European Committee for Standards – CEN. In the area of medical devices, many such examples exist, such as surgical implants, pacemakers, and in vitro diagnostics. For such products, a system of controlling bodies exists to ensure the standards are complied with.

The medical devices directive has not been applied to healthcare software products, e.g. electronic healthcare records and messaging. Also, no mandatory compliance to standards exists from a safety perspective. However, there is European legislation on public procurement. This means that any organization largely funded by public means (which includes most European healthcare) should apply certain rules for procuring products or services. These includes referencing standards when such exist. Given the strong legal position of European standards, this means that CEN standards should be used for health informatics in Europe. However, the interpretation of these is difficult and not yet fully understood. Therefore, many systems are bought without reference to standards.

The main emphasis for promoting standards in health informatics is that they facilitate, not that they are mandatory.

Table 1: CEN's members

Austria
Belgium
Czech Republic
Denmark
Finland
France
Germany
Greece
Iceland
Ireland
Italy
Luxembourg
Malta
Netherlands
Norway
Portugal
Spain
Sweden
Switzerland
United Kingdom

CEN/TC 251, the technical committee on medical informatics, was formed in 1990 (with the name changed to health informatics in 1997). This committee has a very broad scope, covering most aspects of health informatics, unlike some of the other more specialized organizations. This committee als provided a way to make use of the results of the extensive European joint research program in health telematics. Large funds have been allocated to the projects of this program for developing new methods of using IT and telecommunications in health. In several cases, submitted project results submitted regarding formal standardizations were discussed further and finally matured into technical standards (or pre-standards).

Scope of CEN/TC 251

Standardization in the field of Health Information and Communications Technology (ICT) is aimed at achieving compatibility and interoperability between independent systems. This includes requirements on the structure of health information to support clinical and administrative procedures, technical methods to support interoperable systems as well as requirements regarding safety, security and quality.

This scope is very similar to that of the more recently formed ISO/TC 215 committee, which largely covers the same ground, but has emphasized the objective to not always develop new specifications, but rather to endorse solutions developed by other bodies.

Different stakeholder views

The healthcare sector is one of the largest soietal sectors, accounting for some 8-14 % of the Gross Domestic Product. The main parties interested in standards for health informatics are the *organizations providing healthcare services*, in other words, those buying and operating health information and communications systems, and *their*

industrial suppliers. The suppliers of health information system solutions have been rather nationally oriented (with the exception of device related systems), but multi-national actors are increasingly appearing.

Since all people are potential patients at some stage in their life, *every citizen* has a concern for the effectiveness of the health care service system. This applies both when it is used directly for themselves as well as when it is used for others that are close. For the citizens, as payers of services through insurance fees, taxation, or direct payment mechanisms, the efficiency of resource utilization is an issue.

The payment bodies are another important stakeholder in this sector. *Payment bodies*, in many countries private or public insurance organizations, or a regional or national governmental body, are important users of health information, with connections to all types of health service providers, and often directly to the patients/citizens.

The *pharmaceutical industry*, with a truly international market and the need to compile information from clinical trials in different countries, is another stakeholder in health information standardization. Although this stakeholder has not played a very active role in health informatics standards so far, its interest is of growing importance.

Healthcare professionals and other *caregivers* have other interests in the development of this sector and the use of technology to change the working environment, in particular to provide new patterns of collaborative work.

The *national governments*, with responsibility for public health planning is also an important user of health information, which comes from many different sources, and thus is an important stakeholder of standards.

While the patients/citizens have not been directly represented in the standardization activities in this area, there is a growing awareness that patient views are important. In ISO/TC 215 a special ad hoc group has been formed to analyze consumer health issues in relation to the technical standards.

Requirements for standards in patient care

The overall purpose of health services is to provide increasingly good quality care to patients/citizens not only in their home environment, but increasingly to those traveling to other parts of the country or region, such as within Europe, and to some extent globally (although resource constraints make this an impossible luxury for very few). The present lack of standardized ICT communication, which prevents inappropriate access to health records, may result in important clinical risks for patients. This is an important safety issue that has not been recognized sufficiently. E.g. a number of adverse drug reactions could have been prevented if information had been made available on-line that existed elsewhere in another health institution. It is also well recognized that appropriate decision support systems with standard interfaces to the clinical routine situation, e.g. for drug therapy, can decrease suboptimal drug use and reduce costs.

Citizens are increasingly demanding that professional health information related to their case should be available from whatever point of care source, wherever this may be.

Health Information and Communication Systems are essential to improve efficiency by enabling effective integration and co-operation of health professional resources over time and space. ICT systems are required to manage the processes of quality management and control involved in public authority activities, as well as actions within provider organizations and research institutions. The aggregated health monitoring information should also be made available to the citizens/ patients, as described in the Community's proposed strategy for health.

Implemented standards are often crucial for any communication, They are especially important in open and very complex health care systems, which are made up of many different organizations and units, most often equipped with information systems from different suppliers and providing different parts of the overall ICT support.

Suppliers/developers of ICT systems are the primary users of our standards, but some standards are used directly by the healthcare IT management, e.g. for security and safety issues. The suppliers generally welcome standards that enable modular systems solutions and a well-defined market. However, in many areas of health information standardization, the suppliers alone cannot be the driving force. In this case, it is a task for the health professionals, healthcare service providers and authorities.

ICT solution buyers often want to refer to existing relevant standards when requesting proposals from suppliers according to the public procurement directive. Technical standards enable a better working market with competing offers from suppliers active in several countries. However, healthcare information systems, in many cases, need national adaptation. Standards on the market will decrease costs for ICT support, particularly when the requirements to integrate different systems are considered. Integration through communication is a key factor for improving the health systems.

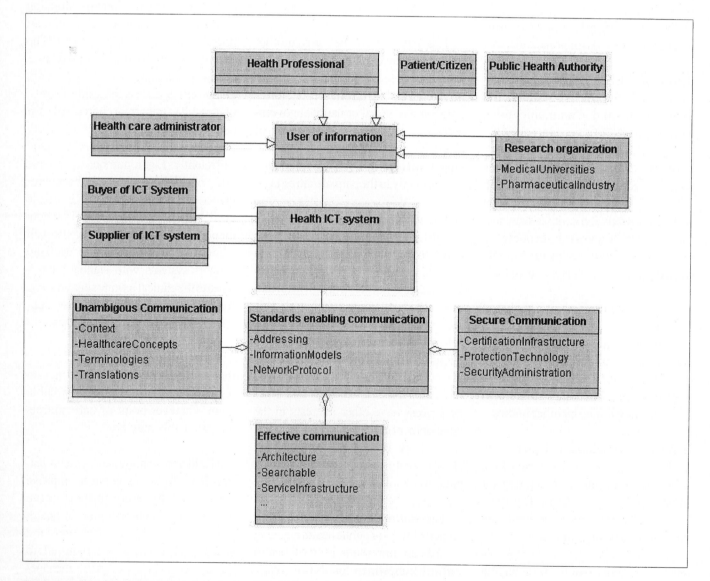

Fig.1. A model of the stakeholders of standards and the main classes of standards

Information models for healthcare processes

A major activity of CEN/TC 251 has been and will remain the specification of detailed information models for various healthcare processes. These correspond to the various clinical documents in the paper world, such as referrals, medical prescriptions, lab reports and healthcare records. A good example is the European standard for Electronic prescriptions completed in 1999.

However, available standards need refinement based on available experiences and the process of global harmonization. Also, there are a large number of healthcare processes for which information models have not yet been standardized.

Syntax specific implementation guidelines are required. In Europe, we are currently in the process of switching from EDIFACT to XML.

Standardized concept representation for processable medical content

Available European standards require additional support in many areas to enable safe and unambiguous communication. The medical content of communication must be *processable*, not just viewed on a screen. This is crucial, because it enables added value use of the information for administrative follow up, improves quality of care, and supports medical research. Defined information structures and concepts are also required for the use of intelligent context-dependent decision support in the clinical situation when treating the individual patient.

Information should be represented by controlled terminologies based on concepts that are well defined by their relations. *Reference terminologies* should be developed nationally or by cross-national specialist groups. An important use of advanced terminology services is the mapping between different terms and codes used by different institutions and professional groups.

This is very useful for the aggregation of data, e.g. for pharmaceutical trials.

Mapping surgical deeds and outcomes to a reference terminology allows cross-border comparison of surgical outcomes, enabling the European citizen to make an informed choice of treatment.

National terms mapped to a reference terminology enable translation between national languages.

Security is essential for health-on-line

The use of ICT can also introduce new, not yet well-controlled risks. While medical devices are controlled through the implementation of directive 93/42, medical software systems and information directly targeting citizens and available on the Net are without proper quality controls. Actions are needed, both to investigate and define proper amendments to European and national legislation, and to introduce measured means for improving the present situation without disturbing the need for innovation and recognition of the importance of "in-house" solutions, which are not available on the market and, therefore, not covered by such legislation.

The eEurope action plan 2000 includes, as its first priority, work for Community action an initiative to ensure a quality certification for medical Websites. CEN has started to work on technical standards supporting this process. A first work item is aimed at defining a Metadata structure to describe the intended scope and quality assurance process of the presented information.

CEN/TC 251 has established important security standards for technical protection mechanisms and for supporting security management. Continued sector specific activities in close collaboration with inter-sector developments are important to ensure secure, broadest interoperability, and to

ensure the special privacy concerns of the sector are supported by technical measures, as well as security management guidelines and *certification infrastructures*. CEN is already working on a standard for Data Protection Contract Guidance to assist meeting the European requirements for communicating personal health information to countries outside of Europe. Standards are essential to establish certification procedures that ensure the safety and privacy concerns in relation to health information systems when necessary.

Summary of Targets

Standards should **exist**,

- **be validated**,
- **well known** and
- **implemented by major actors** to enable:

- The transfer of most types of patient centered information between all European healthcare organizations including complete health records, medical prescriptions, referrals and results of all types of investigations performed.

- Support of multimedia communication for the above purposes, including direct videoconferencing

- The safe integration of wireless medical devices of all types, both those capable of information provision (measurements) and those requiring computer control from external health systems.

- The integration of various knowledge sources into patient centered health information systems. These knowledge bases should be available across borders in multilingual form.

- Processing of medical content to support clinical research and intelligent behavior of information systems, including medical alerts and other forms of decision support.

- Meeting the security requirements for confidentiality, integrity (including electronic signatures added to various document parts), availability and accountability.

- Interoperability and bridging policies which ensure that security services can be provided, including access control between healthcare organizations across borders. This should allow pan-European recognition of digital certificates of professional qualifications and registration. This should also allow the patient using the Internet and appropriate security techniques at home to have direct access to health professionals and their personal health data.

- The build up of appropriate quality control measures in certain cases with appropriate third party testing and certification of health information systems to protect patient safety and to ensure interoperability of products

Work areas and organization

In 1997, CEN/TC 251 restructured its work into the following four working groups, shown in Figure 2 with the corresponding ISO/TC 215 working groups.

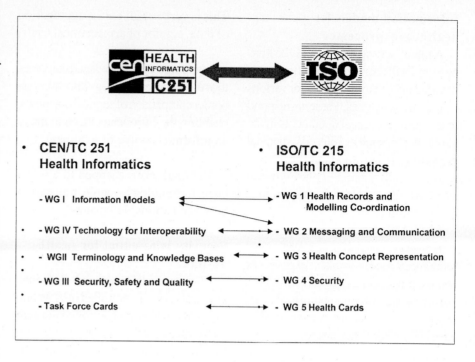

Figure 2. CEN/TC 251 and ISO/TC 215 working groups

Highlights of CEN results

ENV/CR/ No. year	Title/Acronym	Use of the standard
CR **1350** 1993	CEN Report: Investigation of syntaxes for existing interchange formats to be used in healthcare - **MEDIF**	This has guided CEN/TC 251 as well as a large number of message developers in various European countries. However, it is now out of date, since XML is not included.
ENV **1613** 1995	Medical informatics - Messages for laboratory information exchange - **LABMES**	This is the basis of national profiles and large-scale implementations at least in Denmark (50 % of all lab reports are sent using it), the UK and Norway.
ENV **12018** 1997	Identification, administrative, and common clinical data structure for Intermittently Connected Devices for use in healthcare (including machine readable cards) - **DCICD-HC**	This has been the basis for all major European and international healthcare specifications. Through the G8 countries collaboration the US government has used a further development of it. It is presently the basis for the ISO/TC 215 joint development with CEN, according to the Vienna agreement.
ENV **12443** 1998	Medical informatics - Medical informatics healthcare information framework - **HIF**	This is a framework for standardization activities in the field and not intended for direct implementation by industry. The standard is now undergoing major revision.
ENV **12538** 1997	Medical informatics - Messages for patient referral and discharge - **MPRD**	This message standard, with further national implementations in EDIFACT, has been used in national large scale implementations and in Denmark and in several smaller projects in different countries. Currently revised.

ENV **12539** 1997	Medical Informatics - Request and report messages for diagnostic service departments **DIAMES**	This message standard, with further national implementations in EDIFACT, has been used in national large scale implementations and in Denmark and in several smaller projects in different countries. Currently revised.
CR **12587** 1996	CEN Report: Medical Informatics - Methodology for the development of healthcare messages - **METHODOL**	This standard has played an important role for a lot of CEN and EBES-EG9 work and has also had major influence on HL7 in the US. The basic idea has jointly been developed further and is now a CD in ISO/TC 215.
ENV **12612** 1997	Medical Informatics - Messages for the exchange of healthcare administrative information - **ADMES**	This message standard, with further national implementations in EDIFACT, has been used in national large scale implementations and in Denmark and in several smaller projects in different countries. Currently revised.
ENV **13606-1** 1999	Health Informatics - Electronic healthcare record communication - Part 1: Extended architecture – **EHCR-EA**	This is series of standards for the representation of a healthcare record, and is a milestone without international competition. It is, however, complicated and implementation requires national guidelines and considerable work. National strategies intending to use this are underway in the UK, Sweden, Denmark, Norway, Scotland and the Netherlands. It is presently being considered in Belgium for national implementation. Companies that have implemented it include Siemens and Tieto-Enator. Part of this standard is also used in the national Australian record specification under the name GEHR.
ENV **13606-2** 1999	Health Informatics – Electronic healthcare record communication - Part 2: Domain term list – **EHCR-DT**	This is an important part of the record structure that gives meaning to the headings of the record. National guidelines required.
ENV **13606-3** 1999	Health Informatics – Electronic healthcare record communication - Part 3: Distribution Rules – **EHCR-DR**	This part is used less than other data structures.
ENV **13606-4** 1999	Health Informatics – Electronic healthcare record communication - Part 4: Messages for information exchange – **EHCR-ME**	This is a summary message using all the structural elements used in parts 1 –3. This part is actually what is implemented in products. A DTD for an XML implementation is included and used in the products mentioned above.
ENV **13607** 1999	Health Informatics - Messages for information exchange on medical prescriptions– **DRUGPRES**	This is implemented in Denmark in EDIFACT and in Sweden, Netherlands and the UK in XML versions with national adaptations.
ENV **13609-2** 1999	Health informatics - Messages for maintenance of information support in healthcare systems - Part 2: Updating of medical laboratory-specific information – **SUPINFMES2**	This is used by many laboratories in Denmark

ENV 13730-1 2000	Health informatics - Blood transfusion related messages – Part 1: Subject of care related messages Part 2: Production related messages	This is quite recent but is being implemented in France by the national blood transfusion service
ENV **1068** 1993	Medical Informatics – Healthcare information interchange - Registration of coding schemes - **RCS**	This standard was implemented with the World Health Organization as the registration authority, but then put on hold to await a general ISO procedure. It has now been revived and is to become an EN.
ENV **1614** 1995	Healthcare informatics - Structure for nomenclature, classification and coding of properties in clinical laboratory sciences - **PROCT-L**	This is the basis for the major international classification scheme maintained by IUPAC used in many, but not all, European countries.
ENV **1828** 1995	Medical informatics - Structure for classification and coding of surgical procedures - **PROCT-S**	This has been the basis for the French national classification of surgical procedures while other countries have maintained older less structured systems.
ENV **12381** 1996	Health care informatics - Time standards for health care specific problems - **TSMI**	This is being forwarded to an EN without change and will provide a basic common concept system for standards and other specification work.
ENV **12435** 1999	Medical informatics - Expression of the results of measurements in health sciences - **UNITS**	This is being forwarded to an EN without change and will provide a basic common concept system for standards and other specification work.
ENV **12610** 1997	Medical informatics - Medicinal product identification - **CDRUGS**	This is being revised to an EN in collaboration with the European Medicines Evaluation Agency, EMEA
ENV **12611** 1997	Medical informatics - Categorical structure of systems of concepts - Medical Devices - **TCMD**	This vocabulary structure is used in standards works, but not yet in other contexts to our knowledge
ENV **13940** 2000	Health informatics – System of concepts to support continuity of care - **CONTSYS**	This rather recent standard is being implemented nationally with health authorities in the Scandinavian countries and is guiding the development of a number of IT products not yet released. It has also been translated into Dutch and will be the basis for discussions about continuity of care.
ENV **14032** 2000	Health informatics - System of Concepts to Support Nursing - **NURSYS**	This is a step towards international harmonization of Nursing terminology and is the basis for an ISO/TC 215 work item developed in liaison with the International College of Nursing Professional Societies.
ENV **12388** 1996	Medical Informatics - Algorithm for Digital Signature Services in health care - **ADDS**	This standard algorithm (RSA) has been the basis for most trials and implementations of systems for digital signatures in European countries, e.g. in France, Germany, Belgium, Sweden, Norway, Finland and Greece.
ENV **12924** 1997	Medical Informatics - Security Categorization and Protection for Healthcare Information Systems - **COMPUSEC**	This standard guide to information security has been used in training and management mainly in France, the UK and the Netherlands, but it has also influenced regional and local policies in other countries. It is now considered a candidate for an ISO standard.

ENV 13608-1 1999	Health Informatics - Security for healthcare communication - Part 1: Concepts and terminology – **SEC-COM1**	Part 1 of the SECOM series is used in several countries to guide requirement analysis and specification work. France is probably the leader here. It is also an important basis for much of other TC 251 security work.
ENV 13608-2 1999	Health Informatics - Security for healthcare communication - Part 2: Secure data objects – **SEC-COM2**	Part 2 specifies a profile of the well-known IETF standard for secure messaging. Most modern healthcare security protection schemes using a PKI are in fact implementing this standard. Known examples are in France, Germany, Belgium, UK, Sweden and Norway
ENV 13608-3 1999	Health Informatics - Security for healthcare communication - Part 3: Secure data channels – **SEC-COM3**	Part 3 specifies a profile of the well-known IETF standard for secure web access. Most modern healthcare security protection schemes using a PKI are in fact implementing this standard. Known examples are in France, Germany, Belgium, UK, Sweden and Norway
ENV 12251 1999	Health Informatics - Secure user identification for healthcare - management and security of authentication by passwords (Healthcare oriented security functionality classes) – **SEC-ID/PASS**	This standard is not very well known, but the principles specified are followed by the industry in many countries
ENV 13729 1999	Health Informatics - Secure user identification - Strong authentication using microprocessor cards – **SEC-ID/CARDS**	This standard specifies the basic principles of using microprocessor cards and has been followed in the major projects using such cards in e.g. France, Germany and Sweden. Will need an update now that more generic standards are available.
FM-HSP/FR	Health Informatics - Framework for formal modeling of healthcare security policies	This CR provides a basis for further work but is not directly implemented by industry
SAFE-ID	Health Informatics - Safety procedures for identification of patients and related objects	This CR has generated considerable interest for addressing these important safety problems. In the pharmaceutical area, this CR provides a conceptual foundation of the European DRIVE project which involves the pharmaceutical industry as well as hospital pharmacies and information system solution suppliers. EN work has been proposed as a follow-up, but has not yet started.
ENV 1064 1993	Medical informatics - Standard communication protocol - Computer-assisted electrocardiography – **SCP-ECG**	This standard has been taken up by most major companies producing ECG machines not only in Europe but also worldwide. It has now been revised and is forwarded to an EN.
ENV 12052 1997	Medical Informatics - Medical imaging communication - **MEDICOM**	This and ENVs 12623 and 12922-1 are European contributions and endorsements of the world leader in imaging standards for health, DICOM. The global DICOM specs now incorporate European contributions and a revised standard for EN as a general endorsement is being prepared.
ENV 12967-1 1998	Medical Informatics - Healthcare Information System Architecture - Part 1: Healthcare middleware layer - **HISA**	This provides the basis for one successful commercial product (DHE) from Italy which is used in several countries. The standard is now undergoing major revision.

ENV 13728 1999	Health informatics - Instrument interfaces to laboratory information systems – **INTERMED**	This standard, developed with major industries in Europe and the US, has now been agreed on to be fast-tracked as an ISO standard parallel to the EN process under the Vienna agreement.
ENV 13734 1999	Health informatics -Vital Signs Information Representation– **VITAL**	This standard and ENV 13735 has been developed with major industries in Europe and the US, working in IEEE, and has now been agreed on to be fast-tracked as an ISO standard (in two parts) parallel to the EN process under the Vienna agreement
ENV 13735 1999	Health informatics - Interoperability of patient connected medical devices	See above (ENV 13734). Now fast-tracked as an ISO standard parallel to the EN process under the Vienna agreement

ISO/TC 215

In August 1998, ISO/TC 215 "Health Informatics" was started with a scope similar to that of CEN/TC 251. These international efforts have been welcomed by Europe. An active collaboration between the European and international level is encouraged and has been started. A general co-operation agreement exists between ISO and CEN, the Vienna Agreement regulating how close collaboration can be achieved, avoiding different solutions but often allowing CEN results to be processed as formal ISO standards, possibly modified after international review.

In general, the ISO committee is still somewhat in a phase of trying to define its role. Relatively few work items have been formally approved, although a number projects have been started. To date only two technical specifications (corresponding to prestandards) have been approved by the ISO committee: quality criteria for controlled health vocabularies, and public key infrastructure respectively. The first formal standard in the pipeline is scheduled for publication mid 2002. It is called: Health Informatics - Clinical analyzer interfaces for laboratory information systems - Use profiles based on a previous European pre-standard.

A number of device related standards, developed by CEN and IEEE, have also been submitted to become formal standards in ISO, with necessary refinements.

While the general scopes of the ISO and CEN committee overlap, the major emphasis of international efforts has focused on some basic aspects of health informatics in which global consensus is probably achievable in a near future. This includes, but is not restricted to, methodology for message development (but not messages) and vocabulary of terminological systems.

In a few areas, more specific standards where there is already a clear international market of products such as in the area of medical device communication and where an informal collaboration already existed, European and US previous results and new development are now replacing regional efforts. However, at least in the beginning of the ISO work, it has been decided to leave many specific areas of standardization closely related closely to different business practices and standards heritage outside of the ISO work. Notably, for instance, in both Europe and e.g. the US, a large use of standardized healthcare messages already exists that can not be converted to a common global structure easily.

However, the enthusiasm is great, with over 30 countries participating. Many interesting but difficult projects have been started in various areas, including the security field and health cards, where much common global understanding already exists.

IEEE

IEEE – the Institute of Electrical and Electronics Engineers has been developing standards in its areas for more than 100 years. In what is now called point-of-care medical device communication (the 1073 committee) a considerable history of developing standards for device communication can be looked back on, the most famous being the "Medical Information Bus" standard. For more information see http://www.ieee1073.org.

IEEE has had a long and very lively collaboration with CEN/TC 215. Together, much work has been channelled to ISO/TC 215 for consideration as international standards.

DICOM

The American College of Radiology (ACR) and the National Electrical Manufacturers Association (NEMA) decided to form a joint committee in order to create a standard method for the transmission of medical images and their associated information in 1983. The first version was published in 1985. The release of version 3.0 in 1993 saw a name change, to Digital Imaging and Communications in Medicine (DICOM). For more information see: http://medical.nema.org/dicom.html

Scope

The DICOM Standards Committee exists to create and maintain international standards for communicating bio-medical diagnostic and therapeutic information in disciplines that use digital images and associated data. The goals of DICOM are to achieve compatibility and to improve workflow efficiency between imaging systems and other information systems in healthcare environments worldwide. DICOM is a cooperative standard. Therefore, connectivity works, because vendors cooperate in testing via scheduled public demonstration per Internet and during private test sessions. Major diagnostic medical imaging vendors worldwide have incorporated the standard into their product design. Most actively participate in the enhancement of the standard. The majority of the professional societies throughout the world supports and participates in the enhancement of the standard. DICOM is used, or will soon be used, by virtually every medical profession that utilizes images within the healthcare industry, such as cardiology, dentistry, endoscopy, mammography, opthalmology, orthopedics, pathology, pediatrics, radiation therapy, radiology, surgery, etc. DICOM is even used in veterinary medical imaging applications.

Table 2. DICOM Working Groups

WG 1 (Cardiac and Vascular Information)
WG 2 (Digital X-Ray)
WG 3 (Nuclear Medicine)
WG 4 (Compression)
WG 5 (Exchange Media)
WG 6 (Base Standard)
WG 7 (Radiotherapy)
WG 8 (Structured Reporting)
WG 9 (Ophthalmology)
WG 10 (Strategic Advisory)
WG 11 (Display Function Standard)
WG 12 (Ultrasound)
WG 13 (Visible Light)
WG 14 (Security)
WG 15 (Digital Mammography)
WG 16 (Magnetic Resonance)
WG 17 (3D)
WG 18 (Clinical Trials and Education)
WG 19 (Dermatologic Standards)
WG 20 (Integration of Imaging and Information Systems)
WG 21 (Computed Tomography)

HL7

HL7 was founded in 1987 in the US as a developer of healthcare messages. It developed its own syntax for representing information in a rather simple structure of named segments and fields (each of which has a defined data type). This has been further developed and covers a large number of different clinical and some administrative areas. Much of the focus has been placed on communication needs within organizations, such as hospitals. This specification is used particularly in US and Canadian hospitals in various forms of the version 2 (version 2.4 is approved, but most use version 2.3 or 2.2).

For more information on HL7 see http://www.hl7.org.

HL7 is now an American National Standards Institute (ANSI) approved Standards Developing Organization (SDO) and has its main base in the US. In recent years, it has, however, greatly expanded its international presence. Affiliated organizations exist in the following countries: Argentina, Australia, Canada, China, Czech Republic, Finland, Germany, India, Japan, Korea, Lithuania, the Netherlands, New Zealand, Southern Africa, Switzerland, Taiwan, Turkey and the United Kingdom. In most of these countries, some parts of HL7 version 2 have been adapted and are used with national implementation guides in some contexts.

In 1997, it was realized that the development model of HL7 had serious problems in achieving consistency between different parts. It was also noted, which is still a great problem, that different HL7 compliant implementations are not fully compatible since they choose to use options in different ways.

HL7 was influenced by European standardization work regarding building of object-oriented information models separate of implementation syntax. HL7 began the work towards version 3, which at the time of writing, fall of 2001, is not yet finished. That is no messages for implementation have been approved, and, even if installations conforming to this may begin to appear in 2002, it will take considerable time before version 2 is actually replaced.

The work of HL7 with version 3 has resulted in great improvements of the principles of message development. Also, the methodology developed has largely been accepted by CEN, and is about to become an ISO standard. The Reference Information Model (RIM) is the cornerstone of the HL7 Version 3 development process. An object model created as part of the Version 3 methodology, RIM is a large pictorial representation of the clinical data (domains) and identifies the life cycle of events a message or group of related messages will carry. It is a shared model between all domains and, as such, is the model from which all domains create their messages. Explicitly representing the connections that exist between the information carried in the fields of HL7 messages, RIM is essential to our ongoing mission of increasing precision and reducing implementation costs.

While the principle of a reference information model is sound, it is far from trivial to achieve consensus on the most useful model for healthcare information. The HL7 RIM has been revised completely several times, and is now very concise and abstract. This is elegant, but requires agreements on health specifics on another level. In HL7, this is done as part of message development with so called CMETs, Common Message Element Types. This partly corresponds with what the CEN group is working on, the so-called General Purpose Information Components.

In March 2000, a memorandum of understanding between CEN/TC 251 and HL7 was signed hich recognizes:

"There has been a number of fruitful exchanges between experts of the two organizations in the past years, with, e.g., US experts participating in CEN project teams, European experts participating in HL7 meetings, and the CEN principles for message development were adopted and further developed by HL7 in its work on Version 3.0. The organizations have fundamental common goals and many similarities in their solutions, and it is clear that the present incompatibility between the major European and US set of standards is neither beneficial nor desirable from a long term and global perspective. The need for a global family of standards has been apparent for some time, and both CEN TC251 and HL7 agree that collaboration and co-operation is the most effective way to approach this goal.

CEN/TC 251 and HL7 agree to collaborate in the spirit of mutual appreciation, respect and openness to seek pragmatic solutions to obtain unification of their set of standards for healthcare communication and to make the results globally available to ISO."

Since this agreement for collaboration was made, a lot of fruitful interchange has taken place, and CEN has decided to use part of the HL7 RIM achievements in its restructuring of message standards. It has, however, not been possible to agree on the more healthcare business related areas, and the working modes of the US dominated organization. For HL7, it is very important to encompass the old HL7 Version 2 content in the new messages, but other requirements from the European side have been difficult to accommodate. A particular problem relates to the complex structures of the Electronic Healthcare Record Architecture, which has not at all been taken up by HL7, even if an interest group was formed recently to push this aspect. In a NHS sponsored Project, the UK decided to develop their own GP to GP record transfer model using the HL7 RIM but deeming the construction of record containers necessary, and based on the thinking of the European standard ENV 13606.

CEN, on the other hand finds the record structure essential in health informatics and has decided to collaborate with the Open Electronic Healthcare Record Foundation, taking onboard important Australian contributions to the CEN architecture.

Conclusions

Standards now exist from several sources that cover many requirements for health information exchange. They deserve to be used much more, even if they are not perfect, and are in a stage

of global development and harmonization. Procurers of health IT solutions should request standard conformant products for their domains, and industrial suppliers of solutions must consider the benefits of standards to meet customer requirements and to enable the construction of modular solutions.

The major bodies having an international impact in this area, CEN, HL7, IEEE and DICOM, all collaborate in different ways, and with ISO/TC 215. It is a long-term process and probably will never completely end, as different standards bodies learn from each other and gradually harmonize wherever possible. The users of standards eventually decide which standards to use. In several European countries, special governmental committees have been formed with the aim to clarify which standards should be used in their healthcare domain for different purposes if there are several candidates to choose from. However, to a large extent, the different standards initiatives complement each other more than they compete.

References

CEN/TC 251: www.centc251.org contains results and ongoing work for a review of the work done 1991-2001 see: doc N01-022 under TC documents 2001.
ISO/TC 215: http://isotc.iso.ch/livelink/livelink?func=11&objId=529137&objAction=browse&sort=name
HL7: http://www.hl7.org
IEEE: http://www.ieee1073.org
DICOM: http://medical.nema.org/dicom.html

Adress of the author:
Gunnar O. Klein
Centre for Health Telematics
Karolinska Institute
Stockholm, Sweden
E-mail: gunnar@klein.se

M.J. Ackerman

U.S. National Library of Medicine
Bethesda, MD, USA

Review

Visible Human Project®: From Data to Knowledge

In 1989, the U.S. National Library of Medicine (NLM) Board of Regents empowered an ad hoc panel of experts to recommend the position that NLM should take in the rapidly evolving field of electronic imagery. They recommended that NLM proceed with the proposed Visible Human Project (VHP) [1]. In August of 1991, the University of Colorado School of Medicine was awarded a contract that resulted in the acquisition of the NLM Visible Human Project male and female data sets. NLM made the data sets available under a no-cost license agreement over the Internet (Figure 1). The VHP male data set contains 1971 digital axial anatomical images obtained at 1.0-mm intervals (15 Gbyte) [2]. The VHP female data set contains 5189 digital anatomical images obtained at 0.33-mm intervals (39 Gbyte). Since the introduction of the data sets, NLM has signed over 1400 licenses with participants in 43 countries. In addition, three VHP Conferences have been hosted by the NLM [3]. These Conferences have highlighted research and applications based on the Visible Human data sets.

Despite the unprecedented detail in the VHP data sets and its demonstrated utility in conveying information about gross anatomy, deficiencies in the data compromise its use in the focused teaching of specific areas of human anatomy. In February 1998, a workshop sponsored jointly by NLM and National Institute of Dental and Craniofacial Research explored the growing needs of the research

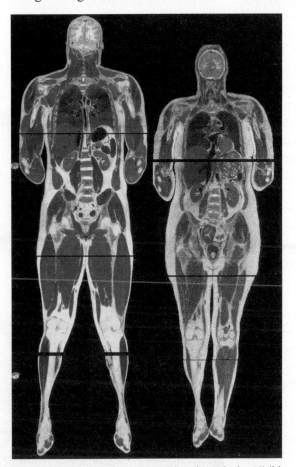

Fig. 1. Reconstructed frontal section through the Visible Human male and female.

and education community for more powerful digital tools and higher resolution models of human anatomy [4]. The workshop focused on an in-depth analysis of the existing male Visible Human data, specifically on the anatomy of the head and neck.

The workshop participants recommended the development of a multimedia, web deployable head and neck atlas created from the existing male data set as a proof of educational and technical concept, the pursuit of advanced image processing software tools to accommodate future higher resolution data, and the development of better tissue fixation and staining techniques to minimize tissue artifacts and maximize the visibility of anatomical objects.

The NLM in partnership with six other U.S. government agencies is sponsoring research and development which will further the core goals of the VHP in three areas:

1) the creation of a Visible Human Project Atlas of the Head and Neck; 2) the development of a software tool kit (Insight) capable of automatically performing many of the basic data handling functions required for using Visible Human data in applications, e.g., segmentation and alignment; and 3) the development of better tissue fixation and staining techniques to rectify the anatomical problems associated with the tissue methods used during the creation of the Visible Human data sets.

Visible Human Project Atlas of the Head and Neck

The purpose of this project is to develop a public domain NLM hosted web site portraying human anatomy based primarily on the VHP male data set. The goal is to create a landmark functional and clinical anatomy atlas of the head and neck human body regions - a prototype for a new wave of educational applications based on the integration of the VHP data sets with other ancillary human imagery sources. The project is designed to demonstrate the utility of the existing data and will provide a platform for new directions in education and medical research. The NLM commissioned the VHP Head and Neck Atlas to the University of Colorado Health Sciences Center through a competitive, peer-reviewed contracting process.

A series of clinically relevant functional anatomy modules are being created as part of the Atlas. These educational modules are being designed to demonstrate the functional processes involved in facial expression, mastication and deglutition, phonation, hearing, and vision. The Atlas web site will allow the user to interact with the appropriate imagery in order to demonstrate functionality,

for example, the function of the muscles that control and move the mandible bone during the chewing (mastication) reflex. Magnetic resonance interferometry (MRI), computerized axial tomography (CAT), and other radiology image modalities as well as conventional anatomic graphic materials will be integrated into each module. The modules will demonstrate normal musculo-skeletal system function as well as abnormal functional deficits including clinical signs and symptoms. They will illustrate neurovascular relationships through the interactive dissection of anatomic structures and fly-through views. For example, the student will be able to experience a walking tour of the optic nerve and view of the distribution of the ophthalmic artery and its tributaries. These web accessible modules will emphasize interactivity over passivity (Figure 2).

Equally important to the educational success of this project is the achievement of an element of novel entertainment quality that will form

a creative prototype to stimulate and encourage the interactive learning process. The Atlas web site is being designed to meet the needs of a wide ranging audience including: medical, dental, and nursing students with an emphasis on normal anatomic structure and function; practicing heath care professionals with an emphasis on clinical relevance; and the general public's need for reference materials to better understand a health concern.

Insight Software Research Consortium

The initial emphasis of this effort is to provide public software tools in 3D segmentation and deformable and rigid registration for medical images Visible Human Project data. The goal is for the consortium to provide the cornerstone of a self-sustaining software community in 3D, 4D and higher dimensional data analysis. The consortium is committed to public, open-source software code including

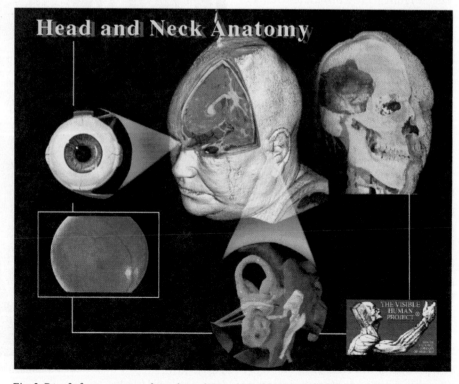

Fig. 2. Proof of concept page from the web based Visible Human Atlas of the Head and Neck.

open interfaces supporting connections to a broad range of visualization and graphic user interface platforms. The goal is the development of a public domain software resource that will serve as a foundation for future medical image understanding research. The intent is to leverage the investment being made through the VHP and other medical image analysis programs by reducing the re-invention of basic imaging algorithms.

The Insight Software Research Consortium which includes partners in academia and in industry has been formed to carry this work forward. The Consortium has completed the design and development of an initial version of a public medical image segmentation and registration toolkit known as the *Insight ToolKit* (ITK). The goal is to create an application programmer's interface (API) which can be used by developers of medical programs and software products wherever the problems of image or volume segmentation and registration exist (Figure 3). Unlike previous software development efforts, the goal is specifically NOT to create a single monolithic program, but rather a software foundation from which a broad range of programs can be supported.

The ITK API has undergone continuous review and modification by the expert developers on the programming team. The software toolkit is being designed to support a variety of visualization and/or rendering platforms and to be easily integrated into existing processing, visualization and presentation systems. The completed software toolkit, including all source code and

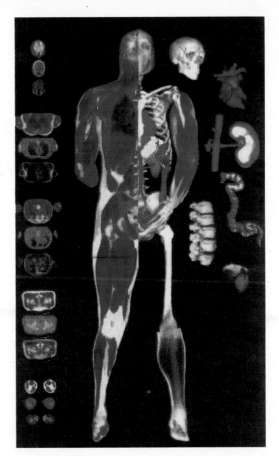

Fig. 3. Current bitmap version of the Visible Human data set (data) on the left versus the future object version (knowledge) on the right.

extensive documentation consisting of manuals, tutorials and examples, will be made available in the public domain by the NLM through a controlled Internet site.

Visible Human Project Anatomical Methods

This initiative is directed at the methods that were utilized to stabilize the anatomical materials used in making the Visible Human data sets. The work is focused on three methodological areas. The first concentrates on the elimination of the freezing and embalming artifacts that can be seen in the data set images. Methods need to be found through which tissue can be fixed without deformation, swelling or misalignment. The second will identify histological staining and wide-spectrum

methods that will enhance the contrast between nerves and their surrounding tissues. This will allow the visualization of the branching of nerves as they reach their target organs. The third involves the identification of vascular structures by the application of dye materials, or by the injection of materials for vascular luminal filling adapted to VHP cryosectioning methodology.

References

1. National Library of Medicine (U.S.) Board of Regents. *Electronic imaging: Report of the Board of Regents*. U.S. Department of Health and Human Services, National Institutes of Health (1990). NIH Publication 90-2197.
2. Spitzer V, Ackerman MJ, Scherzinger AL and Whitlock D. The Visible Human Male: A technical Report. *JAMIA*, 3(2):118-130, 1996.
3. National Library of Medicine (U.S.). *Proceedings of the Third Visible Human Project Conference*. R. A. Banvard, ed. October 5-6, 2000, Bethesda, MD: US Department of Health and Human Services, Public Health Service, National Institutes of Health. (2000). (http://www.nlm.nih.gov/research/visible/vhpconf2000/MAIN.HTM)
4. National Institute of Dental and Craniofacial Research (U.S.). *Summary Report: Virtual Head and Neck Anatomy Workshop*. February 25, 1998, Bethesda, MD: US Department of Health and Human Services, Public Health Service, National Institutes of Health (1998). (http://www.nidcr.nih.gov/news/strat%2Dplan/headneck/contents.htm)

Address of the author:
Michael J. Ackerman, Ph.D.
U.S. National Library of Medicine
Lister Hill National Center
for Biomedical Communications
8600 Rockville Pike
Bethesda, MD 20894, USA

Review Paper

W. L. Nowinski

Medical Imaging Lab
Kent Ridge Digital Labs
Singapore

Review

Model-enhanced neuroimaging: clinical, research, and educational applications

1. Introduction

During the past 30 years medical imaging has been propelled by advances in the computational, biomedical, and physical sciences. Modern medical imaging technologies offer unprecedented views into the human body's structure, function, metabolism, hemodynamics, and pathology. Our ability to generate images is much greater than our ability to understand and interpret them. Processing of medical images involves image acquisition, display, analysis, and interpretation. Deformable body models along with warping techniques facilitate analysis of medical images. Deformable brain atlases in particular are useful for analysis and interpretation of brain scans.

Medical imaging covers numerous areas, including image acquisition and formation, image processing and enhancement, segmentation, analysis, registration, visualization, modeling, compression, picture archiving and communication systems, computer-aided diagnosis, computer-aided surgery, and on-line medical imaging. We briefly review some of them from the point of view of neuroimaging, and focus on four groups of model-enhanced applications for education, medical research, diagnosis, and treatment. We illustrate these applications by the systems and technologies developed in our lab.

2. Medical imaging

Medical imaging has come a long way since 1895, when Roentgen discovered X-rays and produced an image of the bones of his wife's hand. Today's medical imaging modalities are based not only on X-rays but also on a variety of other energy sources including ultrasound, nuclear magnetic resonance, radionuclides, electrons, light, and lasers. The images obtained are characterized by their spatial, contrast, and temporal resolutions. Medical imaging covers a wide range of areas. We briefly review image acquisition, segmentation, registration, visualization, and modelling from the point of view of neuroimaging.

2.1 Image acquisition

Medical imaging modalities, such as X-rays, Computed Tomography (CT), Magnetic Resonance Imaging (MRI), ultrasound (US), Single Proton Emission CT (SPECT), and Positron Emission Tomography (PET) provide views of human anatomy, pathology, and function. Conventional X-ray images are still the most commonly used. An X-ray is a projection image showing the distribution of tissue attenuation of X-rays passing through the body. CT images show a spatial distribution of the tissue attenuation coefficients reconstructed mathema-

tically from multiple X-ray projections. Conventional CT acquires projections in parallel axial planes. Spiral CT allows the projections to be acquired along a spiral trajectory providing high-resolution volumetric images. X-rays and CT use ionizing radiation, as opposed to MRI which is non-invasive. MRI is based on the magnetic resonance phenomenon and uses a magnet and radio signals to generate multi-modal images. Conventional MRI studies exploit the concentration of water protons (i.e., proton density PD) and two relaxation times, T1 (spin-lattice relaxation rate) and T2 (spin-spin relaxation rate). T1-weighted studies demonstrate normal and abnormal anatomy particularly well. T2-weighted studies are particularly sensitive to the detection of pathological processes. US is based on the interaction of acoustic energy with tissue, which provides a signal containing information on tissue properties. US systems vary in terms of the range of acoustic frequencies and energies, and beam divergence. Low cost and real-time scanning make US popular. SPECT is able to detect functional and pathological changes. It shows the distribution of injected or inhaled radiopharmaceuticals that emit protons upon decay. SPECT images are reconstructed from multiple projections, similar to CT, recorded by gamma cameras. PET demonstrates glucose and oxygen consumption as well as metabolic abnormalities. PET images show the distribution of positron-emitting radionuclides administered to the patient.

Vasculature can be examined by using Digital Subtraction Angiography (DSA), CT Angiography (CTA), MR Angiography (MRA), and X-ray rotational angiography. In MRA, a variety of subtraction methods are available to differentiate rapidly moving protons in blood from the relatively static protons in surrounding tissues.

Magnetic Resonance Spectroscopy (MRS) is a biochemical tool for the identification of variety of metabolites in tissue. It can serve as a non-invasive tissue biopsy. Brain connections can be traced by Diffusion Tensor Imaging (DTI).

Functional neuroimaging, with functional magnetic resonance imaging (fMRI), PET, and magnetoencephalography (MEG), has been used exten-sively to identify brain regions associated with motor, sensory, visual, auditory, and cognitive tasks. Functional brain mapping has tremendous potential as a tool for basic neuroscientific investigation as well as the diagnosis of stroke and tumors, and presurgical planning.

2.2. Segmentation

Segmentation refers to the partitioning of the image into components that are homogeneous with respect to some feature(s). Segmentation is an important step in applications involving quantitative analysis, registration, visualization, compression, and computer-aided surgery. Segmentation methods can be broadly divided into interactive (manual), semiautomatic, and automatic, see examples in Figures 1 and 3. Segmentation algorithms operate on the intensity or texture variations of the image using a variety of techniques including thresholding, region growing, edge detection, deformable models, pattern recognition (neural networks and fuzzy clustering), or combination of some of them [14], [23], [73]. Deformable models are curves or surfaces defined within the image that can move under the external forces computed from the image data and the internal forces coming within the model itself [46]. The model is drawn towards the edges by external forces and the internal forces keep the model together and restrain it from bending too much. Deformable models, being able to represent complex shapes and a wide range of shape variability, overcome many of the limitations of the traditional low-level image segmentation techniques.

An accurate segmentation of brain images is a challenging task. Hybrid methods combining image-processing and model-based techniques are particularly effective for brain segmentation [4], [33].

a)   b)

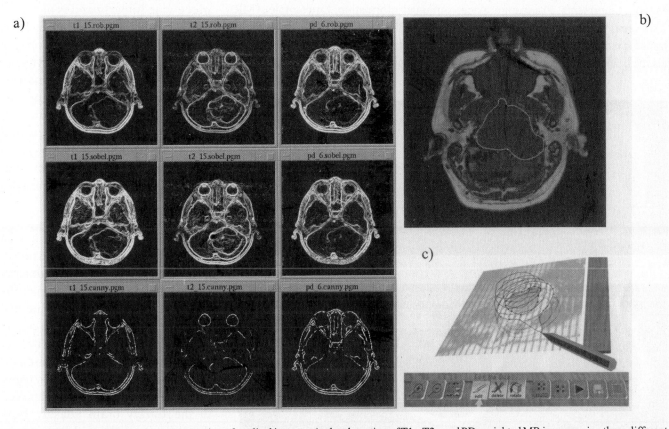

c)

Fig. 1. Image-based and interactive segmentation of medical images: a) edge detection of T1-, T2-, and PD-weighted MR images using three different edge detectors: Roberts, Sobel, and Canny; note that none of them is able to delineate the tumor completely; b) interactive segmentation of a brain tumor in a 2D case; c) interactive segmentation in a 3D case by using a customized 3D contour editor.

Image segmentation may be preceded by image enhancement to accentuate certain features in the image. Image enhancement usually suppresses the noise or increases the image contrast.

2.3. Registration

Registration, also termed as matching or alignment, involves a spatial transformation that maps locations in one image to their corresponding locations in another image or model. These two images may be acquired by different imaging modalities, be taken for the same patient at a different time, correspond to two different patients, or correspond to a patient and a model. Registration usually involves translating, rotating, scaling, and possible non-linear warping of one image into the other. As the images once registered can be compared or combined, registration is useful for:

· model-based segmentation and labeling
· fusion of multi-modal data.

A registration process may involve up to four components: 1) a feature space, 2) a search space of the allowed transformations (such as rigid, affine, or elastic), 3) a similarity or difference measure between the matched images, and 4) a search strategy used to determine the transformation which maximizes the similarity measure or minimizes the difference measure.

There are numerous non-linear registration methods, such as [5], [9], [11], [12], [13], [15], [24], [88], [95], [96], [98], [99], [100]. A general overview of registration methods can be found in [10], while [42] overviews medical image registration. These methods are usually divided into two groups: feature-based and voxel-based. A simple feature may be the set of corresponding points in the registered images. These points may be internal anatomical landmarks or external markers attached to the patient. More complicated features may include the corresponding curves (such as edges, ridges, or crest lines) or surfaces. Voxel-based methods use the full contents of the images and exploit features such as grey values, correlation, and, recently mutual information. An example of MRI and CT registration by using a fast maximization of mutual information approach [99] is shown in Figure 2.

Despite their advantages and tremendous potential, non-linear registration methods have several limitations that make them difficult to use in today's clinical setting. Homologous landmark matching suffers from the need for a large number of landmarks and a subjectivity in selecting them. Iterative methods are often initial guess-dependent, which may not be acceptable in a clinical environment. The registration accuracy of boundary-based methods decreases when one moves away from the boundary. The major practical limitation, however, is a prohibitively large computational time required, as compared in [68].

A practical and clinically accepted registration method overcoming these limitations is the Talairach proportional grid system transformation [85]. It normalizes brains piecewise linearly and is based on the Talairach point landmarks: two internal landmarks lying on the midsagittal plane and six external landmarks lying on the smallest bounding box encompassing the cortex. The Talairach transformation can be performed in real time using hardware-assisted texture mapping [60] or in near real-time when implemented optimally [58], [61].

The Talairach approach can further be speeded up by using a new, equivalent set of landmarks [64]. These new (Talairach-Nowinski) landmarks are defined in a more constructive way and can be easier identified automatically. Figure 3 illustrates registration-based segmentation of MR images by using the Talairach transformation applied to the *Cerefy* brain atlases. Note that this approach is able to segment small brain structures that are not discernible in the image data.

a)

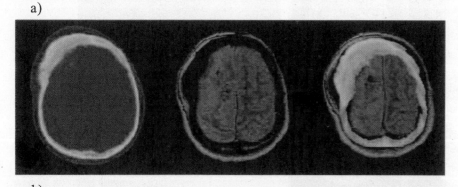

b)

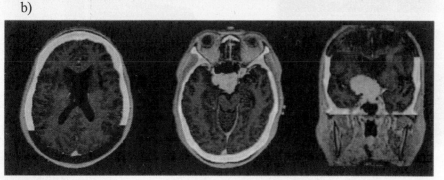

Fig. 2. Registration of MRI and CT brain images in the presence of pathology: a) from left to right: CT, MRI, and fused axial images; b) axial and coronal fused images.

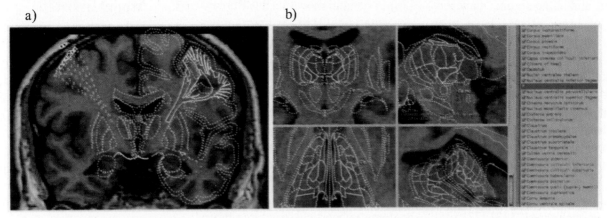

Fig. 3. Atlas-based segmentation. a) Gross anatomy is segmented by using the atlas in contour representation. b) The subcortical structures are segmented on axial, coronal, sagittal, and triplanar views. The structure of interest, i.e. the nucleus centralis magnocelluralis of the thalamus is highlighted and labeled.

2.4. Visualization

CT and MRI data sets have traditionally been interpreted and displayed as cross-sectional images. Recent advances in diagnostic imaging, such as multi-detector CT, faster MRI acquisitions, and rotational X-ray angiography, result in the routine acquisition of large, high-resolution volumetric datasets the effective interpretation of which requires the use of volume visualization. An efficient visualization of these datasets is also becoming a critical step in planning and performing therapeutic interventions.

Numerous 2D and 3D techniques have been developed for visualization, such as multiplanar reformatting, maximum intensity projection, surface rendering, and volume rendering. Multiplanar reformatting includes orthogonal, oblique, and curved reformatting. Surface rendering requires the rendered object(s) to be segmented first. Then standard computer graphics techniques, such as hidden surface removal, lighting, and shading, are used. One of the most popular iso-surface extraction techniques is *Marching Cubes* [41]. Volume rendering techniques, such as [18], [40]

provide direct visualization of the complete volumetric data. Prior segmentation is not required explicitly, however, the color and transparency of the image data are determined by the transfer functions [52]. Several approaches have been proposed to accelerate volume rendering, including adaptive methods, shell rendering, volume encoding, and the most efficient hardware-assisted 3D texture mapping [97]. Figures 4, 5cd, and 9 show examples of volume visualization techniques, while multiplanar reformatting is illustrated in Figures 7 and 10.

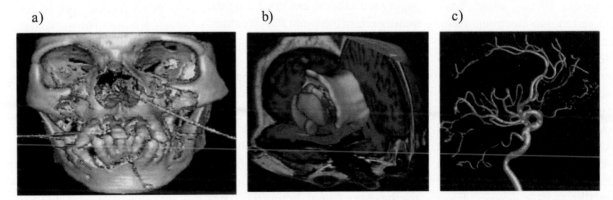

Fig. 4. Volume visualization: a) surface rendered skull from CT data of a car-accident victim; b) hybrid volume and surface rendering of MRI head and the 3D atlas represented as polygonal models; c) volume rendering of cerebral angiographic data.

2.5. Human body modeling

Human body modeling provides the means for prediction, evaluation, simulation, validation, and for enhancing the outcomes of diagnosis and treatment. When models are adapted to the patient, information that is

inherent in them is then automatically mapped to the patient-specific data. This is achieved via registration, which in its simpler form is rigid and in a more complex form is deformable.

Making maps, the collections of which form atlases, is an ancient art-

science. The map represents, organizes, and communicates data on the object of interest. Throughout history man has been producing maps of objects around him, initially the land and sea, later on other planets and solar systems, and most recently the human genome and human brain. Numerous types of brain atlases have been constructed varying in the material used as well as their functionality and applications. A taxonomy of brain atlases with the associated tools is presented in [57].

Printed atlases. A number of brain atlases have been published, such as [16], [19], [21], [37], [47], [48], [49]. In addition, several stereotactic brain atlases have been constructed since the 1950s, including [2], [3], [72], [75], [76], [83], [84], [85], [86], [92].

Electronic stereotactic atlases. Deformable electronic atlases overcome several limitations of the printed atlases and open new possibilities. In addition to atlas warping, they offer new features not available in printed atlases, such as interactive labeling of scans, flexible ways of presentation in 2D and 3D (or even in *n*-dimensional space capturing dynamic changes or multi-modal atlases), defining regions of interest, mensuration, searching capabilities, and integration of information from multiple sources.

To combine the widely accepted stereotactic printed atlases with the capabilities offered by electronic atlases, several printed atlases have been converted into electronic form, including: Schaltenbrand-Bailey atlas [29], [34], [101]; Schaltenbrand-Wahren atlas [32], [51], [53), [81]; Talairach-Tournoux atlas [29], [53]; Referentially Oriented Talairach-Tournoux atlas [53]; Ono *et al* atlas [54]; Afshar *et al* atlas [50] and Van Buren-Borke atlas [29]. Computerized versions of printed atlases may vary substantially from a simple, direct digitization of the original material to a sophisticated, fully segmented, labeled, enhanced, and three-dimensionally extended deformable atlas.

Other electronic brain atlases. Many other types of brain atlases have been developed. They include MRI-based atlases [30], [35], [39], [79]; cryosection-based atlases [8], [17],

[28], [89]; multi-modal Visible Human-derived atlases [31], [77]; brain animations [82]; probabilistic anatomical atlases [20], [44], [45], [87], [91]; surface-based atlases [93]; surface-based probabilistic atlases [94]; and probabilistic functional atlases constructed from microrecordings [66].

***Cerefy* electronic brain atlas database**. The *Cerefy* electronic brain atlas database, [54], [62], [63] contains complementary atlases with gross anatomy, subcortical structures, brain connections, and sulcal patterns. It was derived from the classic printed brain atlases edited by Thieme:

- *Atlas for Stereotaxy of the Human Brain* by Schaltenbrand and Wahren [76];
- *Co-Planar Stereotactic Atlas of the Human Brain* by Talairach and Tournoux [85];
- *Atlas of the Cerebral Sulci* by Ono, Kubik, and Abernathey [72];
- *Referentially Oriented Cerebral MRI Anatomy: Atlas of Stereotaxic Anatomical Correlations for Gray and White Matter* by Talairach and Tournoux [86].

We digitized these complementary printed atlases and then enhanced, segmented, labeled, extended, aligned, and organized them into atlas volumes, Figure 5.

The anatomical index has about 1000 structures per hemisphere and more than 400 sulcal patterns. The electronic atlas images were pre-labeled to speed up structure labeling in atlas-based applications. About 17,000 labels were placed manually for the entire *Cerefy* brain atlas database. Three-dimensional extensions of the atlases were also constructed. In addition, all 2D and 3D atlases were mutually co-registered.

The *Cerefy* brain atlas database is applicable to neurosurgery [55], [56], [60], [65]; neuroradiology [61], [63], [67], [69]; brain mapping [59], [68]; and neuroeducation [70].

3. Model-assisted neuroeducation

Electronic atlases are commonly used in neuroeducation. Pioneering applications include *ADAM* [1], *BrainStorm* [17], *Digital Anatomist* [82], *VOXEL-MAN* [30], and several other reviewed in [54]. Most existing electronic brain atlases are teaching programs for education. They are typically HyperCard type systems, based on a collection of planar images. The *Digital Anatomist*, as opposed to 2D systems, contains animated 3D images of the human brain. Most of these atlases use predefined images and fixed animations, and offer limited visualization capabilities. Those limitations are overcome by constructing 3D brain atlases based on radiological images (CT, MRI) or Visible Human Data, such as the *VOXEL-MAN* [30], *Anatomy Browser* [25], and some other listed in the previous section. The limitations of these 3D atlases include lack of registration capabilities and a coarse anatomical parcellation of cerebral structures.

The *Cerefy Student Brain Atlas* [70] is a user-friendly application on CD-ROM for wide use in neuroeducation. It is useful for medical students, residents, and teachers. This application contains MRI and atlas images of gross anatomy and related textual materials. It also provides testing and scoring capabilities for exam preparation, as illustrated in Figure 6.

The *Cerefy Student Brain Atlas* is a comprehensive, powerful, extensible yet simple tool. Its novelty includes:

- atlas-assisted localization of cerebral structures on radiological images
- atlas-assisted interactive labeling simultaneously on axial, coronal, and sagittal planes
- atlas-assisted testing against location and name of cerebral structures
- saving of the labeled images suitable for preparing teaching materials.

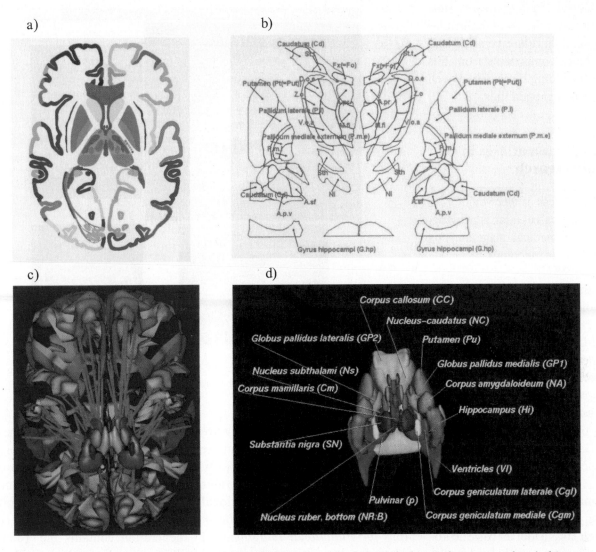

Fig. 5. *Cerefy* electronic brain atlas database: a) 2D axial atlas image with color-coded subcortical structures and cortical areas; b) 2D coronal contour image labeled with subcortical structures; c) 3D atlas with cortical areas, subcortical structures, and brain connections; d) 3D atlas labeled with subcortical structures.

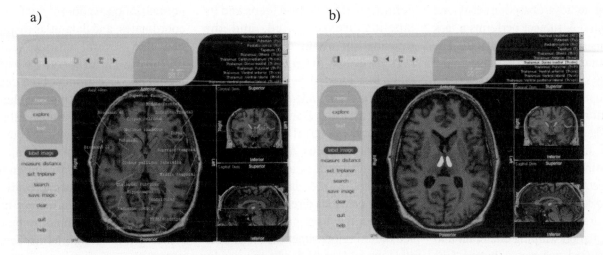

Fig. 6. The *Cerefy Student Brain Atlas*: a) interactive labeling of brain structures on the orthogonal MRI images; b) localization of the cerebral structure selected from the anatomical index (the thalamic dorso-medial nucleus is highlighted).

The *Cerefy Student Brain Atlas* exploits a part of the *Cerefy* brain atlas database and its future versions will include more components from this database (including 3D models) as well as more imaging modalities.

4. Use of brain atlases in medical research

The usefulness of electronic brain atlases in medical research is growing, particularly in medical image analysis and human brain mapping.

4.1. Medical image analysis

The gold standard in medical image analysis is the *ANALYZE* system from the Mayo Clinic [74]. This is a powerful, comprehensive visualization tool for multi-dimensional display, processing, and analysis of biomedical images from multiple imaging modalities. To facilitate analysis of brain images, the *Cerefy* brain atlas has been integrated with *ANALYZE*, Figure 7.

4.2. Human brain mapping

Human brain mapping has tremendous potential as a tool for basic neuro-scientific investigation. Its goal for the normal human brain is to clarify how the brain works in general rather than for any particular individual. Human brain mapping studies are based on behavioral conditions. A subject performs a task while his or her brain is imaged. The human brain varies across subjects and no single study can fully characterize a mental operation and its location in the population. Therefore, processes of knowledge discovery require combining studies from various sources. To compare individual brains, it is necessary to: (*i*) establish a standard, reference brain representation into which the results will be transformed; (*ii*) determine a transformation warping one brain into the standard reference brain; (*iii*) establish a coordinate system for specifying positions within the brain.

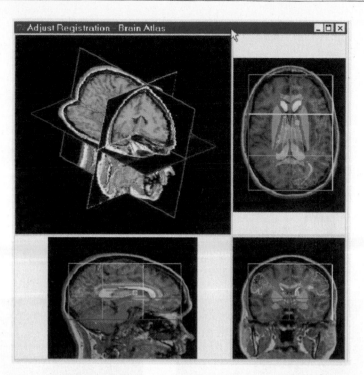

Fig. 7. The *Cerefy* atlas inside Mayo's *ANALYZE*. The Talairach grid is displayed allowing the user to warp interactively the atlas against the data by using the Talairach transformation.

There are numerous software packages for functional image generation as reviewed in [26], [59]. None of them, however, provides atlas-assisted analysis of functional images. *BrainMap* [22] and the *Brain Atlas for Functional Imaging* [59] allow for labeling of functional images. *BrainMap* is an Internet application that does not provide direct access to the atlas. The definition of activation locus and its labeling are separated, and the information about the activation regions is lost during labeling. To label loci located beyond the atlas structures, *BrainMap* uses a so-called Talairach Daemon [38] that looks for the cortical area closest to the activation locus, and the label of this cortical area is assigned to the locus. The *Brain Atlas for Functional Imaging* provides direct access to the atlas and the user can display the activation regions superimposed on the atlas, and place and edit the marks corresponding to activation regions to have them labelable.

Besides providing labeling, the *Brain Atlas for Functional Imaging* has numerous features supporting localization analysis of functional images. None of the existing software packages for functional image generation contains the Talairach-Tournoux atlas, which is the gold standard in human brain mapping research. In addition, it provides numerous functions such as fast data normalization, readout of the Talairach coordinates, and data-atlas display. It has also several unique features including interactive warping, facilitating fine tuning of the data-to-atlas fit, backtracking mechanism compensating for missing Talairach landmarks and enhancing the outcome of the overall process of data analysis, multi-atlas multi-label labeling, navigation on the triplanar formed by the data and the atlas, multiple-images-in-one display with atlas-anatomy-function blending, loci editing in terms of content and placement, fast locus-controlled generation of results, and reading and saving of the loci list, see Figure 8.

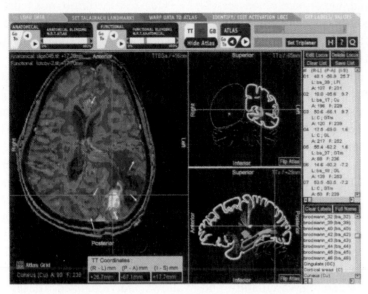

Fig. 8. The *Brain Atlas for Functional Imaging*. The MRI anatomical dataset is fused with a color-coded functional dataset. The region of the tumor is labeled by using the atlas.

- increased neuroradiologist confidence in terms of anatomy and spatial relationships by providing interactive multiple labeling of the scan on the orthogonal planes and triplanar display with one plane from the scan and the other two from the atlas;
- potentially reduced cost by providing some information from mutually co-registered atlases which otherwise has to be acquired from other modalities;
- reduced time in learning neuro-anatomy and scan interpretation by providing 3D and triplanar displays and labeling of multi-modal scans.

5. Model-enhanced diagnosis

Early studies showed a considerable optimism regarding the capabilities of computers and artificial intelligence to automatically generate complete diagnosis. From several categories of systems, such as fully automatic computer diagnosis, interactive computer diagnosis, and computer-supported diagnosis, only the last has survived. Currently, it generally understood is that the computer should provide a physician with the necessary information to make a diagnosis rather than to act as a diagnostician.

To our best knowledge, the only model-enhanced application for neuroradiology used globally is our Internet-enabled *Cerefy Neuroradiology Atlas* [69]. This application assists the neuroradiologist in speeding up scan interpretation by rapid labeling of morphological and/or functional scans, displaying the underlying anatomy for functional studies, and facilitating multi-modal fusion.

The understanding of underlying anatomy in the scan is easy for a neuroradiologist, but communicating this knowledge to others may be tedious and time-consuming. The *Cerefy*

Neuroradiology Atlas which contains a deformable and labeled atlas is well suited for an efficient transfer of this knowledge to other clinicians, such as neurosurgeons, neurologists, referring physicians, and to medical students. It allows the neuroradiologist to annotate the scan with text, regions of interest and measured distances, and then label the structures of interest. The annotated and labeled scan can be saved in Dicom and/or XML formats, giving the neuroradiologist the possibility to store the atlas-enhanced scan in a PACS and to use it in web-enabled applications. In this way, the scan interpretation done by the neuroradiologist can easily be communicated to other clinicians and medical students. As illustrated in [63], [67], the advantages of the use of brain atlases in neuroradiology include:

- reduced time in image interpretation by providing interactive multiple labeling, triplanar display, higher parcellation than the scan itself, multi-modal fusion, and display of underlying anatomy for functional images;
- facility to communicate information about the interpreted scans from the neuroradiologist to other clinicians and medical students;

6. Model-enhanced neurosurgery

The successful use of flight simulators has inspired their application to surgical training and planning. Advances in computer graphics, tissue modeling, haptic instrumentation, and computer capabilities have enabled the development of computer-based surgical simulators. Before performing a neurosurgical procedure on a real patient, the neurosurgeon is able to practice on high-fidelity computer models of patient-specific data to simulate the intervention. In this way, safer and more effective surgical approaches can be planned, requiring less time in an operating room.

Computer-based surgical simulation is useful for education, training, pre-operative planning, and skill assessment. Virtual reality-based surgical simulators only recently have become available due to the complexity of anatomy and the demanding performance to interact directly with volumetric, usually multi-modal, images. A virtual reality simulator should be able to simulate surgical procedures, such as cutting, drilling, grasping, sucking, suturing, and knot tying. Requirements for this type of simulator include: real-time interaction; realism to represent the accurate and detailed shape of patient's organ; quantitative deformation; haptic feedback; and simulation of a variety of surgical operations.

Two types of models are used in computer-aided systems for brain intervention:

· those directly derived from patient-specific data by using segmentation and modeling techniques
· pre-defined ones, such as brain atlases, which are matched to the patient-specific data by using registration techniques.

The first type of model is used in our two applications, *VIVIAN* and *NeuroCath*. The second type of model is used particularly in stereotactic and functional neurosurgery systems.

VIVIAN, or Virtual Intracranial Visualization And Navigation [36], is a system developed for preoperative neurosurgical planning and simulation. It is used to plan complicated cases such as tumor resection in the skull base region, vascular malformation, and separations of craniopagus twins. By using 3D, two-hand intuitive interaction, the neurosurgeon interacts with multi-modal images of a patient's

skull, brain, tumor, and blood vessels fused together and displayed as a single 3D virtual object. The surgeon simulates bone and tissue removal in the image to plan the optimal entry path for tumor resection. *VIVIAN* provides 3D interactive segmentation tools to extract and model critical objects of a patient's anatomy and pathology.

NeuroCath is a computer environment for planning interventional neuroradiology procedures [71]. It supports the extraction of vasculature from patient-specific data, models the physical behaviors between the interventional devices and cerebral vasculature, and provides the tactile apparatus that gives the clinician the sense of touch during intervention planning and training, as shown in Figure 9.

The first stereotactic brain atlases in printed form, such as [75], [84], were constructed in the 1950s. It took about two decades to make the first brain atlases in electronic form available in clinical settings [7]. After another two decades, at the end of the 1990s, electronic brain atlases have become commonplace in stereotactic and functional neurosurgery [29], [60], [66].

Our *Cerefy* brain atlas database [54], [62], [63] has become the standard in stereotactic and functional neurosurgery. It has already been integrated with major image guided surgery systems including the *StealthStation* (Medtronic/Sofamor-Danek), *Target* (BrainLab), *SurgiPlan* (Elekta), *SNN 3 Image Guided Surgery System* (Surgical Navigation Network), and a neurosurgical robot *NeuroMate* (Integrated Surgical Systems). One of the simplest atlas-assisted approaches is to use *The Electronic Clinical Brain Atlas* on CD-ROM [53]. It allows individualized atlases to be generated without loading the patient-specific data. This is useful for anatomical targeting. The planning procedure for stereotactic and functional neurosurgery by using this CD-ROM was proposed in [56]. The atlas is conformed to the patient's scan by means of a 2D local deformation done by matching the atlas' rectangular region of interest to the corresponding data region of interest.

The *NeuroPlanner* is another application developed by us for stereotactic and functional neurosurgery, as illustrated in Figure 10.

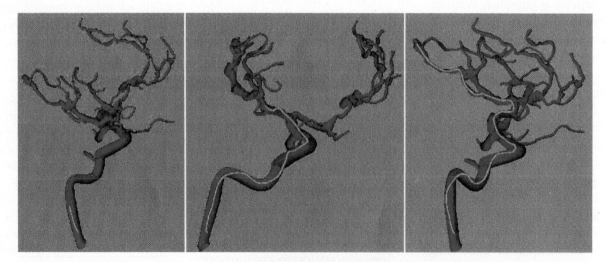

Fig. 9. Interventional neuroradiology simulation: subsequent stages of interventional device navigation. The interventional neuroradiologist can interactively insert the guidewire and the catheter, and manipulate the cerebral vascular model along with the interventional devices by rotating and zooming them.

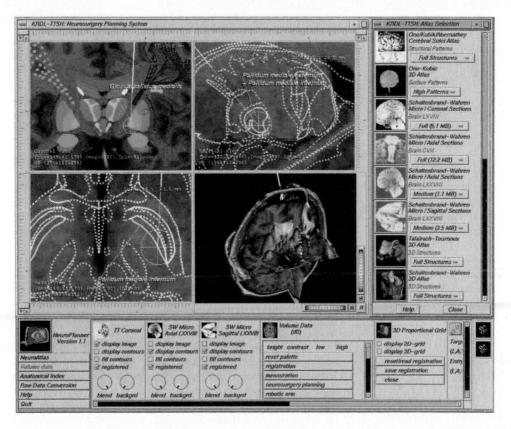

Fig. 10. The *NeuroPlanner*. Functional neurosurgery planning using multiple atlases in multiple orientations. (Center): four views showing the orthogonal data sections registered with the atlases in image and contour representations, and the data-atlas triplanar registered with the 3D atlas. The target structure is highlighted and labeled. The stereotactic trajectory (the thin line) along with the current position of the microelectrode (the thick line) are displayed in all views. (Right): atlas selection panel with multiple atlases in multiple resolutions. (Bottom): control panel with the surgery planning modules and atlas controls.

It supports preoperative planning and training, intraoperative procedures, and postoperative follow-up [60]. It comprises mutually co-registered atlases from the *Cerefy* brain atlas database including their 3D extensions [54]. The *NeuroPlanner* provides four groups of functions: data-related (data interpolation, reformatting, image processing); atlas-related (atlas-to-data interactive 3D warping, 2D and 3D interactive multiple labeling); atlas-data exploration-related (interaction in three orthogonal and one 3D views, continuous data-atlas exploration); and neurosurgery-related (targeting, path planning, mensuration, simulating the insertion of a microelectrode, simulating therapeutic lesioning). The advantages of using the *Cerefy* brain atlases for stereotactic and functional neurosurgery are summarized in [62].

The *BrainBench* [80] is a virtual reality-based surgical planning system for stereotactic frame neurosurgery. It contains a suite of neurosurgery supporting tools and the *Cerefy* brain atlas. The *BrainBench* helps the neurosurgeon to prepare faster plans; have more accurate anatomical targeting; improve the avoidance of critical structures; have fewer sub-optimal frame attachments and speedier, more effective planning and training.

Our recent development in functional neurosurgery is a probabilistic functional atlas constructed from microrecordings collected during the treatment of hundreds of Parkinson's disease patients. This atlas along with the method for its generation will be delivered to the neurosurgeons via an Internet portal [66].

Acknowledgment

Numerous individuals and institutions contributed to this multiple year work. *The Electronic Clinical Brain Atlas* was a joint development with Prof. R. N. Bryan of the Johns Hopkins Hospital, USA. The *Brain Atlas for Functional Imaging* was developed in consultation with Dr. D. N. Kennedy of Massachusetts General Hospital, USA. The integration of the atlas with *ANALYZE* was done by the Mayo Clinic, USA and Figure 7 is courtesy of Prof. R. A. Robb of Mayo. The *NeuroPlanner* was developed within a joint project with Dr. T. T. Yeo of Tan Tock Seng Hospital/National Neuroscience Institute, Singapore. The construction of the probabilistic functional atlas is ongoing joint work with Prof. A. L. Benabid, France. *NeuroCath* is a joint development with Prof. J. Anderson of Johns Hopkins Hospital. The development of *NeuroPlanner* and *Brain Bench/VIVIAN* was supported by grants from the National Science and Technology

Board, Singapore. Key contributors to the development of applications described here include D. Belov, C. K. Chui, A. Fang, L. Jagannathan, R. A. Kockro, H. Ng, L Serra, A. Thirunavuukarasuu, Y. P. Wang, and G. L. Yang.

References

1. A.D.A.M. Animated Dissection of Anatomy for Medicine. Users's Guide. A.D.A.M. Software Inc.; 1994.

2. Afshar E, Watkins ES, Yap JC. Stereotactic Atlas of the Human Brainstem and Cerebellar Nuclei. New York: Raven Press; 1978.

3. Andrew J, Watkins ES. A Stereotaxic Atlas of the Human Thalamus and Adjacent Structures. A Variability Study. Baltimore: Williams and Wilkins; 1969.

4. Atkins MS, Mackiewich B. Fully automatic segmentation of the brain in MRI. IEEE Trans Med Imaging 1998;17(1):98-107.

5. Bajcsy R., Lieberson R. and Reivich M. A computerized system for elastic matching of deformed radiographic images to idealized atlas images. J Comput Assist Tomogr 1983;7(6):618-25.

6. Bajcsy R, Kovacic S. Multiresolution elastic matching. Computer Vision, Graphics and Image Processing, 1989;46:1-21.

7. Bertrand G, Olivier A, Thompson CJ. Computer display of stereotaxic brain maps and probe tracts. Acta Neurochir Suppl 1974;21:235-43.

8. Bohm C, Greitz T, Eriksson L. A computerized adjustable brain atlas. Eur J Nucl Med 1983;15:687-9.

9. Bookstein F. Principal warps: thin-plate splines and the decomposition of deformations. IEEE Trans. Pattern Analysis and Machine Intelligence 1989;11(6):567-85.

10. Brown LG. A survey of image reconstruction techniques. ACM Computing Surveys 1992;24(4):325-76.

11. Collins DL, Neelin P, Peters TM, Evans AC. Automatic 3D intersubject registration of MR volumetric data into standardized Talairach space. J Comput Assist Tomogr 1994;18(2):192-205.

12. Collins DL, Evans AC. Animal: validation and application of non-liner registration-based segmentation. International Journal of Pattern Recognition and Artificial Intelligence 1997;11:1271-94.

13. Christensen GE, Joshi SC, Miller MI. Volume geometric transformations for mapping anatomy. IEEE Trans Med Imaging 1997;16:864-77.

14. Clarke LP, Velthuizen RP, Camacho MA, Heine JJ, Vaidyanathan M, Hall LO, Thatcher RW, Silbiger ML. MRI segmentation: methods and applications. Magn Reson Imaging 1995;13(3):334-68.

15. Davatzikos C. Spatial transformation and registration of brain images using elastically deformable model. Comput Vis Image Underst 1997;66(2):207-22.

16. DeArmond SJ, Fusco MM and Dewey MM. Structure of the Human Brain. A Photographics Atlas. 3rd ed. New York: Oxford University Press; 1989.

17. Dev P, Coppa G. P. and Tancred E. BrainStorm: desiging an interactive neuroanatomy atlas. Radiology 1992;185(P):413.

18. Drebin R, Carpenter L, Harrahan P. Volume rendering. Comput Graph (ACM) 1988;24(4):64-75.

19. Duvernoy H.M. The Human Hippocampus: an Atlas of Applied Anatomy. Bergman, Munch; 1988.

20. Evans AC, Collins DL, Milner B. An MRI-based stereotactic brain atlas from 300 young normal subjects. Proceedings of the 22nd Symposium of the Society for Neuroscience; Anaheim. 1992:408.

21. Fix JD. Atlas of the Human Brain and Spinal Cord. Rockville: Aspen;1987.

22. Fox PT, Mikiten S, Davis G, Lancaster JL. BrainMap: a database of human functional brain mapping. In: Thatcher RW, Hallett M, Zeffiro T, John ER, Huerta M, editors. Functional Neuroimaging: Technical Foundations.; 1994. p. 95-106.

23. Fu KS, Mui JK. A survey of image segmentation. Pattern Recognition 1981;13(1):3-16.

24. Gee JC, Reivich M, Bajcsy R. Elastically deforming an atlas to match anatomical brain images. J Comput Assist Tomogr 1993;17(2):225-36.

25. Golland P, Kikinis R, Halle M, Umans C, Grimson WE, Shenton ME, et al. Anatomy Browser: a novel approach to visualization and integration of medical information. Comput Aid Surg 1999;4:129-43.

26. Gold S, Christian B, Arndt S, Zeien G, Cizadlo T, Johnson DL, et al. Functional MRI statistical software packages: a comparative analysis. Hum Brain Mapp 1998;6:73-84.

27. Grachev D, Berdichevsky D, Rauch SL, Heckers S, Kennedy DN, Caviness VS, et al. A method for assessing the accuracy of intersubject registration of the human brain using anatomic landmarks, Neuroimage 1999 Feb;9(2):250-68.

28. Greitz T, Bohm C, Holte S et al. A computerized brain atlas: construction, anatomical content, and some applications. J Comput Assist Tomogr 1991;15(1):26-38.

29. Hardy TL, Deming LR, Harris-Collazo R. Computerized stereotactic atlases. In: Alexander III E, Maciunas RJ, editors. Advanced Neurosurgical Navigation. New York: Thieme; 1999. p. 115-24.

30. Höhne KH. VOXEL-MAN, Part 1: Brain and Skull. Heidelberg: Springer-Verlag; 1995.

31. Höhne KH, Pflesser B, Pommert A, Riemer M, Schubert R, Schiemann T, et al. A realistic model of human structure from the Visible Human data, Methods Inf Med 2001:83-9.

32. Kall BA. Computer-assisted stereotactic functional neurosurgery. In: . Kelly PJ, Kall BA, editors. Computers in Stereotactic Neurosurgery. Boston: Blackwell; 1992. p.134-42.

33. Kapur T, Grimson WEL, Wells III WM, Kikinis R. Segmentation of brain tissue from magnetic resonance images. Med Image Anal 1996;1(2):109-27.

34. Kazarnovskaya MI, Borodkin SM, Shabalov VA, Krivosheina VY, Golanov AV. 3-D computer model of subcortical structures of human brain. Comput Biol Med 1991;21(6):451-7.

35. Kikinis R, Shenton ME, Iosifescu DV, et al. A digital brain atlas for surgical planning, model-driven segmentation, and teaching. IEEE Transactions on Visualization and Computer Graphics 1996;2(3):232-41.

36. Kockro RA, Serra L, Yeo TT, Chan C, Sitoh YY, Chua GG, et al. Planning and simulation of neurosurgery in a virtual reality environment. Neurosurgery 2000;46(1):118-37.

37. Kraus GE, Bailey GJ. Microsurgical Anatomy of the Brain. A Stereo Atlas. Baltimore: Wiliams & Wilkins; 1994.

38. Lancaster JL, Woldorff MG, Parsons LM, Liotti M, Freitas CS, Rainey L, et al. Automated Talairach atlas labels for functional brain mapping. Hum Brain Mapp 2000;10(3):120-31.

39. Lehmann ED, Hawkes D, Hill D, Bird CF, Robinson GP, Colchester AC, et al. Computer-aided interpretation of SPECT images of the brain using an MRI-derived neuroanatomic atlas. Med Inform 1991;16:151-66.

40. Levoy M. Display of surfaces from volume data. IEEE Computer Graphics and Applications 1988;8(5):29-37.

41. Lorensen W, Cline H. Marching cubes: a high resolution 3D surface construction algorithm. Comput Graph 1987;21:163-9.

42. Maintz JBA, Viergever MA. A survey of medical image registration. Med Image Anal 1998;2(1):1-36.

43. Martin J. Neuroanatomy. Text and Atlas. Norwalk: Appleton & Lange;1989.

44. Mazziotta JC, Toga AW, Evans AC, Fox P, Lancaster J. A probabilistic atlas of the human brain: theory and rationale for its development. NeuroImage 1995;2:89-101.

45. Mazziotta JC. Imaging: window on the brain. Arch Neurol 2000;57(10):1413-21.

46. McInerney T, Terzopoulos D. Deformable models in medical image analysis: a survey. Med Image Anal 1996;1(2):91-108.

47. McMinn RMH, Hutchings RT, Pegington J, Abrahams P. Color Atlas of Human Anatomy. 3rd ed. Mosby Year Book. St. Louis; 1993.

48. Netter FH. The CIBA Collection of Medical Illustrations. Vol 1: Nervous System. CIBA; 1991.

49. Nieuwennhuys R, Voogd J, van Huijzen C. The Human Central Nervous System. A Synopsis and Atlas. 2nd ed. Berlin: Springer-Verlag; 1981.

50. Niemann K, van den Boom R, Haeselbarth K, Afshar F. A brainstem stereotactic atlas in a three-dimensional magnetic resonance imaging navigation system: first experiences with atlas-to-patient registration. J Neurosurg 1999;90(5):891-901.

51. Niemann K, van Nieuwenhofen I. One atlas - three anatomies: relationships of the Schaltenbrand and Wahren microscopic data. Acta Neurochir (Wien) 1999;141(10):1025-38.

52. Nowinski WL, Ho WC. Generalized transfer functions and their use for three-dimensional neuroimaging. Proc SPIE Medical Imaging 1994: Image Capture, Formatting, and Display, Newport Beach, CA, USA, February 1994, SPIE Vol. 2164. p. 34-45.

53. Nowinski WL, Bryan RN, Raghavan R. The Electronic Clinical Brain Atlas. Multiplanar Navigation of the Human Brain. New York – Stuttgart: Thieme; 1997.

54. Nowinski WL, Fang A, Nguyen BT, Raphel JK, Jagannathan L, Raghavan R, et al. Multiple brain atlas database and atlas-based neuroimaging system. Comput Aid Surg 1997;2(1):42-66.

55. Nowinski WL Anatomical targeting in functional neurosurgery by the simultaneous use of multiple Schaltenbrand-Wahren brain atlas microseries. Stereotact Funct Neurosurg 1998;71:103-16.

56. Nowinski WL, Yeo TT, Thirunavuukarasuu A. Microelectrode-guided functional neurosurgery assisted by Electronic Clinical Brain Atlas CD-ROM. Comput Aid Surg 1998;3(3):115-22.

57. Nowinski WL. Analysis of medical images by means of brain atlases. Computer Graphics and Vision 1999:8(3);449-468.

58. Nowinski WL, Thirunavuukarasuu A. Methods and apparatus for processing medical images. Patent application PCT/SG00/00185; 2000.

59. Nowinski WL, Thirunavuukarasuu A, Kennedy DN. Brain Atlas for Functional Imaging. Clinical and Research Applications. New York – Stuttgart: Thieme; 2000.

60. Nowinski WL, Yang GL, Yeo TT. Computer-aided stereotactic functional neurosurgery enhanced by the use of the multiple brain atlas database. IEEE Trans Med Imaging 2000;19(1):62-9.

61. Nowinski WL, Thirunavuukarasuu A, Srinivasan R. Brain atlas for neuroradiology. Scientific Program, 86th Radiological Society of North America Annual Meeting, Nov-Dec 2000, Chicago, IL, USA, Supplement to Radiology, 217 (P). p. 620.

62. Nowinski WL Computerized atlases for surgery of movement disorders. Seminars in Neurosurgery 2001;12(2):183-94.

63. Nowinski WL. Electronic brain atlases: features and applications. In: Caramella D, Bartolozzi C, editors. 3D Image Processing: Techniques and Clinical Applications. Medical Radiology series, Heidelberg: Springer-Verlag; 2002.

64. Nowinski WL. Modified Talairach landmarks. Acta Neurochir 2001;143(10): 1045-57.

65. Nowinski WL. Computer-aided brain surgery: present and future. In: Caramella D, Bartolozzi C, editors. 3D Image Processing: Techniques and Clinical Applications. Medical Radiology series, Heidelberg: Springer-Verlag; 2002.

66. Nowinski WL, Benabid AL. New directions in atlas-assisted stereotactic functional neurosurgery. In: Germano IM, editor. Advanced Techniques in Image-Guided Brain and Spine Surgery. Thieme, New York: Thieme; 2002.

67. Nowinski WL, Thirunavuukarasuu A. Electronic atlases show value in brain studies. Diagnostic Imaging Asia Pacific 2001;8(2):35-9.

68. Nowinski WL, Thirunavuukarasuu A. Atlas-assisted localization analysis of functional images. Med Image Anal 2001;5(3):207-20.

69. Nowinski WL, Thirunavuukarasuu A, Belov A, Yang YJ. Web-based atlas for neuroradiology. Proc American Society of Neuroradiology 39th Annual Meeting ASNR2001, 23-27 April 2001, Boston, MA, USA. p.500. Available from http://www.cerefy.com

70. Nowinski WL, Thirunavuukarasuu A Bryan RN. Cerefy Student Brain Atlas. KRDL, Singapore: KRDL; 2001.

71. Nowinski WL, Chui CK. Simulation of interventional neuroradiology procedures. Proc Medical Imaging and Augmented Reality MIAR2001, Hong Kong, 10-12 June 2001. IEEE Computer Society Press. p. 87-94.

72. Ono M, Kubik S, Abernathey CD. Atlas of the Cerebral Sulci. Stuttgart - New York: Georg Thieme Verlag/Thieme Medical Publishers; 1990.

73. Pal NR, Pal SK. A review of image segmentation techniques. Pattern Recognition 1993;26(9):1227-49.

74. Robb RA, Hanson DP. The ANALYZE software system for visualization and analysis in surgery simulation. In: Lavallee S, Tayor R, Burdea G, Mosges R, editors. Computer Integrated Surgery. Cambridge MA: MIT Press;1995. p. 175-90.

75. Schaltenbrand G, Bailey. Introduction to Stereotaxis with an Atlas of the Human Brain. Stuttgart: Georg Thieme Verlag; 1959.

76. Schaltenbrand G, Wahren W. Atlas for Stereotaxy of the Human Brain. Stuttgart: Georg Thieme Verlag; 1977.

77. Schiemann T, Freudenberg J, Pflesser B, Pommert A, Priesmeyer K, Riemer M, et al. Exploring the Visible Human using the VOXEL-MAN framework. Comput Med Imaging Graph 2000;24(3):127-32.

78. Schitzlein HN, Murtagh FR. Imaging Anatomy of the Head and Spine. A Photographic Color Atlas of MRI, CT, Gross, and Microscopic Anatomy in Axial, Coronal, and Sagittal Planes. 2nd ed. Baltimore: Urban & Schwarzenberg; 1990.

79. Schmahmann JD, Doyon J, McDonald D, Holmes C, Lavoie K, Hurwitz AS, et al. Three-dimensional MRI atlas of the human cerebellum in proportional stereotaxic space. Neuroimage 1999;10(3 Pt 1):233-60.

80. Serra L, Nowinski WL, Poston T, Hern N, Meng LC, Guan CG, et al. The Brain Bench: virtual tools for stereotactic frame neurosurgery. Med Image Anal 1997;1(4):317-29.

81. Sramka M, Ruzicky E, Novotny M. Computerized brain atlas in functional neurosurgery. Stereotact Funct Neurosurg 1997;69(1-4 Pt 2):93-8.

82. Sundsten JW, Brinkley JF, Eno K, Prothero J. The Digital Anatomist. Interactive Brain Atlas. CD ROM for the Macintosh, University of Washington, Seattle; 1994.

83. Szikla G, Bouvier G, Hori T, Petrov V. Angiography of the Human Brain Cortex: Atlas of Vascular Patterns and Stereotactic Localization. Berlin: Springer-Verlag; 1977.

84. Talairach J, David M, Tournoux P, Corredor H, Kvasina T. Atlas d'Anatomie Stereotaxique des Noyaux Gris Centraux. Paris: Masson; 1957.

85. Talairach J, Tournoux P. Co-Planar Stereotactic Atlas of the Human Brain.

Stuttgart - New York: Georg Thieme Verlag/Thieme Medical Publishers; 1988.

86. Talairach J, Tournoux P. Referentially Oriented Cerebral MRI Anatomy. Atlas of Stereotaxic Anatomical Correlations for Gray and White Matter. Stuttgart - New York: Georg Thieme Verlag/Thieme Medical Publishers; 1993.

87. Thompson PM, Woods RP, Mega MS, Toga AW. Mathematical/computational challenges in creating deformable and probabilistic atlases of the human brain. Hum Brain Mapp 2000;9(2):81-92.

88. Thirion JP. Image matching as a diffusion process: an analogy with Maxwell's demons. Med Image Anal 1998;2:243-60.

89. Toga AW, Ambach KL, Schluender S. High-resolution anatomy from in situ human brain. Neuroimage 1994;1(4):334-44.

90. Toga AW, editor. Brain Warping. San Diego: Academic Press; 1998.

91. Toga AW, Thompson PM. Maps of the brain. Anat Rec 2001;265(2):37-53.

92. Van Buren JM, Borke RC. Variations and Connections of the Human Thalamus. New York: Springer-Verlag; 1972.

93. Van Essen DC, Drury HA. Structural and functional analyses of human cerebral cortex using a surface-based atlas. J Neurosci 1997;17(18):7079-102.

94. Van Essen DC, Lewis JW, Drury HA, Hadjikhani N, Tootell RB, Bakircioglu M, et al. Mapping visual cortex in monkeys and humans using surface-based atlases. Vision Res 2001;41(10-11):1359-78.

95. Wang Y, Staib LH. Physical model-based non-rigid registration incorporating statistical shape information. Med Image Anal 2000;4:7-20.

96. Wells WM, Viola P, Atsumi H, Nakajima S, Kikinis R. Multi-modal volume registration by maximization of mutual information. Med Image Anal 1997;1(1):35-51.

97. Westermann R, Ertl T. Efficiently using graphics hardware in volume rendering applications. Proc SIGGRAPH'98, Computer Graphics Proceedings, July 1998, Orlando, FL. p. 169-78.

98. Woods RP, Mazziotta JC, Cherry SR. MRI-PET Registration with Automated Algorithm. J Comput Assist Tomogr 1993;17:536-46.

99. Xu MH, Srinivasan R, Nowinski WL. A fast mutual information method for multi-modal registration. Lecture Notes in Computer Science, Vol. 1613, Proc Information Processing in Medical Imaging, 16th International Conference IPMI'99, June 28- July 2, Visegrad, Hungary. p. 466-71.

100. Xu MH, Nowinski WL. Talairach-Tournoux brain atlas registration using a metalforming principle based finite element method. Med Image Anal 2001;5(4):271-9.

101. Yoshida M. Three-dimensional maps by interpolation from the Schaltenbrand and Bailey atlas. In: Kelly PJ, Kall BA, editors. Computers in Stereotactic Neurosurgery. Boston: Blackwell; 1992. p. 143-52.

Address of the author:
Wieslaw L. Nowinski, DSc, PhD
Medical Imaging Lab
Kent Ridge Digital Labs
21 Heng Mui Keng Terrace
119613 Singapore
wieslaw@krdl.org.sg

J.F. Brinkley, C. Rosse

Structural Informatics Group
Department of Biological Structure
University of Washington
Seattle, USA

Review

Imaging Informatics and the Human Brain Project: the Role of Structure

1 The intersection of imaging informatics, structural informatics and neuroinformatics

The human brain is arguably the most complex and least understood of all organs in the body, yet relatively recent technological advances are rapidly opening up entirely new avenues for understanding its structure and function. Primary among these new technologies are images, not only of structure, but also of function, which provide increasingly detailed views of the thinking brain. These and other technologies have led to an explosion of research results in neuroscience, such that over 15,000 abstracts are presented at the annual meeting of the Society for Neuroscience (http://www.sfn.org).

As in other biomedical fields this proliferation of data has led to an information glut that makes it impossible for any one individual to comprehend more than a small fraction of the available results. Yet it is often argued that the only way we will truly understand the brain is to develop an integrated view that ties together data at levels ranging from genes to behavior.

As a response to this dilemma the Human Brain Project (HBP) [1-3] was initiated in 1993 as a result of an Institute of Medicine Report [4]. The goals of the HBP are to 1) develop reusable, generalizable and widely-available software tools that are specialized for neuroscience data and knowledge, 2) develop methods for integrating diverse forms of raw and processed neuroscience information, 3) develop Internet-based methods for sharing and disseminating the integrated information to promote knowledge discovery and the development of distributed, large scale models of brain function, and 4) apply these tools and information systems to research, clinical medicine and education. The hope is that by applying informatics tools and techniques to the fragmented data and knowledge that currently characterize neuroscience, it will be possible to regain a sense of wholeness from the ever-diversifying parts. The aggregate research endeavor that results from these and similar goals is called *neuroinformatics* [5].

One of the many neuroinformatics research questions that arise from these goals is how to integrate diverse forms of raw and processed information. Neuroscience data collected from humans alone come in multiple forms (e.g., sequence, image-based, electrophysiological, behavioral) at multiple levels (gene, molecular, ultrastructural, cellular, neural circuit, whole brain), and from multiple individuals. The fact that data come from multiple individuals is particularly difficult to address since no two human brains are exactly alike, let alone the brains of non-human species from which a large amount of data are obtained. Much of the research effort in the HBP and other neuroscience labs deals with the problem of relating multiple brains.

Anatomy is the common frame of reference for nearly all HBP efforts at integration, since anatomy in its broadest definition embraces all levels of structure from the molecular to the macroscopic [6]. (Neuro)anatomy not only provides an understanding of the physical organization of the brain, it also can serve as a framework for organizing all forms of neuroscience data. This postulate is consistent with a central tenet of modern biology, namely that function can only be understood in terms of the physical structure that underlies it.

This central role of anatomy is not limited to neuroscience. In fact, an understanding of the structure of the body is essential for virtually all biomedical endeavors since both normal and abnormal functions can be regarded as attributes of anatomical structures. We therefore argue that anatomy is a prime candidate for organizing and integrating not only neuroscience information but virtually all other biomedical information as well.

In order to develop such an anatomical (or structural) information framework many informatics research problems must be solved in areas such as representation, analysis, management, visualization and dissemination of anatomical information. Solutions to these problems require the application and invention of new methodologies rooted in computer science. These problem areas include, for instance, knowledge representation, image understanding, graphics, visualization, databases and user interfaces.

The richness of these problem areas, their broad applicability, and the commonality of anatomical patterns at multiple levels of organization have prompted us to define *structural informatics* as a field for dealing with the broad range of issues arising from the representation, management and use of information that pertains to the physical organization of the body [7]. We use the term *structural* as opposed to *anatomical* informatics to avoid the connotation of the term "anatomy" which, despite its definition to the contrary, is often limited to the macroscopic (gross) level.

The subject of this edition of the Yearbook is *imaging informatics* [8], which can be defined as the development of methods for organizing, managing, retrieving, analyzing and visualizing images. Images of all sorts obtained from any or all regions of the body are the central focus of imaging informatics.

From the point of view of structural informatics images are only one source

(though probably the most important one) of data about anatomical structures. Other sources include, for example, gene sequences, nuclear magnetic resonance spectroscopy, X-ray crystallography, the physical exam, endoscopy, and auscultation.

The focus of *neuroinformatics* is understanding the brain in all its aspects – anatomy, pathology, function (including behavior). Thus, images and anatomy are important components of neuroinformatics research, but they are not the only ones. Others include, for example, genetics, biochemistry, physiology, psychology, pathology, neurology, radiology and neurosurgery.

The subject of this review is the intersection of these three fields (structural-, imaging- and neuro informatics) within the context of the HBP. Of the 26 projects currently listed on the HBP research grants page (http://www.nimh.nih.gov/neuroinformatics/researchgrants.cfm) 19 use images as a primary source of data. We limit our review primarily to these and related projects because 1) we are most familiar with HBP work, 2) the HBP provides exemplary research projects in many relevant areas, 3) the HBP represents the primary national effort in the application of informatics to neuroscience, and 4) we wish to make the wider informatics community more aware of the HBP. However, we point out that a large amount of image related research deals with the brain, as evidenced by any issue of journals such as *IEEE Transactions on Medical Imaging*, and a large amount of non-HBP neuroscience research involves the use of images and anatomical information.

The paper is organized into three basic sections: structural imaging, functional imaging, and image-based brain information systems. Structural imaging provides the anatomical

substrate on which the functional data can be mapped, analogous to geographic information systems, which map various kinds of data to the earth. However, for brain mapping the problem is complicated by the fact that no two brains are alike.

2 Imaging the structure of the brain

Images are almost exclusively the source of data for visualizing and reconstructing the anatomy of the brain. Different imaging modalities provide complementary and often highly detailed anatomical information. All modalities are either inherently digital or can be converted to digital form by film scanning.

Traditional image sources are photographs of gross dissections, or microscopic sections that may be frozen (cryosections) or histochemically stained to emphasize certain structural components such as myelin [9]. Electron microscopy reveals the ultrastructure of the brain at the level of synaptic connections and cytoplasmic inclusions [10]. Immunocytochemical and DNA-hybridization techniques depict the distribution of specific proteins or messenger RNA, thereby allowing the expression of specific genes to be observed in different parts of the brain during development, maturity and senility [11]. From the image processing point of view all these image sources can be regarded as 2-D image sections.

In the living brain, computed tomography (CT) distinguishes different structures by virtue of their radiodensity, magnetic resonance imaging (MRI) distinguishes structures by their differential response to radio frequency pulses applied within a graded magnetic field, and magnetic resonance venography (MRV), and arteriography

(MRA) emphasize veins and arteries by altering the parameters of the radio frequency pulses [12]. An HBP-funded effort at Caltech is developing advanced methods for *in vivo* MR microscopic imaging that is being used to generate high resolution images of the developing embryo [13].

Traditional image sources provide 2-D views of parts of the brain. However, because the brain is three-dimensional, the most informative data come from techniques that either directly or indirectly image the entire 3-D volume of interest. Therefore, most current brain imaging research is concerned with 3-D image volume data.

Informatics issues that arise when dealing with 3-D structural brain images include image *registration, spatial* representation of anatomy, *symbolic* representation of anatomy, integration of spatial and symbolic anatomic representations in *atlases*, anatomical *variation*, and *characterization* of anatomy. All but the first of these issues deal primarily with anatomical structure, and therefore fall in the field of structural informatics. They could also be thought of as being part of imaging informatics and neuroinformatics. Depends on the point of view.

2.1 Image registration

Image volume data are represented in the computer by a 3-D volume array, in which each *voxel* (volume-element, analogous to *pixel* in 2-D) represents the image intensity in a small volume of space. In order to accurately depict brain anatomy, the *voxels* must be accurately *registered* (or located) in the 3-D volume, and separately acquired image *volumes* from the same subject must be *registered* with each other.

2.1.1 Voxel registration

Technologies such as CT, MRI, MRV and MRA (section 2) are inherently 3-D: the scanner generally outputs a series of image slices that can easily be reformatted as a 3-D volume array, often following alignment algorithms that compensate for any patient motion during the scanning procedure. Confocal microscopy [14], which generates a 3-D image volume through a tissue section, is also inherently 3-D, as is electron tomography, which generates 3-D images from thick electron-microscopic sections using techniques similar to those used in CT [15].

Two-dimensional images can be converted to 3-D volumes by acquiring a set of closely spaced parallel sections through a tissue or whole brain. In this case the problem is how to align the sections with each other. For whole brain sections (either frozen or fixed) the standard method is to embed a set of thin rods or strings in the tissue prior to sectioning, to manually indicate the location of these *fiducials* on each section, then to linearly transform each slice so that the corresponding fiducials line up in 3-D [16]. A popular current example of this technique is the Visible Human, in which a series of transverse slices were acquired, then reconstructed to give a full 3-D volume [17].

It is difficult to embed fiducial markers at the microscopic level, so intrinsic tissue landmarks are often used as fiducials, but the basic principle is similar. However, in this case tissue distortion may be a problem, so non-linear transformations may be required. For example Fiala and Harris [18] have developed an interface that allows the user to indicate, on electron microscopy sections, corresponding centers of small organelles such as mitochondria. A non-linear transformation (warp) is then computed to bring the landmarks into registration.

An approach being pursued (among other approaches) by the National Center for Microscopy and Imaging Research (http://ncmir.ucsd.edu/) combines reconstruction from thick serial sections with electron tomography [19]. In this case the tomographic technique is applied to each thick section to generate a 3-D digital slab, after which the slabs are aligned with each other to generate a 3-D volume. The advantages of this approach over the standard serial section method are that the sections do not need to be as thin, and fewer of them need be acquired.

An alternative approach to 3-D voxel registration from 2-D images is stereo-matching, a technique developed in computer vision that acquires multiple 2-D images from known angles, finds corresponding points on the images, and uses the correspondences and known camera angles to compute 3-D coordinates of pixels in the matched images. The technique is being applied to the reconstruction of synapses from electron micrographs by a HBP collaboration between computer scientists and biologists at the University of Maryland [20].

2.1.2 Volume registration

A related problem to that of aligning individual sections is the problem of aligning separate image volumes from the same subject, that is, *intra-subject* alignment. Because different image modalities provide complementary information, it is common to acquire more than one kind of image volume on the same individual. For example, in our own HBP work, we acquire an MRI volume dataset depicting cortical anatomy, an MRV volume depicting veins, and an MRA volume depicting arteries [21]. By "fusing" these separate modalities into a single common frame of reference (anatomy, as given by the MRI dataset), it is possible to gain information that is not apparent from one of the modalities alone. In our case the fused datasets are used to generate a visualization of the brain surface as it appears at neurosurgery, in which the veins and arteries provide prominent landmarks.

When intensity values are similar across modalities, linear alignment can be performed automatically by intensity-based optimization methods [22, 23]. When intensity values are not similar (as is the case with MRA, MRV and MRI), images can be aligned to templates of the same modalities that are already aligned [24,25]. Alternatively, landmark-based methods can be used. The landmark-based methods are similar to those used to align serial sections, but in this case the landmarks are 3-D points. The Montreal Register Program [26] (which can also do non-linear registration, as discussed in section 2.5.1) is an example of such a program.

2.2 Spatial representation of anatomy

The reconstructed 3-D image volume can be visualized directly using volume rendering techniques [27]. It can also be given as input to image-based techniques for warping the image volume of one brain to other, as described in section 2.5.1. However, more commonly the image volume is processed in order to extract an explicit *spatial* (or quantitative) representation of brain anatomy. Such an explicit representation permits improved visualization, quantitative analysis of brain structure, comparison of anatomy across a population, and mapping of functional data. It is thus a component of most research involving brain imaging.

Extraction of spatial representations of anatomy, in the form of 3-D surfaces or volume regions, is accomplished by segmenting (or isolating) brain structures from the 3-D image volume. Fully automated segmentation is an unsolved problem, as attested to by the number of papers about this subject in *IEEE Transactions on Medical Imaging*. However, because of the high quality of

MRI brain images, a great deal of progress has been made in recent years; in fact, several software packages do a credible job of automatic segmentation, particularly for normal macroscopic brain anatomy in cortical and sub-cortical regions [28-34]. The HBP-funded Internet Brain Segmentation Repository [35] is developing a repository of segmented brain images to use in comparing these different methods.

Popular segmentation and reconstruction techniques include reconstruction from serial sections, region-based methods, edge-based methods, model or knowledge-based methods, and combined methods.

2.2.1 Reconstruction from serial sections

The classic approach to extracting anatomy is to manually or semi-automatically trace the contours of structures of interest on each of a series of aligned image slices, then to "tile" a surface over the contours [36]. The tiled surface usually consists of an array of 3-D points connected to each other by edges to form triangular facets. The resulting 3-D *surface mesh* is then in a form where it can be further analyzed or displayed using standard 3-D surface rendering techniques [37].

Neither fully automatic contour tracing nor fully automatic tiling has been satisfactorily demonstrated in the general case. Thus, semi-automatic contour tracing followed by semi-automatic tiling remains the most common method for reconstruction from serial sections, and reconstruction from serial sections itself remains the method of choice for extracting microscopic 3-D brain anatomy [18].

2.2.2 Region-based and edge-based segmentation

This and the following sections primarily concentrate on segmentation at the macroscopic level.

In region-based segmentation voxels are grouped into contiguous regions based on characteristics such as intensity ranges and similarity to their neighbors [38]. A common initial approach to region-based segmentation is first to classify voxels into a small number of tissue classes such as gray matter, white matter, cerebrospinal fluid and background, then to use these classifications as a basis for further segmentation [39, 40]. Another region-based approach is called region-growing, in which regions are grown from seed voxels manually or automatically placed within candidate regions [21, 41]. The regions found by any of these approaches are often further processed by mathematical morphology operators [42] to remove unwanted connections and holes [43].

Edge-based segmentation is the complement to region-based segmentation: intensity gradients are used to search for and link organ boundaries. In the 2-D case contour-following connects adjacent points on the boundary. In the 3-D case isosurface following or marching cubes [44] connects border voxels in a region into a 3-D surface mesh.

Both region-based and edge-based segmentation are essentially low-level techniques that only look at local regions in the image data.

2.2.3 Model- and knowledge-based segmentation

The most popular current method for medical image segmentation, for the brain as well as other biological structures, is the use of deformable models. Based on pioneering work called "Snakes" by Kass, Witkin and Terzopoulos [45], deformable models have been developed for both 2-D and 3-D. In the 2-D case the deformable model is a contour, often represented as a simple set of linear segments or a spline, which is initialized to approximate the contour on the image. The contour is then deformed according to a cost function that includes both intrinsic terms proscribing how much the contour can distort, and extrinsic terms that reward closeness to image borders. In the 3-D case a 3-D surface (often a triangular mesh) is deformed in a similar manner. There are several examples of HBP-funded work that use deformable models for brain segmentation [28, 30, 31, 41].

An advantage of deformable models is that the cost function can include knowledge of the expected anatomy of the brain. For example, the cost function employed in the method developed by MacDonald [30] includes a term for the expected thickness of the cortical sheet. Thus, these methods can become somewhat knowledge-based, where knowledge of anatomy is encoded in the cost function.

An alternative knowledge-based approach explicitly records shape information in a geometric constraint network (GCN) [46], which encodes local shape variation based on a training set. The shape constraints define search regions on the image in which to search for edges. Found edges are then combined with the shape constraints to deform the model and reduce the size of search regions for additional edges [47, 48]. One potential advantage of this sort of model over a pure deformable model is that knowledge is explicitly represented in the model, rather than implicitly represented in the cost function.

2.2.4 Combined methods

Most brain segmentation packages use a combination of methods in a sequential pipeline. For example, in our own recent work we first use a GCN model to represent the overall cortical "envelope", excluding the detailed gyri and sulci [32]. The model is semi-automatically deformed to fit the cortex, then used as a mask to remove non-

cortex such as the skull. Isosurface following is then applied to the masked region to generate the detailed cortical surface. The model is also used on aligned MRA and MRV images to mask out non-cortical veins and arteries prior to isosurface following. The extracted cortical, vein and artery surfaces are then rendered to produce a composite visualization of the brain as seen at neurosurgery.

MacDonald et al. describe an automatic multi-resolution surface deformation technique called ASP (Anatomic Segmentation using Proximities), in which an inner and outer surface are progressively deformed to fit the image, where the cost function includes image terms, model-based terms, and proximity terms [30]. Dale et al. describe an automated approach that is implemented in the FreeSurfer program [28, 49]. This method initially finds the gray-white boundary, then fits smooth gray-white (inner) and white-CSF (outer) surfaces using deformable models. Van Essen et al. describe the SureFit program [31], which finds the cortical surface midway between the gray-white boundary and the gray-CSF boundary. This mid-level surface is created from probabilistic representations of both inner and outer boundaries that are determined using image intensity, intensity gradients, and knowledge of cortical topography. Other software packages also combine various methods for segmentation [33, 41, 50, 51].

2.3 Symbolic representation of anatomy

Given segmented brain structures, whether at the macroscopic or microscopic level, and whether represented as 3-D surface meshes or extracted 3-D regions, it is often desirable to attach labels (names) to the structures. If the names are drawn from a controlled terminology they can

be used as an index into a database of segmented structures, thereby providing a qualitative means for comparing brains from multiple subjects.

If the terms in the vocabulary are organized into symbolic qualitative models ("ontologies") of anatomical concepts and relationships, they can support systems that manipulate and retrieve segmented brain structures in "intelligent" ways. For example, a dynamic scene generator could assemble 3-D scenes of various segmented brain structures, overlaying them with anatomic names [52, 53].

If the anatomical ontologies are linked to other ontologies of physiology and pathology they can provide increasingly sophisticated knowledge about the *meaning* of the various images and other data that are increasingly becoming available in online databases (section 4) It is our belief that this kind of knowledge (by the computer, as opposed to the neuro-scientist) will be required in order to achieve the seamless integration of all forms of data envisioned by the HBP.

As in other biomedical fields the HBP has recognized the need for controlled vocabularies and ontologies to relate multiple sources of data. This recognition is evidenced by the keynote speeches at the 2001 spring meeting of the HBP [54, 55]. As in the spatial case it is commonly accepted that neuroanatomy provides the most logical organizational framework; in this case, however, neuroanatomy is represented symbolically rather than spatially.

At the most fundamental level Nomina Anatomica [56] and its recent successor, Terminologia Anatomica [57] provide a classification of officially sanctioned terms that are associated with macroscopic and microscopic brain structures. This canonical term list, however, has been substantially expanded by synonyms that are current in various fields of the neurosciences, and has also been augmented by a large number of new terms that designate structures omitted from Terminologia Anatomica. Many of these additions are present in clinical controlled terminologies (MeSH [58], SNOMED [59], Read Codes [60], GALEN [61]). Unlike Terminologia, which only exists in hard copy, these vocabularies are entirely computer-based, and therefore lend themselves for incorporation in HPB related applications.

The most complete primate neuroanatomical terminology is NeuroNames, developed by Bowden and Martin at the University of Washington [62]. NeuroNames, which is included as a knowledge source in the National Library of Medicine's Unified Medical Language System (UMLS) [63], is primarily organized as a part-of hierarchy of nested structures, with links to a large set of ancillary terms that do not fit into the strict part-of hierarchy. Other neuroanatomical terminologies have also been developed [64-67]. A challenge for the HBP is to either come up with a single consensus terminology or to develop Internet tools that allow transparent integration of distributed but commonly-agreed on terminology, with local modifications.

Classification and ontology projects to-date have focused primarily on arranging the terms of a particular domain in hierarchies. As we noted with respect to the evaluation of Terminologia Anatomica [68], insufficient attention has been paid to the relationships among these terms. Terminologia, as well as anatomy sections of the controlled medical terminologies, mix -is a- and -part of- relationships in the anatomy segments of their hierarchies. Although such heterogeneity does not interfere with using these term lists for keyword-based retrieval, these programs will fail to support higher level knowledge (reasoning) required for knowledge-based applications.

In our own Structural Informatics Group at the University of Washington we are addressing this deficiency by developing a Foundational Model of Anatomy (FMA), which we define as a comprehensive symbolic description of the structural organization of the body, including anatomical concepts, their preferred names and synonyms, definitions, attributes and relationships [6, 69].

The FMA is being implemented in Protégé-2000, a frame-based knowledge acquisition system developed at Stanford [70, 71]. In Protégé anatomical concepts are arranged in class-subclass hierarchies, with inheritance of defining attributes along the *isa* link, and other relationships (e.g., parts, branches, spatial adjacencies) represented as additional slots in the frame. The FMA currently consists of over 60,000 concepts, represented by 85,000 terms arranged in 75 types of relationships that represent all structures except the brain visible to 1 mm, and many microscopic and molecular structures as well. We are currently in the process of integrating NeuroNames with the FMA as a Foundational Model of Neuroanatomy (FMNA) [72].

Our belief is that the FMNA, as an integral component of the FMA for the entire body, will prove useful for symbolically organizing and integrating neuroscience information. But in order to answer non-trivial queries in neuroscience and to develop "smart tools" that rely on deep knowledge, additional ontologies must also be developed, among other things, for physiological functions mediated by neurotransmitters, pathological processes and their clinical manifestations as well as radiological appearances, with which they correlate. The relationships that exist between these concepts and anatomical parts of the brain must also be explicitly modeled. Next generation HBP efforts that link the FMNA and other anatomical ontologies with separately developed functional ontologies such as the biophysical description markup language (BDML) being developed at Cornell [73] will be needed in order to accomplish this type of integration.

2.4 Atlases

Spatial representations of neuroanatomy, in the form of segmented regions on 2-D or 3-D images, or 3-D surfaces extracted from image volumes, are often combined with symbolic representations to form digital atlases. A digital atlas (which for this review refers to an atlas created from 3-D image data taken from real subjects, as opposed to artists' illustrations) is generally created from a single individual, which therefore serves as a "canonical" instance of the species. Traditionally, atlases have been primarily used for education, and most digital atlases are used the same way.

For example, the Digital Anatomist Interactive Atlas of the brain [74] was created by outlining regions of interest on 2-D images (many of which are snapshots of 3-D scenes generated by reconstruction from serial sections) and labeling the regions with terminology from NeuroNames. The atlas, which is available both on CD-ROM and on the web, permits interactive browsing, where the names of structures are given in response to mouse clicks; dynamic creation of "pin diagrams", in which selected labels are attached to regions on the images; and dynamically-generated quizzes, in which the user is asked to point to structures on the image [75].

An example of a 3-D brain atlas created from the Visible Human is Voxelman [76], in which each voxel in the Visible Human head is labeled with the name of an anatomic structure in a "generalized voxel model" [77], and highly-detailed 3-D scenes are dynamically generated. Several other brain atlases have also been developed primarily for educational use [78, 79].

In keeping with the theme of anatomy as an organizing framework, atlases have also been developed for integrating functional data from multiple studies [65, 80-85]. In their original published form these atlases permit manual drawing of functional data, such as neurotransmitter distributions, onto hardcopy printouts of brain sections. Many of these atlases have been or are in the process of being converted to digital form. The Laboratory of Neuroimaging (LONI) at UCLA has been particularly active in the development and analysis of digital atlases [86], and the Caltech HBP has recently released a web-accessible 3-D mouse atlas acquired with micro-MR imaging [87].

The most widely used human brain atlas is the Talairach atlas, based on post mortem sections from a 60-year-old woman [88]. This atlas introduced a proportional coordinate system (often called "Talairach space") which consists of 12 rectangular regions of the target brain that are piecewise affine transformed to corresponding regions in the atlas. Using these transforms (or a simplified single affine transform based on the anterior and posterior commissures) a point in the target brain can be expressed in Talairach coordinates, and thereby related to similarly transformed points from other brains. Other human brain atlases have also been developed [89-93].

2.5 Anatomical variation

Brain information systems often use atlases as a basis for mapping functional data onto a common framework, much like geographic information systems (GISs) use the earth as the basis for combining data. However, unlike GISs, brain information systems must deal with the fact that no two brains are exactly alike, especially in the highly folded human cerebral cortex. Thus, not only do neuroinformatics researchers have to develop methods for representing individual brain anatomy, they also must develop methods for relating the anatomy of multiple brains. Only by developing methods for relating multiple brains will it be possible to generate a common anatomical frame of reference for organizing neuroscience data. Solving this problem is currently a major focus of work in the HBP.

Two general approaches for quantitatively dealing with anatomic variation can be defined: 1) warping to a template atlas, and 2) population-based atlases. Variation can also be expressed in a qualitative manner, as described in section 2.6.1.

2.5.1 Warping to a template atlas

The most popular current quantitative method for dealing with anatomic variation is to deform or warp an individual target brain to a single brain chosen as a template. If the template brain has been segmented and labeled as an atlas (section 2.4), and if the registration of the target brain to the template is exact, then the target brain will be automatically segmented, and any data from other studies that are associated with the template brain can be automatically registered with the target brain by inverting the warp [94, 95]. Such a procedure could be very useful for surgical planning, for example, since functional areas from patients whose demographics match that of the surgical patient could be superimposed on the patient's anatomy [96].

The problem of course comes with the word, "exact". Since no two brains are even topologically alike (sulci and gyri are present in one brain that are not present in another) it is impossible to completely register one brain to another. Thus, the research problem, which is very actively being pursued by many HBP researchers [94], is how to register two brains as closely as possible. Methods for doing this can be divided into volume-based warping and surface-based warping.

Volume-based warping. Pure volume-based registration directly registers two image volumes, without the pre-processing segmentation step. Whereas intra (single)-patient registration (section 2.1.2) establishes a linear transformation between two datasets, inter (multiple)-patient registration establishes a non-linear transformation (warp) that takes voxels in one volume to corresponding voxels in the other volume. Because of the great variability of the cerebral cortex pure volume-based registration is best suited for sub-cortical structures rather than the cortex. As in the linear case there are two basic approaches to non-linear volume registration: *intensity-based* and *landmark-based*, both of which generally use either physically-based approaches or minimization of a cost function to achieve the optimal warp.

The intensity-based approach uses characteristics of the voxels themselves, generally without the segmentation step, to non-linearly align two image volumes [29, 95, 97, 98]. Most start by removing the skull, which often must be done manually.

The *landmark-based* approach is analogous to the 2-D case: the user manually indicates corresponding points in the two datasets (usually with the aid of three orthogonal views of the image volumes). The program then brings the corresponding points into registration while carrying along the intervening voxel data. The Montreal Register program [26] can do non-linear 3-D warps, as can the Edgewarp-3D program [99], which is a generalization of the Edgewarp program developed by Bookstein [100].

A variation of landmark-based warping matches curves or surfaces rather than points, then uses the surface warps as a basis for interpolating the warp for intervening voxels [101, 102].

Surface-based warping. Surface-based registration is primarily used to register two cortical surfaces. The surface is first extracted using techniques described in section 2.2, then image-based or other functional data are "painted" on the extracted surface where they are carried along with whatever deformation is applied to the surface. Since the cortical surface is the most variable part of the brain, yet the most interesting for many functional studies, considerable research is currently being done in the area of surface-based registration [103].

It is very difficult if not impossible to match two surfaces in their folded up state, or to visualize all their activity. (The cerebral cortex gray matter can be thought of as a 2-D sheet that is essentially crumpled up to fit inside the skull). Therefore, much effort has been devoted to "reconfiguring" [31] the cortex so that it is easier to visualize and register. A prerequisite for these techniques is that the segmented cortex must be topologically correct. The programs FreeSurfer [28], Surefit [31], ASP [30] and others all produce surfaces suitable for reconfiguration.

Common reconfiguration methods include *inflation, expansion to a sphere*, and *flattening. Inflation* uncrumples the detailed gyri and sulci

of the folded surface by partially blowing the surface up like a balloon [31, 33, 49]. The resulting surface looks like a lissencephalic (smooth) brain, in which only the major lobes are visible, and the original sulci are painted on the surface as darker intensity curves. These marks, along with any functional data, are carried along in the other reconfiguration methods as well.

Expansion to a sphere further expands the inflated brain to a sphere, again with painted lines representing the original gyri and sulci. At this point it is simple to define a surface-based coordinate system as a series of longitude-latitude lines referred to a common origin. This spherical coordinate system permits more precise quantitative comparison of different brains than 3-D Talairach coordinates because it respects the topology of the cortical surface. The surface is also in a form where essentially 2-D warping techniques can be applied to deform the gyri and sulci marked on the sphere to a template spherical brain.

The third approach is to *flatten* the surface by making artificial cuts on the inflated brain surface, then spreading out the cut surface on a 2-D plane while minimizing distortion [31, 49, 104]. Since it is impossible to eliminate distortion when projecting a sphere to a plane, multiple methods of projection have been devised, just as there are multiple methods for projecting the earth's surface [94]. In all cases, the resulting flat map, like a 2-D atlas of the earth, is easier to visualize than a 3-D representation since the entire cortex is seen at once. Techniques for warping one cortex to another are applicable to flat maps as well as spherical maps, and the warps can be inverted to map pooled data on the individual extracted cortical surface.

The problem of warping any of these reconfigured surfaces to a template surface is still an active area of research because it is impossible to completely match two cortical surfaces. Thus, most approaches are hierarchical, in which larger sulci such as the lateral and central sulcus are matched first, followed by minor sulci.

2.5.2 Population-based atlases

The main problem with warping to a template atlas is deciding which atlas to use as a template. Which brain should be considered the "canonical" brain representing the population? The widely used Talairach atlas is based on a 60 year-old woman. The Visible Human male was a convict and the female was an older women. What about other populations such as different racial groups? These considerations have prompted several groups to work on methods for developing brain atlases that encode variation among a population, be it the entire population or selected sub-groups. The International Consortium for Brain Mapping (ICBM), a collaboration among several brain mapping institutions headed by Mazziotta at UCLA (http://www.loni.ucla.edu/ICBM), is collecting large numbers of normal brain image volumes from collaborators around the world [105]. To date several thousand brain image volumes, many with DNA samples for later correlation of anatomy with genetics, are stored on a massive file server. As data collection continues methods are under development for combining these data into population-based atlases.

A good high-level description of these methods can be found in a review article by Toga and Thompson [94]. In that article three main methods are described for developing population-based atlases: *density-based, label-based* and *deformation-based* approaches.

In the *density-based* method, a set of brains is first transformed to Talairach space by linear registration. Corresponding voxels are then averaged, yielding an "average" brain that preserves the major features of the brain, but smoothes out the detailed sulci and gyri. The Montreal average brain, which is an average of 305 normal brains [106], is constructed in this way. Although not detailed enough to permit precise comparisons of anatomical surfaces, it nevertheless is useful as a coarse means for relating multiple functional sites. For example, in our own work we have mapped cortical language sites from multiple patients onto the average brain, allowing a rough comparison of their distribution for different patient subclasses [107].

In the *label-based* approach, a series of brains are segmented, and then linearly transformed to Talairach space. A probability map is constructed for each segmented structure, such that at each voxel the probability can be found that a given structure is present at that voxel location. This method has been implemented in the Talairach Demon, an Internet server and Java client developed by Fox et al. as part of the ICBM project [108]. A web user inputs one or more sets of Talairach coordinates, and the server returns a list of structure probabilities for those coordinates.

In the *warp-based* method, the statistical properties of deformation fields produced by non-linear warping techniques (section 2.5.1) are analyzed to encode anatomical variation in population subgroups [109, 110]. These atlases can then be used to detect abnormal anatomy in various diseases.

2.6 Characterization of anatomy

The main reason for finding ways to represent anatomy is to examine the relationship between structure and function in both health and disease. For example, how does the branching pattern of the dendritic tree influence the function of the dendrite? Does the pattern of cortical folds influence the distribution of language areas in the brain? Does the shape of the corpus callosum relate to a predisposition to schizophrenia? Can subtle changes in brain structure be used as a predictor for the onset of Alzheimer's disease? These kinds of questions are becoming increasingly possible to answer with the availability of the methods described in the previous sections. However, in order to examine these questions methods must be found for characterizing and classifying the extracted anatomy. Both qualitative and quantitative approaches are being developed.

2.6.1 Qualitative classification

The classical approach to characterizing anatomy is for the human biologist to group individual structures into various classes based on perceived patterns. This approach is still widely used throughout science since the computer has yet to match the pattern recognition abilities of the human brain.

An example classification at the cellular level is the 60-80 morphological cell types that form the basis for understanding the neural circuitry of the retina (which is an outgrowth of the brain) [111]. At the macroscopic level Ono has developed an atlas of cerebral sulci that can be used to characterize an individual brain based on sulcal patterns [112].

If these and other classifications are given systematic names and are added to the symbolic ontologies described in section 2.3 they can be used for "intelligent" index and retrieval, after which quantitative methods can be used for more precise characterization of structure-function relationships.

2.6.2 Quantitative classification.

Quantitative characterization of anatomy is often called *morphometrics* [113] or *computational neuroanatomy* [114]. Quantitative characterization permits more subtle classification schemes than are possible with qualitative methods, leading to new insights into the relation between structure and function, and between structure and disease [94, 115].

For example, at the ultrastructural level *stereology*, which is a statistical method for estimating from sampled data the distribution of structural components in a volume [116], is used to estimate the density of objects such as synapses in image volumes reconstructed from serial electron micrographs [18].

At the cellular level Ascoli et al. are developing the L-neuron project, which attempts to model dendritic morphology by a small set of parameterized generation rules, where the parameters are sampled from distributions determined from experimental data [114]. The resulting dendritic models capture a large set of dendritic morphological classes from only a small set of variables. Eventually the hope is to generate virtual neural circuits that can simulate brain function.

At the macroscopic level landmark-based methods have shown changes in the shape of the corpus callosum associated with schizophrenia that are not obvious from visual inspection [117]. Probabilistic atlas-based methods are being used to characterize growth patterns and disease-specific structural abnormalities in diseases such as Alzheimer's and schizophrenia [118]. As these techniques become more widely available to the clinician they should permit early diagnosis and hence potential treatment for these debilitating diseases.

3 Imaging the function of the brain

Perhaps a greater revolution than structural imaging has come about with methods that reveal the functioning of the brain, particularly cognitive function at the macroscopic level (i.e., the thinking brain). It is now routinely possible to put a normal subject in a scanner, to give the person a cognitive task, such as counting or object recognition, and to observe which parts of the brain light up. This unprecedented ability to observe the functioning of the living brain opens up entirely new avenues for exploring how the brain works.

Functional modalities can be classified as *image-based* or *non-image based*. In both cases it is taken as axiomatic that the functional data must be mapped to the individual subject's anatomy, where the anatomy is extracted from structural images using techniques described in the previous section. Once mapped to anatomy, the functional data can be integrated with other functional data from the same subject, and with functional data from other subjects whose anatomy has been related to a template or probabilistic atlas. Techniques for generating, mapping and integrating functional data are part of the field of Functional Brain Mapping, which has become very active in the past few years, with several conferences [119] and journals [120, 121] devoted to the subject.

3.1 Image-based functional brain mapping

Image-based functional data generally come from scanners that generate relatively low resolution volume arrays depicting spatially-localized activation. For example, positron emission tomography (PET) [122, 123] and magnetic resonance spectroscopy (MRS) [124] reveal the uptake of various metabolic products by the functioning brain; and functional magnetic resonance imaging (fMRI) reveals changes in blood oxy-genation that occur following neural activity [123]. The raw intensity values generated by these techniques must be processed by sophisticated statistical algorithms to sort out how much of the observed intensity is due to cognitive activity and how much is due to background noise.

As an example, one approach to fMRI imaging is the boxcar paradigm applied to language mapping [125]. The subject is placed in the MRI scanner and told to silently name objects shown at 3 second intervals on a head-mounted display. The actual objects ("on" state) are alternated with nonsense objects ("off" state), and the fMRI signal is measured during both the on and the off states. Essentially the voxel values at the off (or control) state are subtracted from those at the on state. The difference values are tested for significant difference from non-activated areas, then expressed as t-values. The voxel array of t-values can be displayed as an image.

A large number of alternative methods have been and are being developed for acquiring and analyzing functional data [126]. The output of most of these techniques is a low-resolution 3-D image volume in which each voxel value is a measure of the amount of activation for a given task. The low-resolution volume is then mapped to anatomy by linear registration to a high-resolution structural MR dataset, using one of the linear registration techniques described in section 2.1.2.

Many of these and other techniques are implemented in the SPM program [127], the AFNI program [128], the Lyngby toolkit [129], and several commercial programs such as Medex [51] and BrainVoyager [33]. The FisWidgets project at the University of Pittsburgh is developing a set of Java wrappers for many of these programs that allow customized creation of graphical user interfaces in an integrated desktop environment [130].

3.2 Non-image based functional mapping

In addition to the image-based functional methods there are an increasing number of techniques that do not directly generate images. The data from these techniques are generally mapped to anatomy, then displayed as functional overlays on anatomic images.

For example, cortical stimulation mapping (CSM) is a technique for localizing functional areas on the exposed cortex at the time of neuro-surgery. In our own work the technique is used to localize cortical language areas so that they can be avoided during the resection of a tumor or epileptic focus [131]. Following removal of a portion of the skull (craniotomy) the patient is awakened and asked to name common images shown on slides. During this time the surgeon applies a small electrical current to each of a set of numbered tags placed on the cortical surface. If the patient is unable to name the object while the current is applied the site is interpreted as essential for language and is avoided at surgery. In this case the functional mapping problem is how to relate these stimulation sites to the patient's anatomy as seen on an MRI scan.

Our approach, which we call visualization-based mapping [21, 32], is to acquire image volumes of brain anatomy (MRI), cerebral veins (MRV) and cerebral arteries (MRA) prior to surgery, to segment the anatomy, veins and arteries from these images, and to generate a surface-rendered 3-D model of the brain and its vessels that matches as closely as possible the cortical surface as seen at neuro-surgery. A visual mapping program then permits the user to drag numbered tags onto the rendered surface such that they match those seen on the intraoperative photograph. The program projects the dragged tags onto the reconstructed surface, and records the xyz image-space coordinates of the projections, thereby completing the mapping.

The real goal of functional neuro-imaging is to observe the actual electrical activity of the neurons as they perform various cognitive tasks. fMRI, MRS and PET do not directly record electrical activity. Rather, they record the results of electrical activity, such as (in the case of fMRI) the oxygenation of blood supplying the active neurons. Thus, there is a delay from the time of activity to the measured response. In other words these techniques have relatively poor temporal resolution. Electro-encephalography (EEG) or magnetoencephalography (MEG), on the other hand, are more direct measures of electrical activity since they measure the electro-magnetic fields generated by the electrical activity of the neurons. Current EEG and MEG methods involve the use of large arrays of scalp sensors, the output of which are processed in a similar way to CT in order to localize the source of the electrical activity inside the brain. In general this "source localization problem" is under constrained, so information about brain anatomy obtained from MRI is used to provide further constraints [132].

4 Image-based brain information systems

The goal of many of the techniques described in the previous sections is to develop methods for integrating structural and functional brain image data through spatial and symbolic representations of anatomy. As described in section 1 this is one of the major goals of the HBP. Another goal described in that section is to develop Internet-based methods for sharing and disseminating the integrated information.

One way information can be shared is through remote visualization and manipulation of raw and processed images. For example, in our own work we have created a web-based visualization applet that permits 3-D viewing of the results of our visualization-based approach to brain mapping [133]. Similar remote image viewers are being developed by other members of the HBP [134-137].

Two groups permit Internet control of expensive microscopy systems. The Iscope project at the University of Tennessee permits control of a light microscope for viewing slides of a mouse brain atlas [83], whereas the National Center for Microscopy and Imaging Research is implementing web control of an electron microscope [138].

A more comprehensive way for sharing information is to develop backend database systems that allow Web-based queries of the processed and integrated data. As these systems are developed the hope is that links can be established between individual brain information systems so as to promote knowledge discovery and the development of distributed, large-scale models of brain function that will help establish a "wholeness" in neuroscience.

This research area is also active in the HBP, but not as much progress has been made as in the other areas of tool development and methods for integrating data. There seem to be four main reasons for this: 1) the development of information systems depends on progress in tool development and on methods for integrating data in a common anatomical framework, 2) not enough informatics and database experts have become involved in the HBP, 3) not enough content has yet been made available for database experts to "play" with, and 4) the development of information systems raises additional non-trivial issues related to security and intellectual property.

As shown in the previous sections a large amount of effort is going into solving the first problem (tools and integration). We believe that the second problem (not enough informatics experts) arises partly because informatics and computer science investigators are not sufficiently aware of the rich set of problems posed by the HBP. Hopefully, this review article will help in this area. The third problem (not enough content) is also slowly being addressed by ongoing efforts. More content will help attract more database and informatics experts. The fourth problem (security and intellectual property), which is very familiar to clinical informatics workers, is starting to be addressed by those who are developing brain information systems. That this problem is not at all trivial has been noted in several recent articles about the HBP [139, 140].

The information systems that are currently in active development in the HBP can more or less be classified as experiment management systems for local data, systems for handling published results, and raw data repositories analogous to GenBank for gene sequences [141]. This last is the most controversial. A listing of many of the current neuroscience database systems is available [142].

4.1 Experiment Management Systems

In our work we use the term, "Experiment Management System" (EMS) to refer to an information system that keeps track of the results and protocols for specific experiments of interest to an individual or lab [143]. At the least such a system should permit organization of and access to data of interest to the local individual or group. An EMS usually evolves from a collection of computer files or paper records that has become too unwieldy for even local management. An EMS can therefore be appealing to neuroscientists because it solves an immediate problem of interest to them. If the data are made available on the web, and if appropriate safeguards are implemented to prevent unauthorized access to the data, an EMS can permit data sharing among distributed collaborators. In addition, if at least some of the data integration methods described in the previous sections are implemented, the local EMS will be more amenable to wider sharing in a federated database.

Our HBP work follows this approach: we are developing image processing tools and an EMS of interest to a specific set of neuroscience users, while developing or incorporating integration methods that will later permit more widespread data sharing. We believe that this "bottom-up" approach is a viable complement to the top-down approaches of other HBP efforts if the tools and methods can be "cloned" for use by other groups, and if "hooks" can be provided for later integration of these and other efforts in federated information systems.

The main idea of an EMS is that metadata (data about data) provide indices into individual data files, such as images or segmented anatomy, which are the input or output of various image-processing tools. A simple spreadsheet is often the first place where these metadata are stored. As the need for better search becomes evident the spreadsheet may be imported into a local database such as Microsoft Access, and as the need for remote sharing and more robust data management becomes clear the data may be imported to a higher-end database system that is interfaced to the web. Many commercial database systems provide web-accessible views of the database.

In our own work we have developed an open source Experiment Management System Building Environment

(EMSBE), and have used the toolkit to implement an EMS for our HBP work [143, 144]. The toolkit, which is called WIRM (Web Interfacing Repository Manager) is a set of perl APIs that can be interfaced to any back-end relational database, and that can be called by a perl programmer to dynamically generate web views of metadata and associated datafiles [145]. Any of the extensive set of perl modules in the comprehensive perl archive network (CPAN, www.cpan. org) can be used in conjunction with WIRM to provide extensive backend processing of data, including image conversion, import of spreadsheet data, and XML parsing. When coupled with Java applets for viewing 3-D or time varying data located on the server, the resulting systems can provide remote access, visualization, and manipulation of most data of interest to neuroscientists. A similar open source toolkit called Zope (www.zope.org) [146], which is written in Python as opposed to perl, is the basis for a project to develop an open source medical record system (www.freepm.org).

We have used WIRM to create a web-accessible experiment management system for organizing, visualizing and sharing language map data, much of which is in the form of 2-D and 3-D images [143, 147]. The system is currently in use in three widely scattered labs at the University of Washington.

A similar EMS called SUMS (Surface Management System) is being developed at Washington University to handle images processed by the Surefit and Caret programs [31], and a system being developed by Wong et al. at UCSF handles images and other data associated with neurosurgical treatment of epilepsy [148].

Another example of what we call an EMS (our terminology) is the Brain Image Database (BRAID) [137, 149, 150] being developed at Johns Hopkins for management and evaluation of "Image-based clinical trials" [150]. The system, like some others in the HBP [151, 152], is implemented in the Illustra (now Informix now IBM) object-relational database system, which permits the development of specialized "datablades" for image processing and analysis. BRAID is being developed to facilitate lesion-deficit studies in large clinical trials. Patient MR image volumes are warped to one of several labeled human atlases [102], thereby permitting automatic identification of anatomical structures (subject to the limitations discussed in section 2.5). Lesions from patient MR images are manually delineated and stored in the database, along with the warped and labeled images. Analytical tools embedded in the database, and accessed through extended SQL, permit rapid computation of structure-function correlations, as for example, a correlation between lesions in the optic radiations and contra lateral visual field defect [149], or a correlation between traumatic injuries to the right putamen and an increase in attention deficit disorders in children [153].

Other groups in the HBP are also developing what we call EMS's, but these generally do not involve images to much extent [73, 154, 155]. Of particular relevance for eventual data sharing is the electrophysiological EMS under development by Gardner et al. [73]. As part of that effort Gardner has proposed BDML (Biophysical Description Markup Language), an XML-based common format for data exchange. Although initially in use for sharing of electrophysiological data, BDML was designed from the start to encompass other kinds of brain data, including images. A few other HBP groups have begun experimenting with BDML to see if it is relevant to their own data.

There are also some initial efforts to develop federated database systems that can tie together individual EMS's [156], although there appear to be few if any published efforts to explore advanced database issues such as intelligent retrieval or content-based retrieval. We believe that these kinds of efforts represent the next stage of the HBP. They will become more widespread as individual EMSs are developed, as the thorny problems of data integration and intellectual property become ironed out, and as mainstream database experts become interested in the HBP.

4.2 Published results

At the other end of the spectrum from individual EMSs are efforts to essentially index published literature in more meaningful ways than simple term searches in Medline. Like individual EMSs, which deal only with data that the individual researcher wants to share with his or her collaborators, this kind of effort is not controversial because it simply provides enhanced access to public data. The enhancements generally make use of some of the integration methods described in section 2.5 to provide anatomically based queries based on a template atlas, often coupled with a controlled vocabulary.

An early example of such an atlas-based system was the Brain Browser, a Mac HyperCard application that permitted scientists to map experimental results onto a rat brain atlas template [65]. A more recent effort is the Mouse Brain Library at Tennessee, which contains atlas sections and metadata from inbred mouse strains, for use in mapping genetic data [83].

An early, and still one of the few Web-accessible atlas systems that includes mapped data as well as images, is the BrainMap database developed by Fox et al. at the University of Texas [157]. In this system data are integrated primarily according to Talairach coordinates, which are in turn linked to anatomical names. Web forms are used to enter a query as a Boolean combination of constraints such as Talairach coordinates, anatomical names, publication source, laboratory of origin, and imaging protocol. The system returns references to published literature that meet the search constraints. Registered users can retrieve experimental data associated with the data, and an author mode permits authors to input their published results into the system.

The Fox database uses linear Talairach coordinates to integrate data. In contrast, the Bowden brain information system uses the Bookstein landmark-based nonlinear registration method [100] to warp 2-D images from the literature to a brain atlas template, which has been labeled by terms from NeuroNames [62]. The template atlas takes the place of the earth in a commercial Geographic Information System (GIS) [158]. When complete the system will permit a web user to type a NeuroName or click on an area of the template atlas to specify a given structure, to add additional constraints such as neurotransmitter type, and to retrieve all maps that have been warped to the template. These maps in turn will contain links to the original articles.

4.3 Data repositories

The most controversial HBP efforts are aimed at the establishment of raw data repositories that are widely accessible, in analogy to highly successful bioinformatics efforts such as GenBank [141] or the protein data bank (PDB) [159]. One reason for the controversy is that brain data are seen by most neuroscientists as being much more complex than the relatively simple linear sequences or 3-D coordinate files represented in GenBank or PDB, and in fact it is not even clear how the data should be represented and which data should be shared. As evidenced by section 2.5 it is not clear how to relate data from multiple subjects, let alone at different levels of anatomical granularity. In addition many neuroscientists express concern that public data will not have adequate quality control, and that data will not be adequately protected from unauthorized use.

Perhaps because of these issues there are only a few attempts to establish raw data repositories. One example of such an attempt is the Dartmouth fMRI Data Center [152], which is being developed as a repository for organizing fMRI image datasets submitted by multiple authors. When the project was first discussed it was proposed that authors of articles to certain journals be required to submit their fMRI images to the repository as a condition of publication, again in analogy with the requirement for authors of papers about gene sequences to submit their sequences to GenBank. This proposal generated a fierce reaction from other HBP and neuroscience researchers [140], with the result that most journals retracted the requirement. Nevertheless, there are many researchers, including the director of the HBP [139], who feel strongly that neuroscience must begin to share raw data if the field is to advance. It may be that more advanced database methods, such as federated databases [156] or peer-to-peer databases ala Napster [160], will be required in order to achieve this goal.

5 Achieving the promise of the Human Brain Project

In this review we have tried to summarize many of the projects in the Human Brain Project, emphasizing the ubiquity of images in most of them. The resulting imaging informatics problems of image generation, management, processing and visualization are not unique to the brain, yet because of the variety and sheer numbers of brain images, the problems are at least as varied and challenging as any that arise from other areas of the body. Therefore, solutions to these problems should have widespread applicability outside the brain or even biomedicine.

Similarly, we hope we have demonstrated the central role that neuro-anatomy plays as an organizational framework, not only for brain images, but also for most other neuroscience data as well. As we noted earlier, a case for this central role of anatomy can be made throughout all of biomedicine, which has prompted to us to define structural informatics as a sub field of biomedical informatics for dealing specifically with information about the physical organization of the body.

As noted in section 1 the brain presents very challenging research problems in structural informatics, in the areas of spatial and symbolic representation, brain segmentation, and especially anatomic variation, yet considerable progress has been made in these areas by HBP and other brain researchers. Since a central tenet of structural informatics is that patterns of physical organization repeat themselves throughout the hierarchy from macroscopic anatomy to molecules, it is highly likely that these results will find use in other areas of the body. One of the main reasons to define a field is to promote this kind of cross-fertilization of techniques.

This potential for cross-fertilization is one of the main motivators for defining the field of neuroinformatics, which is the field that has the most interest in achieving the goals of the HBP. The goals of the HBP to "database the brain" [2] are so ambitious as to practically dwarf the goals of the Human Genome Project. Many have argued (and they may be right) that the goals are too ambitious to be practical, and that resources would be better spent on specific neuroscience-driven projects that involve the use of computers. But the critics may also be wrong. Whether we get to the moon or not may be less important than the side effects that can result from such an endeavor. Just as medical informatics has evolved to promote cross-fertilization among informaticists and health scientists, so too could neuroinformatics promote cross-fertilization among informaticists and neuroscientists. National initiatives such as the HBP can foster these kinds of collaborations by funding interdisciplinary projects that bring together experts in areas such as imaging informatics, structural informatics, neuroscience, radiology, computer science, and information science.

For these kinds of efforts to succeed each kind of expert needs to become educated in the research problems of the other field, in enough detail so that they see how the problems apply to their own field. This paper is as much as anything an attempt to educate the wider biomedical and health informatics community, and the computer scientists and other technology experts that are associated with this community, in just a few of the informatics and computer science challenges associated with this, the problem of understanding the most complex entity known. The paper will have succeeded if it inspires just a few of them to become involved in this grand challenge for the 21st century.

6 Acknowledgements

This work was funded by Human Brain Project grant MH/DC02310. In preparing this review we found several web sites to be of particular use as starting points for further exploration. These sites are the HBP home page http://www.nimh.nih.gov/neuroinformatics/index.cfm, the HBP list of funded grants http:// www.nimh.nih.gov/neuroinformatics/researchgrants.cfm, a list of software tools developed by Brain Project grantees, maintained by David Kennedy at Harvard http://www.cma.mgh.harvard.edu/tools/index.php, and a list of neuroscience databases maintained by Rolf Kotter at Düsseldorf, for publication in the autumn 2001 issue of the Philosophical Transactions of the Royal Society, Series B: Biological Sciences http://www.hirn.uni-duesseldorf.de/rk/neurodat.htm.

References

1. Koslow SH, Huerta MF, editors. Neuroinformatics: an overview of the Human Brain Project. Mahwah, New Jersey: Lawrence Erlbaum; 1997.
2. Chicurel M. Databasing the brain. Nature 2000;406:822-5.
3. Kahn J. Let's make your head interactive. Wired 2001 August:107-15.
4. Pechura C, Martin J. Mapping the brain and its functions: integrating enabling technologies into neuroscience research. Institute of Medicine Pub 91-108: National Academy Press; 1991.
5. Heurta M, Koslow S. Neuroinformatics: opportunities across disciplinary and national borders. Neuroimage 1996;4:S4-S6.
6. Rosse C, Mejino JL, Modayur BR, Jakobovits RM, Hinshaw KP, Brinkley JF. Motivation and organizational principles for anatomical knowledge representation: the Digital Anatomist symbolic knowledge base. J Am Med Inform Assoc 1998;5(1):17-40.
7. Brinkley JF. Structural informatics and its applications in medicine and biology. Acad Med 1991;66(10):589-91.
8. Kulikowski CA. Medical imaging informatics: challenges of definition and integration. J Am Med Inform Assoc 1997;4(3):252-3.
9. Ambrogi L. Manual of Histologic and Special Staining Techniques. 2nd ed. New York: Mc-Graw-Hill; 1960.
10. Peters A, Palay S, Webster H. The Fine Structure of the Nervous System: Neurons and their Supporting Cells. 3rd ed. New York: Oxford Press; 1991.
11. Crusio WE, Gerlai RT, editors. Handbook of molecular-genetic techniques for brain and behavior research. Amsterdam; New York: Elsevier; 1999.
12. Zimmerman RA, Gibby WA, Carmody RF, editors. Neuroimaging: clinical and physical

13. Jacobs RE, Ahrens ET, Dickenson ME, Laidlaw D. Towards a microMRI atlas of mouse development. Comput Med Imaging Graph 1999;23(1):15-24 http://waggle.gg.caltech.edu/hbp/index.html.

14. Wilson T. Confocal Microscopy. San Diego: Academic Press Ltd.; 1990.

15. Perkins G, Renken C, Martone ME, Young SJ, Ellisman M, Frey T. Electron tomography of neuronal mitochondria: Three-dimensional structure and organization of cristae and menbrane contacts. J Struct Biol 1997;119(3):260-72.

16. Prothero JS, Prothero JW. Three-dimensional reconstruction from serial sections IV. The reassembly problem. Comput Biomed Res 1986;19(4):361-73.

17. Spitzer VM, Whitlock DG. The Visible Human Dataset: the anatomical platform for human simulation. Anat Rec 1998;253(2):49-57.

18. Fiala JC, Harris KM. Extending unbiased stereology of brain ultrastructure to three-dimensional volumes. J Am Med Assoc 2001;8(1):1-16.

19. Soto GE, Young SJ, Martone ME, Deerinick TJ, Lamont SL, Carragher BO, et al. Serial section electron tomography: a method for three-dimensional reconstruction of large structures. Neuroimage 1994;1:230-43 http://ncmir.ucsd.edu/abstracts.html#Neuroimage_1.

20. Agrawal M, Harwood D, Duraiswami R, Davis LS, Luther PW. Three-dimensional ultrastructure from transmission electron micropscope tilt series. In: Proceedings, Second Indian Conference on Vision, Graphics and Image Processing. Bangalore, India; 2000. http://www.umiacs.umd.edu/~mla/tem/icvgipfinal.pdf.

21. Modayur B, Prothero J, Ojemann G, Maravilla K, Brinkley JF. Visualization-based mapping of language function in the brain. Neuroimage 1997;6:245-58.

22. Collins DL, Neelin P, Peters TM, Evans AC. Automatic 3-D intersubject registration of MR volumetric data in standardized Talairach space. J Comput Assist Tomogr 1994;18(2):192-205.

23. Woods RP, Cherry SR, Mazziotta JC. Rapid automated algorithm for aligning and reslicing PET images. J Comput Assist Tomogr 1992;16:620-633.

24. Woods RP, Mazziotta JC, Cherry SR. MRI-PET registration with automated algorithm. J Comput Assist Tomogr 1993;17:536-46.

25. Ashburner J, Friston KJ. Multimodal image coregistration and partitioning - a unified framework. Neuroimage 1997;6(3):209-17.

26. MacDonald D. Register: McConnel Brain Imaging Center, Montreal Neurological Institute; 1993.

27. Lichtenbelt B, Crane R, Naqvi S. Introduction to Volume Rendering. Upper Saddle River, N.J.: Prentice Hall; 1998.

28. Dale AM, Fischl B, Sereno MI. Cortical surface-based analysis. I. Segmentation and surface reconstruction. Neuroimage 1999;9(2):179-94.

29. Collins DL, Holmes DJ, Peters TM, Evans AC. Automatic 3-D model-based neuroanatomical segmentation. Hum Brain Mapp 1995;3:190-208.

30. MacDonald D, Kabani N, Avis D, Evans AC. Automated 3-D extraction of inner and outer surfaces of cerebral cortex from MRI. Neuroimage 2000;12(3):340-56.

31. Van Essen DC, Drury HA, Dickson J, Harwell J, Hanlon D, Anderson CH. An integrated software suite for surface-based analysis of cerebral cortex. J Am Med Inform Assoc 2001;8(5):443-59. http://stp.wustl.edu.

32. Hinshaw KP, Poliakov AV, Martin RF, Moore EB, Shapiro LG, Brinkley JF. Shape-based cortical surface segmentation in a workflow environment for visualization brain mapping.2001 http://sig.biostr.washington.edu/publications/online/hinshawbrain01.pdf

33. Brain Innovation B.V. BrainVoyager. http://www.BrainVoyager.de/; 2001.

34. Ng Y, Shiffman S, Brosnan TJ, Links JM, Beach LS, Judge NS, et al. BrainImageJ: A java-based framework for interoperability in neuroscience, with specific application to neuroimaging. J Am Med Inform Assoc 2001;8(5):431-42.

35. Kennedy D. Internet Brain Segmentation Repository. http://neuro-www.mgh.harvard.edu/cma/ibsr/; 2001.

36. Prothero JS, Prothero JW. Three-dimensional reconstruction from serial sections: I. A portable microcomputer-based software package in Fortran. Comput Biomed Res 1982;15:598-604.

37. Foley JD. Computer graphics: Principles and Practice. Reading, Mass.: Addison-Wesley; 2001.

38. Shapiro LG, Stockman GC. Computer Vision. Upper Saddle River, N.J.: Prentice Hall; 2001.

39. Choi HS, Haynor DR, Kim Y. Partial volume tissue classification of multichannel magnetic resonance images - a mixel model. IEEE Trans Med Imaging 1991;10(3):395-407.

40. Zijdenbos AP, Evans AC, Riahi F, Sled J, Chui J, Kollokian V. Automatic quantification of multiple sclerosis lesion volume using stereotactic space. In: Proc. 4th Int. Conf. on Visualization in Biomedical Computing. Hamburg; 1996.

p. 439-48.

41. Davatzikos C, Bryan RN. Using a deformable surface model to obtain a shape representation of the cortex. IEEE Trans Med Imaging 1996;15(6):785-95.

42. Haralick RM. Mathematical Morphology: University of Washington; 1988.

43. Sandor S, Leahy R. Surface-based labeling of cortical anatomy using a deformable atlas. IEEE Trans Med Imaging 1997;16(1):41-54.

44. Lorensen WE, Cline HE. Marching cubes: a high resolution 3-D surface construction algorithm. Comput Graph (ACM) 1987;21(4):163-9.

45. Kass M, Witkin A, Terzopoulos D. Snakes: active contour models. International Journal of Computer Vision 1987;1(4):321-31.

46. Brinkley JF. Hierarchical geometric constraint networks as a representation for spatial structural knowledge. In: Proceedings, 16th Annual Symposium on Computer Applications in Medical Care; 1992. p. 140-4.

47. Brinkley JF. Knowledge-driven ultra-sonic three-dimensional organ modelling. PAMI 1985;PAMI-7(4):431-41.

48. Brinkley JF. A flexible, generic model for anatomic shape: application to interactive two-dimensional medical image segmentation and matching. Comput Biomed Res 1993;26:121-42.

49. Fischl B, Sereno MI, Dale AM. Cortical surface-based analysis. II: Inflation, flattening, and a surface-based coordinate system. Neuroimage 1999;9(2):195-207.

50. Wellcome Department of Cognitive Neurology. Statistical Parametric Mapping. http://www.fil.ion.ucl.ac.uk/spm/; 2001.

51. Sensor Systems Inc. MedEx. http://medx.sensor.com/products/medx/index.html; 2001.

52. Brinkley JF, Wong BA, Hinshaw KP, Rosse C. Design of an anatomy information system. Computer Graphics and Applications 1999;19(3):38-48.

53. Wong BA, Rosse C, Brinkley JF. Semi-automatic scene generation using the Digital Anatomist Foundational Model. In: Proceedings, American Medical Informatics Association Fall Symposium. Washington, D.C.; 1999. p. 637-41.

54. Rosse C, Tuttle MS. Explaining the brain to a computer. In: Human Brain Project Annual Meeting; 2001. http://www.nimh.nih.gov/neuroinformatics/rosse2001.cfm.

55. Gardner D, Abato M, Knuth KH, DeBellis R, Gardner EP. A functional ontology for neuroinformatics. In: Human Brain Project Annual Meeting; 2001.

http://www.nimh.nih.gov/neuroinformatics/gardner2001.cfm.

56. International Anatomical Nomenclature Committee. Nomina Anatomica. 6th ed. Edinburgh: Churchill Livingstone; 1989.

57. Federative Committee on Anatomical Terminology. Terminologia Anatomica. Stuttgart: Thieme; 1998.

58. National Library of Medicine. Medical Subject Headings - Annotated Alphabetic List. Bethesda, MD: U.S. Department of Health and Human Services, Public Health Service; 1999.

59. Spackman KA, Campbell KE, Cote RA. SNOMED-RT: A reference terminology for health care. In: Masys DR, editor. Proceedings, AMIA Annual Fall Symposium. Philadelphia: Hanley and Belfus; 1997. p. 640-4.

60. Schultz EB, Price C, Brown PJB. Symbolic anatomic knowledge representation in the Read Codes Version 3: Structure and application. J Am Med Inform Assoc 1997;4:38-48.

61. Rector AL, Nowlan WA, Glowinski A. Goals for concept representation in the GALEN project. In: Safran C, editor. Proceedings of the 17th Annual Symposium on Computer Applications in Medical Care (SCAMC 93). New York: McGraw Hill; 1993. p. 414-8.

62. Bowden DM, Martin RF. Neuronames brain hierarchy. Neuroimage 1995; 2:63-83.

63. Lindberg DAB, Humphreys BL, McCray AT. The unified medical language system. Methods Inf Med 1993;32 (4):281-91.

64. Paxinos G, Watson C. The rat brain in stereotaxic coordinates. San Diego: Academic Press; 1986.

65. Bloom FE, Young WG. Brain Browser. New York: Academic Press; 1993.

66. Swanson LW. Brain maps: structure of the rat brain. Amsterdam; New York: Elsevier; 1992.

67. Franklin KBJ, Paxinos G. The mouse brain in stereotactic coordinates. San Diego: Academic Press; 1997.

68. Rosse C. Terminologia Anatomica; considered from the perspective of next-generation knowledge sources. Clin Anat 2000;14:120-33 http://sig.biostr.washington.edu/share/pubs/CRTAnat.pdf.

69. Rosse C, Shapiro LG, Brinkley JF. The Digital Anatomist foundational model: principles for defining and structuring its concept domain. In: Proceedings, American Medical Informatics Association Fall Symposium. Orlando, Florida; 1998. p. 820-4.

70. Musen MA. Domain ontologies in software engineering: use of Protege with the EON architecture. Methods Inf Med 1998;37(4-5):540-50.

71. Mejino JLV, Noy NF, Musen MA, Brinkley JF, Rosse C. Representation of structural relationships in the foundational model of anatomy. In: Proceedings, AMIA Fall Symp. Washington, DC; 2001. p. 973.

72. Martin RF, Mejino JLV, Bowden DM, Brinkley JF, Rosse C. Foundational model of neuroanatomy: implications for the Human Brain Project. In: Proc AMIA Fall Symp. Washington, DC; 2001. p. 438-42.

73. Gardner D, Knuth KH, Abato M, Erde SM, White T, DeBellis R, et al. Common data model for neuroscience data and data model exchange. J Am Med Assoc 2001;8(1):17-33.

74. Sundsten JW, Conley DM, Ratiu P, Mulligan KA, Rosse C. Digital Anatomist web-based interactive atlases. http://www9.biostr.washington.edu/da.html; 2000.

75. Brinkley JF, Bradley SW, Sundsten JW, Rosse C. The Digital Anatomist information system and its use in the generation and delivery of Web-based anatomy atlases. Comput Biomed Res 1997;30:472-503.

76. Höhne KH, Pflesser B, Riemer M, Schiemann T, Schubert R, Tiede U. A new representation of knowledge concerning human anatomy and function. Nat Med 1995;1(6):506-10.

77. Höhne K, Bomans M, Pommert A, Riemer M, Schiers C, Tiede U, et al. 3-D visualization of tomographic volume data using the generalized voxel model. The Visual Computer 1990;6(1):28-36.

78. Stensaas SS, Millhouse OE. Atlases of the Brain. http://medstat.med.utah.edu/kw/brain_atlas/credits.htm; 2001.

79. Johnson KA, Becker JA. The Whole Brain Atlas. http://www.med.harvard.edu/AANLIB/home.html; 2001.

80. Swanson LW. Brain Maps: Structure of the Rat Brain. 2nd ed. New York: Elsevier Science; 1999.

81. Martin RF, Bowden DM. Primate Brain Maps: Structure of the Macaque Brain. New York: Elsevier Science; 2001.

82. Fougerousse F, Bullen P, Herasse M, Lindsay S, Richard I, Wilson D, et al. Human-mouse differences in the embryonic expression of developmental control genes and disease genes. Hum Mol Genet 2000;9(2):165-73.

83. Rosen GD, Williams AG, Capra JA, Connolly MT, Cruz B, Lu L, et al. The Mouse Brain Library @ www.mbl.org. In: Int. Mouse Genome Conference 14; 2000. p. 166. http://www.nervenet.org/papers/MBLabst2000.html.

84. Toga AW, Ambach KL, Schluender S. High-resolution anatomy from in situ human brain. Neuroimage 1994;1(4):334-44.

85. Toga AW, Santori EM, Hazani R, Ambach K. A 3-D digital map of rat brain. Brain Res Bull 1995;38(1):77-85.

86. Toga AW. UCLA Laboratory for Neuro Imaging (LONI). http://www.loni.ucla.edu/; 2001.

87. Dhenain M, Ruffins SW, Jacobs RE. Three-dimensional digital mouse atlas using high-resolution MRI. Dev Biol 2001;232(2):458-70 http://mouseatlas.caltech.edu/.

88. Talairach J, Tournoux P. Co-planar stereotaxic atlas of the human brain. New York: Thieme Medical Publishers; 1988.

89. Van Essen DC, Drury HA. Structural and functional analysis of human cerebral cortex using a surface-based atlas. J Neurosci 1997;17(18):7079-102.

90. Schaltenbrand G, Warren W. Atlas for Stereotaxy of the Human Brain. Stuttgart: Thieme; 1977.

91. Drury HA, Van Essen DC. Analysis of functional specialization in human cerebral cortex using the visible man surface based atlas. Hum Brain Mapp 1997;5:233-7.

92. Höhne KH, Bomans M, Riemer M, Schubert R, Tiede U, Lierse W. A volume-based anatomical atlas. IEEE Computer Graphics and Applications 1992:72-8.

93. Caviness VS, Meyer J, Makris N, Kennedy DN. MRI-based topographic parcellation of human neocortex: an anatomically specified method with estimate of reliability. J Cogn Neurosci 1996;8(6):566-87.

94. Toga AW, Thompson PW. Maps of the brain. Anat Rec 2001;265:37-53.

95. Christensen GE, Miller MI, Vannier MW. Individualizing neuroanatomical atlases using a massively parallel computer. IEEE Computer 1996;29(1):32-8.

96. Kikinis R, Shenton ME, Iosifescu DV, McCarley RW, Saiviroonporn P, Hokama HH, et al. A digital brain atlas for surgical planning, model-driven segmentation, and teaching. IEEE Trans Visualization and Computer Graphics 1996;2(3):232-41.

97. Gee JC, Reivich M, Bajcsy R. Elastically deforming 3D atlas to match anatomical brain images. J Comput Assist Tomogr 1993;17(2):225-36.

98. Kjems U, Strother SC, Anderson JR, Law I, Hansen LK. Enhancing the multivariate signal of ^{15}O water PET studies with a new nonlinear neuroanatomical registration algorithm. IEEE Trans Med Imaging 1999;18:301-19 http://hendrix.imm.dtu.dk/software/kjemswarp/kjemswarp.html.

99. Bookstein FL, Green WDK. Edgewarp 3D: A preliminary manual. ftp://brainmap.med.umich.edu/pub/edgewarp3.1/manual.html; 1998.

100. Bookstein FL. Principal warps: thin-plate splines and the decomposition of deformations. IEEE Trans Pattern Anal Mach Intell 1989;11(6):567-85.

101. Thompson P, Toga AW. A surface-based technique for warping three-dimensional images of the brain. IEEE Trans Med Imaging 1996;15(4):402-17.

102. Davatzikos C. Spatial transformation and registration of brain images using elastically deformable models. Comput Vis Image Underst 1997;66(2):207-22 http://ditzel.rad.jhu.edu/papers/cviu97.pdf.

103. Van Essen DC, Drury HA, Joshi S, Miller MI. Functional and structural mapping of human cerebral cortex: solutions are in the surfaces. Proc Natl Acad Sci 1998;95:788-95.

104. Hurdal MK, Stephenson K, Bowers P, Sumners DW, Rottenberg DA. Coordinate systems for conformal cerebellar flat maps. Neuroimage 2000;11(5):S467 http://www.pet.med.va.gov:8080/papers/abstracts_posters/HBM2000/mhurdal_HBM2000.html.

105. Mazziotta J, Toga A, Evans A, Fox P, Lancaster J, Zilles K, et al. A four-dimensional probabilistic atlas of the human brain. J Am Med Inform Assoc 2001;8(5):401-30.

106. Evans AC, Collins DL, Neelin P, MacDonald D, Kamber M, Marrett TS. Three-dimensional correlative imaging: applications in human brain mapping. In: Thatcher RW, Hallett M, Zeffiro T, John ER, Heurta M, editors. Functional Neuroimaging: technical foundations. San Diego: Academic Press; 1994. p. 145-62.

107. Martin RF, Poliakov AV, Mulligan KA, Corina DP, Ojemann GA, Brinkley JF. Multi-patient mapping of language sites on 3-D brain models. Neuroimage 2000;11(5):S534.

108. Lancaster JL, Woldorff MG, Parsons LM, Liotti M, Freitas CS, Rainey L, et al. Automated Talairach atlas labels for functional brain mapping. Hum Brain Mapp 2000;10(3):120-31 http://ric.uthscsa.edu/projects/talairachdaemon.html.

109. Thompson PM, Toga AW. Detection, visualization and animation of abnormal anatomic structure with a deformable probalistic brain atlas based on random vector field transformations. Med Image Anal 1997;1:271-94.

110. Christensen GE, Rabbitt RD, Miller MI. Deformable templates using large deformation kinematics. IEEE Trans Image Process 1996;5(10):1435-47.

111. Dacey D. Primate retina: cell types, circuits and color opponency. Prog Retin Eye Res 1999;18(6):737-63.

112. Ono MS, Kubik S, Abernathy CD. Atlas of the Cerebral Sulci. New York: Thieme Medical Publishers; 1990.

113. Bookstein FL. Biometrics and brain maps: the promise of the morphometric synthesis. In: Koslow SH, Huerta MF, editors. Neuroinformatics: An Overview of the Human Brain Project. Malwah, New Jersey: Lawrence Erlbaum; 1997. p. 203-54.

114. Ascioli GA. Progress and perspectives in computational neuroanatomy. Anat Rec1999;257(6):195-207 http://www.krasnow.gmu.edu/ascoli/CNG/TNA/index.htm.

115. Toga AW. Brain Atlases. http://www.loni.ucla.edu/Research_Loni/atlases/index.html; 2001.

116. Weibel WR. Stereological Methods. New York: Academic Press; 1979.

117. DeQuardo JR, Keshavan MS, Bookstein FL, Bagwell WW, Green WDK, Sweeney JA, et al. Landmark-based morphometric analysis of first-episode schizophrenia. Biol Psychiatry 1999;45(10):1321-28.

118. Thompson PM, Mega MS, Toga AW. Disease-specific brain atlases. In: Mazziotta JC, Toga AW, editors. Brain Mapping III: The Disorders. New York: Academic Press; 2001. http://www.loni.ucla.edu/~thompson/PDF/DisChptWeb.pdf.

119. Organization for Human Brain Mapping. Annual Conference on Human Brain Mapping. Brighton, United Kingdom; 2001 http://www.academicpress.com/www/journal/hbm2001/.

120. Toga AW, Frackowiak RSJ, Mazziotta JC, editors. Neuroimage: A Journal of Brain Function. New York: Academic Press; 2001.

121. Fox PT, editor. Human Brain Mapping. New York: John Wiley & Sons; 2001.

122. Heiss WD, Phelps ME, editors. Positron emission tomography of the brain. Berlin; New York: Springer-Verlag; 1983.

123. Aine CJ. A conceptual overview and critique of functional neuroimaging techniques in humans I. MRI/fMRI and PET. Crit Rev Neurobiol 1995;9:229-309.

124. Ross B, Bluml S. Magnetic resonance spectroscopy of the human brain. Anat Rec 2001;265(2):54-84.

125. Corina DP, Steury K, Poliakov AV, Martin RF, Mulligan KA, Maravilla K, et al. A comparison of language function derived from cortical stimulation mapping and fMRI: data from object naming. Submitted 2001.

126. Frackowiak RSJ, Friston KJ, Frith CD, Dolan RJ, Mazziotta JC, editors. Human Brain Function. New York: Academic Press; 1997.

127. Friston KJ, Holmes AP, Worsley KJ, Poline JP, Frith CD, Frackowiak RSJ. Stastical parametric maps in functional imaging: a general linear approach. Hum Brain Mapp 1995;2:189-210 http://www.fil.ion.ucl.ac.uk/spm/.

128. Cox RW. AFNI: Software for analysis and visualization of functional magnetic resonance neuroimages. Comput Biomed Res 1996;29:162-73 http://afni.nimh.nih.gov/afni/index.shtml.

129. Hansen LK, Nielsen FA, Toft P, Liptrot MG, Goutte C, Strother SC, et al. Lyngby - modeler's Matlab toolbox for spatio-temporal analysis of functional neuroimages. Neuroimage 1999;9(6): S241 http://www.pet.med. va.gov:8080/distrib/lyngby.html.

130. Cohen JD. FisWidgets. http://neurocog.lrdc.pitt.edu/fiswidgets/; 2001.

131. Ojemann G, Ojemann J, Lettich E, Berger M. Cortical language localization in left, dominant hemisphere. J Neurosurg 1989;71:316-26.

132. George JS, Aine CJ, Mosher JC, Schmidt DM, Ranken DM, Schlitz HA, et al. Mapping function in human brain with magnetoencephalography, anatomical magnetic resonance imaging, and functional magnetic resonance imaging. J Clin Neurophysiol 1995;12(5):406-31.

133. Poliakov AV, Albright E, Corina D, Ojemann G, Martin RF, Brinkley JF. Server-based approach to web visualization of integrated 3-D medical image data. In: Proc AMIA Fall Symp; 2001. p. 533-7.

134. Hurdal MK. A demonstration of cortical flat mapping. http://www.pet.med.va.gov:8080/incweb/circlepack/; 2001.

135. Drury H, West B, Van Essen D. CARET daemon. http://stp.wustl.edu/CARETdaemon/CARETdaemon.html; 1997.

136. Sereno MI. Webcortex: Web interface to cortical surface database. http://cogsci.ucsd.edu/~sereno/webcortex.html; 2001.

137. Herskovits EH. BRAID: Brain imaging database. http://braid.rad.jhu.edu/; 2001.

138. Hadida-Hassan M, Young SJ, Peltier ST, Wong M, Lamont S, Ellisman MH. Web-based telemicroscopy. J Struct Biol 1999;125:235-45 http://ncmir.ucsd.edu/CMDA/jsb99.html.

139. Koslow SH. Should the neuroscience community make a paradigm shift to sharing primary data? Nat Neurosci 2000;3(9):863-5.

140. Nature Neuroscience Editorial. A debate over fMRI data sharing. Nat Neurosci 2000;3(9):845-6.

141. Benson DA, Karsch-Mizrachi I, Lipman DJ, Ostell J, Rapp BA, Wheeler DL. GenBank. Nucleic Acids Res 2000;28(1):15-8.

142. Kotter R. Neuroscience databases - tools for exploring brain structure-function relationships. Philos Trans R Soc Lond B Biol Sci. In Press 2001 http://www.hirn.uni-duesseldorf.de/rk/neurodat.htm.

143. Jakobovits R, Soderland S, Taira RK, Brinkley JF. Requirements of a web-based experiment management system. In: Proceedings, AMIA Symposium 2000. Los Angeles; 2000. p. 374-8.

144. Jakobovits RM, Brinkley JF, Rosse C, Weinberger E. Enabling clinicians, researchers, and educators to build custom web-based biomedical information systems. In: Proc AMIA Fall Symp 2001. p. 279-83.

145. Jakobovits R. WIRM: A perl-based application server. Web Techniques 2000(September):97-100 http://www.webtechniques.com/archives/2000/09/jakobovits/.

146. Pelletier M, Latteier A. The Zope Book: New Riders; 2001 http://www.zope.org/Members/michel/ZB/.

147. Brinkley JF, Jakobovits RM. UW Brain Project Language Map Experiment Management System. http://tela.biostr.washington.edu/cgi-bin/repos/bmap_repo/main-menu.pl; 2001.

148. Wong STC, Hoo KS, Knowlton RC, Laxer KD, Cao X, Hawkins RA. Design and applications of a multimodality image data warehouse framework. J Am Med Assoc. In Press 2001.

149. Letovsky SI, Whitehead SHJ, Paik CH, Miller GA, Gerber J, Herskovits EH, et al. A brain-image database for structure-function analysis. Am J Neuroradiol 1998;19:1869-77.

150. Herskovits EH. An architecture for a brain-image database. Methods Inf Med 2000;39(4-5):291-7.

151. Arbib M. Neural plasticity: data and computational structure. http://www-hbp.usc.edu/; 2001.

152. Gazzaniga MS. The fMRI data center. http://www.fmridc.org/; 2001.

153. Herskovits EH, Megalooikonomou V, Davatzikos C, Chen A, Bryan RN, Gerring JP. Is the spatial distribution of brain lesions associated with closed-head injury predictive of subsequent development of attention-deficit/hyperactivity disorder? Analysis with brain-image database. Radiology 1999;213(2):389-94.

154. Beeman DE, Bower JM, De Schutter E, Efthimiadis EN, Goddard N, Leigh J. The GENESIS simulator-based neuronal database. In: Koslow SH, Huerta MF, editors. Neuroinformatics: An Overview of the Human Brain Project. Malwah, New Jersey: Lawrence Erlbaum; 1997. p. 57-81. http://www.bbb.caltech.edu/hbp/

155. Miller PL, Nadkarni P, Singer M, Marenco L, Hines M, Shepard G. Integration of multidisciplinary sensory data: a pilot model of the Human Brain Project approach. J Am Med Assoc 2001;8(1):34-48 http://ycmi-hbp.med.yale.edu/senselab/.

156. Dashti AE, Ghandeharizadeh S, Stone J, Swanson LW, Thompson RH. Database challenges and solutions in neuroscientific applications. Neuroimage 1997;5(2):97-115.

157. Fox PT, Mikiten S, Davis G, Lancaster JL. BrainMap: A database of human functional brain mapping. In: Thatcher RW, Hallett M, Zeffiro T, John ER, Heurta M, editors. Functional Neuroimaging. San Diego: Academic Press; 1994. p. 95-106. http://ric.uthscsa.edu/projects.

158. Bowden DM, Robertson JE, Martin RF, Dubach MF, Wu JS, McLean MR, et al. Web-tools for neuroscience based on NeuroNames, a template brain atlas, edgewarp and geographic information systems software. In: Fifth international conference on functional mapping of the human brain. Heinrich-Heine University, Dusseldorf, Germany; 1999. http://braininfo.rprc.washington.edu/.

159. Berman HM, Westbrook J, Feng Z, Gilliland G, Bhat TN, Weissig H, et al. The Protein Data Bank. Nucleic Acids Res 2000;28:235-42.

160. Bly BM, Rebbechi D, Grasso G, Hanson SJ. A peer-to-peer database for brain imaging data. In: Hum Brain Mapp; 2001. http://www.academicpress.com/www/journal/hbm2001/11785.htm.

Address of the authors:
James F. Brinkley, Cornelius Rosse
Structural Informatics Group
Box 357 420
Department of Biological Structure
University of Washington
Seattle, WA 98195, USA
http://sig.biostr.washington.edu

Research and Education Section

Biomedical Computation at Stanford University: A Larger Umbrella for the Future

Russ B. Altman, M.D., Ph.D.

The explosion of biological data and knowledge from genomic sequencing, microarray analysis, clinical data warehouses, electronic publishing, and other new sources of high throughput data has made clear the importance of informatics in biology and medicine. Nevertheless, many institutions find themselves with pockets of excellence in biomedical computation, but no centralized organization that allows investigators and students to respond to large, interdisciplinary research and training challenges. Stanford University, with its long history of contributions to biology, medicine, computing, engineering and their intersection, is now mapping out a plan for integrating these efforts to allow a more concerted response to the scientific challenges at the intersection of biomedicine and computer/information science.

The balance between what new technologies offer and what current practice requires must be reassessed constantly.

Here, we report on the thinking behind some of the models for how biomedical computation can be organized. Much of the formal training in biomedical computation at Stanford has focused on the interdisciplinary Biomedical Informatics Training Program (formerly known as the Medical Information Sciences Training program), whose students have worked on research projects university-wide. Other students from disciplinary departments such as computer science, electrical engineering, genetics, and chemistry (among others) have also made important contributions in the field of biomedical computation. Despite the distributed excellence in the applications of computer science and information science to biology and medicine, significant challenges exist in creating a program that integrates efforts throughout the university.

Computational Challenges

The chief computational challenges involve the creation of:

- Standard vocabularies and structured representations for the exchange of biological data and knowledge from person to person, person to computer, and computer to computer. The legacy of natural language literature, while immensely valuable, has created a barrier to using automated methods for analysis and retrieval of this information.
- Accessible databases and knowledge bases of both primary data, and new knowledge elements learned from these data.
- Algorithms for extracting new knowledge automatically from new data. The use of standard vocabularies, and efficient storage of information are useful only if algorithms exist to extract and store new propositions about how things work.
- Faithful simulations of biological systems at scales ranging from Angstroms (molecular dynamics of macromolecules) to microns (cellular apparatus) to meters (full organism simulations). The best way to demonstrate a complete understanding of the roles and interactions of biological systems is to faithfully simulate processes in a computer.
- Software to link information and knowledge systems to the outside, manipulatable physical world. Biology and medicine of the future will mix sensing of data with ability to manipulate biological and medical systems through software-controlled robotic devices.
- Software to support the education and maintenance of professional competency for physicians and scientists in a world where the number of facts available greatly exceeds the ability of any practitioner (even the most exceptional) to remember these facts.

The Changing Climate for Funding

The importance of these challenges has not been lost on biomedical research funding sources, and priorities have been changed to ensure biomedical science of the 21st century has the necessary computational infrastructure to enable progress. The NIH recently started the Biomedical Information Science and Technology Initiative (BISTI) (http://grants.nih.gov/grants/bistic/bistic_news.cfm), which aims to create centers of excellence in biocomputation to train the next generation of biomedical computational scientists, and will provide focus points

The cover of the Winter 2000 Stanford faculty retreat brochure depicts six focus areas. From top left, clockwise: data modeling and informatics, biomechanical simulation, image analysis, networked education, computer-assisted interventions, and structural/functional informatics.

for shared infrastructure and collaborative interdisciplinary research. The National Science Foundation is also supporting the creation of databases and algorithms to accelerate progress in biology and computer science (http://www.

nsf.gov/). The Department of Energy has supported computational applications in biology (www.sc.doe.gov/production/ober/msd_bio_eng.html). The Defense Advanced Research Projects Agency (DARPA) announced its intention to look into the interface of computation and biology from a strategic point of view (www.darpa.mil/DSO/solicitations/00/index.htm).

Philanthropic foundations have also shown great interest in supporting biomedical computation, including the Keck Foundation, which awarded many university grants; the Burroughs-Wellcome Foundation, which created programs supporting computational approaches to functional genomics; the Whitaker Foundation supports computation especially in the context of engineering; and the Howard Hughes Medical Institute recently funded several investigators with a primary presence in the area of computational biology. The Sloan Foundation has supported the training of students and post-doctoral fellows in biomedical computation, and recently expressed interest in creating Master's degrees in areas of biomedical computation.

Most remarkable is the recognition by many U.S. states that biomedical computation may be an area for new competition and technology development and transfer. Several state governors support efforts to build up the biomedical computation capabilities of state universities in order to provide a competitive advantage in recruiting young faculty, new students, and grant funds.

Creating an Umbrella Organization

Since the challenges to computation and information science in biology and medicine are so broad, does it make sense to bring investigators together? Or is it perhaps better to allow computation expertise to infiltrate all areas of biology and medicine, and not to centralize it? While it is true that computational and information scientists must interact closely with (and often become) application area experts, there are reasons to also bring them together. At Stanford, there are three reasons to do this:

Shared infrastructure. Unlike experimental biologists and clinicians, biomedical computation scientists live in a (mostly) dry world of computers, dis-

plays, hard disks, and peripherals. Attempting most of the challenges described earlier requires large computers, databases, and very fast networks that are simply beyond the budget of any single research project. Collaboration is also needed in the creation and maintenance of general-purpose software libraries for numerical analysis, string comparison, data mining and discrete time simulations.

Collaborative interdisciplinary research. Many research challenges require a multi-disciplinary approach, and no single investigator has sufficient expertise to address the technical challenges in all areas. As departments are not interdisciplinary, they rarely have the full set of talents required to solve difficult problems in biomedical computation. Thus, it is critical to have some forum where

---

Most remarkable is the recognition by many U.S. states that biomedical computation may be an area for new competition and technology development and transfer.

---

investigators from a variety of disciplines can seek collaborators and colleagues within the area of biomedical computation. During research, if biologists or physicians recognize they may have a biomedical computational problem, they usually are not sure what kind of expertise is required. A network of at least loosely organized investigators helps catalyze progress.

Shared training. Although the application areas within biomedical computation are diverse, we believe a core set of principles should be taught to all students working in this field. These principles relate to the nature of biological and medical data (fuzzy, incomplete, based on wet-systems), the critical importance of sequence and string analysis in molecular biology, the issues of mathematical modeling of complex physical systems in all areas of biomedical research, and the importance of understanding the biomedical "pipeline" of knowledge—from molecular biology, to cell biology, to physiology, and to population biology.

Areas of Biomedical Computation

The research vision for such centers of biomedical computation is the most critically important justification for their creation. At Stanford, a retreat of over 70 faculty members from the Schools of Medicine, Engineering, Humanities and Sciences, and the Stanford Linear Accelerator Center was held in January of 2000. The abstract book from this retreat is available at http://neurosurgery.stanford.edu/bits/arch/docs/biocomp-retreat.pdf. The areas of biomedical computation that divided these investigators were defined by the organizing committee (see Figure). All areas had representatives from more than one department, and usually more than one school. There were representatives from the application areas and enabling computation and information science areas. Each group articulated its scientific vision, and corresponding computational goals as summarized here:

Structural and functional genomics. The vision is to understand and compute with the molecular objects in biology, and define the common mechanisms that underlie molecular processes of life at the atomic level of detail. The computational goal is to develop data representations and algorithms that allow the explosion of molecular data to be managed and converted into biological knowledge. A sample application is the use of expression microarrays to reconstruct the network of interactions among genes in a single living cell.

Biomechanical simulation. The vision is to allow simulation of biomedical systems to be accurate, fast and relevant to biomedical research and clinical practice. The computational goals are to create robust simulation methods ranging from cellular to organismal to population levels and to elucidate the principles by which these simulations should be created. A sample application is the use of dynamic fluid flow modeling to predict the efficacy of bypass grafts in the setting of atherosclerotic disease.

Computer assisted interventions and robotics. The vision is to link physical devices to software systems allowing both research experiments and clinical interventions to be automated and controlled for efficiency and reproducibility. The computational challenges are in robotic planning, image-reality fusion, and closed-loop control systems. A sample application is the use of display technologies to augment the surgical field, and allow advanced haptics to be used to aid surgeon-controlled microscopic operating fields.

Image acquisition and analysis. The vision is to create new visualization modalities applicable in both basic research and clinical medicine to improve insight and outcomes. The computational challenges are the management of large data sets, the extraction of features, and the indexing and retrieval of images in rapid and relevant manner. A sample application is the use of 3D reconstructed MRI to create a "virtual colonoscopy" digitally, and make the detection of colonic lesions less invasive and more accurate.

Informatics, data modeling, and statistics. The vision is to create an information infrastructure that allows biomedical information and knowledge to be stored, retrieved, and analyzed, efficiently and extensibly. The computational challenges are the creation of robust data models that are sufficient to enable efficient data and knowledge acquisition, data mining, and statistical analysis for new knowledge. A sample application is the creation of a knowledge base that links genomic, laboratory, and clinical data about how variation in human genetics correlates to variation in response to medications (pharmacogenomics) and the creation of clinical decision support systems to deliver this information to the point of care.

Networked and computer-aided education. The vision is to create computational infrastructure to support training and professional continuing education systems that are cost-effective, efficient, and maintainable. The computational challenges are the creation of capabilities in the next generation Internet to support remote training/education, the development and evaluation of methods for interacting with virtual physical systems, and the delivery of these capabilities to the learning environments in which they are most useful and relevant. A sample application is the creation of surgical training software including haptic feedback, real-time instruction, and evaluation.

Nontrivial Challenges

Failure to address the following nontrivial logistical and philosophical challenges can doom efforts to create a useful focus of attention for biomedical computation.

Physical vs. knowledge systems. To organize biomedical computation at Stanford, we divided into six areas. Later we noted that some focus areas, like biomechanical simulation, are primarily concerned with physical systems, whereas others, like informatics, are primarily concerned with cognitive or knowledge structures for the organization of information, and others, like structural and functional genomics, are concerned with both. To create a symmetry in the training environment that mirrors the dichotomy among the research focuses, we may augment our current Biomedical Informatics training program with an additional program focusing on biomedical physical systems computing.

....

The challenge of unifying biomedical computation is sufficiently profound, difficult, and exciting that faculty leaders have been willing to work with the inevitable difficulties that arise.

....

Engineering vs. medicine cultures. We operate at the interface between two very different schools, medicine and engineering, and the frequent clashes between those driven to make contributions in an application area and those driven to make technological innovation is no surprise. The differences in each school's academic culture (modes of publication, expectation for trainees, and traditional sources of funding) can make it challenging for faculty to interact. Finally, variations in financial models for funds flow in each academic unit provide challenges. The solution involves continued contact between the relevant faculty members, so to understand and work within the constraints imposed by different cultures. It is not wise to attempt to re-engineer entire organizations the size of a university or a granting agency, and so compromises must be sought to advance the mission under mostly existing rules.

The organization of biomedical computation may begin by dividing all projects into application and technology goals, and then have members of the collaborative team identify themselves by a primary activity, but recognize and understand the importance of the other. Thus, a collaboration between engineering and surgical groups may be driven by the realities and needs of surgery, but may have a number of technological innovations emerge that cause current surgical practice to be reassessed. The balance between what new technologies offer and what current practice requires must be reassessed constantly. The dual model of application groups and enabling technology groups that mix and match to form relevant projects has been used since 1998 at the National Partnership for Advanced Computational Infrastructure (NPACI) (www.npaci.edu).

Conclusions

We are designing an umbrella organization for biomedical computation allowing us to benefit from shared research infrastructure, shared curriculum and research training, and facilitated interdisciplinary research. Current efforts at Stanford fall within six focus areas with long-range vision, which enables us to define the medium-term set of computational challenges. Faculty participation from multiple schools and departments is a critical element to successfully mobilizing interest and commitment to this organization. The challenge of unifying biomedical computation is sufficiently profound and exciting that faculty leaders have been willing to work with the inevitable difficulties that arise. The long-term success of these efforts will be gauged by the ability to support novel science leading to important contributions to biomedicine.

Acknowledgments

RBA is supported by NIH LM-05652, LM-06422, GM-61374, NSF DBI-9600637, and grants from Burroughs Wellcome Foundation and Sun Microsystems. ●

Russ B. Altman, M.D., Ph.D., Associate Professor of Medicine (and Computer Science, by courtesy), is Director of the Biomedical Informatics Training Program at Stanford University

**M. Fieschi, D. Fieschi,
J. Gouvernet, M. Joubert,
G. Soula**

LERTIM Faculté de Médecine
Université de la Méditerranée Marseille,
France

Research and Education

Education and Research in Health Informatics at the Faculty of Medicine of Marseille, Laboratory for Education and Research in Medical Information Processing (LERTIM)

Abstract: This paper is a brief review of the research and training programs offered in Medical Informatics at the Faculty of Medicine of Marseille (LERTIM). Our laboratory teaches medical informatics and bio-statistics in the medical training curriculum, and prepares for specialised degrees and provides continuing medical education. The research projects developed by our team fall into four groups: clinical decision systems, health information systems, medical education systems, integration systems.

Introduction

The LERTIM laboratory is part of the Faculty of Medicine, a division of "Université de la Méditerranée" including several campuses in Marseille and Aix-en-Provence, France. The Faculty of Medicine, the Faculty of Pharmacy, and the School of Odontology are located on a common campus next to the largest teaching hospital in downtown Marseille.

Our group is approximately 18 strong, including 2 secretaries and 5 PhD students. Some of the LERTIM members (6 in all) have two sets of responsibilities, because of the way French medical schools and teaching hospitals are organized: they have teaching and research activities both in the Faculty of Medicine and the teaching hospital. Their faculty activities deal with research on medical informatics topics and fundamental aspects, and their hospital activities with practical ones.

Teaching activities proceed within the framework of compulsory studies and cover University degrees within the teaching hospital and continuing education facilities.

Research activities in the Faculty of Medicine, are concerned with the application of new information and communication technologies (decision support systems, information indexing and retrieval, modelling and access to knowledge bases, health information systems etc.). The main research goal in the teaching hospital is clinical research in various medical fields.

We shall describe the teaching curriculum and the main research aspects our laboratory is involved in. Most of these descriptions are already available (in French) on our web site http://cybertim.timone.univ-mrs.fr/cybertim/.

Education

In the French medical curriculum, the three first years are dedicated to fundamental medical and biological sciences. The next three years prepare students for internships and residencies.

Our LERTIM laboratory teaches bio-statistics, the methodology of clinical epidemiology, evidence-based medicine, new technologies of information and communication (NTIC), and medical informatics throughout the medical education process. The laboratory covers the complete medical curriculum, from the first year to internship, and even later, in continuing medical education, as summarised in Figure 1.

A medical informatics handbook, co-authored by Patrice Degoulet and translated into several languages [1], summarizes the different aspects of medical informatics as taught by our group.

Bio-statistics teaching

Bio-statistics and clinical epidemiology are mainly taught over the first three years of the medical training program. We teach a compulsory bio-statistics course during the first year. This 30-hour course is dedicated to medicine, odontology, and physiotherapy curricula and is taught to 1700 students. Less than 350 students

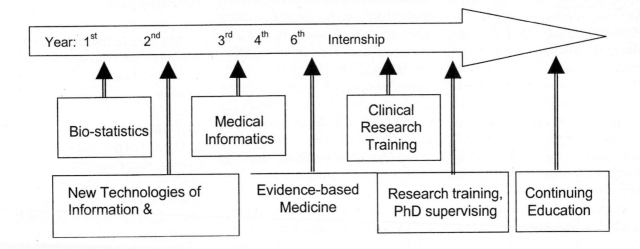

Fig. 1. LERTIM laboratory involvement in medical education curriculum at the Faculty of Medicine of Marseille.

(210 for medicine) are selected in the three disciplines with a competitive examination at the end of the year. The statistics being taught are basic and include descriptive methods used to evaluate everyday clinical data and activities.

New Technologies of Information and Communication training (NTIC)

NTIC training (20 hours) is provided to students in their second year of medical curriculum. They must practice the basic software currently used: operating system environment, word processing, spreadsheet processing, information retrieval and Internet browsing. Two hours are dedicated to scientific documentation research on the Internet. This training is compulsory.

Degrees in Medical Informatics and Evidence-based Medicine

Once their year of first medical curriculum has been completed, students may decide to take advanced degrees. Individual degree training lasts approximately 100 hours. Our laboratory is responsible for two of those.

The first one (Certificate in Medical Informatics and Communication Tech-

nology) surrounds Medical Informatics, including conceptual modelling, database management, multimedia systems, health care information systems and networks, decision support and artificial intelligence applications.

The second one deals with evidence-based medicine, including meta-analysis principles and practice, statistics tools and models, medical information retrieval. Clinicians from the faculty and from the teaching hospital present case studies in various medical specialties, including infectious diseases, cardiology, oncology, dermatology, etc.

Pedagogic Web server project of the Faculty of Medicine

The introduction of computer technologies may support a wide range of learning activities and enlarge pedagogic approaches. These technologies also encourage active learning, support cultural changes and increase resource sharing. Consequently, the development of new pedagogic initiatives needs to be integrated with other forms of learning, i.e. on-site traditional training and courses, discussions and comments regarding case studies in small groups, general clinical training and practice, problem-based learning,

virtual situations and simulations, on-site and/or on-line tutoring.

We have been experimenting along those lines with a pedagogic Web site intended for use by our medical school students (http://medidacte.timone.univ-mrs.fr) since 1999.

A designated Web server, MEDIDACTE, was preliminarily and partially implemented. This server integrates teaching strategy. It was designed according to a general approach, in which technology can be used to supplement and enhance medical education. Significant efforts were made to:

- train teachers in pedagogic aspects of Web technology,
- recognize their involvement in e-learning.

The MEDIDACTE e-learning environment includes three workspaces implemented for users, including students, visitors, and faculty. The most suitable educational resources are suggested in the student workspace, according to their profiles with identification and access rights attributes. The visitor workspace offers access to pedagogic projects by medical specialty. The faculty member workspace being envisioned has three functions:

- managing projects (developing a course, selecting course tools, organizing courses by topics, etc.),
- applying teaching scenarios,
- Assessing projects and follow-up.

More than 30 educational projects, covering different disciplines, included in the training curriculum were compiled in one year. Traditional pathology laboratory operations were, for example, replaced with virtual ones using digital images. This change was unanimously required by the pathology teachers and generally well accepted by the students.

In 2000, with the support of the Dean of the Faculty of Medicine, we decided to design and experiment with an evidence-based medicine degree course in French using Internet facilities and taking the new paradigms emerging in medical education into account.

National training program in Medical Informatics

We are taking part in a national training program for PhDs in cooperation with the universities Paris V, VI and Rennes. This is a DEA (Advanced Research Diploma) in Medical Informatics and is taught in Paris. We are involved in teaching knowledge representation and artificial intelligence applications for decision support in medicine (25 hours), as well as cognitive approaches for knowledge transfer and learning (10 hours).

Continuing education in the hospital

Our group is also involved in continuing education in two different fields including:
- the use of statistics in clinical research with the associated software
- medical language, indexing and retrieving information (Medline queries included).

The courses are given in the hospital environment to healthcare professionals only.

Research

Our research topics have included medical decision support and artificial intelligence applications in medicine for many years now. In the eighties, we designed, developed and experimented with expert systems based on symbolic and fuzzy logic (SPHINX [2] and PROTIS [3]). We also developed expert systems for investigating knowledge representation, decision modelling and knowledge evaluation.

Our current research activity is still centred on decision support and guidelines in medical practice; these are integrated into health information systems to provide "knowledge coupled tools" that are usable in real practice. This must include:
- various researches in medical concepts representation, artificial intelligence and cognitive psychology methods, reasoning models, cognitive man-machine interaction models;
- the development of software components for the representation, treatment and communication of information and knowledge, as well as using multimedia technologies.

We have 5 to 7 students (PhDs, DEA and other researchers) involved in the various projects.

The current research activities of the LERTIM (Medical Informatics Laboratory) are summarised in Figure 2 below.

The ARIANE project

The aim of the ARIANE project is to provide healthcare professionals with efficient access to information sources helpful to their daily practice [4-12]. This means the users need quick and seamless access to the expected level of information. Information sources may either be integrated in their institution network (intranet), or on an Internet site. In the first case, the engineers controlling the quality of information supervise the efficiency of access to those databases integrating information sources within the institution's intranet. Whenever a source of information is located outside an institution's network, questions arise as to how the quality of its contents can be guaranteed and how users can have efficient access to this source. In any case, ARIANE is not only intended to

Main research topics	Medical information and knowledge: decision aids, education			Semantic interoperability
Projects	EsPeR project Guideline-based decision support	ASTI project Guideline-based drug prescription	Learnet project Education and hypermedia knowledge	ARIANE project Medical ontology and language, information system architectures
	Health Information Systems			
	"UMVF" project Virtual French-speaking medical university			

Fig. 2. Synopsis of LERTIM research activities in Medical Informatics.

connect users with servers, but above all, to query servers, and then connect users with those servers at the point of result delivery.

In this framework, we have designed, are currently developing, and will experiment with a complete middle-ware architecture composed of:
- a conceptual interface that helps end-users express their queries,
- a broker identifying relevant inform-ation sources and suggesting access to them
- mediators able to express end-user queries in the languages of re-sources and send them.

This architecture uses the NLM's Unified Medical Language System, knowledge sources and an "Internet Sources Catalog" describing the contents of the information sources and how to access them.

A project named WRAPIN recently accepted (June 2001) by the European Commission aims to integrate both ARIANE results and the currently existing information retrieval and indexing tools developed by the Health On the Net (HON) foundation in Geneva, Switzerland.

The Learnet project

This project is intended to design develop and evaluate interactive environments to optimise decisions and acquire medical knowledge in an NTIC background [13-17]. The courseware allows greater student autonomy; it can individualise the educational pro-cess and may contribute to the various phases of the pedagogical process, i.e. presenting information, repetition, control, and usage on simulations or in real situations. The project takes the educational and cognitive aspects, knowledge bases and their methods of access into account. Its goal is to provide teachers with the means to integrate knowledge bases into their own educational projects.

The project takes several problems inherent to the acquisition and spread of medical knowledge into account:
- identifying the level of knowledge to be spread: superficial, extensive etc.
- modelling and representing the knowledge to be spread,
- developing tools for faculty to integrate NTIC in their educational projects,
- identifying objects and metaphors available to students for accessing knowledge.

Coupling encyclopaedic knowledge and educational projects should help teachers better adjust NTIC and lead to an evolution in medical education.

Partnership projects

The UMVF ("Université Médicale Virtuelle Francophone") project is funded by the French Ministry for Research and is based on a federation of resources either existing or currently being developed in several French Medical Schools. The objectives of this project are not only to share experiences across the country but also to integrate several resources while using NTIC to support new pedagogical approaches for medical students and also to continue medical education [18]. This project includes:
- a virtual Medical Campus securely accessed from several sites,
- the integration of new interactive resources, based on pedagogical methods,
- the implementation of new indexing and search engines, based on medical vocabularies and ontologies,
- the definition of general and specific portals, as well as a system evaluation for ergonomics and contents.

Those French medical faculties not initially involved will evaluate the results of this project.

The EsPeR ("Estimation Personna-lisée du Risque") project is based on rules and guidelines and features an Internet server [19]. We developed this project in cooperation with the Paris VI University's Medical Information Group (Pr P. Degoulet).

This project has two main objectives:
- Providing a tool for physicians to evaluate the risks of death according to patients' individual symptoms,
- Offering suggestions and guidelines for preventive measures that take individual patient risks into account.

A probability based method covering pathologies for which preventive measures exist has been developed to help physicians objectively assess the main causes of death of their patients.

The ASTI ("Aide à la Stratégie Thérapeutique Informatisée") project deals with drug prescriptions that are often inadequate in the hospital or ambulatory setting. We collaborated with the Paris V (Pr. A. Venot) and Paris VI (Pr. JF. Boisvieux) Medical Informatics Groups to conduct this project. Although computer-based physician ordering systems already exist and provide effective drug-centred checks, their optimisation of the patient-centred therapeutic strategy overall is poor. Although evidence-based clinical guidelines were devel-oped to disseminate state-of-the-art and strategic therapeutic knowledge, they are not used very often in daily practice. The ASTI project is intended to design a guideline-based decision support system to help general practitioners avoid prescription errors and comply with best therapeutic practices.
- A « critical mode » is applied as a background process without modi-fying the physician's entry habits and corrects his /her prescriptions with elementary rules that are auto-matically triggered and take indivi-dual recommendations into account.
- A « guided mode » is selected by the physician to browse through the comprehensive guideline knowledge represented as a decision tree and to access the best treatment.

A first prototype is currently under development and applies the manage-ment of hypertension. General practi-tioners will validate the results.

EasyCare was a project developed by an industrial partner for whom LERTIM team members acted as expert consultants. It was used to process the results of the European STAR project involving health scientists from several countries (France, United Kingdom, Ireland, Italy and the Netherlands). EasyCare was designed to provide modelling and implementation tools for an information system that describes health supplies in a given area (region, country, continent (Europe)). This supply system is open to both laymen and healthcare professionals via querying and navigation applications. The results are:

- a conceptual model,
- a telematics infrastructure for continuity of care,
- navigation tools within resources,
- available health services within a geographical area,
- communication and information services.

Its first application is a "Yellow Pages" service for health professions.

Health Information systems

L. Weed [20] said "We would all like to live in a society where the logic and actions of everyone are based on the best available knowledge and analyses of the day"; but we know that this does not happen most of the time. To meet this objective, the designers of new-generation hospital information systems must be compelled to effectively couple medical knowledge and action. Our group is working on architectures and models for better integration of standardised knowledge in health care information systems.

Bio-statistics and clinical research

A LERTIM research group, composed of methodologists and bio-statisticians, commonly handles clinical or public health studies on request by healthcare practitioners. We provide physicians with methodological advice for their research design and the statistical analysis of their data. We are associated usually as authors in the resulting, indexed articles.

Two fields are currently being prioritised. The first one is a fundamental study on survival data analyses and models undertaken in cooperation with McGill University in Canada, and the Faculty of Dijon in France. The second one is related to melanoma in cooperation with dermatology experts [21-22].

The first research tasks mainly cover survival analysis and, particularly, relative survival analysis. We performed an assessment of the two relative regressive survival models frequently used (Hakulinen's and Esteve's method) and gave practical advice to users. We also developed two new relative regressive survival models: the first one uses B-spline functions to accommodate the variation of prognostic factors over time, and the second one, which is being assessed, is based on Markov Chain's Monte Carlo methods applied to perform relative Bayesian survival analyses.

Conclusion

Modern, quality-oriented medicine requires rational management of medical information. The goal of the medical informatics graduation program is for students to learn how to analyse and evaluate health care information and related systems. One must train those students in the daily use of information technologies in the clinical environment. These courses should help students improve the quality of their healthcare using these technology resources.

We shall continue, on the one hand, to focus our research on various areas including integrated systems, decision support and clinical informatics and, on the other hand, to strengthen the biostatistics research groups. Our aim is to enhance cooperative medical informatics research projects between our own group and other national and international institutions.

Acknowledgement

The authors wish to thank all current and past members of the department for their contributions.

References

1. Degoulet P, Fieschi M. Introduction to Clinical Informatics. New-York: Springer-Verlag; 1997.
2. Fieschi M, Joubert M, Fieschi D, Roux M. SPHINX, a system for computer-aided diagnosis. Methods Inf Med 1982;21 (3):143-8.
3. *Vialettes B, Soula G, Thirion X, San Marco JL, Roux M. PROTIS, an expert system* applied to the treatment of non-insulin-dependent diabetes. Evaluation of its efficacy. Presse Med 1985;14(41):2085-8.
4. Joubert M, Miton F, Fieschi M, Robert JJ. A conceptual graphs modelling of UMLS components. Proc. Medinfo. 1995. p. 90-4.
5. Joubert M, Robert JJ, Miton F, Fieschi M. The project ARIANE: conceptual queries to information databases. Proc AMIA Annu Fall Symp. 1996. p. 378-82.
6. Volot F, Joubert M, Fieschi M, Fieschi D. A UMLS-based method for integrating information databases into an Intranet. Proc AMIA Annu Fall Symp. 1997. p. 495-9.
7. Joubert M, Fieschi M, Robert JJ, Volot F, Fieschi D. UMLS-based conceptual queries to biomedical information databases: an overview of the project ARIANE. J Am Med Inform Assoc 1998;5(1):52-61.
8. Joubert M, Aymard S, Fieschi D, Volot F, Staccini P, Fieschi M. ARIANE: integration of information databases within a hospital intranet. Int. J Med Inf 1999;49(3):297-309.
9. Joubert M, Volot F, Fieschi D, Fieschi M. Conceptual integration of information databases into an Intranet. Medinfo. 1998:161-5.
10. Aymard S, Volot F, Fieschi D, Joubert M, Fieschi M. Towards interoperability of information sources within a hospital Intranet. Proc AMIA Symp. 1998. p. 638-42.
11. Joubert M, Aymard S, Fieschi D, Fieschi M. Quality criteria and access characteristics of Web sites: proposal for the design of a health Internet directory. Proc AMIA Symp. 1999. p. 824-8.
12. Aymard S, Joubert M, Fieschi D, Fieschi

M. Mediation services with health information sources. Proc AMIA Symp. 2000. p. 37-41.

13. Soula G, Moulin G, Delquie P, Bartoli JM, Fieschi M, Kasbarian M. Handling information and knowledge in the FORUM hypermedia authoring system: application to uterine magnetic resonance imaging. Medinfo. 1995. p. 1214-7.

14. Bernard JL, Soula G, Vitton O, Puccia J, Boeuf CL, Fieschi M. Top-Forum: an interactive multimedia knowledge database to improve quality of care in pediatric oncology. Bull Cancer 1996;83(11):901-9.

15. Soula G, Delquie P, Vitton O, Bartoli JM, Fieschi M. Designing medical hypermedia: the FORUM project. Stud Health Technol Inform 1997:712-6.

16. Pagesy R, Soula G, Fieschi M. Improving knowledge navigation with adaptive hypermedia. Med Inform Internet Med 2000;25(1):63-77.

17. Pagesy R, Soula G, Fieschi M. DI2ADEM: an adaptive hypermedia designed to improve access to relevant medical information. Proc AMIA Symp. 2000. p. 635-9.

18. Le Beux P, Le Duff F, Fresnel A et all. The French Virtual Medical University. Stud Health Technol Inform 2000;77:554-62.

19. Giorgi R, Gouvernet J, Jougla E, Chattelier G, Degoulet P, Fieschi M. The use of the personalized estimate of death probabilities for medical decision making. Comput Biomed Res 2000;33(1):75-83.

20. Weed LL. Knowledge coupling - New Premises and New tools for Medical Care and Education. New-York: Springer-Verlag; 1991.

21. Richard MA, Grob JJ, Avril MF, Delaunay M, Gouvernet J, Wolkenstein P, et al. Delays in diagnosis and melanoma prognosis (I): The role of patients. International Journal of Cancer 2000;89:271-9.

22. Richard MA, Grob JJ, Avril MF, Delaunay M, Gouvernet J, Wolkenstein P, et al. Delays in diagnosis and melanoma prognosis (II): The role of doctors. International Journal of Cancer 2000;89:280-5.

Address of the first author:
Marius Fieschi
LERTIM
Faculté de Médecine
27 boulevard Jean Moulin
F - 13385 Marseille Cedex 5
E-mail: MFIESCHI@mail.ap-hm.fr

G. Kozmann

Department of Information Systems,
Veszprém University, Veszprém,
Hungary

Research and Education

Education in medical informatics on the basis of the information technology curriculum at the Veszprém University

Introduction

Historically, medical informatics developed as an application of information technology, and, as a matter of course, is based on it even today, but - with regard to its importance and growing size - it can be considered more and more as an independent field of informatics. We have seen this growing independence as it became accepted in developed countries with a strengthening of the literature and institutional background of the field. There is high demand for related educational activities with both health and technical emphases. There are numerous publications and projects such as the "concerted action" EU EDUCTRA (Education and Training in Health Informatics), which began in 1992 under the supervision of the AIM (Advanced Informatics in Medicine) program [1]. It may be said that the educational requirements and the essential thematic characteristics of a health informatics program have taken shape by today. Since medical informatics applications overlap with other disciplines such as economics, management and law it is also necessary to teach such relevant subjects. In Hungary, the demand for

education in medical informatics arose from the computerization of the family doctor system years ago and was significantly accelerated by a World Bank program assisting hospital informatics. According to preliminary surveys, parallel to the modernization of public health, approximately 500 to 1000 health information technologists trained at the university level will be needed in the long run to meet the requirements of the 150 Hungarian hospitals, basic health care providers, the organizations operating, supervising and managing public health (OEP, ÁNTSZ, etc.), health research, and the institutions responsible for health care development and distribution. The above estimate includes the number of experts able to occupy application-oriented job positions, develop systems and elaborate on new methods. In practice we feel that the former should be trained in health sciences institutions of higher learning while the latter are best trained in technical universities. Obviously, it would be an advantage to coordinate the two paths of training. In the present paper we give a brief overview of the philosophy and practice of education based on the information technology curriculum at Veszprém University.

Background for medical informatics curricula at Veszprém University

Veszprém University, as the first in Hungary, started a graduate level health informatics module based on the Information Technology program. It was formed in 1991 under the direction of Professor Tamás Roska, a member of the Hungarian Academy of Sciences. Initially, the module included three and later four optional subjects, which were supplemented by medical topics in the courses of "Self-guided study", "Engineering project work" and "Self-guided laboratory" for advanced students [2]. After five years' experience with such a scheme, the Engineering Faculty at Veszprém University decided that education in medical informatics would be carried out within the Information Technology curriculum as a specialization starting from the academic year 1998/99. This specialization is supervised by the Department of Information Systems. Its aim is to train information technologists who are ready for engineering level research and development work for medical health applications. We also have a PhD sub-program in this field, not detailed here, for those who want to develop advanced research and development experience.

The Information Technology program of Veszprém University runs on a credit system: 300 credits must be accumulated in the 9+1 semesters of training. 240 credits come from core professional subjects, 30 from subjects revolving around language, cultural and communication skills and 30 from a master thesis which is the first major independent engineering task. Taking into consideration only the narrower group of professional subjects, 62% of the 240 credits come from the basic, introductory and core courses and professional subjects, 13% from self-study in laboratory work and engineering project work, and approximately 25% from special (elective) subjects. For choosing material involving 60 credits (25%), a selection of 253 credits, totaling 79 subjects, was available in the academic year 1999/2000.

Embedding Medical Informatics in the Information Technology Curriculum

As we began developing the Medical Informatics Specialization which is embedded in the Information Technology program, the starting point was that the training must fit into the group of special (elective) subjects. According to our design, those students who besides their informatics engineer degree want to also get a certificate for their medical informatics specification, are required to take a group of seven obligatory subjects representing the core (beginning in the 5th semester). This core is worth 24 credits, while the subjects of the remaining 36 credits are optional, though as guidance we provide a few

groups of subjects which are considered to be especially useful from the point of view of a medical informatics educational program [3]. For medical informatics students, just as before, further training options are available through subjects involving "Self-guided laboratory work", "Engineering project work" and "Self-guided study", which can be filled with content in compliance with the interests of the individual student. A maximum of 32 credits in total for these can be obtained, though 19 credits are more realistic. Based on all this, the structure of the topics taught is shown in Figure 1. The structure of one of the oldest European training programs, developed by the University of Heidelberg jointly with the School of Technology Heilbronn, is also shown in the figure. The similarity is conspicuous, the difference being a higher proportion of mathematical-physical subjects taught at Veszprém [1].

The core of medical informatics involves 7 subjects. They can be found on the first 7 lines of the training schedule shown in Table 1. The first subject of the group is "Physiology for engineers", which lays a foundation of medical interdisciplinary knowledge for

the information technologists. It is essential to acquire this knowledge not only for the knowledge's sake but also to learn the special language of health care. "Medical measurement theory" systematically deals with the principles of medical measurements, starting from measuring simple biophysical signals to the underlying physical and mathematical background for modern imaging processes. The first semester of the subject "Health information systems" provides knowledge about the requirements for basic and specialized health care, starting from small units to hospital information systems. Teaching is based on the governing thought that the essential element of modern health care will become a standardized electronic patient record capturing the longitudinal history of a patient which will be in principle available to all authorized users from any location in the country. This electronic patient record can also provide basic data for modules serving the economic operation of the health care system [4]. In the first semester of the subject, the laboratory practice, with the help of special educational programs and based on the MATLAB system, teaches how to solve typical

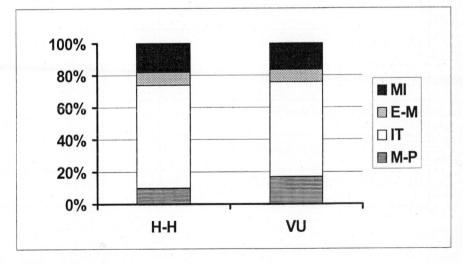

Figure 1. Normalized quantity of basic and specialized subjects taught at the University of Heidelberg and School of Technology Heilbronn (H-H) as well as at the Veszprém University (VE) in the framework of Medical Informatics [1]. (M-P: Mathematics-Physics, IT: Information Technology, E-M: Economy, Management, MI: Medical Informatics)

Table. 1. Compulsory subjects (1-7 lines) in the Medical Informatics specialization at Veszprém University, with examples of optional subjects recommended for the specialization.

Item	Subject	5. semester	6. semester	7. semester	8. semester	9. semester	credit
1.	Physiology for engineers	4+0					4
2.	Medical measurement theory		4+0				4
3.	Health information systems			2+2	0+2		2/4
4.	Statistical decision support				2+1		3
5.	Biological modeling					2+2	4
6.	The finance of health care		2+0				2
7.	Medical code systems			2+1			3
8.	Organizational theory				2+0		2
9.	Micro economics					2+0	2
10.	Image processing	4+0					4
11.	Cellular neural networks		2+0				2
12.	Computer graphics			2+1			3
13.	Use of colors in computer programs			2+0			2
14.	Multimedia systems				2+2		4
15.	Artificial intelligence				3+0		3
16.	Theory of databases				4+0		4
17.	Database applications					4+0	4
18.	Virus protection			2+2			4

medical signal and image evaluation problems. The second semester is exclusively practical work from topics of hospital information systems. It is taught in close co-operation with trainers from SMS Hungary Ltd. and using the CLINICOM systems installed by SMS Hungary Ltd. The next two subjects cover two broad groups of methods for the computer-based evaluation of clinical data, namely statistical analysis (statistical decision support) and modeling (biological modeling). When derived from the electronic patient record, computer-aided decision making could be a corner stone for health care in the future, and these two subjects provide an introduction to this. Subjects on "The finance of health care" and "Medical coding systems" deal with important operational questions of health care by teaching the essence of the financing systems and the coding processes used in health care. The remaining lines of Table 1 show examples of possible subject groups, in which economical, organizational subjects and widely needed subjects such as image evaluation, computer graphics, data bases, and artificial intelligence can be found. Recently, in accordance with the plans and possibilities of the host department, emphasis is placed on topics such as: foundations of communication, mobile communication, and internet applications. Growing interest in these directions is signaled by the number of master thesis topics developed in these areas recently.

Closing remarks

A basic view of the organizers of university education is that this education should provide important, hopefully longterm, valid knowledge and methods. Besides this, the level of demand for medical informatics experts must be given a thought at all times. An education that is over-specialized can risk restricting the jobs for which students are best suited. We do not believe that such a danger of over-specialization exists for those taking our program since the proposed approach to topics covers certain subjects in depth, but permits all aspects of information technology to be dealt with comprehensively for a specific health-related problem.

So hopefully, we have a program in which the methods and tools acquired by the student in the basic and special subjects become familiar and well-practiced, as a result of applying them with strong motivation to a realistically diverse set of problems and solutions in medical informatics.

References

1. Hasman A, Albert A, Wainwright P, Klar R, Sosa M, editors. Education and Training in Health Informatics in Europe. Amsterdam: IOS Press; 1995.
2. Roska T. Forming an Information Department in Turbulent Times. IEEE Commun Mag 1992 Nov:51-7.
3. Kozmann G. Egészségügyi informatika oktatás a Veszprémi Egyetemen [Medical Informatics Education at the University of Veszprém], Kórház 1998;5(5):44-6.
4. van Bemmel JH, Musen MA, editors. Handbook of Medical Informatics. Heidelberg: Springer; 1997.

Address of the author:
György Kozmann
University of Vesprém
Department of Information Systems
Egytem u. 12
H-8200 Veszprém, Hungary
E-mail: kozmann@almos.vein.hu

Y.-C. Li

Graduate Institute of Medical Informatics
Taipei Medical University
Taipei, Taiwan

Research and Education

The Evolving Biomedical Informatics Programs in Taipei Medical University

1. Introduction

Computer literacy has been an important issue to the medical students in Taipei Medical University (TMU). However, not until 1995 did this 40-year-old university start to realize the benefit of applying information technology to clinical care. True multidisciplinary research/education programs in medical informatics are among the latest developments in TMU's rapid expansion during the past six years. The number of faculties and graduate programs doubled in the process of expanding from an independent medical college to a university that consists of five medically-related colleges.

In 1995, a team of IT engineers and physicians were assembled to form the Center for Biomedical Informatics (CBI). Besides studying computer applications in biomedicine as its name indicated, it was also responsible for the design and deployment of the campus computer network. Starting relatively late, it was able to take advantage of the latest network technology and install ample optic fibers for the campus. A high-speed ATM (Asynchronous Transfer Mode) network was installed as the backbone and a Fast Etherswitches were used to link to most of the desktop PCs. The

backbone was later upgraded to Gigabit Etherswitches. Thanks to the flourishing IC and PC industries in Taiwan, since 1996, we were able to allocate at least one networked PC to every teacher and employee at very affordable prices. Intensive training was given to all users to familiarize them with the networked environment. Crucial applications and information were put on the school's website to attract more usage. This arrangement proved to be one of the most important steps to transform a conservative medical college to an innovative e-campus in which faculties and students are eager to harness the power of information technology.

Although computers and information systems were generally available in the business sector, computerization of hospitals and clinics was not prevalent in Taiwan until 1995 when the National Health Insurance (NHI) agent went into operation. With a 300-billion NT annual budget (about 9 billion US dollars), the NHI covers almost all of the twenty-three million people in Taiwan and has become the single largest payer for most of the healthcare expenses. For the purpose of quality control and cost containment, it demanded that all claims be submitted electronically. This decision led to the

rapid computerization of all 670 hospitals and more than 80% of the 17,000 clinics in Taiwan. The dramatic change, in turn, called for much more medical informatics research and attracted many more IT professionals into the healthcare industry.

Between 1995 and 1998, CBI played a major role in helping to computerize our campus and the two university teaching hospitals. However, we still felt a need to provide specialized training programs for this emerging multi-disciplinary domain. After several years of preparation, TMU started the first graduate program of medical informatics in Taiwan under the Graduate Institute of Medical Informatics (GIMI) in 1998. The establishment of this program turns out to be as challenging as it is rewarding to the school. The final approval for GIMI by the Ministry of Education made medical informatics one of the academically recognized disciplines in Taiwan, which also started the trend of multidisciplinary research and training in medical schools around the country.

Besides education and research works, GIMI also oversees the IT departments of the two university teaching hospitals, namely Taipei Medical University Hospital and

Wanfang Hospital. These two hospitals have a total capacity of 1000 acute inpatient beds and 1.6 million outpatient visits a year. Capitalizing on the resources provided by this rich clinical computing environment, GIMI's faculty and students were able to undertake a wide variety of applied research ranging from building electronic health records, managing/analyzing medical images to building knowledge-based systems for clinical decision support.

The evolution of the medical informatics program took another turn in the year 2000 when the draft of the complete human genome was released. The fast-growing biotechnology industry demanded more computational power and innovative algorithms for genomics and proteomics research. GIMI responded to this development with a new bioinformatics curriculum and a new center dedicated to bioinformatics research in 2001. This center, dubbed Bioinformatic Computing Center or BCC, gathered scholars from biochemistry, computer science, biostatistics, mathematics, clinical medicine and medical informatics. Together, they identified crucial problems in genomics and proteomics that can be dealt with by computational methodologies. Developing data mining techniques for microarray analysis and building neural networks for protein-protein interaction prediction were among the first batch of projects in this center.

The current biomedical informatics education and research programs in TMU are supported by GIMI, CBI, BCC and scholars from outstanding research institutes within or outside of our campus. It took time to orchestrate cooperation among highly-specialized inter-disciplinary people, but the rewards are very much worthwhile.

2. Education

TMU consists of five colleges with a total of 4500 undergraduates and 500 graduate students. GIMI offers a series of undergraduate-level courses related to computer applications in biomedicine for all the colleges, as well as a full set of graduate-level curriculum for its own fifty-four Master students and four Ph.D. students. In GIMI, most of the course work is often completed within the first school year. Research projects and theses writing occupies most of the time in the years that follow. Generally speaking, a Master student would need two years and a Ph.D. student five years to complete his degree while a thesis is required for all degrees. A proposal defense is required before a student proceeds to his research for thesis. This approach greatly reduces the chance of having an unqualified thesis at the final oral defense.

The GIMI graduate students came from a diverse range of undergraduate training backgrounds. Among them, approximately 25% were computer-related while the remaining 75% were medical professionals. Half of the GIMI medical professionals were physicians, most of them board-certified specialists, including neurosurgeons, gastroenterologists, nephrologists, oncologists, dermatologists, ophthalmologists, psychia-

trists, etc.. The heterogeneous student composition is crucial to the way our faculty conducts its classes. There are often intriguing questions and arguments raised by students that stir stimulating debate from very different perspectives.

We have designed a highly flexible curriculum to accommodate students from such diverse backgrounds, and with different career plans. A Master student must complete twenty-four credit hours of coursework before proceeding to the thesis defense. Generally speaking, a credit hour is equivalent to sixteen hours of class per semester. Together with adjunct faculty members from other TMU colleges and outstanding institutions in Taiwan, we offer an eighteen credit hour core course complemented by sixty-nine credit hours of elective courses. In order to complete all of the required credit hours, a Master student must take at least six credit hours of the elective course work, in addition to the core course. A Ph.D. student is on a different scheme and requires a total of only eighteen credit hours before thesis defense. The core course is composed of classes like seminars, healthcare information systems, introduction to medical informatics, introduction to biomedical engineering, database management systems and medical decision making (Table 1). The elective courses cover topics in four major

Table 1. Core courses in the Graduate Institute of Medical Informatics

Course	Credit Hours
Healthcare Information Systems	2
Medical Informatics	4
Database Management Systems	2
Graduate Seminars	4
Biomedical Engineering	2
Practical Training - Healthcare Information Systems	2
Medical Decision Making	2

research areas, namely medical decision support, biomedical signal processing, bioinformatics and knowledge discovery in medicine. Although most of our students came with at least basic computer and medical knowledge, two sets of complementary courses, namely basic computer course and basic medical course, are organized into the elective courses for students with different academic backgrounds. Students from a non-medical background are suggested to take the basic medical course with classes such as medical terminology and physiology. On the other hand, the basic computer course, which covers classes such as programming language and algorithms, is recommended to all students without formal computer science training.

3. Research

GIMI is committed to advancing medical care and biomedical research through the use of innovative information technology. A campus-wide Gigabit Ethernet and ATM network connecting the colleges, two university teaching hospitals, as well as two supporting centers (CBI and BCC), provides GIMI with a wealth of resources for biomedical informatics research. In the past six years, our students and faculty have conducted a wide range of research projects. Most of their efforts fit into the following areas: medical decision support, knowledge discovery and data mining, eLearning and eHealth, national Health Information Network project and Distributed Computing in Bioinformatics. Examples of research projects in these areas are described below.

3.1 Medical Decision Support:

One of our long-term projects is to develop a distributed multi-domain medical decision support system on the Web. This system will support multiple knowledge base (KB) mainte-

nance in a distributed fashion, that is, multiple groups of users can collaborate on the Internet to maintain different KBs. The resultant "cluster" of knowledge bases can be used to support different kinds of medical decisions independently, or they can work in tandem to support "multi-domain" decisions. For example, a KB for auto-immune disease can be used to support diagnostic decisions in the autoimmune diseases domain. It can also be used in conjunction with a generalized blistering disease KB to support difficult diagnostic decisions for autoimmune diseases with generalized blisters (e.g. Bullous Systemic Lupus Erythematosus).

A Web-based probabilistic knowledge platform called PIEW (Probabilistic Inference Engine on the Web) is currently available for this purpose (Figure 1). It is equipped with a dictionary editor, a knowledge frame editor, a Bayesian calculator and a consultation interface for decision support. Two knowledge bases were developed and tested on this platform;

one is to help diagnose generalized blistering diseases, while the other was designed to help diagnose autoimmune diseases [1]. "Multi-domain" inference will soon be implemented using our newly developed approximation algorithms for KBs with different knowledge domains.

3.2 Knowledge Discovery and Data Mining

We are working on several clinical databases with neural networks and various data mining techniques to uncover hidden associations among variables. For example, a national Traumatic Brain Injury (TBI) database with more than 50,000 patients was used to investigate factors contributing to the treatment strategy and outcome of patients with TBI [2]. Another example is the 400GB per year national health insurance database that stores health claims of over 300 million outpatient visits and 8 million inpatient stays a year. This database is now anonymized and released for research purpose. A plethora of questions are

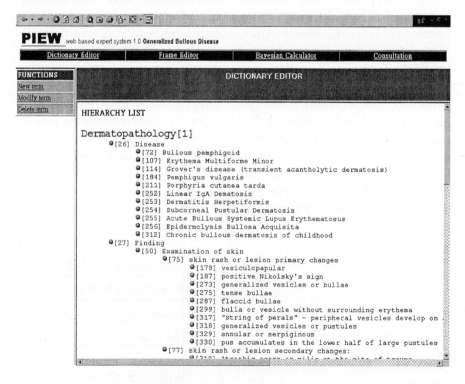

Fig. 1. A screen snapshot of the Dictionary Editor in PIEW. Eleven non-infectious generalized blistering diseases are listed in the data dictionary.

being asked against this huge database using customized data mining software tools developed by our faculty members. Interesting reports are now being published in areas such as drug-drug interactions and physician practice patterns. Neural networks are also heavily used to analyze ECG patterns to predict the risk of myocardial infarction in one of our faculty members' research [3].

3.3 eLearning and eHealth

In light of the fast development of broadband technology and the Internet, Web-based distance learning and its implications in medical education were investigated. One of the most ambitious projects would be the Virtual Medical Campus (VMC) campaign initiated by the TMU and two other leading medical schools in Taiwan. VMC set out to provide a multi-center, multi-disciplinary

information infrastructure for medical education and research. In VMC, virtual libraries, classrooms, laboratories, and teaching hospitals are all connected to a multi-modality, broadband and ubiquitous information network. All multimedia objects (including image, text, sound, video and 3D models) and their associated metadata are stored in a heterogeneous, ultra-high capacity data warehouse. Clusters of high-performance graphics workstations will provide enough computing resources for intensive 3D animation and even real-time simulation. With the vision of VMC in place, we have continuously developed component projects to fill in the big picture. Examples include a Virtual Microscope for Pathology and Histology that uses streaming images to teach pathology and histology [4], a Visible Parasite Web site for teaching medical parasitol-

ogy [5], a Virtual Clinical Pathology Conference Web site that provides high resolution clinical and pathology images for special cases [6], and a Medical Multimedia Resource Locator project for storing multimedia objects.

On the eHealth side of the research, our vision is to build a Virtual Health Community (VHC) that represents an information infrastructure for the general public to access all consumer health information, as well as personal health records securely and conveniently [7, 8]. VHC is also covering related services, ranging from online patient support groups, online pharmacy, tele-consultation to online bookstores. The purpose of VHC is to harness the power of the virtual community, while providing a one-stop-shopping environment for consumer health and wellness needs on the Internet (Figure 2).

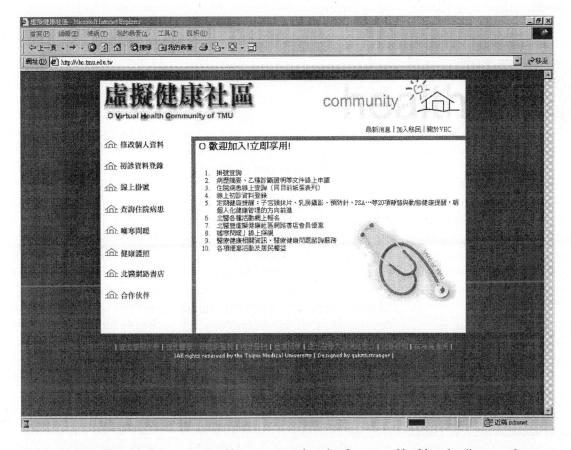

Fig. 2. The Virtual Health Community provides a one-stop shopping for personal health and wellness needs.

3.4 National Health Information Network

The Health Information Network (HIN) is one of the most important medical informatics projects directly supported by the Ministry of Health with an annual budget of several million US dollars. It covers a range of research projects that built a health information infrastructure for all hospitals in Taiwan to facilitate secure exchange of patient information. GIMI students and faculty members play a major part in the HIN project by leading one of its critical segments, the MIEC (Medical Information Exchange Center) [9, 10]. There are six component projects under MIEC, namely "Mechanisms for information exchange among heterogeneous healthcare information systems", "Development of patient-centered information retrieval systems", "Development and deployment of physician workstations in a clinical setting", "Information presentation for electronic patient records", "Extranet clinical information systems" and "Secure medical information link everywhere-SMILE". Undertaking these projects has brought us to the issue of standards such as HL7 and DICOM, as well as security issues similar to those raised by HIPAA (Health Information Portability and Accountability Act) in the United States. In the course of resolving these issues, GIMI also helped found HL7 Taiwan – one of the first official health information standards development organizations in this country.

3.5 Distributed Computing in Bioinformatics

By utilizing PC farms and Peer-to-Peer distributed computation, we are actively developing smart algorithms for genetic and proteomic search/prediction. With the help of staff from BCC, we were able to devote a significant proportion of our students and faculty to bioinformatics research.

A number of data mining techniques are now being reformulated to accommodate distributed computing and are being applied to microarray and proteomic data analysis. Some distributed genetic algorithms for choosing the fittest neural networks are being developed for prediction of specific protein-protein interactions. Molecular biology research groups from within and outside the TMU campus are collaborating with our bioinformatics team to unlock more protein functions and biological pathways for diseases such as asthma and atopic dermatitis.

3.6 Others

Some of our students and faculty are also involved in research topics such as biomedical signal processing and evidence-based medicine. As a young and energetic research institute in TMU, new areas are continuously being explored and new issues debated. This helps GIMI stay innovative and creative.

---

4. Future

As a new and exciting area in our country, medical informatics is becoming one of the most important academic disciplines in medical schools, while also attracting attention of IT industry leaders. Three major factors can be identified that were responsible for the dramatic change observed in the past few years: knowledge-based economy initiative, national health insurance policy and the rapid development of biotechnology. A knowledge-based economy initiative was proposed to the government last year that resulted in significant budget allocations to areas that can "create profit from knowledge itself". Healthcare was considered an area that can potentially contribute to this initiative due to its heavy use of patented technologies and its direct link to the

lucrative pharmaceutical market. A national conference concluded that medical informatics, with its strategic use of information technology, should be heavily invested to further the knowledge-based economy of healthcare.

The second factor is the national health insurance policy which began in 1995. It started as a fee-for-service type of reimbursement and has gradually transformed into a hybrid model that mixes Capitation and Integrated Delivery Systems. As described in the first section, NHI single-handedly forced the computerization of most healthcare organizations in Taiwan, because it accepted only electronic claims. Its continuing accumulation and selective release of anonymized electronic claim data, and its sinuated rules for claim rejections, contributed greatly to the study of healthcare information systems. The emphasis of quality of care in the coming years may again trigger another wave of research and implementation of electronic health record systems.

The third factor is the rapid development of biotechnology and bioinformatics. Reignited by the announcement of a draft of the human genome map from both the public (Human Genome Project) and the private (Celera) sectors in the year 2000, biotechnology is becoming one of the most important topics of the century. The wide implications of technologies, such as Genetically Modified Organisms (GMO) and human cloning further sparks a global debate of what can be done and what should be done. Controversy aside, biotechnology industry could become the largest segment of the worldwide market in the future and no country wants to be left behind in this cut-throat competition of research and development. This brings us to a point where medical informaticians need to decide whether bioinformatics is something worth pursuing or not. In GIMI, we recognized that the multidisciplinary nature of bioinformatics has its similarity to medical informatics and there are many techniques/experiences that can be borrowed from previous accomplishments in the field of medical informatics. On the other hand, no medical informatician is readily a bioinformatician by training. We need to incorporate more expertise from molecular and cellular biology, mathematics and biostatistics into this area. By doing so, we are making medical informatics a much more complete scientific field, since almost every medical problem is now also a genetic problem. In this country, the significance of medical informatics is becoming more eminent by the awareness raised by biotechnology and bioinformatics.

Prestigious medical schools around the world are starting to realize the clear benefit of having multidisciplinary programs, such as medical informatics and bioinformatics. In TMU, we are fortunate enough to have evolved from a small team of physicians and IT professionals into a flourishing biomedical informatics program with scholars from many different disciplines. The next challenge would be to have medical informatics and bioinformatics researchers work towards a common goal. We believe that the convergence of medical informatics and bioinformatics will eventually bring us to the next generation of personalized healthcare, where information from the cellular level is integrated with clinical information for the optimal care of each patient.

References

1. Chang YJ, Shiue HS, Li YC, Liu HN. A web-based dermatopathological diagnostic decision support system for non-infectious generalized blistering diseases. In: Proceedings of the American Academy of Dermatology 59th Annual Meeting. Washington D.C., United States; 2001.
2. Li YC, Li L, Chiu WT, Jian WS. Neural Network Modeling for Surgical Decisions on Traumatic Brain Injury Patients. International Journal of Medical Informatics 2000;57:1-9.
3. Yang TF, Devine B, Macfarlane PW. Use of artificial neural networks within deterministic logic for the computer ECG diagnosis of inferior myocardial infarction. Journal of Electrocardiology. 1999;27:188-93.
4. Surgical pathology teaching slides under virtual microscope. Taipei medical university. Available at: http://pathology.tmu.edu.tw/. Accessed Sep 1, 2001.
5. Parasitology electronic atlas. Taipei medical university. Available at: http://parasite.tmu.edu.tw/. Accessed Sep 1, 2001.
6. Virtual Clinical Dermatopathology Conference. Taipei medical university. Available at: http://cpc.tmu.edu.tw/. Accessed Sep 1, 2001.
7. Virtual Health Community. Taipei medical university. Available at: http://www.vhc.org.tw/. Accessed Sep 1, 2001.
8. Wu JS, Li YC, Jian WS. Consumer Health Information Website in Taiwan. J Formos Med Assoc. 2000;99:663-6.
9. Li YC, Kuo HS, Jian WS, Tang DD, Liu CT, Liu L, et al. Building a Generic Architecture for Medical Information Exchange among Healthcare Providers. International Journal of Medical Informatics. 2001;61:241-6.
10. Liu CT, Long AG, Li YC, Tsai KC, Kuo SS. Sharing patient care records over the World Wide Web. International Journal of Medical Informatics 2001; 61:189-205.

Address of the author:
Yu-Chuan Li
Graduate Institute of Medical Informatics
Taipei Medical University
Taipei, Taiwan
E-mail: Jack@tmu.edu.tw

W. McPhee

Centre of Medical Informatics
Monash Institute of Health Services
Research, Monash University
Melbourne, Australia

Research and Education

Education Downunder (Centre of Medical Informatics, Monash University)

Introduction

This paper describes the methods used by the Centre of Medical Informatics (CMI) to deliver health informatics education to a wide range of medical and health care workers in the undergraduate, postgraduate, health professional and general practice environment. The Centre of Medical Informatics seeks to demonstrably benefit the delivery of health care by: providing the highest calibre health informatics education at undergraduate and postgraduate levels, extending knowledge of health technologies through innovative research and development, furthering understanding of health informatics in real contexts, through quality evaluation, process methodologies and contributing to the development of effectual policy at national and international levels, continuing to collaborate with multiple organisations from a wide range of disciplines in recognition of the multi-faceted nature of informatics research, and to promote effective use of informatics to health bodies, academia and the wider community.

Undergraduate Teaching

First year students are lectured in medical informatics in the first semester of medicine. As a result of surveys conducted in 1991 and 1995 the increase in the knowledge of keyboard expertise, concepts/terms and practical ability have made it unnecessary to teach basic application skills such as word-processing, spreadsheets etc. The aim of the Centre is to equip students with long lasting tools that can be applied throughout their six years of medical training. These include such skills as Email, the Internet (World Wide Web), literature search mechanisms (i.e. OVID), and an overview of the type of working environment that they will face when they graduate. Medical Informatics is a compulsory subject that is assessed by the completion of hurdle tasks that are delivered via the World Wide Web.

Fourth year students are offered the opportunity to interrupt their normal studies for a year to pursue an honors program in one aspect of a medical discipline to gain an extra qualification: the Bachelor of Medical Science. CMI had its first Bachelor of Medical Science in Medical Informatics student in 1995, and has continued to do so each year to date. Theses written include topics such as: "Emerging Trends in General Practice: Complementary Therapies, the Internet and the General Practitioner" (L.Carter, 1997) and "A new information system for the Neonatal Intensive Care Unit at Monash Medical Centre" (H.Rodda, 2001).

Fourth year and final year students use an extensive range of computer assisted learning packages that have been developed by CMI and that are available at the many satellite sites of Monash University and teaching hospitals.

Bachelor of Biomedical Science, Faculty of Medicine first year students have lectures on subjects including: informatics and clinical health care, medical data, networks in health care, medical imaging, security and confidentiality and technology in practice. Health Informatics within the biomedical science degree is an examinable subject.

Bachelor of Radiography & Medical Imaging and the Bachelor of Nutrition & Dietetics are also degrees in which the Centre delivers basic health informatics principles to future health professionals.

General practice, health care workers and educationalists

The Centre has several educational computer programs available for downloading from our Web site. These include the HIV Hypermedia Medical Education package that is designed to teach the fundamental concepts of HIV management and to provide reference material on all aspects of HIV disease. The program Technology in Medical Education (TechME) is a comprehensive web site for developers of educational technology in medical education. This site covers many aspects, including basic pedagogy, design methodology, interface design and links to relevant resources. What's the Hype? is a set of four interactive computer based packages for adolescent patient education, covering asthma, drugs and alcohol, body image and HIV/AIDS. Information regarding these resources are available at the site www.med.monash.edu.au/informatics/resources/

Postgraduate Teaching

PhD students have been participating in our program since 1995, students have covered a wide spectrum of health informatics topics such as: "The Affective Impact of Virtual Patients: Communication Skills, Narrative and the Student Experience" (M. Bearman, 2001). CMI is also involved in the Faculty of Medicine teaching program for PhD students.

Graduate Certificate of Health Informatics is a successful educational program that demonstrates the use of information technologies applied to Health Informatics. This is delivered as a flexible approach to learning via distance education. The course is a collaborative distance education program offered jointly between the Peninsula School of Network Computing: Faculty of Computing, the Centre of Medical Informatics and the School of Nursing: Faculty of Medicine. It is endorsed by the Australian Computing Society and the Health Informatics Society of Australia and

attracts Continuing Medical Education points from relevant professional bodies, including the Royal Australian College of General Practitioners and the Australian College of Surgeons.

The objective of the course is to give the students the expertise needed to be effective developers, users and managers of health information resources. Students learn to identify information needed by doctors, nurses, hospital administrators, government planners and other healthcare professionals and will understand how data is used to make effective healthcare decisions.

A CD-ROM provides the student with the course content, required readings, relevant Internet links, email and a forum for communication. Information is provided using various forms including PowerPoint, scanned abstracts and readings, graphics, audio and video files. This course is taught using flexible delivery mode via distance. The students while either in their home or working environment have the opportunity to work through the content in a fashion that they have more control over. This increases the scope for individual learning styles, for example reflective linear learning with appropriate hyperlinks for further information.

This course was offered for the first time in semester 1, 1999. To date, in August 2001 over sixty students have completed the course. Currently fifty five students are enrolled, with a mixture of national and international students.

The course, together with the student's expectations of the course was evaluated in the first semester and second semester of 1999 and again in 2001. The results show that the

program is successful in content, mode of delivery, student's preconceived expectations, together with the quality of teaching. Results are available at the site: www.med.monash.edu.au/informatics.

The Graduate Diploma in Health Informatics builds on the Graduate Certificate year. This year of teaching was introduced in 2001 and is also delivered in flexible learning distance education mode. On completion of the Graduate Diploma it is expected that the graduates be competent to play a number of roles in the health and allied health arenas in a technologically advanced and information rich society, have an understanding and experience of research in preparation to enhance a career in which Health Informatics research and development will be a key component, be able to use sophisticated information technology and information management techniques to improve the quality of care provided by the health service and to graduate with a detailed understanding of information technology and of the particular issues involved in the development of technology for use in healthcare.

The Graduate Diploma year uses a variety of teaching tools such as: the world wide web for week-to-week notes and guides, assessment, internet links, readings and a component of core teaching, textbooks, Web CT is used for threaded discussion and chat groups and a handbook of essential dates and university forms. As with the Graduate Certificate in Health Informatics, the Graduate Diploma in Health Informatics' enrolments have substantially increased each year. It is now necessary to place quotas on enrolments to ensure quality of teaching.

Master in Health Informatics by research and coursework is the final year of the Centre's postgraduate coursework and will be offered for the first time in 2003.

Short Courses: Contempory Issues in Health Informatics: The Centre offers a range of short and long courses delivered entirely on CD-ROM, catering for the health professional with a specific interest in the areas of: Internet technologies, Evaluation in Health Informatics, Contemporary Issues in Clinical Care, Electronic Health Record and Project Management. Each short course has recognised credit points towards either the Graduate Certificate/Diploma in Health Informatics. The student is assessed by assignment that is returned to the supervisor via email and receives certification upon completion.

Conclusion

Over the past six years CMI has significantly increased its range of delivery of health informatics postgraduate and undergraduate education. As each new year approaches all programs are reviewed and evaluated to ensure that the content is current and in keeping with the ever changing dynamics of information technology in our field. The model of offering a postgraduate course with exit levels of a Graduate Certificate, Graduate Diploma and Masters degree has proven to be highly sought after by students, allowing the flexibility of exit points and therefore allowing for the consideration of personal and work demands and the necessary commitment needed to study. At each exit point the student is able to reenrol in the next level within seven years without penalty. As with all successful programs the Centre would not be able to maintain the high level of quality of teaching without the passionate dedication of our valued staff. Further information regarding the teaching programs described above is available at the site www.med.monash.edu.au/informatics.

Address of the author:
Wendy McPhee
Centre of Medical Informatics
Monash Institute of Health Services Research
Monash Medical Centre
246 Clayton Road
Clayton, 3168 Victoria
Australia
E-mail: Wendy.McPhee@med.monash.edu.au

**E.H. Shortliffe,
S.B. Johnson**

Department of Medical Informatics,
College of Physicians and Surgeons,
Columbia University,
New York, New York, USA

Research and Education

Medical Informatics Training and Research at Columbia University

Introduction

The medical informatics training and research environment at Columbia University has evolved considerably since we last wrote about our program for the Yearbook of Medical Informatics in 1995 [1]. In this article we provide a summary of the current state of the research and educational programs, beginning with their historical base, proceeding to the philosophical perspective on which the department is built, and closing with a discussion of the degree programs and curriculum.

Departmental Roots and Growth

Columbia's Department of Medical Informatics was formed in 1994, emerging from the previous Center for Medical Information Science that had been created in the late 1980s when Dr. Paul Clayton had been recruited to Columbia from LDS Hospital and the University of Utah. Under Dr. Clayton's leadership, the Center had attracted IAIMS funding from the National Library of Medicine [2, 3] and, by the early 1990s, had developed a systems architecture and had implemented a clinical

information system that was in routine use by clinicians at Columbia Presbyterian Medical Center [4]. Our faculty and staff were also major contributors to research projects such as the Arden Syntax for Medical Logic Modules [5], the Unified Medical Language System [6, 7], and the Health Level 7 standard for medical data interchange [8].

As the Center matured as an organization for academic research and training as well as for clinical service, its faculty grew in number and breadth of expertise. Beginning in 1993, we began enrolling our post-doctoral students in courses of study leading to the MA, M Phil, and PhD degrees in Medical Informatics, and in 1995 we enrolled our first group of pre-doctoral students. By 1994, it was reasonable to propose the creation of a formal department and of a degree program to grant masters and PhD degrees in medical informatics. At the time of our previous article, this degree program had just been established and we had begun converting our training program to one that began to emphasize formal degree training rather than post-doctoral fellowships. We developed a curriculum in medical informatics and graduated our first PhD student, Dr. Justin Starren (now a member of our faculty), in 1997. Our first MA degree[1]

was granted that same year. The department constitutes one of only a handful of university informatics departments in the US (it was the second when it was formed in 1994) and the only formal medical informatics education program in the New York Metropolitan Area.

An important feature of our department has been our link to the Clinical Information Services of the Columbia Presbyterian Medical Center (one campus of the New York Presbyterian Healthcare System since the merger of our hospital with Cornell Medical College's hospital in 1995). The department chair serves as Director of this hospital service, and our faculty members contribute innovations for the hospital's clinical information systems. A number of faculty members have full-time responsibility for operational systems. This close link is a major strength of our setting, for it allows trainees the opportunity to develop and evaluate projects in the context of a working hospital information system.

Since early 2000, several additional training changes have taken place as a result of the recruitment of Dr. Edward Shortliffe as Professor and Chair of the department. He assumed the position that Dr. Clayton had vacated when he returned to Utah in 1998. Dr. Shortliffe had created

---

[1] Columbia's Graduate School of Arts and Sciences offers MA rather than MS degrees.

the graduate training program in medical informatics at Stanford University in 1983, and therefore brought with him almost 20 years of experience in directing and evolving the degree program at that institution. The Columbia training program now reflects many changes in philosophy and organization that Dr. Shortliffe has instituted, including a requirement that essentially all trainees, including health-professional post-doctoral students, be formal degree candidates. Dr. Stephen Johnson continues as Director of Graduate Training, working closely with Dr. Shortliffe to implement the changes we have made and that we describe below. They are aided by a Training Executive Committee that oversees all educational programs in the department.

A Perspective on Medical Informatics

The Department of Medical Informatics (referred to as the DMI hereafter) has developed a reputation as a major center for research and education in clinical applications of informatics methods. One of Dr. Shortliffe's goals, with its implementation already underway, is to broaden the training and faculty expertise to include other areas of application. We view the phrase *medical informatics* as describing a set of methods, techniques and theories that have broad applicability in biomedicine (see Figure 1). Some people prefer to call the field *biomedical informatics* (choosing a term that seems to be more inclusive of the biological sciences), whereas others use the term *health informatics* (to use a term that is less tied to physicians and the traditional medical model of disease and treatment). But regardless of the terminology adopted, we are referring to an underlying science with associated methods and techniques. Thus a researcher or graduate student in our department is expected to develop new knowledge at that level – typically new methods that may be motivated by a single problem in biomedicine but that may in turn have broad applicability in other areas of biomedicine or even in totally different

fields. Scholarly work in medical informatics is inherently motivated by problems encountered in a set of applied domains in biomedicine. Perhaps the first of these historically has been clinical care (including medicine, nursing, dentistry, and veterinary care), areas of activity that demand patient-oriented informatics applications. We refer to this area as *clinical informatics* and recognize that it is the field in which our department has had its greatest activities and impact in the past.

Closely tied to clinical informatics is *public health informatics* (Figure 1), in which similar methods are generalized for application to populations rather than to single individuals. Thus clinical informatics and public health informatics share many of the same methods and techniques. We also identify two other large areas of application that overlap in some ways with clinical informatics and public health informatics. These include *imaging informatics* (and the set of issues developed around both radiology and other image-management and

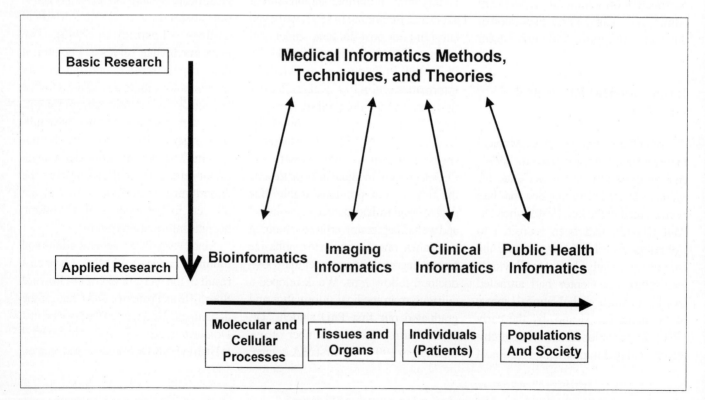

Fig. 1. The relationship of Medical Informatics to its Areas of Application

image-analysis domains such as pathology and dermatology). Finally, there is the burgeoning area of *bioinformatics*, which at the molecular and cellular level is offering challenges that draw on many of the same informatics methods as well.

As is shown in Figure 1, there is a spectrum as one moves from left to right across these application domains. In bioinformatics, workers deal with molecular and cellular processes in the application of informatics methods. At the next level, workers focus on tissues and organs, which tend to be the emphasis of imaging informatics work. Progressing to clinical informatics, the focus is on individual patients, and finally to public health, where researchers address problems of populations and of society. Thus there is a natural spectrum as suggested in the diagram, and informatics has important contributions to make across that entire spectrum. We accordingly believe that training in medical informatics requires a basic education in all four of these areas of application, followed by opportunities for specialization in one of them. Our redesigned curriculum reflects this plan, as do our current activities in faculty recruitment and departmental reorganization.

We emphasize that we see medical informatics as more than medical computer science. Good work in informatics does often contribute new knowledge to computer science, and medical informatics researchers have sometimes developed generalized computational methods and techniques that have had broad applicability, even outside the area of biomedicine. But there are other component sciences as well, including mathematics/statistics and decision science, cognitive science, information science, and management science. Properly exposing students to these diverse fields, while assuring that they become especially competent in at least one, is a major challenge in informatics curriculum design.

Collaborations at Columbia

Columbia Presbyterian Medical Center (CPMC) is one of the largest voluntary hospital centers in the country, with over 1100 beds. It is located in the Washington Heights/Inwood section of northern Manhattan and is the only major medical center in this area. The population served is disproportionately composed of racial and ethnic minorities and the poor. The DMI is a department in the College of Physicians and Surgeons, one of the four schools in the Health Sciences Division of Columbia University, all of which are co-located with the hospitals and clinics of CPMC. We have close ties with programs and individuals in all the other Health Science schools:

- *School of Dentistry and Oral Surgery* - John Zimmerman, DDS, is one of our faculty members and oversees the dental informatics component of our training program.
- *School of Nursing* - Suzanne Bakken, RN, DNSc is jointly appointed in our department and is closely involved with both our research and teaching programs.
- *School of Public Health* - Rita Kukafka, DrPH, MA, is jointly appointed in DMI and the Division of SocioMedical Sciences in the School of Public Health; she is taking the lead in designing the public health informatics components of our curriculum.
- In addition, we have an active, ongoing relationship with the *Columbia Genome Center*. Our first bioinformatics faculty member, Andrey Rzhetsky, PhD is jointly appointed in the Genome Center and has his laboratory space in that building. We are recruiting three more faculty members in bioinformatics to work at the interface between DMI and the Genome Center. All faculty, plus their students, will be located in the Genome Center so that they can work closely with other scientists there.

- We also coordinate closely with the *Computer Science Department* in the Fu School of Engineering on the main Morningside Heights campus of Columbia University. Dr. Shortliffe has an appointment in that department, and we cross-list some of our courses in order to expose computer scientists and undergraduates to medical informatics topics. There are also several collaborative research projects between members of the two departments, including a large digital libraries project on which the principal investigator is Kathy McKeown, PhD (Chair of Computer Science) and for which several collaborators and experimental sites are drawn from the DMI and the health sciences campus.
- There are strong ties between the DMI and the *Department of Psychiatry*, with joint training opportunities and research collaborations. Our Division of Decision Making and Cognition, directed by Vimla Patel, PhD, sits at the interface between these two departments (in which she holds joint appointments), and her research group is actively involved in both research and education related to psychiatry and informatics.
- Our department is the home for Columbia's *Center for Advanced Technology* (CAT) *in Information Management*, funded by the State of New York through the NY State Office of Science, Technology, and Academic Research (NYSTAR). This program funds 15 centers in the state, each devoted to technology transfer activities aimed at creating new economic opportunities in New York. Dr. Shortliffe is director of Columbia's CAT, with Dr. James Cimino from DMI and Prof. Kathy McKeown from computer science as the co-directors. The deputy director, Dr. Vincent Tomaselli, oversees the day to day operation of the CAT, including its internal grants

program. Because the CAT is a collaboration among the DMI, Computer Science Department, and the Columbia Genome Center, it is an explicit indication of the active cross-disciplinary links that characterize our research and training environment.

- We have a close and important relationship with the Office of Scholarly Resources and the Health Sciences Library on our campus. Directed by Pat Molholt, MLS, PhD, the Office of Scholarly Resources has major research projects in educational visualization and provides an important site for projects by our students. Dr. Molholt and her colleagues, Dr. Hilary Schmidt and Dr. Celina Imielinska, have also been important contributors to our educational programs.

- We also have forged new but promising relationships with the New York Academy of Medicine (NYAM). The NYAM is the regional medical library for our part of the country, and it also has an active research program in urban health. With a large continuing education program and well-established ties into the community, including the public schools, the Academy is a promising site for collaborative research applying information technology to problems in urban health and information delivery to clinicians. Our newest faculty member, Dr. Maxine Rockoff, is based at the NYAM and leads the informatics research programs there.

- Finally, we have close ties with many of the clinical departments in the College of Physicians and Surgeons. Many of our faculty members have joint appointments in other medical school departments including Medicine, Anesthesiology, Psychiatry, and Radiology. Furthermore, since Dr. Shortliffe sits on the committees for the chairs of clinical departments, he interacts regularly with the chairs of all the other clinical departments on our campus. Interestingly, he also sits on the committees for basic science chairs because the DMI, unlike most clinical departments, has a strong graduate training mission. This has allowed opportunities for frequent interactions with basic scientists, leading to the ties to the Columbia Genome Center and to computational biologists at Columbia.

The Columbia Program Today

The training program at Columbia has been funded by the National Library of Medicine since 1992. Initially aimed solely at support of post-doctoral trainees, the NLM support was broadened since 1997 to include pre-doctoral trainees as well. Our program is large (we currently have 51 degree candidates), and many of our students are not supported by the NLM training grant. The grant has played an important role in attracting eligible applicants and in facilitating their ability to pursue innovative research topics once they arrive at Columbia.

The design of our program reflects our belief that the evolution of the field of medical informatics, the need for trained informatics professionals, and the unique opportunities available at Columbia make it incumbent upon us to accept a wide range of responsibilities for training students in this area. Our decision to require formal degree programs of almost all trainees reflects a philosophical commitment to the development of medical informatics as a scholarly academic discipline as well as a field of practical importance in biomedicine. We believe that research leaders in the field will require broad formal course exposure in addition to intense research training.

Working with Leslie Perreault, MD, a graduate of the Stanford informatics training program, Dr. Shortliffe has collaborated with Drs. Gio Wiederhold and Lawrence Fagan to publish the second edition of a textbook in medical informatics [9]. This book was developed in response to the need for an introductory text in the field and has been adopted as the principal text for our first course for graduate students.

Our core faculty, all of whom have primary or secondary appointments in the Department of Medical Informatics include:

Edward H. Shortliffe, MD, PhD, (Professor and Chair)

George Hripcsak, MD, MS (Associate Professor and Vice Chair)

Suzanne Bakken, DSc, RN (Professor; also in School of Nursing)

Randolph C. Barrows Jr., MD, MS (Assistant Professor)

James J. Cimino, MD (Associate Professor)

Bruce H. Forman, MD (Assistant Professor)

Carol Friedman, PhD (Professor; also Professor of Computer Science at Queens College)

Celina Imielinska, PhD (Associate Research Scientist)

Robert A. Jenders, MD, MS (Assistant Professor)

Stephen B. Johnson, PhD (Associate Professor)

David Kaufman, PhD (Associate Research Scientist)

Rita Kukafka, DrPH, MA (Assistant Professor)

Yves Lussier, MD (Assistant Professor)

Pat Molholt, MLS, PhD (Senior Lecturer; Associate Vice President for Scholarly Resources)

Vimla L. Patel, Ph.D. (Professor; also Medical Psychology in Department of Psychiatry)

Maxine L. Rockoff, Ph.D. (Senior Lecturer)

Andrey Rzhetsky, PhD (Assistant Professor; also Investigator in Columbia Genome Center)

Soumitra Sengupta, PhD (Assistant Professor)

Justin Starren, MD, PhD (Assistant Professor)

David Wajngurt, MD, MA (Assistant Professor)

John L. Zimmerman, DDS (Associate Professor; also in School of Dentistry)

We also have several participating faculty who teach in our courses, work closely with students, and/or perform research that attracts our trainees to their laboratory:

Conrad Gilliam, PhD (Professor, Genetics; also Director, Columbia Genome Center)

Richard Goldstein, MD (Assistant Professor, Medicine)

Donald P. Harrington, M.D. (Consulting Professor; Professor and Chair, Department of Radiology, SUNY Stony Brook)

Barry Honig, PhD (Professor, Biochemistry and Molecular Biophysics)

Desmond Jordan, MD (Associate Professor, Anesthesiology)

Andrew F. Laine, DSc (Associate Professor, Biomedical Engineering and Radiology)

Kathleen R. McKeown, PhD (Professor and Chair, Computer Science)

William S. Noble, PhD (Assistant Professor, Computer Science; also Investigator in Columbia Genome Center)

Burkhard Rost, PhD (Associate Professor, Biochemistry and Molecular Biophysics)

Hilary J. Schmidt, PhD (Assistant Vice President for Scholarly Resources; Assistant Professor, Psychiatry)

Lynn Vogel, PhD (Adjunct Assistant Professor in DMI; Vice President, Information Technology, New York Presbyterian Healthcare System)

Our students are free to identify other research mentors from any part of the university, and many have attracted the supervision of faculty from other parts of the medical school or the engineering school.

In recent years, an increasing number of trainees have developed interests in biomedical imaging and have wished to pursue research and dissertations in this area. We have accordingly developed a more formal track in imaging informatics, building on cooperation between our department and the new Department of Biomedical Engineering, which was created in the last year as a joint department between the engineering school and the medical school. Our program has also collaborated closely with other departments in the health sciences and the engineering school to develop a new Center for Computational Biology and Bioinformatics. We

have a dynamic and growing environment for bioinformatics research and education, with three additional faculty recruitments underway in this area. Finally, in an effort to build a program in public health informatics, we have partnered with the School of Public Health to recruit a new faculty member, Dr. Rita Kukafka, with a joint appointment between that school and the DMI.

The Training Program

It is our goal that Columbia help shape the evolving discipline of Medical Informatics by establishing a rigorous, academically-oriented training program that offers complementary exposures to real-world systems, in clinical settings here at CPMC, in public health projects in the community, and in the biological sciences. Our training program seeks to further the development of the field, and the quality of future research, by demonstrating to its students, and to the biomedical community, that medical informatics addresses fundamental issues of biomedical knowledge and information, their representation, and their biomedical application. We have accordingly developed a curriculum that assures that our graduates will be familiar with a broad range of pertinent topics in the field. Each trainee then selects an area of subspecialization, with the established tracks being clinical informatics, public health informatics, imaging informatics, or bioinformatics. Our degrees generally require a minimum of two years for the MA and four years for the PhD, although most students take longer as described below.

We offer two types of MA degrees. Some students take an Applied MA (AMA), which principally consists of course work followed by a final project. Trainees in the AMA program are often employed outside the University, and participate in the degree program on a part-time basis. They may take 2-3 years to complete their training. We

offer a second MA degree, referred to as our Research MA (RMA), which requires a full-time commitment to study and approximately half-time involvement in research from the time of entry into the program. Students generally require three years to obtain this degree. The majority of our post-MD post-doctoral trainees have been RMA degree candidates. Research training is a key element in our program's design for RMA and PhD candidates.

We put heavy emphasis on written and verbal presentation of research results, including experience adapting such descriptions to varied audiences. Our weekly student seminars are given by trainees, as are many research colloquia. In addition, RMA and PhD students typically write several papers before they graduate.

All students (both RMA and AMA trainees before graduation, and PhD students before they can apply for doctoral candidacy in their third year) are required to take a DMI oral examination, generally at the end of their second year. This exam is designed to assure that the student has synthesized the diverse topics of the DMI's curriculum and can relate them to one another, has developed verbal skills and can effectively discuss broad topics in biomedical informatics, and has picked up practical knowledge of the field.

Approximately six months into their third year, all PhD candidates are required to present an hour's seminar in which they present proposed research in response to a mock "request for proposals" (RFP) that is prepared in collaboration with their research advisor. This exam is meant to be an exercise in researching a topic thoroughly and presenting a cogent plan for how one might attack the problem in a formal research project. The RFP topics are selected to correspond to the trainee's developing area of research interest and to help the student to gather background and experience that will be pertinent to their formal dissertation proposal.

All PhD candidates are expected to submit a formal thesis proposal (generally a written document of 75-100 pages), ideally by the end of their third year. Each doctoral thesis in Medical Informatics must balance the three following goals: provide significant innovative insights and new results that add to the knowledge of medical informatics; implement an information system that illustrates the practical applicability of the ideas; and evaluate the system to demonstrate generalizability or impact on the intended users.

They then defend their proposal before their thesis committee and in a public forum. The formal thesis proposal defense is intended to occur when the student's research is beginning to mature and become well defined, but when there are still 10-12 months left before completion of the dissertation is expected. This serves two purposes: (a) it establishes a required intermediate milestone that helps assure that the student keeps on schedule for completion of the PhD in 4-5 years, and (b) it allows for intensive review of research plans by the dissertation committee and "mid-course correction" while there is still substantial time left before completion of the degree. A final University-mandated thesis defense is then presented at the end of PhD training, at approximately the same time that the dissertation document is submitted to the university.

All RMA candidates are required to complete a research project before graduation. The research is not considered complete until the student has finished a formal paper on the topic, one that the research preceptor believes is suitable for submission to a peer-reviewed journal. Students are taught that biomedical informatics papers must be more than system descriptions; they are encouraged to extract general lessons and principles and to communicate what they have learned in a form so that others in the field may draw on their results.

Medical Informatics Curriculum

The Medical Informatics curriculum is designed to meet the needs of a wide range of students with different backgrounds and career goals, while providing a uniform foundation in the essentials of the field. The educational objectives addressed by the curriculum fall into four

Table 1. Number of courses required to meet educational objectives in each program

	Objective		AMA	RMA	PhD
Basic	**Biomedical Knowledge**	Is conversant with concepts, terminology, institutions, professionals, and methods of biomedical domain	1	2	2
	Data Management	Can apply computational techniques to organize and manage large collections of data	1	1	1
	Software Engineering	Can apply computational techniques to develop integrate and test software systems	1	1	1
	Statistics	Can apply mathematical techniques to analyze data	1	1	1
Core	**Overview**	Is familiar with theories, methods, and results in Medical Informatics	1	1	1
	Data Representation	Can analyze, develop, and apply representations of biomedical data	1	1	1
	Information Systems	Can analyze, develop, deploy and manage complex information systems	1	1	1
	Formal Models	Can analyze, develop, and apply formal models of biomedical objects and processes	0	1	1
	Information Presentation	Can analyze, develop, and deploy visual presentations of biomedical information	0	0	1
	Decision Making	Can analyze, develop, and apply formal models of biomedical decision making	0	0	1
	Evaluation	Can analyze, plan and carry out formal evaluations of information systems	0	0	1
General	**Research**	Can conduct independent research in Medical Informatics	1	4	6
	Teaching	Can prepare educational materials, deliver lectures, and evaluate students	0	2	2
Specialized	**Application**	Can apply theories and methods of Medical Informatics to area of specialization	2	2	5
			10	**17**	**25**

main areas: basic, core, general, and specialized (described below). Table 1 lists objectives within these areas, and indicates the number of courses related to each objective in the three degree programs (AMA, RMA, and PhD).

The *basic objectives* relate to fundamental areas of biomedicine, computer science and mathematics that are prerequisites for further study in Medical Informatics. A few students may enter the program meeting all of these objectives, but most will lack one or more areas. The basic objectives ensure that students coming from very different backgrounds obtain the necessary breadth to continue study in the field.

Core objectives define the essential skills required by all Medical Informatics students. All students must obtain working familiarity with the field of Medical Informatics, and an ability to work with representations of biomedical data and complex information systems. RMA and doctoral students must understand these systems through various formalisms. Doctoral students must also be able to develop visual representations, to model decision processes, and formally to evaluate such systems.

General objectives include the ability to conduct research and participate in the educational activities of the field. Current courses that support basic, core, and general objectives are listed in Table 2.

Specialized objectives concern the application of general methods and theories in four different areas: bioinformatics, imaging informatics, clinical informatics, and public health informatics. This portion of the curriculum is still evolving, and detailed objectives have not yet been defined. Courses in the four tracks are listed in Table 3. Courses that must be taken by all students in a track are marked as required, while optional courses are marked as elective.

Table 2. Current courses that support educational objectives

Objective	Relevant Courses
Biomedical Knowledge	G6300/G6301 Biochemistry and Molecular Biology of Eukaryotes, G4011 Acculturation to Medicine, E3001/3002 Quantitative Physiology, P6313 Physiology, P6400 Epidemiology, P6530 Issues and Approaches in Health Policy and Management
Data Management	W4111 Database Systems
Software Engineering	W4156 Software Engineering
Statistics	P6104 Introduction to Biostatistical Methods
Overview	W4001 Introduction to Computer Applications in Health Care and Biomedicine
Data Represenation	G4020 Representation and Coding of Medical data
Information Systems	G4040 Health Information Systems Architecture, P8534 Introduction To Information Management
Formal Models	G4002 Methods in Medical Informatics
Information Presentation	G4030 User Interfaces in Medicine, G4031 Understanding Visual Information
Decision Making	G4050 Quantitative Models For Medical Decision Making, G4051 Clinical Decision Support, P8740 Social and economic factors in clinical decision making, W4701 Artificial Intelligence, G5043 Cognitive Science and Medical Informatics
Evaluation	G4060 Evaluation Methods in Medical Informatics, P8116 Design of medical experiments
Research	G6001 Projects In Medical Informatics
Teaching	G8010 Teaching Experience

Table 3. Existing (numbered) and proposed courses in the four areas of specialization

	Bioinformatics	Bioimaging	Clinical Informatics	Public Health Informatics
Required	G4012 Introduction to Genomics	E4894 Biomedical Imaging	G4061 Economics of Informatics	P6513 Hospital Organization & Management
	E4761 Computational Genomics	E6400 Analysis and quantification of medical images	M8018 Project Management	P6781 The use of large scale national health care data sets
	Sequence Analysis	E440 Wavelet applications in bio-medical image and signal processing		
Elective	Statistical Genetics	G4031 Understanding Visual Information	M8122 Inter-active Health Communication	P6710 Health Communications
	Phylogenetic Inference	E4410 Ultrasound in Diagnostic Imaging	M8120 Informatics for Evidence-based Practice	P6503 Introduction To Health Economics
	Protein Folding	E6480 Computational Neural Modeling and Neuroengineering	M8123 Introduction to Databases and Data Mining	P8514 Healthcare E-Commerce
	Micro Arrays and Regulatory Networks	MRI and MRS Imaging		Social and Behavioral Founda-tions for Informatics
	Biological Databases	Graphics and Visualization		Information Ethics

Conclusion

The program in Medical Informatics at Columbia has matured from a loose confederation of courses in multiple departments to a highly integrated curriculum with a large number of courses taught by core departmental faculty. The initial focus on patient care and clinical applications has been expanded to embrace the entire biomedical spectrum, from the molecular level to whole populations. The faculty has diversified as well to implement this vision, and to forge new alliances with other schools and departments. We have also formalized the educational objectives for the curriculum across our three degree programs, with specialization in one of the four biomedical tracks. These objectives elucidate how the Medical Informatics program is distinct from programs in Computer Science, Public Health, Nursing, Engineering, and Biology, while clarifying points of overlap, which provide opportunities for interdisciplinary training and research. In this way, the training program is a step towards articulating a framework for the field as a whole, and provides guidance for its future practitioners.

Acknowledgement

Columbia's training program in medical informatics is supported by the National Library of Medicine under grant LM-07079.

References

1. Cimino J, Allen B, Clayton P. Medical informatics training at Columbia University and the Columbia-Presbyterian Medical Center. In: van Bemmel J, McCray A, editors. IMIA Yearbook of Medical Informatics. Stuttgart: Schattauer; 1995. p. 125-9.

2. Johnson S, Clayton P, Fink D, Sengupta S, Shea S, Bourne P, et al. Achievements in Phase III of an Integrated Academic Information Management System. Proceedings of the Seventh World Congress on Medical Informatics. Geneva, Switzerland: International Medical Informatics Association; 1992.

3. Clayton P. Integrated Advanced Medical Information Systems (IAIMS): Payoffs and problems. Methods Inf Med 1994;33(4):351-7.

4. Johnson S, Forman B, Cimino J, Hripcsak G, Sengupta S, Sideli R, et al. A technological perspective on the computer-based patient record. In: Steen E, editor. Proceedings of the First Annual Nicholas E. Davies CPR Recognition Symposium. Washington, DC: Computer-Based Patient Record Institute; 1995. p. 35-51.

5. Hripcsak G, Ludemann P, Pryor T, Wigertz O, Clayton P. Rationale for the Arden Syntax. Comput Biomed Res. 1994;27:291-324.

6. Cimino J. Auditing the Unified Medical Language System with semantic methods. J Am Med Inform Assoc 1998;5:41-51.

7. Cimino J. Using the Unified Medical Language System in patient care at the Columbia-Presbyterian Medical Center. Methods Inf Med 1995;34:158-64.

8. Sideli R, Johnson S, Weschler M, Clark A, Chen J, Simpson R, et al. Adopting HL7 as a standard for the exchange of clinical text reports. In: Miller R, editor. Proceedings of the 14th Annual Symposium on Computer Applications in Medical Care. Washington, DC: IEEE; 1990. p. 226-9.

9. Shortliffe EH, Perreault LE, Wiederhold G, Fagan LM, editors. Medical Informatics: Computer Applications in Health Care and Biomedicine. New York: Springer; 2000.

Adress of corresponding author:
Edward H. Shortliffe, MD, PhD
Professor and Chair
Department of Medical Informatics
622 West 168th Street, VC-5
New York, NY 10032-3720
212-305-6896
Fax: 212-543-8788
E-mail: shortliffe@dmi.columbia.edu

Challenges in Medical Informatics

183 Lun KC.

Inaugurational address.

187 Haux R, Knaup P, Bauer AW, Herzog W, Reinhardt E, Uberla K, van Eimeren W, Wahlster W.

Information processing in healthcare at the start of the third Millennium: potential and limitations.

Methods Inf Med. 2001 May;40(2):156-62.

194 Musen M, van Bemmel JH.

Challenges for Medical Informatics as an Academic Discipline: Workshop Report.

K.C. Lun

School of Biological Sciences
Nanyang Technological University
Singapore

Challenges in Medical Informatics

Inaugural Address

delivered by Dr K C Lun
President, International Medical Informatics Association
at the Closing Ceremony of MEDINFO 2001
10th World Congress on Health and Medical Informatics
London, Wednesday 5 September 2001

Dr Jan van Bemmel, out-going IMIA President, Honoured Guests, Distinguished Participants, Ladies and Gentlemen:

In the International Medical Informatics Association (IMIA), we have a tradition. The end of a MEDINFO conference marks the beginning of a three-year term for a new IMIA President. The British has an expression for this exercise. It is called the "Changing of the Guard".

Completing the term as IMIA Vice-President (MEDINFO)

As I complete my term as IMIA Vice-President (MEDINFO), I wish to record my sincere gratitude to the people who have given me their unfailing support and the immense pleasure of doing this job. In particular, I wish to thank Ms Jean Roberts and the members of her London Organizing Committee, Dr Arie Hasman and Dr Hiroshi Takeda, the co-chairs of the Scientific Programme Committee and their Committee Members, the Editorial Committee comprising Dr Vimla Patel, Dr Reinhold Haux and Dr Ray Rogers. I am also grateful for the support given to me by the IMIA MEDINFO Steering

Committee comprising the IMIA President, Dr Jan van Bemmel, the IMIA Treasurer, Ms Ulla Gerdin and the IMIA Executive Director, Mr Steven Huesing.

As I take on my new IMIA role as President, I am reminded of yet another British expression, "Uneasy lies the head that wears the crown". In case you think that from hereon, I want to be known as 'His Majesty', let me quickly change the expression to, "Uneasy lies the head that wields the IMIA gavel". I am aware of the big responsibility that lies ahead of me over the next three years and I am honoured to have been given the trust and confidence of my IMIA colleagues from all over the world to handle this job. And I was especially glad that the decision taken at the IMIA General Assembly in 1999 to appoint me as President-elect was unanimous. We did not have to resort to a Florida-style vote recount.

Some Singapore Trivia

As you all know, I come from Singapore but you would be amazed that there are still many people who do not know where Singapore is. For example, a year ago, I was invited to speak at an international conference somewhere in

the western world and I was visibly shocked when I was handed the conference badge. The badge listed me as coming from "Singapore, China"! Hence, when I delivered my plenary paper the next day, I began the presentation with a short lesson in geography for the audience, telling them the exact geographical location of my country. Singapore, as I am sure many of you already know, is geographically located at the southern tip of peninsular Malaysia, just north of the equator. It has been an independent republic since 1965. The main island is about 42 kilometres from east to west and 23 kilometres from north to south and so it is shaped like a diamond or a top. The total land area is about 648 square kilometers (or 253 square miles) and within this area lives a population of some 3.8 million people. The population is cosmopolitan, comprising 75% Chinese, 15% Malays, 7% Indians and 3% of other races. Singapore is also a highly wired country with the highest net penetration in Asia.

About IMIA

Now, let me talk about the International Medical Informatics Association. For those of you who are attending MEDINFO for the first time, this

World Congress is a major IMIA event which is held once every three years. IMIA is an international organization that comprises some 50 national member societies, 12 corporate and 13 academic institutional members. Currently, it has three regional groups viz. the European Federation of Medical Informatics (EFMI), the IMIA-Latin American and Caribbean countries (IMIA-LAC) and the Asia Pacific Association for Medical Informatics (APAMI) of which I was the founding president from 1994-7.

It is auspicious that I hold office as the 10th IMIA President at the 10th World Congress of Medical Informatics. I am also honoured to join a very distinguished company of individuals who had served as IMIA Presidents before me, and the second Asian to hold this high office (Figure 1).

As you can see from Figure 1, the term of each IMIA President is associated with a major accomplishment that each is best remembered for.

All of my IMIA predecessors have big shoes to be filled by someone who wears only size 6! If there is one slogan that I would like my successor to describe what I have accomplished four years from now, it is "Bridging the Medical Informatics Divide". This will be of highest priority in my "Agenda of Action" as the new IMIA President.

Coming from a third world country that has only recently transitioned to a first, I am conscious of the need to assist developing countries to break into medical informatics as one of the means to achieve healthcare delivery standards of the first world. Therefore, to "Bridge the Informatics Divide", I will help steer IMIA on two major initiatives: (1) convening Helina 2002, the pan-African Conference on Medical Informatics in Cairo in 2002

International Medical Informatics Association

IMIA Presidents

- Francois Gremy, France, IMIA President 1968-75
  - Starting the Movement
- Jan Roukens, The Netherlands, IMIA President 1975-1980
  - Transforming the Organization
- David B. Shires, Canada, IMIA President 1980-1983
  - Building International Membership
- Hans Peterson, Sweden, IMIA President 1983-1986
  - Surviving Financial Crisis
- Shigekoto Kaihara, Japan, IMIA President 1986-1989
  - Coping with Political Disruption
- Jos L. Willems, Belgium, IMIA President 1989-1992
  - Preparing for IMIA's Future
- Marion Ball, USA, IMIA President 1992-1995
  - Moving from Theory to Practice
- Otto Rienhoff, Germany, IMIA President 1995 - 1998
  - Towards a Sustainable IMIA Electronic Infrastructure: www.imia.org
- Jan van Bemmel, The Netherlands, IMIA President 1998-2001
  - Entering the Twenty-First Century
- K C Lun, Singapore, IMIA President 2001-2004
  - Bridging the Medical Informatics Divide

Fig.1. IMIA Presidents

and (2) promoting a Virtual University for Medical Informatics to be driven by IMIA WG1 on "Health and Medical Informatics Education".

Bridging the Medical Informatics Divide: Helina 2002

It is my hope that Helina 2002 will serve as a catalyst for more medical informatics activities in Africa. Helina, as a conference, is not new. The first Helina conference took place in Nigeria in 1993. Since then, Helina conferences had been held in South Africa in 1996 and in Zimbabwe in 1999. We know that one positive outcome as a result of increased medical informatics activities in Africa will be an improvement in the standard of healthcare delivery through timeliness of data using infocommunications technology. It is my goal to have the Helina conference serve as a catalyst for the formation of an African regional group of IMIA, coming after EFMI, APAMI and IMIA-LAC by the time I complete my term as IMIA President in 2004.

In reaching out to developing countries to help bridge the Medical Informatics Divide, we can draw on the experience of Informedica 2000, the 1st Iberoamerican Virtual Congress of Medical Informatics which was very successfully held last November under the able leadership of Dr Nora Oliveri, our Chair for IMIA Working Group 9.

Bridging the Medical Informatics Divide: Virtual University for Medical Informatics

It would be wrong to apply the term, "Medical Informatics Divide" only to address the disparity between developed and developing countries. In my opinion, it should also be applied to all countries, organizations and institutions that do not, as yet, have an awareness of medical informatics. I would like to borrow a quotation from the e-Testimony to the Web-based Commission on Education to the President and Congress of the USA, "There is no going back, the traditional classroom has been transformed". The message is clear – we have to look beyond the traditional transfer of knowledge in the physical classroom.

To this end, I would like to strongly support, during the term of my presidency, an initiative on the Virtual University for Medical Informatics, to be launched by IMIA Working Group 1, led by its two co-chairs Dr Evelyn Hovenga of Australia and Dr John Mantas of Greece with the collaboration of Dr Jim Turley of the USA. It is an IMIA initiative which will not only spread medical informatics knowledge and practice far and wide but will also provide a value-added benefit to our IMIA academic institutional members as they will provide the skills and teaching resources to this global programme through distance education.

Meeting the Challenges of the Life Sciences

IMIA will also need to respond to the growing emergence of life sciences, a discipline which is bringing winds of change to the global economy. Those of you who heard Dr Casimir Kulikowski's invited presentation on bioinformatics would have appreciated the need for medical informatics to position itself for the new and exciting research opportunities that come hot on the heels of the mapping of the human genome and the growth of bioinformatics.

Many governments, academic and research organizations have already recognized the importance of the new biotech economy and are committing major investment and resources to tap the opportunities that follow the decoding of the human genome. It is also for this reason that I have recently left my job of 26 years at the National University of Singapore to help start a life sciences initiative at the Nanyang Technological University in Singapore.

Working in a technological university, with a very strong engineering tradition that is also starting to grow the development of life sciences, will offer many exciting opportunities for me to explore the relevance and applications of medical informatics to the life sciences, particularly with respect to its convergence with bioinformatics.

Within IMIA we have also given recognition to the new challenges that the growing emergence of the life sciences will bring to the field of medical informatics. Already, IMIA has convened two workshops on "Challenges in Medical Informatics", one in Madrid in March this year and the other here in London to address this and other issues. These were led by Dr Mark Musen and Dr Jan van Bemmel. In addition, IMIA hopes to convene a conference on Clinical Bioinformatics in Singapore in March 2003 to further address the convergence of medical informatics with bioinformatics.

IMIA resources – its Working Groups and Special Interest Group

You would have noticed that in my inaugural address I have made references to the work of our IMIA Working Groups and SIG on Nursing. To me, the WGs and our SIG on Nursing (Figure 2) are our source of strength and there is a wealth of global talent and resources within IMIA which the organization can leverage on to help "Bridge the Medical Informatics Divide".

In addition, within IMIA, we also have an extensive network of national and corresponding members, corporate and academic institutional members. We need to build better "skyways", "subways" and "linkways" to foster closer strategic partnerships between these members on the one hand and IMIA WGs and the SIG on Nursing on the other.

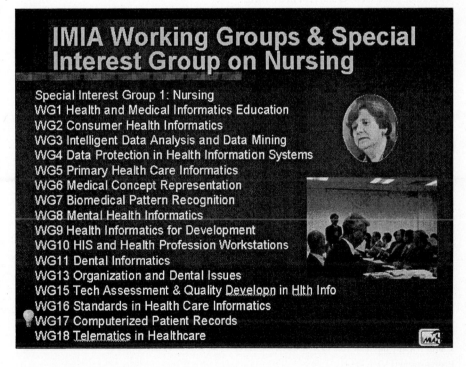

Fig. 2. IMIA Working Groups and Special Interest Group on Nursing

Dream Teams

In carrying out my job, I am very fortunate to have a team of excellent and very capable people that will serve with me on the IMIA Board (Figure 3).

I have an equally exciting team from the American Medical Informatics Association (AMIA), chaired by Dr Edward Shortliffe, who will be bringing you the next MEDINFO in 2004 in San Francisco. MEDINFO 2004 promises to be the best MEDINFO ever and I look forward to greeting everyone again in San Francisco three years from now.

Acknowledgements

Before I end my Inaugural Address, I should acknowledge the generosity of the Singapore International Foundation for honouring me with a *Singapore Internationale* Award to deliver this Inaugural Address. I also wish to thank my new employer, the Nanyang Technological University, for providing me with the conference leave and funding support to attend MEDINFO 2001. I also wish to acknowledge the global community of IMIA colleagues for their trust and confidence in me to lead the organization over the next three years.

Finally, to borrow a quotation from the great British statesman, Sir Winston Churchill, I wish to thank all of you for sharing with me, "My Finest Hour"

Thank you.

KC Lun
IMIA President

Address of the author:
Kwok Chan Lun
Professor and Vice Dean
School of Biological Sciences
Nanyang Technological University
Singapore
E-mail: kclun@ntu.edu.sg

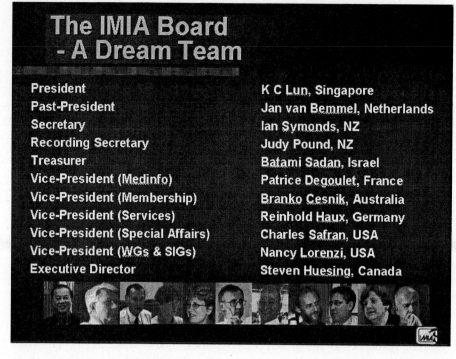

Fig. 3. Members of the IMIA Executive Board

The IMIA Board - A Dream Team

President	K C Lun, Singapore
Past-President	Jan van Bemmel, Netherlands
Secretary	Ian Symonds, NZ
Recording Secretary	Judy Pound, NZ
Treasurer	Batami Sadan, Israel
Vice-President (Medinfo)	Patrice Degoulet, France
Vice-President (Membership)	Branko Cesnik, Australia
Vice-President (Services)	Reinhold Haux, Germany
Vice-President (Special Affairs)	Charles Safran, USA
Vice-President (WGs & SIGs)	Nancy Lorenzi, USA
Executive Director	Steven Huesing, Canada

R. Haux[1], **P. Knaup**[1],
A. W. Bauer[2], **W. Herzog**[3],
E. Reinhardt[4], **K. Überla**[5],
W. van Eimeren[6], **W. Wahlster**[7]

[1] Institute for Medical Biometry and Informatics, University of Heidelberg
[2] Institute for the History of Medicine, University of Heidelberg
[3] University Hospital for Internal Medicine, University of Heidelberg
[4] Division for Medical Engineering, Siemens AG, Erlangen
[5] Institute for Medical Informatics, Biometry and Epidemiology, University of Munich
[6] Medis-Institute for Medical Informatics and Systems Research, GSF-Research Center for Environment and Health, Neuherberg
[7] German Research Center for Artificial Intelligence (DFKI), Saarbrücken, Germany

Information Processing in Healthcare at the Start of the third Millennium: Potential and Limitations

Abstract: The 21st century is said to be a century of the information society. We should be aware that continuing progress in information processing methodology (IPM) and information and communication technology (ICT) is changing our societies, including medicine and health care. At the start of the third Millennium we should ask ourselves, what progress can we expect from modern IPM/ICT for healthcare in the coming decade, what concerns does the information society have to face, and what steps have to be taken. These questions were addressed by clinicians, researchers and industrial representatives in a panel discussion at the joint conference ISCB-GMDS-99 of the International Society of Clinical Biostatistics and the German Society for Medical Informatics, Biometry and Epidemiology. Important aspects raised by the panelists and in the subsequent discussion were: (1) the main goal of expanding IPM/ICT should be to further improve quality of care, while maintaining reasonable costs; (2) with the support of modern IPM and ICT the boundaries between inpatient and outpatient care will fade away enabling a more efficient, patient-centered health care; (3) cooperation between health-care professionals will increase; there will be different ways of communication between them and with the patient, including modern ICT and the Internet; (4) society must be concerned with achieving equal opportunities in being informed about and in using new ICT; (5) misuse of data will remain a serious problem and can become an obstacle to progress.

Keywords: Medical Informatics, Health Informatics, Information Processing Methodology, Information and Communication Technology, Healthcare.

1. Introduction

"Hardly a word needs to be said about the miracle of modern medicine. Those who are involved, since the turn of the century, are witnessing a process which is incomparable in the history of medicine. The process of progress in medical knowledge, slowly beginning in the 17th century, accelerated by the middle of the 19th century, and speeded up since 50 years in a breathtaking manner. The reason for this progress is research in the natural sciences, ranging from the exact sciences to biology" [1][1]. These words are from Karl Jaspers, a philosopher and physician, who was a member of the RUPRECHT-KARLS University of Heidelberg most of his working life. They are taken from a speech he gave in 1958 at the 100th Conference of the Association of German Scientists and Physicians.

In the sense of Jaspers statement we can recognize that in the 19th century many of our societies were characterized by power-producing industry and

---

[1] Original German text: "Über das Wunder der modernen Medizin bedarf es kaum eines Wortes. Wer seit der Jahrhundertwende dabei war, weiß sich als Zeitgenosse eines Vorgangs, der ohne Vergleich in der Geschichte der Medizin ist. Dieser Fortschrittsprozess ärztlichen Könnens, langsam begonnen seit dem 17. Jahrhundert, seit der Mitte des 19. Jahrhunderts schneller, hat seit 50 Jahren einen atemberaubenden Gang genommen. Der Grund dieses Fortschritts ist die naturwissenschaftliche Forschung, von den exakten Wissenschaften bis zur Biologie".

industrial production. The idea of communicating and processing data by means of computers and computer networks was emerging from the second half of the 20th century onwards, at the latest. Nowadays, we are accustomed to speak of the 21st century as being the century of information and communication technology, the century of an 'information society'. It is supposed to become a century in which informatics will be of crucial importance. Information, tied to a medium of matter and energy but largely independent of place and time, shall be made available to man at any time and in any place conceivable. Information shall clear its path to man and not vice versa.

We have to be aware that, nowadays, more computers are sold than cars and that the Internet has already considerably transformed our way of working. As a consequence, globalisation of labour has already started a significant change of our world. When we look back we have to recognize, that 50 or even 30 years ago, our world of work and leisure looked substantially different.

Regarding medicine and healthcare as important parts of our societies, we have to realize that (cf. [2]):

1. Progress in information processing methodology (IPM) and information and communication technology (ICT) is changing medicine and healthcare as well as our societies.
2. The amount of health and medical knowledge is increasing at a phenomenal rate. We cannot store, organize and retrieve this knowledge without using appropriate, modern IPM and ICT.
3. Significant economic benefits can be obtained by using ICT to support medicine and healthcare.
4. Similarly, the quality of healthcare can be enhanced by systematic application of IPM and ICT.
5. It is expected that these developments will continue, most likely at least at the same pace as can be observed today.

At ISCB-GMDS-99, which was a joint international conference of the International Society for Clinical Biostatistics (ISCB) and the German Society for Medical Informatics, Biometry and Epidemiology (GMDS) a panel discussion on the future of information processing in health care in the next decade took place. It was chaired and organized by the first and summarized by the second author. The aim of the panel was to discuss the consequences of the last, fifth statement, the 'quintessence': What is the potential, what are the limitations of IPM and ICT in medicine and health care at the start of the third Millennium? In particular, the following questions were raised:

'Perspectives'. What progress can we expect from modern IPM and ICT for medicine and healthcare in the coming decade?

'Concerns'. What concerns does the information society have to face with respect to the increasing 'informatisation'?

'Next steps'. What decisions have to be made in healthcare politics and for planning and stimulating medical and healthcare research?

Outstanding German personalities accepted to be a member of the panel; their answers to these questions are summarized in this paper. Their contributions reflect a variety of views of different professions and disciplines that are concerned with IPM and ICT in health care:

– ICT industry,
– health care and clinical research,
– medical informatics, biometry and epidemiology,
– history, theory and ethics in medicine,
– computer science and artificial intelligence,
– telematics in healthcare.

The statements of the panelists are published here in the same order as they were presented at the conference.

2. Perspectives, Concerns and Next Steps from the Viewpoint of ICT Industry

Statement by Erich Reinhardt, electrical engineer and adjunct professor at the University of Stuttgart, President of the Siemens Division for Medical Engineering, with its headquarter located in Erlangen. The division is one of the largest ICT enterprises in the healthcare field worldwide.

2.1 Perspectives

Germany is internationally recognized for its high-quality healthcare. But, in comparison to other European countries, it has the highest health expenditure per capita. Thus, it is the aim of ICT solutions for health care to decrease the costs while preserving the quality of health care. Internationally seen, the competition is very hard. To provide better and cheaper solutions, intensity of innovation and efficiency in development and manufacturing have to increase continuously. Therefore, organizational structures must become more process-oriented. This enables a fast and flexible response to the demands of patients and in the offer of new products and solutions. Optimizing processes will increase the efficiency of healthcare. New technologies for information and communication are the basis but all healthcare professionals have to work towards realizing this aim. We identify four steps for optimizing processes, with the patient at the center of care:

– Central archiving of images and documents. Fast access from various places to these documents is a prerequisite for fast and comprehensive diagnosis.
– Optimizing workflow by new ICT, mainly with regard to cost, quality and patient satisfaction. The patient process has to be regarded as a whole.
– Further development of disease management. Processes will be optimized to target diseases. Specialized treatment of individual diseases will be further developed.
– Comprehensive care management by means of a central patient record. If the patient agrees, life-long data on prevention, therapy etc. will be made available by a central patient record which is accessible from various places.

2.2 Concerns

The perspectives of ICT dominate the concerns from ICT industry's point of view. It can be assumed that the demand for healthcare services will continue to increase. A major concern is that life expectancy is still increasing while the birth rate is decreasing. That means that healthcare has to improve considerably so that it can still be financed by the caring society. A solidarity-based healthcare system can only be competitive if the processes are optimized such that quality management is transparent and efficiency can be increased. ICT is the prerequisite to achieve this.

2.3 Next Steps

Financial incentives must be established. The allocation criteria for reimbursement payments must be adjusted according to process optimization, increase of efficiency, quality of care, patient satisfaction, and cost effectiveness. Optimizing the process of patient care as a whole is of major importance in the sense of increased quality and reduced costs.

3. Perspectives, Concerns and Next Steps from the Viewpoint of Healthcare and Clinical Research

Statement by Wolfgang Herzog, professor of internal medicine and psychosomatics at the University of Heidelberg, one of the directors of the Heidelberg University Hospital for Internal Medicine. His research centers on psychosomatc medicine and organizational aspects of healthcare. As head physician he routinely practices patient care.

ICT is a medium of fundamental innovation. Its inventions do not only have an added value but they have already changed (and will continue to do so) the social structure of our society. This is also true for the medical field and opens new perspectives in the field of communication. But it also involves concerns.

3.1 Perspectives

Four main perspectives are distinguished:
- Medical knowledge is available fast (up-to-date), comprehensible and for everybody. Especially the last point means a completely new situation for the treating physician: The knowledge is also available in an understandable form for the patient. During a patient encounter the physician is increasingly confronted with the patients' knowledge. Physicians have to adjust to this situation.
- Patient data will be available much more flexibly and completely, independent of the origin of the document. The data will be aggregated and accessible, not only within one institution. This involves great potential from the medical point of view.
- ICT also leads to new pathways of learning and education. Comparable to the education of pilots, medical education will be increasingly supported by appropriate simulators. The challenge is to develop appropriate simulation models. Sophisticated simulation models will also influence patient care, regarding e.g. multimorbidity: If the mechanisms of the single diseases are well understood, the combination of their occurrence could be simulated and could lead to high-quality decision support.
- A hospital information system stores much information on the processes in the hospital. This should be used to a broader extent as internal evidence and for quality management purposes.

3.2 Concerns

Despite these perspectives, concerns from the medical viewpoint must not be neglected:
- First of all there is the danger of wasting resources such as time, money and physical energy. A simple example of this is the constant stream of new releases of application software products which have to be installed and adapted, and the users have to familiarize themselves with them.
- Obviously, misuse of data is an ongoing problem in the healthcare area. But technology offers the possibility of misuse on an enormous scale. The success of new ICT in medicine will largely depend on to what extent the confidentiality of patient data can be guaranteed.
- Another risk is the abundance of data. An accompanying problem may be that data are used for purposes for which they were not originally intended. For example, a statistic on the frequency of diagnoses which occur in a hospital is not a real indicator for performance and outcome of the hospital.
- Last but not least, it is a concern that electronic media may disturb the personal physician-patient relationship. Equally, it can be seen as a challenge for the physician to integrate these new technologies in a trusting and sensitive way in his daily work with the patient.

3.3 Next Steps

Steps that have to be taken in order to achieve the perspectives despite the concerns are:
- The patient's rights must be adequately discussed. This involves informing the patient, education and data protection. The patient has the right to know the consequences of the performed medical actions and what is happening with hus/her data.
- New methods and tools of medical informatics (which are normally accompanied by new structures in healthcare) have to keep in mind that the basis of medical behavior is a trusting physician-patient relationship.
- Currently, healthcare in Germany is divided in sectors such as hospitals, outpatient departments, general practitioners, insurance companies, authorities, etc. Through ICT and innovative communication processes the boundaries between these sectors should be overcome so that efficient networks can be established.

4. Perspectives, Concerns and Next Steps from the Viewpoint of Medical Informatics, Biometry and Epidemiology

Statement by Karl Überla, physician and psychologist, professor of medical informatics, biometry, and epidemiology at the University of Munich and director of that institute. Since his time as President of the German 'Bundesgesundheitsamt', a position similar to that of the Commissioner of the FDA, he has continued to strongly influence medical progress by initiating advances in therapy research, public health, and epidemiology.

Progress in healthcare in the next decade will depend on three factors:
- Which questions will finally be under investigation?
- Which new technologies will be provided by industry in the field of hardware and software?
- Which resources will be available to promote new developments?

It can be assumed that healthcare worldwide will be completely restructured during the next decade. But it cannot be foreseen how this will materialize. Generally, it can be stated:
- Medical knowledge is complicated, incomplete and inconsistent. It is changing and expanding continuously. In order to give a correct prognosis, we have to learn to cope with these characteristics of medical knowledge.

– New technologies and new knowledge in healthcare should be available for the community at large. It should not be the property of a company or a state. We have to demand equality of opportunities worldwide.

– Main objective of progress in healthcare is outcome quality. It should be evaluated with empirical methods e.g., by indicators such as life expectancy and quality of life.

4.1 Perspectives

Having these general aspects in mind, the following perspectives can be mentioned:

– Main objective of progress in healthcare should be to speed up the transfer of new knowledge on diagnosis and therapy. Currently it takes about 5 years before new knowledge is applied in patient care as a standard strategy.

– Telemedicine will enable high-quality healthcare in certain areas e.g. asthma and diabetes.

– Communication and cooperation with the patient will become increasingly more important in the care process.

– Educating health-care professionals will change with regard to new methods e.g., case-based learning and new technologies like multimedia.

– It is an important task to evaluate and improve the quality of knowledge on the Web. Guideline activities and the Cochrane collaboration will expand. But it has to be remembered that evidence-based medicine will still be prohibitively expensive.

– Regional healthcare networks will be established and the borders between inpatient and outpatient care will be opened up further.

– Patients will seek advice on the Internet where they can get services of the highest quality, or where they can get a second opinion. Teleadvising may also be a growing area.

4.2 Concerns

A major concern is the quality of information on the Internet. There have to be strategies how low quality or even wrong information can be avoided. Questions like: How expensive is wrong information and who is liable for it, have to be solved. We have to be aware that more information does not automatically lead to scientifically sound knowledge and a change of behavior. Even ethical questions such as which information should be excluded from the Internet (e.g. instructions for suicide) have to be discussed.

There is the risk of having no equality of opportunities. If ICT opens a knowledge gap it may lead to medical care on different levels of quality.

Worry about data protection may become a severe obstacle for progress in healthcare, although there are technical solutions. It is important to have ongoing evaluation of existing effects.

4.3 Next Steps

Political demands will not be discussed at this stage. New federal laws in healthcare cannot be foreseen. It is important that university hospitals become a moving force for innovation. Therefore, they should not need to work with a limited budget and they should have enough flexibility to invest in personnel and ICT resources.

5. Perspectives, Concerns and Next Steps from the Viewpoint of History, Theory, and Ethics in Medicine

Statement by Axel W. Bauer, physician, professor of history, theory and ethics in medicine at the University of Heidelberg. Many of his books and journal articles deal with the questions of values and their role in medicine and healthcare.

5.1 Perspectives

ICT has changed the face of healthcare in the last decade. Therefore, a physician of the 21st century should be able to work with new technologies in several main areas, which are: information systems in healthcare, medical documentation, medical signal- and image processing, and knowledge-based decision support.

One important example is the electronic patient record. It should comprise personal data, diagnosis, drugs, notes of the physician and, in more complex systems, all medical results including images. The advantage will be easy access to all these data and the chance to avoid multiple examinations. There are already several examples in the field of image processing (e.g. tomography) where benefit, costs and appropriateness should be carefully analyzed. In the field of therapeutics we also have several examples for all stages of therapy, such as surgery planning, construction of implants, navigation during surgery, and robotics. The interaction with the surgeon is of great importance.

Educating physicians has to be flexibly adapted to these developments much faster than it used to be in previous years.

5.2 Concerns

A major concern is the complexity of methods and tools of information processing. It must be possible to plan, control and manage even complex information systems for the benefit of the patient and the hospital. Progress must not be too expensive and too time-consuming. In case of doubt, the complexity of architectures and tools should be reduced.

Methods and tools of medical informatics and health economy enable to evaluate diagnostic and therapeutic procedures and to give information on costs and services of a hospital. Outcome quality is often measured by means of survival time and quality of life. It is important that these data are analyzed, not only taking into account a certain population but also the individual patient. Otherwise, there is a danger that questions may arise, such as:

– Is it preferable to perform two kidney transplantations or to crown 200 teeth?

– Is it preferable to provide an alcoholic with acute liver failure with costly but life-preserving intensive care, or to provide several hundred rheumatic patients with symptomatic pain therapy?

Another danger in the same context is not adequately considering:

– disabled persons because they are assumed to have a lower quality of life

– elderly people because they have a lower remaining life expectancy.

Concerns are also inherent to computer-aided surgery, because finally it always is the physician who controls the situation, who decides and who has the responsibility. Robots should only be used when it is obvious that the benefit for the patient is higher than the risk. The problem who is liable in case of claim for damage has not yet been solved. Intelligent robots, such as wheelchairs are for example controversial, because they may take over too many decisions from the patients.

Finally, ICT may intensify a two-class society between highly developed and developing countries, where low quality medical technology may involve even more dangers than advantages.

5.3 Next Steps

There is an enormous demand for high technological medical care. Since resources are limited, cost-effective analyses have to be performed carefully. This is especially important in Germany, where healthcare costs are not based on market-economy lines, due to the social policy.

The problem of providing a precise and fair health-insurance system for such a powerful medical care is not yet solved. Political and ethical values are defined for a certain time and a certain task; they are unstable and changeable, but they require consensus. Everybody has an influence on future values and norms in his/her society. Thus, information processing in health care will have to face four principles in the future:
– charity (beneficence)
– damage avoidance (nonmaleficence)
– justice
– respect for autonomy of the patient.

The challenge is that these principles can conflict with each other: charity considerations can restrict the right of self-determination, or justice considerations may have a harmful effect on certain patients.

6. Perspectives, Concerns and Next Steps from the Viewpoint of Computer Science and Artificial Intelligence

Statement by Wolfgang Wahlster, professor of computer science, Director of the German Research Center for Artificial Intelligence (DFKI), Chair of the European Coordination Committee of Artificial Intelligence (ECCAI), President of the Association for Computational Linguistics (ACL) .

6.1 Perspectives

Advanced ICT will be a key factor driving medical progress in the 21st century. It will transform the nature and practice of healthcare. In particular, augmented reality technology, mobile medical computing and wireless monitoring, pedagogical Internet agents, computational ontologies, and intelligent multimodel user interfaces have the potential to improve the current health system dramatically:

Augmented reality, an evolution of virtual reality, will play a key role in advanced telemedicine. It superimposes and integrates computer-generated images with images of the real world. The image fusion of medical imaging data with live video sources is the first practical use of augmented reality for telesurgery. It combines methods from image understanding, virtual reality and adaptive visualization. The intraoperative integration of all imaging modalities by look-through technology combined with minimally invasive procedures and an intuitive visualization of the stereotactic position of instruments relative to the patient's anatomy will support the future surgeon.

Mobile medical computing will change healthcare dramatically. With low-cost high quality technology it will become possible to constantly monitor patients anytime and anywhere via mobile Internet access. Mobile Internet phones with WAP technology make medical advice and knowledge ubiquitous. A personalized never-to-be-switched-off mobile agent for constant individual health consultation is a concrete vision. Bluetooth technology provides low-cost, short range radio links to network PDAs, medical equipment and clinical workstations, so that reconfigurable closed-loop knowledge-based systems in intensive care units or emergency medicine can be realized efficiently. These new wireless communications and monitoring technologies support treatment of patients comfortably from their own homes.

Web-based medical training systems will be augmented by software agents, that serve as pedagogical agents. Animated personae will enrich distance learning, making it both more interactive and engaging. Such pedagogical agents monitor students as they examine a virtual patient on their computers. If the student performs an action that is inconsistent with standard practice, the virtual agent interrupts and suggests an action to perform instead. These life-like characters tailor the information presentation to the individual medical student exploiting explicit user models.

Computational ontologies for medicine will become a necessity for knowledge-based systems, softbots and netbots for knowledge management or information extraction, and advanced machine learning or data and text mining applications. Consequently, there is a strong demand for expressive ontological languages, modular ontologies and distributed tools for collaborative ontological engineering capturing the essence of medical knowledge. These formal ontologies can be used for the XML-based documentation of biomedical knowledge and the definition of high-level communication protocols among software agents processing medical information.

The speaker-independent understanding of spontaneous speech coordinated with deictic gestures will provide intuitive access to medical information systems and online decision support systems. Intelligent multimodal interfaces will provide comfortable access to health-system intranets and medical knowledge repositories. The seamless integration of multiple communication modes will lead to high-bandwidth telemedicine. User-adaptive and resource-sensitive information presentation combining intelligent visualization methods with flexible text and speech synthesis will lead to a new generation of dialog systems.

6.2 Concerns

Medical applications need robust and fault-tolerant systems, but the current medical software is often quite fragile. Fragility is manifested as unreliability, lack of security, performance lapses, errors, and difficulty in debugging, maintenance and upgrading. New deductive methods for generating provably correct software must be established as a standard in medical information processing. Other critical issues include the privacy and security of patient records on the Internet and the development of mechanisms for creating trust between patient and physician in an online environment.

6.3 Next Steps

Increased public funding is needed for long-term, high-risk fundamental research combining advanced computer science and medical information processing to adapt our health system to the needs and potentials of the 21st century.

7. Perspectives, Concerns and Next Steps from the Viewpoint of Telematics in Healthcare

Statement by Wilhelm Van Eimeren, professor, physician and psychologist as well as head of Germany's largest research institute in medical informatics, the MEDIS Institute for Medical Informatics and Systems Research in Neuherberg near Munich. As member of the 'Sachverständigenrat für die Konzertierte Aktion im Gesundheitswesen' (Advisory Board for the Concerted Action in Healthcare) of the German Ministry of Health, he significantly influenced the structure of the German healthcare system, among others, by promoting telematics for healthcare.

7.1 Perspectives

The major tendencies in healthcare delivery and the related telematics contributions can be summarized as follows:
- Evidence-based medicine can be supported by appropriate methods of knowledge presentation. Especially in the case of frequent diseases and diagnostic groups, productivity can be increased by clinical practice guidelines.

- Managed care can be considerably supported by the electronic patient record. Prerequisites for this are adequate contracts, networks, and fading borders between inpatient and outpatient care. This is currently not a problem of technology, mechanisms of encoding of data and digital signature are already available. Pilot projects with the Health Professional Card (HPC) will soon start in Germany. This technology should be used to decrease bureaucratic tasks like admission, transmission, medical reports, and electronic prescriptions.
- However, we still have to face a growing bureaucracy, but we should try to map these tasks isomorphic to the computer, as is already done with online banking, where almost no staff are involved anymore.
- We need telematic solutions to cope with the professional overstress e.g., through information overload; 600 images of a computer tomogram (CT) cannot be analyzed by a single physician.
- Since medical knowledge is increasing and becoming increasingly complex we still have to face growing specialization in medicine. Even university hospitals have to accept that they cannot be experts in every field; therefore, the relevance of telemedicine and distance advice increases.

7.2 Concerns

Any healthcare system in Europe faces the dilemma of keeping three goals in focus and balance:
- providing high quality of care and enabling innovation,
- financial sustainability,
- access with equal opportunities for everybody.

Health telematics can evidently contribute to get a better, cheaper and more easily accessible health service when (and only when) it is used to strengthen the strengths and overcome the weaknesses in the system. But we have to be aware that the opposite can occur. For example, despite the ever-expanding Internet (even in private homes) and its influence on healthcare, currently only 0.5% of people aged over 60 years have Internet access, whereas this is our largest group of patients.

7.3 Next Steps

Healthcare systems in Europe facing this dilemma will strengthen the central monitoring of clinical practice (clinical performance) while allowing within this structure elements of more competitive behavior. The regulated market as an internal market therefore also needs national consensus on those telematics standards that should be implemented to achieve integration (interoperability).

8. Concluding Remarks

These different views on the potential and limitations of information processing in health care in the next decade may have shown the outstanding role of modern IPM and ICT for our societies, and last, but not least, for all persons needing care for their health problems.

Major aspects raised by the panelists and in the subsequent discussion, included:
1. The leading goal of expanding IPM and ICT in healthcare should be to further improve the quality of care. However, it is also necessary to keep the costs of health care at a reasonable level.
2. With the support of modern IPM and ICT the boundaries between inpatient and outpatient care will fade away and provide for a more efficient and patient-centered (not institution-centered) healthcare.
3. The cooperation between healthcare professionals will increase. There will be different ways of communication between them and with the patient, including the use of modern ICT and, particularly, the Internet.
4. Information is power. Society in general and all professionals in the field of medical informatics, biometry and epidemiology in particular must be concerned to achieve equality of opportunities for the different groups of healthcare professionals and for patients in being informed and in using new ICT.
5. Misuse of data will remain a serious problem and can become an obstacle to progress. Organizational efforts and reliable security systems, accepted by the public, to prevent misuse of data have to be provided.

When we consider these aspects it becomes obvious that the patient, not technology, is the focus of the development of IPM and ICT in healthcare. This is true for the perspectives, for the concerns, and for the next steps that have to be taken. We can see that for medical informatics, biometry and epidemiology, although they are technical and formal disciplines, the individual and his/her health have top priority.

This should be understood in the sense in which Karl Jaspers described the role of faculties in medicine (and health sciences, as he would probably say today). It is part of his book on 'The idea of the university', he was able to publish in 1946 after overcoming hard times including 8 years of prohibited lectureship. "Medicine is dealing with the health of man, its preservation, promotion and recovery, on the basis of knowledge, which is understanding the

---

[2] Original German text: "In der Medizin handelt es sich um die Gesundheit des Menschen, ihre Erhaltung, Förderung und Wiederherstellung aufgrund eines Wissens, das die Natur des Menschen begreift. ... [Grundlage] ist für das gesamte Tun ... ein nicht wissenschaftlicher Boden. ... In der Medizin ist der Boden der Wille zur Förderung des Lebens und der Gesundheit jedes Menschen als Menschen in seiner Artung. Es gibt keine Einschränkung".

nature of man: ... [Foundation] for the whole doings is ... a non scientific base. ... In medicine the base is the will to promote life and health of every person as a person in her or his nature. There is no restriction" [3][2].

REFERENCES
1. Jaspers K. Der Arzt im technischen Zeitalter (The Physician in the Technical Age). Klinische Wochenschrift, November 1958. Cited from: Jaspers K. Der Arzt im technischen Zeitalter. Munic: Piper 1986; 39.
2. International Medical Informatics Association, Working Group 1: Health and Medical Informatics Education. Recommendations of the International Medical Informatics Association (IMIA) on Education in Health and Medical Informatics. Method Inform Med 2000; 39: 267-77. http://www.imia.org/wg1.
3. Jaspers K. Die Idee der Universität (The Idea of the University). Berlin: Springer 1946. Cited from the reprint of 1980; 79-80.

Addresses of the authors:
Prof. Dr. Axel W. Bauer,
University of Heidelberg,
Institute for the History of Medicine,
Im Neuenheimer Feld 327,
D-69120 Heidelberg,Germany,
E-mail: q44@ix.urz.uni-heidelberg.de

Prof. Dr. Reinhold Haux, Dr. Petra Knaup,
University of Heidelberg,
Institute for Medical Biometry and Informatics,
Department of Medical Informatics,
Im Neuenheimer Feld 400,
D-69120 Heidelberg, Germany,
E-mail: {Reinhold_Haux, Petra_Knaup} @med.uni-heidelberg.de

Prof. Dr. Wolfgang Herzog,
University of Heidelberg,
University Hospital for Internal Medicine,
Department of General Clinical
and Psychosomatic Medicine,
Bergheimer Straße 58,
D-69115 Heidelberg, Germany,
E-mail: Wolfgang_Herzog@med.uni-heidelberg.de

Prof. Dr. Erich Reinhardt,
Siemens AG, Medical Solutions,
Henkestraße 127, D-91052 Erlangen, Germany,
E-mail: erich.reinhardt@med.siemens.de

Prof. Dr. Karl Überla,
University of Munich, Institue for Medical
Informatics, Biometry and Epidemiology,
Marchioninistr. 15, D- 81377 Munich, Germany,
E-mail: ibe@ibe.med.uni-muenchen.de

Prof. Dr. Wilhelm van Eimeren,
GSF-Research Center for Environment
and Health,
Medis-Institute for Medical Informatics
and Systems Research,
Ingolstädter Landstraße 1,
D-85764 Oberschleißheim
E-mail: ve@gsf.de

Prof. Dr. Dr. h.c. Wolfgang Wahlster,
German Research Center for Artificial
Intelligence (DFKI),
Stuhlsatzenhausweg 3,
D-66123 Saarbrücken, Germany,
E-mail: Wahlster@dfki.de

M.A. Musen[1],
J.H. van Bemmel[2]

[1]Stanford Medical Informatics, Stanford
University School of Medicine
Stanford, CA, USA
[2]Department of Medical Informatics
Erasmus University, Rotterdam
The Netherlands

Challenges in Medical Informatics

Challenges for Medical Informatics as an Academic Discipline: Workshop Report

Origins of the Workshop

In March 2001, twenty members of the informatics community gathered in Madrid, Spain, to discuss the state of our field as an academic discipline and the challenges that university-based workers in health informatics face. This meeting received considerable support from Erasmus University Rotterdam and the Spanish Society for Health Informatics (SEIS), and was designated as an IMIA Satellite Working Conference. The two-and-a-half day meeting took place in conjunction with the SEIS national conference and the meeting of the IMIA board of directors.

The workshop was motivated by observations that members of our community have made in recent years. Although the validity of some of these observations is debatable - and certainly was debated at the workshop - there has been concern that:

· Membership in professional societies for medical informatics, for the most part, remains flat.
· Recognition of medical informatics as a coherent academic discipline - especially by workers outside of medical informatics - has not been abundantly forthcoming.
· Many investigators within the

medical informatics community are perceived to have difficulty articulating the underlying theories and principles that guide their work.
· Many prominent leaders in medical informatics recently have left academia completely in favor of work in the commercial sector.
· It remains difficult to fill available academic positions with well-qualified candidates.
· Many academicians are abandoning work in clinical informatics in favor of work in bioinformatics, which seems to have considerably more cachet.

These observations seem paradoxical at a time when governments and health-care organizations are loudly articulating the need for information technology to improve patient safety, to guide clinical decision making, and to eliminate inequities in the distribution of medical services. They seem worrisome at a time when the vendor community should be relying on the results of university-based research to help frame the next round of industrial innovation. It thus seemed appropriate to take stock as a community of where our field is heading and of how we can address the underlying structural problems that may be impeding our progress.

Participants of the workshop submitted position papers that were distributed among the group in advance of the meeting. Some of these position papers have been expanded, and appear in the January 2002 issue of *Methods of Information in Medicine*. Some of the participants at the workshop also summarized their positions at a special session at Medinfo 2001 in London. There is a hope that the open discussion at Medinfo and the journal publication of the position papers will initiate a broad dialog among members of the health informatics community regarding the issues discussed in Madrid.

The State of Medical Informatics

The format for the workshop allowed the participants to present their positions briefly, followed by considerable discussion among the group. We will not attempt to abstract the positions of each contributor in this report, since most of the corresponding papers are now available in published form and the statements of each participant are best read in context. We believe it is more useful to summarize the key observations made by the group and to enumerate the points of debate.

Much of the discussion focused on the nature of medical informatics itself. One fundamental question centered on whether informatics is some sort of a science or whether it is an engineering discipline. To many, it seemed almost pejorative to describe informatics as engineering, and yet the workshop participants agreed that the scientific underpinnings of the field are not well articulated in our textbooks or by our professional societies. If informatics is a science, then surely it is not a natural science concerned with the elucidation of truths about the natural universe. If it is a "science of the artificial," to use the expression coined by Newell and Simon, then there are open questions about what are the hypotheses that workers in medical informatics are attempting to test, what are the theories that unify our approach, and what are the generic methods that allow us to validate our work empirically. In the absence of a clear expression of an agreed-upon underlying theory, it was difficult for many of the participants to feel comfortable with the description of informatics as a scientific discipline. At the same time, there was a nearly universal sentiment that academic work in informatics is indeed reflective of some sort of science. In the setting of this uncertainty, perhaps the most significant challenge to emerge from the workshop was a desire for our community as a whole to be more active in enunciating the theory that we believe drives our work and to be more precise about stating the hypotheses that we are attempting to test. If all of our theory is to be borrowed from traditional computer science, from information science, or from bio-statistics, for example, we are left with the open question of what might remain at the academic core of informatics that we can claim to be our own.

Despite the problems of defining a core theory for our discipline, the workshop participants rejected the suggestion that academic medical informatics was simply the application of information technology in health care. Although terms such as "computers in medicine" provide an easy-to-understand slogan, the participants believed that such descriptions only confuse the outside world (as well as our own community) about the essence of medical informatics. They pointed out that the word *informatics* increasingly is being used to connote nearly anything that has to do with computers, and that the emphasis on hardware and software obscures the centrality of *information* as a first-class object of study.

Although medical informatics may not be the same thing as "medical computer science,"it is clear that workers in medical informatics frequently serve as "brokers" who can mediate among biomedical professionals, computer scientists, and end users. Conference participants noted that communication skills are very important in our line of work, and that an important contribution of our community is the ability to develop solutions to problems posed in a variety of professional frameworks. Nevertheless, there was a strong belief that research in informatics involves much more than the provision of translation services among the various stakeholders and the application of known computational principles to a particular domain. The challenge for our field, of course, is to be able to articulate better what that unique contribution is.

Attempts to define the "correct" relationship between academic informatics and institutional service led to considerable discussion at the meeting. It is obvious that workers in informatics may fill critical service roles within their organizations - both in the clinical and basic-science arenas. As a consequence, they may manage an information environment that offers them opportunities both for the integration and evaluation of new technologies and for the collection of significant data sets with which to test their computational methods. There was consensus among the conference participants that academic work in informatics involves goals and methods that are inherently different from those of applied work to manage an institution's information infrastructure. There was not agreement, however, whether scholarly activities and service activities are best performed by the same people. The group leaned toward the conclusions that service and scholarship require different training and different aptitudes. Nonetheless, there are clear synergies when a single organization can include individuals who can take on these respective roles.

Attention to Emerging Fields

Much discussion centered on the surfacing of new fields that build on the basic techniques studied by workers in medical informatics. The new, heightened importance of bio-informatics and computational biology was mentioned by many of the participants. Although the generalizability of our work may be obvious to *us*, our field's traditional grounding in the health-care domain often makes it difficult for outsiders to appreciate that many of our basic techniques can translate into support for work in basic science. Again, the conversation focused on the need to clarify basic principles of *informatics* (without an adjective such as "medical" or "bio") that can lead to applications in both health care and basic biology. There was agreement that the boundaries between clinical informatics and bio-informatics are not terribly distinct - particularly as health-care practices increasingly will incorporate knowledge of patients' genetic condition and work in basic biology requires phenotypic information available in electronic patient record systems.

Although they are not receiving nearly as much attention - or funding - as is bioinformatics, other health-related disciplines are trying to carve out special pieces of the informatics pie. In particular, consumer health represents a burgeoning area of interest where information technology can play a key role. While recognizing the importance of such application areas, the group believed strongly that academic research in informatics needs to be able to transcend application areas. Thus, although consumer health and other disciplines can be extremely important driving forces for work in clinical informatics, our fundamental methodologies should not necessarily careen as new application areas are perceived to have greater or lesser importance to the health-care community.

The Role of Education and Training

A major challenge for the informatics community lies in the training of the next generation of researchers and practitioners. There is enormous variability in the curricular goals implemented by different training programs. There are few textbooks in our field and each one has its own definition of medical informatics. Once again, the lack of well articulated principles for the discipline make it difficult to know what core competencies our trainees need for success in their careers.

The group identified a need for better professional leadership to help set standards for training in informatics and to define the appropriate scope of formal curricula. Although IMIA and other societies have advocated guidelines for medical informatics education, there does not exist a perception - either from within the informatics community or from the outside - that there is an agreed-upon, circumscribed

set of learning objectives in force within all training programs in informatics. The group stopped short of advocating accreditation of informatics training programs or certification or credentialing of informatics professionals. The participants noted, however, that accreditation and certification are important objectives for professional societies in other fields, clarifying the core concepts of the discipline and making the statement that certified individuals have unique knowledge and skills. The group believed that organizations such as IMIA can play a key role in supporting the education of trainees and in advertising the qualifications of people with formal training in informatics to the outside world. Such activities, however, would require a new level of leadership in our professional societies. Attaining these objectives also would require our community to reach consensus concerning the boundaries of our discipline.

Where to Draw the Line

A central issue that kept reemerging in the discussion concerned the scope of medical informatics itself. Ours has always been an inclusive discipline, and we have gained strength from the interactions that occur when we bring together people who have a variety of viewpoints. We always have involved both basic scientists and practitioners in our discussions, and our journals and conferences can take advantage of contributions from many different perspectives. We have never worried about what is - and what is not - medical informatics, believing that our field benefits from diversity. As the participants of the workshop struggled to define underlying principles for medical informatics and a core curriculum for our students, however, it became increasingly unclear how inclusive our field ought to be. It is

impossible to define learning objectives or desirable skill sets without drawing boundaries that determine what is "in" and what is "out"; it is impossible to begin to discuss the credentialing of practitioners of medical informatics without some notion of what the core competencies are. Many of the challenges facing academic informatics seemed to stem from a lack of crispness in defining what the field really is. Past monikers such as "computers in biomedicine" have done little to clarify the situation. The vagueness also has made it particularly difficult for our community to argue that workers in medical informatics have special skills, since the boundaries of those skill sets are not defined.

The result is a dilemma: We can clarify the core dimensions of medical informatics - its theory, its principles, its applicability - and have a foundation for designing curricula, for credentialing practitioners, and for defining the place of informatics as an academic discipline. To clarify these dimensions, however, inherently will disenfranchise important members of our community. To paraphrase Kuhn, all paradigm shifts in science redefine the relationship of each academic to the discipline, forcing some investigators to the center and others to the periphery. In medical informatics, we have not done a particularly good job of defining a prevailing paradigm in the first place. This vagueness has served us well, allowing many of us to move between quite theoretical research and pragmatic applications, between laboratory experiments and large-scale deployment of information systems. The problem is that, although we and our particular health-care environments may have benefited individually from this lack of clarity, our discipline overall has not acquired any more coherence.

The workshop participants acknowledged that applications of informatics often address very broad user needs and must embrace a wide range of perspectives. Inclusivity is essential if informatics is to succeed as an engineering discipline. At the same time, there needs to be a sharpening of our focus if medical informatics is to be considered a science. We need to define our paradigm, and to demonstrate how our research collectively builds on a common theory. Of course, articulating that theory remains a major academic challenge for all of us.

Acknowledgments

All the participants at the Madrid workshop contributed ideas that appear in this report. The authors take responsibility for the manner in which they are presented here. An edited version of this workshop report appears as an editorial introducing the workshop papers in the January 2002 issue of *Methods of Information in Medicine*. The workshop in Madrid would not have been possible without the expert assistance of Ms. Desiree de Jong.

Address of the authors:
Mark A. Musen
Stanford Medical Informatics
Stanford University School of Medicine
251 Campus Drive, Room X-215
Stanford, CA 94305-5479, USA
E-mail: Musen@SMI.Stanford.EDU

Jan H. van Bemmel
Department of Medical Informatics
Erasmus University Rotterdam
PO Box 1738
NL-3000 DR Rotterdam
The Netherlands
E-mail: vanbemmel@mi.fgg.eur.nl

Special Section:

Reprinted by kind permission of:
Elsevier Science (201, 238)
Lippincott Williams & Wilkins (218)
Mary Ann Liebert, Inc. (259)
The Institute of Electrical and Electronical Engineers, Inc. (248)

An algorithmic overview of surface registration techniques for medical imaging

Michel A. Audette[a,*], Frank P. Ferrie[b], Terry M. Peters[c]

[a]*Montreal Neurological Institute (McGill University), 3801 University, Montreal, Quebec, Canada H3A 2B4*
[b]*McGill Center for Intelligent Machines (McGill University), Montreal, Canada*
[c]*The John P. Roberts Research Institute, London, Ontario, Canada*

Received 24 September 1998; received in revised form 1 July 1999; accepted 27 August 1999

Abstract

This paper presents a literature survey of automatic 3D surface registration techniques emphasizing the mathematical and algorithmic underpinnings of the subject. The relevance of surface registration to medical imaging is that there is much useful anatomical information in the form of collected surface points which originate from complimentary modalities and which must be reconciled. Surface registration can be roughly partitioned into three issues: choice of transformation, elaboration of surface representation and similarity criterion, and matching and global optimization. The first issue concerns the assumptions made about the nature of relationships between the two modalities, e.g. whether a rigid-body assumption applies, and if not, what type and how general a relation optimally maps one modality onto the other. The second issue determines what type of information we extract from the 3D surfaces, which typically characterizes their local or global shape, and how we organize this information into a representation of the surface which will lead to improved efficiency and robustness in the last stage. The last issue pertains to how we exploit this information to estimate the transformation which best aligns local primitives in a globally consistent manner or which maximizes a measure of the similarity in global shape of two surfaces. Within this framework, this paper discusses in detail each surface registration issue and reviews the state-of-the-art among existing techniques. © 2000 Elsevier Science B.V. All rights reserved.

Keywords: Registration, Feature, Free-form surface, Surface model, Appearance

1. Introduction

The registration of 3D surfaces is dealt with extensively in machine vision and medical imaging literature. Its applications vary from building terrain maps, in the context of providing autonomy to a planetary rover (Hebert et al., 1989), and depth maps of a sea floor for oceanographic studies (Kamgar-Parsi et al., 1991), to the recognition of objects from a CAD database (Fan et al., 1989), and of course, to reconciling various imaging modalities in biomedical imaging (Collignon et al., 1993). The goal of this paper is to provide a detailed overview of surface registration techniques which have been, or could potentially be, applied to anatomical surfaces.

This problem is a subset of the general medical image registration problem, as surveyed recently by Maintz and Viergever (1998), who also discuss landmark and volume registration, but we emphasize algorithmic details, with a view to providing some motivation for each technique. Surfaces provide more redundancy than landmarks, and this redundancy may be particularly advantageous for characterizing non-rigid motion. Moreover, we can make a distinction between landmarks automatically extracted from surfaces, which can be seen as feature point-based surface registration and are included in this survey, and manually identified landmarks, which may be tedious to determine and less repeatable than the former. Furthermore, a surface-based approach is likely to be less affected than volumes if the two modalities of interest cover parts of the anatomy which overlap only partially, for example if one modality represents a small subset of the anatomy

---

*Corresponding author.
E-mail address:* maudette@bic.mni.mcgill.ca (M.A. Audette).

which appears in the second modality. In other words, we can usually register a subpatch with a larger surface patch, on the basis of local and global surface shape, as will be seen later. Finally, in medical imaging literature, anatomical surfaces are usually explicitly identified within tomographic data such as MRI and CT and are often closed (Herman and Liu, 1979; Udupa, 1982). We expand on this definition by including range images of anatomical structures, such as those obtained by laser-based triangulation, which have a particular relevance to image-guided surgery (Audette and Peters, 1999; Simon et al., 1994b; Kikinis et al., 1994) and which are typically open.

Registration, between modalities A and B, is the *estimation of a mapping between coordinate systems* Ref_A and Ref_B associated with each modality:

$$x_B = T(x_A), \tag{1}$$

where $x_A = (x_A, y_A, z_A)$ and $x_B = (x_B, y_B, z_B)$ are points in coordinate systems Ref_A and Ref_B respectively which correspond to the same anatomical point, and where the quality of this mapping can be quantified by a global measurement based on fitting residuals. In an ideal, noise- and distortion-free environment where the same anatomy is imaged by two modalities of like scale, the computation of the transformation from point pairs matched on the basis *local* information would produce a relation which is also *globally* consistent. In other words, the resulting transformation would exactly align all pairs of homologous points. In practice, the data contain noise and distortion, and the anatomy itself may distort between images. Therefore the optimal relation (especially if a rigid transformation assumption is maintained) is that which reconciles local homologous point alignment and global consistency in some optimal manner.

Surface registration can be roughly partitioned into three stages, as illustrated in Fig. 1: **choice of transformation**,

elaboration of **surface representation** and **similarity criterion**, and **matching and global optimization**. The first issue concerns the assumptions made about the *nature of relationships* between the two modalities, e.g. whether a rigid-body assumption applies, and if not, what type and how general a relation optimally maps one modality onto the other. The second issue determines *what type of information* we extract from the 3D surfaces, which typically characterize their local or global shape, and *how we organize this information* into a representation of the surface which will lead to improved efficiency and robustness in the last stage. The last issue pertains to *how we exploit this information* to estimate the transformation which best aligns local primitives in a globally consistent manner or which maximizes a measure of the similarity in global shape of two surfaces. Within this framework, this paper discusses each surface registration issue in detail and reviews the state-of-the-art among existing techniques.

2. Choice of transformation

The first stage is the formalization of the assumptions about the type of relation T between the two 3D surfaces which is appropriate for mapping points x_A onto x_B. In most registration problems, T is a transformation between the same anatomy imaged either by different modalities or by one modality at different times. In this context, a **rigid-body transformation** is applicable provided that the deformations sustained by the anatomy are negligible compared with the required accuracy of the transformation. If the deformations between surfaces are significant, and especially if these deformations are caused by factors other than noise and distortion within the modality, then a **nonrigid transformation** must apply. Moreover, one can further classify nonrigid transformations based on whether they are specified by a global or piecewise local fitting.

2.1. Rigid-body transformation

A general rigid-body transformation can be expressed as combination of a rotation and a translation:

$$x_B = R_{AB}x_A + t_{AB}. \tag{2}$$

Consequently, rigid-body registration typically seeks the values of R and t which minimize

$$\min_{R,t} \sum_{i=1}^{N} \|x_{B_i} - (Rx_{A_i} + t)\|^2, \tag{3}$$

given 3D point correspondences x_{A_i} and x_{B_i}. The problem can be reformulated in a manner which decouples the computation of t from that of R by referring the coordinates *to the respective centroids of each point set*, leading to the minimization

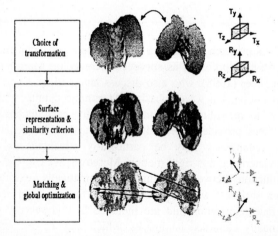

Fig. 1. 3D surface registration framework, featuring the choice of transformation between two anatomical surfaces (and of the search space for transformation parameters); the representation of the surface in terms of matching primitives (e.g. regions of consistent curvature); and finally, the matching of surface primitives and computation of the "best" transformation.

$$\min_{R,t} \sum_{i=1}^{N} \| x'_{B_i} - (Rx'_{A_i}) \|^2$$

where $x'_{A_i} = x_{A_i} - \dfrac{1}{N} \sum_{j=1}^{N} x_{A_j}$

and $x'_{B_i} = x_{B_i} - \dfrac{1}{N} \sum_{j=1}^{N} x_{B_j}$ \hfill (4)

The translation is given by the difference of centroids:

$$t = \frac{1}{N} \sum_{j=1}^{N} x_{B_j} - R \frac{1}{N} \sum_{j=1}^{N} x_{A_j}. \tag{5}$$

We review four common representations for rotation, as well as a fifth model which represents both translation and rotation. The relevance of choosing one particular representation is that it may lead to more efficient and/or numerically stable estimation of its parameters than others, or may be better suited to a particular surface representation. It is worth noting that these techniques are applicable not only to the registration of surfaces, but also to any set of explicit point pairs. Furthermore, while they may not have been published in a medical imaging context, they are still applicable to anatomical data.

The **orthonormal matrix** representation consists of a 3×3 matrix, which can be viewed as a mapping from reference frame A to frame B, once the translation between their origins is compensated, where each element R_{ij} is a *direction cosine* [i.e. the projection of one axis of reference frame A onto one axis of reference frame B (Craig, 1989)]. Arun et al. (1987) obtain rotation by first computing the *singular value decomposition* (Press et al., 1992) of the matrix $H = \sum_{i=1}^{N} x'_{B_i} x'^{T}_{A_i}$ determined from centroid-referred coordinates:

$$H = UDV^T, \tag{6}$$

where D is diagonal and U and V are orthonormal. The rotation is given by the expression $R = VU^T$.

We briefly address two interesting representations, the **Euler angles** and **axis-angle** models, although we emphasize less the techniques that employ them, because they are iterative rather than closed-form. We can express rotation as the product of three successive rotations (γ, β, α) of a predefined *fixed* coordinate system about axes $\hat{x}$, $\hat{y}$ and $\hat{z}$, or equivalently, as a succession of rotations about $\hat{z}$, $\hat{y}$ and $\hat{x}$ *moving* axes (Craig, 1989). Huang et al. (1986) use this Euler angle representation to design a 3D iterative motion estimation scheme that is a sequence of well-behaved 2D minimizations involving the projections of (partially rotated) points on the $x-z$, $y-z$ and $x-y$ planes. Moreover, a rotation can also be completely specified by a unique vector whose *direction is the rotation axis* and whose *norm is the rotation angle about this axis* (Ayache, 1991). Lin et al. (1986) adopt the axis-angle representation for a Fourier space approach to rigid-body motion estimation which does not require explicit correspondences.

A widely used representation of rotation is based on

quaternions (Faugeras and Hebert, 1986; Horn, 1987). A quaternion can be thought of as a *generalization of a complex number*, with *a real part* and *three imaginary parts*, or as *a composite of a 3-vector in* $\mathbb{R}^3$ *and a scalar in* $\mathbb{R}$. Moreover, the rotation quaternion can also be interpreted in terms of the axis-angle representation by the *Euler Symmetric Parameters* (Walker et al., 1991): $\dot{q} = [\sin \theta/2 n, \cos \theta/2]^T$. In other words, the orientation of the 3-vector component specifies the axis of rotation, and the norm of the 3-vector and the scalar component are related to the rotation angle about this axis. Horn casts the search for the optimal rotation parameters as a *maximization* based on quaternion components (in contrast to the minimization of Faugeras and Hebert (1986)). His objective function is optimized with respect to rotation by finding the eigenvector corresponding to the largest positive eigenvalue of a matrix N (see Horn, 1987) determined from centroid-referred point coordinates.

The motivation for the **dual quaternion**[1] rigid transformation estimation technique of Walker et al. (1991) is that other rigid transformation estimation techniques first determine optimal orientation and then use this solution to obtain the translation (e.g., Arun et al., 1987), resulting in the accumulation of error in this computation. The dual quaternion technique solves for both relative orientation and position by minimizing a single cost function. The underlying model views the transformation between two coordinate frames as a *translation of the original coordinate frame along a direction* n *by a distance* d, *followed by a rotation by an angle* θ *with respect to a line having* n *as its direction and passing through a point* p, as illustrated in Fig. 2. Walker reports similar accuracy to Arun's SVD technique for estimating rotation, but improved accuracy for estimating translation, across identical sets of point correspondences.

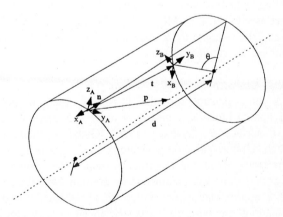

Fig. 2. Illustration of the dual quaternion model for rigid transformation (Walker et al., 1991) (reproduced with the permission of R.A. Volz, copyright Academic Press, 1991).

---

[1] A *dual number* $\hat{a} = a + \varepsilon b$ is defined as a combination of two real numbers a and b, with a special multiplication rule given for ε given by $\varepsilon^2 = 0$, such that, e.g. $(a + \varepsilon b)(c + \varepsilon d) = ac + \varepsilon(ad + bc)$.

2.2. Nonrigid transformations

In the event that surface deformations must be accounted for in the transformation, a nonrigid approach must be adopted. The simplest classes of nonrigid transformations are basically *generalizations of the rigid body transformation*. A more general formulation is one where a *global polynomial function* maps surface *A* to surface *B*. To make the mapping even more general, a global polynomial can be replaced by *piecewise polynomial relations*, or *splines*, and such functions can be seen as either *interpolating*, whereby the transformation they express is directly determined by the motion between two sets of primitives (and as such is sensitive to errors in the data), or *approximating*, whereby the agreement between the local motion of any pair of matches is reconciled with global consistency, in some optimal manner.

2.2.1. Generalization of rigid body motion: the affine transformation

The generalization of the rigid body transformation relevant to 3D surface matching is the *affine* transformation. The general **affine** class of transformations is characterized by the expression

$$x_B = A_{3\times3}x_A + b_{3\times1}, \qquad (7)$$

where there is no orthogonality constraint on the elements a_{ij} of matrix A as there is in Eq. (2). Affine transformations do not in general preserve angles or lengths, but parallel lines remain parallel (Foley et al., 1990). The affine transform relating two 3D surfaces is solved by Feldmar and Ayache (1994a), whose method matches "closest" points of compatible shape. This ensures that the solution to the minimization $\min_{A,b} (1/N) \sum_{i=1}^{N} \|Ax_{A_i} + b - x_{B_i}\|^2$ tends to a stable solution. Moreover, Henri et al. (1991) determine the translation, rotation and nonuniform scaling which maps stereotactic frame coordinates to corresponding CT or MR voxel values, prior to superimposing stereoscopic DSA images on the equivalent projections of the volumetric scan.

2.2.2. Global polynomial functions

A more general formulation is one where a global polynomial function, typically of order 2–5, maps surface *A* to surface *B* (Lavallée, 1996). Global methods use matched point pairs to generate a single optimal transformation, based on a sufficient number of points to (over)determine the parameters of the transformation, via either approximation or interpolation. Polynomial transformations are typically expressed in either cartesian or spherical coordinates. Moreover, global polynomial transformations are only useful to account for low-frequency distortions because of their unpredictable behaviour when the degree of the polynomial is high (Brown, 1992). This component of inter-surface motion is typically computed after an initial rigid alignment.

Approximation is the search for transformation parameters which map matched points or features *as closely as possible globally, but not necessarily perfectly individually*, whereas interpolation finds the transformation which maps two 3D surfaces so that *matched control points are exactly satisfied*. In the former case we assume that some noise or unwanted distortion exists and should not be accounted for in the transformation. For large numbers of control points, this choice makes sense because matches likely include inaccuracies, but taken together they contain sufficient statistical data to make the transformation reliable. Interpolation is more appropriate for a few accurately-matched control points, since it involves an independent parameter for each control point match, which may result in unexpected undulation for a high-order fit.

For a *cartesian* formulation, the global polynomial transformation in three dimensions can be stated as follows:

$$x_B = \sum_{ijk} a_{ijk} x_A^i y_A^j z_A^k,$$

$$y_B = \sum_{ijk} b_{ijk} x_A^i y_A^j z_A^k,$$

$$z_B = \sum_{ijk} c_{ijk} x_A^i y_A^j z_A^k, \qquad (8)$$

where a_{ijk}, b_{ijk} and c_{ijk} are the constant polynomial coefficients to be determined. If interpolation is used, these coefficients express a system of $3N$ unknowns which can be determined by N control points. In a least squares approximation, the sum over all matched feature/point pairs of the squared difference between the left and right-hand side of these equations is minimized, for example by setting the partial derivatives associated with these equations to zero.

Jacq and Roux (1993) implement a trilinear interpolation (i.e. where the summation indices i, j and k each go from 0 to 1, and where $i + j + k \leqslant 3$), determined by eight reference distortion values which span the volume to be warped. Subsol et al. (1994) register skulls and cortical surfaces to build a 3D atlas, by first rigidly matching crestlines and then using an iterative closest point algorithm (both techniques are discussed in Section 3) on crestline points to determine a global second order polynomial to describe the relation between iteratively transformed surface *A* and surface *B*. This results in a 2^n-order polynomial transformation, based on *n* iterations.

For closed surfaces that can be modelled as functions on a sphere, some authors prefer to work in spherical coordinates (Coppini et al., 1987; Chen et al., 1994). For example, **spherical harmonic** surfaces are closed surfaces on a sphere that can be decomposed into a set of orthogonal functions. To represent an arbitrary shape, the radius $r(\theta, \phi)$ in the spherical coordinate system (centered on the centroid) can be written as a linear sum of spherical harmonic basis functions:

$$r(\theta, \phi) \approx \sum_{n=1}^{N} \sum_{m=0}^{n} [A_{nm} U_{nm}(\phi, \theta) + B_{nm} V_{nm}(\phi, \theta)], \qquad (9)$$

where A_{nm} and B_{nm} are basis coefficients computed from the data points from a 3D object or surface and N represents the order of the fitting. The basis functions are:

$$U_{nm}(\theta, \phi) = \cos(m\phi) P_{n,m}(\cos(\theta))$$

$$\text{and } V_{nm}(\theta, \phi) = \sin(m\phi) P_{n,m}(\cos(\theta)), \qquad (10)$$

where $P_{n,m}(x) = (1 - x^2)^{m/2} \, d^m/dx^m \, P_n(x)$ and $P_n(\cdot)$ is the Legendre polynomial of degree n (Press et al., 1992). In other words, surfaces S_A and S_B, and the displacement between them, can be seen as functions on a sphere, represented by a set of real coefficients A_{nm} and B_{nm}. Because the shape is approximated as a sum of different harmonics, in theory this representation can reconstruct high-frequency surface detail.

Coppini et al. (1987) model the epicardial stretch tensor, based on tracked vascular bifurcations, by performing a third-order spherical harmonic fitting over individual displacements $r_A(\theta_i, \phi_i) - r_B(\theta_i, \phi_i)$, after correction for translation and rotation. Chen et al. (1994) adopt a similar method, but first characterize global shape with **superquadric** surfaces (Barr, 1981; 1984; Bajcsy and Solina, 1987), prior to characterizing local shape variation with spherical harmonics.

2.2.3. Local nonrigid transformations: piecewise polynomials

Global mapping functions do not always adequately capture deformations of anatomical structures, which are often intrinsically local (Lavallée, 1996; Bookstein, 1989). *Piecewise polynomial functions* produce a more general relation. In general, the relative density and reliability of the data determine whether an interpolation or an approximation scheme is used.

One well-documented interpolating scheme is the **thin-plate spline** (Duchon, 1976; Bookstein, 1989). The thin-plate spline over a 2D domain can be expressed as $z(x, y) = U(r) = r^2 \log r^2$, where $r = \sqrt{x^2 + y^2}$, and as such U is a fundamental solution of the biharmonic equation. The interpolant $f(p)$ is optimal in that it has *minimum bending energy* amongst all functions which pass exactly through points $x_i = (p_i, z(p_i))$; i.e.

$$\iint_{\mathbb{R}} \left[\left(\frac{\partial^2 f}{\partial x^2} \right)^2 + \left(\frac{\partial^2 f}{\partial x \partial y} \right)^2 + \left(\frac{\partial^2 f}{\partial y^2} \right)^2 \right] dx dy \qquad (11)$$

is minimized. This type of interpolation function can then be applied to modelling nonrigid motion. Instead of having $f(p)$ represent a displacement in the z-direction over the $p = (x, y)$ domain, it can express the x-component of a deformation. Likewise functions $g(p)$ and $h(p)$ can express the y- and z-components of a deformation (Bookstein, 1989; Evans et al., 1991), where now $p = (x, y, z)$. This method presupposes the use of relatively sparse point matches in order to determine a set of local polynomials or spline functions exactly, when in fact it may be useful to consider denser displacement information to describe a fundamentally underdetermined relationship. Moreover, the notion of minimum bending is better suited to deformation over a 2D, rather than 3D, domain.

Another useful piecewise polynomial representation is the **B-spline**, particularly in the context of *smoothing* (regularizing) and *least-squares* spline approximation (Dierckx, 1995). Given a set of displacement data $d(x_r, y_r, z_r)$, and three sets of knots λ_i, $i = 0, \ldots, f + 1$, μ_j, $j = 0, \ldots, g + 1$, and ν_k, $k = 0, \ldots, h + 1$, we can compute the least-squares pth order volumetric spline

$$u(x, y, z) = \sum_{i,j,k} u_{i,j,k} B_i(x) B_j(y) B_k(z), \text{ where, e.g.}$$

$$B_i(x) = \sum_{l=i}^{i+p+1} \frac{(\lambda_l - x)^p}{\lambda_l - \lambda_i} \quad \text{if } x \in [\lambda_i \lambda_l] \text{ and}$$

$$B_i(x) = 0 \quad \text{elsewhere}, \qquad (12)$$

and such that $\delta = \Sigma_r \, (w_r(\|d_r - u(x_r, y_r, z_r)\|))^2$ is minimized. Here, the determination of B-spline coefficients of $u_{i,j,k}$ is by the least-squares solution of an overdetermined linear system. For a smoothing spline approach, the problem is to find the function $u_p(x, y, z)$ minimizing a smoothing norm which is a function of the B-spline coefficients, subject to $\delta < S$. Szeliski and Lavallée (1996) model the nonrigid transformation between two anatomical surfaces as a first order spline in x, y and z, which is constrained by zeroth and first order stabilizers. This approach penalizes large variations of the spline coefficients, while also enforcing agreement with displacement data. We (Audette and Peters, 1999) have recently demonstrated the use of 2D *recursive* splines (Unser et al., 1993a, 1993b) to efficiently characterize nonrigid cortical motion undergone during brain surgery, as captured by a time sequence of range images.

Lastly, a few other ways of characterizing nonrigid motion appear in the literature. Goldgof and Mishra classify the nonrigid motion of surfaces in terms of how it affects their mean and Gaussian curvature properties, namely as *rigid, isometric, homothetic, conformal* and *general nonrigid*[2] (Goldgof et al., 1988a; Mishra et al., 1991). Moreover, Feldmar and Ayache (1994b) determine *locally* affine transformations for individual surface points $(A_{A,i}, b_{A,i})$ by a weighted sum of the rigid transformation

---

[2]Conformal motion is characterized by *proportionality* of the coefficients of the first fundamental form (do Carmo, 1976):

$$\frac{E_A}{E_B} = \frac{F_A}{F_B} = \frac{G_A}{G_B} = \eta(u, v).$$

This function $\eta(u, v)$ becomes a *constant* over (u, v) for homothetic motion, and *identity* for isometric motion.

parameters of locally neighbouring matched surface points $(\boldsymbol{R}_{A,k}, \boldsymbol{t}_{A,k})$, where $k \neq i$.

3. Surface representation and similarity criterion

The second stage of registration consists of computing a surface representation and defining a matching criterion based on it. In general, the surface representation should be stable over the two modalities or over the time sequence considered. It should afford a similarity criterion which is sufficiently discriminating to associate homologous points unambiguously and efficiently, if the application dictates that algorithmic performance is an issue. There are four approaches to representing a surface for the sake of registration: **feature**, **point**, and **model-based** methods as well as techniques based on **global similarity**. The definition of the similarity criterion is typically closely related to the choice of matching primitive. Furthermore, the criteria for selecting a particular primitive are application-specific, depending for example on whether the anatomy of interest is smooth, such as the cranium, or highly angular, such as a vertebra. Other factors which influence this choice include the size of the transformation to be computed (i.e. whether the two surfaces are separated by an arbitrarily large transformation or roughly aligned), and whether the transformation is rigid or non-rigid.

The feature-based method attempts to express surface morphology as a set of features which are extracted by a preprocessing step. Such features provide a *compact description of the surface shape* (at the expense of losing information), which is quantifiable by stable, discriminating scalar measurements. The similarity criterion is then an outgrowth of this feature characterization: it consists of a comparison of scalar measurements. The point and model-based methods do not attempt to reduce the surface representation to a more compact description, rather they use *all, or a large subset of all, points*. Generally, for the point-based method, the primitive used is often the surface point itself, and the similarity criterion is a distance to be minimized between a pair of surface points. For model-based approaches, often an implicit criterion is used, such as an external force or halting condition driven by two sets of image data, with which an evolving deformable surface model must be reconciled. Finally, a new class of registration methods matches surfaces typically on the basis of their *global* similarity. While there are currently few anatomical applications, the relevance of these methods stems from the feasibility of precomputing a number of training views of a surface generated from a patient's tomographic data, and from the desirability of computing arbitrarily large transformations for smooth, relatively featureless surfaces.

The feature-based and global approaches are potentially more discriminating than point- or model-based techniques, and can therefore resolve a large motion or transformation. On the other hand, most point and model-based methods may be attractive in the case of small or iteratively estimated motion, because they exploit large redundancy of information, which is especially useful for estimating locally nonrigid transformations, as these are inherently underdetermined.

3.1. Feature-based representations

Feature-based matching is largely founded on the use of differential geometry to describe local surface shape (do Carmo, 1976; Besl and Jain, 1986). According to Bonnet's fundamental existence and uniqueness theorem, if two surfaces S_A and S_B possess equivalent fundamental forms I and II (or equivalent Gaussian and Mean curvatures K and H), then there exists an appropriate translation and rotation such that S_A and S_B coincide exactly (Besl and Jain, 1986). In general, feature-based matching is applied to computing *rigid* transformations.

Features used for surface registration fall into three categories: (sparse) *point features* (distinct from dense point-based schemes, also referred to as free-form surface registration), *curves* and *regions*. Point features are salient, well-localized, sparse loci of important geometric significance, such as extrema of curvature: local peaks, pits, saddle points where the two principal curvatures are most pronounced, or where K is at a local minimum or maximum. The second type of feature corresponds to contiguous lines or curves, consisting typically of differential structures such as ridges or boundaries between regions. Regions, in turn, are areas possessing some homogeneous characteristic, such as consistent curvature sign. Each feature in surface S_A can be matched with its homolog in S_B by first characterizing each feature in either surface by parameters expressing its respective topology, and looking for a compatible vector of parameters in the other surface. If there is more than one suitable candidate for a given feature, the match can be disambiguated by assuming that neighbouring features on the same surface which are matched one-to-one should undergo motion consistent with the ambiguous candidate. False candidates can then be eliminated on the basis of motion inconsistency.

Moreover, *accuracy* issues related to feature extraction include the use of the neighbourhood information around each surface point to stabilize the computation of its differential properties (Sander and Zucker, 1990; Ferrie et al., 1993) and the sensitivity to noise statistics of a given numerical method for estimating derivatives and surface curvature (Flynn and Jain, 1989; Abdelmalek, 1990; Roth and Levine, 1993). Finally, another relevant area of research is the application of *recursive* infinite impulse response filters (Proakis, 1996), particularly near-Gaussian exponential filters (Shen and Castan, 1986; Deriche, 1987; Deriche, 1990) to speed up the smoothing stage prior to feature extraction (Monga et al., 1992; Thirion, 1994).

Point features can be matched on the basis of their intrinsic information, such as surface curvature values, as well as position relative to *neighbouring* point features. One such feature is the *extremum of principal curvatures*, computed by Thirion (1994) within volumetric data by detecting the zero-crossings of two "extremality" functions. The first function is discussed later in this section, and is used to detect *ridge lines*, or lines of locally maximal higher principal curvature, while the second function finds a local extremum of the lesser principal curvature within each ridge line. The scalar measurements used in the matching include the type of extremal point, which depends on the sign of the principal curvatures, the response of the extremality functions, the principal curvature values, and the distances and orientations of vectors to neighbouring points. An alternate representation, used by Goldgof et al. (1988b) in terrain matching but nonetheless applicable to anatomical surfaces if they possess sharp corners, is the *extremum of Gaussian curvature* (K), detected on the basis of a threshold on the value of K.

A somewhat less compact way of representing surface shape is as a collection of **curves**. One particularly relevant curvilinear feature in medical images is the *ridge or crest line* (e.g. the trough of a sulcus or the maximum height of a gyrus). As pointed out by Maintz et al. (1996), there are many ways to define a ridge, and consequently many ways to detect one. Monga et al. (1992) and Monga and Benayoun (1995) look for a contiguous set of loci of a surface where the largest principal curvature κ_1 is locally maximal. These correspond to the zero-crossings of the extremality function $e_1 = \nabla\kappa_1 \cdot t_1$, where $\nabla\kappa_1$ is the directional derivative of the largest principal curvature, and t_1 is the principal direction corresponding to κ_1.

Maintz et al. (1996) propose two operators of their own which stem from the consideration of the gradient w of a smoothed surface and its right-handed normal v in the proximity of a ridge. The gradient at any non-ridge position *points towards* the ridge, but at a ridge position the gradient is *aligned with* the ridge. A consequence of this geometry is that the directional derivative along v of a surface is characterized by a highly concave profile at a ridge point in comparison with other points. Maintz then detects a ridge point either as a minimum of the *second derivative of the surface*, or as a maximum of the derivative of the *direction of the gradient*, along v. An alternative to a ridge-based curve is the *distance contour* (Radack and Badler, 1989), which could be applied to anatomical data, and which is the set of points of constant distance from a highly salient point.

Guéziec and Ayache (1994) present an elegant technique for characterizing and matching curves, which in turn is based on the curve matching algorithm of Kishon et al. (1990). Kishon addresses the problem of finding the longest matching subcurve appearing in two curves. This uses local, rotationally and translationally invariant, stable shape signatures, namely *curvature* $\kappa(s)$ and *torsion* $\tau(s)$,

of smoothed curves[3]. Each shape signature is represented as a *hash table* (see Section 4), where entries are associated with pairs of curvature–torsion values (κ, τ). The improvements introduced by Guéziec and Ayache relate to the approximation of the curves, to the hash table and to the statistical analysis of various invariants for matching, particularly in directly determining a 3D transformation from homologous points on matched curves.

Regions constitute an even denser feature-based representation. They are typically characterized either by the homogeneity of their local surface shape or as being circumscribed by some boundary. One advantage is that the notion of neighbourhood between regions is natural (Toriwaki and Yokoi, 1988), and leads to the characterization of a surface as an adjacency graph. Matching is then carried out as an exercise in finding the maximal *clique* of compatible subgraphs (see (Radig, 1984) and the references therein). Here, groups of regions are matched based on neighbourhood topology as well as local region characteristics. One definition of homogeneity used to segment surfaces into regions or surface patches is the *K/H sign combination* (Besl and Jain, 1986; Kehtarnavaz and Mohan, 1989). Surfaces can be subdivided into patches according to surface type: elliptic and outwardly bulging $(K > 0/H < 0)$, elliptic and inwardly bulging $(K > 0/H > 0)$, parabolic and outwardly bulging $(K = 0/H < 0)$, parabolic and inwardly bulging $(K = 0/H > 0)$, planar $(K = 0/H = 0)$ and hyperbolic or saddle shaped $(K < 0/H \neq 0)$. In practice, a small nonzero threshold is used to determine sign. An illustration of a K/H surface representation for a range image of a femur epiphysis appears in Fig. 3.

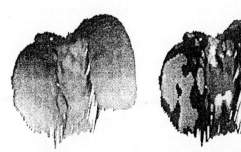

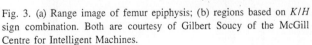

Fig. 3. (a) Range image of femur epiphysis; (b) regions based on K/H sign combination. Both are courtesy of Gilbert Soucy of the McGill Centre for Intelligent Machines.

---

[3]For a curve $\alpha\colon I = (a, b) \to \mathbb{R}^3$, parametrized by arclength s, *curvature* $\kappa(s)$ is the scalar $\|\alpha''(s)\|$. It is a measure of how rapidly the curve pulls away from the *tangent* line $t(s)$. The direction of $\alpha''(s)$ is given by the unit *normal* $n(s)$, and the unit vector $b(s) = n(s) \times t(s)$ is called the *binormal* vector. Torsion $\tau(s)$ corresponds to $\|b'(s)\|$, and it is a measure of how quickly the curve pulls away from the *osculating plane* at s spanned by n and t (do Carmo, 1976).

3.2. Point-based methods

Point-based methods register surfaces on the basis of relatively dense point sets brought into correspondence, where these point sets constitute all, or a significant subset of, the available surface point samples. An alternate name for surface matching based on dense point sets is **free-form** surface matching (Besl and McKay, 1992; Zhang, 1994). The two point sets are generally assumed to be relatively close to being aligned, and are usually registered by *iteratively* minimizing a global function such as the sum of squared distances between mutually closest points between (possibly transformed) surface S_A and surface S_B, as expressed by Eq. (3). Differences between many of these methods exist strictly at the level of the choice of distance metric and of the methods of optimally finding a match based on this metric (described in detail in Section 4). An illustration of this technique appears in Fig. 4.

One common distance metric is the distance from a point x_B in set $X_B = \{x_B\} \subseteq S_B$ to the (transformed) point set $X_A = \{x_A\} \subseteq S_A$:

$$d(x_B, R_k x_{A,min} + t_k) = \min_{x_A \in X_A} d(x_B, R_k x_A + t_k). \qquad (13)$$

Besl and McKay (1992) propose the *Iterative Closest Point* (ICP) method to determine the closest point pairs according to Eq. (13), then compute the transformation from these pairs with a quaternion technique. The positions of the surface points S_A ("data shape") are then updated: $X_{A,k} = R X_{A,k-1} + t$ and the process iterates until the mean-square distance, or point matching error, stabilizes to within some tolerance. An accelerated variant of the ICP method (discussed in Section 4) is also proposed. The method is better adapted to registering comparable patches, but a subpatch can also be put into correspondence with a larger patch, at the cost of considering several "initial translation states".

Zhang (1994) and Lavallée and Szeliski (1995) adopt an objective function identical to that proposed by Besl, except for weighting factors to accomodate measurement

noise, and in the case of Zhang, to exclude outliers. They also introduce execution efficiencies: Zhang uses *k-D trees* to make the search for closest points more efficient, and Lavallée dispenses with this search altogether by pre-computing a *distance map*, which unfortunately does not provide explicit point pairs and thus still entails a search for optimal transformation parameters. Simon et al. (1994a, 1994b) apply this technique to intrasurgical registration of a range image of the head with a surface extracted from tomographic data and address the issue of sensitivity to the perturbation of individual points. We (Audette and Peters, 1999) also use a free-form surface technique to characterize intrasurgical non-rigid cortical motion, where we refine the distance map proposed by Lavallée: a *closest-point map* is produced, which provides explicit point pairs suitable for closed-form transformation computation.

Other point-based techniques, which differ from those discussed above in terms of the distance metric which is minimized, have been proposed by Chen and Medioni (1991), by Pelizzari et al. (1989) by Soucy and Ferrie (1997), and by Rangarajan et al. (1997). Chen uses a subset of *control points* in relatively smooth areas, leading to an iterative technique with very good convergence properties. For each surface normal $n_{A,i}$ defined at a control point $x_{A,i}$, its intersection $x_{B,i}$ with surface S_B is found. Next, defining $s_{B,i}$ the plane tangent to S_B at $x_{B,i}$, the global transformation which minimizes the sum of squared distances between the set of transformed $x_{A,i}$ with their corresponding *tangent planes* $s_{B,i}$ on S_B is computed. Pelizzari fits a "hat" or external surface, consisting of relatively sparse points from the scalp as imaged by the modality of lesser resolution or coverage, to a "head" constituted by the set of 2D contours extracted on a slice-by-slice basis from the higher coverage/resolution modality. The residual which is minimized is the sum of distances from each hat point to the head surface, along a direction from the former point to the head centroid. Soucy proposes an iterative technique which takes local surface shape into account. It matches small surface patches (as small as 3×3 pixels) by minimizing a similarity functional which enforces compatible local shape and piecewise-smooth motion. Rangarajan matches points with a technique (demonstrated on 2D autoradiograph slices but equally applicable to 3D surfaces) which imbeds the search for match pairs and for optimal transformation parameters, as well as the explicit exclusion of outliers, into *one* elegant minimization, which makes the method more robust to initial transformation estimation than the ICP technique.

Finally, Feldmar and Ayache (1994a,b) do not attempt strictly to find closest points, but to find closest **feature vectors**. This approach is a comparison of 8 parameters, namely the coordinates of each point (x, y, z), the components of its normal (n_x, n_y, n_z) and the principal curvatures κ_1 and κ_2 of the surface at that point. They

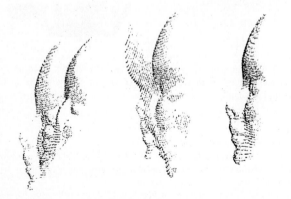

Fig. 4. Iterative point-based registration of phantom face range data (courtesy of S. Lavallée, R. Szeliski and L. Brunie, copyright MIT Press, 1986 [Lavallée et al., 1996]).

determine a *globally affine* transformation and then possibly a set of *locally affine* transformations, by extended Kalman filtering (see Section 4), based on point-pairs which minimize the following expression:

$$d(\boldsymbol{v}_{A,i}, \boldsymbol{v}_{B,j}) = \alpha_1(x_{A,i} - x_{B,j})^2 + \alpha_2(y_{A,i} - y_{B,j})^2$$
$$+ \alpha_3(z_{A,i} - z_{B,j})^2 + \alpha_4(n_{xA,i} - n_{xB,j})^2$$
$$+ \alpha_5(n_{yA,i} - n_{yB,j})^2 + \alpha_6(n_{zA,i} - n_{zB,j})^2$$
$$+ \alpha_7(\kappa_{1A,i} - \kappa_{1B,j})^2 + \alpha_8(\kappa_{2A,i} - \kappa_{2B,j})^2, \quad (14)$$

where α_i are weights determined by minimum and maximum data values. In other words, the closest point to $x_{A,i}$ on S_B is one which best fulfills a compromise between 3D distance, difference in normal orientation, and difference of principal curvatures.

3.3. Model-based representations

Deformable surface modelling consists of expressing surface identification (segmentation) in one volume or surface tracking over a volume sequence, as a model which reconciles the likely shape and/or dynamic behaviour of the surface, according to some **physically-based** or **surface evolution** expression, with raw image data. With some exceptions (Amini and Duncan, 1992; Sclaroff and Pentland, 1993), such methods generally compute curve and surface motion not by explicit matching, but by implicit consideration of image motion in the form of virtual forces that tend to make the model agree with shifts in strong image gradients. Because the thrust of active surface models is mostly on segmentation, only influential techniques and those which emphasize registration are described in detail. For more on active contour and surface models, the reader is referred to McInerney and Terzopoulos (1996) for physically-based models and to Sethian (1996b) and to Kimmel et al. (1997) for surface evolution models. One important issue in segmentation which has an impact on the accuracy of the registration is **anisotropic filtering**, whereby smoothing which is required for surface extraction is carried out tangentially to the surface, without washing out image features in the direction normal to it (Perona and Malik, 1990; Alvarez et al., 1992; Kimia and Siddiqi, 1996).

For physically-based deformable surface models, the basic idea is to model an object which is tracked over time as being in, or quickly reaching, an equilibrium between internal and external virtual forces. **Internal forces** include inertia, damping and strain, and are typically determined by the current state which is assumed for a 3D object. **External forces** are typically determined by image data. The relative motion undergone by the various parts of a surface is a result of the interaction of these two sets of forces, according to formal physical principles.

Important early research includes Kass' *snakes* paper (Kass et al., 1987), Terzopoulos' symmetry-seeking 3D shape model (Terzopoulos et al., 1988) and Bajscy's multiresolution elastic matching (Bacjsy and Kovacic, 1989). Kass casts the 2D contour detection and tracking problem of intensity images as a minimization of the following energy functional:

$$E_{\text{snake}} = \int_0^1 E_{\text{int}}(\boldsymbol{v}(s)) + E_{\text{image}}(\boldsymbol{v}(s)) + E_{\text{con}}(\boldsymbol{v}(s)) \, ds, \quad (15)$$

which is a controlled-continuity spline under the influence of *image* forces and *external constraint* forces. Terzopoulos' model is expressed as

$$\mu \frac{\partial^2 \nu}{\partial t^2} + \gamma \frac{\partial \nu}{\partial t} + \frac{\delta \mathscr{E}(\nu)}{\delta \nu} = f(\nu), \quad (16)$$

and consists of a deformable sheet of elastic material, which is rolled to form a tube, through which passes a deformable spine, also of elastic material. *Coupling* forces try to make the shape retain its axial symmetry, and *extrinsic* forces constrain the shape to be consistent with one or more 2D image projections. The Bajscy model is

$$\mu \nabla^2 u_i + (\lambda + \mu) \frac{\partial \theta}{\partial x_i} + F_i = 0, \quad i = 1, 2, 3, \quad (17)$$

where θ is the *dilatation*[4] at a point on the body, and μ and λ are *Lamé's constants*, which define the elastic properties of the model. The *external forces* $\boldsymbol{F} = (F_1, F_2, F_3)^T$ bring similar regions of two 3D objects into correspondence by enforcing grey-level value correlation and edge alignment between blurred volumes (in a multiresolution framework).

Research conducted separately by Pentland (Pentland and Sclaroff, 1993; Essa et al., 1993) and by Terzopoulos (Terzopoulos and Metaxas, 1991; McInerney and Terzopoulos, 1995) proposes a finite-element model approach to the numerical solution of deformable surface models, and consequently these surface models are based on the *finite-element equilibrium equation*, which has the form

$$M\ddot{U} + C\dot{U} + KU = R, \quad (18)$$

where M, C and K are virtual *mass*, *damping* and *stiffness* matrices, U is the displacement of the FEM nodes, and R is the sum of external forces, determined by image data. Pentland and Terzopoulos use a hybrid representation featuring a superquadric ellipsoid upon which is grafted a displacement function, which in turn is estimated by finite-element modelling. In a static segmentation context, this displacement function represents the difference between the simple superquadric shape and the final, more general shape which is more in keeping with image forces. In a surface tracking context, a general shape at t_k is used as a

---

[4]This is the change in volume per unit initial volume under small strains and sum of principal strains in general (Malvern, 1969).

first estimate towards the final shape at t_{k+1}, and the displacement is just $U_{k+1} - U_k$.

Significant improvements to the static model are suggested by Cohen et al. (Cohen and Cohen, 1990; Cohen, 1991; Cohen et al., 1992b), and by Metaxas et al. (Metaxas and Kakadiaris, 1996; DeCarlo and Metaxas, 1996). If the model is not initialized close enough to the desired surface, short-range image forces may be unable to attract it. To alleviate this problem, Cohen (Cohen and Cohen, 1990; Cohen, 1991) uses a *pressure force* to inflate the model towards the object surface. In (Cohen et al., 1992b), the surface produced by a physical model is characterized in terms of its differential structure, and the model is then expanded to enforce the agreement of the surface's *normal orientation* with that estimated by a Monga–Deriche edge detector (Monga et al., 1991). Metaxas devises methods for adaptively estimating *virtual material properties* (Metaxas and Kakadiaris, 1996), and for using *blending functions* in order to merge two simple (e.g. superquadric) shapes to express more complex surfaces (DeCarlo and Metaxas, 1996).

Improvements relating to surface tracking are proposed by Nastar and Ayache (1993) and by Sclaroff and Pentland (1993). If physically based models can be viewed as virtual masses on the surface with *springs* relating them to their neighbours, this viewpoint can be extended over time to a spring between a boundary point at t_1 and its closest neighbour at t_2, as pointed out by Nastar. Moreover, salient feature points such as curvature extrema are used to anchor the dynamic behaviour of the model, by attaching particularly stiff springs between feature point pairs. Sclaroff suggests that FEM numerical estimation can benefit from a change of basis from *nodal* to *modal* displacements ϕ, where $U = \phi \sin[\omega(t - t_0)]$ and ω represents a virtual frequency of vibration, based on object shape, corresponding to each mode (see also the section in (Bathe, 1982) on mode superposition). This change of basis is justified not on the grounds of expected periodic motion, but because it decouples the system of Eq. (18), which is now expressed as the eigenproblem (neglecting damping by taking $C = 0$):

$$K\Phi = M\Phi\Omega^2, \quad \text{where } \Phi = [\phi_1 | \cdots | \phi_P]$$

$$\text{and } \Omega^2 = \begin{bmatrix} \omega_1^2 & & \\ & \ddots & \\ & & \omega_P^2 \end{bmatrix}. \tag{19}$$

The matrix Φ has an interesting interpretation: its vector entries ϕ_i can be ordered according to increasing corresponding eigenvalue ω_i^2. In this case Φ is an orthogonal, frequency-ordered description of on object's shape and its natural deformations, somewhat like a Fourier series. An important consequence of this representation is that it leads to an *explicit* matching algorithm, after an initial rigid alignment, where low-order nonrigid modes ϕ_i are used as

a coordinate system, and two shapes are nonrigidly registered on the basis of modal feature vectors.

In contrast to the preceding models, those developed independently by Malladi et al. (1995) and by Caselles et al. (1992) have a geometric, rather than physical, interpretation, and are generally based on a *curve or surface evolution equation*, a partial differential equation of the Hamilton-Jacobi type (Levesque, 1992, Kimmel et al., 1997). These techniques are attractive for registration because they inherently compute contour or surface shape parameters, and possess other advantages, such as robustness to initialization as well as the capacity for a contour or surface to split or to merge. Here, a contour or surface is viewed as the zero level of a higher-dimensional function. For example, to identify a contour in 2D, a 3D hypersurface is initially placed completely inside (or outside) such a shape, and then made to flow outward (or inward) with a speed dependent on the strength of the image gradient $g(I)$, on surface curvature $\mathrm{div}(\nabla u / \|\nabla u\|)$ and on a constant advection term ν which acts as an inflation (or deflation) force:

$$\frac{\partial u}{\partial t} = g(I)\|\nabla u\|\left[\nu + \mathrm{div}\left(\frac{\nabla u}{\|\nabla u\|}\right) \right]. \tag{20}$$

The factor $\mathrm{div}(\nabla u / \|\nabla u\|)$ is the curvature κ of the level-set contour in 2D. In 3D, it is the mean curvature H of the level-set surface. The image gradient-based factor acts as a halting criterion which binds the level-set surface to intensity discontinuities. Recent improvements include a *doublet* term (Caselles et al., 1995, 1997; Kichenassamy et al., 1995) which prevents the surface from overshooting past image gradients, and the application of the *fast marching* level sets algorithm (Sethian, 1996a; Malladi and Sethian, 1998).

Lastly, the model of Amini and Duncan (1992) uses 3D surface points as its raw data, and views the local surface shape as a bending energy from an idealized thin flat plate $\varepsilon_{be}(u, v) = \kappa_1^2 + \kappa_2^2$. It seeks to match surface points of consistent energy and therefore of consistent principal curvature. Moreover, their model also has a stretching energy term which penalizes *non-conformal* motion (i.e. motion where the proportionality of the various coefficients of the first fundamental form, E, F and G, are not maintained). Consequently, the following energy measure is minimized over two surfaces:

$$\lambda_{be}\{(\kappa_{1A} - \kappa_{1B})^2 + (\kappa_{1A} - \kappa_{1B})^2\}$$
$$+ \lambda_{st}\left\{ \left(\frac{E_A}{E_B} - \frac{F_A}{F_B}\right)^2 + \left(\frac{F_A}{F_B} - \frac{G_A}{G_B}\right)^2 + \left(\frac{E_A}{E_B} - \frac{G_A}{G_B}\right)^2 \right\}. \tag{21}$$

The tracking model of Cohen et al. (1992a) is similar to Amini's in that it is characterized by a functional that minimizes curvature differences, between two 2D contours at comparable arclength parameters, while enforcing smooth motion along arclength. The zero arclength value on each contour corresponds to a matched feature point. They propose an extension to 3D surface tracking in the same paper.

3.4. Techniques based on global shape

The feature, point and model-based algorithms discussed so far can be broadly described as relying on local information to register surfaces. However, there are a few recently-published algorithms which register surfaces on the basis of global surface geometry, that do not rely on a rough prior estimation of the transformation and that may be able to deal with relatively featureless patches. We are alluding to the **spinmap** representation of Johnson and Hebert (1998) and to the **eigenshape** or **appearance-based** methods for registering 3D surfaces (Campbell and Flynn, 1999).

The spinmap representation is a set of 2D footprints conveying global surface shape in the neighbourhood of selected *oriented points* (Johnson and Hebert, 1998), as illustrated in Fig. 5. A 3D oriented point consists of a point p and a surface normal n estimated at that point. In order to describe its neighbouring topology, a 2D basis is formed. To define this basis, Johnson first defines a line L through p whose direction is along n, and a tangent plane P through p. The two coordinates of the bases are α, the perpendicular distance of a neighbouring point to line L, and β, the perpendicular distance of this point to plane P. A spinmap S_O is the function which maps 3D neighbouring points x to the 2D coordinates of a basis corresponding to an oriented point O:

$$S_O(x) \rightarrow (\alpha, \beta) = \left(\sqrt{\|x - p\|^2 - (n \cdot (x - p))^2}, (n \cdot (x - p))\right).$$

(22)

The term spinmap comes from the cylindrical symmetry of the oriented point basis. Given this basis, the 3D shape of the neighbouring surface points can be reduced to a 2D snapshot of global shape, which is a representation invariant to a rotation about its central axis L. 3D surface point correspondences can then be established on the basis of a *2D correlation* between their respective spin maps. The applicability of the technique to anatomical surfaces is demonstrated with skull and bone data sets. The use of points matched by spinmap correlation to determine the transformation between two surfaces is comparable to feature-point matching, as addressed in Section 4.

Early work on appearance-based techniques mostly deals with face recognition in 2D intensity images, and is based on projecting face images onto a feature space that spans the significant variations among known face images (Turk and Pentland, 1991). Murase and Nayar (1995) apply a similar framework to recognize 3D objects, whose model is stored in a CAD database, from 2D images, as well as estimate the transformation between the two. This in turn is the basis for the eigenshape technique of Campbell and Flynn (1999) for object recognition and pose estimation of range images.

In Murase's application, the basic idea is to take several training views of an object, which rests on a turntable. The object pose is varied by rotating the turntable by an angle θ in increments of a few degrees. Each $N \times N$ image $I(i, j)$ corresponding to a training view is represented as an N^2-vector

$$\hat{x} = [I(1, 1) \cdots I(1, N) I(2, 1) \cdots I(2, N) \cdots I(N, N)]^T,$$

(23)

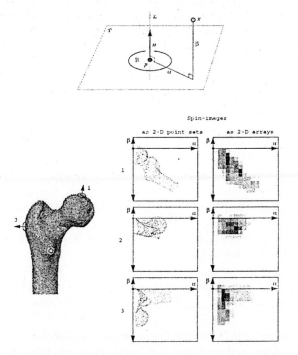

Fig. 5. (a) An illustration spinmap geometry; (b) points distributed on the surface of a femur bone, shown with three point bases and their corresponding spinmaps, appearing as point sets and grey-scale images (courtesy of A.E. Johnson).

obtained by concatenating the rows of the image and taking the transpose. An image is then equivalent to a point in a huge N^2-dimensional space. Fortunately, most of the variation in the images can be accounted for by a subspace spanned by just a few vectors, as in **principal component analysis** (or Karhunen-Loeve expansion) (Fukunaga, 1990). Each vector corresponding to a distinct training view constitutes a column of an *object image set*

$$X_{N^2 \times m} = [\hat{x}_1, \ldots, \hat{x}_m],$$

(24)

where m is the number of training views. A covariance matrix is then defined from the image set:

$$Q_{N^2 \times N^2} = XX^T.$$

(25)

The eigenvectors $[e_1 \cdots e_k]$ corresponding to the k largest eigenvalues are computed (Murase lists three algorithms for doing this efficiently), where $\lambda_i e_i = Q e_i$, comprising a *parametric eigenspace*.

Thereafter, the set of training views projected onto the parametric eigenspace constitutes samples of a *smoothly varying manifold*. If $k = 3$ this manifold is a closed curve whose arclength is a one-to-one function of θ in the 3D space spanned by $[e_1 e_2 e_3]$, which in turn can be fitted with cubic splines. Given a new image, its pose can be estimated by projecting it onto the parametric eigenspace. For example, if $k = 3$, this can be achieved by finding the position of its projection within the cube spanned by $[e_1 e_2 e_3]$) and by finding the closest point on the manifold to this projection. The pose can then be estimated by interpolation along arclength between the two closest discrete poses.

Now, for surface registration (Campbell and Flynn, 1999), we are dealing with more than one pose parameter (i.e. not just θ corresponding to turntable rotation), but the framework is the same (and this could applied to registering an open anatomical surface with a closed surface extracted offline from tomographic data). The steps are (the first three can be implemented offline):

- compute training views of the anatomy at sufficient increments of each pose parameter;
- compute the parametric subspace which captures enough of the shape variation across all poses;
- project back the training views to this subspace to generate a manifold (which may then be smoothed);
- and for a new open surface, project it also onto the parametric subspace and obtain its transformation by interpolating the projections of discrete training poses.

4. Matching, optimization and transformation computation

The third stage comprises the search for corresponding points or feature pairs, based on the surface representation of the second stage, and the computation of the optimal transformation as idealized in the first stage. The search for a match can be either a *succession of comparisons* of discrete candidates, as is frequently the case for feature pairs, or an *iterative minimization* of an objective function, as usually occurs with point- and model-based schemes. The subsequent transformation computation depends on the assumptions made in the first stage. It comprises a closed-form computation or an iterative search for the six or more parameters which best align feature pairs. Alternately, a *Kalman filtering* approach presents advantages to tracking surface points over an extended time sequence, as this estimation of transformation parameters is optimal for the noise characteristics of the whole sequence yet is recursive over time. As for the techniques based on global shape, points whose spinmaps correlate well are used to (over-)determine a transformation in the same manner as discrete feature points (discussed below). The special case of appearance-based matching was fully described in the previous section.

4.1. Discrete feature matching and transformation computation

Feature matching generally determines a rigid transformation, due the relative sparseness of features, and involves a comparison in terms of shape parameters, such as surface curvature values at extrema, curvature and torsion values of curvilinear features, and shape type, averaged properties and size for regions. In the event a particular matching technique does not imbed a transformation computation, most of the rigid-body motion representations reviewed in Section 2.1 lead to a closed-form expression for estimating rotation and translation. Early techniques include **pose clustering** (also known as generalized Hough transform), **sequential hypothesis and test** (also known as prediction and verification and alignment), and **geometric hashing**. We also review the **eigenvector** technique of Shapiro and Brady (1992) for matching point features.

Pose clustering matches like simple or compound structures and derives a transformation from *each* such correspondence. This approach involves quantizing the space of relevant transformations and using it as an accumulator in which each match increments a corresponding cell. A globally acceptable transformation is detected as a cluster in the space of all such candidate transformations (Stockman, 1987).

Sequential hypothesis and test consists of picking a set of feature pairs which are consistent and which determine a transformation, validating these hypothesized matches based on how other features from the two spaces agree with the putative transformation, then possibly backtracking and proceding anew with a new set of consistent feature pairs (Bolles and Horaud, 1986; Chen and Huang, 1988).

Geometric hashing involves precomputing local matching information, which is rotationally and translationally invariant, and storing it in the form of a *hash table*, where each entry is associated with a simple or compound feature to which a local coordinate system (or basis) can be unambiguously assigned, for surface A. Subsequently, a feature or set of features in surface B is similarly characterized. Finally, given the transformation between the two local bases, the consistency of the mapped non-basis features is evaluated, where consistent feature pairs validate this transformation by voting for it (Lamdan and Wolfson, 1988; Kishon et al., 1990).

Shapiro and Brady (1992) match feature points on the basis of consistent same-space distances by an elegant eigenanalysis technique, following the inter-image distance-based matching technique of Scott and Longuet-Higgins (1991). Shapiro suggests accounting for global structure, and proposes that each image or surface be represented by a proximity matrix H of *intra-image* (or intra-surface) distances. The eigenvalues of each matrix are then computed, resulting in a *modal matrix V* whose columns correspond to the eigenvectors of H. Each row of V can be thought of as a feature vector F_i containing the modal coordinates of a feature i. The final stage consists of correlating the two sets of feature vectors $F_{i,A}$ and $F_{j,B}$.

In general, techniques involving some sort of voting or accumulation, such as pose clustering and geometric hashing, are likely to be the most robust, particularly to missing information (such as a partial overlap between different modalities, i.e. registering a sub-patch with a larger surface patch).

4.2. Closest point finding and global optimization

Free-form surface matching involves a closest-point finding stage, which may or may not benefit from some form of preprocessing (k-D trees, distance maps), and frequently a global optimization stage which is used either to compute the best current transformation T_k based on the latest closest-point pairs, or to accelerate the convergence of these fundamentally iterative techniques towards a definitive result.

Classical techniques can be used to implement the minimization of Eq. (13), and generally are of the **unconstrained nonlinear optimization** type (Luenberger, 1984). These approaches are based on the conditions that, for a minimum, the objective function must have a null gradient and a positive semidefinite Hessian matrix. Starting at some initial point, one determines, according to a fixed rule, a direction of movement in the domain, then one moves in that direction to a relative minimum of the objective function along that line. At that point, a new direction is determined and the process is repeated, until some termination condition is met. These techniques include the *method of Steepest Descent, multivariate Newton's, Conjugate-Gradient* and *Quasi-Newton methods*, and related methods (Luenberger, 1984).

These methods are also used, once point-matches are determined, to iteratively *compute optimal transformation parameters*. Lavallée and Szeliski use a Levenberg-Marquardt technique, which is a hybrid of the Steepest Descent and multivariate Newton's Method (Luenberger, 1984), to iteratively compute both rigid (Lavallée and Szeliski, 1995) and non-rigid (Szeliski and Lavallée, 1996) transformations. Besl and McKay's accelerated ICP technique involves a series of line searches in a seven-parameter space spanned by rotation quaternion and translation (Besl and McKay, 1992). The unaccelerated stage finds closest point pairs and uses a quaternion technique to find the current iteration's least-squares registration. Each such iteration is equivalent to a small step in 7-space, and the accelerated stage fits an interpolant in the direction of this step (from the last 7-vector), whereupon the convergence can be improved by a line search for the minimum. Special switching logic determines whether a linear or parabolic interpolant is used.

The **k-D tree** (Zhang, 1994) is a sequence of bisections in a space of k dimensions (here $k=3$). Each successive cut plane passes through a point chosen such that it divides the remaining points into clouds of roughly equal numbers of points, producing a left and a right son. Each son is split into two grandsons by choosing the appropriate plane parallel to $x-z$, followed by a plane parallel to $x-y$, and so on, while alternating the cut plane orientation, until sufficient divisions occur such that no resulting rectangular parallelopiped contains a data point. Such a cut is termed a "leaf". Each node ν of the 3-D tree is characterized by a point $x_{A,i}(\nu)$ through which it passes, and a parameter $t(\nu)$ indicating the orientation of the cut plane. The search for the closest point via a 3-D tree calls a recursive procedure that begins at the root of the 3-D tree assigned to X_A, and exploits the tree structure, branching off into one son or the other depending on the signs of the distance components, to zero-in on the best candidate.

A **distance map** can be precomputed off-line, to determine for each voxel in a volume containing a surface S_B, the closest point on that surface and the distance to it. Thereafter, for a surface S_A falling within this mapped volume, each of its points inherits the closest point precomputed for the voxel on which it falls. In the case of an *octree spline* implementation (Lavallée and Szeliski, 1995), the representation is carried out by a classic octree subdivision (Foley et al., 1990). For each corner vertex of all terminal cubes, the signed distance to its closest point on the surface is computed. The determination of the distance to the closest point on S_B is achieved by interpolation. Alternate techniques for computing the distance map of a surface are by *fast marching level sets* (Sethian, 1996a; Kimmel et al., 1996), where distance is the arrival time of a moving front starting from the initial surface, and by various local mask-based *distance transforms* (Borgefors, 1984, 1986; Paglieroni, 1992).

Alternately, each match pair $\hat{x}_k \equiv (x_{A,k}, x_{B,k})$ can be viewed as a measure $\hat{x}_k$ of a match x_k resulting from the application of the true transformation relating the two surfaces, corrupted by a random error v_k. This leads to an **extended Kalman filtering** (EKF) (Kalman, 1960; Sorenson, 1980) formalism for recursively estimating the optimal (with respect to noise statistics) transformation parameters. The application of EKF to tracking surface points over time is an issue of expressing a relationship between positions or feature vectors of the matched pairs and the transformation parameters as a *measurement equation* that can be linearized, and for which the linear Kalman filter can recursively compute the best transformation estimate. This is the technique used by Feldmar and Ayache (1994c) for estimating the global affine transformation relating matched feature vector pairs. Because it is recursive, it presents advantages for tracking surface points over time. Only the new measurements and the statistics and transformation parameters of the previous iteration need to be considered, in computing the parameters which are optimal for the noise statistics of the whole sequence.

4.3. Model-based motion estimation

The method of estimating motion from surface models depends on the nature of the model. As seen in the discussion of Section 3.3, many physically-based models segment the surface explicitly, but surface motion is often just the difference between consecutive shapes at a given surface coordinate (u, v), particularly when the shape at time t_k is used to initialize the shape estimation at t_{k+1} (Terzopoulos et al., 1988; McInerney and Terzopoulos, 1995). The application of surface evolution models to motion estimation is still in its infancy, but as emphasized by Audette and Peters (1999), this framework can be exploited not only to extract a surface reliably, but also to alleviate an explicit search for matches in a subsequent point-based registration scheme.

Finite element modelling is the most prevalent technique for computing physically based models (Essa et al., 1993; Terzopoulos and Metaxas, 1991). Here, the displacement FEM represents a surface as a mesh of 2D simple polygonal elements whose global behaviour (where a surface reaches equilibrium between internal and external forces) can be characterized by an element-by-element analysis of the dynamics involved. The global mass, damping and stiffness matrices are summations of the corresponding element matrices, as are non-concentrated load matrices. In practice, the integration of expression (18) is simplified by neglecting either mass (Terzopoulos and Metaxas, 1991), leading to the *explicit first-order Euler integration*[5] $U^{(t+\delta t)} = U^{(t)} + \delta t(C^{(t)})^{-1}(R^{(t)} - KU^{(t)})$, or damping, leading to the change of basis to modal coordinates and the expression (19), which can also be integrated numerically.

The Amini surface tracking technique finds closest points in a manner similar to free-form surface registration techniques (Amini and Duncan, 1992). For each point of surface A, the point on surface B that minimizes expression (21) is selected. This ensures that the match is most similar in local surface shape and that its relative movement is nearest to being conformal. The result is a 3D flow field, which may be noisy, defined over the first surface. Thereafter, a *vector smoothing* technique (Horn and Schunck, 1981) is applied to components of each flow vector, and flow estimates are propagated over other regions of the surface.

Other formulations have also been proposed for computing or tracking deformable model points. The change of basis of expression (19) allows Sclaroff and Pentland (1993) to adapt Shapiro's *modal matching* technique to explicitly match FEM surface nodes. Pentland and Horowitz (1991), Metaxas and Terzopoulos (1993) and

Terzopoulos and Szeliski (1992) also apply a *Kalman filter* formalism to estimate 3D motion from a physical model. Cohen (1991) suggests a *finite-differences* based technique for finding the energy-minimizing contour of his balloon model. Moreover, surface evolution models are implemented with a combination of central and *upwind* (Osher and Sethian, 1988; Levesque, 1992) finite-differences (Malladi et al., 1995; Kimmel et al., 1997). For alternative approaches to estimating deformable contours and surfaces, see (Terzopoulos and Szeliski, 1992; McInerney and Terzopoulos, 1996).

5. Conclusion

This paper has presented a survey of surface registration techniques, particularly those which apply to anatomical surfaces, with an emphasis on their mathematical or algorithmic foundations. We chose to represent the process of registration as the succession of three stages: choice of transformation representation, choice of surface representation and similarity criterion, and matching per se and global optimization. According to Section 2, transformations can be categorized as rigid and non-rigid. Several different representations for rigid-body transformations have been surveyed, while non-rigid transformations can be further categorized into global and local polynomial representations, and according to the choice of coordinates (cartesian or otherwise), which is best suited for the problem.

We saw in Section 3 that a feature, point, global shape or model-based approach can be employed to represent a surface for the purpose of registration, and that each has certain advantages. Feature-based and global shape-based techniques can determine an arbitrarily large rigid transformation. A point-based technique is best suited for bringing two surfaces into very close alignment, given a good starting point for the final transformation, particularly if we wish to quantify non-rigid motion, while a model-based approach is advantageous if identifying the surface within a volume must be accomplished prior to registration. Furthermore, we discussed three categories of features: sparse points, curves and regions. We demonstrated that dense point-based techniques vary according to their definition of proximity between points and according to their means of estimating the closest point to a surface. Finally, we pointed out that models for identifying and possibly registering surfaces are either based on physical or surface evolution equations. We identified which techniques compute surface motion implicitly, from the evolution over time of a 3D model, and which explicitly establish correspondences between surface points.

Next, in Section 4 we offered a survey of the main numerical estimation schemes or algorithms for matching features (and points correlated on the basis of spinmaps),

---

[5] Based on virtual time steps which need not related to the time lapse separating two surfaces.

points and model coordinates (matching on the basis of appearance was concluded in the discussion on representation). Features are typically matched by discrete comparisons, in a manner which may imbed the computation of the resulting transformation in the matching process. Since the transformation specified by these matches is usually rigid-body and the robustness of each match is typically very good (due to the discriminating ability of features), the global registration parameters can then be obtained by a closed-form expression. In contrast, matching and registration for point-based techniques are imbedded into a highly iterative process, with the matching characterized either by a classical optimization technique or by a more efficient procedure requiring offline preprocessing, such as a k-D tree or distance map. The registration may also require an optimization or Kalman filtering procedure for finding the best-fitting transformation parameters in the global sense. Lastly, for physical model-based approaches, surface motion computation frequently amounts to identifying the surface over consecutive volumetric scans. This identification is usually implemented with the finite-element model, where a surface at t_1 initializes that at t_2. In contrast, surface evolution models are less prevalent in registration, and typically estimated by finite differences.

In conclusion, the design choices, namely how to model the transformation, whether to use a feature, point, global shape or model-based technique (as well as how to preprocess the data) and how to optimally compute the transformation, are very context-specific. There are instances, e.g. when dealing with rigid tissue, when a rigid-body transformation will suffice, and others, such as tracking soft tissue deformations, where a spline-based non-rigid transformation model is necessary. In between these two poles, there is a whole spectrum of situations where a rigid model may be too constrictive, but an approach based on splines may also be inapplicable, by being underdetermined or inappropriate for a given noise distribution, for example. Likewise, the choice of surface representation is influenced by the size of the transformation (e.g. whether surfaces are already roughly aligned or not), by the smoothness, noise distribution, and mutual overlap of the data, as well as by time constraints. Moreover, establishing correspondences between two sets of primitives is basically an outgrowth of the formalization of the transformation and the choice of primitives, and consequently is also highly related to the situation at hand.

Acknowledgements

The authors wish to thank E.A. Johnson, S. Lavallée, R. Szeliski, L. Brunie, G. Soucy and R.A. Volz, for contributing images and for granting permission to duplicate illustrations for this paper, as well as K. Siddiqi, G. Dudek, S. Zucker and R. Kimmel for stimulating discussion.

References

Abdelmalek, N., 1990. Algebraic error analysis for surface curvatures of 3-D range images obtained by different methods. In: IEEE Proc. ICPR, pp. 529–534.

Alvarez, L., Lions, P.L., Morel, J.-M., 1992. Image selective smoothing and edge detection by nonlinear diffusion. II. SIAM J. Numer. Anal. 29 (3), 845–866.

Amini, A.A., Duncan, J.S., 1992. Differential geometry for characterizing 3D shape change. Proc. SPIE Math. Methods in Med. Imag. 1768, 170–181.

Arun, K.S., Huang, T.S., Blostein, S.D., 1987. Least-squares fitting of two 3-D point sets. IEEE Trans. PAMI 9 (5), 698–700.

Audette, M.A., Peters, T.M., 1999. Level-set surface segmentation and registration for computing intrasurgical deformations. Proc. SPIE 3661 Medical Imaging, to appear.

Ayache, N., 1991. Artificial Vision for Mobile Robots: Stereo Vision and Multisensory Perception. MIT Press, Cambridge, MA.

Bacjsy, R., Kovacic, S., 1989. Multiresolution elastic matching. CVGIP 46, 1–21.

Bajcsy, R., Solina, F., 1987. Three dimensional object representation revisited. In: Proc. IEEE Int. Conf. Comp. Vision. pp. 231–240.

Barr, A.H., 1981. Superquadrics and angle-preserving transformations. IEEE Comp. Graph. Appl. 1, 11–23.

Barr, A.H., 1984. Global and local deformations of solid primitives. Comp. Graph. 18 (3), 21–30.

Bathe, K.-J., 1982. Finite Element Procedures in Engineering Analysis. Prentice-Hall, Englewood Cliffs, NJ.

Besl, P.J., Jain, R.C., 1986. Invariant surface characteristics for 3D object recognition in range images. CVGIP 33, 33–80.

Besl, P.J., McKay, N.D., 1992. A method for registration of 3-D shapes. IEEE Trans. PAMI 14 (2), 239–256.

Bolles, R.C., Horaud, P., 1986. 3DPO: a three-dimensional part orientation system. Int. J. Rob. Res. 5 (3), 3–26.

Bookstein, F.L., 1989. Principal warps: thin-plate splines and the decomposition of deformations. IEEE Trans. PAMI 11 (6), 567–585.

Borgefors, G., 1984. Distance transformations in arbitrary dimensions. CVGIP 27, 321–345.

Borgefors, G., 1986. Distance transformations in digital images. CVGIP 34, 344–371.

Brown, L.G., 1992. A survey of image registration techniques. ACM Comp. Surveys 24 (4), 326–376.

Campbell, R.J., Flynn, P.J., 1999. Eigenshapes for 3D object recognition in range data. In: Proc. IEEE Conf. Computer Vision and Pattern Recognition.

Caselles, V. et al., 1992. A geometric model for active contours in image processing. CEREMADE report no. 9210.

Caselles, V., Kimmel, R., Sapiro, G., 1995. Geodesic active contours. In: IEEE Proc. Int. Conf. Comp. Vision. pp. 694–699.

Caselles, V. et al., 1997. Minimal surfaces: a three dimensional segmentation approach. Numer. Math. 77 (4), 423–451.

Chen, C.W., Huang, T.S., Arrott, M., 1994. Modeling analysis, and visualization of left ventricle shape and motion by hierarchical decomposition. IEEE Trans. PAMI 16 (4), 342–356.

Chen, H.H., Huang, T.S., 1988. Maximal matching of 3-D points for multiple-object motion estimation. Patt. Rec. 21 (2), 75–90.

Chen, Y., Medioni, G., 1991. Object modelling by registration of multiple range images. In: IEEE Proc. Conf. Rob. and Auto, pp. 2724–2729.

Cohen, L.D., 1991. On active contour models and balloons. CVGIP: Image Under. 53 (2), 211–218.

Cohen, L.D., Cohen, I., 1990. A finite element method applied to new active contour models and 3D reconstruction from cross sections. In: IEEE Proc. Int. Conf. Comp. Vision. pp. 587–591.

Cohen, I., Ayache, N., Sulger, P., 1992a. Tracking points on deformable objects using curvature information. INRIA Tech. Report No. 1595.

Cohen, I., Cohen, L.D., Ayache, N., 1992b. Using deformable surfaces to segment 3D images and infer differential structures. CVGIP: Image Under. 56 (2), 242–263.

Coppini, G. Demi, M., d'Urso, G., L'Abbate, A., Valli, G., 1987. Tensor description of 3D time varying surfaces using scattered landmarks: an application to heart motion. In: Cappellini, V. (Ed.), Time-Varying Image Processing and Moving Object Recognition. North-Holland, Amsterdam, pp. 158–163.

Craig, J.J., 1989. Introduction to Robotics: Mechanics and Control. Addison-Wesley, Reading, MA.

Collignon, A., Vandermeulen, D., Suetens, P., Marchal, G., 1993. Surface based registration of 3D medical images. Proc. SPIE 1898: Med. Imag., pp. 32–42.

DeCarlo, D., Metaxas, D., 1996. Blended deformable models. IEEE Trans. PAMI 18 (4), 443–448.

Deriche, R., 1987. Using Canny's criteria to derive a recursively implemented optimal edge detector. Int. J. Comp. Vision 1 (2), 167–187.

Deriche, R., 1990. Fast algorithms for low-level vision. IEEE Trans. PAMI 12 (1), 78–87.

Dierckx, P., 1995. Curve and Surface Fitting with Splines. Clarendon, Oxford.

do Carmo, M.P., 1976. Differential Geometry of Curves and Surfaces. Prentice-Hall, Englewood Cliffs, NJ.

Duchon, J., 1976. Interpolation des fonctions de deux variables suivant le principe de la flexion des plaques minces. R.A.I.R.O Analyse Numérique 10, 5–12.

Essa I., Sclaroff, S., Pentland, A., 1993. Physically based modelling for graphics and vision. In: Martin, R. (Ed.), Directions in Geometric Computing. Information Geometers, Winchester, UK, pp. 161–218.

Evans, A.C., Dai, W., Collins, L., Neelin, P., Marrett, S., 1991. Warping of a computerized 3-D atlas to match brain image volumes for quantitative neuroanatomical and functional analysis. Proc. SPIE 1445 Med. Imag. V: Image Proc., 236–246.

Fan, T.J., Medioni, G., Nevatia, R., 1989. Recognizing 3-D objects using surface descriptions. IEEE Trans. PAMI 11 (11), 1140–1157.

Faugeras, O.D., Hebert, M., 1986. The representation, recognition, and locating of 3-D objects. Int. J. Rob. Res. 5 (3), 27–52.

Feldmar, J., Ayache, N., 1994a. Rigid and affine registration of free-form surfaces, using differential properties. In: Proc. Euro. Conf. Comp. Vision. pp. 397–406.

Feldmar, J., Ayache, N., 1994b. Locally affine registration of free-form surfaces. In: IEEE Proc. Conf. Comp. Vision and Patt. Rec. pp. 496–501.

Feldmar, J., Ayache, N., 1994c. Rigid, affine and locally affine registration of smooth surfaces. INRIA Technical Report No. 2220.

Ferrie, F.P., Mathur, S., Soucy, G., 1993. Feature extraction for 3-D model building and object recognition. In: Jain, A.K., Flynn, P.J. (Eds.), Three-Dimensional Object Recognition Systems. Elsevier, Amsterdam, pp. 57–88.

Flynn, P.J., Jain, A.K., 1989. On reliable curvature estimation. In: IEEE Proc. Conf. Comp. Vision and Patt. Rec. pp. 110–116.

Foley, J.D., van Dam, A., Feiner, S.K., Hughes, J.F., 1990. Computer Graphics – Principles and Practice. Addison-Wesley, Reading, MA.

Fukunaga, K., 1990. Introduction to Statistical Pattern Recognition, 2nd Edition. Academic Press, Boston.

Goldgof, D.B., Lee, H., Huang, T.S., 1988a. Motion analysis of nonrigid surfaces. In: Proc. Conf. Comp. Vision and Patt. Rec. pp. 375–380.

Goldgof, D.B., Lee, H., Huang, T.S., 1988b. Feature extraction and terrain matching. In: Proc. Conf. Comp. Vision and Patt. Rec. pp. 899–904.

Guéziec, A., Ayache, N., 1994. Smoothing and matching of 3-D space curves. Int. J. Comp. Vision 12 (1), 79–104.

Hebert, M., Caillas, C., Krotkov, E., Kweon, I.S., Kanade, T., 1989. Terrain mapping for a roving planetary explorer. IEEE Proc. Int. Conf. Rob. and Auto. pp. 997–1002.

Henri, C.J., Collins, D.L., Peters, T.M., 1991. Multimodality image integration for stereotactic surgical planning. Med. Phys. 18 (2), 167–177.

Herman, G.T., Liu, H.K., 1979. Three-dimensional display of human organs from computed tomograms. Comp. Graph. and Image Proc. 9 (1), 1–21.

Horn, B.K.P., 1987. Closed-form solution of absolute orientation using unit quaternions. J. Opt. Soc. Am. A 4 (4), 629–642.

Horn, B.K.P., Schunck, B.G., 1981. Determining optical flow. Art. Intel. 17, 185–203.

Huang, T.S., Blostein, S.D., Margerum, E.A., 1986. Least-squares estimation of motion parameters from 3-D point correspondences. In: IEEE Proc. Conf. Comp. Vision and Patt. Rec. pp. 198–201.

Jacq, J.J., Roux, C., 1993. Automatic registration of 3D images using a simple genetic algorithm with a stochastic performance function. In: IEEE Proc. Eng. Med. and Biol. Soc. pp. 126–127.

Johnson, A.E., Hebert, M., 1998. Surface matching for object recognition in complex three-dimensional scenes. Image and Vision Computing 16, 635–651.

Kalman, R.E., 1960. A new approach to linear filtering and prediction problems. Trans. AMSE J. Basic Eng. 820, 35–45.

Kamgar-Parsi, B., Jones, J.L., Rosenfeld, A., 1991. Registration of multiple overlapping range images: scenes without distinctive features. IEEE Trans. PAMI 13 (9), 857–871.

Kass, M., Witkin, A., Terzopoulos, D., 1987. Snakes: active contour models. Int. J. Comp. Vision 1 (4), 321–331.

Kehtarnavaz, N., Mohan, S., 1989. A framework for estimation of motion parameters from range images. CVGIP 45, 88–105.

Kichenassamy, S., Kumar, A., Olver, P., Tonnenbaum, A., Yezzi, A., 1995. Gradient flows and geometric active contour models. In: Proc. IEEE Int. Conf. Comp. Vision. pp. 810–815.

Kikinis, R., Gleason, P.L., Lorensen, W., Wells, W., Grimson, W.E.L., Lozanc-Perez, T., Ettinger, G., White, S., Jolesz, F., 1994. Image guidance techniques for neurosurgery. In: Proc. SPIE 2359: Visualization in Biomedical Computing. pp. 537–540.

Kimia, B.B., Siddiqi, K., 1996. Geometric heat equation and nonlinear diffusion of shapes and images. Computer Vision Image Understanding 64 (3), 305–322.

Kimmel, R., Kiryati, N., Bruckstein, A.M., 1996. Distance maps and weighted distance transforms. J. Math. Imag. Vision 6, 223–233.

Kimmel, R., Kiryati, N., Bruckstein, A.M., 1997. Analyzing and synthesizing images by evolving curves with the Osher-Sethian method. Int. J. Comp. Vision 24 (1), 37–56.

Kishon, E., Hastie, T., Wolfson, H., 1990. 3-D curve matching using splines. In: Proc. Euro. Conf. Comp. Vision. pp. 589–591.

Lamdan, Y., Wolfson, H.J., 1988. Geometric hashing: a general and efficient model-based recognition scheme. In: IEEE Proc. Int. Conf. Comp. Vision. pp. 238–249.

Lavallée, S., 1996. Registration for computer-integrated surgery: methodology, state of the art. In: Taylor, R.H., Lavallee, S., Burdea, G.C., Mosges, R. (Eds.), Computer-Integrated Surgery – Technology and Clinical Applications. MIT Press, Cambridge, MA, pp. 77–97.

Lavallée, S., Szeliski, R., 1995. Recovering the position and orientation of free-form objects from image contours using 3D distance maps. IEEE Trans. PAMI 17 (4), 378–390.

Lavallée, S., Szeliski, R., Brunie, L., 1996. Anatomy-based registration of three-dimensional medical images, range images, X-ray projections, and three-dimensional models using octree-splines. In: Taylor, R.H., Lavallee, S., Burdea, G.C., Mosges, R. (Eds.), Computer-Integrated Surgery – Technology and Clinical Applications. MIT Press, Cambridge, MA, pp. 115–143.

Levesque, R.J., 1992. Numerical Methods for Conservation Laws, 2nd Edition. Birkhäuser Verlag, Basel.

Lin, Z.C., Lee, H., Huang, T.S., 1986. A frequency-domain algorithm for determining motion of a rigid object from range data without correspondences. In: IEEE Proc. Conf. Comp. Vision and Patt. Rec., pp. 194–198.

Luenberger, D.G., 1984. Linear and Nonlinear Programming, 2nd Edition. Addison-Wesley, Reading, MA.

Maintz, J.B.A., Viergever, M.A., 1998. A survey of medical image registration. Med. Image Anal. 2 (1), 1–36.

Maintz, J.B.A., van den Elsen, P.A., Viergever, M.A., 1996. Evaluation of ridge seeking operators for multimodality medical image matching. IEEE Trans. PAMI 18 (4), 353–365.

Malladi, R., Sethian, J.A., 1998. A real-time algorithm for medical shape recovery. In: Proc. IEEE Int. Conf. Comp. Vision. pp. 304–310.

Malladi, R., Sethian, J.A., Vemuri, B.C., 1995. Shape modeling with front propagation: a level set approach. IEEE Trans. PAMI 17 (2), 158–175.

Malvern, L.E., 1969. Introduction to the Mechanics of a Continuous Medium. Prentice-Hall, Englewood Cliffs, NJ.

McInerney, T., Terzopoulos, D., 1995. A dynamic finite element surface model for segmentation and tracking in multidimensional medical images with application to cardiac 4D image analysis. J. Comp. Med. Imag. and Graph. 19 (1), 69–83.

McInerney, T., Terzopoulos, D., 1996. Deformable models in medical image analysis: a survey. Med. Image Anal. 1 (2), 91–108.

Metaxas, D., Kakadiaris, I.A., 1996. Elastically adaptive deformable models. In: Proc. Euro. Conf. Comp. Vision. pp. 550–559.

Metaxas, D., Terzopoulos, D., 1993. Shape and nonrigid motion estimation through physics-based synthesis. IEEE Trans. PAMI 15 (6), 580–591.

Mishra, S.K., Goldgof, D.B., Huang, T.S., 1991. Motion analysis and epicardial deformation estimation from angiography data. In: IEEE Proc. Conf. Comp. Vision and Patt. Rec. pp. 331–336.

Monga, O., Benayoun, S., 1995. Using partial derivatives of 3D images to extract typical surface features. Comp. Vision and Image Under. 61 (2), 171–189.

Monga, O., Deriche, R., Rocchisiani, J.-M., 1991. 3D edge detection using recursive filtering: application to scanner images. CVGIP: Image Under. 53 (1), 76–87.

Monga, O., Benayoun, S., Faugeras, O.D., 1992. From partial derivatives of 3D density images to ridge lines. In: IEEE Proc. Conf. Comp. Vision and Patt. Rec. pp. 354–359.

Murase, H., Nayar, S.K., 1995. Visual learning and recognition of 3-D objects from appearance. Int. J. Computer Vision 14, 5–24.

Nastar, C., Ayache, N., 1993. Fast segmentation, tracking, and analysis of deformable objects. In: IEEE Proc. Int. Conf. Comp. Vision. pp. 275–279.

Osher, S., Sethian, J.A., 1988. Fronts propagating with curvature-dependent speed: algorithms based on Hamilton-Jacobi formulations. J. Comp. Phys. 79, 12–49.

Paglieroni, D.W., 1992. Distance transforms: properties and machine vision applications. CVGIP: Graph. Models and Image Proc. 54 (1), 56–74.

Pelizzari, C.A. et al., 1989. Accurate three-dimensional registration of CT, PET, and/or MR images of the brain. J. Comp. Ass. Tomog. 13 (1), 20–26.

Pentland, A., Horowitz, B., 1991. Recovery of nonrigid motion and structure. IEEE Trans. PAMI 13 (7), 730–742.

Pentland, A., Sclaroff, S., 1993. Closed-form solutions for physically based shape modelling and recognition. IEEE Trans. PAMI 13 (7), 715–729.

Perona, P., Malik, J., 1990. Scale-space and edge detection using anisotropic diffusion. IEEE Trans. PAMI 12 (7), 629–639.

Press, W.H., Chui, H., Mjolsness, E., Pappin, S., Daviachi, L., Goldman-Rakic, P., Duncan, J., 1992. Numerical Recipes in C: The Art of Scientific Computing, 2nd Edition. Cambridge University Press, Cambridge.

Proakis, J.G., 1996. Digital Signal Processing: Principles, Algorithms, and Applications. Prentice Hall, Upper Saddle River, NJ.

Radack, G.M., Badler, N.I., 1989. Local matching of surfaces using a boundary-centered radial decomposition. CVGIP 45, 380–396.

Radig, B., 1984. Image sequence analysis using relational structures. Patt. Rec. 17 (1), 161–167.

Rangarajan, Flannery, B.P., Teukolsky, S.A., Vetterling, W.T., 1997. A robust point-matching algorithm for autoradiograph alignment. Medical Image Analysis 1(4), 379–398.

Roth, G., Levine, M.D., 1993. Extracting geometric primitives. CVGIP: Image Understanding 48 (1), 1–22.

Sander, P.T., Zucker, S.W., 1990. Inferring surface trace and differential structure from 3-D images. IEEE Trans. PAMI 12 (9), 833–854.

Sclaroff, S., Pentland, A., 1993. Modal matching for correspondence and recognition. M.I.T. Media Lab. Perceptual Computing Section Tech. Rep. No. 201.

Scott, G.L., Longuet-Higgins, H.C., 1991. An algorithm for associating the features of two images. Proc. Royal Soc. London B 244, 21–26.

Sethian, J.A., 1996a. A fast marching level set method for monotonically advancing fronts. Proc. Natl. Acad. Sci. USA 93, 1591–1595.

Sethian, J.A., 1996b. A review of the theory, algorithms, and applications of level set methods for propagating interfaces. Acta Numerica 5, 309–395.

Shapiro, L.S., Brady, J.M., 1992. Feature-based correspondence: an eigenvector approach. Image Vision Comput. 10 (5), 283–288.

Shen, J., Castan, S., 1986. An optimal linear operator for edge detection. In: IEEE Proc. Conf. Comp. Vision and Patt. Rec. pp. 109–114.

Simon, D.A., Hebert, M., Kanade, T., 1994a. Real-time 3-D pose estimation using a high-speed range sensor. In: Proc. IEEE Int. Conf. Rob. and Auto. pp. 2235–2241.

Simon, D.A., Hebert, M., Kanade, T., 1994b. Techniques for fast and accurate intra-surgical registration. In: Proc. Int. Symp. Med. Rob. and Comp. Assis. Surg. pp. 90–97.

Sorenson, H.W., 1980. Parameter Estimation: Principles and Problems. Marcel Dekker, New York.

Soucy, G., Ferrie, F.P., 1997. Surface recovery from range images using curvature and motion consistency. Comp. Vision and Image Under. 65 (1), 1–18.

Stockman, G., 1987. Object recognition and localization via pose clustering. CVGIP 40, 361–387.

Subsol, G., Thirion, J.Ph., Ayache, N., 1994. Non rigid registration for building 3D anatomical atlases. In: IEEE Proc. IEEE Int. Conf. Patt. Rec. pp. 576–578.

Szeliski, R., Lavallée, S., 1996. Matching 3-D anatomical surfaces with non-rigid deformations using octree-splines. Int. J. Comp. Vision 18 (2), 171–186.

Terzopoulos, D., Metaxas, D., 1991. Dynamic 3D models with local and global deformations: deformable superquadrics. IEEE Trans. PAMI 13 (7), 703–714.

Terzopoulos, D., Szeliski, R., 1992. Tracking with Kalman snakes. In: Blake, A., Yuille, A. (Eds.), Active Vision. MIT Press, Cambridge, MA, pp. 3–20.

Terzopoulos, D., Witkin, A., Kass, M., 1988. Constraints on deformable models: recovering 3D shape and nonrigid motion. Artificial Intelligence 36, 91–123.

Thirion, J.-Ph., 1994. Extremal points: definition and application for 3D image registration. In: IEEE Proc. Conf. Comp. Vision and Patt. Rec. pp. 587–592.

Toriwaki, F.I., Yokoi, S., 1988. Voronoi and related neighbors on digitized two-dimensional space with applications to texture analysis. In: Toussaint, G.T. (Ed.), Computational Morphology. North-Holland, Amsterdam.

Turk, M., Pentland, A., 1991. Eigenfaces for recognition. J. Cognitive Neuroscience 3 (1), 71–86.

Udupa, J.K., 1982. Interactive segmentation and boundary surface formation for 3-D digital images. Comp. Graph. and Image Proc. 18 (3), 213–235.

Unser, M., Aldroubi, A., Eden, M., 1993a. B-spline signal processing: Part I – theory. IEEE Trans. Signal Proc. 41 (2), 821–833.

Unser, M., Aldroubi, A., Eden, M., 1993b. B-spline signal processing: Part II – efficient design and applications. IEEE Trans. Signal Proc. 41 (2), 834–848.

Walker, M.W., Shao, L., Volz, R.A., 1991. Estimating 3-D location parameters using dual number quaternions. CVGIP: Image Understanding 54 (3), 358–367.

Zhang, Z., 1994. Iterative point matching for registration of free-form curves and surfaces. Int. J. Comp. Vision 13 (2), 119–152.

Planning and Simulation of Neurosurgery in a Virtual Reality Environment

Ralf A. Kockro, M.D., Luis Serra, Ph.D.,
Yeo Tseng-Tsai, M.D., Chumpon Chan, M.D.,
Sitoh Yih-Yian, M.D., Chua Gim-Guan, B.Sc.,
Eugene Lee, B.Sc., Lee Yen Hoe, M.Sc.,
Ng Hern, M.Sc., Wieslaw L. Nowinski, D.Sc., Ph.D.

Biomedical Laboratory (RAK, LS, CG-G, EL, LYH, NH, WLN), Kent Ridge
Digital Laboratories; Departments of Neurosurgery (RAK, YT-T) and Radiology (SY-Y),
National Neuroscience Institute; and Department of Neurosurgery (CC),
Singapore General Hospital, Singapore

OBJECTIVE: To report our experience with preoperative neurosurgical planning in our stereoscopic virtual reality environment for 21 patients with intra- and extra-axial brain tumors and vascular malformations.

METHODS: A neurosurgical planning system called VIVIAN (*V*irtual *I*ntracranial *Vi*sualization and *N*avigation) was developed for the Dextroscope, a virtual reality environment in which the operator reaches with both hands behind a mirror into a computer-generated stereoscopic three-dimensional (3-D) object and moves and manipulates the object in real time with natural 3-D hand movements. Patient-specific data sets from multiple imaging techniques (magnetic resonance imaging, magnetic resonance angiography, magnetic resonance venography, and computed tomography) were coregistered, fused, and displayed as a stereoscopic 3-D object. A suite of 3-D tools accessible inside the VIVIAN workspace enabled users to coregister data, perform segmentation, obtain measurements, and simulate intraoperative viewpoints and the removal of bone and soft tissue.

RESULTS: VIVIAN was used to plan neurosurgical procedures primarily in difficult-to-access areas, such as the cranial base and the deep brain. The intraoperative and virtual reality 3-D scenarios correlated well. The VIVIAN system substantially contributed to surgical planning by 1) providing a quick and better understanding of intracranial anatomic and abnormal spatial relationships, 2) simulating the craniotomy and the required cranial base bone work, and 3) simulating intraoperative views.

CONCLUSION: The VIVIAN system allows users to work with complex imaging data in a fast, comprehensive, and intuitive manner. The 3-D interaction of this virtual reality environment is essential to the efficient assembly of surgically relevant spatial information from the data derived from multiple imaging techniques. The usefulness of the system is highly dependent on the accurate coregistration of the data and the real-time speed of the interaction. (Neurosurgery 46:118–137, 2000)

Key words: Brain imaging, Cranial base surgery, Neurosurgical planning, Neurosurgical simulation, Skull base surgery, Three-dimensional reconstruction, Virtual reality

A neurosurgical procedure is a planned intervention in a highly complex three-dimensional (3-D) space. A comprehensive understanding of the spatial relationships between intracranial anatomy and pathological features is therefore imperative for successful neurosurgical planning. Such planning usually relies on the study of data generated from preoperative radiological examinations, such as magnetic resonance imaging (MRI), computed tomography, digi-

tal x-ray angiography, and, increasingly, magnetic resonance angiography (MRA) or computed tomographic (CT) angiography. With the exception of MRA and CT angiography, this information is represented in two-dimensional (2-D) imaging series, each technique providing detailed information about different structures. To plan a surgical approach, the neurosurgeon has to mentally integrate this variety of information into a 3-D concept. The difficulty of this mental transforma-

---

The original paper contained coloured figures.

---

tion increases with the complexity of spatial relationships of intracranial structures and is additionally complicated by the fact that the imaging series vary in slice thickness, scale, and patient orientation.

Several research groups have introduced the use of computers to assist the surgeon with these tasks by providing 3-D reconstructions of the imaging data. 3-D neurosurgical planning started in the early 1980s, when computer technology was sufficiently developed to allow acceptable rendering of graphics. Although pioneering attempts faced long processing times and were restricted to CT data, they were found to be useful in enhancing the surgeons' 3-D perception. The 3-D reconstructions were presented as static screen photographs from different angles (3, 5, 26, 49, 51).

Since the late 1980s, MRI data have been included in 3-D neurosurgical planning systems, and several techniques for data segmentation (6, 7, 9, 22, 24, 27, 31) and data coregistration (17, 18, 28, 30, 36, 48, 53) have been described. Computed tomography-based 3-D reconstructions have been successfully used to plan craniofacial surgery (29, 35, 50, 52), and the 3-D renderings of data from MRA and CT angiography have become increasingly valuable in planning vascular neurosurgery (13–15, 20, 32).

Several groups have evaluated the usefulness of a variety of neurosurgical planning programs that combine on-line interaction with 3-D imaging data to varying degrees (10, 21, 23, 32, 55). However, common to all these planning systems is the fact that interaction with the increasingly sophisticated 3-D data sets is still achieved in a rather nonintuitive, 2-D, fashion; that is, by moving a screen-bound cursor with a mouse. We believe that the three-dimensionality of a neurosurgical procedure should be reflected during the planning. Therefore, the ideal neurosurgical planning environment should present a 3-D computer-generated reconstruction of the imaging data in a 3-D space and allow interaction in a natural, easy, and direct manner. The system should allow the physician to work directly in 3-D; in particular, to specify distances between points that do not necessarily lie on the same plane, to simulate intraoperative viewpoints, and to specify the extent of tissue removal and bone work needed.

We have developed a neurosurgical planning system called VIVIAN (*Virtual Intracranial Visualization and Navigation*) that integrates the information derived from different imaging techniques and accommodates the intrinsic three-dimensionality of the resulting data set. It is based on the Dextroscope (formerly the Virtual Workbench), a virtual reality environment for fine and precise 3-D interaction previously developed by our group (37, 38, 42, 44, 45). This system enables the physician to interact directly with complex computer-generated 3-D graphics by reaching into them in a manner resembling the way one interacts with real objects. Patient-specific CT and MRI data can be coregistered and displayed as a single 3-D object. The system allows real-time manipulation of the multitechnique 3-D data and provides a suite of segmentation and planning tools, including tools for simulating bone drilling (CT data) and soft tissue removal (MRI data). The VIVIAN system was used to plan neurosurgical procedures in areas in which the spatial relationships between anatomic and abnormal structures are most complex: the cranial base, the deep brain, and the central cortex. This article describes our experiences with VIVIAN in preoperative neurosurgical planning for 21 patients and evaluates the clinical usefulness of this system.

PATIENTS AND METHODS

Patient series

From September 1997 to March 1999, we used the VIVIAN system to carry out preoperative surgical planning for 21 patients with complex neurosurgical anatomy. The clinical data for these patients (10 males and 11 females, ranging in age from 11 to 66 years) are summarized in *Table 1*. The clinical diagnoses included 10 meningiomas (in the region of the olfactory groove, the sphenoidal and the petroclival ridge, the sphenoid planum, the tentorium, and the cerebellopontine angle), three large vestibular schwannomas, two arteriovenous malformations, one cavernous angioma, one high-grade and one low-grade glioma, one intraorbital granulomatous lesion, one jugular foramen schwannoma, and one large clival chordoma.

Data acquisition

MRI studies were acquired on a Siemens Expert 1.0-T unit (Patients 1–3, 5, 7) (Siemens, Stuttgart, Germany), a Siemens Vision 1.5-T unit (Patients 4, 8, 11, 17, 18), or a General Electric Signa 1.5-T unit (Patients 6, 9, 10, 12–16, 19–21) (General Electric Medical Systems, Milwaukee, WI). First, MRA was performed in a 3-D time-of-flight mode with the following imaging parameters: for the General Electric unit, TR = 36 ms, TE = 6.9 ms, flip angle = 25 degrees, field of view (FOV) = 24 cm, matrix = 512 × 512, and slice thickness = 1.2 mm with a 0.6-mm overlap; for the Siemens unit, TR = 30 ms, TE = 6.4 ms, flip angle = 20 degrees, FOV = 24 cm, matrix = 512 × 512, and slice thickness = 2 mm with a 1-mm overlap. Subsequent contrast-enhanced MRI studies were obtained as a 3-D fast gradient-recalled-echo sequence covering the whole brain (for the General Electric unit: TR = 10 ms, TE = 2 ms, flip angle = 15 degrees, FOV = 24 cm, matrix = 256 × 256, and slice thickness = 2 mm; for the Siemens unit, a T1-weighted magnetization-prepared rapid gradient-echo sequence was used: TR = 9.7 ms, TE = 4 ms, flip angle = 12 degrees, FOV = 24 cm, matrix = 256 × 256, and slice thickness = 2 mm).

In selected patients (Patients 5, 13, 15, 16, 18–21), magnetic resonance venography (MRV) was performed subsequently in time-of-flight mode (for the General Electric unit: TR = 37 ms, TE = 6.9 ms, flip angle = 60 degrees, FOV = 24 cm,

TABLE 1. Patient Series[a]

Patient No.	Age (yr)/Sex	Diagnosis	Scanning Technique[b]	Spatial Information Gained in Planning Session[c]	Surgical Approach
1	51/F	Vestibular schwannoma	MRI, MRA	Relationship to brainstem, basilar artery, PICA, AICA, and Cranial Nerve V	Suboccipital
2	46/F	Right medial temporo-occipital low-grade glioma	MRI, MRA	Relationship to PCA, cerebral peduncle, basal ganglia; simulation of transtemporal and occipital supratentorial approach	Transtemporal
3	47/F	Large tuberculum meningioma	MRI, MRA	Relationship to A1, A2, Acom, and optic nerve	Pterional
4	66/M	Petroclival meningioma	MRI, MRA, CT	Relationship to PCA, basilar artery, and brainstem; simulation of suboccipital, petrosal, and subtemporal approach	Suboccipital and subtemporal (two sessions)
5	47/F	Intra- and extra-cranial jugular schwannoma	MRI, MRA, MRV, CT	Relationship to vertebral artery, sigmoid sinus, internal jugular vein, ICA, and PICA; simulation of retrosigmoid craniotomy and transmastoid approach with transposition of the facial nerve	Combined suboccipital and transmastoid
6	53/M	Large olfactory groove meningioma	MRI, MRA, CT	Relationship to ACA and trifurcated A2 (one encased, two splayed over the tumor, bony spur from cribriform plate indenting the tumor)	Subfrontal
7	49/F	Medial sphenoidal ridge meningioma	MRI, MRA, CT	Relationship to ICA, A1, and MCA (encased by tumor), simulation of sphenoid bone work	Pterional
8	64/M	Frontotemporoparietal astrocytoma	MRI, MRA	Comprehension of tumor extension; relationship to MCA and ACA	Transcortical
9	44/M	Giant medial sphenoidal ridge meningioma	MRI, MRA, CT	Relationship to ACA, MCA, (stretched over the tumor) and optic nerves; simulation of sphenoid bone work	Pterional
10	52/F	Vestibular schwannoma	MRI, MRA, CT	Relationship to vertebral artery and brainstem; simulation of translabyrinthine bone work	Translabyrinthine
11	11/M	Intra/retro-orbital granulomatous lesion	MRI, MRA, CT	Spatial intra- and retro-orbital extension, relationship to ophthalmic artery and optic nerve	Fronto-orbital
12	60/M	Large vestibular schwannoma	MRI, MRA, CT	Relationship to vertebral artery, tentorium, and brainstem; simulation of bone drilling of internal auditory canal	Suboccipital
13	61/F	Giant occipital meningioma	MRI, MRA, MRV	Site of craniotomy, relationship to transverse and sagittal sinuses and PCA	Occipital
14	35/M	Left-sided precentral, subcortical AVM	MRI, MRA	Relationship to brain surface; site and size of craniotomy	Transcortical
15	45/F	Large pineal region meningioma	MRI, MRA, MRV	Relationship to deep cerebral veins, PCA, superior cerebellar artery, tentorium, falx cerebri, brainstem, temporal and occipital cortices	Combined supra- and infratentorial
16	46/F	Right-sided parietal, subcortical AVM	MRI, MRA, MRV	Relationship to gyri and sulci of the brain surface	Transcortical

TABLE 1. (*Continued*)

Patient No.	Age (yr)/Sex	Diagnosis	Scanning Technique[b]	Spatial Information Gained in Planning Session[c]	Surgical Approach
17	28/M	Clival/midfacial chordoma	MRI, MRA, CT	Relationship to maxilla, sphenoid bone, petrous bone, clivus, right and left ICA, basilar artery, right Cranial Nerve V, and optic nerves	Transmaxillar
18	55/F	CP angle meningioma	MRI, MRA, CT, MRV	Relationship to sigmoid sinus, basilar artery, internal auditory canal, and jugular bulb	Suboccipital
19	52/M	Large septal cavernous angioma	MRI, MRA, MRV	Relationship to the fornices, ventricles, and internal cerebral veins	Transcallosal, transventricular
20	48/F	Petroclival meningioma	MRI, MRA, MRV, CT	Relationship to basilar artery, right and left PCA, and tentorium; simulation of retrosigmoid, petrosal, and subtemporal approach	Combined petrosal, retrosigmoid, and subtemporal
21	56/M	Large trigonal intraventricular meningioma	MRI, MRA, MRV	Relationship to tentorium, basal ganglia, PCA, and deep cerebral veins	Two stages: transparietal and transcallosal

[a] A1 and A2, anterior cerebral artery parts 1 and 2, respectively; ACA, anterior cerebral artery; Acom, anterior communicating artery; AICA, anteroinferior cerebellar artery; AVM, arteriovenous malformation; CP, cerebellopontine; CT, computed tomography; ICA, internal carotid artery; MCA, middle cerebral artery; MRI, magnetic resonance imaging; MRA, magnetic resonance angiography; MRV, magnetic resonance venography; PCA, posterior cerebral artery; PICA, posteroinferior cerebellar artery.

[b] Coregistered and fused scanning techniques used for three-dimensional reconstruction.

[c] As compared with the planning done with separate, conventional two-dimensional imaging series.

matrix = 512 × 512, and slice thickness = 2 mm; for the Siemens unit: TR = 27 ms, TE = 9 ms, flip angle = 50 degrees, FOV = 25 cm, matrix = 512 × 512, and slice thickness = 2 mm). The patient's head was fixed firmly throughout the imaging procedure.

If an additional CT study was required, 8 to 10 skin fiducial markers serving as landmarks for data fusion were attached to the patient's head before the scanning sessions and remained attached during the MRI and CT examinations. The CT data were obtained as axial, contiguous 1.5-mm slices (FOV = 24 cm, matrix = 256 × 256) on a GE scanner (Patients 4, 5, 7, 11, 17, 18) or a Picker 2000 scanner (Picker, Cleveland, OH) (Patients 6, 9, 10, 12, 20).

The scanning of the patients was scheduled 1 to 3 days before surgery, and the imaging data were transferred by Ethernet to the Dextroscope installed at the hospital or via optical disks and digital audiotapes to the Dextroscope at Kent Ridge Digital Laboratories.

The Dextroscope

Set-up

In the Dextroscope, a computer-generated stereoscopic image is displayed on a monitor (1024 × 768 pixels) and reflected via a mirror into the user's eyes (*Fig. 1A*). The monitor and the mirror are carried by a table-mounted plastic frame, and the user works from a seated position, with forearms positioned on comfortable armrests (*Fig. 1B*). Wearing liquid

crystal display shutter glasses (Crystal Eyes, Stereographics, Inc., San Rafael, CA), which are synchronized with the time-split display, the user looks into the mirror and sees a stereoscopic virtual image that seems to float behind the mirror.

The user reaches with both hands behind the mirror into the floating 3-D image (*Fig. 1C*). Electromagnetic sensors (FasTrack; Polhemus, Inc., Colchester, VT) on both hands convey the interaction to the computer. In one hand (typically the left), the user holds an ergonomically shaped handle with a switch. When the switch is pressed with the forefinger, the 3-D image can be moved freely as if it were an object held in real space (*Fig. 2*). When the switch is released, the spatial position of the 3-D image freezes. The other hand holds a pen-shaped sensor (stylus) with a switch, which appears as a computer-generated virtual instrument inside the virtual reality workspace and can be used to perform detailed manipulations. The position of the virtual instrument and the stylus in the user's hand is calibrated so that the user perceives them to be in the same spatial position and orientation (*Figs. 1C and 2*).

The VIVIAN virtual interface

Neither the mouse nor the keyboard is used. The 3-D reconstruction of the imaging data seems to float above a computer-generated virtual toolrack consisting of sliders and buttons (*Figs. 2D and 3*). The virtual toolrack automatically appears when the stylus in the user's hand touches the bottom of the workspace inside the Dextroscope (*Fig. 2, C and D*). In all interactions with the 3-D virtual structures, the approach is

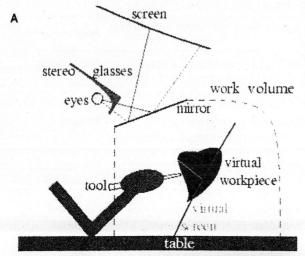

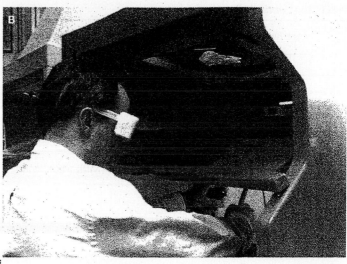

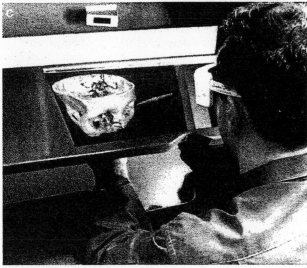

FIGURE 1. The set-up of the Dextroscope. *A,* the stereoscopic image on the monitor screen is reflected by a mirror. The user, looking into the mirror and wearing liquid crystal display shutter glasses, perceives the image as a virtual 3-D structure behind the mirror and reaches into it with his hands. *B,* photograph taken during interaction with the Dextroscope. The user holds electromagnetically tracked devices in his hands. The ergonomically shaped device in the left hand controls the object movements, and the stylus in the right hand interacts with the 3-D object and the virtual 3-D interface. *C,* a semitransparent mirror illustrates the user's perception of the 3-D data. The stylus in the user's hand appears as a virtual stylus (in *blue*) inside the virtual workspace. The spatial positions of the real and the virtual stylus seem to be identical.

to reach for the object of interest and press the switch on the stylus to interact with it. When the tip of the virtual instrument enters into the volume of an object, the object signals by discrete color change that it is ready to be manipulated.

By depressing labeled buttons on a virtual toolrack menu at the bottom of the workspace, tools for data fusion, segmentation, and surgical planning can be activated. By operating sliders, the user can scale the whole head ensemble or adjust the image resolution. A list of all available objects (scanning data and their subsegments) is overlaid on the display at the top-left corner, providing feedback on the status of the objects (i.e., visible or hidden, active or inactive for interaction).

Data loading

As the data become available in digital form from the various scanners, they are converted into stacks of images in red-green-blue format. These tomographic images are then accessed and presented through a 2-D interface for optional processing (e.g., deleting defective or dispensable slices, cropping, or adjusting resolution, contrast, and brightness) and stored as studies (CT scans, MRI studies, etc.). Finally, the

virtual reality image is built by means of a Virtual Reality Modeling Language 2.0 format file, generated automatically from the available studies.

3-D rendering

3-D rendering is achieved by a technique known as direct volume rendering. In this method, rays are traced from the viewer's eye through the screen pixels onto the data (the volume), and the contribution from each volume element (voxel) is composed to produce the final image. Simultaneously, polygonal iso-surfaces can be displayed.

Data coregistration and fusion

Because MRI, MRA, and MRV data sets originate from the same scanning session with identical FOV and spatial slice orientation, automatic coregistration and fusion is possible. Shifts caused by patient movement during the scanning procedure can be corrected by using a set of tools that allow direct transformations on an object, such as translation, scaling, and rotation. To coregister CT and MRI data, a tool based on an *n*-point alignment was developed. The algorithm re-

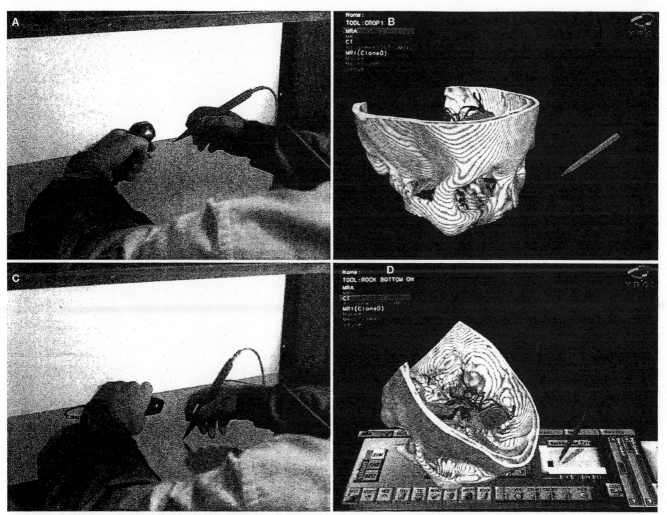

FIGURE 2. 3-D interaction with the 3-D image. *Panels B* and *D* are screen shots reflecting the user's view into the virtual workspace. The positions of the hands in *Panel A* correspond with the positions of the 3-D objects in *Panel B,* and the position of the hands in *Panel C* correspond with the position of the 3-D objects in *Panel D.* The stylus in the user's hand is reflected as a computer-generated virtual stylus in the 3-D workspace (*blue* in *Panel B* and *red-blue* in *Panel D*). Movement of the left hand (*Panel C*) results in a corresponding movement of the 3-D imaging data (*Panel D*). By touching the bottom of the Dextroscope with the stylus in the right hand (*Panel C*), the virtual toolrack appears (*Panel D*). It contains computer-generated buttons and sliders, which can be operated with the virtual stylus. Tools for visualization, image coregistration, segmentation, measurement, and simulation can be activated.

quires at least four corresponding landmarks from source and destination objects. Least-squares error minimization estimates the transformation (scaling/rotation matrix, and translation vector), which relates corresponding voxels of the separate volumes. The VIVIAN system allows manual specification of landmarks directly against the volume. Landmarks can be either skin fiducials attached to the patient before imaging or anatomic structures visible in both data sets (17). To compensate for MRI-inherited distortions (2), the MRI data sets are coregistered with the dimensions of the CT data sets as the reference.

We have recently implemented a fast and automatic image registration algorithm (54) that is based on the integration of mutual image information (49). The CT and MRI studies of Patient 20 in our series were successfully coregistered using

this method. The actual image fusion of the coregistered volumetric data sets was achieved by capitalizing on the multi-sampling mask option available in Silicon Graphics workstations (Silicon Graphics, Mountain View, CA).

Segmentation

Structures that are demarcated clearly by their outstanding intensity on the gray scale (like contrast-enhancing meningiomas) are segmented by semiautomatic adaptation of the color-adjustment table (*Fig. 3*). When a significant gray-scale threshold is not detectable, an outlining tool is used to define the extent of a lesion manually. In this interface, the lines are drawn on the MRI planes inside the virtual environment of

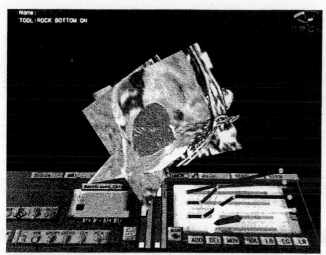

FIGURE 3. Segmentation with the 3-D color-adjustment table. The meningioma (in *green*) in the 3-D MRI reconstruction is interactively segmented by using the color-adjustment table. With the virtual pen (in *red-blue*), the user can interact with the graph, controlling transparency. The graphs for red, green, and blue intensity adjustments are seen behind. The original MRI image is displayed in cross sectional planes.

the Dextroscope with a virtual pen (*Fig. 4*), which generates a polygonal iso-surface. For the segmentation of cranial nerves, a tube "editor" was developed to quickly trace cranial nerves (or any other tubular structures) by drawing virtual tubes of on-line adjustable diameters inside the MRI data set (*Fig. 5*) (38).

Visualization and surgical planning

The system provides a generic set of tools for volume exploration of the fused multitechnique data set. A 3-D color-adjustment table (*Fig. 3*) allows individual color and transparency adjustments of all displayed structures to any degree. A cut-box tool removes an adjustable quarter of the volume to provide a mixed orthogonal and volumetric view. Crop and clip tools control the positions of the six orthogonal bounding planes that define each of the volumes. They also control the position and orientation of up to six arbitrary orientation clipping planes. The imaging data sets, or the segmented subvolumes, can be displayed as 3-D objects or as three orthogonal planes that can be moved by "touching" and "sliding" them (*Figs. 6, A and E, and 7*). A virtual fork allows one to pick a segmented object and uncouple it from its surroundings for closer inspection of the object itself or the area left behind.

The roaming tool allows one to move a box inside the multitechnique data set by cropping all the displayed data simultaneously and in real time along the side planes of the box. In this way, the volumetric shape of structures inside the box, as well as a cross section of all the structures along the side planes of the box, can be studied simultaneously (*Fig. 6B*). An outline of the head can be automatically generated from the silhouette on the MRI study, providing an orientation frame of reference (*Fig. 7A*).

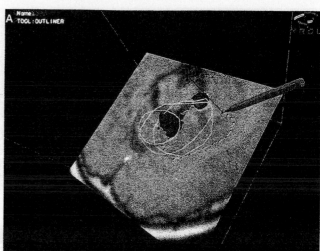

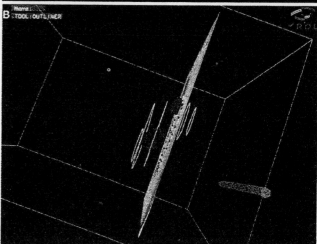

FIGURE 4. Manual 3-D segmentation of a spherical structure (astrocytoma). With the computer-generated 3-D pen (in *green*), the user is outlining the volume of the planned resection (*Panel A*). The two bright contrast-enhancing parts of the tumor were segmented with the color-adjustment table and are displayed in *green*. The lines can be drawn on planes (here, an axial MRI image), which can be freely moved and slid up and down with the left hand while the outlining is performed with the right hand. The completed lines are displayed on top of each other and are therefore continuously forming a 3-D structure while the drawing procedure is in progress. Especially while moving the 3-D data (*Panel B*), the spatial extension of the outlined volume becomes perceivable.

The VIVIAN system provides a drawing tool that produces line segments with their lengths displayed at one end that enables the user to measure and mark distances between points in 3-D space (*Figs. 6C and 7*). The end points of the lines can be adjusted by reaching into them with the virtual stylus and shifting them to a new position. The segments either connect two points in a straight line or mold to the surface of an object (e.g., to the MRI surface, which is equivalent to the skin surface). The system also provides a voxel-editing tool to

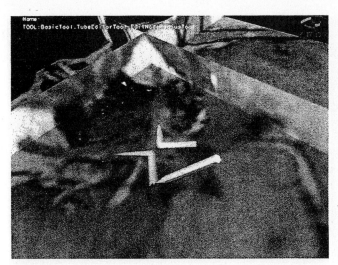

FIGURE 5. Manual 3-D segmentation of a tubular structure (optic nerve). With the tip of the virtual pen, tubular structures, such as (in this case) the optic nerves, can be traced on the tomographic imaging planes (here, the axial MRI plane). A tube is generated while the pen progresses, and its diameter and transparency are adjustable on-line.

change the properties of voxels (3-D pixels) in real time. This selectively allows one to turn voxels transparent (for simulating a drilling or a suctioning tool), to paint them in a different color (for marking purposes), or to restore their original values (for correcting interaction errors). The user can select the shape of the voxel editor and can control its size. A spherical shape was chosen to simulate bone drilling with CT data, a cylindrical or conical shape to simulate suctioning with MRI data. By introducing the tool into the volume, the voxels covered by the shape of the tool are transformed immediately (*Figs. 6, D* and *F; 8, B* and *D;* and *9, A, C,* and *E*). To simulate the magnified view through the microscope, a window with a central cross wire, which appears when the object is moved, can be generated. The surface point on the virtual object targeted by the cross wire becomes the center of rotation and scaling.

Implementation

The Dextroscope provides real-time volume rendering by using 3-D textures. The software that drives the VIVIAN system was developed in Kent Ridge Digital Laboratories and is called the BrixMed C++/OpenGL Software Toolkit (43). The system runs on a desk-side Silicon Graphics Onyx2 workstation and relies on hardware-assisted texture mapping.

Data analysis

A report was written about each planning session. Each report was divided into two parts. One part recorded the size of the data set, the time needed for fusion and segmentation, the average system performance in frames per second, and the planning and simulation tools used during the session. The other part was submitted by the neurosurgeon and stated

the additional information gained when using the VIVIAN system as compared with surgical planning using conventionally displayed data (e.g., CT and MRI slices or 3-D reconstructions of MRA and MRV images as provided by the scanner manufacturers).

RESULTS

Data loading, coregistration, and segmentation

The loading of the images, the conversion to red-green-blue files, and the subsequent generation of the virtual reality image took 5 to 10 minutes for each data set. Coregistration of MRI, MRA, and MRV images originating from the same scanning session was usually achieved instantly and with submillimeter accuracy. The landmark-based coregistration of CT and MRI data sets typically took about 30 minutes; however, our recently implemented automatic coregistration algorithm (54) has reduced this time to 5 minutes. The landmark-based registration accuracy (root-mean-square displacement) between corresponding anatomic landmarks varied from 0.9 to 3.1 mm, with a mean of 1.9 mm and a standard deviation of 0.6 mm. The registration accuracy increased with the number of landmarks specified. The registration accuracy of the automatic image fusion (Patient 20) was about 1 mm.

The data segmentation took between 15 and 30 minutes, depending on the complexity of the data. Tumors with a bright and homogeneous contrast enhancement were segmented semiautomatically by color table adjustments (Patients 3, 4, 6, 7, 9, 13, 15, 18, 20, 21). Tumors without an intensity threshold were manually outlined (Patients 1, 2, 5, 8, 10–12, 17). Surgically relevant cranial nerves could be segmented in six cases by using the 3-D tube editor (Patients 1, 3, 5, 9, 11, 17). The loading and coregistration of the data were usually performed by a radiographer or a software engineer, the segmentation by a radiologist or a neurosurgeon.

Planning and simulation

We obtained an average performance of 10 frames per second in stereo, with the data sets occupying 50% of the screen space (1024 × 768 pixels). In addition to the time spent for segmentation, the neurosurgeons spent, depending on the case, 10 to 45 minutes planning and discussing the surgery. The neurosurgeons involved in the respective procedures stated that the VIVIAN system substantially contributed to surgical planning primarily by 1) providing a faster and better understanding of the intracranial 3-D anatomic and abnormal spatial relationships, 2) optimizing the craniotomy and the required cranial base exposure through a rehearsal of bone removal, and 3) simulating intraoperative views. *Table 1* presents an overview of the additional information gained by using the VIVIAN system over that derived from conventional planning.

The basic features of the system (zooming, color and transparency adjustments, cropping, and straight measuring) were used in all cases. In the area of the cranial base, reliance solely on 3-D renderings to depict the relationships among bone, tumor, blood vessels, and cranial nerves was sometimes

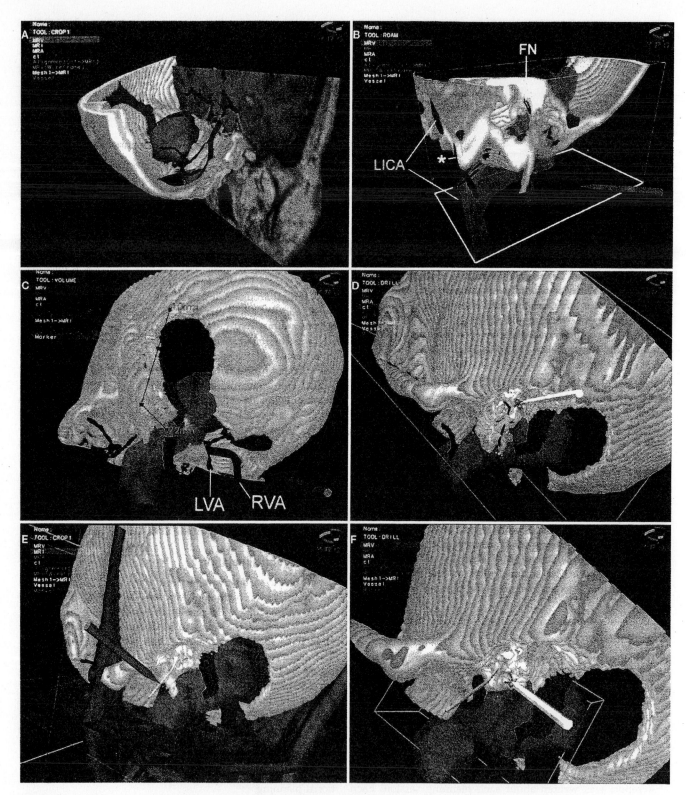

FIGURE 6. Patient 5, left-sided intra- and extracranial jugular schwannoma. *A,* overview of the posterior fossa. The tumor is in *blue* (segmented from MRI data), the transverse/sigmoid sinus in *pink* (from MRV data), and the vertebral/basilar/posterior cerebral arteries in *red* (from MRA data). The MRI is blended in as a movable coronal plane. *B,* roaming box mode to explore the data, left anterolateral view. The left lateral plane of the roaming box is cutting sagittally through the temporal bone at the level of the styloid process. Parts of the tumor are visible through the mastoid air cells. The extracranial part of the left

found to be insufficient. In such cases, an understanding of the detailed relationships, especially between structures that are encapsulated into others, requires a cross sectional view. The roaming box was useful in these cases, because it allows simultaneous visualization of the surface of objects inside the box as well as a cut through all scanning techniques along the box's side planes (*Fig. 6B*).

The simulation of bone removal (based on CT data) was useful to estimate the extent of bone work in cranial base approaches. We simulated pterional (Patients 7 and 9), subfrontal (Patient 6), transmaxillar (Patient 17), fronto-orbital (Patient 11), subtemporal (Patients 4 and 20), transmastoidal (Patient 5), translabyrinthine (Patient 10), suboccipital (Patients 4, 5, 12, 18, and 20), and petrosal (Patients 4 and 20) approaches. The simulation of soft tissue removal was helpful in planning the process of tumor removal with respect to surrounding structures; however, the information obtained was limited owing to the fact that physical tissue properties and intraoperative tissue movements are not reflected in the planning system.

Maintenance of real-time speed of interaction was highly critical for all visualization and planning procedures. Especially during the simulation of bone drilling, fine hand movements need to be rendered with a speed of at least eight frames per second. Below a speed of three frames per second, interaction becomes difficult. This problem arose in very large data sets, in which the workstation's Raster Manager capacity was exceeded.

REPRESENTATIVE CASE REPORTS

Four cases are presented to illustrate the planning sessions and the information gained from them. *Figures 6–9* are snapshots of the screen taken during the sessions (unfortunately, much of the depth information is lost in these 2-D reproductions).

Patient 5

Jugular schwannoma

A 47-year-old woman presented with unstable gait and dysphagia. The CT and MRI studies revealed a dumbbell-shaped mass with intra- and extracranial components straddling the jugular foramen. The intracerebral component extended into the left cerebellopontine angle, causing deformity of the pons and medulla. The extracranial components extended inferiorly along the carotid artery.

Two days preoperatively MRI, MRA, MRV, and CT studies were obtained, and the data were then coregistered in the VIVIAN system. The tumor was segmented by outlining it manually, since its low contrast enhancement offered no consistent threshold for semiautomatic segmentation. The infratemporal part of the facial nerve was outlined on the basis of the visible bony canal on the CT scan (*Fig. 6, B and D*). Surgical planning with the VIVIAN system revealed the close relationships between tumor, internal carotid artery (ICA), basilar artery, posteroinferior cerebral artery, sigmoid sinus, and internal jugular vein. Parts of the ICA and the internal jugular vein were seen to be embedded in the tumor (*Fig. 6, B–F*).

Inspection of the 3-D data revealed that the mass was accessible in a combined retrosigmoid (suboccipital) and transmastoid approach. A retrosigmoid craniotomy and a cortical mastoidectomy with lowering of the facial ridge were simulated. The extension of the craniotomy and the depths from the tip of the mastoid process to the proximal and distal tumor surfaces were measured (*Fig. 6C*). Skeletization of the facial nerve was simulated (*Fig. 6D*) as well as its transposition anteriorly (*Fig. 6E*). The carotid artery was partly laid open in the carotid canal (*Fig. 6F*). The tympanic plate was virtually drilled down, and the tumor was then fully exposed. The approach was rehearsed under a simulated intraoperative perspective, and the simulation suggested that complete removal of the tumor could be achieved safely by using this approach. Preoperatively, the perception of the spatial extent of the tumor and its relationship to the facial nerve and the temporal part of the carotid artery and their depths in the operative field was significantly improved. The "park bench" position was determined to be the optimal head position. The measurements of the retrosigmoid craniotomy on the virtual head were duplicated on the bone surface intraoperatively (with the mastoid process as a landmark), which facilitated carrying out the craniotomy in respect to the sigmoid sinus. The intraoperative findings correlated well with the preoperative simulation, and the tumor was completely removed. The patient continues to have mild dysphagia, owing to a palsy of Cranial Nerves IX and X, and is without signs of tumor regrowth 10 months postoperatively.

Patient 15

Pineal region meningioma

A 45-year-old woman presented with decreased visual acuity and dizziness. The CT and MRI studies revealed a large meningioma in the pineal region on both sides of the tentorial edge, compressing the midbrain and causing an obstructive hydrocephalus. After an emergency ventriculostomy of the third ventricle, the size of the ventricles returned to normal and the vision improved. MRI, MRA, and MRV data were three-dimensionally reconstructed and coregistered in the VIVIAN system. The contrast-enhancing meningioma and parts of the tentorium were segmented semiautomatically. It was evident that

---

ICA (*LICA*) is embedded in the tumor. The middle meningeal artery (*asterisk*) is cut by the anterior coronal plane of the roaming box in the foramen spinosum. The facial nerve (*FN*) is cut tangentially in the temporal bone. *C*, retrosigmoid craniotomy is completed. The sigmoid sinus (in *pink*) runs through the tumor. The left and right vertebral arteries are visible (*LVA* and *RVA*, respectively). From the tip of the mastoid bone, the distances to the most superior part of the craniotomy as well as the most direct distance to the tumor surface are measured. *D*, simulation of the mastoidectomy. The *red sphere* at the tip of the virtual drill is removing bone (CT data). The canal of the facial nerve could be visualized in the CT data, and the facial nerve was segmented and is displayed (in *dark blue*). The second genu of the facial nerve is laid open, whereas the vertical part is partly covered by bone. *E*, after its vertical part is exposed, the facial nerve (now in *gray*) is transposed anteriorly by grasping and moving it with the virtual pen. The three planes of the MRI are blended in to study the surrounding soft tissue. *F*, the craniotomy is being completed with the virtual drill. The carotid artery (in *red*) has been partly exposed in the carotid canal and is shown to be embedded in the anterior portion of the tumor.

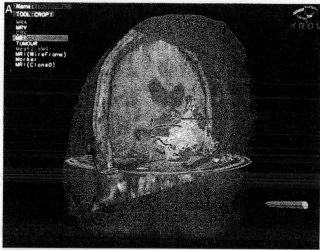

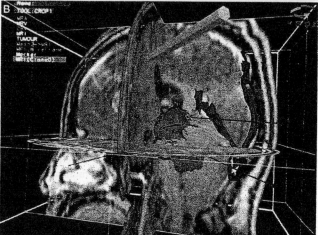

FIGURE 7. Patient 15, large meningioma of the pineal region. *A,* view from left occiput; *B,* lateral view. Tumor (in *blue*) and tentorium (in *yellow*) are both segmented from MRI data; the sagittal, straight, and transverse sinuses (in *purple*) are segmented from MRV data; the posterior cerebral artery and superior cerebellar artery (in *red*) are stretched over the tumor (from MRA data). The possible supra- and infratentorial surgical trajectories and their lengths are marked in *red*. In *Panel A,* the silhouette of the head is displayed semitransparently. The movable MRI planes help the viewer understand the spatial relationships to the surrounding soft tissue structures, such as the basal ganglia, the midbrain, and the brainstem. It was concluded that a combined supra- and infratentorial approach was necessary to achieve total excision of this tumor. In *Panel B,* the user is moving the coronal MRI plane with the virtual pen by touching it.

the lesion was very extensive in both the supra- and infratentorial compartments and that it was embedded in a mesh of blood vessels (*Fig. 7*). The posterior cerebral artery and the superior cerebellar artery were stretched laterally over the tumor with multiple smaller branches apparently feeding into it.

The skin to tumor distances were measured along possible infra- and supratentorial surgical approaches (*Fig. 7*). The brain tissue was visualized by blending in the three movable MRI orthogonal planes

(*Fig. 7*). The planning suggested that a combined supra/infratentorial approach to this large tumor was necessary. Indeed, intraoperatively, it was found that the occipital transtentorial approach alone was insufficient to facilitate removal of the infratentorial portion of the tumor. Unfortunately, the tumor was extremely vascular at surgery and could not be totally removed. Postoperatively, the patient has done well and the tumor remnant will possibly be treated with radiosurgery in the future.

Patient 17

Midfacial chordoma

A 28-year-old man presented with a nasal voice, difficulty in breathing through the nose, and decreased smell perception. The clinical neurological examination revealed no detectable deficits. The MRI and CT studies showed a large tumor in the posterior nasal space, occupying the middle and posterior ethmoidal cells and the sphenoidal sinus, eroding into the hard palate as well as into the clivus and right petrous apex and encroaching into the prepontine cistern. MRI, MRA, MRV, and CT data sets were three-dimensionally reconstructed and coregistered in the VIVIAN system 2 days before surgery. The low-contrast-enhancing tumor showed no clear threshold against the surrounding tissue on the MRI studies and was therefore outlined manually. The optic nerves as well as the Vth nerve could be identified on the MRI examinations and were segmented with the tube-editing tools (*Fig. 8A*).

A virtual maxillotomy was performed, which simulated the view that could be obtained intraoperatively by a maxillary swing approach (*Fig. 8, B* and *C*). Simulation of tumor removal showed that most of the superior and posterior parts of the tumor, which extended to the right petrous apex, were in a blind area behind the right orbit (*Fig. 8, E* and *F*). The simulation suggested that these parts should be accessed via an endoscope. The proximity of the tumor to both carotid arteries was apparent, and the tumor appeared to be partly encased in the right carotid artery, in the carotid canal. Intraoperatively, the angled endoscope was used in the suggested area, and the computer-generated and actual intraoperative scenarios were similar. The tumor was completely removed, with the dura left intact. Postoperatively, the patient's smell and taste perception improved, and the nasal airways were free. In an endoscopic examination and control MRI study performed 4 months postoperatively, no tumor regrowth was detected.

Patient 20

Petroclival meningioma

A 48-year-old woman presented with left-sided weakness, cerebellar dysfunction, dizziness, and mild left-sided palsy of Cranial Nerves V, VII, IX, X, and XI. CT and MRI examinations showed a large right-sided petroclival meningioma extending inferiorly to the lower clivus and compressing the midbrain and the brainstem. One day before surgery, the CT, MRI, MRA, and MRV data were three-dimensionally reconstructed and fused using the VIVIAN system. The tumor as well as parts of the tentorium were segmented semiautomatically. The brainstem was three-dimensionally segmented by using the manual outlining tool. Cranial nerves were not visible on the MRI study. The VIVIAN system revealed the spatial infra- and supratentorial tumor extensions with the tumors bulging out of the incisura. The cerebral peduncles, midbrain, and brainstem were highly compressed. The right posterior cerebral artery was stretched superiorly over the meningioma and was partly embedded in it. The 3-D reconstruction of the MRV data showed the position of the transverse, sigmoid, straight, and superior petrosal sinuses.

By simulating the craniotomy and the necessary bone work, it was possible to consider various surgical approaches. An extensive mastoidectomy, with exposure of the full length of the sigmoid sinus as low as the jugular bulb, as well as removal of the posterior wall of the petrous pyramid, was simulated (*Fig. 9, B* and *C*). With the voxel-removing tool, the volume-rendered tumor was removed under various viewpoints and its relationship to the brainstem and the vascular tree became clear (*Fig. 9E*). It was concluded that a combined subtemporal, transpetrosal, suboccipital approach would be most suitable for the removal of this large tumor. This was indeed the approach used during the operation, and gross total excision of the tumor was achieved. Postoperatively, the patient has done well, and the left hemiparesis has improved.

DISCUSSION

Great progress has been made in the field of computer-integrated neurosurgery. 3-D visualization of various imaging techniques has been widely explored to enhance the comprehension of volumetric data for diagnosis and surgical planning (1, 41, 47). It has been shown that the main prerequisites for a 3-D multitechnique neurosurgical planning system are high image resolution, accurate coregistration of data obtained from different imaging techniques (17, 18, 28, 30, 36, 48, 53), and software tools for data segmentation to extract surgically relevant structures (6, 7, 9, 22, 24, 27, 31).

3-D multitechnique data sets are complex organizations consisting of various subsegments (tumor, cranial nerves, parts of the brain) of the different scanning methods. The ability to use the software to manipulate the data is therefore crucial for the success and efficacy of neurosurgical planning. Our goal in the development of a computerized neurosurgical planning system was to create an environment that allows optimized exploitation of information from a multitechnique 3-D data set and that enables direct and on-line manipulation of the 3-D data, derived from CT and MRI studies, to simulate the removal and restoration of bone and soft tissue, respectively. To accomplish this goal, we found three elements to be essential: 1) the ability to detach the 3-D data from the monitor screen and to interact with it by reaching into it with natural 3-D hand movements; 2) the capability to perform high-speed rendering (at least 10 frames per second) to allow real-time interaction; and 3) the means to display the multitechnique data stereoscopically to achieve the greatest depth cues. Given the current state of computer technology, these features can only be adequately embodied in the environment by driving the system with a high-end graphics computer workstation that is capable of sustaining a fast display update sufficient to generate smoothly interactive graphics.

The manipulative capabilities of common input devices, like a mouse and keyboard, are poorly matched to the volumetric manipulation and visualization tasks of a complex 3-D data set. However, controlling a 3-D object displayed on a desktop screen by a mouse is proposed by most of the groups that have developed an interactive neurosurgical planning system (10, 21, 23, 32, 55). With our data sets, we found the conventional means of interaction to be nonintuitive, leading to object behavior that is hard to predict, since the movements of the screen-bound cursor have to be mentally translated into

3-D object movements. This becomes most obvious in manipulations along the z axis (orthogonal to the screen surface). Measuring distances with the mouse along, or oblique to, the z axis requires either that the object be rotated to bring the distant point within reach of the surface-bound cursor or that the operator use a combination of mouse clicks to simulate cursor movements in the depths of the screen. The simulation of bone drilling or tissue removal as a procedure mainly along the z axis of the object demands 3-D interaction, since hand movements directly determine the depth and extent of the operation.

We found the set-up of the Dextroscope to be well suited for fine and intuitive 3-D interaction (37, 38, 42–45) and developed the VIVIAN system as the Dextroscope's graphical interface for neurosurgical planning. Because the virtual object is reflected behind a mirror, the system allows the user to directly manipulate the object by reaching with the hands to where the object appears to be without obscuring it. The fact that object and hand movements take place in the same apparent position allows for careful, dexterous work with 3-D objects and adds the sensation of hand-eye coordination as another depth cue. In contrast to head-mounted displays, in which the appearance of the image is related to head or body movements (39, 46), the Dextroscope set-up, similar to the operative scenario, allows the user to sit down comfortably, rest the arms, and look naturally downward toward one's hands, where the virtual image appears. The user works with the full resolution of the monitor screen (most of the liquid crystal display monitors in head-mounted displays offer unsatisfactory resolution), and visual access to the data set is not restricted to one user only. We found it important to remain within the virtual environment during the entire planning procedure and not to have to reach outside for the keyboard and mouse. Once the data are transferred to the workstation, all subsequent steps of data fusion, segmentation, planning, and simulation are performed using 3-D tools within the virtual environment of the VIVIAN system.

3-D interaction in computer-integrated surgical planning has been addressed by only a few groups. Globe et al. (11) described an approach in which the user manipulates a 3-D image on a desktop screen by holding an electromagnetically tracked doll's head in one hand (representing the volumetric data) and a plastic plate or pointer in the other. The arbitrary cuts or trajectories of the 3-D MRI data are determined by the relative position of the plastic plate or pointer to the doll's head. We have conducted similar experiments by controlling a 3-D stereoscopic image on a desktop monitor with handheld Polhemus devices and experienced a strange feeling of remote control, as the controlling hand movements take place in front of the virtual image, which seems to be inside the monitor. Moreover, the user's hands occasionally obscured the line of sight to the image, resulting in loss of control.

Cutler et al. (8) described a device called the Responsive Workbench, in which a stereoscopic image is projected on a horizontal screen and interaction is achieved via hand-tracked instruments. Besides having applications for architectural planning and automotive engineering, this apparatus is useful for teaching anatomy with life-sized interactive 3-D models

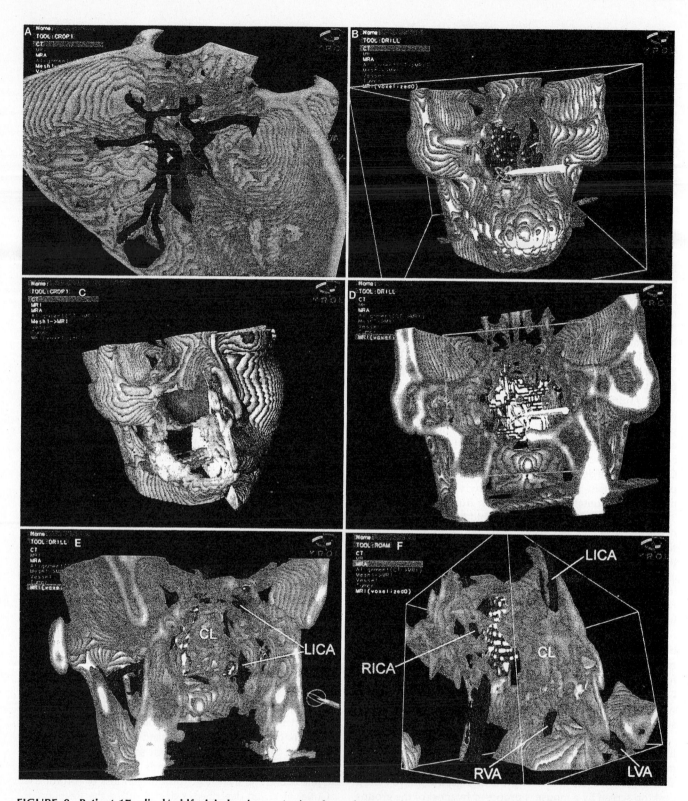

FIGURE 8. Patient 17, clival/midfacial chordoma. *A*, view from above to the cranial base. Bone (in *yellow*) was segmented from CT data, blood vessels (in *red*) from MRA data, tumor (in *green-blue*) from MRI data. The two optic nerves as well as both trigeminal nerves were segmented from the MRI data and are displayed as *gray tubes*. Note the close relationship of the tumor to the right carotid artery. *B*, anterior view. Beginning of the simulation of a right maxillotomy. *C*, MRI and CT data are coregistered. The now-completed virtual maxillotomy simulates the view that is intraoperatively obtained by a maxillary

and for 3-D sonographic visualization in cardiology (25). A mirror-based set-up similar to the Dextroscope was presented as a suitable environment for interaction with 3-D data sets by several other groups (4, 12, 19); however, it was never embedded in the clinical routine to plan surgical procedures with patient-specific imaging data.

Our experience is that the efficiency and quality of perception of 3-D spatial relationships between the displayed structures are directly related to the mode of interaction. The effect of holding and moving the 3-D data with one's hand proved to be very intuitive for viewing structures from any angle and for gaining an overview within a few minutes. The stereoscopic display enhances the 3-D perception substantially. In interactive neurosurgical planning systems described previously (10, 21, 23, 32), the 3-D depth appearance of the computer-generated structures is achieved through a combination of perspective projection, surface shading, and parallax stereoscopic cues. The latter requires image rotation for depth perception. Our approach uses stereoscopic rendering, which provides a strong sense of depth perception even on static images. The drawback of stereoscopic rendering is that the whole data set always has to be rendered twice (right- and left-eye projections), which imposes heavy demands on the hardware to maintain real-time interaction. Another drawback is that an effective stereoscopic image cannot be rendered in print; snapshots of the planning procedure that could be used for intraoperative guidance can appear only in 2-D format (like the images in this article), thereby losing much of the 3-D information.

The visualization and manipulation capabilities of the VIVIAN system were most useful in the area of the cranial base, in which the computer-generated 3-D surgical area of interest usually consists of multitechnique imaging information, depicting soft tissue (MRI), blood vessels (MRA and MRV), and bone (computed tomography). The 3-D perceptions of the shape and extent of tumors and their relation to the vascular tree, the cranial base, and, if extractable from the MRI data, the cranial nerves and tentorium, represented significant improvements over planning in conventional 2-D imaging planes. In cases in which 3-D segmentation was difficult, as for the brainstem, the midbrain, the basal ganglia, and the sylvian fissure, it was useful to inspect the 3-D structures and the sliding 2-D cross sectional MRI planes simultaneously. The 3-D structures and the structural information provided in the 2-D MRI planes were complementary, and the presence of each type of image enhanced the interpretation of the other (*Figs. 6, A and E, and 7*).

The technique of direct volume rendering allows one to remove individual voxels or blocks of voxels by making them transparent. In the VIVIAN system, the size and shape of the active voxel-removing volume at the tip of the virtual instrument is adjustable (spherical, conical, cubical, etc.), and a restoring mode allows one to correct interaction errors or to repeat the procedure. We used this technique to simulate bone removal by interacting with the virtual bone derived from CT data. For example, for sphenoidal ridge meningiomas, we found it helpful to simulate preoperatively the drilling of the sphenoidal ridge and the anterior clinoid process with respect to the optic nerves and the carotid artery. In tumors of the cerebellopontine angle, we could simulate the craniotomy in relation to the sigmoid sinus; in vestibular schwannomas, we simulated the required bone work to reveal the intrameatal tumor parts. In the case of petroclival meningiomas, the simulation of the retrosigmoid, temporal, and petrosal bone work helped us determine the route of the approach.

Translabyrinthine or transmastoid approaches (*Fig. 6*) could be simulated by considering the facial nerve and the inner ear structures. A limitation, however, was that 3-D segmentation of these fine nerve structures from the MRI or CT data was difficult, time-consuming, and partially incomplete. Compared with the simulation of bone removal, the simulated soft tissue removal was less realistic. This was mainly due to missing or insufficient information about details of tissue structure, microvasculature, and physical tissue properties. The brain-tumor interface, which is a major visual guide during the surgery of both intra- and extra-axial lesions, is seldom captured reliably by MRI and is therefore difficult to represent realistically as a 3-D image. However, we found it useful to simulate the tumor debulking of cranial base lesions from an intraoperative viewpoint, especially in combination with the necessary bone work. This revealed the position of some relevant surrounding structures (such as the blood vessels and the brainstem in Patient 20, *Fig. 9*) and the angle from which they might be encountered during surgery. The computer-simulated intraoperative perspectives were well remembered by the surgeons and contributed intraoperatively to the surgical strategy. For the neurosurgical residents, the simulation of bone and soft tissue removal and the consideration of different surgical approaches through interaction with 3-D imaging data had excellent training and teaching effects.

Nevertheless, with the degree of detail possible still somewhat limited, the VIVIAN system provides only a rough approximation of the actual anatomy and pathological features. Many structures, such as the cranial nerves and small blood vessels, are beyond the current resolution of MRI or CT technology and therefore cannot be segmented and displayed as 3-D structures. Unfortunately, they often play a major role in determining the surgical approach. Some structures that are visible with MRI, like the silhouette of the brainstem, the

swing approach. *D,* simulation of tumor removal with the voxel-editing tool. *E,* right anterior view into the tumor cavity toward the clivus (*CL*). Most of the middle and left-sided parts of the tumor are removed (*LICA,* left ICA). The right superior part of the tumor, which is stretching toward the right petrous apex (see *Panel A*), is located in a blind area behind the right orbit. *F,* simulation of operative view from left inferoanterior position toward the tumor parts in the blind area at the right petrous apex. This view was intraoperatively obtained with an angled endoscope. *RICA,* right ICA; *LICA,* left ICA; *RVA,* right vertebral artery; *LVA,* left vertebral artery; *CL,* clivus.

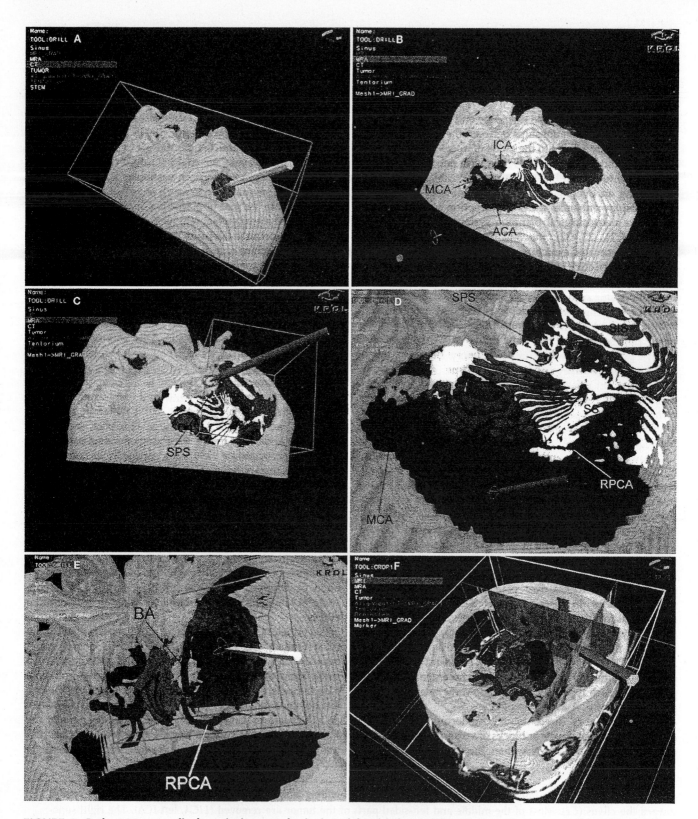

FIGURE 9. Patient 20, petroclival meningioma. *A,* beginning of the simulated right-sided craniotomy, seen from the actual surgical viewpoint, as on the operating table. Sigmoid sinus (in *pink*) was segmented from MRV data. *B,* combined retro/presigmoid and temporal craniotomy. Tumor (in *blue*) and tentorium (in *white*) were both segmented from MRI data; right ICA, middle cerebral artery (*MCA*), and anterior cerebral artery (*ACA*) (in *red*) were segmented from MRA data. *C,* the

basal cisterns, the basal ganglia, or the sylvian fissure, are hard to segment semiautomatically because of their geometrical complexity and the difficulty in determining the correct threshold that defines them (10, 22, 31). Manual segmentation of structures of almost any shape is theoretically possible with VIVIAN's manual contouring and tube-editing tools, but time constraints limit the feasibility of this application.

To achieve 3-D representation of the basal ganglia in cases of brain distortion caused by tumors, we are working on patient-specific deformation of our Electronic Clinical Brain Atlas (33, 34). Intracranial vasculature could be displayed with a high level of detail by integrating 3-D reconstructions of x-ray angiograms (16). With the recent introduction of rotational x-ray angiographic scanners, which provide fast and accurate 3-D reconstructions of 2-D digital subtraction angiographic rotational data (Advantx LCN+ Biplane Neuroangiography System; General Electric), high-resolution volumetric vascular imaging data are available. These data are still superior to those provided by MRA, especially for the visualization of arteriovenous malformations and tumor vascularity. We are currently working on the integration of these data into the VIVIAN environment.

Even if the 3-D depiction of anatomic structures were perfected, the assessment of the feasibility of different neurosurgical approaches would still be dependent on more than the size of the craniotomy, the required bone work, and the arrangement of 3-D structures. Of at least equal importance is the prediction of the physical properties of the soft tissues, such as their intraoperative flexibility and mobility. These physical properties should ideally be reflected in a preoperative 3-D planning and simulation environment, but they are defined by innumerable parameters that are difficult or impossible to extract from the preoperative scanning data. We have experimented with a haptic feedback device (Phantom; Sensable Technologies, Cambridge, MA), but even for bone, we found it very difficult to adjust the device to give a realistic simulation of tissue properties. In addition, we thought that the device restricted the user's freedom of movement. We concluded that, at this point, the haptic feedback device does not add significant value to the planning of a neurosurgical procedure based on patient-specific imaging data. However, haptic feedback might be useful in the field of surgical training with non-patient-specific anatomic models (19, 40). In this environment, it is not necessary to adjust the device to different clinical data sets, and its response can be fine-tuned to the models and to specific tasks. The haptic device might improve the perception of spatial structures, especially when dealing

with detailed models, and might provide the means for sophisticated dexterity training.

The successful integration of the VIVIAN system into daily clinical practice depends to a large extent on time constraints and requires a well-trained and coordinated team of radiographers, radiologists, and neurosurgeons. The system should be linked directly to the CT and MRI scanners, and data transfer and data loading should be highly automated. The landmark-based data coregistration turned out to be rather time-consuming, especially in patients who were scanned without skin fiducials. We have recently implemented an automatic registration algorithm (54) based on integration of mutual image information (53) that substantially increases the speeds of data coregistration, and we are currently extending it to coregister functional MRI data. However, the 3-D segmentation of surgically relevant structures is highly dependent on the anatomic knowledge and image interpretation skills of the neurosurgeons and radiologists and will therefore be difficult to automate completely.

Currently, the 3-D information generated by the VIVIAN system is, apart from prints carried to the operating room, not directly available during surgery. We are therefore exploring the feasibility of injecting the stereoscopic data of VIVIAN into both optical channels of a microscope. Coregistered with the intraoperative findings seen through the microscope, the stereoscopic images of VIVIAN (including landmarks, measurements, and trajectories placed by the surgeon during the planning session) could serve for intraoperative image guidance, providing a 3-D computer-generated representation of the surgical field and the surrounding structures.

CONCLUSION

We have developed a neurosurgical planning system that coregisters MRI, MRA, and CT data into a fused stereoscopic 3-D data set; provides segmentation, planning, and simulation tools; and allows 3-D interaction in real time in a virtual reality environment. Our experience has shown that the more complex a 3-D data set is, the easier the mode of interaction needs to be to efficiently extract surgically useful information. To achieve this goal, the data have to be displayed in an interactive virtual reality environment that allows one to handle a computer-generated 3-D object in a manner similar to how one would handle a real object. The VIVIAN system provides a precise, fast, and easy way of handling complex 3-D patient scanning data, resulting in instant and comprehensive 3-D information about spatial relationships of surgi-

mastoidectomy and the removal of the posterior wall of the petrous pyramid are being simulated with the virtual drill. The *red sphere* at the top of the virtual instrument is the drill size, which is the active volume in which voxels are turned transparent and thus appear to be removed. *SPS*, superior petrosal sinus. *D*, close-up view of the operative site. The posterior wall of the petrous pyramid is removed; *SPS*, superior petrosal sinus; *SS*, straight sinus; *MCA*, branches of the middle cerebral artery; *RPCA*, right posterior cerebral artery; *SIS*, sigmoid sinus. *E*, parts of the tumor are being removed with the voxel-editing tool. The spatial relationships between tumor, cranial base, blood vessels, and brainstem are clearly visible. *BA*, basilar artery; *RPCA*, right posterior cerebral artery. *F*, overview from above, as the craniotomy is being completed. The virtual stylus is moving the coronal MRI plane. The proximal parts of the posterior cerebral arteries are embedded in the tumor, and the left PCA is stretched over the tumor. Note the compression of the brainstem (in *brown*).

cally relevant structures. Especially in cranial base surgery, the simulation of bone and tumor removal in combination with the simulation of views that would be seen through the operating microscope decreased the pre- and intraoperative guesswork and increased the surgeon's confidence in carrying out complex procedures. Currently, a costly high-end computer platform is needed to drive this system; however, with rapidly improving computer technology, it will be more accessible in the near future.

ACKNOWLEDGMENTS

We gratefully acknowledge the support and valuable contributions of Benjamin Carson, M.D., and Tushar Goradia, M.D. (Johns Hopkins Hospital, Baltimore); Prem Pillay, M.D. (Pillay Brain Spine Nerve Centre, Singapore); Peter Jannetta, M.D. (University of Pittsburgh); Hans J. Reulen, M.D. (Ludwig Maximilians University of Munich, Germany); Alvin Hong, M.D., Mathew Tung, M.D., Winston Lim, M.D., Christopher Goh, M.D., Low Wong Kein, M.D. (Singapore General Hospital); Seow Wan Tew, M.D., Peter Hwang, M.D., Ng Puay Yong, M.D., Robert Tien M.D., Violet Chua (National Neuroscience Institute, Singapore); as well as Terry Lim, Norsalawati Salamat, and Peter Kellock.

This work was supported by grants from the Singapore National Science and Technology Board, Singapore General Hospital, and the German Ministry of Education and Research.

Received, April 21, 1999.
Accepted, August 20, 1999.
Reprint requests: Ralf Alfons Kockro, M.D., Biomedical Laboratory, Kent Ridge Digital Laboratories, 119613 Singapore.

REFERENCES

1. Alexander E III, Maciunas RJ (eds): *Advanced Neurosurgical Navigation*. New York, Thieme, 1999.
2. Alexander E III, Kooy HM, van Herk M, Schwarz M, Barnes PD, Tarbell N, Mulkern RV, Holupka EJ, Loeffler JS: Magnetic resonance image-directed stereotactic neurosurgery: Use of image fusion with computerized tomography to enhance spatial accuracy. J Neurosurg 83:271–276, 1995.
3. Batnitzky S, Price HI, Lee KR, Cook PN, Cook LT, Fritz SL, Dwyer SJ III, Watts C: Three-dimensional computer reconstructions of brain lesions from surface contours provided by computed tomography: A prospectus. Neurosurgery 11:73–84, 1982.
4. Blackwell M, O'Toole RV, Morgan F, Gregor L: Performance and accuracy experiments with 3D and 2D image overlay systems, in *Proceedings of MRCAS 95*. Philadelphia, Wiley & Sons, 1995, pp 312–317.
5. Chalif DJ, Dufrense CR, Ransohoff J, McCarthy JA: Three-dimensional computed tomographic reconstructions of intracranial meningiomas. Neurosurgery 23:570–575, 1988.
6. Cline HE, Lorensen WE, Kikinis R, Jolez FA: Three-dimensional segmentation of MR images of the head using probability and connectivity. J Comput Assist Tomogr 14:1037–1045, 1990.
7. Cline HE, Lorensen WE, Souza SP, Jolez FA, Kikinis R, Gering G, Kennedy TE: 3D surface rendered MR images of the brain and its vasculature. J Comput Assist Tomogr 15:344–351, 1991.
8. Cutler LD, Froehlich B, Hanrahan P: Two-handed direct manipulation on the Responsive Workbench, in *Proceedings of the 1997 Symposium on Interactive 3D Graphics*. New York, Association for Computing Machinery, 1997, pp 107–114.
9. Ehricke HH, Laub G: Integrated 3D display of brain anatomy and intracranial vasculature in MR imaging. J Comput Assist Tomogr 14:846–852, 1990.
10. Gandhe AJ, Hill DLG, Studholme C, Hawkes DJ, Ruff CF, Cox TC, Gleeson MJ, Strong AJ: Combined and three-dimensional rendered multimodal data for planning cranial base surgery: A prospective evaluation. Neurosurgery 35:463–471, 1994.
11. Globe JC, Hinckley K, Pausch R, Snell JW, Kassell NF: Two-handed spatial interface tools for neurosurgical planning. IEEE Comput 28:20–26, 1995.
12. Green PS, Hill JW, Jensen JF, Shah A: Telepresence surgery. IEEE Eng Med Biol 3:324–329, 1995.
13. Harbaugh RE, Schlusselberg DS, Jeffery R, Hayden S, Cromwell LD, Pluta D: Three-dimensional computerized tomographic angiography in the diagnosis of cerebrovascular disease. J Neurosurg 76:408–414, 1992.
14. Harbaugh RE, Schlusselberg DS, Jeffery R, Hayden S, Cromwell LD, Pluta D: Three-dimensional computed tomographic angiography in the preoperative evaluation of cerebrovascular lesions. Neurosurgery 36:320–326, 1995.
15. Harrison MJ, Johnson BA, Gardner GM, Welling BG: Preliminary results on the management of unruptured intracranial aneurysms with magnetic resonance angiography and computed tomographic angiography. Neurosurgery 40:947–955, 1997.
16. Hildebrand A, Grosskopf S: 3D reconstruction of coronary arteries from X-ray projections, in *Proceedings of the Conference of Computer Assisted Radiology*. Berlin, Springer, 1995, pp 201–207.
17. Hill DL, Hawkes DJ, Crossman JE, Gleeson MJ, Cox TC, Bracey EE, Strong AJ, Graves P: Registration of MR and CT images for skull base surgery using point like anatomical features. Br J Radiol 64:1030–1035, 1991.
18. Hill DL, Hawkes DJ, Gleeson MJ, Cox TC, Strong AJ, Wong WL, Ruff CF, Kitchen ND, Thomas DG, Sofat A, Crossman JE, Studholme C, Gandhe AJ, Green SEM, Robinson GP: Accurate frameless registration of MR and CT images of the head: Applications in planning surgery and radiation therapy. Radiology 191:447–454, 1994.
19. Hill JW, Holst PA, Jensen JF, Goldman J, Gorfu Y, Ploeger DW: Telepresence interface with applications to microsurgery and surgical simulation, in Westwood JD, Hoffman HM, Stredney D, Weghorst SJ (eds): *Medicine Meets Virtual Reality*. Amsterdam, IOS Press, 1998, pp 96–102.
20. Hsiang JN, Liang EY, Lam JM, Zhu XL, Poon WS: The role of computed tomographic angiography in the diagnosis of intracranial aneurysms and emergent aneurysm clipping. Neurosurgery 38:481–487, 1996.
21. Hu X, Tan KK, Levin DN, Galhotra S, Mullan JF, Hekmatpanah J, Spire JP: Three-dimensional magnetic resonance images of the brain: Application to neurosurgical planning. J Neurosurg 72:433–440, 1990.
22. Kapur T, Grimson WE, Wells WM III, Kikinis R: Segmentation of brain tissue from magnetic resonance images. Med Image Anal 1:109–127, 1996.
23. Kikinis R, Gleason L, Moriarty TM, Moore MR, Alexander E III, Stieg PE, Matsumae M, Lorensen WE, Cline HE, Black P, Jolesz FA: Computer-assisted interactive three-dimensional planning for neurosurgical procedures. Neurosurgery 38:640–651, 1996.

24. Kikinis R, Jolesz FA, Gerig G, Sandor T, Cline HE, Lorensen WE, Halle M, Benton SA: 3D morphometric and morphologic information derived from clinical brain MR images, in Hoehne KH, Fuchs H, Pizer SM (eds): *3D Imaging in Medicine: Algorithms, Systems, Applications*. Berlin, Springer, 1990, pp 441–454.

25. Krueger W, Bohn CA, Froehlich B, Schueth H, Strauss W, Wesche G: The Responsive Workbench: A virtual work environment. **IEEE Comput** 28:42–48, 1995.

26. Lansky LL, Batnitzky S, Price HI, Cook PN, Dwyer SJ III: Application of three-dimensional computer reconstruction from computerized tomography to intracranial tumors in children. **J Neurooncol** 1:347–356, 1983.

27. Levin DN, Hu X, Tan KK, Galhotra S: Surface of the brain: Three-dimensional MR images created with volume rendering. **Radiology** 171:277–280, 1989.

28. Levin DN, Pelizzari CA, Chen GT, Chen CT, Cooper MD: Retrospective geometric correlation of MR, CT, and PET images. **Radiology** 169:817–823, 1988.

29. Lo LJ, Marsh JL, Vannier MW, Patel VV: Craniofacial computer-assisted surgical planning and simulation. **Clin Plast Surg** 21:501–516, 1994.

30. Maintz JBA, Viergever MA: A survey of medical image registration. **Med Imag Anal** 2:1–36, 1998.

31. Mohamed FB, Vinitski S, Faro SH, Gonzalez CF, Mack J, Iwanaga T: Optimization of tissue segmentation of brain MR images based on multispectral 3D feature maps. **Magn Reson Imaging** 17:403–409, 1999.

32. Nakajima S, Atsumi H, Bhalerao AH, Jolesz FA, Kikinis R, Yoshimine T, Moriarty T, Stieg PE: Computer-assisted surgical planning for cerebrovascular neurosurgery. **Neurosurgery** 41:403–410, 1997.

33. Nowinski WL, Bryan RN, Raghavan R: *The Electronic Clinical Brain Atlas: Multiplanar Navigation of the Human Brain*. New York, Thieme, 1997.

34. Nowinski WL, Fang A, Nguyen BT, Raphel JK, Jagannathan L, Raghavan R, Bryan RN, Miller GA: Multiple brain atlas database and atlas-based neuroimaging system. **Comput Aided Surg** 2:42–66, 1997.

35. Patel VV, Vannier MW, Marsh JL, Lo LJ: Assessing craniofacial surgical simulation. **IEEE Comput Graph Appl** 16:46–54, 1996.

36. Pelizzari CA, Chen GTY, Spelbring DR, Weichselbaum RR, Chen CT: Accurate three-dimensional registration of CT, PET and MR images of the brain. **J Comput Assist Tomogr** 13:20–26, 1989.

37. Poston T, Serra L: Dextrous virtual work. **Commun ACM** 39:37–45, 1996.

38. Poston T, Serra L, Lawton W, Chua BC: Interactive tube finding on a virtual workbench, in *Proceedings of MRCAS 95*. Philadelphia, Wiley & Sons, 1995, pp 119–123.

39. Robb RA, Hanson DP, Camp JJ: Computer-aided surgery planning and rehearsal at Mayo Clinic. **IEEE Comput** 29:39–47, 1996.

40. Salisbury JK, Srinivasan MA: Phantom-based haptic interaction with virtual objects. **IEEE Comput Graph** 17:6–10, 1997.

41. Satava RM: Virtual reality, telesurgery, and the new world order of medicine. **J Image Guid Surg** 1:12–16, 1995.

42. Serra L, Ng H, Chua BC, Poston T: Interactive vessel tracing in volume data, in *Proceedings of the 1997 Symposium on Interactive 3D Graphics*. Nanterre, EC2, 1997, pp 131–137.

43. Serra L, Ng H, Fairchild KM: Building virtual realities with bricks, in *Proceedings of Informatique 93*. New York, Association for Computing Machinery, 1993, pp 101–109.

44. Serra L, Nowinski WL, Poston T, Ng H, Lee CM, Chua GG, Pillay PK: The brain bench: Virtual tools for stereotactic frame neurosurgery. **Med Image Anal** 1:317–329, 1997.

45. Serra L, Poston T, Ng H, Heng PA, Chua BC: Virtual space editing of tagged MRI heart data, in *Proceedings of the First International Conference of Computer Vision, Virtual Reality and Robotics in Medicine*. Berlin, Springer, 1995, pp 71–76.

46. Tanaka H, Nakamura H, Tamaki E, Nariai T, Hirakawa K: Brain surgery simulation using VR technology and improvement of presence, in Westwood JD, Hoffman HM, Stredney D, Weghorst SJ (eds): *Medicine Meets Virtual Reality*. Amsterdam, IOS Press, 1998, pp 150–154.

47. Taylor RH, Lavallee S, Burdea GC, Mosges R: *Computer-Integrated Surgery*. Cambridge, MIT Press, 1995.

48. van Herk M, Kooy HM: Automatic three-dimensional correlation of CT-CT, CT-MR and CT-SPECT using chamfer matching. **Med Phys** 21:1163–1178, 1994.

49. Vannier MW, Gado MH, Marsh JL: Three-dimensional display of intracranial soft-tissue structures. **AJNR Am J Neuroradiol** 4:520–521, 1983.

50. Vannier MW, Marsh JL, Warren JO: Three-dimensional CT reconstruction images for craniofacial surgical planning and evaluation. **Radiology** 150:179–184, 1984.

51. Virapongse C, Shapiro M, Gmitro A, Sarwar M: Three-dimensional computed tomographic reformation of the spine, skull, and brain from axial images. **Neurosurgery** 18:53–58, 1986.

52. Weingaertner T, Hassfeld S, Dillman R: Virtual Jaw: A 3D simulation for computer assisted surgery and education, in Westwood JD, Hoffman HM, Stredney D, Weghorst SJ (eds): *Medicine Meets Virtual Reality*. Amsterdam, IOS Press, 1998, pp 329–335.

53. Wells WM III, Viola P, Atsumi H, Nakajima S, Kikinis R: Multimodal volume registration by maximization of mutual information. **Med Image Anal** 1:35–51, 1996.

54. Xu M, Rajagopalan S, Nowinski WL: A fast mutual information method for multi-modal registration, in *Proceedings of the XVI International Conference on Information in Medical Imaging, IPMI 99*. Berlin, Springer, 1999, pp 466–471.

55. Zahao J, Colchester ACF, Henri CJ, Hawkes D, Ruff C: Visualisation of multimodal images for neurosurgical planning and guidance, in *Proceedings of the First International Conference of Computer Vision, Virtual Reality and Robotics in Medicine*. Berlin, Springer, 1995, pp 40–46.

COMMENTS

I commend the authors on the technological advancements described in this article. They review a virtual reality environment called VIVIAN (Virtual Intracranial Visualization and Navigation), which is essentially a neurosurgical planning system. The authors emphasize that the three-dimensional (3-D) nature of a procedure should be considered during the planning phase, and they therefore used this format in the creation of their system, which was developed for the Dextroscope. Unfortunately, the system is limited by the same problems as those in previously described surgical planning programs. Essentially, coregistration and segmentation continue to be the limiting factors. Identification of cranial nerves and microvasculature from magnetic resonance imaging (MRI), magnetic resonance angiography, and computed tomography remains extremely difficult and is still done on a manual basis by users of this system. The effect of this is a less than completely accurate image in the computer simulation process. As someone experienced with surgical planning programs, I believe they are extremely useful in surgical planning; however, the neurosurgeon must be fully aware of the limitations of the computer programs. In addition, this system does not provide any new information on the properties and intraoperative movement of tissue.

I find the system unique in its 3-D presentation of data and in the advantages this format provides preoperatively to a neurosurgeon. The authors readily admit that the information rendered from bone images is much better than that garnered from soft tissue images. Thus, I suspect that the program is quite effective for selecting a surgical approach but, since the microvessels cannot be identified preoperatively, it is certainly difficult to plan for and model them and to translate these data into real-time information.

Finally, the cost of these programs is exorbitant. The computer networks and systems are extensive and limited to institutions with large research budgets. We are still a long way from having systems like this readily available. I commend the authors on their advancement of the technology and look forward to further reports from this group.

Philip E. Stieg
Boston, Massachusetts

Kockro et al. describe a virtual reality environment for preoperative neurosurgical planning (the VIVIAN system) that provides a unique 3-D representation of preoperative imaging data for surgical planning within an interactive simulation program. But the machine does not simulate the feel or texture that a surgeon senses during an operation. Sensory feedback is very important to a neurosurgeon for a true virtual reality experience.

A surgical planning device should do something useful with the data generated in preoperative planning, such as transfer the information to the actual operation. However, there is no correlation between the virtual reality patient and the real patient on the operating table, and we have nothing more than a bunch of pretty pictures. In addition, the system wastes time for an engineer and a neurosurgeon in requiring data manipulation before its use. This will "grow old" very quickly in a busy practice. Finally, the device is more suited to planning a surgical approach to extra-axial cranial base lesions than to intra-axial lesions, and intra-axial lesions are far more common than cranial base lesions in clinical practice.

The VIVIAN system does not integrate data from digital subtraction angiography, something other systems have done for years. Accurate and detailed angiographic information may be important in preoperative surgical planning of lesions located in proximity to important vascular structures, such as cranial base meningiomas and the carotid artery, or temporal gliomas and the vein of Labbé. We do not agree that MRI does not reliably define the brain-tumor interface. If this were true, we should abandon the idea of imaged-guided tumor resection. MRI is the best technique we have available for this purpose.

The VIVIAN system is, presumably, a costly device. Is it worth the money? Is there evidence that preoperative planning based on computer-assisted imaging leads to shorter operating times, fewer days in the hospital, overall cost reduction, or improved patient care? Without answers to these questions, few neurosurgeons will be able to afford this technique in these days of diminishing reimbursement. Nonetheless, the device displays the 3-D anatomic relationships of abnormal and normal anatomy. Clearly, this is important, and such simulation devices may be useful in the training of residents or neurosurgeons unfamiliar with a particular surgical approach. Furthermore, surgeons using this device may be able to preoperatively evaluate various surgical approaches and choose the best or most direct one, determine the optimal head position, and decide whether endoscopy is feasible. We encourage the authors to expand the system for accurate transfer and interactive display of virtual reality patient information to the real-world environment of the surgical field.

Patrick J. Kelly
Jeffrey Weinberg
New York, New York

This is an outstanding paper and here's why: the work it reports—surgical simulation—is conceptually of extreme importance (especially from the long-term perspective), it represents a great deal of excellent technical development, and it describes its extension into sufficient clinical experience to verify its usefulness. This last point is made even in this early implementation of the technology. The evolution in surgical training and preparation through such means will without question prove to be dramatic within this generation of neurosurgeons. I have had an opportunity to visit these investigators and to actually use an earlier prototype of their device: the team and the implementation are at the forefront of this technology and exemplify the superb multidisciplinary collaboration that is advancing computer-assisted surgery.

David W. Roberts
Lebanon, New Hampshire

The authors describe an interesting virtual reality environment called VIVIAN and discuss their experience with surgical planning for 21 patients to date. The system is used concurrently with the Dextroscope, which allows the operators to place their hands within the virtual field while using stereoscopic lenses. The article is informative and well written and provides an interesting description of a tool that could be of significant future use with regard to the practice of approaches in the perioperative period, most specifically for physician training. A number of interesting case discussions have been included to allow the reader to understand appropriate scenarios for its use.

Obviously, the most important consideration regarding this technology is its applicability to the physician's education and to potential applications with regard to patient care. The initial information sources required for the 3-D reconstructions to be used in the working environment will continue to be streamlined, both with advances in hardware (specifically, MRI and computed tomography) and software.

Specific enhancements in software should allow further rapid integration and registration of multiple imaging techniques, without the need for smoothing or data loss, in a timely fashion. The obvious constraints with regard to applications for patient care are the same as those that have been well documented for frameless stereotaxy and need not be discussed here. An interesting consideration would be the integration of haptic feedback systems with this current technology. Through correspondence with the authors in the review of this manuscript, it is obvious that, to date, haptic feedback systems have not lent themselves well to the current technology. In fact, the use of haptics in physician training has been minimal, at best, to date, with the most obvious examples being in the training of suturing techniques, lumbar puncture, and thoracentesis. As we become more sophisticated with regard to our ability to correlate haptic feedback with additional reconstructive imagery, I believe that this will eventually become a positive addition to this technology.

The importance of this article is that it defines an early step, which I believe is in the right direction, with regard to the utilization of this technology. Clearly, the costs and processing requirements at this time are most likely appropriate only in a university setting. With improvements in software and hardware, in addition to data transmission, this technology should become much more affordable and potentially one that could be most appropriately used for resident training and patient care at some time in the future.

Michael L. Levy
Los Angeles, California

Automatic labelling of the human cortical surface using sulcal basins ☆

Gabriele Lohmann*, D. Yves von Cramon

Max-Planck-Institute of Cognitive Neuroscience, Stephanstrasse 1a, 04103 Leipzig, Germany

Received 30 November 1998; received in revised form 1 June 1999; accepted 27 August 1999

Abstract

Human brain mapping aims at establishing correspondences between brain function and brain anatomy. One of the most intriguing problems in this field is the high interpersonal variability of human neuroanatomy which makes studies across many subjects very difficult. The cortical folds ('sulci') often serve as landmarks that help to establish correspondences between subjects. In this paper, we will present a method that automatically detects and attributes neuroanatomical names to the cortical folds using image analysis methods applied to magnetic resonance data of human brains. We claim that the cortical folds can be subdivided into a number of substructures which we call *sulcal basins*. The concept of sulcal basins allows us to establish a complete parcellation of the cortical surface into separate regions. These regions are neuroanatomically meaningful and can be identified from MR data sets across many subjects. Sulcal basins are segmented using a region growing approach. The automatic labelling is achieved by a model matching technique. © 2000 Elsevier Science B.V. All rights reserved.

Keywords: Medical image analysis; Cortical topography; Model matching

1. Introduction

The folding of the cortical surface of the human brain varies dramatically from person to person. However, the folding pattern is not completely arbitrary. In fact, the cortical folds (also called 'sulci') often serve as landmarks for referencing brain locations, and the more pronounced sulci have names that are well established in the neuroanatomical literature (Ono et al., 1990).

In this paper, we will present image analysis methods applied to T1-weighted magnetic resonance data sets that automatically segment and attribute neuroanatomical names to these folds. More precisely, we subdivide each fold into a number of substructures which we call *sulcal basins*, and attach labels to these substructures. The reason why we introduce the concept of a sulcal basin is that we believe that sulcal basins have a lower degree of inter-

personal variability than entire sulci. Our belief is based on the findings of a twin study which showed that the deepest parts of the sulci are more strongly genetically predetermined than the more shallow ones (Lohmann and von Cramon, 1999a). The same study also shows that sulcal variability decreases with depth in the general population. The work we present here is an extension of our earlier work (Lohmann and von Cramon, 1998a,b).

The method uses two stages. During the first stage, sulcal basins are segmented using morphological and region growing techniques. The second stage is a model matching procedure that automatically attributes neuroanatomical labels to the segmented basins. The model against which basins are matched is based on a volumetric shape representation of basins as well as on a model of spatial variation.

Our method is important in the context of human brain mapping. Human brain mapping aims at establishing correspondences between brain function and brain anatomy. One of the most intriguing problems in this field is the high interpersonal variability of human neuroanatomy which makes studies across many subjects difficult.

☆ A preliminary version of this article was presented at the Workshop on Biomedical Image Analysis, held in Santa Barbara (USA) in June 1998.

*Corresponding author.

E-mail address: lohmann@cns.mpg.de (G. Lohmann).

Most previous attempts at solving this problem are based on various methods of image registration where MR data sets are registered and warped onto a brain atlas (Maziotta et al., 1995; Thompson and Toga, 1996; Thompson et al., 1997; Rizzo et al., 1997; Sandor and Leahy, 1997). A related approach is that by Guéziec and Ayache (1994) and also Declerck et al. (1995) who presented methods for extracting and matching lines in multiple MR data sets. New approaches to the problem of intersubject registration of sulcal patterns can be found in a number of references (Vaillant and Davatzikos, 1999; Caunce and Taylor, 1999; Goualher et al., 1999; Chui et al., 1999). Warping methods depend on establishing local correspondences between structures found in the image and in the atlas. Mismatches may lead to significant errors.

The approach presented in this paper allows interpersonal comparisons without having to resort to image warping. Our concept of sulcal basins allows us to establish a complete parcellation of the cortical surface into separate regions. These regions are neuroanatomically meaningful and can be identified from MR data sets across many subjects. At the same time, the parcellation is detailed enough to be useful for brain mapping purposes.

The work closest in spirit to ours is that by Mangin et al. (1995), Manceaux-Demiau et al. (1997) and Regis et al. (1995) who also seek to obtain a structural description and generic model of the cortical topography. It differs from ours in a number of respects. Most importantly, their concept of 'sulcal roots' is based on a structural decomposition of sulcal skeletons. In contrast, our approach does not use sulcal skeletons but is based on a volumetric concept of sulcal indentations. This conceptual difference leads to different cortical parcellations. For instance, their parcellation would usually regard junctions between sulci as separations. However, sulcal junctions are often the deepest areas within sulci and are therefore at the heart of a basin in our model rather than at a boundary.

The paper is organized as follows. We begin by defining the concept of a sulcal basin and present an algorithm for extracting sulcal basins from MR images of the human brain. We then introduce a sulcal basin model and a matching procedure for identifying basins. Finally, we present some experiments.

2. Sulcal basins

2.1. Definition

We have previously introduced the notion of a sulcal basin (Lohmann and von Cramon, 1998a,b). In the following, we will summarize our definition and our method of extracting sulcal basins from MR images.

Fig. 1(a) shows a volume rendering of an MR data set depicting a top-right view of a healthy subject's brain. The sulci are clearly visible as dark valleys. Fig. 1(b) shows the top part of the same brain. This time, however, we removed the grey matter so that the white matter surface becomes visible and the sulci become more pronounced. Corresponding locations in both images are indicated by labels.

Note that the fold labelled 'sprc-sfs (superior precentral/ superior frontal sulcus)' which appears to consist of one large part in the volume rendering decomposes into three separate concave basins in Fig. 1(b). In fact, all sulci decompose into several such substructures, which we call 'sulcal basins'.

More precisely, sulcal basins are defined to be concavities in the white matter surface which are bounded by convex ridges that separate one basin from the next so that adjacent sulcal basins meet at the top of the ridge. Fig. 1(c) illustrates this definition. The entire white matter surface is covered by such concavities so that a decomposition into sulcal basins yields a complete parcellation of the surface.

There are two principal advantages in introducing the concept of a sulcal basin. Firstly, in subdividing sulci we obtain a spatially more precise definition of brain loci. As we are ultimately interested in intersubject comparisons, this is an important consideration. Secondly, the high interpersonal variability in sulcal patterns can at least be partly attributed to different forms of groupings of sulcal basins. The two sets of sulcal basins below for instance can be easily matched, even though the two groups formed in each set cannot be matched:

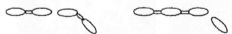

The postcentral sulcus, for instance, usually consists of

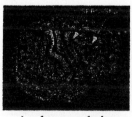

a) volume rendering

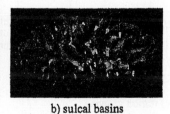

b) sulcal basins

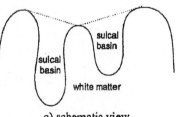

c) schematic view

Fig. 1. Sulcal basins.

two basins, a superior and an inferior basin. In some brains, these two basins are connected to form a continuous sulcus. In others, they are completely disconnected. Thus, sulcal basins may be much more useful as entities for matching than entire sulci.

2.2. Automatic detection of sulcal basins from MR data

In the following, we will describe our algorithm for extracting sulcal basins from MR images. Sulcal basins are concavities in the white matter surface, so that in principle it would be possible to detect sulcal basins by simply computing curvature properties of the white matter surface. However, the white matter surface is highly convoluted and the MR data sets have a limited spatial resolution, so that the computation of second-order differentials becomes quite inaccurate. As a consequence, we found that curvature computations are not feasible for our purpose.

Therefore, we use a different approach which is not based on curvature properties. The method consists of a sequence of image analysis steps which are illustrated in Fig. 2. The input data set [Fig. 2(a)] is first subjected to a white matter segmentation which separates white matter from other tissue classes [Fig. 2(b)]. This step helps to make the sulcal indentations more pronounced and thus more easily identifiable.

A large number of segmentation algorithms are known from the literature. Any suitable segmentation procedure can be used here. A general segmentation algorithm that produces satisfactory results for all types of input data does not exist at this point, so that the choice of a suitable

algorithm and its parameters still very much depends on the type of data at hand. In our experiments, we used both simple thresholding techniques, as well as a new algorithm based on region growing (Lohmann, 1997).

We then close the sulci using a 3D morphological closing filter (Maragos and Schafer, 1990) to obtain an idealized smoothed surface [Fig. 2(c)]. We use a structuring element of spherical shape with a very large diameter. The exact size of the diameter is not critical as long as it is large enough. We subtract the white matter from the morphologically closed image so that only the sulcal interiors remain [Fig. 2(d)].

At this point in the procedure, the processed image contains the union of all sulcal basins. We now need to separate the individual basins by trying to find the ridges between them. These ridges can be viewed as 'watersheds' so that an approach reminiscent of a watershed segmentation is applicable.

The basic idea is to first identify a locally deepest region at the bottom of each basin, and then to allow each such region to grow until all sulcal interiors are filled up.

We define sulcal depth using a 3D distance transform with respect to the morphologically closed image depicted in Fig. 2(c). The distance transform attaches a distance label to each white voxel in Fig. 2(c) which encodes its 3D Euclidean distance towards the nearest black voxel. In our application, we are only interested in the depth of each sulcal interior voxel. Note that this depth might sometimes be underestimated if measured along a path that traverses white matter. Therefore, we use a variation of the ordinary distance transform called 'constrained distance transform'

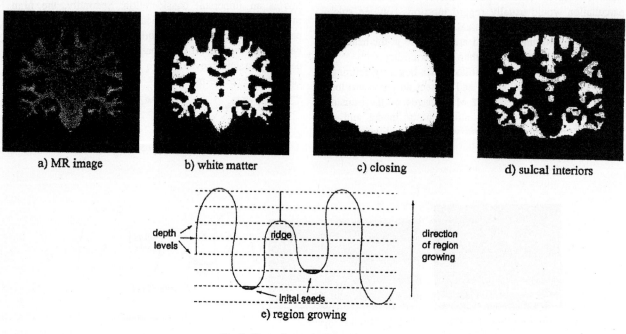

a) MR image   b) white matter   c) closing   d) sulcal interiors

e) region growing

Fig. 2. The major steps of the algorithm.

(Verbeek et al., 1986; Verwer et al., 1989) which allows us to explicitly prohibit measuring the length of paths that lead through the white matter.

Once each voxel is depth-encoded, we search for locally deepest points by moving a search window of size $n \times n \times n$ across the image where typically $n = 7$. Adjoining deepest points that are of almost equal depth and are close are merged into one larger patch so that perturbations due to noise are eliminated. In our experiments we used a 3D morphological closing filter with a sphere-shaped structuring element with a diameter of 3 voxels to achieve this.

We then let each initial island grow in a manner similar to region growing until a separating ridge is encountered. During region growing, successively higher levels are processed so that at each stage in the procedure, only voxels at the current depth level are added to a sulcal basin [Fig. 2(e)].

Note that the parcellation of the cortex induced by this algorithm is complete as each voxel in a sulcal interior is a member of some depth level and is therefore processed at some point and assigned to some basin. A pseudocode version of the region growing procedure is listed in Table 1.

This algorithm is used to segment the lateral sulcal basins. The Sylvian fissure cannot be well segmented by the algorithm described above because of its more complicated shape. Note that the ventricles are also cavities in the white matter and might therefore be falsely segmented as basins. However, the ventricles are very much deeper than the lateral sulci and can therefore be easily excluded by using a depth threshold, which in our experiments was set to 3 cm.

In a final postprocessing step, adjacent regions are merged if the ridge that separates them is not high enough. The height of a ridge is given through the depth encoding discussed earlier. More precisely, let $depth(R)$ and $depth(S)$ denote the depths of two basins R and S, where the depth of a basin is defined as the depth of its deepest voxel. The depth of a ridge denoted by $depth(R, S)$ is defined as the depth of the deepest voxel that is adjacent to both R and S.

In our experiments, two basins R, S were merged if $depth(R) - depth(R, S) < threshold$ and $depth(S) - depth(R, S) < threshold$ where $threshold$ was set to about 1

Table 1
Region growing algorithm

```
currentdepth ← maxdepth
while currentdepth > 0 {
  for each voxel v in sulcal interior {
    if depth(v) < currentdepth {
      if v is not yet assigned to a region {
        assign v to the region to which it is closest
      }
    }
  }
  currentdepth ← currentdepth − decrement
}
```

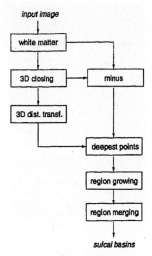

Fig. 3. Flow diagram.

mm. The above considerations induce a concept of adjacency between basins that will be used again later on.

Fig. 3 shows a data flow diagram of the entire basin segmentation procedure. Fig. 4 shows the result of a segmentation. To allow a better view into the deepest parts of the sulci, several layers of depth are morphologically eroded.

3. Automatic labelling of sulcal basins

In the following, we will describe a method of automatically attaching neuroanatomical labels to the sulcal basins that have been segmented using the procedures described in the previous sections. It is based on a model matching procedure that employs a point distribution model for describing spatial variations as well as shape similarity measures.

3.1. The shape model

Our anatomical model contains both a volumetric description of the 'mean' shape of each sulcal basin as well as a model which describes possible variations in the location of basins.

We identified 38 left-hemispheric basins that could be located across most subjects. Neuroanatomical labels for these 38 basins are listed in Appendix A.

The mean shape of these basins are obtained by averaging across a set of training images. More precisely, we segment basins from several MR images and manually attach anatomical labels to all basins found in each image. Basins for which no meaningful label can be found are given a special null label which by convention is set to $k = 1$.

In order to obtain a characterization of the mean shape for basins we simply perform a pixelwise average as

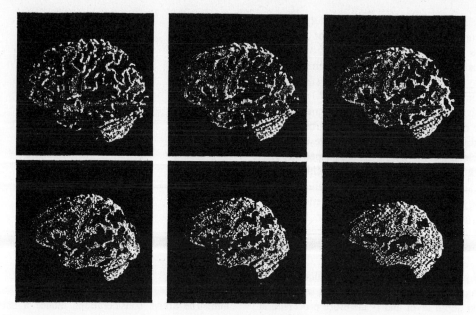

Fig. 4. Segmentation of sulcal basins. Several depth layers are eroded to permit a better view into the sulcal fundi.

follows. First we rotated and translated all data sets into a common coordinate system with AC (anterior commissure) at the origin of the system. We also performed a linear scaling along all three coordinate axes to compensate for differences in brain size.

Let $i = 1, \ldots, N$ denote the training images, and $k = 2, \ldots, n$ denote the basin labels, and let $x_i^k \in R^3$ denote the center of gravity of the kth basin in the ith data set. Then the mean location of basin k is calculated as

$$\bar{m}_k = \frac{1}{N} \sum_{i=1}^{N} x_i^k.$$

In order to correct for overall brain shape differences – in particular for variations in the locations of major sulci – we first shift each basin separately into its mean location as

defined above. We do not, however, correct for rotational variations of sulci as the orientation is quite characteristic of sulci and should be preserved. At each pixel location in stereotactic space we record the number of images in which this pixel is occupied by each basin label. A voxel is defined to belong to the mean shape of basin k if this number is larger than a given threshold. In our experiments, we used a threshold of $t = 5$ out of 15 training data sets.

The mean shape captures the average position as well as the average geometrical outline. Fig. 5(a) shows the resulting mean shapes for all 38 basins with the exception of basins belonging to the Sylvian fissure.

Note that the Procrustes mean shape as described in Goodall (1991) and Bookstein (1997) would not have been suitable in our context. The Procrustes mean shape does

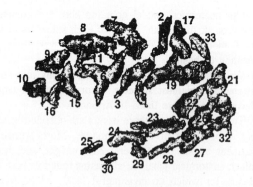

a) Mean shapes of basins.

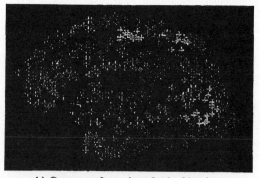

b) Centers of gravity of sulcal basins

Fig. 5. (a) The model shapes of sulcal basins. These were obtained by averaging basins segmented from 15 training data sets. (b) The centers of gravity of the training set basins.

not capture rotational and translational characteristics of the shape. However, in our domain, the orientation (i.e. rotation) and position are crucial aspects of the mean shape.

3.2. The spatial distribution model

In order to represent allowable variations in the location of sulcal basins we use the point distribution model as introduced by Cootes et al. (1995). Point distribution models (PDMs) require sets of landmark points as training data. In our application, the landmark data are entire volumetric objects, namely the sulcal basins that have been segmented and hand-labelled from MRI data.

In order to be able to employ the point distribution approach, we only use the centers of gravity of each basin as landmarks. Fig. 5(b) shows the location of these points. We can then estimate the average location of sulcal basins as well as variations in their location as follows (see also (Cootes et al., 1995)).

Let N be the number of training data sets, and let n be the number of basins contained in the model. Further, let $x_i \in R^{3n}$ denote the locations of all n basins in the ith data set. Then the mean location is calculated as

$$\bar{x} = \frac{1}{N} \sum_{i=1}^{N} x_i.$$

Note that this time the mean location is calculated across all basins and all training images. For each training set, the deviation from the mean location is calculated using

$$d_i = x_i - \bar{x},$$

with the $3n \times 3n$ covariance matrix given by

$$S = \frac{1}{N} \sum_{i=1}^{N} d_i \, d_i^{\mathsf{T}}.$$

The main modes of variation in the location of the training points are determined by a principal component analysis such that the first eigenvector of the covariance matrix describes the most significant variation.

Each training instance x can be recovered from the covariance matrix and the mean location vector as a linear combination of eigenvectors using

$$x = \bar{x} + Pb,$$

where $P = (p_1, \ldots, p_t)$ is the matrix of the first t eigenvectors and $b = (b_1, \ldots, b_t)$ is a vector of weights. New instances of the model can be constructed by allowing the parameters b_k to vary within acceptable ranges.

Fig. 6 illustrates the first two modes of variation applied to a sulcal line representation of one individual data set. Sulcal lines are polygonal representations of the cortical folding as described in (Lohmann, 1998).

3.3. Model matching

Matching the model to an individual data set requires us to find a vector b of weights that yields a new instance x of the PDM model that corresponds more closely to the individual data set. This task can be cast into an optimization problem.

The goal function that we seek to minimize is defined as follows. Consider the raster image shown in Fig. 2(d) containing the sulcal interiors. It is obtained by a subtraction of the white matter segmentation from the morphological closure as explained before. We now perform a 3D distance transform on this image (Borgefors, 1984; Saito and Toriwaki, 1994) such that each black voxel obtains a distance label that encodes its distance towards the nearest white voxel.

The goal function is obtained by adding all distance values which are covered by a non-zero voxel of the model basins. More precisely, let $j = 1, \ldots, m$ denote voxel sites in stereotactic space with m being the number of voxel sites. For the individual data set whose basins we want to label, let $dist_j$, $j = 1, \ldots, m$, denote the distance of the voxel at position j towards the nearest white voxel where the distance is obtained as described above.

For the model image containing the model basins, let $\chi_j = 1$ iff the voxel at position j in the model image belongs to some basin in the deformed model, and $\chi_j = 0$

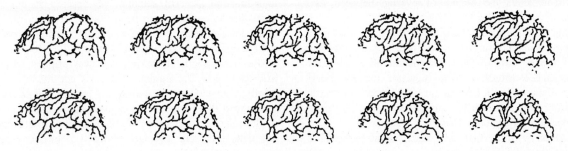

Fig. 6. The two main modes of variation. The top row shows the variation pertaining to the first eigenvector. Its main anatomical characteristic appears to be a variation in the size of the frontal brain versus the posterior brain. The second row shows the variation pertaining to the second eigenvector. The variation ranges between $-\sqrt{\lambda_k}$ and $+\sqrt{\lambda_k}$, $k = 0,1$ with eigenvalues λ_k, $k = 0,1$.

if it does not belong to any basin. Then the quality of the match is defined as

$$\sum_{j=1}^{m} \chi_j \mathrm{dist}_j.$$

Thus, large discrepancies between the model image and the sulcal interior image are penalized.

The optimization process seeks to find a weight vector $b = (b_1, \ldots, b_t)$ that generates an instance

$$x = \bar{x} + Pb$$

of the PDM model that minimizes the goal function where $P = (p_1, \ldots, p_t)$ is the matrix of the first t eigenvectors of the PDM covariance matrix. Note that x defines new centers of gravity for all model basins. Thus, it describes translations of the model basins, their shape, however, is not altered.

We use Powell's optimization method (Press et al., 1992) to solve this optimization problem. In order to avoid local minima, a number of different starting values are tested.

3.4. Assignment of labels

Once the model is deformed to an individual data set, we can use it to attribute anatomical labels to sulcal basins. However, this task is not trivial as the model basins will not completely overlap with the basins found in the individual data set. Therefore, we need a shape similarity measure for identifying the best match.

We use the Hausdorff distance metric (Huttenlocher et al., 1993) for this purpose. The Hausdorff metric is defined as follows. Let $A = \{a_1, \ldots, a_p\}$ and $B = \{b_1, \ldots, b_q\}$ be two sets of points in R^3. Then the Hausdorff distance between A and B is defined as

$$H(A,B) = \max(h(A,B), h(B,A)),$$

where

$$h(A,B) = \max_{a \in A} \min_{b \in B} \|a - b\|.$$

The function $h(A,B)$ ranks each point of A with respect to its distance to B, and uses the largest distance as the result. Thus, it captures the degree of overlap between two shapes.

Using the Hausdorff metric we measure the distances between basins of the individual data set towards the shifted model basins. Thus, we obtain an assignment matrix $X_{kl} \in R$ where $X_{kl} \in R$ indicates the Hausdorff distance between basin l in the individual data set towards the shifted model basin k. We can now simply attribute the label that has the smallest Hausdorff distance.

Occasionally, more than one match might be possible for some basin. In order to resolve such ambiguities we use Sinkhorn's assignment procedure as described by Gold and Rangarajan (1996). This procedure amounts to an iterative update of the matching matrix until the match becomes unique.

3.4.1. Composite basins

In some cases, the basin segmentation procedure fails to detect a ridge between two basins. For instance in about 10% of the cases, the central sulcus was not segmented into two basins but into just one. Note, however, that the absence of a basin or the merger of two basins does not necessarily indicate a segmentation error. Such an event may also be due to anatomical variation. In order to distinguish between the two, we compute depth images such as the one shown in Fig. 4. An erroneous segmentation is present if two basins are segmented as one basin even though they appear separate in at least one depth level. In fact, a truly erroneous segmentation occurred in only one basin of one data set out of 37 data sets. In the remainder of the cases, the separating ridges were either not present or they were below the spatial resolution of our MRI data.

In order to deal with merged basins, we additionally use 'composite' basins which are composed of two or more model basins. At present we use four composite basins: a basin representing the central sulcus (composed of basins 2 and 3), a basin representing the postcentral sulcus (basins 17 and 19), and a basin representing the superior temporal sulcus (basins 22, 23 and 24).

These composite basins enter the assignment procedure just like any other basin. In cases where the segmentation was too coarse they provide a better match.

4. Experiments and results

Our input data consisted of 37 T1-weighted magnetic resonance images (MRI) of healthy volunteers. The spatial resolution between planes was approx. 1.5 mm and the within-plane resolution was set to approx. 0.95 mm×0.95 mm. The images were subsequently resampled to obtain isotropic voxels of size 1 mm×1 mm×1 mm so that each data set contained 160 slices with 200 × 160 pixels in each slice. As noted before, all data sets were rotated into a standard stereotactic coordinate system and linearly scaled to a uniform size. In addition, we applied an automatic procedure to extract brain from non-brain material. For a more detailed description of our preprocessing procedure see (Kruggel and Lohmann, 1997).

Our basin segmentation method was applied to all 37 MR data sets. The model graph was acquired by hand-labelling the sulcal basins extracted from 15 of these data sets, and a PDM model was derived as described above.

The matching procedure was then applied to all remaining data sets. On average, about 1.5 basins received incorrect labels. Note that the number of basins varies across subjects. The assignment procedure prevented multiple matches. Only the null label was allowed to be assigned to several basins. Large major basins never received a null label. The assignment of the null label to a small basin was not counted as an error because those assignments are problematic in any case.

Most errors occurred in areas where interindividual variability is largest. Particular problem areas were the intermediate frontal sulcus which was sometimes confused with either the superior or the inferior frontal sulcus. Most

errors involved only small parts of secondary or tertiary sulci. In each case, the correctly labelled area equalled much more than 90% of the entire labelled area.

The Sylvian fissure and insula, however, cannot be adequately segmented with our present approach. This is due to the fact that the watershed mechanism does not really capture the complex shape of these structures. Therefore, the Sylvian fissure is not suitably represented in

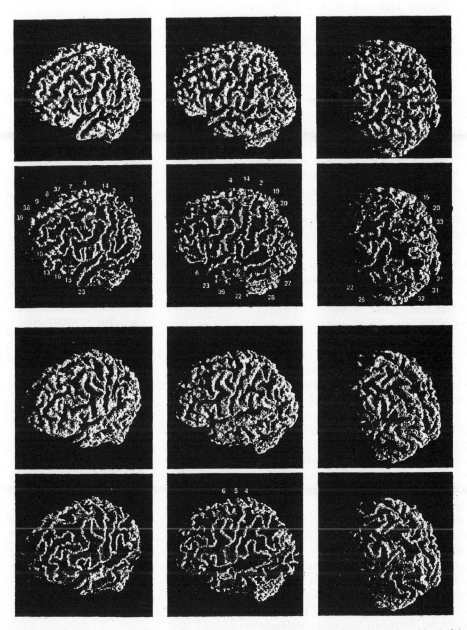

Fig. 7. Results of the basin labelling procedure applied to two data sets. The top rows show the white matter segmentation with sulcal depth color-coded in shades of blue. The bottom rows show the labelling results. The colors correspond to nodes in the model graph. Note that corresponding basins can be identified in both brains. However, there are basins that appear in one data set, but not in the other (e.g. basin 5).

our basin model. We are currently in the process of developing methods that specifically address this problem.

The computation time for the basin segmentation was approximately 4:30 min on an SGI Unix workstation. The model matching algorithm also takes about 4:30 min per data set. Fig. 7 shows the result of the sulcal labelling applied to two data sets. The white matter segmentations are also shown to provide better visual clues.

5. Conclusion and future work

We have presented a method that automatically detects and attributes neuroanatomical names to substructures of the cortical folds which we call sulcal basins using magnetic resonance data of healthy human brains.

The labelling process is cast as a model matching process involving a point distribution model and a label assignment process using the Hausdorff distance metric and Sinkhorn's assignment algorithm. The PDM model is used here in a somewhat unusual manner. Normally, PDM models are used to describe shape contours, whereas here we use it to model locations of volumetric objects. However, it is quite well suited for this task as it yields a spatial model that is specific enough to exclude illegal instances but general enough to permit all possible variations.

Currently, our model covers the entire lateral surface of the left hemisphere where it provides a complete parcellation of the cortex. Future work will aim at expanding the model to include both hemispheres, as well as the medial and basal surfaces of the brain.

The experiments have shown that sulcal basins can indeed be segmented and labelled reliably and reproducibly. However, the correctness of a labelling cannot be easily assessed as even human experts do not always agree on the assignment of neuroanatomical labels. This is particularly true for small tertiary sulci for which no well-established anatomical names exist. But even some parts of secondary sulci such as the superior frontal sulcus are often difficult to identify visually. Therefore, quantitative assessments of the classification accuracy are somewhat dubious. The numbers given in the preceding section are based on visual inspection by a human expert.

Future work will include a refinement of the basin segmentation. So far, sulcal basins are rather large, and will have to be subdivided into smaller units.

The most important aspect of our future work will be however to provide a neuro-psychological validation for our concept of sulcal basins. Of particular interest are correlations between sulcal basin labellings and functional activations measured by functional magnetic resonance imaging (fMRI) studies. We expect to find that functional activations fall into equivalent basins across subjects.

Some preliminary experiments indicate that this may indeed be the case (Lohmann and von Cramon, 1999b).

Appendix A

In Table 2 a list of neuroanatomical labels is given. The identification numbers correspond to the numbers given in Figs. 5 and 7.

Table 2

Id	Neuroanatomical name
1	Unknown
2	Superior central sulcus
3	Inferior central sulcus
4	Superior precentral sulcus
5	Medial precentral sulcus
6	Inferior precentral sulcus
7	Superior frontal sulcus 1
8	Superior frontal sulcus 2
9	Superior frontal sulcus 3
10	Superior frontal sulcus 4 (anterior portion)
11	Intermediate frontal sulcus
12	Intermediate frontal sulcus
13	Intermediate frontal sulcus
14	Marginal sup. basin (posterior)
15	Inferior frontal sulcus
16	Lateral orbital sulcus
17	Superior postcentral sulcus
18	Inferior postcentral sulcus
19	Intraparietal sulcus (ascending branch)
20	Intraparietal sulcus (horizontal branch)
21	Intraparietal sulcus (descending branch)
22	Superior temporal sulcus 1 (posterior portion)
23	Superior temporal sulcus 2
24	Superior temporal sulcus 3
25	Superior temporal sulcus 4 (polar portion)
26	Medial temporal sulcus
27	Inferior temporal sulcus 1 (posterior portion)
28	Inferior temporal sulcus 2
29	Inferior temporal sulcus 3
30	Inferior temporal sulcus 4 (anterior portion)
31	Occipital basin
32	Inferior occipital sulcus
33	Transverse parietal basin
34	Sylvian fissure (anterior)
35	Sylvian fissure (medial)
36	Sylvian fissure (posterior)
37	Marginal sup.frontal basin
38	Marginal sup. frontal basin
39	Marginal sup. frontal basin

References

Bookstein, F.L., 1997. Shape and the information in medical images: a decade of morphometric synthesis. Comput. Vision and Image Understanding 66 (2), 97–118.

Borgefors, G., 1984. Distance transforms in arbitrary dimensions. Comput. Vision, Graphics and Image Proc. 27, 321–345.

Caunce A., Taylor, C.J., 1999. Using local geometry to build 3D sulcal models. In: Int. Conf. on Information Processing in Medical Imaging (IPMI 99). Visegrad, Hungary, 28 June–2 July, pp. 197–209.

Chui, H., Rambo, J., Duncan, J., Schultz, R., Rangarajan, A., 1999. Registration of cortical anatomical structures via robust 3D point matching. In: Int. Conf. on Information Processing in Medical Imaging (IPMI 99). Visegrad, Hungary, 28 June–2 July, pp. 169–181.

Cootes, T.F., Taylor, C.J., Cooper, D.H., Graham, J., 1995. Active shape models–their training and application. Comput. Vision and Image Understanding 61 (1), 38–59.

Declerck, J., Subsol, G., Thirion, J.-P., Ayache, N., 1995. Automatic retrieval of anatomical structures in 3D medical images. In: Proc. Computer Vision, Virtual Reality and Robotics in Medicine, (CVRMed 95). Nice, France, April 1995, pp. 153–162.

Gold, S., Rangarajan, A., 1996. A graduated assignment algorithm for graph matching. IEEE Trans. Pattern Anal. and Machine Intell. 18 (4), 377–388.

Goodall, C., 1991. Procrustes methods in the statistical analysis of shape. J. Roy. Stat. Soc. B53 (2), 285–339.

Goualher, G.L., Procyk, E., Collins, D.L., Venugopal, R., Barillot, C., Evans, A.C., 1999. Automated extraction and variability analysis of sulcal neuroanatomy. IEEE Trans. Med. Imaging 18 (3), 206–217.

Guéziec, A., Ayache, N., 1994. Smoothing and matching of 3-D space curves. Int. J. Comput. Vision 12 (1), 79–104.

Huttenlocher, D.P., Klanderman, G.A., Rucklidge, W.J., 1993. Comparing images using the Hausdorff distance. IEEE Trans. Patt. Anal. and Machine Intell. 15 (9), 850–863.

Kruggel, F., Lohmann, G., 1997. Automatic adaptation of the stereotactical coordinate system in brain MRI data sets. In: Int. Conf. on Information Processing in Medical Imaging (IPMI 97). Poultney, VT, USA, 9–13 June, 1997.

Lohmann, G., 1997. A new approach to segmenting white matter from magnetic resonance images of the human brain. Technical Report. Max-Planck-Institute of Cognitive Neuroscience, Leipzig, Germany.

Lohmann, G., 1998. Extracting line representations of sulcal and gyral patterns in MR images of the human brain. IEEE Trans. Med. Image Anal. 17 (6), 1040–1048.

Lohmann, G., von Cramon, D.Y., 1998a. Automatic detection and labelling of the human cortical folds in magnetic resonance data sets. In: ECCV (European Conference on Computer Vision). 2–6 June, 1998, Freiburg, Germany.

Lohmann, G., von Cramon, D.Y., 1998b. Sulcal basins and sulcal strings as new concepts for describing the human cortical topography. In: Workshop on Biomedical Image Analysis (WBIA). 26–27 June, 1998, Santa Barbara, CA.

Lohmann, G., von Cramon, D.Y., 1999a. Sulcal variability of twins. Cerebral Cortex 9, 754–763.

Lohmann, G., von Cramon, D.Y., 1999b. Using sulcal basins for analyzing

functional activations patterns in the human brain. In: 2nd Int. Conf. on Medical Image Computing and Computer-assisted Intervention (MICCAI). September 1999, Cambridge, UK, pp. 487–497.

Manceaux-Demiau, A., Mangin, J.F., Regis, J., Pizzato, O., Frouin, V., 1997. Differential features of cortical folds. In: Proc. CVR Med 97. Grenoble, France.

Mangin, J.-F., Frouin, V., Bloch, I., Régis, J., López-Krahe, J., 1995. From 3-D magnetic resonance images to structured representations of the cortex topography using topology preserving deformations. J. Math. Imaging and Vision 5 (4), 297–318.

Maragos, P., Schafer, R.W., 1990. Morphological systems for multidimensional signal processing. Proc. IEEE 78 (4), 690–709.

Maziotta, J.C., Toga, A.W., Evans, A., Fox, P., Lancaster, J., 1995. A probabilistic atlas of the human brain: theory and rationale for its development. Neuroimage 2, 89–101.

Ono, M., Kubik, S., Abernathy, C.D., 1990. Atlas of the Cerebral Sulci. Georg Thieme Verlag, Stuttgart, New York.

Press, W.H., Teukolsky, S.A., Vetterling, W.T., Flannery, B.P., 1992. Numerical Recipes in C, 2nd Edition. Cambridge University Press.

Regis, J., Mangin, J.F., Frouin, V., Sastre, F., Peragut, J.C., Samson, Y., 1995. Generic model for the localization of the cerebral cortex and preoperative multimodal integration in epilepsy surgery. In: Proc. of the Meeting of the American Society for Stereolactic and Functional Neurosurgery. Marina del Rey, pp. 72–80.

Rizzo, G., Scifo, P., Gilardi, M.C., Bettinardi, V., Grassi, F., Cerutti, S., Fazio, F., 1997. Matching a computerized brain atlas to multimodal medical images. Neuroimage 6 (1), 59–69.

Saito, T., Toriwaki, J.-I., 1994. New algorithms for Euclidean distance transformation of an n-dimensional digitized picture with applications. Patt. Recog. 27 (11), 1551–1565.

Sandor, S., Leahy, R., 1997. Surface-based labeling of cortical anatomy using a deformable atlas. IEEE Trans. Med. Imaging 16 (1), 41–54.

Thompson, P., Toga, A.W., 1996. A surface-based technique for warping three-dimensional images of the brain. IEEE Trans. Med. Imaging 15 (4), 402–417.

Thompson, P., MacDonald, D., Mega, M.S., Holmes, C.J., Evans, A.C., Toga, A.W., 1997. Detection and mapping of abnormal brain structure with a probabilistic atlas of cortical surfaces. J. Comput. Ass. Tomography 21 (4), 567–581.

Vaillant, M., Davatzikos, C., 1999. Hierarchical matching of cortical features for deformable brain image segmentation. In: Int. Conf. on Information Processing in Medical Imaging (IPMI 99). Visegrad, Hungary, 28 June–2 July, pp. 183–195.

Verbeek, P.W., Dorst, L., Verwer, B.J.H., Groen, F.C.A., 1986. Collision avoidance and path finding through constrained distance transformation in robot state space. In: Proc. Intelligent Autonomous Systems. Amsterdam, The Netherlands, pp. 634–641.

Verwer, B.J., Verbeek, P.W., Dekker, S.T., 1989. An efficient uniform cost algorithm applied to distance transforms. IEEE Trans. Patt. Anal. and Machine Intell. 11 (4), 425–429.

Rapid 3-D Cone-Beam Reconstruction with the Simultaneous Algebraic Reconstruction Technique (SART) Using 2-D Texture Mapping Hardware

Klaus Mueller* and Roni Yagel

Abstract—**Algebraic reconstruction methods, such as the algebraic reconstruction technique (ART) and the related simultaneous ART (SART), reconstruct a two–dimensional (2-D) or three–dimensional (3-D) object from its X-ray projections. The algebraic methods have, in certain scenarios, many advantages over the more popular Filtered Backprojection approaches and have also recently been shown to perform well for 3-D cone-beam reconstruction. However, so far the slow speed of these iterative methods have prohibited their routine use in clinical applications. In this paper, we address this shortcoming and investigate the utility of widely available 2-D texture mapping graphics hardware for the purpose of accelerating the 3-D algebraic reconstruction. We find that this hardware allows 3-D cone-beam reconstructions to be obtained at almost interactive speeds, with speed-ups of over 50 with respect to implementations that only use general-purpose CPUs. However, we also find that the reconstruction quality is rather sensitive to the resolution of the framebuffer, and to address this critical issue we propose a scheme that extends the precision of a given framebuffer by 4 bits, using the color channels. With this extension, a 12-bit framebuffer delivers useful reconstructions for 0.5% tissue contrast, while an 8-bit framebuffer requires 4%. Since graphics hardware generates an entire image for each volume projection, it is most appropriately used with an algebraic reconstruction method that performs volume correction at that granularity as well, such as SART or SIRT. We chose SART for its faster convergence properties.**

Index Terms—**Algebraic reconstruction technique (ART), computed tomography, cone beam reconstruction, hardware acceleration, simultaneous algebraic reconstruction technique (SART), three—dimensional reconstruction.**

I. INTRODUCTION

THE ALGEBRAIC reconstruction technique (ART), first proposed by Gordon *et al.* [8], tomographically reconstructs a three–dimensional (3-D) object from its projection images. These images may be obtained from any projective imaging modality, such as X-Ray, positron emission tomography, or single photon emission computed tomography. ART is an iterative method and reconstructs the volumetric object by a sequence of alternating volume projections and correction backprojections. The volume projection measures how close the current state of the volume matches the corresponding scanner projection, while in the backprojection step a corrective image is distributed onto the volume. Many such projection/backprojection operations are typically required to make the volume fit all projections in the acquired set. Different ART variants exist: While the original ART corrects the volume on a ray-basis, simultaneous ART (SART) [2] corrects the volume only after a whole projection image has been computed.[1]

In this paper, we concentrate on reconstruction from cone-beam data (parallel-beam reconstruction can be treated as a special case). Although there are no specially designed clinical cone-beam scanners as yet, the advent of 3-D reconstruction angiography using C-arm scanners (see, e.g., [1]) has recently brought cone-beam computed tomography (CT) into the arena of real clinical application. Another recent application of cone-beam CT is in radiotherapy: In an approach termed tomotheraphy [14], the MV radiation unit is not only used to administer and measure the radio-therapeutical dose, it is also employed to collect the necessary data for a 3-D reconstruction of the patient immediately before treatment. Using this 3-D reconstruction one can then register the treatment plan with the patient's position to ensure optimal tumor targeting.

Although the majority of the proposed cone-beam algorithms are based on filtered backprojection (FBP) (refer to, e.g., [22], [25] for comparisons and reviews), more recent research [16] has demonstrated that both ART (with certain modifications) and SART can reconstruct general cone-beam data as well, at high accuracy and even for large cone-angles of up to 60°. But the iterative process is slow [17], and this lack of computational speed has so far prevented ART from being used in real-life clinical applications. This is unfortunate since there are quite a few scenarios in which ART has advantages over the more commonly used FBP. For example, the use of ART seems advantageous when one does not have a large set of projections available, when the projections are not distributed uniformly in angle, or when the projections are sparse or missing at certain orientations [3], [11]. Scenarios of this sort occur in both 3-D reconstruction angiography and tomotheraphy. In the latter, one can simply not obtain a large number of MV projections due to the enormous patient dose, and recent research has shown [20]

Manuscript received May 5, 1999; revised September 6, 2000. The Associate Editor responsible for coordinating the review of this paper and recommending its publication was C. Crawford. *Asterisk indicates corresponding author.*

*K. Mueller was with the Department of Computer and Information Science, Ohio State University, Columbus, OH 43210 USA and Biomedicom, Ltd., Manachet Technology Park Malha, Jerusalem 91487, Israel. He is now with the Department of Computer Science, State University of New York, Stony Brook, NY 11794-4400 USA (e-mail: muellerk@acm.org).

R. Yagel was with the Department of Computer and Information Science, Ohio State University, Columbus, OH 43210 USA and Biomedicom, Ltd., Manachet Technology Park Malha, Jerusalem 91487, Israel. He is now with Insight Therapeutics, Petach Tikva 49170, Israel.

Publisher Item Identifier S 0278-0062(00)10616-0.

[1]For the remainder of this section, we will use the term ART to stand for both variants of algebraic reconstruction methods: ART and SART.

that ART can produce a reconstruction with good feature delineation even with just 24 MV projections. On the other hand, in 3-D reconstruction angiography one may want to reconstruct a four–dimensional (4-D) volume of the coronary arteries in a beating heart, and the number of projections that can be obtained with a safe dose of radio-opaque dye may be limited here as well.

Thus, cone-beam ART has a number of clinical applications for which it appears useful, if only its computational speed could be improved. It was already shown in [16] that two to three iterations with 80 projections are sufficient to reconstruct a low-contrast 3-D object. However, still more than 1.5 hrs are needed on a modern workstation to reconstruct a 128^3 volume from 80 projections. As a remedy, one could build dedicated ART computer boards and incorporate those into the clinical scanners, along with the usual custom digital signal processing (DSP) chips which already run the FBP algorithm extremely fast. However, designing and configuring special chips or boards to implement our ART and SART algorithms would be a rather expensive and tedious task, and it would produce narrow devices with little room for modifications and adaptations of the algorithms, hampering the evolution of technology. Fortunately, today's widely available graphics workstations provide us with another option, as the graphics hardware resident in these workstations is especially designed for fast projection operations, the main ingredients of the algebraic algorithms. A plus of this hardware choice is the growing availability of these machines in hospitals, where they are more and more utilized in the daily task of medical visualization, diagnosis, and surgical planning. The feature of these graphics workstations that we will rely on most is *texture mapping*, a technique that is commonly used to enhance the realism of polygonal graphics objects by painting pictures onto them prior to display. Texture mapping is not always, but often, implemented in hardware, and runs at fill rates of over 100 Megapixels/s. However, hardware texture mapping is not limited to graphics workstations only, many manufacturers offer graphics boards with texture-mapping capabilities that can be added to any modern PC.

In this paper, we will thoroughly investigate the utility and applicability of texture mapping hardware for the purpose of 3-D reconstruction with algebraic methods. Earlier, this hardware was also used by Cabral *et al.* to accelerate the FBP algorithm [5]. Our programs were written using the widely accepted OpenGL application programming interface (API) [21] and can easily be reproduced to run on any medium-range graphics workstation or PC with graphics board. Since graphics hardware generates an entire image for each volume projection, it is most appropriately used with an algebraic reconstruction method that performs volume correction at that granularity as well, such as SART.[2] This constraint does not impose a restriction in terms of the reconstruction result, since it was demonstrated in [16] that both cone-beam ART and SART deliver reconstructions of similar quality at similar convergence rates. We, hence, refer to our proposed approach as texture-mapping hardware accelerated *SART* (or *TMA-SART*).

---

[2]We could have chosen SIRT [7] as well, but its convergence rate is much slower than that of SART.

The outline of the paper is as follows: After a brief introduction to SART in Section II, we describe the general approach of TMA-SART in Section III. Then, in Section IV, we extend the functionality of TMA-SART to improve accuracy and also speed. Finally, Section V presents results, and Section VI discusses the prospects, impact, and future of TMA-SART in light of current graphics hardware trends.

II. PRELIMINARIES

In tomographic reconstruction with algebraic methods it is our goal to solve the following simultaneous equation system[3]:

$$P_i = \sum_{j=1}^{N} w_{ij} v_j \qquad (1)$$

We would like to recover the values v_j of the $N = n^3$ voxels j in the volume, using the values p_i of the pixels i in the scanner images P_φ, where φ is the source/detector orientation at which the projection was taken by the scanner, assuming a planar source/detector orbit (without loss of generality). In (1), a w_{ij} is the weight with which a voxel j contributes its value to a pixel i. SART solves this equation by an iterative procedure, in which the correction/update for a voxel j, to be performed for each volume correction step k, is written as follows:

$$v_j^{(k)} = v_j^{(k-1)} + \lambda \frac{\displaystyle\sum_{p_i \in P_\varphi} \left(\frac{p_i - \displaystyle\sum_{l=1}^{N} w_{il} v_l^{(k-1)}}{\displaystyle\sum_{l=1}^{N} w_{il}} \right) w_{ij}}{\displaystyle\sum_{p_i \in P_\varphi} w_{ij}}. \qquad (2)$$

In (2), λ is a relaxation factor, typically chosen $\ll 1.0$. The collective voxel update procedure of SART can be broken down into several steps, illustrated in Fig. 1.

A line integral can be computed by sampling the volume at equidistant locations using some interpolation kernel (trilinear, Gaussian, or cubic spline) and forming the integral via the trapezoidal rule [2], [10]. Alternatively, one can take an approach in which one thinks of the volume as being decomposed into a field of (overlapping) 3-D interpolation kernels, with one such kernel placed at each voxel location (the grid line intersections) and attenuated by the voxel's value v_j. The weight w_{ij} that a voxel has on a ray r_i is then the line integral of the traversed voxel kernel function [12]. Using this representation, volume projection and backprojection can be performed by a procedure termed *splatting* [26], in which the kernel integrals are preintegrated into tables (so-called *footprints*) and mapped to the image plane where they accumulate into the projection image or retrieve the voxel corrections (more detail is given in [17]). The less discretized integration of the splatting methods yields more accurate weight factors and, as a consequence, more accurate projections/backprojections.

---

[3]We will use the following terminology: the basic elements of the reconstructed volume are the voxels ν while the bins in the projection images are referred to as pixels p.

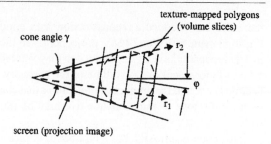

SART algorithm

Initialize volume

Until convergence

  Select a projection P_φ

  Image projection:

    Compute line integrals for all rays r_i starting at pixels p_i of P_φ

    (the $\sum\limits_{l=1}^{N} w_{il} v_l^{(k-1)}$ in (1) are the line integrals, the $\sum\limits_{l=1}^{N} w_{il}$ are closely related to the ray lengths)

  Correction image computation:

    (expression in parentheses in the nominator of (1))

    For all p_i

      Subtract the calculated line integrals from the p_i's in the acquired images

      Normalize by ray length

  Image backprojection:

    Distribute normalized corrections, weighted by w_{ij}, onto voxels

    Normalize accumulated corrections by the sum of weights $\sum\limits_{p_i \in P_\varphi} w_{ij}$

    Scale by λ

Fig. 1. The steps of the SART algorithm.

Although it is possible to simulate the splatting approach in hardware, using polygon-mounted, voxel-weighted texture maps for each voxel's kernel footprint, this approach tends to be rather slow, since the granularity of this approach (on the order of voxels) is too small to be efficient [18]. We now describe an approach with higher granularity (on the order of volume slices) that offers more promise.

III. TMA-SART COMPONENTS

In TMA-SART, some of the blocks in Fig. 1 can be accelerated by the graphics hardware, while others have to be performed on the CPU. We will now describe the basic TMA-SART algorithm in terms of the decomposition of Fig. 1.

A. Projection

TMA-SART decomposes the volume into n slices and treats each slice separately. In volume projection [shown in Fig. 2(a)], each slice is associated with a square polygon that has the volumetric slice content texture-mapped onto it. Rotating this texture-mapped polygon by the scanner orientation angle φ and perspectively projecting it with cone angle γ maps the voxels in this volume slice, properly weighted, onto the image pixels.[4]

Fig. 2(b) illustrates the projection algorithm, in which the slice-to-screen mapping is performed by the graphics hardware, but the accumulation of projections is done in software, due to the limited bit resolution of the framebuffer. After all n texture-mapped polygons have been accumulated in the software buffer, it contains the volume projection at projection angle φ.

Note that the hardware uses a bilinear interpolation kernel to resample the texture image into screen coordinates. Thus, the ray integrals so computed are equivalent to the ray integrals obtained in a software solution that uses a trilinear interpolation filter in conjunction with raycasting and samples the rays only within each volume slice. In this respect, the integration follows the trapezoidal rule and is similar to that obtained by Joseph's

[4]For reconstruction from parallel-beam data one just sets the viewing geometry to parallel projection.

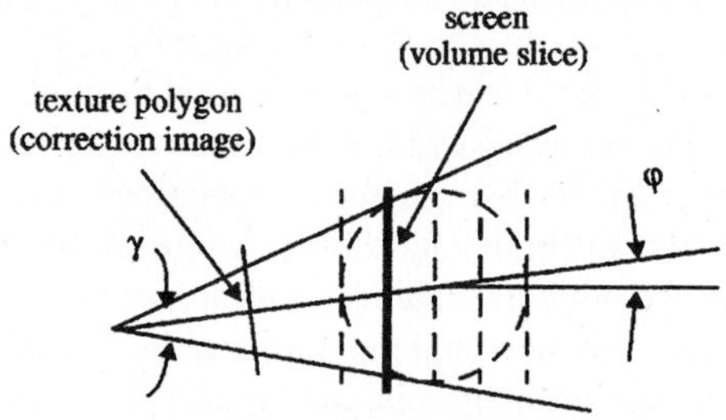

(a)

Fig. 2. Projection with TMA-SART. (a) Projection geometry [two-dimensional (2-D) case shown]. (b) Algorithm pseudocode.

(b)

> **TMA-SART Projection Algorithm**
>
> Initialize software accumulation buffer
>
> For each of the n volume slices
>
>   Rotate associated polygon by orientation angle φ
>
>   Texture map volume slice content onto polygon
>
>   Project texture-mapped polygon onto the screen
>
>   Read projection image from framebuffer
>
>   Add projection image to software accumulation buffer

Fig. 3. Impractical backprojection with TMA-SART (2-D case shown): the main viewing axis is not perpendicular to the screen, and the viewing axis does generally not traverse the volume slices at their center.

algorithm [10]. Continuing this analogy with raycasting, note that if we sample only within the volume slices, then the distance between sample points varies depending on the orientation of a ray with respect to the volume slices. A ray that is perpendicular to the volume slices has a sample spacing Δs of 1.0 [ray r_1 in Fig. 2(b)], while for a nonslice perpendicular ray $\Delta s < 1.0$ [ray r_2 in Fig. 2(b)]. Thus we have to normalize the calculated ray integrals in the projection image for this location-dependent sample spacing. To save these calculations during reconstruction, we instead normalize the images obtained from the scanner by the inverse amount in a preprocessing step. Further, since the hardware can only produce values in the range of $[0.0 \cdots 1.0]$, the acquired images are also scaled to the range $[0 \cdots n]$.

B. Correction Image Computation

After a projection image has been generated, the correction image is computed in software. (A hardware acceleration is not possible, due to the extended value ranges of the images involved.) First, the calculated projection image is subtracted from the acquired projection image. Then the resulting image is divided by the weight image at that orientation. A weight image holds the sum of weights in the denominator of the nominator in (2) for each pixel. Ideally, this sum of weights is equivalent to the intersection distance of a ray with a solid sphere, which could be calculated analytically. However, it is not exactly the same, due to the discretized ray integration and the interpolation round-off errors of the hardware. For this reason, we compute the weight images in the same fashion than the projections, by projecting a volume in which all voxels within the spherical reconstruction region have been set to 1.0 and all others have been set to zero. These weight images can be re-used for all reconstructions that have equivalent image acquisition spacings and cone angles. We simply load them from disk prior to reconstruction.

Finally, since the texture map can only hold values in the range $[0.0 \cdots 1.0]$, but the correction image may have values in the range $[-1.0 \cdots 1.0]$, we must scale and translate the values in the correction image to the $[0.0 \cdots 1.0]$ interval. Note that, in this way, the values in the volume slices are always in the range $[0.0 \cdots 1.0]$.

C. Backprojection

In backprojection, we need to distribute the correction image onto the volume slices. This is achieved by associating each volume slice, one by one, with the screen, onto which the correction image, mapped to a polygon, is rendered. Basically, this is the reverse situation of Fig. 2, with the screen now being a volume slice and the texture-mapped polygon being the correction image. Fig. 3 shows this configuration. We notice, however, that now the main viewing axis is no longer perpendicular to the screen, and neither does it always traverse the center of the screen (i.e., the volume slices). Although OpenGL does allow the viewing axis to be at an oblique angle, it is difficult, if not impossible, to set up the correct projection in presence of the second condition. Hence, a simple reversal of the forward projection to perform the backprojection is not feasible.

We shall now describe an approach that separates the screen from the volume slices, thus avoiding the problems stemming from the misalignment of the viewing axis with the screen center. Our approach uses the projective textures described by Segal *et al.* [23] and works just like a slide projector. Consider Fig. 4(a) where the method is illustrated: In contrast to the direct approach, the correction image is now first perspectively projected onto a polygon, which has been placed at the location of the volume slice that is to receive the backprojected correction. The image projected onto the polygon is then viewed by the framebuffer in parallel (orthographic) projection. In other words, the correction image is a slide (a projective texture) that is projected with a cone-beam "light" source onto a slide screen (the volume slice polygon), and the projected slide is then photographed by a parallel-beam camera (the framebuffer). The image captured in that way is the volume slice correction, properly weighted by bilinear interpolation. Note, however, that we must first scale and translate the values of the screen image back into the $[-1.0 \cdots 1.0]$ range before we can add it to the volume slice in memory. The resulting voxel values are then clamped to an interval of $[0.0 \cdots 1.0]$ and voxels outside the spherical reconstruction region are set to zero.

Let us now explain this slide-projector approach in some more detail, assuming a hardware implementation of OpenGL. In that case, when a polygon is projected onto the screen,

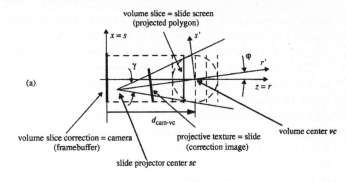

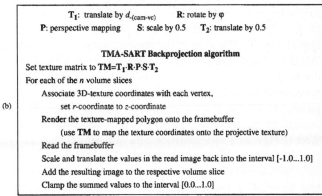

Fig. 4.   Volume backprojection with TMA-SART. (a) Projection geometry (2-D case shown). (b) Algorithm pseudocode.

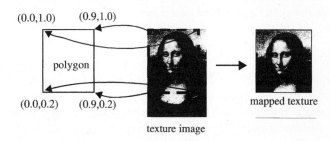

Fig. 5.   Texture mapping an image onto a polygon. The texture coordinates (s, t) assigned to the polygon vertices are given in parentheses.

the coordinates of its vertices are transformed by a sequence of hardware matrix operations, which may include a perspective transform and a perspective divide. (For more detail on these fundamental issues refer to [6] and [21].) A texture is an image indexed by 2–D coordinates in the range $[0.0 \cdots 1.0, 0.0 \cdots 1.0]$. When a texture is mapped onto a polygon, the polygon's vertices are associated with texture coordinates (s, t), as shown in Fig. 5. The viewing transformation (i.e., the world-to-screen mapping) of the polygon vertices yields a closed region on the screen. In a process called *scan conversion*, all pixels inside this region are assigned (via interpolation) texture coordinates within the range assigned to the bounding vertices. These texture coordinates are used to index the texture image. Note that the transformation can lead to a stretching or shrinking of the texture on the screen.

The texture mapping coordinates need not be 2-D. As a matter of fact, they can be up to 4-D (involving a homogeneous coordinate), just like the vertex coordinates. In addition, OpenGL provides a transformation facility, similar to the one supplied for vertex transformation, with which the interpolated texture coordinates can be transformed prior to indexing the texture image. We can use this facility to implement our virtual slide projector.

The algorithm proceeds as follows (see again Fig. 4). First, we create an array of n square texture coordinate polygons with vertex coordinates (s, t, r) and associate them with the volume slice polygons. We set the four (s, t) coordinates to $(n/2, n/2)$, $(-n/2, n/2)$, $(-n/2, -n/2)$, and $(n/2, -n/2)$, with n being the extent of the cubic volume. The r-coordinate is varied between $[d_{\text{cam}-\text{vc}} - n/2, d_{\text{cam}-\text{vc}} + n/2]$ ($d_{\text{cam}-\text{vc}}$ is the distance of the camera to the volume center), depending on the location of the volume slice polygon in camera space. Note, that the (s, t, r) texture coordinate system is aligned with the (x, y, z) spatial coordinate system of the camera, where it has its origin. When a volume slice polygon is parallel (orthographically) rendered to the screen (the framebuffer), the hardware generates the corresponding texture map coordinates. These are first transformed by the texture transformation matrix $\mathbf{TM}$ before indexing the texture image. To achieve the slide-projector effect, $\mathbf{TM}$ is built as a concatenation of a number of matrices [see Fig. 4(b)]. The first sequence of terms, $\mathbf{T_1} \cdot \mathbf{R}$, achieves the coordinate transform from the (s, t, r) volume coordinate system into the (s', t', r') slide-projector coordinate system, which has its origin at the volume center. The term $\mathbf{T_1} \cdot \mathbf{R}$ rotates each texture coordinate polygon about the volume center $\boldsymbol{vc}$ by the viewing angle φ. Next is the perspective mapping, achieved by the perspective matrix $\mathbf{P}$. Here, the distance between slide projector center and volume center is

$$ sc - vc = \frac{n/2}{\sin(\gamma/2)} \qquad (3) $$

and $\mathbf{P}$ is defined such that, after the perspective divide, the texture coordinates of the polygon portions that fall inside the slide projector cone assume values in the range $[-1.0 \cdots 1.0]$. This is the case in the configuration shown in Fig. 4(a). However, since we can only index the texture image within a range of $[0.0 \cdots 1.0]$, we need to scale and translate the perspective texture coordinates prior to the perspective divide and texture indexing. This is achieved by incorporating a scale and translation given by $\mathbf{S} \cdot \mathbf{T_2}$ into $\mathbf{TM}$. Thus, any texture coordinate (s, t, r) generated by viewing the volume slice polygon is transformed by $\mathbf{TM}$

$$ (s', t', r') = (s, t, r) \cdot \mathbf{TM}. \qquad (4) $$

The perspective divide then produces the texture index (s_t, t_t):

$$ s_t = \frac{s'}{r'} \qquad t_t = \frac{t'}{r'}. \qquad (5) $$

Note that this process is not any more expensive than direct texture mapping. Once the texture transformation matrix is compounded, just one hardware vector-matrix multiplication is needed. As a matter of fact, this multiplication is always performed, even if the texture transformation is unity.

IV. EXTENSIONS

In this section, we shall describe some extensions to the basic TMA-SART algorithm, for the benefit of both efficiency and accuracy.

A. Projection Image Accumulation in Hardware

Let us first assume that the framebuffer has 12 bits, as is the case for the SGI Octane. We noted before that the accumulation of the projection image takes place in main memory. This is necessary since the 12 bit framebuffer does not have any extra bits beyond the resolution of the projected image, which has at least 12 bits. Besides the fact that now the CPU must be used to add the n projection images, there are also n rather expensive framebuffer reads. One way to perform accumulations in the framebuffer would be to sacrifice precision (i.e., the lower bits) for speed. This, however, would impede the accuracy of the projection images, which is clearly undesirable.

We will now discuss a scheme that we can use to virtually extend the resolution of the framebuffer. The framebuffer has three color channels, red, green, blue, and alpha. Usually, we are only reconstructing grey level data, so all we utilize is a single color channel, say red, both in texture memory and in the framebuffer. However, if we partition the 12-bit data word into two components, one 8-bit and one 4-bit, and render it into two separate color channels, red and green, then we can accumulate data into the remaining upper 4 bits of the two framebuffer channels. This is illustrated in Fig. 6.

The four extra bits allow us to accumulate up to 16 images, which decreases the number of necessary framebuffer reads by $2/16$ (we now have to read two color channels). Notice, however, that bit_{8-11} of the texture word are not interpolated by the texture mapping hardware in 12 bits, but only in 8 bits. This may cause inaccuracies. To illustrate this problem, imagine the following simple case. Assume a *texel* (a texture element) has a binary value of 1 0000 0000 (only bit_8 is set) and its immediate neighbors are all 0. Thus the red texture channel contains 0, and the green texture channel contains 1 0000. Now let us assume that the texture mapping interpolation of this texel neighborhood yields a binary value of 1000. In the original approach, the framebuffer would contain that value, in the second approach (Fig. 6), however, the framebuffer would contain zero.

B. Extending the Framebuffer Accuracy

The accuracy of TMA-SART is mainly determined by the resolution of the buffer elements in the graphics hardware, i.e., the texture memory and the framebuffer. The texture memory on an SGI Octane has a resolution of 16 bits, while the framebuffer has a resolution of 12 bits. As there is no need to keep the volume data at a higher resolution than the texture memory that projects them, TMA-SART stores the volume data as 16 bit unsigned shorts. On the other hand, the images—those obtained from the scanner, the computed projections, and the weight images—are all stored as 32 bit unsigned integers, since they represent accumulations of many (i.e., n) 16 bit voxel slices. The correction image is stored in 16 bit, since it is normalized to one volume slice prior to backprojection. Thus the precision of the reconstruction process is inherently 16 bit, hampered, however, by

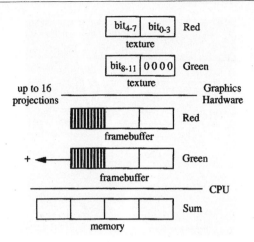

Fig. 6. Rendering a 12-bit data word using two color channels. The shaded upper four bits in the framebuffer can be used for accumulation. After the four upper bits have been filled by 16 projections, we must add the two channels in the CPU. For this purpose, the green channel must be shifted to the left by four bits.

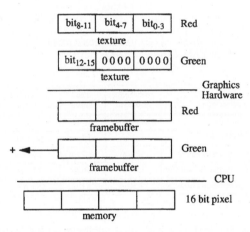

Fig. 7. Increasing the framebuffer resolution from 12 bit to 16 bit by adding up two color channels, properly shifted.

the limited 12 bit resolution of the framebuffer. Although reconstructions with moderate contrast levels should not be affected by this precision-bottleneck, it could cause low-contrast detail to be left unresolved in high-fidelity reconstructions. To alleviate these limitations, we shall now investigate a scheme that extends the framebuffer width in a virtual fashion, without hardware modification.

Consider Fig. 7 where these concepts are illustrated. The lower 12 bits of the volume data (or correction image data) are written to the Red texture channel, while the upper 4 bits of the data are written to the upper 4 bits of the Green texture channel. Rendering is performed as usual, and the Red and the Green framebuffer is read into two software buffers. The 16 bit result is constructed by adding the two software buffers, with the data in the Green buffer shifted to the left by 4 bits.

Note that, similar to the accumulation buffer, the (virtual) 16 bit data in the Green channel are not interpolated in 16 bits, but only in 12 bits. This will have effects similar to the ones outlined in the previous section. Hence, the presented implementation is not a true 16 bit extension to the framebuffer, it is only an

approximation. However, it will still help produce considerably more precise results than the original 12 bit implementation.

If only an 8 bit framebuffer is available, along with 8 bit textures, then we use 12 bit volume data and render the lower 8 bit into the Red framebuffer channel and the upper 4 bit, shifted 4 bits to the left, into the Green framebuffer channel. Combining the channels is done as usual and a 12 bit data word results.

V. Results

All programs were written using the widely accepted OpenGL API (Application Programming Interface) and can easily be reproduced to run on any medium-range graphics workstation or PC with graphics board. Using both the software implementation of SART (discussed in [16] and [17]) and the new hardware-accelerated version, TMA-SART, we reconstructed a simulated brain dataset, the 3-D extension of the Shepp–Logan phantom [24] (described, e.g., in [4], a slice is shown in Fig. 9(a). Projection sets of $S = 80$ cone-beam projections ($\gamma = 40°$) of 128^2 pixels each were obtained by analytical integration of the phantom.[5] These projections were used to reconstruct a 128^3 reconstruction volume in three iterations ($\lambda = 0.1$). To evaluate the effect of the limited framebuffer resolution in TMA-SART, we acquired the brain projection sets at three different feature contrast levels for the 12-bit SGI Octane and at five different levels for the 8-bit SGI O2, a low-end Unix-PC equipped with graphics hardware.[6] The original contrast of the main features in the phantom is 2% of the full dynamic range, while the background contrast of the small tumors in the bottom portion of the slices, shown in Fig. 9(a) is only 0.5%. (Note that, in all images of Fig. 9, the small dynamic range of the features was stretched into the full displayable range in order to make the features visible and to provide equivalent brightness for all contrast levels. The original range is [0.0, 2.0].)

Fig. 9(b) shows a slice [from the same location than that in Fig. 9(a)] across a volume reconstructed with the software implementation of SART described in [17]. This implementation employs splatting with analytically preintegrated Bessel–Kaiser kernels [12]. Next to the reconstructed slice, we show the intensity profile along a line that cuts horizontally across the center of the three small tumor ellipsoids [see Fig. 9(a)]. We observe that very little reconstruction artifacts are present and that the brain features (e.g., the small tumors) can be well discerned.

The software implementation uses both floating point arithmetic and floating point buffers throughout the reconstruction process. TMA-SART, on the other hand, also uses floating point arithmetic but only fixed point buffers. This amounts to some inaccuracies in the reconstruction process, which is demonstrated next. In Fig. 9(c), we show three reconstructions (slices and profile plots) obtained with the basic 12-bit framebuffer TMA-SART, while in Fig. 9(d) we show three reconstructions (slices and profile plots) obtained with the enhanced, 16-bit frame-

---

[5]The phantom was centered on the rotation axis, no noise was added to the projections.

[6]For the purposes relevant to this paper, the O2 graphics hardware is equivalent to the various boards available for PC's. However, computation time is likely to vary and tends to change fast in today's rapidly evolving market.

buffer TMA-SART. The contrast of the imaged phantom doubles in every column from left to right. We observe that the basic TMA-SART produces reconstructions with consistently higher levels of noise-like artifacts than the 16-bit TMA-SART. The difference is particularly striking in the first column for the original contrast. Here, the three small tumors in the lower third of the slice are only discernible in the 16-bit TMA-ART reconstruction. However, the higher the contrast, the lesser the impact of the framebuffer precision. The reconstructions obtained at twice the contrast of the Shepp–Logan phantom are already of acceptable quality. In Fig. 9(c) and (d), we also observe a number of artifacts that do not seem to be dependent on framebuffer resolution. These artifacts are more of a structured nature, as, for example, the dark ripple below the three small tumors. Other similar artifacts can be seen all over the reconstructions and do not decrease with framebuffer resolution.

Fig. 9(e) shows reconstructions obtained with an 8-bit framebuffer that uses the 12-bit enhancement described in Section IV-B. We notice that the reconstructions at twice the original contrast are not of the same quality than those of the true 12-bit framebuffer. This is due to the incomplete 12-bit precision and the use of an 8-bit texture map instead of the 12 bits available on the Octane. However, the reconstruction at four times the original contrast, although still somewhat noisy, already distinguishes the three small tumors rather well. The images at 8 and 16 times the original contrast resemble those for the enhanced 12-bit framebuffer at two and four times the original contrast, respectively, and are of acceptable quality.

Finally, Table I compares the run times for both the software and the various TMA-SART implementations. We see that by utilizing texture mapping hardware for the volume projection and backprojection operations, dramatic speedups can be achieved: a cone-beam reconstruction of a 128^3 volume from 80 projections can now be performed in about 2 min, down from the 1.8 hrs that were required in the software implementation on the same host CPU. This represents a speed-up of over 50.

By using the accumulation buffer enhancement, outlined in Section IV-A, we can reduce the reconstruction time even more to 1.6 min (a speedup of 68 with respect to software-ART). A reconstruction using the increased precision framebuffer, (outlined in Section IV-B, but not the accumulation buffer, takes somewhat longer (3.1 min for a speedup of 49), due to the increased number of framebuffer reads and CPU computations. The time required for reconstruction with our O2, using the 12-bit framebuffer enhancement, was 15.8 min, which amounts to a 6.8 speedup with respect to the software implementation on the Octane. However, the speedup is about eight when compared to the slower runtime of software SART on the O2 itself.

The runtime complexity of the SART algorithm is $O(S \cdot N)$, which indicates that the runtimes given in Table I should scale linearly with increasing S and N. This was verified in experiments conducted on volumes up to 512^3. The SGI Octane texture memory will currently fit 1 MB of texels, so volumes with up to 512^3 voxels (and slices with 512^2 16-bit texels) can be processed as is. For larger volumes, the slices need to be broken up into tiles, with the projection results being merged later, which adds some overhead. The O2 and many other modern graphics boards have unified memory architectures in which the texture

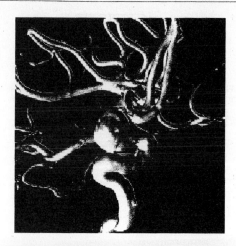

Fig. 8. Reconstructed and volume rendered blood vessel in a human brain. Projection data were obtained by 3-D rotational angiography on a Siemens C-arm scanner.

TABLE I
RUN TIMES FOR ONE ITERATION AS WELL AS FOR A COMPLETE RECONSTRUCTION (THREE ITERATIONS) OF DIFFERENT SART IMPLEMENTATIONS. [THESE TIMINGS WERE NEEDED TO PRODUCE THE IMAGES SHOWN IN FIG. 9(b)–(e).] THE OCTANE HAD A MIPS R10000/195-MHz CPU WITH 640 MB OF RAM. THE O2 HAD A MIPS R10000/175-MHz CPU AND 128 MB OF RAM. BOTH HAD 32-KB PRIMARY DATA CACHE AND 1-MB SECONDARY CACHE

SART implementation	framebuffer resolution	time / iteration	reconstruction time	speedup
software	floating point	36.0 min	1.8 h	-
TMA: basic	12 bits	42.2 sec	2.1 min	52
TMA: accumulation buffer	12 bits	33.2 sec	1.6 min	68
TMA: 16 bit enhanced framebuffer	12 bits	62.0 sec	3.1 min	35
TMA: 12 bit enhanced framebuffer	8 bits	316.0 sec	15.8 min	7- 8

memory is synonymous with main memory, so the texture capacity is far less constrained. Since we store the volume as voxel runs in the volume coordinate that is aligned with the rotation axis, extra cache faults during volume reads and write-backs will rarely occur [19]. Although software-ART has a somewhat more irregular data access [17], which affects its cache behavior, experiments have shown that linear relationships in terms of S and N exist here as well. Thus the speed-up ratios given in Table I remain approximately the same, even for larger S and N.

VI. DISCUSSION AND CONCLUSIONS

In this paper, we have investigated the utility and applicability of widely available graphics hardware with texture mapping capabilities for the purpose of 3-D reconstruction with algebraic methods. Algebraic methods have a number of advantages in certain reconstruction scenarios, but are presently far too slow for routine clinical use. The advantage of employing graphics hardware for reconstruction acceleration is that this equipment is likely to exist in clinical imaging labs anyhow, for image-aided diagnosis and medical procedure planning, and therefore no or little capital effort has to be made to apply the proposed technology.

We first determined that of all the available algebraic methods, SART was the most appropriate one to use. We then

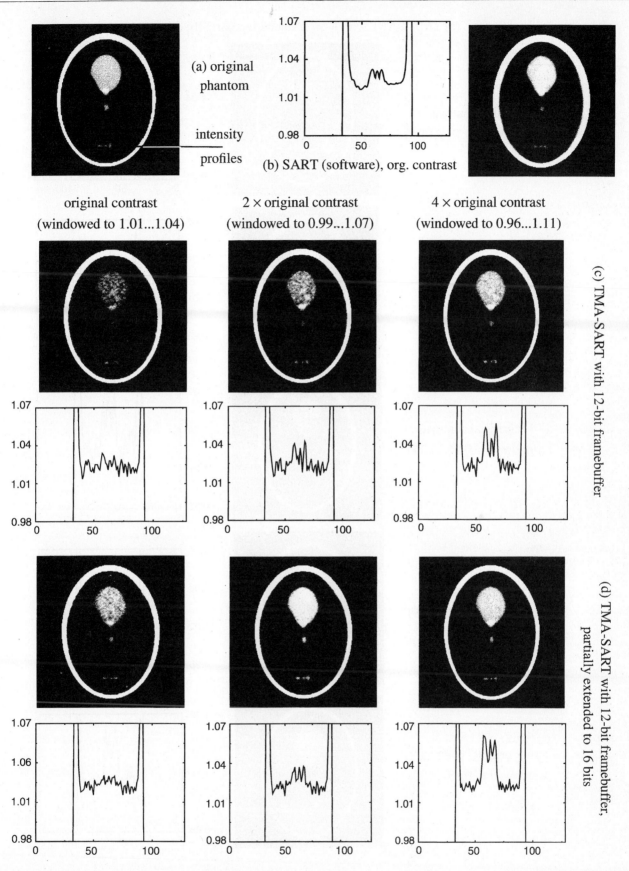

Fig. 9. Slices across reconstruction volumes obtained with different implementations of SART, software and hardware-accelerated. All reconstructions were performed using S = 80 128 x 128 projections of the 3-D extension of the Shepp Logan phantom (cone-angle = 40°, three iterations, a 128 reconstruction grid, λ = 0.1). The plots show the intensity profiles across the center of the three small ellipsoids (tumors) near the bottom of the phantom.

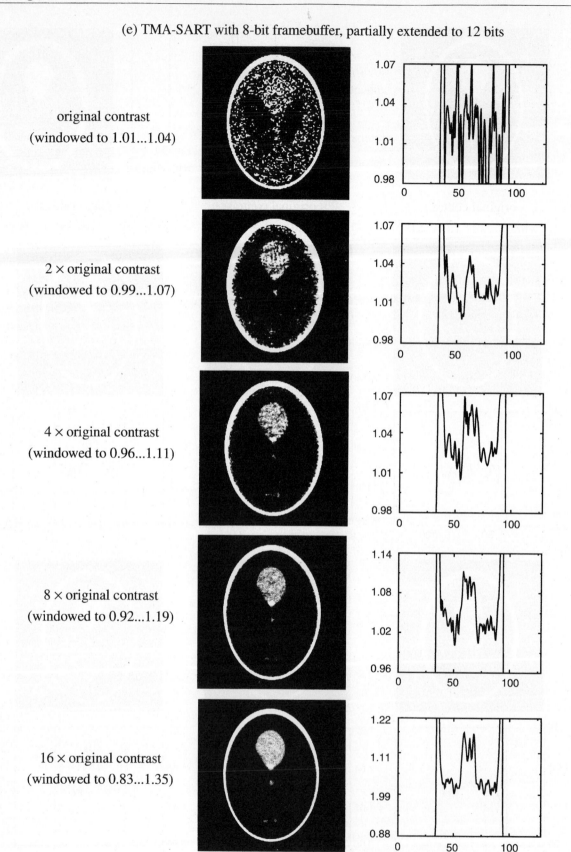

(e) TMA-SART with 8-bit framebuffer, partially extended to 12 bits

original contrast
(windowed to 1.01...1.04)

2 × original contrast
(windowed to 0.99...1.07)

4 × original contrast
(windowed to 0.96...1.11)

8 × original contrast
(windowed to 0.92...1.19)

16 × original contrast
(windowed to 0.83...1.35)

Fig. 9. (Continued) Slices across reconstruction volumes obtained with different implementations of SART, software and hardware-accelerated. All reconstructions were performed using S = 80 128 x 128 projections of the 3-D extension of the Shepp Logan phantom (cone-angle = 40°, three iterations, a 128 reconstruction grid, λ = 0.1). The plots show the intensity profiles across the center of the three small ellipsoids (tumors) near the bottom of the phantom.

partitioned the available graphics architectures into two groups: 1) mid-range graphics workstations (below $25 000), such as the SGI Octane, that have a 12-bit framebuffer, and 2) low-end graphics PCs and graphics boards that currently only have an 8-bit framebuffer. Our experiments indicate that the first group offers speedups between 35 and 68 when compared to a fairly optimized software implementation of SART, running on the same host CPU. The second group was investigated primarily to determine whether an 8-bit framebuffer can provide meaningful reconstructions at all. The timings that were obtained for that group are bound to be outdated very quickly, given the rapid performance growth of today's graphics boards, such as NVidia's GeForce series. We obtained a speedup of about eight on an SGI O2, an entry-level graphics PC with hardware comparable to a last-generation PC graphics board.

Our experiments indicate that the limiting factor in this endeavor is the limited resolution of the framebuffer. To ease this drawback we devised a scheme that partially extends a given framebuffer resolution by 4 bits. This allowed the resolvable contrast to be lowered to half the level that could be resolved without the extension. Using this extension for a 12-bit framebuffer, we found that object features of 1% contrast can already be distinguished well. We also found that the noise levels due to the limited framebuffer resolution are in the 0.5%–1% contrast range. This means that once the features exceed this range, the signal-to-(reconstruction) noise ratio becomes sufficient for a reconstruction of good quality. For an 8 bit framebuffer, partially extended to 12 bit, the noise level is slightly below 2%. Thus features of 2% contrast can be distinguished, but the noise is still well perceivable. If only features of 4% contrast are present then the noise can de-emphasized sufficiently by widening the brightness window.

The software implementation of SART [17] uses high-quality Bessel–Kaiser interpolation kernels that were analytically preintegrated. This provides near-analytical line integration and very accurate weight factors. TMA-SART, on the other hand, must use bilinear interpolation within the volume slices and the trapezoidal rule for integration. Furthermore, the sampling interval is greater than unity for the majority of rays, i.e., all those that are nonperpendicular to the volume slices most parallel to the image plane. The lower quality filter and integrator approximation can cause aliasing artifacts that are independent of framebuffer resolution, and we have observed them as the minor structured artifacts in Fig. 9(c) and (d). One possible way to increase the sampling rate is to interpolate additional, intermittent volume slices prior to a projection step. This interpolation can be done in hardware by blending two adjacent volume slices according to their distance relative to the new slice. Projection would then be based on all volume slices—the original ones and the interpolated ones. Backprojection would occur in the reverse fashion: One would backproject onto all slices, and the contributions of the intermittent slices would be distributed onto the original slices by a separate blending step in hardware.

Although TMA-SART, with present hardware, does not deliver reconstructions that can resolve the low contrasts (0.5%) of a software implementation, it can resolve 1% with a 12-bit framebuffer and 2%–4% with an 8-bit framebuffer, which is not too far from the desired levels. There are in fact a number of CT applications that do not require contrast levels beyond the capabilities of TMA-SART. One example is 3-D reconstruction angiography [1] (see Fig. 8), where the task is to reconstruct an opacified blood vessel from its projections. Another application is the reconstruction of bone structures. Many industrial CT applications may also benefit from TMA-SART. Finally, algebraic methods have also been quite successful in PET and SPECT reconstruction, where contrasts are typically rather high [13].

But nevertheless, an improvement of the framebuffer resolution of inexpensive graphics boards would be ideal. One incentive for board developers to provide wider framebuffers is the circumstance that they enable fast, high-quality motion-blur, a highly desirable effect in graphics and game applications. To achieve motion-blur, a moving object is rendered into the framebuffer a number of times, once for each time step. This calls for an extended framebuffer to allow for the frame accumulations without loss of precision. After a certain number of frames are rendered, the framebuffer is averaged by bit-shifting it to the right, and the motion-blurred scene or object is displayed. These extended framebuffers, called accumulation buffers [9], can also be used to generate soft shadows, depth-of-field effects, as well as high-quality anti-aliasing of polygonal objects [9]. On the other hand, there are also a number of new graphics and volume rendering boards currently being prepared for market introduction (e.g., the VIZARD volume rendering board [15]). One may be able to work with the designers to add mechanisms that would allow a framebuffer word to be changed, via software switch, from three 8-bit RGB slots to a single 24-bit Luminance slot. The added arithmetic would only require a small number of extra logical gates and would enable the TMA-SART accumulator as well.

REFERENCES

[1] "3D reconstruction angiography at General Electric,", Available: http://www.ge.com/medical/xray/msxclnv1.htm.

[2] A. H. Andersen and A. C. Kak, "Simultaneous algebraic reconstruction technique (SART)," *Ultrason. Img.*, vol. 6, pp. 81–94, 1984.

[3] A. H. Andersen, "Algebraic reconstruction in CT from limited views," *IEEE Trans. Med. Imag.*, vol. 8, pp. 50–55, Feb. 1989.

[4] C. Axelson, "Direct Fourier methods in 3-D reconstruction from cone-beam data," master's thesis, Linkoping Univ., Linkoping, Sweden, 1994.

[5] B. Cabral, N. Cam, and J. Foran, "Accelerated volume rendering and tomographic reconstruction using texture mapping hardware," in *1994 Symposium on Volume Visualization*, 1994, pp. 91–98.

[6] J. D. Foley, A. van Dam, S. K. Feiner, and J. F. Hughes, *Computer Graphics: Principles and Practice.* New York: Addison-Wesley, 1990.

[7] P. Gilbert, "Iterative methods for the three-dimensional reconstruction of an object from projections," *J. Theo. Biol.*, vol. 36, pp. 105–117, 1972.

[8] R. Gordon, R. Bender, and G. T. Herman, "Algebraic reconstruction techniques (ART) for three-dimensional electron microscopy and X-ray photography," *J. Theor. Biol.*, vol. 29, pp. 471–481, 1970.

[9] P. Haeberli and K. Akeley, "The accumulation buffer: hardware support for high-quality rendering," *Computer Graphics (Proceedings of SIGGRAPH'90)*, vol. 24, no. 4, pp. 309–318, 1990.

[10] P. M. Joseph, "An improved algorithm for reprojecting rays through pixel images," *IEEE Trans. Med. Imag.*, vol. 1, June 1982.

[11] A. C. Kak and M. Slaney, "Principles of computerized tomographic imaging," . Piscataway, NJ: IEEE Press, 1988.

[12] R. M. Lewitt, "Alternatives to voxels for image representation in iterative reconstruction algorithms," *Phys. Med. Biol.*, vol. 37, no. 3, pp. 705–715, 1992.

[13] S. Matej, G. T. Herman, T. K. Narayan, S. S. Furuie, R. M. Lewitt, and P. E. Kinahan, "Evaluation of task-oriented performance of several fully 3D PET reconstruction algorithms," *Phys. Med. Biol*, vol. 39, pp. 355–367, 1994.

[14] T. R. Mackie, T. Holmes, S. Swerloff, P. Reckwerdt, J. O. Deasy, J. Yang, B. Paliwal, and T. Kinsella, "Tomotherapy: a new concept for the delivery of dynamic conformal radiotherapy," *Med. Phys.*, vol. 20, no. 6, pp. 1709–1719, 1993.

[15] M. Meißner, U. Kanus, and W. Straßer, "VIZARD II: a PCI-card for real-time volume rendering," in *Proc. 1998 Eurographics Workshop Graphics Hardware*, pp. 61–67.

[16] K. Mueller, R. Yagel, and J. J. Wheller, "Anti-aliased 3-D cone-beam reconstruction of low-contrast objects with algebraic methods," *IEEE Trans. Med. Imag.*, vol. 18, pp. 519–537, June 1999.

[17] ——, "Fast implementations of algebraic methods for the 3-D reconstruction from cone-beam data," *IEEE Trans. Med. Imag.*, vol. 18, pp. 538–547, June 1999.

[18] K. Mueller and R. Yagel, "On the use of graphics hardware to accelerate algebraic reconstruction methods," in *Proc. 1999 SPIE Medical Imaging Conf.*, Feb. 1999, Paper 3659–62.

[19] ——, Rapid 3-D cone-beam reconstruction with ART utilizing texture mapping graphics hardware. presented at IEEE Medical Imaging Conf. 1998

[20] K. Mueller, J. Chang, H. Amols, and C. C. Ling, "Cone-beam computed tomography (CT) for a megavoltage linear accelerator (LINAC) using an electronic portal imaging device (EPID) and the algebraic reconstruction technique (ART)," in World Congress on Medical Physics and Biomedical Engineering, July 23–28, 2000, to be published.

[21] J. Neider, T. Davis, and M. Woo, *OpenGL Programming Guide*. Reading, MA: Addison-Wesley, 1993.

[22] P. Rizo, P. Grangeat, P. Sire, P. Lemasson, and P. Melennec, "Comparison of three-dimensional x-ray cone-beam reconstruction algorithms with circular source trajectories," *J. Opt. Soc. Amer. A*, vol. 8, no. 10, pp. 1639–1648, 1991.

[23] M. Segal, C. Korobkin, R. van Widenfelt, J. Foran, and P. E. Haeberli, "Fast shadows and lighting effects using texture mapping," *Computer Graphics (Proceedings of SIGGRAPH'92)*, vol. 26, pp. 249–252, 1992.

[24] L. A. Shepp and B. F. Logan, "The fourier reconstruction of a head section," *IEEE Trans. Nucl. Sci.*, vol. NS-21, pp. 21–43, 1974.

[25] B. Smith, "Cone-beam tomography: recent advances and a tutorial review," *Opt. Eng.*, vol. 29, no. 5, pp. 524–534, 1990.

[26] L. Westover, "Footprint evaluation for volume rendering," *Comput. Graphics (SIGGRAPH)*, vol. 24, no. 4, pp. 367–376, 1990.

Perspective

Three Novel Lossless Image Compression Schemes for Medical Image Archiving and Telemedicine

JIAN WANG, M.Eng., and GOLSHAH NAGHDY, B.Sc., Mphil., Ph.D.

ABSTRACT

In this article, three novel lossless image compression schemes, hybrid predictive/vector quantization lossless image coding (HPVQ), shape-adaptive differential pulse code modulation (DPCM) (SADPCM), and shape-VQ–based hybrid ADPCM/DCT (ADPCMDCT) are introduced. All are based on the lossy coder, VQ. However, VQ is used in these new schemes as a tool to improve the decorrelation efficiency of those traditional lossless predictive coders such as DPCM, adaptive DPCM (ADPCM), and multiplicative autoregressive coding (MAR). A new kind of VQ, shape-VQ, is also introduced in this article. It provides predictive coders useful information regarding the shape characters of image block. These enhance the performance of predictive coders in the context of lossless coding. Simulation results of the proposed coders applied in lossless medical image compression are presented. Some leading lossless techniques such as DPCM, hierarchical interfold (HINT), CALIC, and the standard lossless JPEG are included in the tests. Promising results show that all these three methods are good candidates for lossless medical image compression.

INTRODUCTION

DIGITAL IMAGING TECHNIQUES are becoming increasingly prevalent in medical applications. Consequently, there is a need to find economical ways of storing and transmitting the acquired digital data. Coupled with this need is the requirement to preserve the integrity of medical images after reconstruction. Lossless data compression reduces the massive storage requirement of medical images. The absolute fidelity requirement, however, forces the compression ratio obtained through lossless compression to be inferior to those reported for lossy schemes. Most of the lossless schemes are based on some form of prediction, while the lossy schemes take advantage of such methods as transform and wavelet coding, and vector quantization (VQ).

The lossless variant of DPCM is the most common form of the lossless image compression; the lossless JPEG algorithm is a variant of DPCM. Several variants of DPCM have been reported in the literature.[1] For image data, the effectiveness of DPCM as a coding algorithm stems from the inherent interpixel redundancies. The success of the lossless variant of DPCM depends on the ability of the predictor to model the image data, thereby yielding a low variance of estimation error. In a lossless

School of Electrical, Computer and Telecommunication Engineering, University of Wollongong, Wollongong, NSW, Australia.

coder, this error needs to be encoded as well in order to enable an accurate reconstruction of the data.

The nonstationary nature of the majority of digital images makes straightforward prediction ineffective, especially at edge locations. Model-based approaches have been used to overcome this problem.[2] Recently, context-based and segmentation-based methods have been proposed to predict the pixels in the edge area.[3] In this paper, three novel adaptive hybrid schemes are developed to improve the prediction based on the shape of edge.

This article is organized as follows. Lossless coding and its applications in telemedicine are briefly reviewed. Then, the proposed schemes are introduced. A performance comparison between the new coders and other lossless predictive coders is provided, followed by the conclusion and further development.

LOSSLESS IMAGE CODING AND TELEMEDICINE

In electronic medical recording, images such as x-rays, magnetic resonance imaging (MRIs) computed tomography (CT), etc., are digitized and stored as a matrix of binary digits in the computer memory. The number of medical images stored in digital form has increased significantly in recent years.[4] Attention is, therefore, focused on reducing the electronic storage requirement for archiving or transmitting digital medical images. One way of achieving this goal is through compressing the data before storage and decompressing it after retrieval.

Each digital image is represented by a matrix of digits denoting the light intensity of each picture element called a pixel. The number of pixels per image is dependent on the required spatial resolution, whereas the number of bits per pixel is determined by quantization accuracy needed for the application. For example, a typical image has 256×256 pixels, each requiring eight (8) binary bits for gray level quantization. Storing or transmitting such an image, which is about half a million bits of information, requires extensive memory or bandwidth capacity. In addition, most of medical images are in very high resolution, similar to the

mammograms used in this research, which are around 100 Mbits per image ($4 k \times 2 k \times 12$ bits).

Image compression is primarily used to minimize the number of bits required for storing or transmitting an image. The compressed image is reconstructed to its original form through a reconstruction process. Image compression has extensive applications in various medical fields such as:

- Image transmission for telemedicine, remote sensing via satellite, teleconferencing, teleconsultation, and the like;
- Storage of images produced in CT, MRI, digital radiology, and positron emission tomography (PET); and
- Smart card where the compressed medical history of a patient is stored on a special computer card.

It has been suggested that there are two modes of operation with telemedicine, real-time, and store-and-forward.[5] Image compression technology can provide help with both aspects in terms of time and space. For real-time telemedicine applications, image compression technologies bring great benefits by reducing the size of the information to be sent, hence save the time of transmission. For store-and-forward applications, they save the space of hardware requirement by reducing the bit rate of images. Compression techniques in both modalities can further reduce the cost of telemedicine, which is regarded as a primary barrier to its implementation.[5,6] Therefore, image compression is a major research issue in this field.

Image compression techniques can be divided into two categories, namely lossless and lossy. Those schemes, in which the original and the decompressed images are identical, are referred to as lossless, otherwise they are referred to as lossy. The quality of lossless coding schemes is measured by the ratio of the required bit rate for storing the original image to its compressed form (compression ratio), or the average number of bits required to represent each pixel of the image in compressed form (bit rate). The quality of lossy scheme is measured by the objective and/or subjective quality at a given compression ratio or bit rate.

Ideally, lossless image coding techniques with their total reconstruction fidelity are suitable for medical imaging. These techniques enable the doctors to get the full version of the images, which helps in making an accurate diagnosis, thereby reducing possible legal repercussions that might result from missed information in medical images.

The rate of compression in lossless schemes is relatively low compared to lossy schemes. In lossless schemes, the high compression rate achieved by conventional lossy techniques is sacrificed in order to retain potentially vital information. The trade-off has always been between the rate of compression and reconstruction fidelity. Some researchers have proposed near lossless schemes for medical imaging that is a compromise between the lossy and the lossless schemes.

Due to its unique characteristics and applications in medical and satellite photography, lossless image coding has attracted considerable attention since its introduction. However, because of the uncertainty of image pixels prevalence, a lossless coding scheme can seldom achieve a compression ratio of more than 4:1.

In conventional lossless coders, especially predictive coders that are widely used in lossless coding, the encoder predicts current pixel based on the information from its context. The prediction process performs poorly when there are abrupt changes of pixel values such as edges in images. This explains why lossless coders are not as effective as lossy coders in terms of their compression ratio. The lossless JPEG schemes, which are the combination of simple linear predictive coders, suffer heavily from these abrupt changes.

This article proposes a new, more accurate and efficient method for prediction than conventional schemes. It introduces a novel shape-VQ and combines it with other techniques to overcome the problem incurred by the uncertainty mentioned earlier. These hybrid shape-VQ–based schemes have a unique way of compressing the images with the vital shape information of image blocks provided by shape-VQ. Shape-VQ brings unmatched accuracy and simplicity in depicting image blocks, which includes the occurrence and quantity of edges inside block. The outstanding results achieved through this scheme confirm that this could be a promising way in future lossless image compression.

The most significant aspect of these new techniques is the way they retain the simplicity of the traditional predictive schemes and still produce largely improved compression ratios. There are other methods that address the problems associated with pixels at edge locations. However, the price is usually increased complexity.[3]

HYBRID PREDICTIVE/VQ LOSSLESS IMAGE CODING

The proposed scheme proceeds as in the basic MAR lossless coder, but goes further to exploit the inherent interblock correlation among image blocks. The model coefficients of correlated blocks lie within a close range of each other. It has been found that there is very little difference in the prediction errors generated. In this scheme, instead of coding the coefficients by scalar quantization, VQ is applied.

A VQ encoder consists of a code book generated from a sequence of training vectors. Each vector to be encoded is compared with the code vectors in the code book and the index of the closest (in the minimum-squared-error sense) code vector is transmitted (or stored) instead of the vector.

There are two ways of generating the required code book:

1. A set of model coefficients estimated from an image is used to produce an image adaptive code book.
2. A set of model coefficients from a set of training images is used to generate a universal code book.

The hybrid predictive/VQ encoder (HPVQ) forms the predicted pixel value using the appropriate code vector in the code book. In the adaptive code book case, both the code book and the appropriate indices for each block are transmitted (or stored).

The proposed HPVQ brings saving by using VQ for the prediction coefficients. It cuts the bits for side information by only transmitting the index of VQ, while it also maintains the performance of MAR coder. In addition, it saves the computation of MAR coder where the complex calculation of recursive pseudo-linear regression (RPLR) is required.[2] This is very important for telemedicine because processing time is reduced substantially.

LOSSLESS PREDICTIVE SHAPE-ADAPTIVE DPCM

A new linear prediction scheme, shape-adaptive DPCM (SADPCM), is presented in this section. Its suitability in a lossless DPCM compression algorithm stems from the high-performance prediction and low computational requirement.

The basic DPCM procedure is able to decorrelate pixels in a smooth image region, but performs poorly in areas with low correlation because the pixels are unpredictable. DPCM with constant prediction order will produce nonstationary errors. In the proposed scheme, the coder adjusts the predictor adaptively pixelwise as the correlation of the pixels changes.

Figure 1 depicts eight possible relationships that can exist between a given pixel and its neighbors in a 2×2 region of support (ROS). In Figure 1, "*" denotes the current pixel, $f(i, j)$, to be predicted. Pixels denoted as "•" are $f(i - 1, j)$, $f(i, j - 1)$, and $f(i - 1, j - 1)$ which constitute ROS. The lines joining pixels imply that a high correlation exists among the joined pixels; otherwise, no useful relationship exists between the pixel to be predicted and the predictor pixels. Correlation between two pixels depends on their gray scale values and a high correlation is defined as two pixels having identical or close values.

The structures depicted in Figure 1 are now considered in terms of prediction. In fact the required predictors will change as the correlation between the pixels varies. In Figure 1a, the pixel being predicted has no correlation with the pixels in ROS. For this kind of pixels, a special strategy of prediction based on VQ will be exploited. In Figures 1b to 1d the pixel being predicted has correlation with only one of the pixels in ROS. A first-order predictor is applied in this case:

$$\tilde{f}(i, j) = f(i - p, j - q) \qquad (1)$$

where $p, q \in [0,1]$ and $(p,q) \neq (0,0)$.

In Figures 1e to 1g, the pixels to be predicted are correlated with two pixels in ROS. Under such condition, a second-order predictor is appropriate:

$$\tilde{f}(i, j) = \frac{[f(i - p, j - q) + f(i - r, j - s)]}{2} \qquad (2)$$

where $p,q,r,s \in [0,1]$, $(p,q) \neq (0,0),(r,s) \neq (0,0)$, and $(p,q) \neq (r,s)$.

Finally, for those pixels with a correlation structure as depicted in Figure 1h, a third-order predictor is used:

$$\tilde{f}(i, j) = \frac{[0.95^* f(i, j - 1) + 0.95^* f(i - 1, j) - 0.95^* 0.95^* f(i - 1, j - 1)]}{[0.95^* (2 - 0.95)]} \qquad (3)$$

In this way, the order of prediction switches based on the shape of pixels within the 2×2 ROS; linear prediction is applied adaptively. A higher accuracy of prediction is obtained as only highly correlated pixels are used.

VQ is used as a tool to acquire the local shape of the image blocks. In the proposed scheme, the original image is first divided into nonoverlapping blocks. The mean of each block is computed and removed from the pixel value (mean normalization). This process removes the bias of the block mean and reveals the shape or structure of the block. Therefore, this kind of VQ is called shape-VQ.

The shape vectors can be grouped together using a universal or image adaptive code book. For each input shape vector, the index of the nearest code vector in the code book stores its information. VQ is used in this situation as a quantifier of the shape information of the image blocks. Therefore, the system can easily obtain the information about the local shape without much overhead by shape-VQ.

A universal code block is used in this work because of the low overhead when compared to an image adaptive code book. This is more so because of the premium placed on the use of available bits budget. The adaptive code book leads to less distortion as it more closely models the input vectors. A large universal code book can solve this problem.

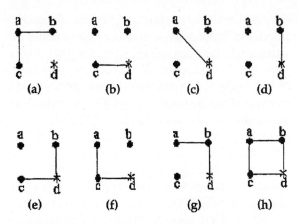

FIG. 1. Eight possible relationships between a given pixel and its region of support (ROS).

At the encoder side of the proposed system, the original image is split into 8×8 nonoverlapping blocks, and the shape vectors are formed by mean normalization. Shape-VQ is applied to each shape vector, and the resulting indices are stored as side information.

In applying SADPCM to each pixel in high activity regions, the shape pixels in the code vector are used. The current pixel and its 2×2 ROS in the code vector are evaluated for correlation. A simple difference calculation is used. For example, using the 2×2 block of Figure 2, the absolute difference between pixel $f(i,j)$ and each of the pixels in ROS in the code vector is calculated as:

$$\overset{\rho}{e}(i, j) = |\overset{\rho}{f}(i, j) - \overset{\rho}{f}(i - p, j - q)| \quad (4)$$

where $\overset{\rho}{e}(i, j)$ is the difference and $p,q \in [0,1]$ $(p,q) \neq (0,0)$.

Here, in Figure 2B, the three differences are 0, 0.5, and 0. Correlation in this context is defined as the difference being less than some threshold. Otherwise there is no correlation.

The threshold here is set to 0.2 as a result of some experimentation. As the threshold increases, pixels with little correlation may be included for the prediction. Decreasing the threshold will exclude those pixels with high correlation. In both cases, the performance of the predictor will be degraded. In the example given, pixel $f(i - 1, j - 1)$ has no correlation with pixel $f(i,j)$. This situation is equivalent to the decision rule given in Table 1 in which the predictor of (2) is used.

If it is found in the code vector in Figure 2C that $f(i,j)$ has no correlation with any of the pixels in ROS, which is the case in Figure 1a, the predictor uses VQ in the following manner. Recall that each element of the shape vector is mean normalized. Then, the four pixels in Figure 2 are related according to:

$$\frac{f(i - 1, j - 1)}{f'(i - 1, j - 1)} = \frac{f(i - 1, j)}{f'(i - 1, j)} =$$

$$\frac{f(i, j - 1)}{f'(i, j - 1)} = \frac{f(i, j)}{f'(i, j)} = \mu_b, \quad (5)$$

where μ_b is the block mean, $f(i - 1, j)$, $f(i, j - 1)$, $f(i - 1, j - 1)$, and $f(i, j)$ are the raw gray scale values of the pixels, which are those in Figure 2A, and $f'(i - 1, j)$, $f'(i, j - 1)$, $f'(i - 1, j - 1)$, and $f'(i, j)$ are the values of the shape vector pixels, which are those in Figure 2C. Using the relationship in equation 5 it is possible to write:

$$\frac{[f(i - 1, j - 1) + f(i - 1, j) + f(i, j - 1)]/3}{[f'(i - 1, j - 1) + f'(i - 1, j) + f'(i, - 1)]/3}$$

$$= \frac{f(i, j)}{f'(i, j)} \quad (6)$$

The ratio on the left-hand side of equation 6 can be interpreted as the ratio of mean of the pixel in ROS of the predictor in both the image domain and the codebook. The predicted pixel value, $\tilde{f}(i, j)$, can now be calculated as:

$$\tilde{f}(i, j) = f'(i, j) * \bar{R} / \bar{C} \quad (7)$$

where $\bar{R}$ is the mean of the pixels in ROS of the predictor in image data, $\bar{C}$ is the mean of the same pixels in the mean normalized codebook, and $f'(i, j)$ is the corresponding value of the pixel being predicted in the codebook.

	A		**B**		**C**	
$f(i-1,j-1)$ $f(i-1,j)$	•	•	1.3	0.8	1.3	1.3
$f(i,j-1)$ $f(i,j)$	•	•	0.8	0.8	1.3	0.8

FIG. 2. Two $2 * 2$ blocks in the original image and their corresponding pixels in the codebook. **A.** The original pixel. **B.** An example of pixels with two correlations. **C.** An example of pixels with no correlation.

The decision rule for selecting the prediction order is listed in Table 1. At the transmitter, not only the errors of prediction but also all the side information, the indices of 8×8 image blocks, need to be sent. At the decoder side, all the pixels can be losslessly recovered by using the errors and the side information. The whole error image is divided into 8×8 blocks, and the code vector for each block is found by the index in the side information. The image can therefore be totally recovered by the same decision rule as introduced before.

The idea of switching the predictor in the hybrid SADPCM coder is by no means new. Several schemes based on this idea have been reported in the literature. The novelty of the scheme presented in this research is that local shape is transmitted without much side information via VQ. VQ simplifies the process of selecting the appropriate predictor based on the decision rule and storing or transmitting the information through the index of the shape vector. Unlike DPCM, sudden changes in the image can be found precisely in SADPCM scheme and the high-activity components can be detected and decorrelated. The proposed hybrid scheme retains the good characteristics of pixel-based ADPCM. The drawback of huge side information is overcome by using VQ. When compared to block-based ADPCM, complex matrix computation is prevented, and prediction performance is improved by switching the predictors more finely on a pixel-by-pixel basis.

SHAPE VQ-BASED LOSSLESS HYBRID ADPCM/DCT CODER

A typical image contains segments that can be described variably as edge and smooth regions. Obviously, these segments should be modeled differently so that an image coder can adaptively take advantage of this segmentation. The strategy adopted in the coder presented in this section is to partition the image into edge areas that can be encoded by DCT, and the other areas that can be encoded by ADPCM.

In shape VQ-based lossless hybrid ADPCM/DCT coder (ADPCMDCT), the whole image is first processed by shape-VQ as introduced in the previous section. The VQ in this stage is thereafter called VQ-I. The variance inside the vector is used to determine its classification, where each shape block is classified into one of two classes, edge or smooth, by a preset threshold δ_T.

For systems using adaptive VQ, δ_T can be chosen adaptively as well. However, this will greatly increase the computational burden. In addition, current δ_T has been tested extensively on images, which makes it optimal for normal images in terms of final decorrelation results. Therefore, in this research, as the universal VQ is applied in all the cases, δ_T is also fixed. The optimum δ_T is generated from several images that include nonmedical and medical images. For mammograms, however, another threshold is used. This improves the performance of the system with a particular group of images like mammograms.

The shape vector brings more accurate classification than raw image blocks because the interference from the image background is eliminated through the mean-normalization. This would further improve the performance of universal code blocks as blocks from different pictures with different background.

The two-dimensional Levinson and modified multichannel version of the Burg algorithm introduced in equation 1 are used to form a set of prediction parameters for ADPCM for each code vector. Thus, the code book of the shape vector includes three parts which are index of the vector, shape vector, and the set of prediction parameters appointed to the vector. This is clearly shown in Figure 3, where S stands for the smooth block and E stands for the edge.

When an image block A comes, it is first mean-normalized, which generates a shape vector $\tilde{A}$. The shape vector is then vector quan-

TABLE 1. DECISION RULES FOR SELECTING THE "OPTIMAL" PREDICTOR

Number of pixels in ROS that have correlation with current pixel	The optimal predictor
None (see Fig. 1a)	VQ-based predictor (See (7))
One (see Fig. 1b–1d)	First-order predictor (See (1))
Two (see Fig. 1e–g)	Second-order predictor (See (2))
Three (see Fig. 1h)	Third-order predictor (See (3))

ROS, region of support.

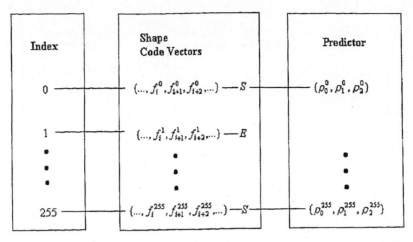

FIG. 3. The codebook of shape VQ-I.

tified. A code vector is found for $\bar{A}$ based on the nearest neighbor rule. If this code vector is assigned as smooth block, ADPCM will be applied to A, and the prediction parameters also can be found in the codebook which is pointed to by the index.

It has been proved in equation 8 that DCT is a good candidate for compressing of edge components. Therefore, it is used in this research for decorrelating edge blocks.

It has been reported that similar shape blocks have close prediction parameter vectors. This is also true for DCT coefficient matrix. The coefficient matrix of DCT represents the variation inside the image block. This variation is a sign of the shape. Therefore, it can be concluded that one shape vector is corresponding to a certain DCT coefficient matrix. Therefore shape-VQ is used to save the complicated calculation in DCT and the side information of the coefficient matrix.

Another universal shape-VQ code book, VQ-II, is set up specifically for the edge blocks. DCT is then applied to each block in the code book. The computation of DCT used in this paper is similar to the lossy coder recommended by JPEG.[9] The resulting matrix is stored, and is pointed to by the index in the codebook. Therefore, the VQ index depicts not only the edge block in the codebook but also the coefficient matrix of this code vector. This is shown in Figure 4.

During the encoding of images, those blocks labeled as edge components are vector quanti-

fied by VQ-II. The errors being the original block and the reversed one are calculated and retained. Also kept is the index of the block.

From the depiction above, it can be seen that for smooth blocks, only 8 bits side information are needed for the whole block, and edge blocks require 8 bits extra for the VQ index. These are all the side-information of the proposed scheme.

SIMULATION AND DISCUSSION

The test images used in assessing the proposed coders (Fig. 5) are medical images. *Abdo, Feet, Head, Pelvis,* and *Skull.* All images are 512×512 pixels with 4,096 gray scale (12 bits per pixel). Compression results with mammograms from Digital Mammogram Library of Lawrence Livermore National Laboratory are also included. The mammograms with various spatial resolutions ranging from approximate 1 k $\times$ 2 k to 2 k $\times$ 5 k, are all in 12 bits per pixel as well. All these image are processed with full bit-depth and full spatial resolution.

A comparison of the performance of the proposed coders against DPCM, HINT, and context-based, adaptive, lossless image coding (CALIC) is presented. The former two are well regarded as popular methods in lossless coding.[1] The last one, CALIC, is recently developed, and appears as the benchmark for lossless coding.[3]

The results quoted here are the first-order entropy of the errors, plus the bits used for side

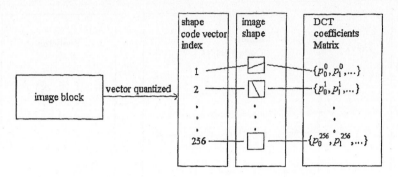

FIG. 4. The proposed shape-DCT/VQ-II encoder.

information, which are in bits per pixel. This enables us to compare all the methods fairly and in the same platform. However, all the proposed schemes can be interfaced with any entropy coding methods because the errors are independent of the prediction (redundancy has been removed).

From the results in Table 2, it can be seen that all three proposed coders outperform DPCM and HINT. The results prove that these systems are more efficient than traditional schemes in terms of lossless coding. Compared to CALIC, SADPCM and ADPCMDCT both show their strength. Although their performance in "simple" images like *Feet* is not as good as that of CALIC, they perform very well in "complex" images. This is mainly attributed to shape-VQ, which generates fine description of the shape information especially edge components. These

edge components are hard to forecast, and often incur large prediction errors. However, in SADPCM and ADPCMDCT, the abrupt change (edge) inside the block can be observed. Not only the location but also the quantities of changes are reflected in shape-VQ. Therefore, schemes based on shape-VQ have promising results in complex medical images. This argument has been further proven by the tests on mammograms, which have huge amount of texture features inside. Results in Table 3 show that both schemes outperform CALIC in mammograms.

HPVQ, however, produces worse results than CALIC. This is mainly due to the direct use of VQ and MAR in the design. However, HPVQ has some advantages due to its simple computation. Results in Tables 4A and 4B verify this. HPVQ well leads in the tests of compression time. In addition, when the decom-

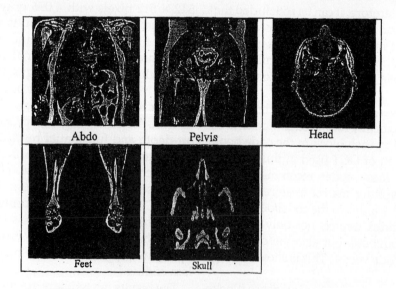

FIG. 5. A mosaic of the test images used in the simulation.

TABLE 2. PERFORMANCE OF SEVERAL SCHEMES ON MEDICAL IMAGES

	DPCM	HINT	CALIC	HPVQ	SADPCM	ADPCMDCT
Abdomen	5.13	5.22	4.70	4.90	4.33	4.30
Head	3.20	3.18	3.10	3.14	2.79	2.69
Pelvis	4.34	4.35	3.97	4.15	3.47	3.54
Feet	2.37	2.53	2.08	2.42	2.31	2.10
Skull	2.60	2.58	2.31	2.51	2.49	2.39

DPCM, differential pulse code modulation; HINT, hierarchical interfold; CALIC, context-based, adaptive, lossless image coding; HPVQ, hybrid predictive vector quantization; SADPCM, shape-adaptive DPCM; ADPCMDCT, shape-VQ–based hybrid ADPCM/DCT.

TABLE 3. PERFORMANCE OF SCHEMES ON MAMMOGRAMS

Mammogram	CALIC	HPVQ	SADPCM	ADPCMDCT
Afrcc	2.68	2.77	2.48	2.54
Aflcc	2.75	2.95	2.53	2.63
Agrcc	2.49	2.54	2.46	2.37
Aglcc	2.49	2.57	2.37	2.45
Ahrcc	2.70	2.90	2.54	2.49
Ahlcc	2.74	2.73	2.44	2.47
Aircc	2.38	2.41	2.10	2.37

CALIC, context-based, adaptive, lossless image coding; HPVQ, hybrid predictive vector quantization; SADPCM, shape-adaptive DPCM.

TABLE 4A. COMPRESSION TIME OF THE SCHEMES

Test Image	CALIC	HPVQ	SADPCM	ADPCMDCT
Afrcc	8.89	8.65	10.26	10.90
Aflcc	9.12	8.90	11.93	11.93
Agrcc	8.76	8.74	11.26	10.89

TABLE 4B. DECOMPRESSION TIMES OF THE SCHEMES

Test Image	CALIC	HPVQ	SADPCM	ADPCMDCT
Afrcc	8.89	2.61	2.71	2.75
Aflcc	9.12	2.61	2.72	2.78
Agrcc	8.76	2.62	2.72	2.74

CALIC, context-based, adaptive, lossless image coding; HPVQ, hybrid predictive vector quantization; SADPCM, shape-adaptive DPCM; ADPCMDCT, shape-VQ–based hybrid ADPCM/DCT.

TABLE 5. PERFORMANCE OF THE BEST OF JPEGs COMPARED TO THOSE OF THE NEW SCHEMES

Mammogram	JPEG	HPVQ	SADPCM	ADPCMDCT
Afrcc	3.79	2.77	2.48	2.54
Aflcc	4.07	2.95	2.53	2.63
Agrcc	3.35	2.54	2.46	2.37
Aglcc	3.85	2.57	2.37	2.45
Ahrcc	4.14	2.90	2.54	2.49
Ahlcc	4.27	2.73	2.44	2.47
Aircc	3.01	2.41	2.10	2.37

HPVQ, hybrid predictive vector quantization; SADPCM, shape-adaptive DPCM; ADPCMDCT, shape-VQ–based hybrid ADPCM/DCT.

pression time of these schemes, which is sometimes more important than compression time in telemedicine, is compared. It is observed that all three are faster than CALIC. This is mainly due to the absence of VQ in the decoding end where the systems can directly find the right predictor through code vector.

Results from lossless JPEG are also included in this study. The schemes are those listed in.[9] Only the best results for each image from JPEGs are shown. From Table 5, it easily can be seen that the proposed schemes outperform JPEG in those complex mammograms. The strength of JPEG lies in its simple implementation and computation that saves time in real-time applications. However, for those non-real-time tasks, the bit-rate is still an important issue in judging performance. Therefore, in telemedicine applications, the new techniques may be regarded as better candidates than JPEG.

CONCLUSION

Three new lossless image coding schemes have been proposed and their performances have been compared to a number of lossless image coding techniques. The results indicate a superior performance in favor of the new methods. The superiority of the new schemes is attributed to their ability to identify local image features especially abrupt changes. The low bit rate and running time achieved by the schemes are crucial in telemedicine in particular in the high-resolution medical images such as digital mammograms. The performance of the schemes in terms of compressed image bit rate and computational complexity makes

them as optimal candidates for lossless medical image compression.

REFERENCES

1. Kuduvalli G, Rangangyyan R. Performance analysis of reversible image compression techniques for high-resolution digital teleradiology. *IEEE Trans Med Imaging* **1992**;11:430–445.
2. Das M, Burgett S. Lossless compression of medical images using two-dimensional multiplicative auto-regressive models. *IEEE Trans Med Imaging* **1993**;12:721–726.
3. Wu X, Memon N. Context-based, adaptive, lossless image coding. *IEEE Trans Commun* **1997**;45:437–444.
4. Wong S, Zaremba L, Goodden D, Huang H. Radiology image compression—A review. *Proc IEEE* **1995**;83:194–218.
5. Lin J. Applying telemedicine technology to health-care delivery. *IEEE Trans Eng Med Biol* **1999**;28–31.
6. Bashshur R. Telemedicine effects: Cost, quality, and access. *J Med Syst* **1995**;19:81–91.
7. Cowman P, Oehler K, Riskin E, Grey R. Using vector quantization for image processing. *Proc IEEE* **1984**;81:1326–1341.
8. Andrew J, Ogunbona P. On the step response of the DCT. *IEEE Trans Circuits Systems II-Analog Digital Signal Processing* **1997**;44:260–262.
9. Wallace G. The JPEG still picture compression standard. *IEEE Trans Consumer Electronics* **1992**;38:xviii–xxxiv.

Address reprint requests to:
Golshah Naghdy, Ph.D.
School of Electrical, Computer and
Telecommunication Engineering
University of Wollongong
Northfield Avenue
Wollongong, NSW, 2500, Australia

E-mail: g.naghdy@elec.uow.edu.au

Section 1:

S. Chu

The University of Auckland,
New Zealand

Synopsis

Information Retrieval and Health/Clinical Management

Introduction

The healthcare industry is one of the most, if not the most, information intensive industries. Medical information/knowledge and clinical data are growing at close to explosive rates each day. Ten years ago, medical publications were added to the world's biomedical journal collections at the rate of approximately 3,000 per month. Today, the volume of bibliographic citations is growing at 1,000 per day in Medline alone [1]. Hospitals also generate huge amounts of healthcare data. It has been estimated that an acute care hospital may generate up to five terabytes of data a year [2]. The volume of information and knowledge available today has far exceeded the cognitive capability of the human brain. However, availability and use of accurate information/knowledge are crucial for delivery of quality healthcare to consumers. The demand by society and professional organizations on use of evidence-based practice to help improve quality of care also adds great pressure on healthcare professionals to regularly access best quality information and knowledge during the processes of healthcare planning, decision and delivery.

Computer-assisted information retrieval and processing provides effective mechanisms to rapidly retrieve and present the relevant information/ knowledge required for supporting quality decision-making and help overcome the human cognitive constraints. Biomedical publications and considerable volumes of clinical data are created and stored as free text documents. However, numerical machines, such as computers, are not designed to process free text effectively and structured query methods, such as SQL (structured query language) cannot be easily employed to manipulate free texts.

The benefits of being able to effectively process free text medical documents and retrieve from them relevant information and knowledge are substantial to meet the needs of healthcare professionals. However, significant technical hurdles still exist. The papers included in the 2002 IMIA Yearbook section on 'Health and clinical management' have examined and proposed some of the techniques of free text processing as useful solutions for health information retrieval. Based on these selected papers, I have categorized the issues related to healthcare information retrieval into those pertinent to (a) searching and retrieval techniques, (b) intelligent information presentation, (c) information retrieval and delivery on the Internet. Within the constraints set for this paper, I have attempted to review each issue as widely as possible and have included some discussions on future directions and developments.

Free Text Searches and Information Retrieval

1 Basic Text Searching by Pattern Matching

A number of text search techniques are available. Major categories commonly involve the application of exact string pattern matching algorithms. In most cases, they fall into the 'brute-force' (or naïve) implementation. The text string to be searched is matched to the texts in the target documents using 'character comparison and slide to next comparisons' approach. It is possible to optimize the pattern matching algorithms to produce quite fast search results [3].

Basic free text searches, either in the form of single keyword searches or text phrase searches, have the major advantage of not requiring the source texts to be pre-processed for fast queries. Commonly used text search/matching algorithms, including the Boyer-Moore-Horspool, have been evaluated by a number of experimental studies as very efficient string matching algorithms [3-5]. These algorithms can play an important role in supporting dynamic searches and retrieval of free text medical data, including clinical progress notes, pathology and radiology reports, and medical imaging reports stored in electronic medical records in which pre-processing is either difficult or not economical.

When utilizing any free text search techniques, the user needs to choose between exact text phrase matching or expanded search (i.e. combining search terms in a text phrase with operators, such as 'and', 'or') strategies. Using the exact match strategy has the benefit of returning documents more relevant to user requirements, but may also face the risk of quite few or zero document hits. The expanded search strategy, on the other hand, can bring back more documents, but has the disadvantage of returning excessively large document sets with varying degrees of relevancy to user requirements.

Morphological differences between the texts in the target documents and the search words used often further hamper the search results [6, 7], and are beyond the technological spectrum of basic free text searching/pattern matching techniques. This issue is particularly problematic in healthcare, in which the biomedical language is packed with many interchangeable terms, such as common cold and coryza, chest pain and angina pectoris, fever and pyrexia, lock-jaw and trismus, arrhythmias and dysrhythmias (although strictly speaking these two terms have quite different meanings), weakness and paresis, and many others. Substantial user frustration when clinicians attempt to search and retrieve free text information from electronic medical records can arise.

2. Indexing and use of Dictionaries/ Thesauri in text searching

To rectify some of the shortcomings of basic free text searching/pattern matching techniques, some form of pre-processing of both the search terms and the target text documents is considered a desirable approach. A number of studies had confirmed the use of indexing systems as a highly effective technique to reduce the search space and query time, hence producing very fast and accurate

searches on the rapidly growing free text document databases [8, 9]. While pattern matching style of free-text searching provide the benefit of search flexibility, search speed often suffers as the document store grows. Search speed and accuracy could be greatly enhanced by the use of indexing systems based on some standard descriptors or dictionaries. Using search terms generated from standard dictionaries also helps resolve the morphological differences problems and thus reduces user frustrations by minimizing the rates of missed-hits/failed searches. The effectiveness of this combined search approach has been confirmed by repeated studies since the early 1970s [10-13].

It is possible to build indexing systems (based on some form of standard terminology/dictionary) that are simultaneously sublinear in search space overhead and in query time [14]. Processing speed can be further enhanced by loading the entire list of indices (or its address space) onto the secondary memory of the document database server. The construction of a standard dictionary, however, presents considerable challenges. For example, the need to resolve morphological differences exists not only between authors and retrievers, but also morphological problems within the biomedical language itself. The biomedical language is loaded with morphologically similar (e.g. leucocytes, leukaemia) and semantically ambiguous (e.g. diaphoresis and diaphysis) morphemes. The shear size of biomedical terminologies and their rapid growth and dynamic nature also make the maintenance of such dictionaries extremely difficult, if not at all impossible.

The morphological segmentation, together with the automated segmentation engine developed by Schulz and Hahn [15], represented an effective interactive tool to automate the pro-

cesses of identifying and linking the semantically identical morphemes. This tool can be trained to automatically segment words imported from source texts and then link semantically identical morphemes to construct a thesaurus/repository of morphologically and semantically related biomedical terms. The technique also provides a solution to facilitate easy, dynamic updates of the dictionary in the environment of rapidly growing biomedical terminologies. The dictionary created can be used to index target free-text documents (publications and electronic healthcare record documents) and to facilitate rapid, more effective searches and information retrieval by users.

Intelligent Information/ Knowledge Search and Presentation

The conventional method of text searching and retrieval returns free text document sets (matching the search terms) to users with little regard to the context of the search terms within the document and the relevancy/precision of the documents to the users. Low relevancy of document sets is a major cause of user dissatisfaction and abandonment of search efforts. Users' inexperience in determining appropriate search terms and strategies often aggravate the stress and add much frustration to the search processes.

Interactive graphical user interfaces today have replaced text-based search screen design as standard interfaces in almost all information retrieval engines, especially those used in libraries. Significant amount of 'smartness' can be built into the graphical interface to provide such functions, like clear display of search descriptors from standard dictionary for users to choose from, visualization of the search query building process, and guiding the user's query modification process through the display of search results or number of hits. In the absence of human information search experts, graphical display of the information with automated query guides as a built-in search engine function produces far better results than basic free text searches that generate thousands of non-specific hits [16, 17].

A simply strategy to improve search result quality is the application of some form of information ranking techniques [18]. This approach typically requires the use of knowledge-bases containing a set of relevance indices and their relative ranking weightings, and an inference engine to manipulate the rules and the values of the ranking indices. The documents retrieved are assigned a relevance value by the inference engine based on the locations and frequencies of the search terms within the documents.

Another approach highly relevant to health/clinical management is the utilization of a categorization tool that dynamically groups and displays the document sets returned from a query under a number of specific and meaningful headings [19]. For example, a query on the concept 'breast cancer' will return a document set that can be dynamically categorized and displayed under the groups of causes, diagnosis, treatment, complications of diagnosis/ treatment, and prognosis, etc. Graphically displayed, the categorized search result becomes contextually meaningful to the user.

It is technically trivial to graphically present search terms (and their semantically related morphemes) from a biomedical dictionary in a tree-like structure. Users can then simply point-and-click to select and combine relevant terms and visualize/refine the construction of the Boolean queries [10]. If such improved search engine can be further enriched by adding a dynamic categorization tool, like the one reported in [19], the quality of search outputs (and hence their usefulness) could be dramatically enhanced.

Information Retrieval and Delivery on the Internet

Explosive developments in the Internet have made Web-based health documents increasingly important resources not only for healthcare professionals, but also for health consumers. The adoption of hypertext markup language (HTML) and extensible markup language (XML) as the de facto standards facilitates easy and rapid development of information delivery and sharing applications.

The use of free text search techniques on HTML pages to perform biomedical literature searches on remote hypertext transport protocol (HTTP) servers is a common practice in nearly all healthcare and education facilities today. It is also possible to search on, and retrieve, medical images using free text search terms submitted via an HTTP form [20]. Intelligent retrieval engine receives the free text search terms from a Web browser, map the search term to a standard term for medical image identification and use the standard term to retrieve the relevant medical image(s). The same technique can be applied to retrieving free text clinical progress notes, pathology and radiological reports.

Rapid advances in, and adoption of, Internet information access/distribution technology raise a number of highly important issues. These issues, especially those related to security and confidentiality, urgently need to be addressed. As the focus of this synopsis is not on the Internet, these issues are only touched upon briefly.

(a) Security and Confidentiality

The Internet has been designed as an open system. As such security is its weakest link. Technological capabilities (especially in the area of security) of many medium- to small- healthcare facilities is still relatively rudimentary. Technology, such as public key infrastructure (PKI), has been considered by many, particularly small clinics, as too expensive and too complicated. The use of a smart card based token (randomly generated security key) combined with user-selected password to produce a use-once only access code is a highly secure, and simple and affordable, authentication solution for all healthcare facilities, big or small. De-identification of clinical data for non clinical use and application of encryption technologies [21], such as the 3-DES (Data Encryption Standard defined encryption technology), are also crucial data protection measures which should not be ignored.

(b) Distributed Data Storage and Access Speed

The volume of Web-based documents is increasing rapidly. They are also distributed across disparate data storage and network systems. Accessing these documents from the distributed sources presents significant technical challenges. A middleware-based directory service offers the most reliable and cost effective solution for multi-organisational/regional information access. But even if the documents are located quickly, pulling large document sets and medical images across the network can create serious network traffic problems necessitating serious planning and considerable investments in network infrastructures.

(c) Reliability Issues

The Internet is essentially an unregulated (or more likely unregulable) environment. Quality of information published on Internet varies widely depending on the information sources.

Some information is potentially harmful rather than beneficial to the consumers. This can post significant risks to the less knowledgeable. One possible solution is the establishment of some international rating organization responsible for the establishment of health information evaluation criteria and publication of ratings of health-related Web sites based on the validated evaluation rules. However, rapid increases and collapses of Web sites make such activity extremely difficult and resources intensive.

Future Directions and Development

Free text biomedical documents contain huge volumes of knowledge embedded within the jungle of unstructured texts constructed by many authors. Conventional retrieval techniques (including those with categorization functions) recall abstracts and documents in their entirety, without ability to process and present the knowledge embedded within the text structures. Knowledge-based information retrieval systems focusing on knowledge acquisition from the documents, knowledge representation, knowledge-base refinement and knowledge retrieval mechanisms are required to fill this rapidly increasing demand.

Research on biomedical knowledge extraction (from medical texts), representation and retrieval using techniques, such as conceptual graph (CG) formalisms has produced promising results [22]. Canonical conceptual graphs are formed with biomedical concepts interlinked by semantic relations. Using graph construction rules, these canonical graphs may be combined to derive new CG that build up an entire sentence structure, and eventually the whole document. CG applications have been used in automated coding of clinical documents, such as patient discharge summaries, pathology and radiology reports [23, 24]. Relations between interventions and outcomes (clinical effectiveness) knowledge can be adequately represented by CG and the coding rules. Efficient clustering (for clustering related CG documents) and graph query techniques have been developed, thus allowing rapid knowledge retrieval from the conceptual graph document sets [25]. The remaining challenges include optimization of the graph query techniques and the development of integrated applications/ software modules for information/ knowledge retrieval and clinical information management systems.

Query agents have been/are being developed to assist users in generating suitable information retrieval queries, and in learning to adjust the queries according to user demand so that the document sets returned are contextually appropriate and best suited to user requirements [26]. The ultimate goal will be the creation of intelligent query agents that can automatically roam the Internet information/knowledge spaces and bring back knowledge relevant to the user based on user's patient profile or clinical problems. Agents could also be designed to poll/mine the clinical databases for relevant intervention-outcome data relations and submit the knowledge for automated clinical guideline improvements.

Conclusion

The papers selected for this section represent some excellent work done in various areas of information retrieval. Achievements in document/information retrieval in the past have contributed significantly to enhancing the use of information in health and clinical care management. The explosive growth in biomedical literature and pressure for knowledge retrieval have set challenging targets for the health informatics community. Already research in knowledge extraction, representation and retrieval using conceptual graphs and intelligent agents has yielded exciting results. The challenge is to further improve these technologies and to build them into integrated software applications to support automated knowledge retrieval relevant to user's patient problem/profile.

References

1. http://www.nlm.nih/gov/pubs/factsheets/ online_databases.html
2. Crowe BL, McDonald JG. Evaluation of developments in storage and retrieval systems for health information systems. Proc HIC'99 – 7th National Health Informatics Conference, Hobart, Australia, 28-31 August 1999.
3. Berry D. Combing Boyer-Moore string search with regular expressions. C/C++ User Journal 2000 June;18(6):32-7.
4. De Moura SE, Navarro G, Ziviani N, Baeza-Yates R. Fast and flexible word searching on compressed text. ACM Transactions on Information Systems 2000 April;18(2):113-39.
5. Lovis C, Baud RH. Fast exact string pattern-matching algorithms adapted to the characteristics of the medical language. J Am Med Inform Assoc 2000 August; 7(4):378-91.
6. Wenzel F. Solution of morphological problems in free text retrieval during segmentation. Nachrichten für Dokumentation 1979 Dec.;30(6):212-8.
7. Doszhocs TE. Implementing an associative search interface in a large online bibliographic database environment. Proc the 39th FID Congress; 1980. p. 295-7.
8. Asokan N, Ranka S, Frieder O. A parallel free-text searching system with indexing. Proc International Conference on Databases, Parallel Architecture and their Applications, LA, USA; 1990. p. 519-21.
9. Cutting D, Pedersen J. Optimizations for dynamic inverted index maintenance. Proc the 13th International Conference on Research and Development in Information Retrieval, NY, USA; 1990. p. 405-12.
10. Xia L. Designing a visual interface for online searching. Proc The 62nd ASIS Annual Meeting NJ, USA; 1999. p.390-5.
11. Ojala M. Research into full-text retrieval. Database 1990 August;13(4):78-80.
12. Henzler RG. Free or controlled vocabularies: some statistical user-oriented evaluation of

biomedical information. International Classification 1978 March;5(1):21-6.

13. King DW, Neel PW, Wood BL. Comparative evaluation of the retrieval effectiveness of descriptor and free text search systems using CIRCOL. Research Report, Westat Research Inc., Rockville, MD, USA; January 1972.

14. Baeza-Yates R, Navarro G. Block addressing indices for approximate text retrieval. J Am Soc Inf Sci 2000 January;51 (1):69-82.

15. Schulz S, Hahn U. Morpheme-based, cross-lingual indexing for medical document retrieval. Int J Med Inf 2000; 8-59:87-9.

16. Faragher J. Questions, questions, question and answer software. Information Age 2001 January; 27-31.

17. Skolnick T. Stack search: a graphical search model. Proc International Conference on Intelligent User Interfaces NY, USA; 1999. p.190-4.

18. Lee J, Grossman D, Frieder O, McCabe MC. Integrating structured data and text: a multi-dimensional approach. Proc International Conference on Information Technology: Coding and Computing NV, USA; March 2000. p.27-9.

19. Pratt W, Fagan L. The usefulness of dynamically categorizing search results. J Am Med Inform Assoc 2000 December;7 (6):605-17.

20. Tang YK, Chiang TT. Intelligent retrieval of medical images from the Internet. Proc of Spie: The International Society for Optical Engineering, USA 1996;2711:440-8.

21. http://www.viacorp.com/crypto.html

22. Volot F, Joubert M, Fieschi M. Review of biomedical knowledge and data representation with conceptual graphs. Methods Inf Med 1998 January;37(1):86-96.

23. Delamarre D, Burgun A, Seka LP, Le Beux P. Automated coding of patient discharge summaries using conceptual graphs. Methods Inf Med 1995 September; 34(4):345-51.

24. Schroder M. Knowledge based analysis of radiology reports using conceptual graphs. Proc the 7th Annual Workshop on Conceptual Graphs, Santa Cruz, USA; 1992. p. 445-70.

25. Chu S, Cesnik B. Knowledge representation and retrieval using conceptual graphs and free text document self-organization techniques. Int J Med Inf 2001 July;62:121-33.

26. Jiang MF, Tseng SS, Tsai CJ. Intelligent query agent for structural document databases. Expert Systems with Applications 1999;17:105-13.

Address of the author:
Stephen Chu, PhD, FACS,
Associate Professor of Health Informatics
Department of Management Science
and Information Systems
University of Auckland
Private Bag 92 019
Auckland, New Zealand
Email: stephen.chu@auckland.ac.nz

Fast Exact String Pattern-matching Algorithms Adapted to the Characteristics of the Medical Language

CHRISTIAN LOVIS, MD, ROBERT H. BAUD, PhD

Abstract   Objective: The authors consider the problem of exact string pattern matching using algorithms that do not require any preprocessing. To choose the most appropriate algorithm, distinctive features of the medical language must be taken into account. The characteristics of medical language are emphasized in this regard, the best algorithm of those reviewed is proposed, and detailed evaluations of time complexity for processing medical texts are provided.

Design: The authors first illustrate and discuss the techniques of various string pattern-matching algorithms. Next, the source code and the behavior of representative exact string pattern-matching algorithms are presented in a comprehensive manner to promote their implementation. Detailed explanations of the use of various techniques to improve performance are given.

Measurements: Real-time measures of time complexity with English medical texts are presented. They lead to results distinct from those found in the computer science literature, which are typically computed with normally distributed texts.

Results: The Boyer-Moore-Horspool algorithm achieves the best overall results when used with medical texts. This algorithm usually performs at least twice as fast as the other algorithms tested.

Conclusion: The time performance of exact string pattern matching can be greatly improved if an efficient algorithm is used. Considering the growing amount of text handled in the electronic patient record, it is worth implementing this efficient algorithm.

■ **J Am Med Inform Assoc.** 2000;7:378–391.

Many, if not most, sources of medical texts are pre-processed and allow fast queries. However, health care providers and scientists are doing more and more literature research and text queries using the Internet. Information that comes through this way is not pre-processed and usually arrives as full-streamed text, in real time, in the user's computer. Clinicians need help filtering the information they receive from Internet sources like MEDLINE. On the one hand, too-specific queries will induce silence that is difficult to detect. On the other hand, too-sensitive queries provide huge numbers of data that cannot be reviewed in clinical settings in a reasonable time. A local filter providing specificity to a sensitive query in real time can answer this problem.

The same needs of filtering streamed data occur when information about patients is received from several electronic patient records (EPRs) and has to be organized in real time. Natural language processing (NLP) technologies are in focus in the literature, especially because of the growing importance of textual medical information.[1-3] The shift in the trend from numeric

Affiliations of the authors: Puget Sound Health Care System, Seattle, Washington (CL); University Hospital of Geneva, Geneva, Switzerland (RHB).

This work was supported by a grant from the University Hospital of Geneva, Switzerland.

Correspondence and reprints: Christian Lovis, MD, University Hospital of Geneva, Division of Medical Informatics, Rue Micheli-du-Crest, CH-1211 Geneva 4, Switzerland; e-mail: ⟨christian.lovis@dim.hcuge.ch⟩.

Received for publication: 10/26/99; accepted for publication: 2/16/00.

data to textual data is one of the paradigms of the modern EPR. Command-line order-entry systems are gaining popularity, and "just-in-time" literature retrieval in the EPR is becoming an essential tool.[4]

The amount of available textual data tends to double at an increasing rate. Powerful commercial document management systems that will enhance this trend are now available. With the expanding computational power at the workplace, the use of free-text data entry systems allows more freedom for physicians while maintaining the capability of further processing. In addition, the EPR extends increasingly to other sources of information, such as online medical textbooks and Internet-based references.[5]

Recent developments made in the EPR at the University Hospital of Geneva have shown the necessity of parsing, analyzing, and organizing medical text of various sources in real time during the clinician's work. A review of the medical informatics literature on that subject shows that little attention has been given to string pattern matching, especially because research in NLP has been highly focused on semantic representation, which is considered the most important and difficult step. Hume and Sunday[6] state that, "partially because the best algorithms presented in the literature are difficult to understand and to implement, knowledge of fast and practical algorithms is not commonplace." Other authors report similar observations.[7,24]

Two very different groups of techniques are known in the domain of string pattern matching. One deals with exact string pattern matching, while the other deals with partial or incomplete string pattern matching. The latter group addresses automatic word correction and the identification of typographic errors. Assuming that the pattern length is no longer than the unit memory size of the machine, the shift-or algorithm is an efficient algorithm that adapts easily to a wide range of approximate string matching problems. This algorithm is based on finite automata theory, such as the Knuth-Morris-Pratt algorithm, and exploits the finiteness of the alphabet, as in the Boyer-Moore algorithm.

In pattern recognition works, genetic algorithms are widely used to identify occurrences of complex patterns, although they are regarded primarily as a problem-solving method. Genetic algorithms are based on ideas from population genetics; they feature populations of genotypes (characteristics of an individual) stored in memory, differential reproduction of these genotypes, and variations that are created in a manner analogous to the biological processes of mutation and crossover. Genetic algorithms are powerful tools for solving complex pattern-matching problems, especially when the matching is incomplete or inexact or when it occurs on repetitive patterns separated by unmatched patterns, as it can be in searches for long DNA sequences that take into account possible alterations, from single deletions or insertions to crossovers.[8,9] However, these issues will not be discussed here.

Most exact string pattern-matching algorithms are easily adapted to deal with multiple string pattern searches or with wildcards. We present the full code and concepts underlying two major different classes of exact string search pattern algorithms, those working with hash tables and those based on heuristic skip tables. Exact string matching consists of finding one or, more generally, all of the occurrences of a pattern in a target. The algorithmic complexity of the problem is analyzed by means of standard measures of the running time and amount of memory space required by the computations.

Text-based applications must solve two kinds of problems, depending on which string, the pattern or the target, is given first. Algorithms based on the use of automata or combinatorial properties of strings are usually implemented to preprocess the pattern and solve the first kind of problem. However, difficulties arise when one tries to recognize a specific pattern in various targets or streams of symbols arriving through a communication channel. In this case, no preprocessing of the target is possible. This contrasts with locating words in a dictionary or an entire corpus of texts that are known in advance and can be preprocessed or indexed. Among all exact text pattern-matching algorithms, those that can be used in real time on continuous streams of data are the focus of this paper. This means that neither the target nor the patterns are known in advance. Therefore, neither preprocessing nor indexing is feasible.

Notation

The term *target* is used to specify the corpus of text to search in, and the term *pattern* to identify the substring of text to search for. The pattern is denoted by $x = x_{0..m-1}$ characters and the target by $y = y_{0..n-1}$ characters. The first character in a target is therefore y_0, and the last one is y_{n-1}, where n and m are, respectively, the length of the target and the pattern. The notation x_i or y_j refers to the characters currently analyzed in both the pattern and the target. By definition, the *alphabet* is the set of all possible symbols that can be used to represent a target or a pattern. The representation $O(mn)$ is used to express the time complexity of the algorithm

Table 1 ■

Effect of Multiple Occurrences on the Number of Iterations before a Correct Fail Occurs

ICD Expression	Segments	Occurrences in ICD-10	Minimum Iterations
dilated cardio-myopathy		1	
	dilated	1	7
	cardiomyopathy	27	378
	cardio	106	636
	myopathy	51	408
	myo	297	891
	pathy	354	1,770

as a function of the sizes of the pattern and the target. Typically, the pattern is small and the target is large, m being much smaller than n.

Morphologic Characteristics of Medical Language

Medical language is characteristic in its wide and frequent use of Latin and Greek roots. This results in many words that have similar suffixes or prefixes. The consequence of frequent use of common roots is that trivial string pattern-matching algorithms, which usually perform their character matching sequentially, have a high rate of unnecessary *fail* iterations.

Our previous work in morphosemantic analysis and representation of medical text demonstrates the high use rate of compound words in medical texts.[10,11] The frequent utilization of common roots implies that, in theory, purely left-to-right or right-to-left algorithms are generally less efficient than algorithms that proceed randomly. Although these roots have a typical length of five to seven characters, their aggregation can lead to much longer repetitive patterns. Table 1

shows an example of a diagnosis found in ICD-10 with the number of occurrences of its different roots. So, for example, an algorithm analyzing strictly from right to left will have to compare the word *cardiomyopathy* 27 times before it will find the first association with *dilated*.

Some frequent patterns can be found within words that are an aggregation of typical common roots, such as *gastroentero* or *colorecto*, and suffixes, such as *ectomy* and *stomy*. The behavior of that kind of typical pattern in medical language is recognized and has been widely studied.[12-15] The overall result is a non-normal distribution of morphologic patterns in texts, which emphasizes the problem of exact string pattern-matching by increasing significantly the number of attempts needed to uniquely identify words when common algorithms are used. An example is shown in Figure 1.

Increasing the performance of exact pattern matching is a complex task. Theoretic good solutions can have high computational costs. For example, because of common prefixes and suffixes, it is interesting, in theory, to perform a pattern comparison in the middle of a potential match to improve the chance of failure in case of mismatch. However, the cost of searching the middle of a word (performing a div 2, for example) appears to be more expensive in time than performing a few additional comparisons, except in the case of long patterns.

Search Algorithms

Major categories and characteristics of exact string pattern matching algorithms have been reviewed by Hume and Sunday[16] and Pirklbauer,[17] among others. Deep and comprehensive understanding of conceptual frameworks and theoretic estimates of time and

```
Looking for hypothyroidism in the sentence.

Attempts pass 1:
The patient suffers from hypothermia probably due to hypothyroidism
                        hypothyroidism
In a conventional algorithm, six successful character matches were done before the first fail
    because of the hypoth common root

Attempts pass 2 :
The patient suffers from hypothermia probably due to hypothyroidism
                                                     hypothyroidism
In a conventional algorithm, the window analyzed goes forward one character at each fail
    comparison, except when it finds the first hypoth. At this position, the window stops and
    comparisons are performed in the word itself until it fails because the 7th letter of
    hypothermia is different than the 7th character of hypothyroidism. The window is then again
    forwarded one character. This shows that, in conventional algorithms, there is a high cost
    (and unnecessary comparisons) each time a common root is found in a word that will not match.
```

Figure 1 Example of exact pattern matching in case of common roots.

space complexity is provided,[18] especially in analyzing the behavior of these algorithms in the worst cases or using randomly generated string targets and patterns. However, there is a lack of data about the average behavior of these algorithms when used with real text corpora that have highly non-normal distributed symbols, such as the medical sublanguage. When neither preprocessing nor indexing is feasible for the target, and only limited preprocessing in space and time is affordable for the pattern, the problem of pattern matching analysis can be roughly divided into two sequences—*comparison* and *slide to next comparison*. Both steps can be optimized.

The comparison step often can be spared by the use of a hashing table.[21] Hashing functions provide an alternative way to compare strings. Essentially, this technique is based on the comparison of string hash values instead of direct character comparison and usually requires the text to be preprocessed. Hashing is a powerful and simple technique for accessing information: Each key is mathematically converted into a number, which is then used as an index into a table. In typical applications, it is common for two different strings to map to the same index, requiring some strategy for collision resolution. With a perfect function, a string could be identified in exactly one probe, without worrying about collisions.

A simple hash function performs calculations using the binary codes of the characters in a key. The record's position in the table is calculated based only on the key value itself, not how many elements are in the table. This is why hash-table inserts, deletes, and searches are rated constant time. However, finding perfect hashing functions is possible only when the set of possibilities is completely known in advance, so that each unique entry in the text has one entry in the hash table. In case of collision, that is, when the hashing value is the same for two different substrings, a formal, character-by-character comparison is performed. If the comparison is a success, a match is found. In our measures, such algorithms behave poorly for medical text, with high costs due to the time spent in the hashing function. It must be emphasized, however, that algorithms using hashing tables perform spectacularly when the target can be preprocessed and can be easily extended to multidimensional pattern matching problems. These problems are common in bioinformatics and imaging.

Use of a skip table that allows a jump of more than one character in the case of failure[20] can optimize the slide step. To understand the use of heuristic skip tables, consider that the target is examined through a window. This window delimits a region of the target and usually has the length of the pattern. Such a window slides along the target from one side to the other and is periodically shifted according to rules specific for each algorithm. When the window is at a certain position on the target, the algorithm checks whether the pattern occurs there or not by comparing symbols in the window with the corresponding aligned symbols of the pattern. If a whole match occurs, the position is reported. During this scan operation, the algorithm acquires information from the target that is used to determine the length of the next shift of the window. This operation is repeated until the end of the pattern goes beyond or reaches the end of the target. It is an effective procedure to optimize time cost during a scan operation that can be used in right-to-left or left-to-right search engines.

The so-called *naive* or *brute force* algorithm is the most intuitive approach to the string pattern-matching problem. This algorithm attempts simply to match the pattern in the target at successive positions from left to right. If failure occurs, it shifts the comparison window one character to the right until the end of the target is reached. In the worst case, this method runs in $O(mn)$ time, but in a practical approach, the expected overall performance is near $O(n + m)$. Despite the theoretic bad performance of this algorithm, our measures show that the naive algorithm is one of the fastest methods when the pattern is a short sequence of characters.

The Knuth-Morris-Pratt method[19] derives an algorithm from the two-way deterministic automata that runs, in the worst case, in $O(m + n)$ time for random sequences. The basic idea behind this algorithm is to avoid backtracking in the target string in the event of a mismatch, by taking advantage of information given by the type of mismatch. The target is processed sequentially from left to right. When a substring match-attempt fails, the previous symbols, which are known, are used to determine how far the pattern can be shifted to the right for the next match attempt.

Boyer and Moore[20] published a much faster algorithm in 1974. The speed of this algorithm is achieved by disregarding portions of the target that cannot, in any case, participate in a successful match.

The Naive Algorithm

The naive algorithm (Figure 2) is the simplest and most often used algorithm. It uses a linear and sequential character-based comparison at all positions in the text between y_0 and y_{n-m-1}, whether or not an occurrence of the pattern x starts at the current position. In case of success in matching the first element of the pattern x_0, each element of the pattern is successively tested against the text until failure or success

```
function naive(const target, pattern : PChar; const lTarget, lPattern : integer) : integer;
var
  i,                                         // main loop
  j     : integer;                           // comparison loop
begin
  result := -1;                              // returns -1 if no match or error
  if lTarget * lPattern = 0 then exit;       // nothing to compare
  for i := 0 to lTarget - 1 do               // main loop
    if pattern[0] = target[i] then
    begin
      for j := 1 to lPattern - 1 do          // comparison loop
        if pattern[j] <> target[i+j] then break;   // failure, exit comparison loop
      if j = lPattern then                   // match found
      begin
        result := i+1;
        exit;
      end;
    end; // for
end; // Naive
```

Figure 2 The Naive algorithm.

```
function Karp_Rabin(const target, pattern : PChar; const lTarget, lPattern : integer) :
  integer;
const
  b = 8;                                     // func for bitwise left rotate
var
  hashPattern,                               // pattern hash value
  hashTarget,                                // target hash value
  Bm,                                        // dummy var for computing the hash
  i,                                         // main loop
  j         : integer;
begin
  result := -1;
  if lTarget * lPattern = 0 then exit;
  Bm := 1;
  hashPattern := 0;
  hashTarget := 0;
                                             // preprocessing of pattern's hash value
  for j := 0 to lPattern-1 do
  begin
    Bm := Bm shl b;
    hashPattern := hashPattern shl b + ord(pattern[j]);
    hashTarget := hashTarget shl b + ord(target[j]);
  end;
                                             // search main loop
  for j := pred(lPattern) to pred(lTarget) do
  begin
    if (hashPattern = hashTarget) then       // match of hash values
    begin
      i := 0;
      while (i < lPattern-1) and (pattern[i] = target[j-lPattern+1 + i]) do inc(i);
                                             // comparison loop
      if i=lPattern - 1 then                 // Match found
      begin
        result := j-lPattern+2;
        exit;                                // if failure, incremental computation
                                             // of the target's hash value
    end else hashTarget := hashTarget shl b - ord(target[j-lPattern+1])*Bm +
ord(target[j+1]);
    end else hashTarget := hashTarget shl b - ord(target[j-lPattern+1])*Bm +
ord(target[j+1]);
  end; // for
end; // Karp_Rabin
```

Figure 3 The Karp-Rabin algorithm.

occurs at the last position. After each unsuccessful attempt, the pattern is shifted exactly one position to the right, and this procedure is repeated until the end of the target is reached.

The naive search algorithm has several advantages. It needs no preprocessing of any kind on the pattern and requires only a fixed amount of extra memory space.

The Karp-Rabin Algorithm

In theory, hashing functions provide a simple way to avoid the quadratic number of symbol comparisons in most practical situations. These functions run in constant time under reasonable probabilistic assumptions. Hashing technique was introduced by Harrison and later fully analyzed by Karp and Rabin. The Karp-Rabin algorithm (Figure 3) is a typical string-pattern-matching algorithm that uses the hashing technique.[21] Instead of checking at each position of the target to see whether the pattern occurs, it checks only whether the portion of the target aligned with the pattern has a hashing value similar to the pattern. To be helpful for the string-matching problem, great attention must be given to the hashing function. It must be efficiently computable, highly discriminating for strings, and computable in an incremental manner in order to decrease the cost of processing. Incremental hashing functions allow new hashing values for a window of the target to be computed step by step without the whole window having to be recomputed. The time performance of this algorithm is, in the unlikely worst case, $O(mn)$ with an expected time performance of $O(m + n)$.

Several different ways to perform the hashing function have been published. The original Karp-Rabin algorithm has been implemented in our system because it is easily adaptable to different alphabet sizes. The comparative measures we performed showed that most of the time is spent during the incremental hashing phase. Therefore, even though the Karp-Rabin algorithm needs fewer symbol comparisons than other algorithms to locate a pattern in a large target text, the cost of computing the hashing function outweighs the advantage of performing fewer symbol comparisons, at least for common medical language.

The Knuth-Morris-Pratt Algorithm

The first published linear-time string-matching algorithm was from Morris and Pratt and was improved by Knuth et al.[22] and others.[23] The Knuth-Morris-Pratt algorithm (Figure 4) is the classical algorithm that implements efficiently the left-to-right scan strategy. The search behaves like a recognition process by automaton, and a character of the target is compared to a character of the pattern. The basic idea behind the algorithm is to avoid backtracking in the target string in the event of a mismatch. This is achieved by the use of a failure function. When a substring match attempt fails, the previous character sequence is known (*the suffix*), and this fact can be exploited to determine how far to shift the pattern to the right for the next match attempt. Basically, if a partial match is found such that $target[i - j + 1..i - 1] = pattern[1..j - 1]$ and $target[i] \neq pattern[j]$, then matching is resumed by comparing $target[i]$ and $pattern[f(j - 1) + 1]$ if $j > 1$, where f is the failure function. If $j = 1$, then the comparison continues with $target[i + 1]$ and $pattern[1]$. An auxiliary step table (heuristic skip table) containing this optimal shift information (failure function) is computed from the pattern before the string is searched.

Two examples of failure function follow:

- Pattern "*abcabcacab*": If we are currently determining whether there is a match beginning at $target[i]$, then if $target[i]$ is not the character "*a*," we can proceed by comparing $target[i + 1]$ and "*a*." Similarly, if $target[i] = $ "*a*" and $target[i + 1] < >$ "*b*," then we may continue by comparing $target[i + 1]$ and "*a*." If $target[i] = $ "*a*" and $target[i + 1] = $ "*b*" $= ab$ and $target[i + 2] < >$ "*c*," then we have the situation:

  $$target: \text{"ab?.."}$$

  where ? means that the character is not yet known.

- Pattern: "*abcabcacab*": The first ? in the target represents $target[i + 2]$ and it is different from the character "*c*." At this point, it is known that the search might be continued for a match by comparing the first character in the pattern with $target[i + 2]$. However, there is no need to compare this character of the pattern with $target[i + 1]$, since we already know that $target[i + 1]$ is the same as the second character of the pattern, "*b*," and that it is not matched with the first character of the pattern, "*a*." Thus, by knowing the characters in the pattern and the position in the pattern where a mismatch occurs with a character in the target we can determine where in the pattern to continue the search for a match without moving backwards in the target.

The worst case performance occurs for normally distributed string patterns. In this case, the algorithm usually runs near $O(mn)$ in time complexity, but it may run in $O(m + n)$. This method performs well for large patterns made of repetitive short substrings.

```
function Knuth_Morris_Pratt(const target, pattern : PChar; const lTarget, lPattern :
  integer) : integer;
var
  step  : array[0..255] of integer;              // failure table
  i,                                             // main loop
  j        : integer;
begin
  result := -1;
  if lTarget * lPattern = 0 then exit;
  i := 0;
  j := -1;
  step[0] := -1;
                                                 // preprocessing the table
  repeat
    if (j = -1) or (pattern[i] = pattern[j]) then
    begin
      inc(i);
      inc(j);
      if pattern[j] = pattern[i] then step[i] := step[j] else step[i] := j;
    end else j := step[j];
  until i = lPattern - 1;
  j := -1;
  i := 0;
                                                 // search main loop
  while i < lTarget do
  begin
    if (j=-1) or (pattern[j] = target[i]) then   // comparison loop
    begin
      inc(i);
      inc(j);
      if j >= lPattern then                      // Match found
      begin
        result := i-j+1;
        exit;
      end;
    end else j := step[j];                       // skips the value found in the table
  end; // while
end; // Knutt_Morris_Pratt
```

Figure 4 The Knuth-Morris-Pratt algorithm.

This situation is rarely met in medical texts. Thus, in practice, the KMP algorithm is not likely to be significantly faster than the other approaches.

The Boyer-Moore-Horspool Algorithm

The Boyer-Moore algorithm (Figure 5) is considered the most efficient string-matching algorithm for natural language. In this method, the pattern is searched in the target from left to right. At each trial position, the symbol comparisons are performed to minimize the number of trials in case of unsuccessful matches while maximizing the pattern shift for the next trial. In a case of mismatch, the BM algorithm combines two different shift functions to optimize the number of characters that can be skipped during the skip process. These two shift functions are called the *bad-character shift* (or *occurrence* heuristic) and the *good-suffix shift* (or *match* heuristic). The latter method is similar to the one used in the KMP algorithm and is based on the pending symbol causing the mismatch. For every symbol of the pattern the length of a safe shift is stored. This shift corresponds to the distance between the last occurrence of that symbol in the pattern and the length of the pattern. The most interesting property of that technique is that the longer the length of the pattern, the longer the potential shifts. The final pattern shift is determined by taking the larger of the values from the two precomputed auxiliary tables. It is important to note that both methods can be preprocessed and kept in tables. Their time and space complexities depend only on the pattern. However, although there is a theoretic advantage in using the BM algorithm, many computational steps in this algorithm are costly in terms of processor instructions. The cost in time of the computational step was not shown to be amortized by the economy of character comparisons. This is particularly true of the function that computes the size comparisons in the skip tables. Horspool proposed a simplified form of the BM algorithm that use only a single auxiliary skip table indexed by the mismatching text symbols.[24] Baeza-Yates showed that the Boyer-Moore-Horspool algorithm (BMH) is the best in terms of average case perfor-

```
function Boyer_Moore_Horspool(const target, pattern : PChar; const lTarget, lPattern :
  integer) : integer;
var
  i,                                         // main loop
  j,                                         // comparison loop
  k      : integer;
  step   : array [0..255] of integer;        // skip table for the alphabet
begin
  result := 0;
  if lTarget * lPattern = 0 then exit;
  // preprocessing
  for k := 0 to 255 do step[k] := lPattern;          // initialize skip table
  for k := 0 to Pred(lPattern) do step[ord(pattern[k])] := lPattern-k;   // skip table for
                                                                          // the pattern

                                                     // search main loop
  k := Pred(lPattern);
  while k <= lTarget do
  begin
    i := k-1;
    j := lPattern-1;
    while target[i] = pattern[j] do                  // comparison loop
    begin
      dec(i);
      dec(j);
    end; // while
    if j = - 1 then                                  // Match found
    begin
      result := i + 2;
      exit;
    end;
    k := k + step[ord(target[k])];                   // if failure, skip the value in skip table
  end; // while
end; // Boyer_Moore_Horspool
```

Figure 5 The Boyer-Moore-Horspool algorithm.

mance for nearly all pattern lengths and alphabet sizes (remember that the French alphabet is somewhat larger than the English alphabe).[25] Yet, among all published algorithms we tested, the BMH algorithm showed the best performance in time, by far. The BMH algorithm will be studied more deeply, as it appears to be the best-choice algorithm in most cases. Because of its low space complexity, we recommend the use of the BMH algorithm in any case of exact string pattern matching, whatever the size of the target. Despite its apparent conceptual complexity, the BMH algorithm is relatively simple to implement. Moreover, it can easily be extended to handle multiple matches by generating events when a match occurs instead of leaving the algorithm as in the following example:

Example of pattern:

a	b	c	d

Example of text:

a	b	d	e	b	c	a	b	d	d	e	a	b	c	d

Construction of the skip table for the pattern:

a	b	c	d	e	f	...	y	z
3	2	1	4	4	4	4	4	4

This means that the distance from any character in the pattern to the last position in the pattern is known and that any character not in the pattern will produce a shift that is the length of the pattern. This table contains an entry for every single symbol present in the alphabet. For usual hardware platforms, it consists of the 256 entries found in an 8-bit ASCII table.

Search process

Loop 1: ◄——————— *right-to-left*

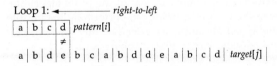

pattern[i] = d is different than *target[j] = e*.
Lookup in skip table for symbol *e* gives value 4; therefore, shift right four characters.

Loop 2: ——————► *left-to-right shift*

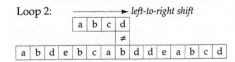

pattern[i] = d is different than *target[j] = b*.
Lookup in skip table for symbol *b* gives value 2; therefore, shift right two characters.

Loop 3:

a	b	c	d
			=

a	b	d	e	b	c	a	b	d	d	e	a	b	c	d

pattern[i] = d is equivalent to *target[j] = d*.
pattern[i − 1] = c is different than *target[j − 1] = d*.
Lookup in skip table for symbol *d* gives value 4; therefore, shift right four characters.

Loop 4:

a	b	c	d
			≠

a	b	d	e	b	c	a	b	d	d	e	a	b	c	d

pattern[i − 1] = d is different than *target[j − 1] = c*.
Lookup in skip table for symbol *c* gives value 1; therefore, shift right one character.

Loop 5 (finish):

a	b	c	d
			=

a	b	d	e	b	c	a	b	d	d	e	a	b	c	d

Full match after four successful comparisons.

The BMH-2 algorithm is a slight variant of the BMH algorithm, which implements a new comparison method. In the BM and BMH algorithms, the comparison loop is entered if the last character of the pattern matches the current target position. In the BMH-2 algorithm, this loop is entered only if both the last and the middle characters of the pattern match with their respective positions in the target. This is a more conservative control of the right-to-left comparison loop. For long medical words, because of the frequent use of common suffixes and prefixes, this preliminary comparison generally allows skipping of several character comparisons and optimizes the left-to-right shift. Although this improvement decreases the number of character comparisons by 80 percent in the best cases, as described under Measures, the overall time complexity is often similar to that of the BMH algorithm. Given the increased time cost, performing the middle comparison becomes cost-effective only for long patterns, usually longer than 20 characters.

Space Complexity of the Tested Algorithms

For all algorithms, space usage of the pattern and the target is the same. The extra space complexity of each algorithm is self-explained in the code by the added variables—4 bytes for the naive algorithm, 12 bytes for the Karp-Rabin algorithm, 516 bytes for the Knuth-Morris-Pratt algorithm, and 518 bytes for the Boyer-Moore-Horspool algorithm. These values have been computed with 32-bit integers. They are constant.

Measures

Method

All algorithms were implemented in Object Pascal using Delphi version 4.03.[26] The tests were conducted on a 400-MHz Pentium II biprocessor PC with 256-Mbytes of 7ns SDRAM so that all tests could be done in memory. We used a biprocessor computer to minimize the variance of time measures caused by alternate system interruptions or operating system processes. All threads used by the test program were forced to run asynchronously on the same processor. Therefore, we expect the measures to be comparable with what could be found in real conditions in applications.

The target text was a corpus of medical texts that has a usual distribution of symbols and words. All tests were done using French and English texts. The French corpus consisted of 1,000 discharge summaries of the surgical depatment of the University Hospital of Geneva. The English corpus was the complete volume II of the World Health Organization's International Classification of Diseases, version 10, which was chosen because it is a stable, well-known, and reproducible source of text. This target text consisted of 197,550 words in 57,742 lines, corresponding to 1,606,861 characters (including spaces and end-of-line separators). All texts were converted to be compatible with the ASCII 8-bit table. The measures we present here were accomplished using the English corpus. Comparable results were found when using the French corpus.

All preprocessing loads were measured within their respective algorithms. The parameters of the function calls of each algorithm used pointers to zero-terminated strings in order to avoid variance due to memory management. All memory for strings was allocated before the calls. The functions, however, were self-contained. All function examples have been implemented using the same function call prototype —**function** *aSearchAlgorithm*(**const** target, pattern : PChar; **const** 1Target, 1Pattern : integer) : integer— where *pattern* and *target* are pointers to zero-terminated strings, *lTarget* and *lPattern* are integers representing the respective lengths of the target and the pattern. The functions return the value −1 in case of error, or else they return the position in the target where the first occurrence of pattern was found. No preprocessing or global variables were needed for their execution. When hashing tables were needed, the computation was done within the function and the time cost allocated to that function. Whenever possible, the functions were optimized for speed, for example, by using bitwise shifts to compute fast multiplications. Time measures were done using the motherboard's high-resolution performance counter. The expected precision is about 0.00083 msec. An overview of the method is shown in Figure 6.

The corpus of text was divided into 150 slices of 3,214 characters, except the last one, which had 39 fewer characters. All measurements were done in an incremental manner for a corpus size growing in 150 steps from the size of one slice to the whole target size. At each of the 150 increases in size, all algorithms were tested for the various patterns. Each measurement was repeated ten times at each increase step. The values reported are arithmetic means of these ten measurements.

If *f* is the position where the pattern can be found in the target, then a regular augmentation of duration will be observed as the size increases. This increase will be observed until the actual size reaches the *f* point. This increase of duration represents the processing cost and is a function of the size of both the pattern and the target. This function is equivalent to $O(f[n, m])$, the complexity in time. In all algorithms tested, this function is linear in time. A linear regression of this function permits comparison of the time complexity of the algorithms. The slope of the regression line corresponds to the average number of characters parsed per milliseconds.

Once the position *f* is reached, further increases of the target size will not continue to influence the time complexity. In the graphical representation of the results, the plot of the data shows a slope almost flat after the *f* position. The slight slopes remaining are due to the increase in space complexity of the target. This flat portion of the plot represents the stability of the algorithm to reach *f* even if the size after *f* continues to grow. The mean abscissa can be used to compare different algorithms with an independent *t*-test.

All the algorithms we considered work with an approximately constant cost in space. In the worst case, the extra space needed for processing is a linear function of the length of the pattern, which is negligible. Moreover, in this analysis, space complexity is similar for all algorithms tested. It must be emphasized that this would not be true for any algorithm. In particular, it excludes most automata based on tree representations that typically have a quadratic cost in space.

Choice of Patterns

All tests were performed using three different patterns. The first pattern tested was *dyspraxia*. This word was chosen because its position is at one third of the target. It is a short word (nine characters), composed

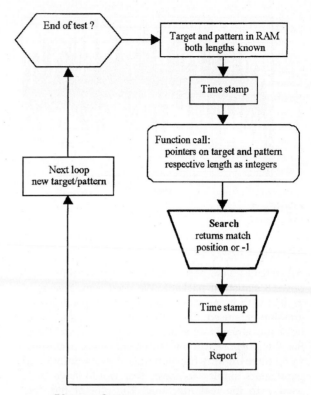

Figure 6 Overview of the test method.

of a very common prefix (*dys*) and a rather uncommon suffix (*praxia*). Such words tend to give an advantage to right-to-left algorithms.

The second pattern tested was *polychondritis*. It is a typical-length word (14 characters) for the medical domain, composed of three Latin/Greek roots (*poly–chondr–itis*). Among these roots, the first and the last are very common in the target corpus. For all types of algorithms, such words tend to increase the number of comparisons that fail. The length of this word tends to give a slight advantage to algorithms that use skip tables.

The last pattern tested was *superficial injuries of wrist and hand*. This sentence represents a typical aggregation of words used in the EPR. It is composed of six words and 37 characters. The length of such a pattern tends to favor algorithms that optimize the skip function. The length also favors algorithms that optimize the comparison loop. The pattern is located at the end of the target and therefore also demonstrates the impact of space complexity on overall performance.

Detailed data of the analysis and the program sources are available at http://www.lovis.net/pub/patterntest.htm

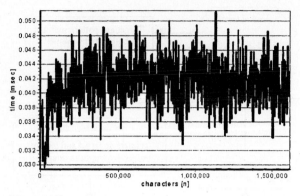

Figure 7 Baseline measures determining the noise of the system.

Statistical Analysis

All statistics were performed using the SPSS for Windows 8 statistical package. We used comparisons of groups with independent samples. Multiple linear regression was used, and all models were adjusted for noise introduced by the precision of the internal timer. For this purpose, 10^{12} measurements were performed using three dummy function calls with conditions and parameters similar to those that would have been used with the real functions. The plot of the data shows an initial increasing region that permitted a precise analysis of time complexity during mismatch phases. Analysis was performed using linear regression with the duration of processing as the predictor of interest and the size the target as the response variable. This made the interpretation of the slope easier. In this case, the slope was the number of characters analyzed in the target for each 1-msec increase of the predictor. Means were compared using an analysis of variance (ANOVA) and an independent two-tailed t-test. Where appropriate, 95% confidence intervals (CI) are given.

Results

Baseline

The baseline measurements of the system are shown in Figure 7. They can be assimilated to the noise of the system. The data are obtained by calling the function with parameters as used in normal conditions but without any action performed. Mean time spent to call function and background noise was 0.0414 ± 0.0032 msec, (95% CI, 0.04136–0.04166). These data are almost normally distributed. It must be emphasized that the cost in time is constant and independent of the size of the tested target, with the exception of a size fewer than 50 thousand characters, for which the cost in time is slightly less. This explains the slight

left skewness of the histogram plot of these data. However, when these algorithms were evaluated in real conditions, this slight skewness appeared to be of negligible importance for the interpretation of the results.

Figure 8 shows an example of the graphical output of the data. The test was performed with the pattern *amnesia nos*. This pattern is found at position 647,906 in the English target (ICD-10). For all algorithms, the data presented the same global pattern. The first phase was a linear increase for duration along with augmentation of the size of the target, as long as the pattern was not present in the part of the target being analyzed. As soon as the pattern was found in the target, the duration remained approximately constant and independent of the size of the target that was after the match position. This figure shows that the time complexity increased linearly or nearly so for each algorithm until the target contained the pattern. On the one hand, analysis of slopes of the regression line before the match for algorithms using the same pattern allowed comparison of the efficiency of the algorithm for different target sizes. On the other hand, use of the same algorithm and different patterns allowed comparison of the efficiency according to the pattern size and provided, therefore, an experimental observation of the $O(f[n, m])$ theoretic evaluation.

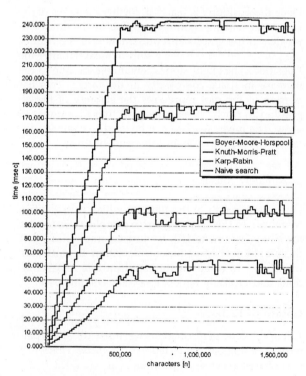

Figure 8 Complexity is linear in time.

Search for *Dyspraxia*

The first test was done using the word *dyspraxia*. This word was found at position 599,410 in the target text.

The difference in performance was highly significant for all group mean comparisons ($p < 0.0001$) except between BMH and BMH-2, where the p value was 0.661 (Table 2). It is worth noting that BMH is 1.68 times faster than the naive algorithm.

Search for *Polychondritis*

The word *polychondritis* was found at position 939,424 in the target text.

Means were very different between all groups ($p < 0.0001$) except BMH and BMH-2, where the p value was 0.99 (Table 3).

Search for *Superficial Injuries of Wrist and Hand*

The phrase *superficial injuries of wrist and hand* was found at position 1,224,835 in the target text.

Means were highly different between all groups ($p < 0.0001$), including BMH and BMH-2 (Table 4). However, the mean difference of 8.11 msec (95% CI, 6.18–10.03) in favor of BMH-2, while significant, was probably negligible in practice, since it represents less than 10 percent improvement.

Performance According to Pattern Size

Algorithms that do not use a skip table to optimize the shift function are rather independent of the pattern size in their time complexity. This was not the case for the two BMH algorithms. In the latter, one sees that the greater the pattern size, the longer the skip shift in case of mismatch and, therefore, the faster the algorithm. However, as illustrated with the word *polychondritis*, when the pattern ends with a suffix that appears frequently in the target, the BMH algorithms lose performance, because the loop comparison is more complex than the one in the naive algorithm. This fact was even more strongly illustrated with the BMH-2 algorithm, as a greater loss in the case of *polychondritis* and a greater win in the case of the longest pattern. Nevertheless, the BMH algorithms were still faster in all three cases (Table 5).

The overall results of all algorithms tested are presented in Figure 9, using the number of characters analyzed per millisecond. In this figure, for each pattern tested, the fastest algorithm received the index value of 1. The other algorithms for the same pattern are represented as fractions of the fastest. For example, for the pattern of nine characters, the KR algo-

Table 2 ∎

Search Results Using the Word "Dyspraxia"

	Slope (char/msec)	Mean (msec)	SD (msec)	95% CI Mean (msec)
Naive	4,694.21	131.93	3.88	131.14–132.72
KMP	2,622.41	229.26	4.43	228.36–230.17
KR	2,008.03	296.63	4.40	295.73–297.53
BMH	8,648.89	77.71	5.83	76.52–78.90
BMH-2	8,051.44	77.30	6.90	75.90–78.71

NOTE: Naive indicates naive algorithm; KR, Karp-Rabin algorithm; KMP, Knuth-Morris-Pratt algorithm; BMH, Boyer-Moore-Horspool algorithm; BMH-2, variant of Boyer-Moore-Horspool algorithm.

Table 3 ∎

Search Results Using the Word "Polychondritis"

	Slope (char/msec)	Mean (msec)	SD (msec)	95% CI Mean (msec)
Naive	4,491.43	199.25	4.45	198.13–200.38
KMP	2,514.84	365.95	4.27	364.88–367.03
KR	2,009.18	462.21	3.33	461.37–463.04
BMH	8,544.54	108.70	5.49	107.32–110.08
BMH-2	7,635.49	108.71	5.54	107.32–110.11

NOTE: Naive indicates naive algorithm; KR, Karp-Rabin algorithm; KMP, Knuth-Morris-Pratt algorithm; BMH, Boyer-Moore-Horspool algorithm; BMH-2, variant of Boyer-Moore-Horspool algorithm.

Table 4 ∎

Search Results Using the Pattern "Superficial Injuries of Wrist and Hand"

	Slope (char/msec)	Mean (msec)	SD (msec)	95% CI Mean (msec)
Naive	4,295.91	273.58	3.28	272.47–274.49
KMP	2,570.51	468.25	3.12	467.19–469.30
KR	1,899.99	632.08	4.66	630.51–633.66
BMH	10,087.08	108.81	4.89	107.15–110.46
BMH-2	11,216.133	100.70	3.12	99.64–101.75

NOTE: Naive indicates naive algorithm; KR, Karp-Rabin algorithm; KMP, Knuth-Morris-Pratt algorithm; BMH, Boyer-Moore-Horspool algorithm; BMH-2, variant of Boyer-Moore-Horspool algorithm.

Table 5 ∎

Slope Variation According to Pattern Size (Characters per Millisecond)

	9 chars/msec	14 chars/msec	37 chars/msec
Naive	4,694.21	4,491.43	4,295.91
KMP	2,622.41	2,514.84	2,570.51
KR	2,008.03	2,009.18	1,899.99
BMH	8,649.89	8,544.54	10,087.08
BMH-2	8,051.44	7,635.49	11,216.133

NOTE: Naive indicates naive algorithm; KR, Karp-Rabin algorithm; KMP, Knuth-Morris-Pratt algorithm; BMH, Boyer-Moore-Horspool algorithm; BMH-2, variant of Boyer-Moore-Horspool algorithm.

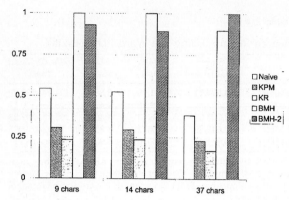

Figure 9 Overall performance of the five algorithms tested.

rithm performs the search at one fourth the speed of the BMH algorithm. This figure emphasizes the extreme speed of the BMH algorithm and the slight advantage to implement an optimized control for the optimization loop for long patterns. It shows also that the naive algorithm, compared with the BMH algorithm, performs less well with long patterns than with short ones.

Reproducibility

There are several limitations to this study. The performance of all algorithms tested may vary with the processors and the way they handle memory accesses, integer manipulation, and floating operations. On a given hardware, algorithms may behave differently according to the language used to implement them. In a given language, different versions of compilers may lead to different results. Finally, the programming style will affect the results. In our experience, however, it seems that the relative performance of each algorithm, one to the other, is stable across all these factors except the programmer's style.

The measures of performance have been performed on various texts in French and English. These texts include ICD-10, MEDLINE abstracts, discharge letters, and several nonmedical texts. The relative performance of all algorithms tested has been similar to that of the algorithms presented in this paper using ICD-10.

Conclusion

The BMH algorithm is a fast and easy-to-implement algorithm. The performance of this algorithm can barely be improved when working with medical lanaguage, except for long patterns. It typically performs better than the naive algorithm, which is mostly used

for string pattern matching. Considering the growing amount of text handled in the EPR, the BMH algorithm is worth implementing in any case. Other algorithms that could theoretically perform better do not, compared with the BMH algorithm under real conditions. If long patterns are used, a more conservative control of the right-to-left comparison loop can slightly improve the time performance of the BMH algorithm.

References ■

1. Friedman C, Hripcsak G, Shagina L, Liu H. Representing information in patient reports using natural language processing and the extensible markup language. J Am Med Inform Assoc. 1999;6(1):76–87.
2. Stein HD, Nadkarni P, Erdos J, Miller PL. Exploring the degree of concordance of coded and textual data in answering clinical queries from a clinical data repository. J Am Med Inform Assoc. 2000;7:42–54.
3. Charlet J, Bachimont B, Brunie V, el Kassar S, Zweigenbaum P, Boisvieux JF. Hospitexte: toward a document-based hypertextual electronic medical record. Proc AMIA Symp. 1998:713–7.
4. Lovis C, Baud RH, Planche P. Power of expression in the electronic patient record: structured data or narrative text? Submitted to Int J Med Inform.
5. Lovis C, Baud RH, Scherrer JR. Internet integrated in the daily medical practice within an electronic patient record. Comput Biol Med. 1998;28:567–79.
6. Hume SC, Sunday D. Fast string searching. Software Practice and Experience. 1991;21(11):1221–48.
7. Sedgewick R. Algorithms. Reading, Mass: Addison-Wesley, 1983;19:241–55.
8. Forrest S. Genetic algorithms: principles of natural selection applied to computation. Science. 1993;261(5123):872–8.
9. Notredame C, Holm L, Higgins DG. COFFEE: an objective function for multiple sequence alignments. Bioinformatics. 1998;14(5):407–22.
10. Baud RH, Lovis C, Rassinoux AM, Scherrer JR. Morphosemantic parsing of medical expressions. Proc AMIA Symp. 1998;760–4.
11. Lovis C, Baud RH, Rassinoux AM, Michel PA. Medical dictionaries for patient encoding systems: a methodology. Artif Intel Med. 1998;14(1–2):201–14.
12. Pacak MG, Norton LM, Dunham GS. Morphosemantic analysis of -itis forms in medical language. Methods Inf Med. 1980(19):99–105.
13. Norton LM, Pacak MG. Morphosemantic analysis of compound word forms denoting surgical procedures. Methods Inf Med. 1983;(22):29–36.
14. Wolff S. The use of morphosemantic regularities in the medical vocabulary for automatic lexical coding. Methods Inf Med. 1984;(23):195–203.
15. Dujols P, Aubas P, Baylon C, Grémy F. Morphosemantic analysis and translation of medical compound terms. Methods Inf Med. 1991(30):30–5.
16. Hume SC, Sunday D. Fast string searching. Software Practice and Experience. 1991;21(11):1221–48.
17. Pirklbauer K. A study of pattern-matching algorithms. Structured Programming. 1992;(13):89–98.
18. Gonnet GH, Baeza-Yates R. Text Algorithms: Handbook of Algorithms and Data Structures in Pascal and C. 2nd edi-

tion. Wokingham, U.K.: Addison-Wesley, 1991(7):251–88.

19. Knuth DE, Morris JH Jr, Pratt VR. Fast pattern matching in strings. SIAM J Comput. 1997;6(1):323–50.

20. Boyer RS, Moore JS. A fast string searching algorithm. Commun ACM. 1977;20(10):762–72.

21. Karp RM, Rabin MO. Efficient randomized pattern-matching algorithms. IBM J Res Dev. 1987;31(2):249–60.

22. Knuth DE, Morris JH Jr, Pratt VR. Fast pattern matching in strings. SIAM J Comput. 1977;6(1):323–50.

23. Horowitz E, Sahni S. Fundamentals of Data Structures in Pascal. 4th ed. Woodland Hills, Calif: Computer Science Press, 1994:86–7.

24. Horspool RN. Practical fast searching in strings. Software Practice and Experience. 1980;10(6):501–6.

25. Baeza-Yates RA. Improved string matching. Software Practice and Experience. 1989;19(3):257–71.

26. Borland International. Delphi, version 4.03. Available at: http://www.borland.com or http://www.inprise.com.

The Usefulness of Dynamically Categorizing Search Results

WANDA PRATT, PHD, LAWRENCE FAGAN, MD, PHD

Abstract Objective: The authors' goal was to determine whether dynamic categorization, a new technique for organizing search results, is more useful than the two existing organizational techniques: relevance ranking and clustering. They define a useful tool as one that helps users learn about the kinds of information that pertain to their query, find answers to their questions efficiently and easily, and feel satisfied with their search experience.

Design: Fifteen patients with breast cancer and their family members completed query-related tasks using all three tools. The authors measured the time it took the subjects to accomplish their tasks, the number of answers to the query that the subjects found in four minutes, and the number of new answers that they could recall at the end of the study. Subjects also completed a user-satisfaction questionnaire.

Results: The results showed that patients with breast cancer and their family members could find significantly ($P < 0.05$) more answers in a fixed amount of time and were significantly ($P < 0.05$) more satisfied with their search experience when they used the dynamic categorization tool than when they used either the cluster tool or the ranking tool. Subjects indicated that the dynamic categorization tool provided an organization of search results that was more clear, easy to use, accurate, precise, and helpful than those of the other tools.

Conclusion: The experiments indicate that dynamic categorization is an effective and useful approach for organizing search results. Tools that use this technique will help patients and their families gain quick and easy access to important medical information.

■ J Am Med Inform Assoc. 2000;7:605–617.

Vast quantities of medical information are now available. MEDLINE alone contains more than 9.2 million bibliographic entries from more than 3,800 biomedical journals, and it adds more than 31,000 new entries each month.[1] This volume of available information has created a problem of information overload. People become frustrated and overwhelmed when their searches yield tens or hundreds of relevant documents, so they abandon their search before they understand the kinds of information that it has returned.

We developed a new approach, called dynamic categorization, and created a corresponding system called DynaCat that attempts to solve this problem by organizing the documents returned from a bibliographic search into meaningful groups that correspond to the query.[2-4] In this paper, we focus on our experiment to determine how useful the approach is in helping users understand and explore their search results. Specifically, we tested the claim that search results organized by dynamic categorization will be more useful to those who have general questions than are search results organized by the two other approaches: relevance ranking and clustering. We define a useful system as one that helps users:

Affiliations of the authors: University of California, Irvine, California (WP); Stanford University, Stanford, California (LF).

This work was supported by grant LM-07033 from the National Library of Medicine and contract N44-CO-61025 from the National Cancer Institute.

Correspondence and reprints: Wanda Pratt, PhD, Information and Computer Science, University of California–Irvine, Irvine, CA 92697-3425; e-mail: <pratt@ics.uci.edu>.

Received for publication: 1/5/00; accepted for publication: 5/3/00.

- Learn about the kinds of information that pertain to their query
- Find answers to their question efficiently and easily
- Feel satisfied with their search experience

For this evaluation, satisfaction includes the users' perception of many attributes, such as the clarity of the organization of search results, the ease of tool use, the usefulness of the organization, and the accuracy of the organization. The complete satisfaction questionnaire appears in the Appendix.

Comparison Systems

In this evaluation, we compared DynaCat with two other systems that organize search results. Each subject used all three organizational tools: 1) a tool that ranks the search results according to relevance criteria (ranking tool), 2) a tool that clusters the search results (cluster tool), and 3) DynaCat (category tool). Although the purpose of all three tools is to help searchers find their requested information, the approach of each tool differs (Table 1). We briefly describe each tool and the differences among them in the following sections.

Relevance-ranking Tool

Relevance-ranking systems create an ordered list of search results in which the order of the documents is based on a measure of similarity between the document and the query. The documents that are most similar to the query are assumed to be the most relevant to the user.[5-7] These techniques typically represent documents using the vector-space paradigm, where each document in the collection is represented by a vector.[8,9] The length of a vector is the number of unique words in the entire set of documents, and the value of each element in a document's vector is calculated on the basis of both how frequently the corresponding word occurs in the document and how many other documents contain that word. Each document's vector acts as the coordinates for that document in a multidimensional space. This paradigm provides a way of viewing documents as positions in space, where the similarity between a document and a query is the distance between their vectors, measured by taking the cosine of the angle between those vectors.

Researchers have studied the effectiveness of many different algorithms for weighting the words in the vector and ranking the results, but no one algorithm appears to be superior in all cases.[10,11] Thus, the recommendations from these studies depend on the characteristics of the domain and the type of search. The relevance-ranking tool for this evaluation used a standard algorithm recommended by Salton and Buckley[10] for this situation, where the queries are short and the vocabulary is technical. We created an interface to the relevance-ranking tool that presents the results as a hypertext file, with an interface that is similar to that of DynaCat (see Figure 1).

Cluster Tool

Document-clustering systems also use a vector-space representation of the documents, but instead of ranking the documents, they group similar documents and label each group (or cluster) with representative words from that group. Like ranking algorithms, clustering systems estimate the similarity between documents by using a measure of the distance between the documents' vectors. A variety of statistical techniques have been used to create document clusters,[12-14] but none has proved superior in all situations.

For our experiments, we used the SONIA document-clustering tool, which was developed as part of Stanford University's Digital Library Project.[15,16] SONIA uses a two-step approach to clustering documents: it uses group-average hierarchic agglomerative clustering (a bottom-up approach) to form the initial set of clusters, then refines the clusters by an iterative method. We provided the search results for each query as a set of hypertext documents, and SONIA provided a set of documents indicating the number of clusters created, the words that described each cluster, and the set of documents that SONIA assigned to each cluster. We used the default settings for SONIA and had it find the maximum number of clusters. We wrote an interface to read its files and to present the results in an interface that is similar to that of DynaCat (see Figure 1).

Table 1 ■

Comparison of Characteristics of the Tools for Organizing Search Results

	Ranking Tools	Clustering Tools	DynaCat
Orders search results	Yes	No	No
Creates groups of search results	No	Yes	Yes
Uses domain knowledge	No	No	Yes
Uses information about user's query	Yes	No	Yes

Category Tool (DynaCat)

Unlike the other two statistical approaches, DynaCat uses a knowledge-based approach to organize the search results.[2,3] Like the clustering systems, it organizes the search results into groups of documents. It dynamically selects pertinent categories, assigns the appropriate documents to each category, and generates a hierarchic organization of those categories. This approach is based on three key premises:

- An appropriate categorization depends on both the user's query and the documents returned from the query.

- The type of query can provide valuable information about both the expected types of categories and the criteria for assigning documents to those categories.

- Taxonomic knowledge about words or word phrases in the document can make useful and accurate categorization possible.

As opposed to relevance-ranking tools, the purpose of DynaCat is not to separate nonrelevant from relevant documents but rather to organize the user's search results so that the organization provides information 1) about what kinds of information are represented in (or are absent from) the search results, by creating document categories with meaningful labels and by hierarchically organizing the document categories; 2) about how the documents relate to the query, by making the categorization dependent on the type of query; and 3) about how the documents relate to one another, by grouping ones that cover the same topic into the same category. This approach can provide such capabilities because it is based on a representation of the documents that is semantically richer than the vector-space representation, which is used by most clustering and relevance-ranking systems.

The semantics in dynamic categorization stem from two types of models: 1) a small query model that contains knowledge about what types of queries users make, and how search results from those queries should be categorized; and 2) a large domain-specific terminology model that connects individual terms (e.g., single words, abbreviations, acronyms, or multiword phrases) to their corresponding general concept or semantic type (e.g., aspirin's semantic type is pharmacologic substance). For a medical terminology model, DynaCat uses the Metathesaurus of the Unified Medical Language System (UMLS), which provides semantic information on more than 500,000 biomedical terms.

We based the query model on an analysis of frequently asked questions from patients in a breast cancer clinic.

The query model maps between the types of queries a user may enter and the criteria for generating categories that correspond to the user's query. Query types are high-level representations of the user queries that are independent of disease-specific terms; therefore, many queries have the same query type. For example, the queries "What are the complications of a mastectomy for breast cancer?" and "What are the side effects of taking the drug Seldane to treat allergies?" both have the same query type: *treatment—adverse effects*—even though they mention different diseases and different treatments. The types of queries represent the intersection of the kinds of medical information that are available in the medical literature and the kinds of questions that users typically ask. Each query type is mapped to the categorization criteria, which specify the conditions that must be satisfied for a document to belong to that type of category.

DynaCat also takes advantage of the keywords or Medical Subject Headings (MeSH) terms that have been assigned to medical journal articles. Because many keywords of a document do not correspond to the user's query, DynaCat must prune the nonrelevant keywords from the list of potential categories. When a keyword satisfies all the categorization criteria, the categorizer component adds the document to the category labeled with that keyword.

As an example, consider a woman who has breast cancer. She is contemplating having a mastectomy and is worried about possible complications. She issues the query "What are the possible adverse effects of a mastectomy?" to DynaCat and specifies her query type as *treatment—problems*. One of the categorization criteria for that query type stipulates that the categories must be keywords specifying a *disease or syndrome*. If DynaCat finds a document titled "Chronic post-treatment symptoms in patients with breast cancer operated in different surgical units" with keywords such as *lymphedema,paresthesia, adult, female, risk factors, mastectomy, surgery department*, and *treatment outcome*, the system categorizes that document under *lymphedema* and *paresthesia* because they match the categorization criteria of having *disease or syndrome* as a semantic type. DynaCat does not categorize the document under the other keywords, because those terms do not match the categorization criteria.

Notice that *lymphedema* and *paresthesia* were not predefined category labels in the query model; rather, they were selected dynamically because they satisfied the categorization criteria in the query model. The resulting categorization hierarchy allows the patient with breast cancer to see immediately that both *lymphedema* and *paresthesia* are adverse effects discussed in her search results and allows her to explore other documents that discuss those adverse effects.

The tested version of DynaCat was implemented in Common LISP and used the Oncology Knowledge Authority to search the CancerLit database and to access the UMLS Metathesaurus.[17] The current JAVA version uses a local copy of the UMLS and accesses MEDLINE through PubMed. In this version, categorizing several thousand search results takes a few minutes.

Methods

For this evaluation, we used methods from the field of human–computer interaction, unlike most evaluations of information-retrieval systems, which use precision and recall measures exclusively. Although no other study is exactly like the one that we designed, we were inspired to use methods from other user-centered studies.[18–20]

Our intent was to measure the effect of the organization of the documents, rather than the effect of individual user interfaces. Thus, we created hypertext interfaces to these three tools and made them as similar as possible. Figure 1 shows examples of the interfaces that we used for each of the three tools.

Because the ranking tool only creates ranked lists, whereas our interface is based on groups, we broke the ranked search results into groups of ten, which is the common point for splitting a ranked list into separate pages. In the following sections, we describe the subjects of the study and the procedure that these subjects followed.

Subjects

The subjects for this study were 15 patients with breast cancer or their family members. We recruited these subjects via the Community Breast Health Project,[21] the Stanford Health Library, and Stanford University's Oncology Day Care Center. Each subject signed a written consent form before participating. Participants knew that the purpose of the study was to investigate the usefulness of three search tools: a category tool (DynaCat), a cluster tool, and a ranking tool. However, they did not know that we had created one of the tools.

Procedures

Every subject used all three organizational tools: the category tool, the cluster tool, and the ranking tool.

In each of the tool's interfaces, the subjects could access any document's abstract by clicking on that document's title. Each subject used the same three queries for the experiment. We randomized the query used with each tool and the order in which the subjects used the tools. Figure 2 illustrates the study design graphically.

Each subject followed this procedure:

1. Filled out a human subjects consent form.
2. Filled out a background questionnaire.
3. Answered the following questions on how much she or he knew about the subject of the queries:
   a. List all the treatments for breast cancer that you can think of.
   b. List all the ways to prevent breast cancer that you can think of.
   c. List all the factors that influence breast cancer prognosis that you can think of.
4. Read and followed the tutorial for each of the three tools for the query "What are the risk factors for breast cancer?" (Notice that only the tutorial used this query.)
5. Given a tool and a query, completed three timed tasks to find specific information.
6. Found as many answers to the original query as possible in four minutes.
7. Found a document that answers a specific question related to the original query, and recorded the time it took to find the answer.
8. Found a document that answers a different, specific question related to the original query, and recorded the time it took to find the answer.
9. Filled out the user-satisfaction questionnaire (see Appendix) for the tool that he or she just used.
10. Repeated steps 5 and 6 for the remaining two tools and queries.
11. Answered the original questions on how much she or he knew about the subject of the queries, not counting his or her original answers from step 3. (Subjects did know that there would be a post-test.)
12. Answered the following questions:
    a. Which tool (ranking tool, cluster tool, or category tool) did you like best? Why?
    b. Which tool (ranking tool, cluster tool, or category tool) did you like least? Why?
    c. Did any of the tools help you learn more about the topic of the question? If so, which one?

The order of the tutorial exposure was the same as the order of tool use. Because each subject used each tool before starting the measured part of the study,

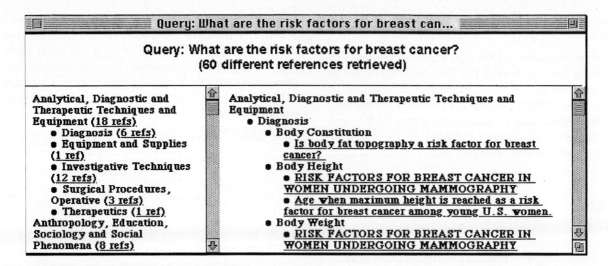

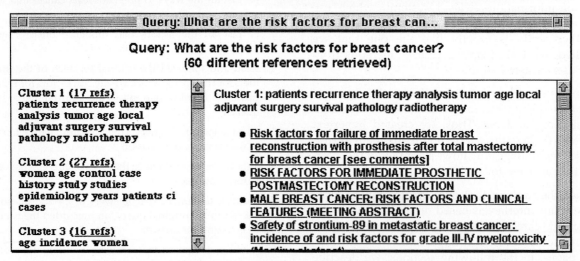

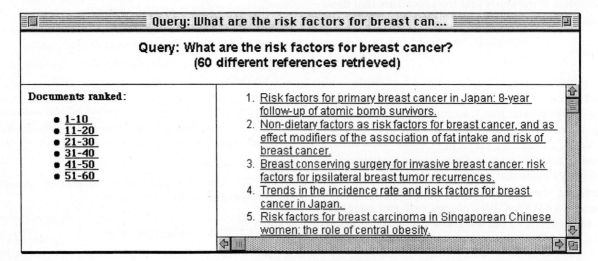

Figure 1 The interfaces to DynaCat *(top)*, the cluster tool *(middle)*, and the ranking tool *(bottom)*. All interfaces are divided into three frames, or window panes. The top window pane displays the user's query and the number of documents found. The left pane provides a table of contents view of the organization of search results. The right pane displays all the document titles using the organization of the scheme of the tool.

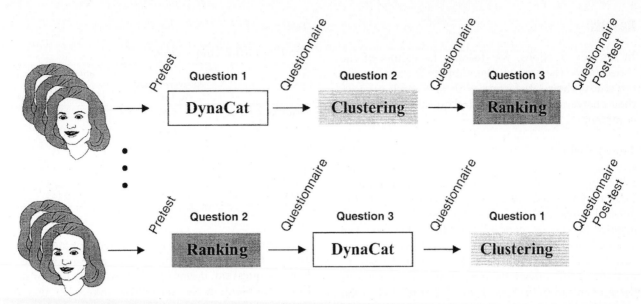

Figure 2 The study design. The 15 subjects were randomly assigned to groups in which the order of tool use and the question-to-tool pairing varied. Every subject used each tool once.

we assumed that the order of tool use would not influence the results.

We generated the search results by querying the CancerLit database through the Oncology Knowledge Authority[22] and limiting the results to documents that were written in English and that contained an abstract. We chose three general queries that represented the kinds of questions that patients typically ask, which were general enough to have multiple answers and thus would be appropriate for an information-exploration tool like DynaCat. The three queries that we used were "What are the prognostic indicators for breast cancer?" "What are the treatments for breast cancer?" and "What are the preventive measures for breast cancer?" We also provided the corresponding query types: *problem—prognostic-indicators*, *problem—treatments*, and *problem—preventive-actions*. We chose these three queries for the evaluation because the number of documents returned were similar (between 78 and 83 documents), and we did not want the number of documents returned to influence tool performance.

To create the specific questions for step 5, we asked an oncologist what he expected a patient to learn after reading documents returned from the different queries. In a pilot study, both of the timed questions came from him. However, for some of his questions, the subject could not determine which documents could answer the question by looking at the title of the documents, even when the abstract of the document contained the answer. In these cases, the

subjects became extremely frustrated when they were using either the cluster tool or the ranking tool. They often gave up before they could find a document that was relevant to the question in their task. No subject experienced this difficulty using DynaCat, because the category labels indicated when a document discussed the topic related to the question.

Even though the results were better with our tool, we decided to use only questions that related to topics that were visible in some document's title for the final study. We made this decision because the subjects became upset when they could not find an answer and because we would have difficulty comparing the timed tasks if people gave up. In the final study, we chose one question from the oncologist and one from the list of frequently asked questions gathered from the Community Breast Health Project.[21] For both questions, we chose the first question that was answered by one of the documents in the search results, that met the criterion of being visible in at least one document's title, and that had either a yes-or-no answer or a simple one-word answer.

We instructed the subjects to answer the timed questions as quickly as they could and promised them that they could use any of the tools after the study if they wanted to examine any articles in more detail or search for other information. We allowed the subjects to experiment with the tool again when they answered the user satisfaction questionnaire, but we cleared the screen before they answered the post-test questionnaire.

Results

In the next sections, we discuss the results of the timed tasks, the amount the subjects learned during the study, their satisfaction with the search process, their answers to the open-ended questions, and their comments.

Timed Tasks

All subjects completed two types of timed tasks. First, they found as many answers as possible to the general question (e.g., "What are the preventive actions for breast cancer?") in four minutes. We counted all the answers that they found in the search results. The second type of task was to find answers to two specific questions (e.g., "Can diet be used in the prevention of breast cancer?") that related to the original, general query. We combined the results of the second type of task into one mean value—the time to answer specific questions. Table 2 summarizes the results for the timed tasks.

To determine whether there was a significant difference among the three tools, we first used a repeated-measures analysis of variance (ANOVA). Using the repeated-measures ANOVA, we found a significant difference ($P = 0.035$) among the tools for the number of answers that the subjects found in four minutes. Because we were interested only in whether DynaCat performed better than the cluster tool or better than the ranking tool, we also used a paired, one-tailed t test to determine the level of significance in comparing DynaCat with the cluster tool and in comparing DynaCat with the ranking tool. When the subjects used DynaCat, the category tool, they found nearly twice as many answers as they did with the other two tools. This difference was significant when we used the paired t test as well. Notice that, although the mean number of answers found with the ranking tool was greater than that found with the cluster tool, the P value was lower in the comparison of DynaCat with the ranking tool than it was in the comparison of DynaCat with the cluster tool. This result occurred because the subjects consistently found fewer answers with the ranking tool than they did with DynaCat, whereas their results with the cluster tool were variable.

There was no significant difference across the tools for the time it took the subjects to find answers to specific questions. As in the pilot study, the time it took subjects to find documents that answered the specific questions varied greatly. In this final study, we noticed two sources of this variability. The first

Table 2 ∎

Results for the Timed Tasks

	Answers Found in 4 min	Time (min) to Find Answers to Specific Questions
DynaCat (D)	7.80	2.15
Cluster Tool (C)	4.53	2.95
Ranking Tool (R)	5.60	2.21
P value:		
D vs C	0.013	0.274
D vs R	0.004	0.448

source was the position of a document containing an answer to the question in the relevance-ranked list. For one question, it was obvious from the title of the first document in the relevance-ranked list that it answered the question, so the time that a subject took to answer that question was very short if she used the ranking tool. Second, we observed that several subjects answered the question on the basis of only the title of the document, whereas most other subjects read the entire abstract before answering the question. Reading the abstract took much longer than simply reading the title, particularly because the terminology in the abstracts was technical and sometimes completely unfamiliar to the subjects. Thus, the time to read the abstract, rather than the time to find a document among the search results, most heavily influenced the time to find an answer.

Amount Learned

To determine the amount that subjects learned during the study, we gave each subject a pretest and a post-test of their knowledge related to the three breast-cancer questions (see steps 3 and 8 in the Procedures section). We measured the number of new answers on the post-test. The mean number of answers learned for DynaCat (2.80) was greater than those for the cluster tool (2.20) and for the ranking tool (2.33); however, this difference was not statistically significant. The largest influence on this measurement was the order in which the subjects looked for answers to the question. Subjects remembered fewer answers to their first question (1.93) than they did answers to their second (2.80) and third (2.60) questions. Using a paired, one-tailed t test, we found the difference between the times of the first and second questions to be significant ($P = 0.04$). However, the difference between the second and third questions was not significant ($P = 0.36$), possibly because the subjects could still remember answers to their second question, about 30 minutes in the past, but had more difficulty

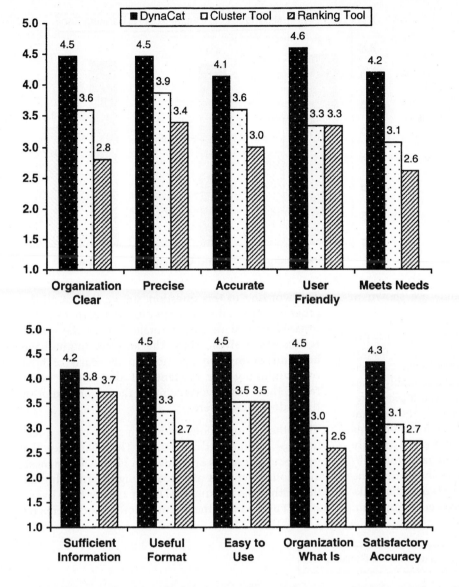

Figure 3 Results from the validated user-satisfaction questionnaire. The mean values across all 15 subjects are shown on the *y* axis. The *x* axis shows a brief summary of the questions asked. (See the Appendix for the full questionnaire.) Subjects answered the questions using a scale from 1 to 5, where 1 meant "almost never" and 5 meant "almost always" (the ideal answer). The difference between DynaCat and the cluster tool was statistically significant ($P < 0.05$) for all five questions, as was that between DynaCat and the ranking tool, with the exception of question 6, about sufficient information, which had a P value of 0.11.

remembering answers to their first question, nearly an hour in the past. The tool used may have had an influence on the amount learned, but the number of answers that the subjects remembered for the post-test was correlated more strongly with how recently the subjects found answers to that question rather than with which tool they used.

User Satisfaction

To measure user satisfaction, we used both a validated satisfaction questionnaire[23] and a questionnaire that we created to measure other important types of satisfaction for this type of tool. The Appendix shows the combined questionnaire that we used. Subjects filled out the questionnaire for each of the three tools.

Questions 1 through 10 were from the validated questionnaire, although we modified questions 3, 5, and 10 slightly to match each tool more closely. Figure 3 shows the results from the validated questionnaire.

The subjects answered the questions using a scale from 1 to 5, where 5 was the most positive answer. The subjects' answers for DynaCat were significantly higher ($P < 0.05$) than those for either the ranking tool or the cluster tool, indicating that the subjects were more satisfied with DynaCat than they were with either the ranking tool or the cluster tool.

We created the remaining 16 questions on the questionnaire. For the first four questions, we provided statements and asked the subjects to rate them on a scale of 1 to 5, where 1 meant "strongly disagree" and 5 meant "strongly agree." Five was the ideal answer for

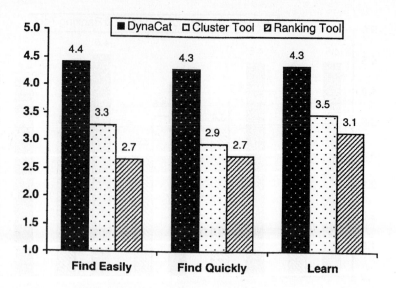

Figure 4 Results from the user-satisfaction questionnaire. The mean values across all 15 subjects are shown on the *y* axis. The *x* axis shows a brief summary of the questions asked (questions 11, 12, and 14; see the Appendix for the full questionnaire.) Subjects rated the statements on a scale from 1 to 5, where 1 meant "strongly disagree" and 5 meant "strongly agree" (the ideal answer). The difference between DynaCat and the cluster tool was statistically significant ($P < 0.01$), as was the difference between DynaCat and the ranking tool.

three of those questions. The results are shown in Figure 4.

For these questions, DynaCat also scored significantly higher than either the ranking tool or the cluster tool, indicating that the subjects found DynaCat better at helping them find information quickly, find information easily, and learn about the topic corresponding to their query. Question 13 ("The amount of information provided in the search results was overwhelming") had an ideal answer of 1 (strongly disagree). For this question, the mean value that subjects assigned to DynaCat (2.40) was lower than the mean values for the cluster tool (2.53) and the ranking tool (2.67), but the difference was not significant.

The wording of this question, unlike that of all the other questions, does not refer to the system or to the organization of results; it refers to only the search results themselves. Thus, the subjects might have been answering the question on the basis of how overwhelming the contents of documents were rather than how overwhelming the organization of those documents were.

The other 12 questions were either yes-or-no questions or open-ended questions. The results for the yes-or-no questions are shown in Figure 5. For these questions, DynaCat also scored significantly higher than either the ranking tool or the cluster tool. Every subject agreed that the organization of documents by

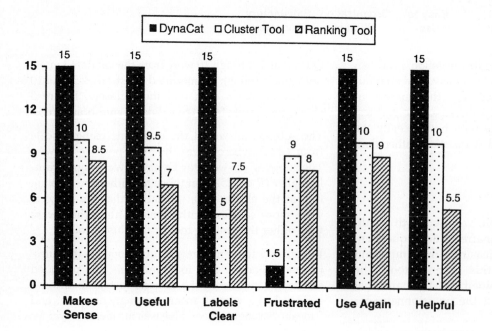

Figure 5 "Yes" responses to the yes-or-no user-satisfaction questions. The labels along the *x* axis summarize questions 15, 17, 19, 22, 24, and 26. (See the Appendix for the full questionnaire.) Some subjects answered "somewhat" instead of "yes" or "no." Such answers were counted as half a "yes" response.

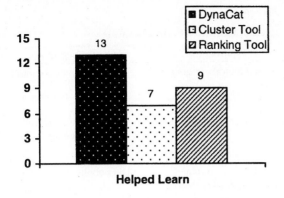

Figure 6 Responses to the final question, "Did any of the tools help you learn more about the topic of the question? If so, which one?"

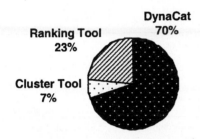

Figure 7 Responses to the question "Which tool did you like best?" One person could not choose between the ranking tool and DynaCat, so we counted her answer as half a vote for DynaCat and half a vote for the ranking tool.

DynaCat made sense, was useful, provided clear labels, and helped them perform their tasks. For the cluster tool and the ranking tool, only two thirds of the subjects or fewer answered those questions positively. Only one subject said that she found the category tool frustrating to use, and one other subject found it somewhat frustrating. Nine subjects found the cluster tool frustrating, and eight found the ranking tool frustrating. All 15 subjects said that they would use the category tool again when they wanted to search the medical literature, whereas only 10 subjects said they would use the cluster tool again, and only 9 said they would use the ranking tool again.

After the subjects finished using all the tools, we asked three more user-satisfaction questions:

- Which tool (ranking tool, cluster tool, or category tool) did you like best? Why?

- Which tool (ranking tool, cluster tool, or category tool) did you like least? Why?

- Did any of the tools help you learn more about the topic of the question? If so, which one?

The results for the final three questions appear in Figures 6 and 7.

Most subjects (87 percent) thought DynaCat helped them learn about the answers to the question, whereas only 60 percent thought the ranking tool helped, and only 46 percent thought the clustering tool helped. Most people (70 percent) chose DynaCat as the best tool, and no one chose DynaCat as the tool that she liked the least. Most subjects expressed a strong opinion about the ranking tool: 23 percent thought it was the best tool, and 67 percent thought it was the worst. In contrast, most subjects seemed indifferent to the cluster tool.

Comments and Answers to Open-ended Questions

We asked several open-ended questions as part of the user-satisfaction questionnaire. It would be difficult to create a quantitative report of these results, but we have included several representative positive and negative quotes from the subjects in Tables 3, 4, and 5.

When the evaluation was over, three subjects asked whether they could look at more information using one of the tools. All three subjects asked to use the category tool (DynaCat).

Discussion

This evaluation provided insights into the strengths and weaknesses of each approach to organizing search results.

Subjects liked the idea of grouping the search results into clusters, but they had many problems with the cluster tool. Subjects indicated that the similarities found by clustering did not always correspond to a grouping that was meaningful to them. They rated the clarity of the cluster labels and the labels' correspondence to the search results as poor. The clustering tools face this limitation because they use only information based on word occurrences. The document groups are labeled by words extracted from the clusters, usually chosen by an information-theoretic measure. Such lists of words may be understandable if the contents of the cluster are cohesive, but a list of words is not as inviting to the general user as a well-selected category label. The results also are unlikely to correspond well to the user's query, because clustering algorithms do not use information about the user's query in forming the clusters.

When subjects assessed the ranking tool, some liked the concept of ordering the documents according to their relevance and found the concept easy to understand. However, they also complained that they did not understand how the ranking was done, nor did they believe that any system would be able to rank the results according to their own personal needs. Another problem with an ordered list is that it does not give the user much information about the similarities or differences in the contents of the documents. For example, without examining every retrieved document and noting the contents of each, the user would not be able to determine that 30 different preventive measures were discussed in the retrieved documents or that 10 documents discussed the same preventive drug. People usually do not have the time or energy to browse all the documents on the list. They may give up examining the documents long before they see all the results, thus missing potentially useful information.

Although the data provide clear evidence that most users prefer the results that were generated by DynaCat, this system has limitations, too. Developing a tool on this knowledge-based approach requires effort to understand the terminology model and to create the query model, whereas the statistical approaches require no such models. The effectiveness of DynaCat also depends on the comprehensiveness and appropriateness of the models. For example, in this study of patients with breast cancer and members of their families, subjects complained about the technical nature of the category labels. If the terminology model incorporated consumer-oriented medical terms rather than the more physician-oriented Metathesaurus terms, DynaCat could choose category labels that matched the needs of targeted user populations. Also, the technique is applicable only if the user's query maps well to one of the query types in the query model.

The current system also provided no easy mechanism to help consumers critically assess the quality of retrieved documents. Yet such quality information could be helpful in the selection of peer-reviewed articles to read and would be very important in a search through unrefereed Web documents. Our future research plans include investigating ways to minimize these limitations. One possibility for reducing the modeling effort is to use machine learning techniques in the generation of the query types and categorization criteria. We are also exploring information visualization techniques for an interactive categorization environment that would allow users to categorize documents along multiple dimensions such as quality, in addition to the main topic.

In summary, we showed that DynaCat is a more useful organizational tool than either the cluster tool or

Table 3 ∎

Subjects' Comments on DynaCat

Positive	Negative
Clear and logical category names	Terminology too technical
Liked hierarchy of categories	Want further classification of large categories
Liked alphabetic organization of categories	Did not like "Other" category
Easy to read and find specific information	
Articles grouped into manageable numbers	

Table 4 ∎

Subjects' Comments on the Cluster Tool

Positive	Negative
Better than no organization	Labels not clear
Easy to skim	Labels don't match articles in cluster
	Not apparent how to find specific information
	Not intuitive

Table 5 ∎

Subjects' Comments on the Ranking Tool

Positive	Negative
Easy to understand the organization and browse	Don't know how the ranking was done
Easy to look at more important information first	Seemingly random order
Logical	No help in looking for specific information
	Waste of time to read every title to find topics
	It can't know what we think are the most important documents

the ranking tool. The results showed that DynaCat is significantly better than the other two tools along two dimensions: 1) users were able to find answers more efficiently and 2) users were more satisfied with the search process.

Measurements of the amount learned were inconclusive; however, many more subjects thought that DynaCat helped them learn about the topic of the query. The subjects indicated that DynaCat provided an organization of search results that was more clear, easy to use, accurate, precise, and helpful than the organization of results provided by the other tools. Because this study involved a small number of queries, more evaluation is needed to justify broader claims. Nevertheless, these initial results suggest that, by using knowledge about users' queries and the kinds of categories that are useful for those queries, DynaCat can help users find information quickly and easily.

Conclusion

The amount of medical literature continues to grow as the content becomes increasingly specialized. At the same time, many patients and their families are becoming proactive in searching the medical literature for information about their medical problems. Medical journal articles can be intimidating for lay people to read; thus, lay readers need tools to help them sift through and understand the information they seek. We have described a new approach to organizing medical search results and have proved that our approach is helpful; our research should lead to the development of tools that will help lay people—both patients and their families—explore the medical literature, become informed about health care topics, and play an active role in making decisions about their own medical care.

Although our system was evaluated with only patients as users, it could be useful for health care workers as well. They also need tools to help them cope with the vast quantities of medical information that they must access to care for their patients or to further medical research. The questions that health care workers ask might be more specific or more varied, but the terminology model and categorization process would remain the same. If tools based on our research were available to health care workers, they might be able to find the needed information quickly enough to use it during a patient visit, when that information is most useful. This research could result in new tools that would help all users (patients as well as health care workers) explore quickly and effectively the information space related to their individualized information needs.

The authors thank Marti Hearst, Edward Shortliffe, and Russ Altman for their feedback on this work. They also thank Mike Walker for helping with the statistics, Lexical Technology, Inc. for providing tools to access their Oncology Knowledge Authority through the Web, and Dr. Bob Carlson and the Community Breast Health Project for helping them recruit subjects.

References ■

1. National Library of Medicine. NLM Online Databases and Databanks. 1999. Available at: http://www.nlm.nih.gov/pubs/factsheets/online_databases.html.
2. Pratt W. Dynamic Categorization: A Method for Decreasing Information Overload [PhD thesis]. Stanford, Calif: Stanford University Medical Information Sciences, 1999.
3. Pratt W, Hearst MA, Fagan LM. A knowledge-based approach to organizing retrieved documents. In: AAAI '99: Proceedings of the 16th National Conference on Artificial Intelligence; Orlando, Florida; 1999.
4. Pratt W. Dynamic organization of search results using the UMLS. AMIA Annu Fall Symp. 1997:480–4.
5. van Rijsbergen CJ. Information Retrieval. London: Butterworths, 1979.
6. Salton G. Automatic Text Processing: The Transformation, Analysis, and Retrieval of Information by Computer. Reading, Mass: Addison-Wesley, 1989.
7. Harman D. Ranking algorithms. In: Frakes WB (ed). Information Retrieval Data Structures and Algorithms. Englewood Cliffs, NJ: Prentice Hall, 1992.
8. Salton G, Wong A, Yang CS. A vector space model for automatic indexing. Commun ACM. 1975;18:613–20.
9. Salton G, McGill MJ. Introduction to Modern Information Retrieval. New York: McGraw-Hill, 1983.
10. Salton G, Buckley C. Term-weighting approaches in automatic text retrieval. Inf Proc Manage. 1988;24(5):513–23.
11. Efthimiadis EN. A user-centred evaluation of ranking algorithms for interactive query expansion. In: SIGIR '93: Proceedings of the 16th Annual International ACM-SIGIR Conference on Research and Development in Information Retrieval. 1993:146–59.
12. Willett P. Recent trends in hierarchic document clustering: a critical review. Info Proc Manage. 1988;24(5):577–97.
13. Rasmussen E. Clustering algorithms. In: Frakes WB (ed). Information Retrieval Data Structures and Algorithms. Englewood Cliffs, NJ: Prentice Hall, 1992:419–42.
14. Hearst MA, Pedersen JO. Reexamining the cluster hypothesis: Scatter/Gather on retrieval results. In: SIGIR '96: Proceedings of the ACM Conference on Research and Development in Information Retrieval. 1996:76–84.
15. Sahami M. Using Machine Learning to Improve Information Access [PhD thesis]. Stanford, Calif: Stanford University Computer Science Department, 1998.
16. Sahami M, Yusufali S, Baldonado MQW. SONIA: A Service for Organizing Network Information Autonomously. Presented at: Digital Libraries 98: Third ACM Conference on Digital Libraries; Pittsburgh, Pa; Jun 24–27, 1998.
17. Tuttle MS, Sherertz DD, Olson NE, et al. Toward reusable software components at the point of care. AMIA Annu Fall Symp. 1996:150–4.
18. Egan DE, Remde JR, Gomez LM, Landauer TK, Eberhardt J, Lochbaum CC. Formative design-evaluation of SuperBook. ACM Trans Inf Syst. 1989;7(1):30–57.
19. Pirolli P, Schank P, Hearst MA, Diehl C. Scatter/Gather Browsing Communicates the Topic Structure of a Very Large Text Collection. Presented at: CHI 96: ACM SIGCHI

Conference on Human Factors in Computing Systems. 1996.

20. Hersh WR, Elliot DL, Hickam DH, Wolf SL, Molnar A, Leichtenstein C. Towards new measures of information retrieval evaluation. In: SIGIR '95: Proceedings of the 18th Annual International ACM-SIGIR Conference on Research and Development in Information Retrieval. 1995:164–70.

21. Community Breast Health Project home page. Stanford Medical Center. 1999. Available at: http://www-med.stanford.edu/CBHP/. Accessed Jun 23, 2000.

22. Tuttle MS, Sherertz DD, Fagan LM, et al. Toward an interim standard for patient-centered knowledge-access. Proc 17th Annu Symp Comput Appl Med Care. 1994:564–8.

23. Doll W, Torkzadeh F. The measurement of end-user computing satisfaction. MIS Q. 1988;12:259–74.

APPENDIX
User Satisfaction Questionnaire

Using the scale below, please answer questions 1–10:

> 1 = Almost never
> 2 = Some of the time
> 3 = Almost half of the time
> 4 = Most of the time
> 5 = Almost always

1. Is the organization of the information clear?

2. Does the system provide the precise information you need?

3. Is the system accurate in assigning documents to categories?

4. Is the system user-friendly?

5. Does the organization of the information content meet your needs?

6. Does the system provide sufficient information?

7. Do you think the information is presented in a useful format?

8. Is the system easy to use?

9. Does the system provide an organization of the information that seems to be just about exactly what you need?

10. Are you satisfied with how well the system assigns documents to categories? [NOTE: This wording is for the category tool. The exact wording of this question depended on the tool that the subjects were assessing. For the cluster tool, the word "clusters" was substituted for the word "categories," and for the ranking tool, the question asked how well the system ranks the documents.]

Using the scale below, please answer questions 11–14:

> 1 = Strongly disagree
> 2 = Disagree
> 3 = Uncertain

> 4 = Agree
> 5 = Strongly agree

11. The organization of the search results makes it easy to find information.

12. The organization of the search results makes it easy to find information quickly.

13. The amount of information provided in the search results was overwhelming.

14. The organization of the search results made it easy to learn about information related to the query.

Please answer the remaining questions in your own words:

15. Does the organization of the documents make sense?

16. How do you think the organization could be improved?

17. Do you find the organization useful?

18. If so, in what way?

19. Do the labels that describe each group of documents make sense?

20. What do you like about the organization of the documents returned?

21. What do you not like about the organization of the documents returned?

22. Were you frustrated when you used the system?

23. If so, why?

24. Would you use the system again when you want to search for medical information?

25. Why or why not?

26. Did the grouping of the documents help you perform your tasks? [NOTE: For the ranking tool, the word "ranking" was substituted for the word "grouping."]

Methods for the Design and Administration of Web-based Surveys

Titus K. L. Schleyer, DMD, PhD, Jane L. Forrest, RDH, EdD

Abstract This paper describes the design, development, and administration of a Web-based survey to determine the use of the Internet in clinical practice by 450 dental professionals. The survey blended principles of a controlled mail survey with data collection through a Web-based database application. The survey was implemented as a series of simple HTML pages and tested with a wide variety of operating environments. The response rate was 74.2 percent. Eighty-four percent of the participants completed the Web-based survey, and 16 percent used e-mail or fax. Problems identified during survey administration included incompatibilities/technical problems, usability problems, and a programming error. The cost of the Web-based survey was 38 percent less than that of an equivalent mail survey. A general formula for calculating breakeven points between electronic and hardcopy surveys is presented. Web-based surveys can significantly reduce turnaround time and cost compared with mail surveys and may enhance survey item completion rates.

■ **J Am Med Inform Assoc. 2000;7:416–425.**

The Web-based survey described in this article was designed to investigate the use of the Internet in clinical practice by 450 dental professionals. The results of the survey itself have been published previously.[1] This paper describes the design and implementation of the survey in detail to assist other researchers who are considering using Web-based surveys. From a review of the background literature and our own experiences, we present issues in sampling for electronic surveys; survey design, programming, testing, and administration; potential problems and pitfalls; and cost comparisons between electronic and hardcopy surveys. We developed several general breakeven calculations based on cost, provided all other variables are equal, to help researchers choose between electronic and traditional mail surveys.

Affiliations of the authors: Temple University School of Dentistry, Philadelphia, Pennsylvania (TKLS); University of Southern California School of Dentistry, Los Angeles, California (JLF).

Correspondence and reprints: Titus K. L. Schleyer, DMD, PhD, Department of Dental Informatics, Temple University School of Dentistry, 3223 N. Broad Street, TU 600-00, Philadelphia, PA 19140; e-mail: ⟨di@dental.temple.edu⟩.

This work was supported in part by grant T15-LM07059 from the National Library of Medicine/National Institute of Dental and Craniofacial Research.

Received for publication: 9/7/99; accepted for publication: 1/31/00.

Background

Several recent publications have reported use of the Internet to conduct survey research.[2-9] Investigators in the fields of medicine, psychology, sociology, dentistry, and veterinary medicine are recruiting participants for their research studies by targeting specific search engines, newsgroups, and Web sites. Participants often answer surveys by returning a completed form by e-mail or by entering their responses directly on a Web site. Commonly cited advantages include easy access, instant distribution, and reduced costs. In addition, the Internet allows questionnaires and surveys to reach a worldwide population with minimum cost and time. Researchers can contact rare and hidden populations that are often geographically dispersed,[3] as well as patient populations different from those typically seen in the clinical or hospital setting.[2,10]

Other reported benefits relate to graphical and interactive design on the Web. Ideally, HTML survey forms enhance data collection, compared with conventional surveys, because of their use of color, innovative screen designs, question formatting, and other features not available with paper questionnaires. They can prohibit multiple or blank responses by not allowing the participant to continue on or to submit the survey without first correcting the response error. This feature is somewhat controversial, because there may be legitimate reasons for not answering questions, and responses such as "don't know" or "prefer not to answer" force an answer when participation and question response is supposed to be voluntary.[11] Regardless of one's view on this issue, the program can provide cues to make sure the respondent does not inadvertently skip a question. In addition, coding errors and data entry mistakes are reduced or eliminated while compilation of results can be automated.[12] Finally, online forms can help minimize costs, facilitate rapid return of information by participants, and allow timely dissemination of results by investigators.[13]

Several examples show how the Internet is used for survey research. Physicians in Germany developed a Web-based patient information system about atopic eczema to attract patients to the Web site and Internet survey.[2] The purpose of the survey was to explore the relations between atopic stigmata and its symptoms, predisposing factors, patient demographics, and associations with other diseases. As an incentive to fill out the survey, an atopy score was calculated and presented to the participant upon completion. Approximately 240 subjects complete the survey each month. Healthy Web surfers serve as controls.[2]

In another study, researchers at Columbia University explored the properties of a new measure of sexual orientation by monitoring network traffic on an intranet over a two-week period and collecting all postings to two newsgroups related to their topic of study.[3] From the formulated list of e-mail addresses, 360 subjects were randomly selected. Subjects were notified of their selection, and those who consented to participate were e-mailed a survey. Of the participants who were contacted, 66.1 percent provided their consent to participate and 56.4 percent of that group returned completed surveys.[3]

Veterinarians conducted research via e-mail and Web pages to investigate causes of dog death in small veterinary practices.[4] In this study, 25 veterinarians submitted case material. On the basis of analysis by region and school attended, the investigators found that participants were representative of the veterinarian population in the United States.

Nursing researchers have found the Internet a valuable vehicle for collecting data from cancer survivors.[7] In this study, three cancer-related newsgroups were used to distribute the Cancer Survivors Survey Questionnaire. This method proved useful for collecting preliminary data, which are often needed to demonstrate the feasibility of conducting a large-scale study and for determining adequate sample size.

Theoretically, conducting research over the Internet has many benefits. However, survey experts and researchers warn that the current online population is not representative of the general population in the United States. Estimates of computer ownership and e-mail access vary depending on how data were gathered, e.g., face-to-face or via telephone, and how it is reported, e.g., household computer ownership vs. "access to" computers.[14,15] For example, in 48,000 face-to-face interviews conducted in 1997, 37 percent of households in the United States reported owning a computer, 19 percent reported online access, and 17 percent reported e-mail access. In comparison, through telephone polls, 67 percent reported having access to a computer and 31 percent had an e-mail address.

While access to e-mail and the Internet grow daily, a "digital divide" exists among age and racial groups, income levels, and geographic settings.[14] Ensuring that each potential respondent has an equal chance of being selected to participate poses a major challenge in conducting a scientifically sound survey. This is especially true in the health sciences, where electronic access to specific provider or patient groups cannot easily be obtained.[9] Currently, not all health professional associations or licensing boards collect e-mail addresses, nor is it possible to estimate the number of individuals with the particular health state of interest who have access to computers and the Internet.[7] However, rigorous sample selection procedures must be followed if results are to be generalized to a population and sources of coverage and sampling error are to be kept to a minimum.[11,16]

Unfortunately, the sampling procedures reported in many electronic surveys reflect unknown samples.[2,3,5,13] When subjects are recruited by targeting newsgroups or search engines, it is nearly impossible to determine the distribution of the sample population. These survey procedures should be used only when sampling and self-selection biases can be tolerated.

Another concern unique to conducting electronic surveys is the variation of the level of computer literacy among respondents and the capabilities of their computers. Internet users tend to be highly educated white men between the ages of 26 and 30 years.[13] Even so, their experience responding to online questionnaires may be limited. Thus, Web-based surveys need to have clear directions on how to perform each needed skill, e.g., how to enter answers with a drop-down box or erase responses from a check box[11] so that responding to the questionnaire does not become a frustrating experience.

Providing specific instructions will assist respondents in accurately completing and returning the survey, provided their computer is capable of receiving it in the first place. Differences among computers, such as their processing power, memory, connection speeds, and browsers, potentially negate some of the benefits purported for using the Web. For example, the use of graphics and animation may increase the attractiveness and novelty of participating. However, advanced Web progamming features, such as Java, JavaScript, DHTML, or XML either may be incompatible with certain browsers or may cause them to respond slowly or crash. In *The Influence of Plain vs. Fancy Designs on Response Rates for Web Surveys*, Dillman et al.[17] showed that such features can actually lower response rates. In this study, a plain questionnaire obtained a higher response rate than one that used tables and colors. The plain design also was more likely to be fully completed in a shorter period of time.

Dillman et al. proposed three criteria and 11 supporting principles for designing respondent-friendly Web questionnaires, some of which were used to guide the development of the study presented in this article.[11] These criteria include:

- Take into account the inability of some respondents to receive and respond to Web questionnaires with advanced programming features that cannot be received or easily responded to because of equipment, browser, and/or transmission limitations.

- Take into account both the logic of how computers operate and the logic of how people expect questionnaires to operate.

- Take into account the likelihood that a Web questionnaire will be used in mixed-mode survey situations.

The next section describes the purpose of the survey described in this article, how the sample was selected, and how the survey was designed, pilot tested, and administered.

Survey Development and Administration

The Study

The Web-based survey described in this article was designed to investigate the use of the Internet in clinical practice by 450 dental professionals. There were three primary reasons for choosing a Web-based survey method. First, the survey population used e-mail, since all participants subscribed to an Internet discussion list. Use of e-mail is not an absolute indicator of Web use; however, since discussions often referenced Web sites, it seemed likely that the majority of individuals used the Web. The survey results confirmed this assumption. Second, because of an imposed deadline, survey development, implementation, and data analysis had to be completed within eight weeks, which made it impossible to conduct a traditional mail survey. Finally, funds or other resources for the production of a hardcopy survey, postage, and data entry were not available.

Sample Selection

A random sample of dentists could not be selected because no comprehensive list of dentists with e-mail addresses was available. Consequently, the largest discussion list for general dentistry (Internet Dental Forum) was identified. Selection of the discussion list permitted identification of the total population and controlled follow-up with nonrespondents, blending a methodologically sound approach with a new method of collecting data. The investigators believed that selection of this convenience sample, although not representative of all dentists with Internet access, was more appropriate than soliciting volunteers from general sites with unknown populations. Dr. D. Dodell, list owner of the Internet Dental Forum and member of the project team, made the list of e-mail addresses available. Institutional Review Board approval for this survey was not sought, since the project was exempt under CFR §46.101 (b) (2).

Survey Design

A 22-question survey instrument with a total of 102 discrete answers was developed. Rather than being presented on a single, lengthy Web page, questions were grouped on 18 sequential screens, for two reasons. First, sequential screens kept transmission time to a minimum and avoided potential server time-outs for respondents with slow modem connections (33 KBps and below). Second, the use of sequential screens allowed questions to be displayed completely and prevented the need for participants to scroll through pages and potentially get lost.

Figure 1 illustrates some of the design features of the survey. All screens were designed to display fully at a screen resolution of 800 × 600 pixels. Most screens contained a single question. The top of the screen displayed a static 6 kb JPEG banner with a small picture (which emphasized the clinical aspect of the survey) and the title of the survey. Each question was displayed in bold. List boxes, radio buttons, and check boxes provided answers for close-ended questions. Text fields were available for answers to open-ended

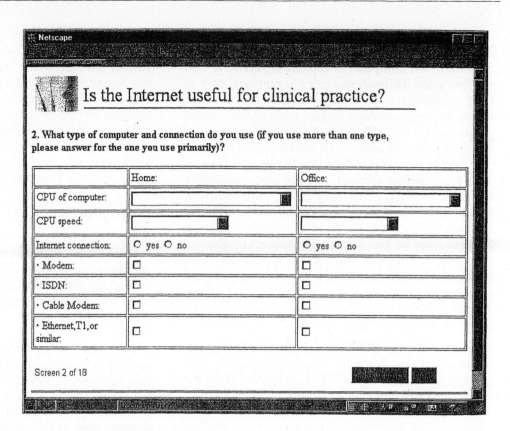

Figure 1 Sample screen of the survey.

questions. Formatting the answers in a table ensured consistency of layout for different browsers, operating systems, and window sizes. The lower left corner of each screen indicated the participant's relative position in the total number of survey screens (in gray). The lower right corner contained buttons to clear the current screen and to move to the next screen. The total file size of each screen averaged about 9 kb.

Several published recommendations and findings for designing survey screens were followed.[11,17,18] The small file size minimized download time. Formatting clearly differentiated questions and answers and de-emphasized secondary screen elements. Consistent layout reduced the number of required cognitive adjustments and allowed participants to concentrate on answering the questions. The "next" button, combined with the relative screen indicator, encouraged a page-turning rhythm that resembled completing a hardcopy survey.

To minimize incompatibilities with browsers, survey pages were compliant with HTML 3.0. Neither JavaScript, which is often employed to validate entry fields on the Web, nor Java, ActiveX controls, and other advanced Web programming concepts were used for the reasons cited above.

The survey was programmed in PL/SQL on an Oracle 8 database server. Programming took approximately 35 hours. Code review and testing added another

eight hours. Since the code was going to be used only once, the programmer neither optimized the code for performance and maintenance nor added detailed comments. The total length of the program was 2,471 lines. During the code review, the program was reviewed line by line. In the testing phase, each question was answered and the corresponding entry checked in the database. Initially, the survey was programmed to validate every screen (e.g., to check that all fields were filled out, that the zip code was formatted correctly). This feature was deactivated on the basis of the results of the pilot test. A second program also was developed to send survey messages to all participants. This program took three hours to develop and test and totaled 895 lines.

Pilot Testing

After programming, the survey was pilot-tested in-house and with several remote participants. The program was tested with two different browsers (Netscape Communicator versions 4.0 and 4.5 and Internet Explorer version 4.0), three operating systems (Windows NT 4.0, Windows 95, and Macintosh OS 7.5), two types of Internet access (high-speed local area network and modem dial-up line), and three different Internet service providers. The pilot test did not uncover any technical problems. However, the wording on some questions was slightly modified, and the validation for required input fields was dropped. Several pilot-testers felt that requiring entries in all fields was too restrictive, especially when they felt that a question did not apply to them personally or when the response choices did not exactly match their expectations.

Survey Administration

Next, a list of participants' e-mail addresses was generated from the list of subscribers to the discussion list. This list was imported into Microsoft Excel and a unique, random four-character survey ID for each participant was generated. The IDs were composed of letters and numbers. Participants entered their IDs to authenticate themselves and access the survey. The list was then imported from the Excel file into the Oracle database.

The main survey page (for introduction and login) was hosted on the discussion list server (idf.stat.com) rather than the Oracle server (heracles.dental.temple.edu). Although this method avoided confusion about the origin of the survey, it prevented the investigators from providing a URL that would have directly logged participants into the Oracle server. To begin data collection and identify any significant problems, a survey message was initially sent to 47 participants. The messages originated on the Oracle server were sent through an SMTP mailer program that spoofed* an e-mail address on the server hosting the discussion list. Participants received a personal message stating the purpose of the survey, who was conducting it, the estimated time required to complete it, the URL of the survey, the survey ID, and who to contact with questions. The survey also instructed them to return duplicate e-mail messages with the subject line "DUPLICATE." Once authenticated through their survey ID, participants could begin answering questions.

The group of individuals who responded to the first mailing did not report any problems. However, several problems were identified when the survey was mailed to the remaining 403 individuals:

- Several individuals stated that they entered their survey ID, pushed submit, and then could not proceed with the survey because of an error message. Unfortunately, the source of this problem could not be tracked down. Most of these participants used America Online as their Internet service provider.

---

*Spoofing is a common technique to fool hardware and software in networked environments. Spoofing an e-mail address, for instance, makes a message appear to be sent from someone else than the actual sender.

Consequently, an ASCII copy of the survey was mounted on the home page to provide an alternative method of answering the survey. Participants were advised to use this method of replying if the Web form failed. At the same time, participants who had had problems were provided with an explanation. A copy of the survey was included in the reply. Completed surveys received through e-mail or fax were entered by hand into the database later.

- Some international users with slow modem connections reported that they received a server timeout when trying to answer the survey. As a result, the timeout period for client responses to the server was increased from 60 seconds to five minutes.

- When typing in their survey ID, several respondents mistook the digit "0" for the letter "O," and the digit "1" for the letter "l" and vice versa. Thus, the server rejected their ID. Since a complete URL could not be provided for respondents to click on to access the survey, and since most participants obviously did not copy and paste their survey IDs into the field, respondents were advised by e-mail of the correct way of entering their survey ID.

- Several users were not aware that they could include the text of the original message in their reply or paste the survey from the Web page into an e-mail message. Instead, they printed the survey and returned the completed hardcopy by fax. Although this was not a major problem, it delayed the entry of approximately ten surveys into the database.

- After receiving approximately 130 surveys, the responses to one question revealed that participants seemed to choose only two of the four responses on a Likert scale. A review of the program revealed an error that stored answers incorrectly. The error was corrected, and the incorrectly stored answers were discarded.

Three additional messages were sent to non-respondents during the following two weeks. Figure 2 shows the dates and times of the messages, the distribution of responses, and the cumulative response rate.

The response rate for surveys entered via the Web was 32.9 percent—144 of 438 (adjusted) participants—after the initial mailing. The first follow-up mailing resulted in receipt of 76 surveys and brought the total response up to 50.2 percent. The second follow-up mailing raised the response rate to 57.1 percent, and the third raised it to 64.4 percent (30 and 32 responses, respectively). The 52 surveys returned by e-mail or fax were entered by hand and increased the final response rate to 74.2 percent (334 of 438 participants). We sent

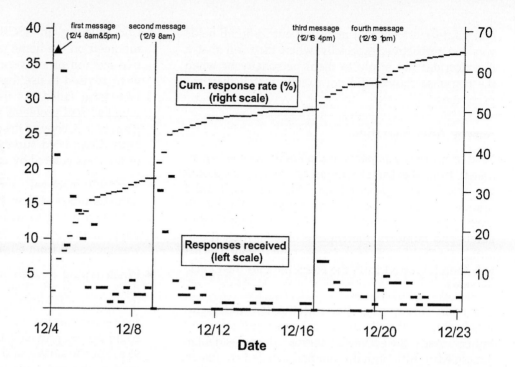

Figure 2 Number of responses received (left scale) and cumulative response rate (right scale, in percents) by date. The graph includes surveys entered through the Web only and indicates when survey mailings were sent.

a total of 1,132 e-mail messages to participants of this survey. To increase the response rate, the survey was directly included in the e-mail message in the second and third follow-up mailings. In addition, while the initial messages and the first follow-up messages were sent from a generic e-mail account (survey@stat.com), the subsequent follow-up messages were sent from the listowner's account directly, with a personal request for a response to the survey.

The next section compares the costs of this survey with costs if the survey had been administered by mail. General breakeven equations for the sample size using Web-based vs. mail surveys are presented. The section concludes with a comparison of characteristics of Web and e-mail/fax respondents.

Cost and Response Pattern Analysis

Costs

Costs were calculated to assess the cost-effectiveness of the Web-based survey method for planning future surveys. Table 1 shows the costs for the Web-based survey compared to the costs of an equivalent mail survey. The comparison excludes costs that are the same regardless of the survey methodology, such as design of the survey instrument and pilot-testing. Also excluded is the cost of obtaining the mailing list.

As Table 1 shows, the total cost of the Web survey was $1,916, comprising the costs for programming and testing the survey, programming the bulk mailer program, and performing limited manual data entry.

If all respondents had completed the Web-based survey successfully, the cost would have dropped by $206. Costs for an equivalent mail survey are calculated both for a non-anonymous survey (our case) and an anonymous survey. The two alternatives differ in their cost of preparing and mailing surveys. In non-anonymous surveys, surveys are prepared for and sent to non-respondents only after the initial mailing. Anonymous surveys require that all participants receive the initial and all follow-up mailings and are thus somewhat more expensive. We present different breakeven calculations (see below) for these two options.

If our survey had been administered as a mail survey, its total cost would have been $3,092, including the cost of preparing 1,132 mailings, mailing costs, postage for returned mailings, and data entry. The Web-survey was 38 percent cheaper than the equivalent (non-anonymous) mail survey. The figures used for the calculations in Table 1 represent local costs for a mail survey of 450 individuals. In other settings, costs might differ on the basis of factors such as sample size, reproduction costs, study requirements, programming costs, and data entry costs. Costs arising from handling technical problems for the Web-based survey (e.g., responding to user questions) were disregarded, since the required time was minimal and an improved design could have avoided most of those problems.

As Table 1 shows, the cost of a Web-based survey is independent of the sample size, whereas the costs of a mail survey vary with the initial sample size as well

Table 1 ■

Cost Comparison of a Web-based Survey and Non-anonymous and Anonymous Mail Surveys

	Web-based Survey			Mail Survey	
				Non-anonymous (1,132 mailings)	Anonymous (1,800 mailings—4 × 450 participants)
Survey preparation	Programming (35 hrs × $30)	$1,050	Printing/duplication of a 7-page survey and the cover letter ($0.08/page)	$724	$1,152
	Testing and code review (8 hrs × $60)	480	Envelopes at $0.055/envelope	62	99
			Business reply envelopes at $0.033/envelope	37	59
Distribution and return	Bulk mailer program (3 hrs × $60)	180	Mailing of surveys at $0.65/envelope ($0.55 postage + $0.10 envelope stuffing)	736	1,170
	Sending e-mail messages	0			
			Return postage on 334 surveys ($0.63/survey)	210	210
Data entry	Entry by participant	0	Entry by investigator/staff member (334 × 6 min × $0.66)	1,323	1,323
	Manual entry of 52 surveys (52 × 6 min × $0.66)	206			
Total		$1,916		$3,092	$4,013

NOTE: The calculations for the non-anonymous survey use actual response rates. The calculations for the anonymous survey assume that each participant receives the mailing four times, whether they replied or not. Personnel costs include fringe benefits (30%).

as with the incremental and the total response rate. Avoiding manual entry of completed surveys generated significant cost savings, a fact that has not been lost on transaction-intensive industries such as airlines and banks.

To assist others in choosing between Web-based and mail surveys on the basis of cost (assuming that all other variables are equal), we use a standard breakeven calculation[19] to determine the sample size for which both types of surveys cost exactly the same. This point is the threshold for which conducting one type of survey becomes more cost-effective than the other.

Equations 1 and 2 in Table 2 are used to calculate the breakeven point for non-anonymous and anonymous surveys, respectively, when the incremental and/or the final response rates can be estimated. When that is not possible, equations 3 and 4 can be used to calculate lower and upper bounds for the breakeven point.

For the described survey, n would have been 245 under the idealistic assumption that all respondents suc-

cessfully answered the survey through the Web. Even if the costs of entering of the surveys manually are included, the breakeven point rises only to 274. Thus, with a sample size of approximately 275 or below, a mail survey would have been more economical than a Web-based survey.

Equation 1 makes two assumptions of practical significance. First, it assumes that exactly as many hardcopy surveys are prepared as needed. In reality, this is rarely possible. Equation 1 thus will often reflect slightly lower costs for a mail survey than are achievable, slanting the comparison in favor of mail surveys. Second, it assumes that incremental and final response rates can be estimated. When this is not possible, we can calculate a range for the breakeven point by approximating the extreme values of equation 1 through equations 3 and 4. Using our costs, the lower bound for the breakeven point would have been 190 and the upper bound 347. This means that for a sample size of 189 or less, a mail survey would have been more economical, and with a sample size of 348 or more, a Web-based survey. In between, the cost advantage would have depended on the actual incre-

Table 2 ∎

Equations to Determine Breakeven Sample Size

Assumptions	Equations		
Incremental and/or final response rates can be estimated:	*Non-anonymous Survey**: $$n = \frac{c_{PR}}{\left(m - \sum_{i=1}^{m-1} r_i\right) \cdot (c_D + c_M) + r_m \cdot c_E}$$ (1)		*Anonymous Survey*†: $$n = \frac{c_{PR}}{m \cdot (c_D + c_M) + r_m \cdot c_E}$$ (2)
	Both types of survey:		
Incremental and/or final response rates cannot be estimated:	Lower bound: $n_l = \dfrac{c_{PR}}{m \cdot (c_D + c_M) + c_E}$ (3)		Upper bound: $n_u = \dfrac{c_{PR}}{m \cdot (c_D + c_M)}$ (4)

NOTE: Equations to determine the breakeven sample size for non-anonymous surveys (equation 1) and anonymous surveys (equation 2). If incremental or final response rates cannot be estimated, equations 3 and 4 can be used to determine the boundaries for the breakeven point. The equations make the assumption that the denominator is not zero and that the Web-based survey is entered successfully by each respondent. In addition, equations 1 and 2 assume that the cumulative response rate never reaches 100% before the last mailing. The variables are as follows: n, breakeven point; n_l, n_u, lower and upper bounds for breakeven point; m, number of mailings; r_1, r_2, ... r_m, cumulative response rate after the 1st, 2nd, ... mth mailing (r_m is the final response rate); c_{PR}, cost of programming the survey; c_D, cost of preparation per survey (duplication, envelopes, etc.); c_M, cost of mailing per survey; c_E, cost of receipt and data entry per survey.
*Repeat mailings of the non-anonymous survey are sent to nonrespondents only.
†Repeat mailings of the anonymous survey are sent to all participants.

mental and final response rates. Equations 3 and 4 thus provide a useful heuristic for determining a range for the breakeven point if basic costs for the two survey methods are known.

Comparison of Web and E-mail/Hardcopy Responses

The goal of using a Web-based survey was to have all respondents complete the questionnaire using the Web. However, we had to provide an alternative method to avoid converting individuals with technical or user problems into non-respondents. Once we allowed participants to answer the survey by e-mail or fax, some may have chosen one of these methods based on personal preference or convenience. The data were reviewed to discern potential patterns that might distinguish Web from hardcopy respondents.

Sixteen percent of the 334 respondents returned the completed survey by e-mail or fax. Although no differentiation was made between e-mail and fax responses, the majority were received by e-mail. America Online users submitted 31 percent of the e-mail/fax responses and 12 percent of the Web responses. E-mail messages about technical problems were received most frequently from America Online users. Thus, at least some of the technical problems were due to incompatibilities with America Online. One reason that some AOL users were successful in submitting the survey through the Web may have been their use of different versions of the AOL client software.

Chi-squared tests ($P = 0.05$) were used to test for independence between the type of response (either Web or e-mail/fax) and the following variables: top-level domain of the participant (either com, net, or other); self-reported computer experience ("not at all comfortable," "not very comfortable," "comfortable," "very comfortable"); self-reported years of Internet experience (1, 2, 3, 4, 5, 6, >6); and, the number of fields left empty on the survey (<21, 21–25, 26–30). Self-reported computer experience showed a significant relationship with the type of response ($X^2 = 10.3$; $df = 2$; $P = 0.006$), indicating that respondents more comfortable with computers tended to be more successful in completing the Web survey. Respondents answering the Web survey also tended to complete more fields on the survey ($X^2 = 37.3$; $df = 2$; $P = 0.001$).

The other two variables showed no relationship to the type of response. Thus, two hypotheses for future studies could be that successful completion of Web surveys is dependent on computer experience and that respondents to Web surveys complete more questionnaire items than e-mail/hardcopy respondents.

Conclusion

Several authors have proposed guidelines on how to conduct Web-based surveys.[11,13,17,18,20] However, few papers report the use of this method, and none describe its procedural aspects in detail.[2–5] One primary reason that the Web is not used frequently for large-scale or general surveys may be that Web access is not a given. Although 19 percent of households in the United States reported being online in 1997, not all members of each household may use the computer.[21] Even in a recent study, the first step in the survey was to find out whether participants used the Internet or not.[17] Although consumer research companies are beginning to tap AOL's 17 million users for market research,[22] it has not been proved that AOL's users are representative of the U.S. population at large. Until the e-mail address becomes as widely used as the postal address, large survey populations cannot be surveyed using the Web or e-mail alone.

As previously mentioned, some authors advocate publishing Web surveys through newsgroups, indexes, and search engines.[13] However, the resulting selection bias makes the results less valid and generalizable. Where defined populations are accessible through the Internet, a Web-based survey can be an effective method of gathering data using rigorous survey methodologies. However, even a relatively large group of Internet users may still represent a convenience sample that allows generalization to only that group.

Several authors have made recommendations for Web-survey design.[11,18] On the basis of our experiences in this case study, some additional recommendations can be made:

- *Consider Web-based surveys software development projects.* Unless an off-the-shelf survey application[23,24] is used, several tools must be integrated (such as HTML forms and PERL scripts). Sometimes survey applications must be custom-programmed. A survey application should be tested thoroughly to reduce the number of software defects and incompatibilities. Depending on the sample population, testing variables may include operating systems, browsers, Internet service providers, and Internet connection types. A systematic approach to identifying all variables and testing can reduce the chance of failure.

- *Usability and survey design should reflect the characteristics of the sample population and its environment.* If the computer literacy of the sample population is not known, the survey should be easy to complete in as few steps as possible. In this case study, simple usability issues became major problems for some participants. Among participants who have a high degree of computer literacy, usability may be less of a issue. Likewise, surveys designed for unknown computing environments should use the lowest common technical denominator. In contrast, a survey application could use advanced programming techniques that match the capabilities of standardized computing environments on an intranet.

- *Pilot-test with a sufficiently large random sample of the sample population.* It is often impossible to test all environments for a survey before its release. Thus, it is very important to pilot-test with a sufficiently large random sample of users. This will, it is hoped, account for computer literacy levels and the range of computer configurations.

- *Scrutinize early returns earlier.* Scrutinizing early returns is important in mail surveys.[25] The potentially immediate response to electronic surveys makes this recommendation even more important. As this example has shown, close monitoring of early returns can identify problems that were not caught during the pilot test, from technical issues to program bugs. Immediate resolution of such problems is required to prevent an unnecessarily large portion of non-respondents or increased measurement error.

This case study has shown that surveys administered through the Web can, compared with mail surveys, potentially lower costs, reduce survey administration overhead, and collect survey data quickly and efficiently. However, it also confirms that a number of variables have the potential to influence survey response and measurement negatively, such as incompatibility with the target computing environment, survey usability, computer literacy of participants, and program defects. In this case study, respondents to the Web survey tended to complete more questionnaire items than respondents who used e-mail or fax. Because of its potential impact on the quality of data collection, this finding should be validated in future studies.

The authors thank Dr. R. Kenney, Dr. D. Dodell, and N. Dovgy for their help in conducting this project, Dr. Sorin Straja for his help with the statistical analysis, Ms. Syrene Miller for her assistance in the literature review, and the reviewers for their helpful suggestions and comments.

References ■

1. Schleyer T, Forrest J, Kenney R, Dodell D, Dovgy N. Is the Internet useful in clinical practice? J Am Dent Assoc. 1999; 130:1502–11.
2. Eysenbach G, Diepgen TL. Epidemiological data can be gathered with World Wide Web. BMJ. 1998;316(7124):72.
3. Sell RL. Research and the Internet: an e-mail survey of sexual orientation. Am J Public Health. 1997;87(2):297.
4. Gobar GM, Case JT, Kass PH. Program for surveillance of causes of death of dogs, using the Internet to survey small animal veterinarians. J Am Vet Med Assoc. 1998;213(2):251–6.
5. Schleyer T, Spallek H, Torres-Urquidy MH. A profile of cur-

rent Internet users in dentistry. J Am Dent Assoc. 1998;129: 1748–53.

6. Lakeman R. Using the Internet for data collection in nursing research. Comput Nurs. 1997;15(5):269–75.

7. Fawcett J, Buhle EL Jr. Using the Internet for data collection: an innovative electronic strategy. Comput Nurs. 1995;13(6): 273–9.

8. Swoboda WJ, Mühlberger N, Weitkunat R, Schneeweib S. Internet surveys by direct mailing. Soc Sci Comput Rev. 1997;15(3):242–55.

9. Hilsden RJ, Meddings JB, Verhoef MJ. Complementary and alternative medicine use by patients with inflammatory bowel disease: an Internet survey. Can J Gastroenterol. 1999; 13(4):327–32.

10. Soetikno RM, Mrad R, Pao V, Lenert LA. Quality-of-life research on the Internet: feasibility and potential biases in patients with ulcerative colitis. J Am Med Inform Assoc. 1997; 4(6):426–35.

11. Dillman D, Tortora RL, Bowker D. Principles for constructing Web surveys. Presented at the Joint Meetings of the American Statistical Association; Dallas, Texas; August 1998.

12. Clark R, Maynard M. Research methodology: using online technology for secondary analysis of survey research data —"act globally, think locally." Soc Sci Comput Rev. 1998; 16(1):58–71.

13. Houston JD, Fiore DC. Online medical surveys: using the Internet as a research tool. MD Comput. 1998;15(2):116–20.

14. National Telecommunications and Information Administration. Falling through the Net: new data on the digital di-vide. Available at: http://www.ntia.doc.gov/ntiahome/net2/falling.html. Accessed Dec 8, 1999.

15. Intelliquest. Latest IntelliQuest survey reports 62 million American adults access the Internet/online services. Available at: http://www.intelliquest.com/press/release41.asp. Accessed Dec 8, 1999.

16. Groves R. Survey errors and survey costs. New York: John Wiley, 1989.

17. Dillman D, Tortora RL, Conradt J, Bowker D. Influence of plain vs. fancy design on response rates for Web surveys. In: Proceedings of the Joint Statistical Meetings, Survey Methods Section. Alexandria, Va: American Statistical Association, 1998.

18. Turner JL, Turner DB. Using the Internet to perform survey research. Syllabus. 1999;12(Jan):55–6.

19. Weygandt J, Kieso D, Kell W. Accounting Principles. 2nd ed. New York: John Wiley, 1990.

20. Turner JL, Turner DB. Using the Internet to perform survey research. Syllabus. 1998;12(Nov/Dec):58–61.

21. Stets D. Who's using computers? Philadelphia Inquirer. 1995 Nov 19, 1995:sect D3.

22. Kranhold K. Foote Cone turns to AOL for online polls. Wall Street Journal. Jul 28, 1999:sect B1.

23. Senecio Software Inc. Online and disk-by-mail surveys. Available at: http://www.senecio.com/. Accessed Dec 8, 1999.

24. Perseus Development Corporation. A survey software package for conducting Web surveys. Available at: http://www.perseus.com/. Accessed Dec 8, 1999.

25. Dillman DA. Mail and Telephone Surveys. New York: John Wiley, 1978.

Morpheme-based, cross-lingual indexing for medical document retrieval

Stefan Schulz [a,b,*], Udo Hahn [a]

[a] *CLIF Computational Linguistics Laboratory, Freiburg University, Werthmannplatz 1, D-79085 Freiburg, Germany*
[b] *Department of Medical Informatics, Freiburg University Hospital, Stefan-Meier-Strasse 26, D-79104 Freiburg, Germany*

Received 31 December 1999

Abstract

The increasing availability of machine-readable medical documents is not really matched with the sophistication of currently used retrieval facilities to deal with a variety of critical natural language phenomena. Still most popular are string-matching methods which encounter problems for the medical sublanguage, in particular, concerning the wide-spread use of complex word forms such as noun compounds. We introduce a methodology for the segmentation of complex compounds into medically motivated morphemes. Given the sublanguage patterns in our data these morphemes derive from German, Greek and Latin roots. For indexing and retrieval purposes, such a morpheme dictionary may be further structured by defining the semantic relations among morpheme sets in order to build up a multilingual morpheme thesaurus. We present a tool for thesaurus compilation and management, and outline a methodology for the proper construction and maintenance of a multilingual morpheme thesaurus. © 2000 Elsevier Science Ireland Ltd. All rights reserved.

Keywords: Medical language processing; Morphological analysis; Information retrieval

1. Introduction

Modern clinical documentation systems, as well as an increasing number of health-related electronic publications and databases available on CD-ROMs, hospital intranets and the Internet have swamped the physician's desktop with large amounts of computer-readable free text. The full utilization of these textual resources, however, is currently hampered by inadequate retrieval facilities.

In a common free-text information retrieval environment, the search for a document relies on an (exact) pattern matching operation between the query term(s) and the document terms. So, a query term such as '*Leukocyte*' retrieves all documents in which this query term occurs literally. Germanic

* Corresponding author. Tel.: +49-761-2036702; fax: +49-761-2033251.
E-mail addresses: stschulz@uni-freiburg.de (S. Schulz), hahn@coling.uni-freiburg.de (U. Hahn).

and Romanic languages, however, are characterized by the morphological process of *inflection*. This introduces grammatically motivated string variants of document terms such that (usually) suffixes are concatenated with a basic word form, e.g. '*Leukocyte* $\oplus$ *s*' ($\oplus$ denotes the string concatenation operator). Furthermore, through the morphological process of *derivation* basic word forms are concatenated with derivational prefixes and suffixes, usually implying a change of the word class (e.g. the noun '*Leukocyte*' changes into the adjective '*leukocyt* $\oplus$ *ic*'). While inflection preserves semantic invariance, derivation is usually accompanied with subtle changes of the core meaning of the stem undergoing derivation. Finally, by means of *composition* several basic word forms are combined to form a complex compound (e.g. the nouns '*Leukocyte*' and '*[H]em* $\oplus$ *o*' join into '*Leuk* $\oplus$ *em* $\oplus$ *ia*', with a tricky omission of the starting character of '*Hemo*', and the use of '*-ia*' as suffix). In the case of transparent composition, this introduces a great deal of systematic semantic refinement such that the core meaning of the head of a compound (usually the rightmost stem) is semantically modified in a significant way by the semantic facets of the other fundamental units within the compound. All the three morphological processes, inflection, derivation and composition, may combine and interact, grammatically as well as semantically. In order to account for the morphological variation of these types, three possibilities arise in a free-text retrieval system:

1. Enumerate, either manually or automatically, all morphological variants of a query term and combine them in a disjunctive query such as in '*Leukocyte*' $\lor$ '*Leukocytes*' $\lor$ '*Leukocyte's*' $\lor$ '*Leuk ocytic*' $\lor$ '*Leukemia*' $\lor$ ..., and let the system perform exact matches with the corresponding document terms.

2. Apply a masking (or truncation) operator (such as '$') to the longest common substring of all morphological variants (a so-called *formal stem*), e.g. '*Leuk*$'. The system will then perform a partial string match between this truncated query term and all document terms whose leftmost substring is identical with '*Leuk*', while the remainder can be any arbitrary string (including ε, the empty string)[1]. Obviously, such a mechanism mimics linguistically based morphological computations by mere string processing approximation.

3. Submit a linguistically motivated basic word form as a query term, e.g. '*Leukocyt*', and let the system automatically cope with morphological variants using a considerable stock of linguistic knowledge of the host language's morphology, and let it perform a search for the documents based on the system-determined variant sets.

Solution (1) often yields incomplete coverage due to missing variants even for linguistically well-trained human searchers (thus, lowering recall); when this is performed by a computational device, the procedure, if feasible at all, is just a generative reversal of analytic principles underlying the third approach. Solution (2) in many non-trivial cases has the tendency to overgenerate, i.e. produce many unintended matches (lowering precision), since the matching process is entirely underconstrained. Considering solution (3), one certainly has to distinguish different methodologies to automatic morphological analysis in order to assess the potential

---

[1] Note that in order to account for notoriously occurring '*K–C–Z*' spelling variants, such as '*Leuko...*' versus '*Leuco...*', one even has to reduce the formal stem to '*Leu*', which increases the number of false positives. In an Internet search, we determined a ratio of 5:1 for both forms (on a hit rate of 10 000 altogether) on English Web pages.

benefits or drawbacks for document retrieval systems. In the information retrieval community, the most common approach to morphological analysis is based on *stemming*, i.e. conflating different morphological variants to a single formal stem. Typically such algorithms (e.g. the Lovins stemmer [1] or the Porter stemmer [2]) refrain from using dictionary information and are solely based on simple string processing routines. Their principal way of operation consists of removing inflectional endings (e.g. plural or genitival or tense suffixes) or derivational suffixes, including some recoding transformations. Some of them, e.g. the Lovins stemmer, follow a one-pass strategy based on right-to-left longest matching plus recoding, others, e.g. the Porter stemmer, employ an iterative multi-pass approach. In fact, there has been some controversy about their contribution to improving the effectiveness of document retrieval systems [3–5]. The key issue for quality improvement seems to be rooted mainly in the presence or absence of some form of dictionary, i.e. a list of content words in some agreed-upon basic lexical format plus, possibly, additional linguistic information concerning parts of speech, gender, number, tense, mood, semantic relations, etc. Empirical evidence has been brought forward that inflectional and/or derivational stemmers augmented by (machine-readable) dictionaries indeed perform substantially better than those without access to lexical repositories [5].

In addition, the above-mentioned stemming algorithms and their many variants benefit from the limited suffix set and rather simple formation rules underlying English inflection. When turning to other languages, e.g. French, Italian, Spanish, or German, no comparable algorithmic standard yet exists, not to mention major Asian languages such as Japanese, Korean and major dialects of Chinese. Many of these languages exhibit a much richer inventory of inflectional suffixes, and also their structural combination is more complex. Evidence for this statement and the implications on text retrieval performance comes from a large variety of highly inflectional and/or agglutinating languages such as Hebrew [6], Finnish [7], or Slovene [8]. Taking the perspective of different languages makes perfect sense here, since routinely generated narratives in medical practice (finding and admission reports, discharge summaries, etc.), no matter whether they appear in a clinical environment or at the practitioner's work place, are written in the medical expert's native language.

Morphological complexity further increases, in structural terms and independent of particular languages, when one looks at derivation and composition (for a survey of German language, cf. [9], for English composition, cf. [10]). There have already been observations on the crucial status of compounds for information retrieval and the problems they cause [7]. This becomes particularly pertinent for the medical domain where a large number of established terms of tremendous morphological complexity yet exist. In Section 3, we present the results of an experiment that elucidates the impact of derivation and composition on medical terminology. Also, medical terminology is characterized by a typical mix of Latin and Greek roots with the corresponding host language (e.g. German)[2] often referred to as *Neo-Latin compounding*. While this is often merely a side issue for general-purpose morphological analyzers, such an observation becomes important for any attempt to cope with medical

---

[2] In contradistinction to other languages, equally characterized by medical terms of Greek/Latin origin (e.g. *duodenal ulcer, ulcère duodénal*), the German medical sublanguage simultaneously includes both varieties either obeying German (*Duodenalulkus*) or Latin (*Ulcus duodeni*) morphological rules.

free-texts in an information retrieval setting (cf. [11]).

In this article, we propose a methodology for morphological analysis that accounts for (a) all the three basic morphological processes, i.e. inflection, derivation, and composition, and (b) the combination of Greek, Latin, and the particular host language (in our case, German). Unlike approaches, which are purely driven by considerations of general natural language processing (NLP), we embed our methodology in the framework of medical information retrieval. We will see that this has implications for (c) the choice of the fundamental unit of morphological analysis, as well as (d) the way in which we conceptually relate these basic units by making reference to well-known medical terminologies. It is this 'light-weight' conceptual foundation that sets our approach apart from all standard NLP methods — typically they do not explicitly link up to particular ontologies. Making full use of a large corpus and computational facilities we are able to provide a general automaton-based methodology that supersedes early pattern-matching-based or string-based proposals in the MLP community in terms of linguistic generality.

2. Discussion of alternative approaches to morphological analysis of medical language

While considerable pessimism has been expressed with respect to a full semantic interpretation of medical compounds [12], several approximations have already been proposed to get around with this intricate problem. The earliest approach to deal with medical terminology by way of morphological analysis is due to Pratt and Pacak [13]. Their approach transforms semantically equivalent adjectival and nominal forms by employing simple suffix trees and transformation rules for recoding morphologically reduced forms. Transformations succeed if a recoded form is matched with an entry in the SNOP nomenclature. Hence, this approach is fully dependent on the existence of a dictionary containing relevant lexical forms of the medical sublanguage.

Follow-up studies of this work by Pacak and Norton [14,15] not only determine a preferred normalized form for several morphological variants but rather compute paraphrase and other semantic relations (such as locative, causative ones). These are implicitly denoted by complex medical compound nouns and can be made explicit by breaking compounds up into their constituent parts. The distributional patterns suggested by Pacak and Norton are based on four top-level conceptual categories, which are directly derived from SNOP/SNOMED codes (viz. topography, (medical) morphology, etiology, and function). A major limitation of this study, however, is due to the restriction of the decompositional analysis to compounds referring to inflammatory processes (indicated by the '-*itis*' ending) or to surgical procedures (indicated, e.g. by '-*ectomy*' or '-*plasty*' endings) only. In a similar vein, Dujols et al. [16] treat '-*osis*' forms only, though in a slightly more sophisticated manner than implied by the Norton/Pacak morphosemantic patterns. These restrictions are somewhat weakened in the study of Wolff [11] both in terms of a larger number of Greco-Latin suffixes being covered, as well as more general compositional patterns of Neo-Latin compounding. However, her approach — by design, a lexical knowledge engineering strategy for augmenting LSP-style lexicons rather than aiming at classical document retrieval applications — diverges from medical orthodoxy, insofar as the conceptual categories she employs refer to the subclass coding principles specifically holding within the Linguistic

String Project (LSP) context (for an overview of the LSP, cf. [17]), rather than to the conventional SNOP/SNOMED-style nomenclature.

Also a part of this study is loosely characterized by a mixture of isolated data structures (e.g. suffix trees) and various procedural heuristics (right-to-left longest matching, floating '*o*' insertion as in '*cyst $\oplus$ o $\oplus$ lith $\oplus$ ectomy*' vs. '*cyst $\oplus$ ectomy*', etc.). In an attempt to formulate the principles of medical word segmentation in a formally more rigid, almost language-independent framework, Wingert [18] chose an automaton-based specification for morphological analysis in terms of augmented transition networks [19]. He, finally, proposes a set of 255 cascading rules to capture the combinatorial regularities of different morpheme classes and, similar to Pratt and Pacak, refers to the entries of the SNOP nomenclature in order to exploit semantic information from the medical domain.

In the last decade, research in morphology has ceased in the medical language processing (MLP) community. Just recently, interest in this topic has revived employing much more sophisticated linguistic and conceptual knowledge. Baud et al. [20–22] use finite-state technology for the decomposition of complex terms into semantically non-decomposable segmentation units they refer to as *morphosemantemes*. A lot of power of their approach derives from the fact that the conceptual correlates of these morphose mantemes no longer refer to flat SNOMED-style categories but rather are formulated in GRAIL, a highly expressive deductive terminological knowledge representation language within the GALEN framework [23]. In order to isolate a morphosemanteme, composite concepts are dissected to their medically plausible conceptual core, using terminological knowledge derived from GRAIL. Baud et al.'s approach fully depends on and is, therefore, limited by the comparatively poor coverage of the medical domain by GRAIL, which, as any of these *deep* knowledge approaches, hardly scales up to reasonably sized, practically-to-use knowledge bases. Also, Baud et al.'s notion of a morphosemanteme is more promiscuous than what we call a *medically relevant morpheme*. More generally, we argue in favor of an automaton for word decomposition whose segmentation capability depends on a stricter though medically bounded sense of morphological atomicity. As we will see, this criterion also eases information retrieval on multilingual platforms.

It is interesting to observe that none of the above-mentioned proposals make use of the state-of-the-art methodologies for morphological analysis in NLP proper at the time of their writing, viz. chart-based approaches in the (early) eighties [24], or, currently, the model of two-level morphology as originally formulated by Koskenniemi [25] and lucidly described in [26]. The reason might be that these pure NLP methodologies still pose too strong requirements on their linguistic resources (e.g. two-level morphology requires elaborate and complete stem and suffix lexicons) and are also too rigid with respect to well-formedness of their input. Also major efforts have been so far directed at deflection only, with only minor attention being paid to derivational (for exceptions to the rule, cf. [27,28]) or compositional morphology (for exceptions to the rule, cf. [29,30]). Even worse, some languages such as German pose particularly weird problems to a two-level machine because of contextual alteration dependencies within words such as umlauts (for a problem statement, cf. [31,32]). The problem of mixed-language input, as evidenced by medical Neo-Latin compounding, has to the best of our knowledge not been considered in this framework so far.

3. An empirical study of the distribution and coverage of complex compounds

In order to collect empirical evidence whether morphological analysis of complex word forms is really an urgent need, we conducted the following experiment. In a random selection of 100 pathology reports (average token count 147.9 per report) we found 895 occurrences of different domain-specific compounds. We then matched these 895 forms with all words contained in a machine-readable version of a comprehensive German-language medical dictionary, the 'Pschyrembel'[3]. The retrieval process was based on exact string match. Surprisingly, 400 out of these 895 compounds did not occur in the dictionary. This reflects the enormous productivity of medical language leading to a large number of ad hoc compounds. A number of examples, both German and English ones, are given in Table 1. Analyzing the rubrics of the English-language coding system ICD-9-CM, we found — to a minor extent — a considerable number of nominal compounds (cf. the English terms in Table 1), thus indicating that this phenomenon is by no means restricted to the German language

only. Generalizing from this study, we find confirmation for the hypothesis that accounting for complex morphological phenomena is highly rewarded in medical retrieval environments.

At least two basic approaches seem to be reasonable. In the first one, the derivational and compositional forms have to be explicitly spelt out for each medical term in the terminology. This causes the size of those thesauri to grow dramatically by the sheer number of different terms. Also, given the speed of terminological growth, the goal of enumerating all morphological varieties can always only be approximated but never fully achieved.

Alternatively, one might want to avoid these scaling problems (and the associated maintenance load) and keep up with continuous terminological dynamics by exploiting basic linguistic regularities through a sophisticated morphological analyzer. We adhere to this second approach, and propose the concept of a morpheme-based dictionary/thesaurus. A repository of morphemes as the smallest meaningful morphological units is expected to be several orders of magnitude below the size of phrasal or fully lexicalized dictionaries, with quite a lower growth rate. Hence, it should also be much easier and cheaper to compile and to maintain. This parsimony must, however, be

---

[3] *Pschyrembel Klinisches Wörterbuch*: for MS Windows 3.1, 3.11 and '95, Walter de Gruyter. Its whole text corpus contains more than 100 000 different entries.

Table 1
Nominal compounds in medical German and English

Kryostatschnittverfahren	Kryo ⊕ stat ⊕ schnitt ⊕ verfahr ⊕ en
Fibroblastenproliferation	Fibro ⊕ blast ⊕ en ⊕ prolifer ⊕ ation
Nierentransplantatgewebe	Niere ⊕ a ⊕ trans ⊕ plant ⊕ at ⊕ geweb ⊕ e
Transitionalzellkarzinom	Transi ⊕ tio ⊕ nal ⊕ zell ⊕ karzin ⊕ om
Schilddrüsenüberschreitung	Schil ⊕ drüse ⊕ n ⊕ über ⊕ schreit ⊕ ung
Neuroencephalomyelopathy	Neur ⊕ o ⊕ encephal ⊕ o ⊕ myel ⊕ o ⊕ path ⊕ y
Pseudohypoparathyroidism	Pseudo ⊕ hypo ⊕ para ⊕ thyroid ⊕ ism
Proctosigmoidoscopy	Proct ⊕ o ⊕ sigm ⊕ oid ⊕ o ⊕ scop ⊕ y
Hyperprebetalipoproteinemia	Hyper ⊕ pre ⊕ beta ⊕ lipo ⊕ protein ⊕ em ⊕ ia
Arterionephrosclerosis	Arteri ⊕ o ⊕ nephr ⊕ o ⊕ scler ⊕ os ⊕ is

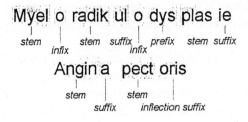

Fig. 1. Example for segmentation of complex words and morpheme classes.

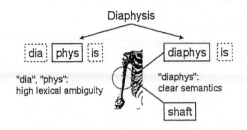

Fig. 2. Task-specific atomicity: incomplete segmentation to avoid lexical ambiguities.

traded against the lack of semantic expressiveness of the entries and an increased computational complexity of the algorithms needed for decomposition and disambiguation. In the following, a tool and a methodology for a morpheme thesaurus will be described and preliminary results obtained by a pilot study are given.

4. Morphological segmentation model

We distinguish the following morpheme classes and define syntactic rules of well-formedness formally encoded in a finite state automaton (we only give some informal and incomplete examples here) for their use within composed words:

- Stems like {*gastr, hepat, nier, leuk, diaphys*...} are the primary carrier of content in a word; they can be prefixed, linked by infixes, and suffixed.

- Prefixes like {*a, de, in, ent, ver, anti, ...*} precede the word's stem(s).
- Infixes (e.g. '*o*' in '*gastr* $\oplus$ *o* $\oplus$ *intestinal*', or '*s*' in *Sektion* $\oplus$ *s* $\oplus$ *bericht*') are just used as a (phonologically motivated) 'glue' between morphemes, typically as a link between stems.
- Derivational suffixes such as {*io, ion, ie, ung, itis, tomie, ...*} usually follow the word's stem(s).
- Inflectional suffixes like {*e, en, s, idis, ae, oris, ...*} appear at the very end of a word following the word's stem(s) or derivational suffixes.
- Eponyms (mostly proper names), digits and acronyms {*AIDS, ECG, ...*} are non-decomposable entities in morphological terms and also undergo no further morphological variation, e.g. by suffixing.

A segmentation of two compounds that is based on these distinctions into morpheme classes is depicted in Fig. 1. In general, however, adequate morphological segmentation for use in an information retrieval environment places restrictions on morphological analysis, which differ from purely linguistic considerations. In effect, it turns out that a balanced notion of morpheme atomicity is crucial for success. While linguists tend to strive for the utmost degree of breaking up complex words into the smallest morphological units possible, from an information retrieval perspective this might be inappropriate. The reason for this lies in a priori meaning assignments to morphological complex forms in a particular domain.

In the example depicted in Fig. 2, the morphologically complex word stem '*diaphys*' has a unique conceptual correlate in the medical domain, viz. the shaft of a long bone. Further segmentation into '*dia*' and '*phys*', though linguistically entirely plausible, would produce ambiguous morphological entities with conceptual correlates, if any, of far lesser specificity, at least in medical terms. Hence, we argue for a conceptually motivated criterion for morphological atomicity, one that is rooted in medical plausibility (similar arguments were already raised in [15,33]).

The following heuristics were considered to be adequate for determining medically motivated morphemes: a lexical string undergoes no further segmentation if an apparently atomic synonymous or quasi-synonymous stem exists (SHAFT in our example) and/or if it points to a basic conceptual entity in the medical domain. Obviously, this view implies a trade-off between compactness (reduced number of morphemes) and expressiveness (reduced semantic specificity of morphemes). This is demonstrated in Fig. 3, where variants of word stems, so-called allomorphs ('leuko', 'leuco', 'leuk', 'leuc') can be generalized up to the longest common substring, viz. 'leu'. While this certainly reduces the size of the morpheme dictionary, an increased number of morphological segmentation ambiguities and, even worse, false positives are likely to be encountered in an information retrieval environment. We refrain from such a solution and subscribe to a modest size growth of the dictionary by the intentional inclusion of allomorphs.

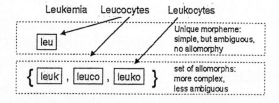

Fig. 3. Allomorphy: set of semantically identical morphemes (allomorphs).

5. MEDSEARCH: an interactive tool for the construction of a morpheme dictionary

On the basis of these considerations, we developed a morphological segmentation engine, MEDSEARCH. The system consists of a morphological parser that builds, on the basis of existing morpheme lexicons, *all* possible parse trees for the input. Morphological segmentation ambiguities are ranked according to the following preference criteria:

1. longest match;
2. minimal number of stems per word;
3. minimal number of consecutive affixes (this criterion penalizes utterly formal segmentations); and
4. relative weight — more specifically, a semantic weight factor $w = 2$ is assigned to all stems and some semantically important suffixes, such as '-tomie', '-itis'; $w = 1$ is assigned to prefixes and derivational suffixes, and $w = 0$ is rendered to inflectional suffixes and infixes.

The MEDSEARCH tools provide a graphical interface for interactive management of the morpheme dictionary, the *MedSearch Morphology Workbench*. In each training cycle, it imports complex words from the source corpora under consideration, performs segmentation on the basis of the morphemes already specified, and displays the analysis results, weighted according to the above mentioned criteria. Fig. 4 gives a glimpse of the user interface and illustrates the result of the segmentation of the nominal compound '*Postgastrektomiesymptomatik*'. Note that many ambiguous analyses are displayed, since the stem '*gastr*' has not yet been specified as a stem. Upper case characters mark morphemes with a weight factor $w = 2$. Every relevant morpheme that is missing can be manually inserted in the appropriate morpheme lists such as it is shown in Fig. 4. By supplying new entries the segmentation capa-

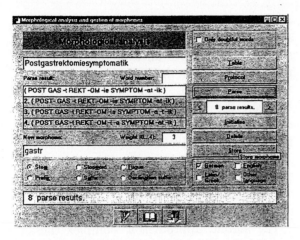

Fig. 4. MEDSEARCH morphology workbench: tool for the incremental construction of the morpheme dictionary.

bility of our tool continuously improves. Prior to storing a new morpheme, attributes concerning morpheme class and language (German, Latin, Greek) have to be supplied.

MEDSEARCH has been implemented using the programming environment of Visual Basic 6.0. Besides the graphical interface, it can be run as a Microsoft component object model (COM) server application, thus exporting its methods within a network.

6. Experience with running MEDSEARCH

In a pilot study, we proceeded in the following way in order to get started. Using the MEDSEARCH Workbench, we first manually supplied an a priori selected set of German and Greco-Latin prefixes, suffixes, and infixes. In particular, no word stems were provided. After this initialization phase, our test corpus was obtained by merging the following sources: the German translation of the 9th and the 10th release of the international classification of diseases (ICD), the German SNOMED, the international classification of procedures in medicine in its German version

OPS301, and, finally, a list of more than 100 000 German language clinical diagnosis phrases. This raw material was automatically segmented by the morphological analyzer without human interaction in a fast batch mode. This led to a huge list of unknown substrings, since except the previously determined affixes no other morphemes were initially known to MEDSEARCH. These unknown substrings were then ranked by frequency. The first 1000 most frequent substrings were checked manually, and the missing word stems were included in the morpheme lexicon.

This bootstrapped morpheme list was then used for another cycle of automatic segmentation and manual workup in which the above-cited rules for domain-specific delimitation were applied once again. The following criteria for the exclusion of word stems were defined, (1) one-time occurrence only; (2) acronyms or proper names (e.g. drug names); (3) non-medical word stems. Applying these rules the analysis of the whole material yielded a core table of 7130 medicine-specific word stems, with 22 369 words or word fragments being excluded.

We also performed a second study in order to estimate the growth behavior of a medical word stem lexicon using 30 000 diagnosis phrases from a clinical documentation system (this constituted a more homogeneous text sample). Applying the above exclusion criteria we obtained a list of 4098 word stems. The growth curve can be approximated by a logarithmic function (cf. Fig. 5)

7. Steps towards a multilingual morpheme thesaurus

In the procedure just described, we already account for morphemes from different languages. In this section, we propose an extension of the emerging multilingual dictionary to a multilingual thesaurus by incorporating semantic relations between the morpheme items (an idea first articulated by Pacak et al. [14]). In order to map between synonymous or quasi-synonymous expressions within the same language, but also between different natural languages, we will discuss two alternative approaches (cf. Fig. 6).

The first approach, a 'simple thesaurus' (cf. Fig. 6, left side), is based on the definition of semantic links within the morpheme thesaurus proper, without any reference to an external ontology. As basic semantic relations between pairs of morphemes, we choose the similarity S and the equivalence E relations. Both S and E are symmetric, but only E is transitive. Hence, E defines sets of semanti-

cally equivalent morphemes, and S links those groups with one another that have a similar meaning. As an example, the E relation holds within the morpheme set $M1 = \{stomach, magen, estomac\}$, as well as between the elements of $M2 = \{heart, cor, cord, herz, coeur\}$. Regarding a third morpheme set $M3 = \{ventric, ventrik\}$, we state a *similarity* relation between $M1$ and $M3$ as well as between $M2$ and $M3$, because 'ventricle' means both the cavity of the heart and the cavity of the stomach.

The second approach, a 'complex thesaurus' (cf. Fig. 6, right side), maps morphemes to sets of elements of an existing terminological system, e.g. the UMLS. The UMLS metathesaurus provides, besides the synonymy relation, hierarchy-inducing relations

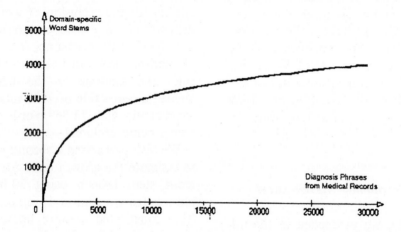

Fig. 5. Growth behavior of a word stem lexicon obtained from diagnosis phrases.

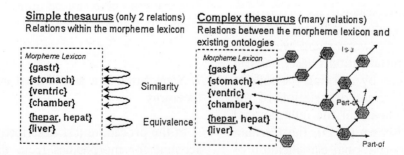

Fig. 6. Two approaches for semantic linkage in a multilingual morpheme thesaurus.

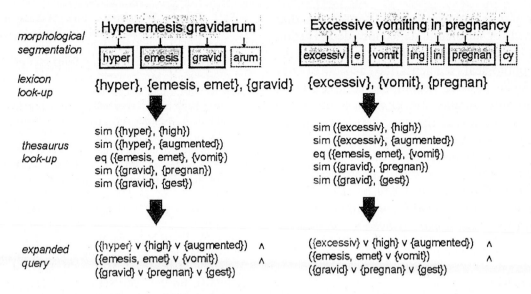

Fig. 7. Query obtained by morpheme-supported expansion of two synonymous surface expressions.

such as broader/narrower or child/parent relationships, and — to a minor extent — semantically more specific relations such as *is-a* or *part-of*.

The advantage of the first approach is that all the knowledge necessary for morphological analysis and efficient retrieval is directly available at the repository level. However, the internal linkage has to be done from the scratch. Even with a relatively small number of dictionary entries, and the restriction to two basic relations only, the decision as to whether two morphemes should be linked in terms of a real synonymy or only a similarity relation will in many cases not always be easy to make and requires much experience in the use of medical language.

The second approach has, in contradistinction, the advantage that all semantic relations are already given. Its difficulties will arise from the task of the adequate mapping of a small set of semantically shallow morphemes to a huge collection — about two orders of magnitude larger in size — of semantically precise concepts. As an example, in the

UMLS metathesaurus there is no concept for the generic notion of *'ventricle'*. A solution may be the subscription to the first approach, but using the UMLS as a support for the thesaurus construction process.

Considering the 'simple thesaurus' approach, a scenario for information retrieval is outlined in Fig. 7. Nearly identical queries are obtained by the morpheme-supported expansion of two synonyms, though lexically entirely different surface expressions were used in the original query.

8. Conclusion

Given the productivity and developmental dynamics of medical terminologies, it seems almost impossible to keep pace with their excessive lexical growth rates. As a way out of this dilemma, we opt for automatic morphological segmentation. In order to support effective free-text retrieval, in this article we proposed a pragmatic methodology that builds on a morpheme thesaurus, a repository of morphologically significant forms, that is used for automatic deflection, dederivation and decomposition. While we stressed the morphological segmentation aspect of our work, i.e. how to decompose complex word forms into simpler morphological units, we have also outlined the next step required viz. how to link these basic morphological units by conceptual relationships. Finally, a retrieval-based evaluation of our framework is still pending. The latter part will be the focus of on-going work, while the operational segmentation tool has already proved to be useful.

References

[1] J.B. Lovins, Development of a stemming algorithm, Mech. Trans. Comput. Linguistics 11 (1/2) (1968) 22–31.

[2] M.F. Porter, An algorithm for suffix stripping, Program 14 (3) (1980) 130–137.

[3] D. Harman, How effective is suffixing?, J. Am. Soc. Inf. Sci. 42 (1) (1991) 7–15.

[4] D.A. Hull, Stemming algorithms: a case study for detailed evaluation, J. Am. Soc. Inf. Sci. 47 (1) (1996) 70–84.

[5] R. Krovetz, Viewing morphology as an inference process, in: R. Korfhage, E. Rasmussen, P. Willett (Eds.), SIGIR'93 — Proceedings of the 16th Annual International ACM SIGIR Conference on Research and Development in Information Retrieval, Pittsburgh, PA, USA, June 27–July 1, 1993, ACM, New York, NY, pp. 191–203.

[6] Y. Choueka, Responsa: an operational full-text retrieval system with linguistic components for large corpora, in: A. Zampolli (Ed.), Computational Lexicology and Lexicography: A Volume in Honor of B. Quemada, Giardini Press, Pisa, 1992.

[7] H. Jäppinen, J. Niemistö, Inflections and compounds: some linguistic problems for automatic indexing, in: Proceedings of the RIAO 88 Conference: 'User-Oriented Content-Based Text and Image Handling', vol. 1, Cambridge, MA, March 21–24, 1988, pp. 333–342.

[8] M. Popovic, P. Willett, The effectiveness of stemming for natural language access to Slovene textual data, J. Am. Soc. Inf. Sci. 43 (5) (1992) 384–390.

[9] J. Toman, Wortsyntax. Eine Diskussion ausgewählter Probleme deutscher Wortbildung, Max Niemeyer, Tübingen, 1987.

[10] J.N. Levi, The Syntax and Semantics of Complex Nominals, McGraw-Hill, New York, 1978.

[11] S. Wolff, The use of morphosemantic regularities in the medical vocabulary for automatic lexical coding, Methods Inf. Med. 23 (4) (1984) 195–203.

[12] A.T. McCray, A.C. Browne, D.L. Moore, The semantic structure of neo-classical compounds, in: R.A. Greenes (Ed.), SCAMC'88 — Proceedings of the 12th Annual Symposium on Computer Applications in Medical Care, IEEE Computer Society Press, Washington, DC, 1988, pp. 165–168.

[13] A.W. Pratt, M.G. Pacak, Identification and transformation of terminal morphemes in medical English, Methods Inf. Med. 8 (2) (1969) 84–90.

[14] M.G. Pacak, L.M. Norton, G.S. Dunham, Morphosemantic analysis of ITIS forms in medical language, Methods Inf. Med. 19 (2) (1980) 99–105.

[15] L.M. Norton, M.G. Pacak, Morphosemantic analysis of compound word forms denoting surgical procedures, Methods Inf. Med. 22 (1) (1983) 29–36.

[16] P. Dujols, P. Aubas, C. Baylon, F. Grémy, Morphosemantic analysis and translation of medical compound terms, Methods Inf. Med. 30 (1) (1991) 30–35.

[17] N. Sager, M. Lyman, C.E. Bucknall, N.T. Nhan, L.J. Tick, Natural language processing and the representation of clinical data, J. Am. Med. Inf. Assoc. 1 (2) (1994) 142–160.

[18] F. Wingert, Morphosyntaktische Zerlegung von Komposita der medizinischen Sprache, Methods Inf. Med. 16 (4) (1977) 248–255.

[19] F. Wingert, Morphologic analysis of compound words, Methods Inf. Med. 24 (3) (1985) 155–162.

[20] C. Lovis, R. Baud, P.-A. Michel, J.-R. Scherrer, Morphosemantems decomposition and semantic representation to allow fast and efficient natural language recognition, in: R. Masys (Ed.), AMIA'97 — Proceedings of the 1997 AMIA Annual Fall Symposium (formerly SCAMC). The Emergence of 'Internetable' Health Care: Systems that Really Work, Nashville, TN, October 25–29, 1997, Hanley & Belfus, Philadelphia, PA (long version on CD-ROM), pp. 873.

[21] R.H. Baud, C. Lovis, A.-M. Rassinoux, J.-R. Scherrer, Morpho-semantic parsing of medical expressions, in: C.G. Chute (Ed.), AMIA'98 —

Proceedings of the 1998 AMIA Annual Fall Symposium. A Paradigm Shift in Health Care Information Systems: Clinical Infrastructures for the 21st Century, Orlando, FL, November 7–11, 1998, Hanley & Belfus, Philadelphia, PA, pp. 760–764.

[22] R.H. Baud, A.-M. Rassinoux, P. Ruch, C. Lovis, J.-R. Scherrer, The power and limits of a rule-based morpho-syntactic parser, in: N.M. Lorenzi (Ed.), AMIA'99 — Proceedings of the 1999 Annual Symposium of the American Medical Informatics Association. Transforming Health Care through Informatics, Washington, DC, November 6–10, 1999, Hanley & Belfus, Philadelphia, PA, pp. 22–26.

[23] A.L. Rector, S. Bechhofer, C.A. Goble, I. Horrocks, W.A. Nowlan, W.D. Solomon, The GRAIL concept modelling language for medical terminology, Artif. Intell. Med. 9 (1997) 139–171.

[24] M. Kay, Morphological analysis, in: A. Zampolli, N. Calzolari (Eds.), Computational and Mathematical Linguistics, Proceedings of the International Conference on Computational Linguistics, vol. 1, Pisa, August 27–September 1, 1973, L.S. Olschki, Firenze, pp. 205–223.

[25] K. Koskenniemi, A general computational model for word formation recognition and production, in: COLING'84 — Proceedings of the 10th International Conference on Computational Linguistics and 22nd Annual Meeting of the Association for Computational Linguistics, Stanford, California, USA, July 2–6, 1984, pp. 178–181.

[26] R. Sproat, Morphology and Computation, MIT Press, Cambridge, MA, 1992.

[27] G.J. Russell, G.D. Ritchie, S.G. Pulman, A.W. Black, A dictionary and morphological analyzer for English, in: COLING '86 — Proceedings of the 11th International Conference on Computational Linguistics, Bonn, August 25–29, 1986, Institut fur angewandte Kommunikations- und Sprachforschung (IKS), Bonn, pp. 277–279.

[28] H. Trost, Coping with derivation in a morphological component, in: EACL'93 — Proceedings of

the 6th Conference of the European Chapter of the Association for Computational Linguistics, Utrecht, The Netherlands, April 21–23, 1993, Assoc. Comput. Linguistics 368–376.

[29] A.W. Black, J. van de Plassche, B. William, Analysis of unknown words through morphological decomposition, in: Proceedings of the 5th Conference of the European Chapter of the Association for Computational Linguistics, Berlin, Germany, April 9–11, 1991, Assoc. Comput. Linguistics 101–106.

[30] L. Karttunen, R.M. Kaplan, A. Zaenen, Two-level morphology with composition, in: COLING'92 — Proceedings of the 15th International Conference on Computational Linguistics, vol. 1, topical papers, August 23–28, 1992, ICCL, Nantes, pp. 141–148.

[31] H. Trost, The application of two-level morphology to non-concatenative German morphology, in: COLING'90 — Papers presented at the 13th International Conference on Computational Linguistics on the Occasion of the 25th Anniversary of COLING and the 350th Anniversary of Helsinki University, vol. 2, Helsinki, Finland, 1990, pp. 371–376.

[32] A. Schiller, P. Steffens, Morphological processing in the two-level paradigm, in: O. Herzog, C.-R. Rollinger (Eds.), Text Understanding in LILOG. Integrating Computational Linguistics and Artificial Intelligence, final report on the IBM Germany LILOG-Project, number 546 in Lecture Notes in Artificial Intelligence, Springer, Berlin, 1991, pp. 112–126.

[33] C. Lovis, P.-A. Michel, R.H. Baud, J.-R. Scherrer, Word segmentation processing: a way to exponentially extend medical dictionaries, in: R.A. Greenes, H.E. Peterson, D.J. Protti (Eds.), MEDINFO '95 — Proceedings of the 8th Conference on Medical Informatics, number 8 in IFIP World Conference Series on Medical Informatics, Vancouver, Canada, North-Holland, Amsterdam, 1995, pp. 28–32.

Section 2:

Reprinted by kind permission of:
American Medical Informatics
Association (340, 365)
Blackwell Science Ltd. (358)
F.K. Schattauer Verlagsgesellschaft
mbH. (332, 377)
The Royal College of General
Practitioners (352)

M. Kimura

Hamamatsu University, School of Medicine
Department of Medical Informatics
Hamamatsu, Japan

Synopsis

What can we currently expect from patient records?

1. What purpose do patient records serve?

Originally, patient records were for maintaining the level of healthcare. Continuation of patient, whether it is by the same healthcare professional or not, is the purpose to which record keeping can contribute. The importance of the record was emphasized as healthcare provision by allied professionals became common.

The information processing system for patient records should be measured using many basic indicators. It should 1) be re-readable, 2) provide prompt display, 3) assure no records can be lost, 4) be easy to use. Without guaranteeing these basics, any added feature systems, such as electronic patient records, are "Trying to walk, before being able to stand". Users are accustomed to the performance of the latest IT systems, high speed CPUs and networks. Handling health information cannot be an excuse, no matter how enormous the amount of information is.

Plus, as advanced indicators, information processing systems of patient records should 5) present information for future users, 6) provide useful search mechanisms, 7) allow access to multiple users in remote locations, and, 8) provide enough security. We have been working hard on this issue, through health information system research, for decades.

2. What more can we expect?

With the above mentioned functions, we have, and can handle, much more health information than ever. These are cumulative laboratory test results from automated analyzers, slices of images from many modalities, long history of prescriptions ordered, etc. Decades ago, many applied artificial intelligence systems[1] were built requiring exhausting data input. We can now import automatically, thanks to the standardization of healthcare data exchange. What can we now expect from patient records, in addition to the basic role of well-kept patient records?

a. Contribution to progress of medical science

For medical science, the size of trials is of primary importance. More power is added by the massive amounts of data collected by statistical or any other retrospective analysis method. Automated methods can even be applied to create hypotheses. Methods used for this purpose include data mining and intelligent information retrieval.

b. Optimization of patient care

The fruits of medical science are to be applied to patient care. The high percentage of patient data, handled by information systems, improves the precision of its application. The more patient data that is acquired at real time, the better planned care can be checked automatically, and the better the timeliness of decision making.

Due to networks, the source of the application can be located remotely. This means, the patient, attending professional, and information system do not have to be in the same place at the same time.

c. Improvement of management by the healthcare provider

Eliminating multiple data input and other unnecessary paperwork (whether on paper or not) dramatically improves the efficiency of the healthcare professional's work. Recognition of hand-written prescription orders is not the professional work to be done by pharmacy professionals.

Moreover, outcome analyses of healthcare provider performance yields many valuable ideas for improvement.

3. Barriers

Electronic patient record (EPR) systems are now being developed in many places, in many ways. Yes, we now have plenty of data. CPUs and networks are amazingly fast and inexpensive. Under these circumstances, it seems like most of the problems that have been carried over are to be solved by the EPR systems.

In 1996, Kameda General Hospital in Awa-Kamogawa, Japan, launched a hospital-wide EPR system. Its user interface is based on 2-dimensional clinical pathway. This case provided us with many lessons. Clinical pathways performed like guidelines and are proven beneficial for less-experienced physicians, acting as check lists. The user interface, used by the professionals for inputting signs and symptoms, was not fluent enough. Above all, it proved that unless data codes, like diagnosis, were standardized, outcome studies cannot be sufficient, especially if analysis is done by comparison with other hospitals.

Let us take another viewpoint. To enjoy the scale merit of available data from many sub-systems and other healthcare providers' information systems, there must be mutual understanding and migration of each data. To transmit any intelligent observations, ideas, decisions, two things must be mutually understandable: the model representing basic structures of the subjects, and the terminology to be used on the model. The latter is now being improved by many efforts to standardize terminology and codes. The difficult part, however, is yet to come. The achievement of the former, where object-oriented methods are promising, is slower than the latter, and is much slower than IT evolution. We see the same old fundamental wisdom now and again: information systems cannot use knowledge that has not been taught and cannot process data that has not been input.

Given the limited materials for successful construction of EPR, we cannot expect all problems can be solved by it. [2] Then, we have to limit our speculations. We have to clarify the purposes of the EPR installation and check feasibility of each. In 2000, Shimane Central Prefectural Hospital in Izumo Japan launched hospital-wide, total-paperless, full order entry EPR. The purpose of this EPR project was not for the EPR itself, but for patient accommodation improvement and outcome studies. The EPR system showed technical improvements of network speed, better user interface, etc., which enabled this huge system to work in reality. Still, however, in areas of less standardization, outcome studies are not satisfactory.

Again we are now in a stage of discriminating between what has been conquered and what still requires efforts, some of which has been described in the papers selected for this section.

---

4. In this section

Six outstanding papers were selected for this section. The first two papers show new methods that contribute to the benefits mentioned above, while the following four papers denote barriers.

a. Data mining

Brosette, et. al. [3] applied novel data mining techniques to hospital laboratory data of cultures of nosocomial infection germs and resistance of antimicrobial agents. Decades ago, antibiotics selection for infections was a good application area of artificial intelligence systems [4][5]. The variety of antibiotics is large and new agents are being introduced everyday. One of the barriers the old applied artificial intelligence systems was the effort of importing lab results. Now, we have them in standardized form. Another barrier was limited understanding and implementation of underlying domain knowledge.

Now, circumstances of this domain must be noted more. The high price of antibiotic medication is targeted. Multi-drug resistant infections, like that by MRSA, VRE, etc., became popular. A colleague antibiotic medication specialist, who taught me to implement domain knowledge, repeatedly predicted and warned about this situation in the late 80's, looking at all the abuse of wide-spectrum antibiotics. He hoped that applied artificial intelligence systems might decrease unnecessary prescriptions. We may or may not have enough time left, but this new technique of data mining, applied to cumulative lab data, will definitely contribute to an improvement of this situation.

b. Information retrieval by semantic terminological models

Brown et al. [6] showed the definite relative effectiveness of semantic terminological models for use in information retrieval of clinical findings. In this paper, the compared methods are: free text retrieval, ICD-10 retrieval, hierarchic retrieval. The last one is based on Read-code.

The semantic terminological method used is to prepare attributes for each concept. For example, "Ectopic pregnancy" is a "pathological process" in "site" of "intrauterine conception structure", "morphology" is "malposition", while "function" is "pregnancy". Obviously, this method is multi-axial, like SNOMED [7], while the ICD and Read-code based methods are single-axial. The advantage is remarkable.

The point is how to control the definition of each attributes [8], which could be solved by using a controlled vocabulary.

c. Concept indexing by UMLS

Nadkarni et al. [9] evaluated the feasibility of concept indexing to medical narrative text using UMLS [10]. It showed 82.6% were true positive matches. Causes of errors are redundant concepts in UMLS, homonyms, acronyms, abbreviations and elisions, concepts missing from UMLS, etc. The authors say that this rate is too low for this method to be used alone.

It has been reported that indexing with words is superior to indexing phrases in a controlled vocabulary. This may not be a perpetual result, as UMLS will be improved in future versions. The authors suggested future improvement directions in their paper. The authors also state that an approach, for example, that combines UMLS concepts with word-indexing will be encouraging.

d. Diagnostic coding tools

Nilsson, et., al. [11] evaluated three versions of Swedish ICD-10 coding tools for primary care: the official book version, a computerized version with the traditional ICD structure, a computerized version with a newly suggested compositional structure.

The paper notes that the viewpoint of primary care is somewhat different with a traditional ICD structure. This motivated the creation of the compositional structure tailored to primary care.

The result showed that all three are almost identical in reliability at code level, while reliability of diagnostic code aggregation was improved by the new compositional structure.

e. Patients with or without their own record

It seems that when patients hold their own healthcare records, see, and show them to their current attending physicians, this results in better care, improved communication, and promotes patient involvement. In obstetric and pediatric care, it was true. Drury et al. tried this for cancer care. [12]

The result is surprising. Supplementary patient-held records for radiotherapy outpatients appeared to have no effect (better or worse) on satisfaction in regard to communication, participation in care, or quality of life.

This report implies many lessons. We call "hospitals for patients", while "patients" are of many kinds. Improvement of the availability of information is not a goal, just a method.

f. EPR and its discontents

In the last paper of this section, Goorman et al. claim the reason why current EPRs frequently show

problems in practice is that they are based on models that often contain projections of nurses' and doctors' work as it should be performed on the ward, rather than depicting how work is actually performed. [13]

This is not only the case for EPR, but also for the order entry system. In Japan, order entry systems are very common. 42% of the hospitals with more than 500 beds have order entry systems. Lessons learned from Japan's situation is, to make matters worse, "the discontents" are different among hospitals. This paper helpfully suggests many proposals to improve this chaotic circumstance.

5. Final remarks: preparating for an unpredictable future

About two decades ago, the introduction of MRI was a smashing hit. It seemed like MRI can image anything invisible by X-CT. Taking X-ray radiation doses into account, it seemed that no X-CT may survive. Now, we have both and good indications for each. We must clearly know what we can expect from the EPR and what we cannot.

Hospital managers want "good data" every time, regardless of the source, from information system or not. Medical informatics professionals predict as far as their imagination reaches. Yet, we cannot predict all of the future. We cannot create a universal model. The least we can do is to prepare healthcare information systems to yield data in an intelligent and standardized way, and prepare good documents to provide a good working environment to future users.

References

1. Fieschi M. Knowledge Processing and Decision Support Systems. Synopsis. 2001 IMIA Yearbook of Medical Informatics. p. 487-9.
2. McDonald CJ. The barriers to electronic medical record systems and how to overcome them. J Am Med Inform Assoc 1997;4:213-21.
3. Brossette SE, Sprague AP, Jones WT, Moser SA. A Data Mining System for Infection Control Surveillance, Method Inform Med 2000;39:303-10.
4. Shortliffe, E H. Computer-Based Medical Consultations: MYCIN, North-Holland; 1976.
5. Kimura, M, et al. Cross-Hierarchy Representation of Medical Knowledge – As Applied in Antibiotic Medication Counseling and Side Effect Information. Proc. of SCAMC;1987. p.207-12.
6. Brown PJB, Sonksen P. Evaluation of the Quality of Information Retrieval of Clinical Findings from a Computerized Patient Database Using a Semantic Terminological Model. J Am Med Inform Assoc 2000;7:392-403.
7. The Systematized Nomenclature of Human and Veterinary Medicine: SNOMED International. College of American Pathologists; 1993.
8. Rector AL. Clinical Terminology: Why is it so Hard? Method Inform Med 1999;38 (4-5):239-52.
9. Nadkarni P, Chen R, Brandt C. UMLS Concept Indexing for Production Databases: A Feasibility Study. J Am Med Inform Assoc 2001;8:80-91.
10. National Library of Medicine, UMLS Knowledge Sources, 9th ed. Bethesda, MD; 1999.
11. Drury M, Yudkin P, Harcourt J, Fitzpatrick R, Jones L, Alcock C, et al. Patients with cancer holding their own records: a randomized controlled trial. British J Gen Practice 2000;50:105-10.
12. Goorman E, Berg M. Modelling nursing activities: electronic patient records and their discontents. Nursing Inquiry 2000;7:3-9.
13. Nilsson G, Petersson H, Ahlfeldt H, Strender L-E. Evaluation of Three Swedish ICD-10 Primary Care Versions: Reliability and ease of Use in Diagnostic Coding. Method Inform Med 2000;39:325-31.

Address of the author;
Michio Kimura
Professor and Director
Medical Informatics Department
Hamamatsu University, School of Medicine
1-20-1 Handayama
Hamamatsu, 431-3192, Japan
E-mail: kimura@mi.hama-med.ac.jp

**S. E. Brossette, A. P. Sprague,
W. T. Jones, S. A. Moser**

A Data Mining System
for Infection Control Surveillance

Department of Pathology
and Department of Computer
and Information Sciences,
The University of Alabama
at Birmingham,
Birmingham, AL, USA

Abstract: Nosocomial infections and antimicrobial resistance are problems of enormous magnitude that impact the morbidity and mortality of hospitalized patients as well as their cost of care. The Data Mining Surveillance System (DMSS) uses novel data mining techniques to discover unsuspected, useful patterns of nosocomial infections and antimicrobial resistance from the analysis of hospital laboratory data. This report details a mature version of DMSS as well as an experiment in which DMSS was used to analyze all inpatient culture data, collected over 15 months at the University of Alabama at Birmingham Hospital.

Keywords: Data Mining, Surveillance, Antibiotic Resistance, Infection Control

1. Introduction

Each year in the United States nosocomial infections affect 2 million patients, cost more than $4.5 billion, and account for half of all major hospital complications [1]. Even more alarming, the number of drug-resistant infections has reached unprecedented levels [2]. Vancomycin-resistant enterococci and extended spectrum beta-lactamase, producing gram-negative rods, are but two examples of highly resistant bacteria that now cause significant morbidity and mortality. While bacterial resistance is a global problem, its origins can be traced to local events. Microenvironments, especially hospital intensive care units, are foci where resistant organisms originate and propagate, only to spread to larger environments as opportunity provides [3-6]. Early recognition of outbreaks and emerging resistance, therefore, requires proactive surveillance at the hospital and sub-hospital levels [3-6]. Extensive analysis of hospital data, however, requires considerable time and resources, both of which few hospital epidemiologists have in reserve. Consequently, these data are underutilized and the patterns they contain go undiscovered.

Traditional hospital infection control surveillance relies on the manual review of suspected cases of nosocomial infections and the tabulation of basic summary statistics, while antimicrobial resistance surveillance consists of the construction of annual or semi-annual, hospital-wide antibiogram summaries. These measures are not timely and often miss emerging, complex patterns [5]. It has been widely recognized that sophisticated, active, and timely intra-hospital surveillance is needed [5, 6].

Historically, computer-assisted infection control surveillance research has focussed on identifying high-risk patients including those on suboptimal antibiotic regimens [7, 8], the use of expert systems to identify possible cases of nosocomial infection [9], and the detection of deviations in the occurrence of predefined events [10]. The Data Mining Surveillance System (DMSS – Patent Pending) was designed to assist traditional infection-control surveillance by automatically detecting useful patterns that would not have been detected by either traditional or existing computer-assisted surveillance methods.

Previous versions of DMSS have been used to analyze relatively small data sets [11, 12]. In this report, we describe significant improvements to DMSS and present experimental results obtained from the analysis of all inpatient culture data from 15 months at the University of Alabama at Birmingham (UAB) Hospital.

2. Methods

2.1 The Data Mining Surveillance System

Significant modifications and improvements have been made to DMSS and the conceptual framework of data mining in epidemiologic surveillance since they were first described [11]. Therefore, a review of definitions and a description of the latest version of DMSS are given.

2.1.1 Definitions

An *item* is a discrete element found in a data set. An *item* set x is a subset of the set of all items. The support of item set x, sup(x), is the number of records in a data set that contain x. If sup(x) ≥ FSST (frequent set support threshold), x is a *frequent set*. For example, in a database where each record describes a single bacterial isolate and the patient from whom it was obtained, the item set {*P. aeruginosa*, SICU, Resistant to Tobramycin} may be found together in 5 records from January. If 5 ≥ FSST, then {*P. aeruginosa*, SICU, Resistant

Table 1 Association rule templates used in the analysis of the UAB data set.

Type	Left (*be1*)		Right (*be2*)	Explanation
Exclude	(R~*Antibiotic*)	⇒	(Anything)	Want antibiotic sensitivity information on the right only.
Exclude	(Anything)	⇒	(Source)	Source of infection is not an outcome. Therefore, exclude all rules with a source on the right.
Exclude	(NS OR Org OR GrMp)	⇒	(NS OR Org OR GrMp)	NS, Org, and GrMp are more informative if kept together in either a group or an outcome.
Exclude	(Loc)	⇒	(Org OR GrMp) AND (R~ *Antibiotic*)	If the Left contains Location, then exclude rules that have Org and R~ Antibiotic or GrMp and R~ Antibiotic.
Include	EmptySet	⇒	(Loc AND NSNosocomial) OR Org	Include empty set rules that are nosocomial and location specific or organism specific.
Include	(Org OR Loc)	⇒	(R~ *Antibiotic* OR GrMp OR Org) AND Not(Loc)	Include rules whose groups are Org or Loc specific and whose outcomes are Antibiotic or GrMp specific.

GrMp = gram stain/morphology (NP-GNR, GPC), R~ = resistant antibiotic, NS = nosocomial status (nosocomial, community), Loc = location, Org = organism.

to-Tobramycin} is frequent in that one-month data set and is, therefore, a frequent set.

An *association rule*, $A ⇒ B$, where A and B are frequent sets and $A \cap B = \emptyset$, is a statement about how often the items of B are found in records with the items of A. The incidence of B in A, or the *incidence proportion* of $A ⇒ B$, is denoted ip $(A ⇒ B)$, and is equal to sup $(A \cup B)/\sup(A)$. This can also be thought of as the conditional probability of B given A, $p(B|A)$. The *precondition support* of association rule $A ⇒ B$ is sup (A), the denominator of the incidence proportion. For example, the association rule {SICU, *P. aeruginosa*} ⇒ {Resistant to-Tobramycin} describes the incidence of Tobramycin resistance

in *P. aeruginosa* isolates from the SICU. If in January, the support of {SICU, *P. aeruginosa*} is 20 and the support of {*P. aeruginosa*, SICU, Resistant to-Tobramycin} is 5, the incidence proportion is 5/20.

The incidence proportion of association rule $A ⇒ B$ in data partition p_i is the number of times outcome B occurs in group A in time t_i. Consequently, a series of incidence proportions for $A ⇒ B$ from partitions $p_1, p_2, ..., p_n$ describes the incidence of the outcome B in group A from t_1 through t_n. Therefore, by analyzing the time-series of incidence proportions of an association rule $A ⇒ B$, it is possible to detect shifts or trends in the incidence of B in A over time.

2.1.2 Generating Association Rules

For each frequent set, all association rules with a precondition support greater than or equal to a preset value, precondition set threshold (PST) are generated. Frequent set discovery and rule generating algorithms are beyond the scope of this paper, but are described in the data mining literature [13-15].

Each association rule generated is compared to a set of user-defined *rule templates* that describe "flavors" of interesting and uninteresting rules. Each rule template is of the form $be_1 ⇒ be_2$ where be_1 and be_2 are Boolean expressions over items and attributes (Table 1). Association rule $A ⇒ B$ satisfies rule template $be_1 ⇒ be_2$ if A satisfies be_1 and B satisfies be_2. For example, the association rule (*Location*_SICU) ⇒ (Resistant to_Ampicillin) satisfies the template (*Location* OR *Organism*) ⇒ (*Antibiotic Result*).

Two types of rule templates are used: *include templates* and *exclude templates*. An association rule $A ⇒ B$ *passes* a set of templates if it satisfies at least one include template in the set and does not satisfy any exclude template in the set. Any number of include and exclude templates can be specified.

Since rule templates contain domain knowledge, domain experts must handcraft them. In general, an expert usually has an idea of some types of rules that are interesting, or may know of some types that are never interesting. Even if this is not known initially, experimental iterations with representative data provide insight.

2.1.3 History

The *history* (H) is a database that holds association rules and their incidence proportions for different data partitions. Only association rules that pass the rule templates are stored in the history. To establish a baseline for each new association rule, the incidence proportions of the rule for previous partitions are obtained and stored in H. Once a rule is stored in H, it is updated for each new partition, regardless of whether or not it is generated in the partition. Therefore, the history has an up-to-date time series of incidence proportions for every association rule it contains.

2.1.4 Events

High-level patterns, called *alerts*, are presented to the user as potentially interesting findings. Low-level patterns, called *events*, are not seen by the user, but are used to construct alerts. Therefore, the search for useful patterns begins with events.

DMSS generates events by analyzing information stored in the history. An *event* describes an interesting change in the series of incidence proportions of an association rule. For example, Table 2 describes the incidence of *Acinetobacter baumannii* in tracheal aspirates obtained from patients in the surgical intensive care unit (SICU) over 6 partitions. Clearly, a shift in incidence occurs between the first 4 months and the most recent 2 months of the series. If the first, second, third, and fourth months are called the *past window*, w_p, and the fifth and sixth the *current window*, w_c, one can ask if there has been a change in incidence between w_p and w_c. To check this, the cumulative incidence proportion for w_p (1/43) and the cumulative incidence proportion for w_c (6/18) are compared by a statistical test of two proportions. If the test returns a p-value less than a prespecified threshold, then there is a *suggestive* change in the incidence of *A. baumannii* in tracheal aspirates obtained from patients in the SICU between w_p and w_c.

Since significance testing is used in DMSS for exploratory purposes only, domain experts determine the ultimate value of each pattern. To this end, the term "suggestive" is used instead of "significant" since "significant" connotes formal assumptions of significance testing and statistical inference that are violated by multiple comparisons inherent to data mining techniques.

For each association rule, DMSS constructs a current window and a past window on the timeseries of incidence proportions, computes the cumulative incidence proportion for each window, compares the two cumulative incidence proportions by a test of two proportions, and generates an event if the difference between the proportions is suggestive ($p \le \alpha = 0.05$). If an event is

not generated, then a different pair of current and past windows is formed and their cumulative incidence proportions are compared. This continues for the same association rule until an event is generated or no more current and past window pairs remain to be formed. The next rule in H is then considered.

Time Windows and the Windowing Schedule

Current and past windows are obtained sequentially from a user-defined *windowing schedule*. Each entry in the schedule is a *window pair* of the form $(|w_p|, |w_c|)$ where $|w_p|$ is the number of partitions in w_p and $|w_c|$ is the number of partitions in w_c. Both w_p and w_c are composed of one or more contiguous partitions, w_c contains the current partition (p_c), and w_p and w_c are disjoint and contiguous. For example, when the schedule (3,1) and (6,2) is used to generate window pairs for the time-series of incidence proportions in Table 3, the two window pairs of Table 4 are created. Each window pair forms the basis for a comparison between the cumulative incidence proportions of the past and current windows.

Cumulative Incidence Proportion

A *cumulative incidence proportion* is computed by "summing" one or more incidence proportions in a time window. The cumulative incidence proportion of a rule $r = A \Rightarrow B$ in a time window w is:

$$cip\,(r, w) = \frac{\sum_{p_i \in w} sup\,(A \cup B, p_i)}{\sum_{p_i \in w} sup\,(A, p_i)}.$$

Simply stated, the numerator of the cumulative incidence proportion is the sum of the numerators of all incidence proportions in w, and the denominator is the sum of the denominators of all incidence proportions in w. For example, the cumulative incidence proportion of w_p for window pair 1 of Table 4, $cip\,(r, w_p)$, is 11/130, and the cumulative incidence proportion of w_c, $cip\,(r, w_c)$, is 9/46. For window pair 2 of Table 4, $cip\,(_r w_p)$ is 13/209 and $cip\,(r, w_c)$ is 16/96.

Testing for a Difference between two Incidence Proportions

Using window pair 1 of Table 4, the incidence of outcome B = {nosocomial, *Enterobacter cloacae*} in group A =

Table 2 An example of an alert generated by DMSS.

Association Rule		p_{c-5}	p_{c-4}	p_{c-3}	p_{c-2}	p_{c-1}	p_c
{SICU, tracheal aspirate}	==> {Acinetobacter baumannii}	0/11	1/10	0/9	0/13	2/9	4/9
		w_p				w_c	

Table 3 A series of 8 incidence proportions for {SICU} $\Rightarrow$ {nosocomial, *Enterobacter cloacae*}.

p_{c-7}	p_{c-6}	p_{c-5}	p_{c-4}	p_{c-3}	p_{c-2}	p_{c-1}	p_c
3/38	1/26	2/32	3/33	1/26	3/54	7/50	9/46

Table 4 Window pairs generated when the windowing schedule is applied to the incidence proportions of Table 3.

Window Pair 1					[]1/26	[]3/54	[]7/50	*9/46
Window Pair 2	[]3/38	[]1/26	[]2/32	[]3/33	[]1/26	[]3/54	*7/50	*9/46

[] => in w_p * => in w_c. Window Pair 1 chi-square is not significant. Window Pair 2 chi-square is significant

Table 5 A set of related events. Bracketed partitions (e.g. []1) are in w_p. Starred partitions (*) are in w_c. NP_GNR = non-pseudomonas Gram-negative rods, R~An = resistant to antibiotic n.

---

1)　　{EmptySet} $\Rightarrow$ {R~A2}

　　[]1: 1/950 | []2: 1/812 | []3: 2/768 | *4: 8/780

2)　　{SICU} $\Rightarrow$ {R~A2}

　　[]1: 0/57 | []2: 1/60 | []3: 2/52 | *4: 7/65

3)　　{SICU, NP_GNR} $\Rightarrow$ {R~A1, R~A2}

　　[]1: 0/23 | []2: 0/20 | []3: 2/18 | *4: 7/21

4)　　{SICU, NP_GNR, nosocomial} $\Rightarrow$ {R~A1, R~A2}

　　[]1: 0/11 | []2: 0/10 | []3: 1/12 | *4: 5/13

5)　　{SICU, NP_GNR, nosocomial, *K. pneumonia*} $\Rightarrow$ {R~A1, R~A2}

　　[]1: 0/5 | []2: 0/5 | []3: 1/6 | *4: 5/7

6)　　{SICU, NP_GNR, nosocomial, *K. pneumonia*, sputum} $\Rightarrow$ {R~A1, R~A2}

　　[]1: 0/5 | []2: 0/4 | []3: 1/4 | *4: 5/6

{SICU} during w_p is $h_1 = 11/130$, and the incidence of B in A during w_c is $h_2 = 9/46$. To compare the two proportions, a p-value for $H_0 : h_1 = h_2$ is computed using this standard statistic based on the 2×2 contingency table [16]:

$$X^2 = \frac{176[(11)(37) - (119)(9)]^2}{(130)(46)(20)(156)} = 3.13.$$

The sampling distribution of this statistic under H_0 is the chi-squared distribution with one degree of freedom (DOF). Since $X^2_{0.05,1} = 3.84$ is the value of chi-squared with one DOF that corresponds to a p-value of 0.05, $X^2 = 3.13$ leads us to conclude that the difference between the two cumulative incidence proportions is not suggestive. For the two cumulative incidence proportions computed from window pair 2 of Table 4, $X^2 = 7.56$ which is greater than $X^2_{0.05,1}$. Therefore, the difference between these two incidence proportions is suggestive, and an event is generated. We refer to a test of two proportions h_1 and h_2 that returns a p-value under $H_0 : h_1 = h_2$ as $ttp(h_1, h_2)$. If the expected values of the 2×2 contingency table are small, then $ttp(h_1, h_2)$ is a Fisher exact test [16].

The choice of α for classifying the result of either test is rather arbitrary and, indeed, this is a general criticism of significance testing [17]. However, since significance testing is used in DMSS for exploratory purposes only, with the value of patterns ultimately determined by experts, the rather arbitrary choice of α is not troublesome as long as the output is manageable and reasonably sensitive. Additionally, no formal claims of statistical inference are made.

2.1.5 Alerts

Consider the set of events in Table 5. This set has several characteristics. First, the left-hand sides of the association rules of events 1 through 5 are each a subset of the left-hand side of the association rule of event 6. Similarly, the right-hand sides of the rules for events 1 through 5 are each a subset of the right-hand side of event 6. Second,

the current window, $w_c = \{4\}$ is the same for all events, as is the past window, $w_p = \{1, 2, 3\}$. Finally, changes in the cumulative support of {SICU, nosocomial, *K. pneumonia*, sputum, R~A1, R~A2} between w_p and w_c, which is the change in the numerator of the cumulative incidence proportion between w_p and w_c in event 6, account for most of the changes in the numerators of the cumulative incidence proportions between w_p and w_c of events 1 through 5. From these characteristics, it is clear that event 6 is responsible for events 1 through 5. Therefore, event 6 contains the pertinent information about all events in the set and is the only event from the set that needs to be presented to the user. Indeed, for this set, event 6 is the *alert* and the entire set is the *event set* of event 6. Construction of event sets is mediated by the subsumption heuristic called *event capture*.

Event Capture

Association rule $A1 \Rightarrow B1$ is a *descendent* of association rule $A2 \Rightarrow B2$ if $A2 \subseteq A1$ and $B2 \subseteq B1$. For any two events x and y, x is said to *capture* y if the association rule of x, $A_x \Rightarrow B_x$, is a descendent of the association rule of y, $A_y \Rightarrow B_y$, (w_p, w_c) of x is equal to (w_p, w_c) of y, and the result of the test of two proportions (ttp):

$$ttp \left(\frac{\sup(Ay \cup By, w_p) - \sup(Ax \cup Bx, w_p)}{\sup(Ay, w_p)}, \right.$$

$$\left. \frac{\sup(Ay \cup By, w_c) - \sup(Ax \cup Bx, w_c)}{\sup(Ay, w_c)} \right) \quad (i)$$

is greater than α. Intuitively, event x captures event y if when x is "removed" from y, y is no longer suggestive.

For example, consider events 3 and 6 from Table 5. First, the rule of event 6 is a descendant of the rule of event 3. Next, (w_p, w_c) of event 3 is equal to (w_p, w_c) of event 6. "Subtracting" 6 from 3 and substituing the appropriate values into expression (1),

$$ttp \left(\frac{2-1}{61}, \frac{7-5}{21} \right) = 0.32.$$

Therefore, without the cases of event 6, event 3 is no longer suggestive since $0.32 > 0.05$. Therefore, event 6 captures event 3. By the same logic, event 6 also captures events 1, 2, 4, and 5.

2.1.6 Event Sets

An *event set x'* is the event *x* and all events that *x* captures. After creating event sets, each event is a member of an event set – some containing only one event, the alert itself, of other events, only one is the alert. Since the alert of an event set contains all pertinent information for the entire set, only alerts are presented to the user; all other events are redundant. This greatly reduces the number of patterns for the user to review.

Alerts and Descriptive Specificity

Alerts ensure that patterns presented to the user are as specific as possible. For example, consider the following alert:

{NP_GNR, nosocomial} ⇨ {R~Piperacillin, R~Ceftazidime, R~Gentamicin} (ii)

[]Sep-96: 0/180 | []Oct-96: 2/124 | []Nov-96: 1/130 | *Dec-96: 6/100 |

How is it known that the change in piperacillin, ceftazidime, and gentamicin resistance did not occur only amongst nosocomial *Klebsiella pneumoniae* isolates? After all, these are nosocomial, non-*Pseudomonas* gram-negative rods. If nosocomial *K. pneumoniae* isolates were responsible for the in-crease in piperacillin, ceftazidime, and gentamicin resistance in NP_GNRs, then (ii) would have been captured by the event with association rule {*K. pneumoniae,* NP_GNR, nosocomial} ⇨ {R~Piperacillin, R~Ceftazidime, R~Gentamicin}, and this event, not event (b), would have been presented to the user. Therefore, since an alert with rule {*K. pneumoniae,* NP_GNR, nosocomial} ⇨ {R~Piperacillin, R~Ceftazidime, R~Gentamicin} was not presented, *K. pneumoniae* isolates were not responsible for event (ii). This can be easily verified by checking the original data.

2.2 Application of DMSS to Inpatient Culture Data

2.2.1 Data

Fifteen months (September 1996 through November 1997) of bacterial culture data and related patient infor-

Table 6 Summary of UAB data and its analysis.

Partition	Records	Rules in H	Events	Alerts	Time(sec)
09/96	677	954	NA*	NA	45
10/96	576	1416	NA	NA	72
11/96	573	1877	NA	NA	85
12/96	475	2126	73	35	75
01/97	597	2582	181	55	218
02/97	521	2862	93	43	128
03/97	511	3109	59	34	145
04/97	524	3272	34	29	95
05/97	504	3477	73	32	109
06/97	496	3650	56	42	173
07/97	605	3815	70	40	101
08/97	550	4084	117	41	215
09/97	576	4272	74	46	99
10/97	537	4358	62	44	123
11/97	535	4461	73	46	98

*NA = not applicable

mation were extracted from the UAB clinical laboratory information system. Each record describes a single bacterial isolate and contains items for the following attributes: organism name, gram stain/morphology, date collected, nosocomial status, source of isolate (e.g., sputum, blood, urine), location of patient in hospital (e.g., Surgical Intensive Care Unit, Medical Intensive Care Unit), and test results Resistant (R~), Intermediate resistance (I~), or Susceptible (S~), according to NCCLS criteria [18] for each member of a set of antimicrobials.

The gram stain/morphology attribute is "GPC" for gram-positive cocci, "NP-_GNR" for non-*Pseudomonas* gram-negative rod, and empty for *Pseudomonas*. The nosocomial status is either "nosocomial" or "community," depending on when the sample was obtained from the patient. If the isolate is from a sample collected on or after the patient's third day in the hospital, then it is classified as "nosocomial,"

otherwise it is classified as "community."

To test the ability of DMSS to identify outbreaks of resistant organisms, the data set was seeded with records describing a nosocomial outbreak of highly resistant *A. baumanii* that occurred in UAB hospital in 1994 [19]. This was done by removing all nosocomial *A. baumanii* records from the corresponding months of the 1997 data set, and replacing them with all nosocomial *A. baumanii* records from the same months in 1994 which contain, but are not limited to the previously identified outbreak.

Duplicate records were removed so that the data set contained no more than one record per patient per organism per month. Additionally, for each record, antimicrobials to which the organism is historically resistant were removed. Since resistance to these antimicrobials is expected, their test results are of little surveillance interest. S~*Antimicrobial* items were then discarded and each I~*Antimicrobial* item was changed to R~*Antimicrobial* simply lumping together intermediate resistant and resistant results. Finally, all records were split into disjoint monthly partitions.

2.2.2 Experimental Design

DMSS analysis of the data set was conducted with frequent set support threshold (FSST) of 3, precondition support threshold (PST) of 8, the association rule templates in Table 1, the windowing schedule (3,1) (6,2) (9,3), and $\alpha = 0.05$. The partitions were processed sequentially and a search for patterns was conducted after each of the December 1996 through November 1997 partitions yielding 12 sets of alerts.

3. Results

Association rule templates (Table 1) reduced the number of rules in the history by 90%, and alerts reduced the number of events for the user to review by half (Table 6). Running times per partition were reasonable with none over 4 minutes and no more than 55 alerts (partition 01/97) were generated by any search (Table 6). The expert reviewer was easily able to inspect each set of alerts in less than a half-hour.

Although not all alerts were interesting, some describe potentially important outbreaks of infection and changes in antimicrobial resistance. Representative examples of the different classes of alerts are shown in Table 7. Section A contains two alerts describing the known nosocomial clonal outbreak of highly resistant *A. baumanii* from

1994. The first isolate was obtained from a patient at autopsy in March of 1994. Subsequently, four additional isolates were discovered, and a cluster was later confirmed [21]. This outbreak was detected by DMSS (Table 7, alert 1). In the following months, additional isolates were discovered suggesting a second outbreak of the same strain in August [21]. This was also detected by DMSS (Table 7, alert 2). This strain subsequently disappeared with stringent infection control and isolation practices.

Table 7 section B contains location-specific alerts not associated with any single microorganism. Alerts of this type suggest possible misuse or overuse of antimicrobial agents with subsequent changes in resistance patterns of resident organisms. Alerts such as these should trigger evaluations of antimicro-

Table 7 Selected Alerts from the UAB Analysis.

#	Association Rule		Sep-96	Oct-96	Nov-96	Dec-96	Jan-97	Feb-97	Mar-97	Apr-97	May-97	Jun-97	Jul-97	Aug-97	Sep-97	Oct-97	Nov-97
Section A																	
1	EmptySet ⇒	*Acinetobacter baumannii,* Noso, LocMICU, CAZ, PIP, TM, GM, AN, CIP, ATM, MZ, TIM, OFX, CTX, SxT				0/477	0/599	0/523	5/511								
2	EmptySet ⇒	*Acinetobacter baumannii,* Noso, CAZ, PIP, TM, GM, AN, CIP, ATM, MZ, TIM, OFX, CTX, SxT									3/506	1/496	1/607	7/550			
Section B																	
3	LocMICU ⇒	Noso, CAZ, PIP, GM, CIP, AN					0/15	0/15	0/23	4/24							
4	LocRNIC ⇒	Noso, CAZ									1/10	0/9	1/15	6/13			
Section C																	
5	*Klebsiella pneumoniae* ⇒ Noso	CTT, CAZ, CXM, CZ, PIP, SxT, CR, TM, GM, TIM, CRO		1/11	0/22	1/23	11/25										
6	*Klebsiella pneumoniae* ⇒ Noso	CTT, CAZ, CXM, CZ, PIP, SxT, CR, TM, GM, TIM, CIP, AN, CRO									0/26	0/26	0/21	3/25			
Section D																	
7	EmptySet ⇒	*Staphylococcus aureus,* LocW9NW, E, CC, OX		0/578	0/575	0/477	4/597										
8	LocDIAL ⇒	*Staphylococcus aureus,* Noso											5/13	1/11	2/8	10/18		
Section E																	
9	*Streptococcus pneumoniae* ⇒ NonNoso	E, P, CRO		1/6	0/9	0/9	4/9										
10	EmptySet ⇒	*Streptococcus pneumoniae*, NonNoso, P, CRO												0/552	0/578	0/539	3/535

Shaded boxes = w_c, Unshaded boxes = w_p Noso = nosocomial; NonNoso = community acquired; AN = Amikacin, ATM = Aztreonam, CAZ = Ceftazidime, CC = Clindamycin, CIP = Ciprofloxacin, CR = Cephalothin, CRO = Ceftriaxone, CTT = Cefotetan, CTX = Cefuroxime, CXM = Cefuroxime; CZ = Cefazolin, E = Erythromycin, GM = Gentamicin, MZ = Mezlocillin, OFX = Ofloxacin, OX = Oxacillin, P = Penicillin, PIP = Piperacillin, SxT = Trimethoprim/Sulfmethoxazole, TIM = Ticarcillin/Clavulanic acid, TM = Tobramycin

bial utilization by the Pharmacy and Therapeutics committee and, if indicated, recommendations to change prescribing habits. None of these patterns were known prior to this analysis.

Table 7 section C contains two alerts that describe substantial changes in the incidence of multi-drug resistant *K. pneumoniae*. The first potential outbreak was in January 1997 and the second in August 1997. These combinations of antimicrobial resistance are uncommon at UAB and would have been investigated. Neither was detected by traditional surveillance at the time.

Table 7 section D contains two location-specific alerts. The number of oxacillin resistant *S. aureus* isolated from location W9NW increased from a baseline of zero to 4 in January 1997 as indicated by alert 7. Another possible outbreak of nosocomial *S. aureus,* this time from the dialysis unit, occurred in October 1997 (alert 8). These patterns were also undetected by traditional surveillance.

The alerts of Table 7 section E demonstrate that DMSS can detect aberrations in known phenomenon such as seasonal changes in the incidence of community acquired *S. pneumoniae*. The strains noted here are from either blood or CSF and are both penicillin and ceftriaxone resistant which is an unusual phenotype for our patient population. This finding suggests that the empiric use of antimicrobials in cases of serious pneumococcal disease could be adjusted, prior to issuing the periodic summary antibiogram months later.

4. Discussion and Conclusions

New and sophisticated analytical tools are needed in both public health and hospital infection control surveillance. As described by Dean et al. [20], the ideal public health surveillance system will include analysis tools that automatically identify, on different time and geographical scales, unusual and interesting patterns from timeslices of raw data. Likewise, infection control systems of the future will require tools that recognize trends in nosocomial infection and antimicrobial resistance in an efficient and timely

manner [6]. DMSS represents the first generation of these tools.

This work is only the beginning of the application of data mining to epidemiologic surveillance. More research is needed. For example, how can the interaction between DMSS and the user or a group of users be improved? A more efficient interaction would be especially valuable for defining association rule templates and facilitating a collaborative interpretation of results. Once templates are satisfactory, i.e., useful results are obtained and the user is not overwhelmed with patterns, can they be made to adapt to the changing perceptions of users over time? Other areas for research include more intuitive information presentation and increasing the expressiveness of association rule templates and windowing schedules. While the windowing strategy coupled with tests of two proportions provides a simple and effective means of identifying useful patterns, additional strategies for detecting trends and outbreaks in time-series data could be investigated.

DMSS could potentially be used in conjunction with other computer-assisted surveillance systems. For example, an expert system like GermWatcher© [9] could select only data that describe significant infections. DMSS could then analyze these data only.

Finally, since comprehensive hospital and public health surveillance practice will likely someday use automated analysis systems such as DMSS, utilization research issues are plentiful. What data are needed for the types of surveillance desired, how can it be collected and cleaned in a timely fashion, and how will results be used to make proactive decisions that will change current practice?

Acknowledgments

This work was supported in part by cooperative agreement U47-CCU411451 with the Centers for Disease Control and Prevention (SAM) and predoctoral research fellowship LM-00057 from the National Library of Medicine (SEB).

REFERENCES

1. Centers for Disease Control and Prevention. Public health focus surveillance: prevention and control of nosocomial infections. Morbidity and Mortality Weekly Report 1992; 41: 783-7.

2. Goldmann DA, Weinstein RA, Wenzel RP, Tablan OC, Duma RJ, Gaynes RP, Schlosser J. Martone WJ. Strategies to Prevent and Control the Emergence and Spread of Antimicrobial-Resistant Microorganisms in Hospitals. A challenge to hospital leadership. JAMA 1996; 275: 234-40.

3. Jones RN. The current and future impact of antimicrobial resistance among nosocomial bacterial pathogens. Diag Microbiol Infect Dis 1992; 15 Suppl 2: 3-10.

4. Koontz FP. A review of traditional resistance surveillance methodologies and infection control. Diag Microbiol Infect Dis 1992; 15 Suppl 2: 43-7.

5. Neu HC, Duma RJ, Jones RN, McGowan JE Jr., O'Brien TF, Sabath LD, Sanders,CC, Schaffner W, Tally FP; Tenover FC, Young LS. Antibiotic resistance: epidemiology and therapeutics. Diag Microbiol Infect Dis 1992; 15 Suppl 2: 53-60.

6. Shlaes DM, Gerding DN, John JF Jr, Craig WA, Bornstein DL, Duncan RA, Eckman MR; Farrer WE; Greene WH; Lorian V; Levy S; McGowan JE Jr; Paul SM; Ruskin J; Tenover FC; Watanakunakorn C. Society for Healthcare Epidemiology of America and Infectious Diseases Society of America Joint Committee on the Prevention of Antimicrobial Resistance: guidelines for the prevention of antimicrobial resistance in hospitals. Clin Infect Dis 1997; 25: 584-99.

7. Evans RS, Pestotnik SL, Classen DC, Clemmer TP, Weaver LK, Orme JF, Lloyd JF, Burke JP. A computer-assisted management program for antibiotics and other anti-infective agents. NEJM 1998; 338: 232-8.

8. Evans RS, Larsen RA, Burke JP, Gardner RM; Meier FA; Jacobson JA; Conti MT; Jacobson JT; Hulse RK. Computer surveillance of hospital-acquired infections and antibiotic use. JAMA 1986; 256: 1007-11

9. Kahn MG, Steib SA, Fraser VJ, Dunagan WC. An expert system for culture-based infection control surveillance. Proceedings of the Annual Symposium on Computer Applications in Medical Care 1993: 171-5.

10. Sellick JA. The use of statistical process control charts in hospital epidemiology. Infection Control and Hospital Epidemiology 1993; 14: 649-56.

11. Brossette SE, Sprague AP, Hardin JM, Waites KB, Jones WT, Moser SA. Association rules and data mining in hospital infection control and public health surveillance JAMIA 1998; 5: 373-81.

12. Brossette, SE, AP Sprague, WT Jones, and SA Moser. Application of knowledge discovery and data mining to intensive care microbiologic data (Abstract). International Conference on Emerging Infectious Diseases. March 8-11, 1998. Atlanta, GA.

13. Agrawal R, Srikant R. Fast algorithms for mining association rules. Proceedings of the 20th International Conference on Very Large Data Bases 1994: 487-99.

14. Bayardo JR. Brute-force mining of high-confidence classification rules. Proceedings of the Third International Conference on Knowledge Discovery and Data Mining 1997: 123-6.

15. Brin S, Rajeev M, Ullman JD, Tsur S. Dynamic itemset counting and implication rules for market basket data. Proceedings of the ACM SIGMOD Conference on Management of Data 1997: 255-63.

16. Brownlee KA. Statistical Theory and Methodology (2nd ed.). Malabar, FL: Rovert E. Kriegler Publishing Co., Inc 1965.

17. Rothman KJ, Greenland S. Modern Epidemiology (2nd ed.) Philadelphia: Lippincott-Raven 1997.

18. NCCLS. Methods for dilution antimicrobial susceptibility tests for bacteria that grow aerobically – Fourth Edition; approved Standard. NCCLS document M7-A4. NCCLS, Wayne, Pennsylvania 1997.

19. Marques MB, Waites KB, Mangino JE, Hines BB, Moser SA. Genotypic investigation of multidrug-resistant Acinetobacter baumannii infections in a medical intensive care unit. J Hosp Infect 1997; 37: 125-35.

20. Dean AG, Fagan RF, Panter-Conner BJ. Computerizing public health surveillance systems. In: Teutsch SM, Churchill RE (ed). Principles and Practice of Public Health Surveillance. New York, NY: Oxford University Press, 1994; 200-17.

Address of the authors:
Stephen A. Moser, Ph.D.,
University of Alabama at Birmingham,
Department of Pathology, P246,
619 19th St., South,
Birmingham, AL 35233-7331,
E-mail: moser@uab.edu

Evaluation of the Quality of Information Retrieval of Clinical Findings from a Computerized Patient Database Using a Semantic Terminological Model

PHILIP J. B. BROWN, MD, MRCGP, PETER SÖNKSEN, MD, FRCP

Abstract   Objectives: To measure the strength of agreement between the concepts and records retrieved from a computerized patient database, in response to physician-derived questions, using a semantic terminological model for clinical findings with those concepts and records excerpted clinically by manual identification. The performance of the semantic terminological model is also compared with the more established retrieval methods of free-text search, ICD-10, and hierarchic retrieval.

Design: A clinical database (Diabeta) of 106,000 patient problem record entries containing 2,625 unique concepts in an clinical academic department was used to compare semantic, free-text, ICD-10, and hierarchic data retrieval against a gold standard in response to a battery of 47 clinical questions.

Measurements: The performance of concept and record retrieval expressed as mean detection rate, positive predictive value, Yates corrected and Mantel-Haenszel chi-squared values, and Cohen kappa value, with significance estimated using the Mann-Whitney test.

Results: The semantic terminological model used to retrieve clinically useful concepts from a patient database performed well and better than other methods, with a mean detection rate of 0.86, a positive predictive value of 0.96, a Yates corrected chi-squared value of 1,537, a Mantel-Haenszel chi-squared value of 19,302, and a Cohen kappa of 0.88. Results for record retrieval were even better, with a mean record detection rate of 0.94, a positive predictive value of 0.99, a Yates corrected chi-squared value of 94,774, a Mantel-Haenszel chi-squared value of 1,550,356, and a Cohen kappa value of 0.94. The mean detection rate, Yates corrected chi-squared value, and Cohen kappa value for semantic retrieval were significantly better than for the other methods.

Conclusion: The use of a semantic terminological model in this test scenario provides an effective framework for representing clinical finding concepts and their relationships. Although currently incomplete, the model supports improved information retrieval from a patient database in response to clinically relevant questions, when compared with alternative methods of analysis.

■ **J Am Med Inform Assoc.** 2000;7:392–403.

Affiliations of the authors: The Guys', King's College, and St. Thomas' Hospitals Medical and Dental School, London, United Kingdom.

Some of the results of this work were presented at the AMIA Annual Symposium, Washington, DC, November 6–10, 1999.

Correspondence and reprints: Philip J. B. Brown, MD, MRCGP, Hethersett Surgery, Great Melton Road, Hethersett, Norfolk NR9 3AB, United Kingdom; e-mail: ⟨pjbb@hicomm.demon.co.uk⟩.

Received for publication: 11/29/99; accepted for publication: 1/31/00.

Clinical data in computer systems have to be accurate if they are to support patient care, research, and health service management, but despite this there is little published literature devoted to measuring this in electronic health care records.[1] Inaccurate data can lead to an underestimate of disease prevalence, with potentially serious consequences for monitoring the success of health care interventions and detrimental effects on decision support protocols and alert systems.[2]

The retrieval of meaningful information is dependent on data being entered in an organized way, and to maximize the benefit of electronic health care records, an underlying structure is required.[3] If data are collected in free text, the text has to be converted to computer-understandable codes and structures to extract meaningful data.[4] It is postulated that the content of the electronic health care record should be provided by a clinical terminology in which concepts and their relationships are formally expressed.[5] Clinical Terms Version 3 (The Read Codes) (CTV3)[6] is a clinical terminology in which concepts are represented according to their meaning (semantically) with reference to standard structured hierarchies of component values, e.g., anatomy and micro-organisms (semantic terminological model). The use of this formal semantic model for describing the intrinsic characteristics (atoms) of concepts in CTV3 has parallels in other schemes such as LOINC[7] and the cross-references available in SNOMED International.[8] The model employed by GALEN uses GRAIL to express sanctioned associations between primitive concepts.[9] Similarly, SNOMED RT uses the KRSS description logic to formally express relationships.[10] Thus, there is an emerging convergence of approaches toward the use of a concept-based clinical terminology with an underlying formal semantic terminological model (STM).

There has been little reported work on the effect of different search methods on the efficacy of data retrieval from clinical records. However, significant efforts have been invested in initiatives in the U.K. with the development of CTV3,[11] in Europe with the GALEN-in-Use project,[12] and in the United States with the development of SNOMED RT.[10] These initiatives have confirmed that considerable resources are required to create and maintain such products, and they are all based on the assumption that a clinical terminology will bring improved data quality. There is, therefore, an urgent need to investigate whether the use of semantic-based terminologies will deliver any practical advantages over simpler existing systems.

This study explores the hypothesis that the use of an STM improves the quality of information retrieval in response to a battery of physician-derived questions from a clinical database. The Diabeta patient database,[13] populated with the CTV3 terminology, has been used to compare retrieval using an STM (semantic differential retrieval) with more established approaches. The experiment measures the strength of agreement between the concepts and records retrieved from the database using the STM with those concepts and records expected clinically by manual identification. The performance of semantic differential retrieval is also compared with more traditional methods, including free-text searching, class retrieval using the CTV3 hierarchy table,[14] and the framework of the International Classification of Diseases and Related Health Problems, 10th revision (ICD-10).[15]

Background

Clinical Terms Version 3

Clinical Terms Version 3 was developed during the Clinical Terms Project to provide a common terminology for electronic health care records.[6,11,16,17] The structure of CTV3 provides a formal framework for representing the meaning and relationship of clinical findings and procedures, allocating each unique clinical concept a Read code.[6,14] Each concept code is labeled with a unique unambiguous preferred term and, where appropriate, synonyms. Concepts are formally arranged in a hierarchy in which those of more narrow meaning appear as "types of" concepts of more general meaning (subtype hierarchy), e.g., bacterial meningitis is a subtype of meningitis (Figure 1). Concepts are also mapped, where appropriate, to ICD-10 and the U.K. surgical procedure classification OPCS-4.[18] These cross-mappings have been subject to independent quality assurance and practical evaluation in use since 1994 and are, therefore, considered to be of high quality.

Semantic Terminology Model

The design of CTV3 employs object-attribute-value triples stored in a template file as a mechanism for defining each core clinical concept in relation to more primitive value concepts, e.g., anatomy, pathological processes, and micro-organisms.[6,19] This feature allows the semantic definition of concepts according to their meaning (Figure 1). The model describing the formal relationship between the core terminology and their constituent values (atoms) is referred to in this paper as the STM (semantic terminology model) to distinguish it from alternative models describing the structure of the record and models of health care. A detailed but provisional STM has been developed within CTV3, describing disorders.[20] This has been extended in this study to provide at least partial representation of other findings, including symptoms and signs (Figure 2).

The provisional STM defined 44.7 percent of the Diabeta concepts completely, with the 55.3 percent remaining concepts containing at least one additional nonrepresented characteristic.[21] Incomplete definitions included concepts such as *Osteogenesis imperfecta, Scleroderma variant, Osteopetrosis*, and *True hermaphrodite*, whose semantic definitions are not amenable to full

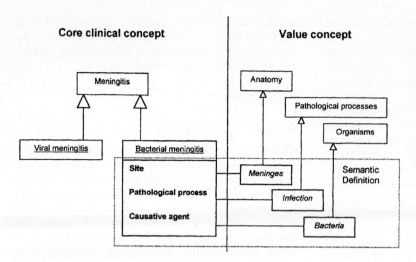

Figure 1 Concepts in Clinical Terms Version 3 are placed in a pure subtype hierarchy. The structure also allows the formal definition of concepts according their meaning (semantic definition); thus, *Bacterial meningitis* is represented by [Site]: Meninges; [Pathological process]: Infection; [Causative agent]: Bacteria. NOTE: The triangle represents a subtype relationship utilizing the notation of the Unified Modelling Language (UML), the Object Management Group (OMG) industry standard (Rational Software Corporation, Cupertino, California, 1995).

representation using the present STM. Characterization of these might be achievable from consideration of more detailed aspects of their embryologic, cellular, and molecular origins, but this would require considerable specialist clinical input, which might not be consistently applicable to other areas.[20] The definition of other classes of concepts, such as *Cicatricial junctional epidermolysis bullosa* is highly dependent on the extensiveness of purely descriptive elements that do not currently exist in the supportive hierarchies.

Despite this level of incompleteness, 818 of these par-

tially defined concepts had unique definitions that did not coincide with others. Thus, within the clinical database examined (Diabeta), the STM provides either a complete (1,175) or unique (818) semantic definition for 76 percent (1,993) of findings, with a residual 24 percent (634) of concepts having incomplete definitions that are shared with other concepts.[22]

Diabeta Database

Diabeta is a computerized clinical record system that has been developed and used with ongoing modifi-

Figure 2 Abridged representation of the provisional semantic terminological model identifying the main characteristics of clinical findings expressed as attributes and applicable value concept hierarchies, with examples. The section mark (§) indicates that the expression of laterality is applied via anatomy.

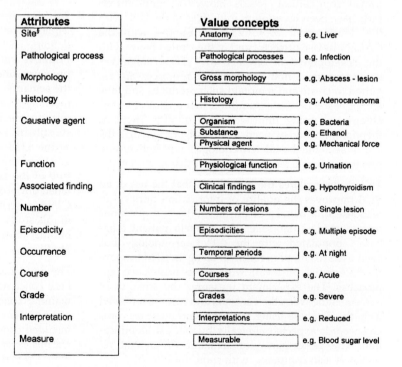

cation since 1973 at St. Thomas' Hospital, London (part of The Guys', King's College, and St. Thomas' Hospitals Medical and Dental School).[13] It is used for supporting the management of patients attending the medical outpatient department, many of whom have diabetes mellitus.[23] The original system (Diabeta 1) allowed, at every encounter between the patient and clinician, the recording of clinical findings as "problems" using a locally created list of reusable free-text term strings. The system thus allowed the collection of a large corpus of clinically relevant terms without any potential restraint of a fixed terminology. This database has been converted to a new database of patient problem records (Diabeta 3), in which every unambiguous clinical finding term string has been matched to an applicable term in CTV3. During the translation process between the existing Diabeta database and CTV3, any clinically important concept or term that was found to be absent was incorporated into the next release of CTV3 and was thus available for the analysis experiment. Consequently, the created Diabeta test database represents a valuable corpus of clinically derived concepts.

The experimental Diabeta database contained 12,696 different term strings (accounting for 106,000 "problem" record entries) mapped to 3,049 unique terms associated with 2,625 unique Read-coded concepts. Mappings to ICD-10 were available for 2,301 concepts (87.7 percent). Those concepts without an ICD-10 map fell into two groups: observations that are not specifically included in ICD-10, e.g., alcohol consumption and persistent microalbuminuria, and classes of concepts based on anatomic regions not accommodated by the axes in the classification, e.g., limb complication and limb infection.

Study Objectives

A key function of a terminology is the support it provides for the retrieval of information from a clinical system.* In practice, the interrogation of a clinical database, to answer a specified question, usually involves two main steps:

- Creating a list of *concepts* for retrieval (in response to a posed question)

- Retrieving *records* containing these identified concepts

The kernel of the problem is to measure how well the concepts (and records) retrieved in response to a clin-

---

*A system in this context refers to the hardware, software and terminology populating the database.

ical question match the expectation of the clinician who posed it. The objective of the study was to measure the strength of agreement between the concepts and records retrieved using an STM from a computerized patient database with those concepts and records expected clinically by manual identification in response to physician-derived questions. It tests the hypothesis that the use of an STM for clinical findings improves the performance of data retrieval in comparison with the more established retrieval methods of free-text search, ICD-10, and hierarchic retrieval.

Methods

Clinical Question Battery

A survey was performed to gather a battery of clinical questions relating to clinical findings that a clinician might want to ask the Diabeta clinical information system. Fifteen copies of a questionnaire were distributed to all grades of medical staff in two clinical academic departments. Eight completed forms were returned, which collectively suggested 47 unique questions relating to clinical findings (Table 1). These questions were then formulated into database queries using the four alternative methods of retrieval.

Methods of Retrieval

A table of the Diabeta clinical term strings mapped to CTV3 was created in an Microsoft Access database together with their frequency in records in the system and the concept (Read code) to which they had each been mapped (e.g. diabetes mellitus| 7463| C10..). A separate table was created, containing the default ICD-10 maps for each concept (Read code) using the mapping table from the October 1997 Read Codes release. Another table expressed the semantic definition of each concept with reference to the attributes expressed in the STM (Figure 3).

The semantic definition table contained an entry for each concept with a separate column for every attribute. The applicable values (atoms) for each concept were entered in the appropriate column field (Figure 4). The database design dealt with the uncommon circumstance in which a concept had an attribute containing more than one value by replicating the line for each value (e.g., *Vulvovaginitis* has a separate row for the attribute [Site]: Vulval structure and Vaginal structure).

These resource tables were then used to retrieve concepts and records in response to each of the 47 clinical questions. The principle adopted was that a user would want to retrieve the chosen clinical concept and

Table 1 ■

Battery of Questions Collected from a Survey of
Physicians, and Their Frequency of Occurrence

Question	Frequency
Absent foot pulses	1
Alcohol consumption	1
Amputations	3
Cataract	1
Chronic pancreatitis	1
Diabetes treated with diet alone	1
Diabetic autonomic neuropathy	1
Diabetic hand syndrome (diabetic cheiroarthropathy)	1
Diabetic ketoacidosis	1
End-stage renal failure	1
Erectile dysfunction	1
Frozen shoulder	1
Gastric paresis/autonomic bowel dyfunction	1
Hyperlipidemia	1
Hypertension	5
Impotence	1
Infection	1
Insulin-dependent diabetes mellitus	3
Insulin-treated diabetes mellitus	2
Ischemic heart disease	2
Limb amputation	1
Limb complications	1
Limb infection	1
Macrovascular complication [IHD, PVD]	1
Major limb amputation	1
Microvascular complication [retinopathy + nephropathy]	1
Myocardial infarction	4
Necrobiosis lipoidica	2
Nephropathy [diabetic nephropathy]	3
Neuropathic foot ulcer	1
Neuropathy	4
Obesity	1
Painful neuropathy	1
Peripheral vascular disease	2
Persistent microalbuminuria	2
Pregnancies	2
Pregnancy complications	2
Problematic hypoglycemia	1
Proteinuria	1
Retinopathy	3
Smokers	1
Stroke	1
Tumor of pancreas	1
Ulcer of foot	2
Ulcers [skin]	1
Unsuccessful diabetic pregnancies	1
Vascular foot ulcer	1

any *subtypes* of that clinical concept, e.g., *Gallstone chronic pancreatitis* was retrieved when searching for cases of *Chronic pancreatitis*. The concepts and records of the experimental Diabeta database were identified and flagged for each question and stored in 47 separate tables using each of the following four approaches:

Free-text Retrieval

Free-text searching was performed using standard Access query methods to find phrases containing the required string, which has previously been found to be effective.[24] For example, record entries of *Frozen shoulder* were retrieved by searching for all strings containing ⟨*froz*⟩ (where * is a wildcard representing any characters). Multiple searches were allowed to identify alternative expressions of the same concept; for example, both ⟨*IHD*⟩ and ⟨*ischaemic heart*⟩ were used to identify records of *Ischaemic heart disease*.

ICD-10 Retrieval

The ICD-10 categories required for retrieval for each question were identified with reference to the ICD-10 (volume 3) index. A single ICD-10 code or list of codes was constructed and its appropriateness to the clinical question validated by an independent clinician. The ICD-10 code (or codes) were then used to retrieve a unique list of Read-coded concepts that were relevant to the question, to identify the concepts with applicable maps, e.g., L92.1 for cases of *Necrobiosis lipoidica*.

Hierarchic Retrieval

The October Read Version 3 browser[25] was used to identify the Read-code node of the hierarchy required for each question. For example, *Myocardial infarction* (Read code X200E) was identified as the superordinate node marking the hierarchy of concepts required, in response to the question "Find all types of *Myocardial infarction*." A unique descent from this identified node was then performed using the "descent" functionality of the Version 3 browser. Occasionally, more than one Read code descent was needed to retrieve the concepts required to answer the clinical question, e.g., *Ischaemic heart disease* and *Peripheral vascular disease*.

Semantic Differential Retrieval

Semantic retrieval was performed by exploiting the "atoms" of concepts in the STM and the formal structuring of the underlying primitive values that have a strict subtype arrangement.[22] For example, to find all "disorders affecting the limbs," a list of concepts was created that had a semantic definition containing [Site]: Limb structure, or a subtype of Limb structure (Figure 5). In the example shown, this would result in the retrieval of two concepts, *Toe infection* ([Site]: Toe structure) and *Ulcer of foot* ([Site]: Foot structure). The described STM of clinical findings contains a large number of attributes, and a more complex query might involve the differential retrieval of concepts that have more than one characteristic in common (semantic differential retrieval). For example, to retrieve all "limb infections," a list of concepts was created

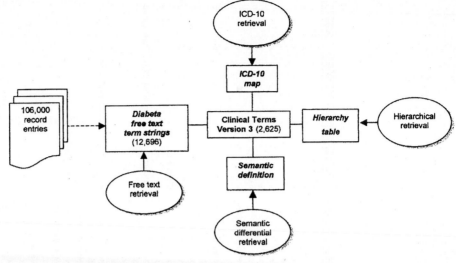

Figure 3 Relationship between the four methods of retrieval, the original Diabeta clinical finding term string and the Clinical Terms Version 3 concepts (with their mapping to ICD-10, hierarchical position represented in the hierarchy table, and semantic definition) in the experimental database.

that had a semantic definition containing [Site]: Limb structure or a subtype and [Process]: Infection (Figure 6). In the example shown, this would result in the retrieval of a single concept, *Toe infection*, but not *Ulcer of foot* (as its semantic definition does not contain the [Process]: Infection).

Gold Standard

To evaluate the retrieval performance of a terminology, comparison against a gold standard is needed. The creation of such gold standards in medical informatics is recognized as problematic.[26] Ideally, such a standard should represent the (perfect) "truth" about the population against which the performance of the information resource can be compared. In the evaluation of the performance of a terminology, the gold standard is the complete subset of concepts from the terminology that all clinicians (with perfect knowledge) would expect to retrieve in response to a particular clinical question. Thus, a separate gold standard is required for each discrete clinical question (and relating to the version of the terminology at the time of the query).

An initial flagged list of concepts was created that one would expect to be retrieved from the total 2,625 concepts in the database, in response to each question posed. The quality of these was then independently assured by a second clinician, who had a good knowledge of the contents of the original Diabeta database. A 10 percent sample was then further validated by a third clinician, to create the final gold standard list of concepts expected to be retrieved from the database for each of the 47 questions.

A table was constructed for each question and search method for all concept database tables (141 fields) and record database tables (168 fields). These tables contained those concepts and records that were *expected* for each question and those that were actually *observed* for each method (Figure 7).

Statistical Analysis

The choice of the statistical method for the evaluation of the retrieval performance of a clinical terminology requires careful consideration.[27] The retrieved concepts and records are nominal data, dictating the use of 2 × 2 contingency tables as the most appropriate method to compare the observed retrieval with that of the gold standard.[17] Individual derived measures and means of performance across all 47 questions were calculated and expressed by the mean detection rate $(TP/(TP + FN))$ and mean positive predictive value $(TP/(TP + FP))$. The likelihood of the association was estimated using the Yates continuity-corrected chi-squared test. This test was chosen because it provides a more robust estimate of the exact probability (compared with the chi-squared test) where the expected and observed numbers are relatively small, e.g., when the clinical questions are specific and generate only small frequencies of retrieved concepts (e.g., *Frozen shoulder*).

The Cohen kappa (κ) has been used as an index of the strength of agreement (between the observed retrieval and the gold standard) against that which might be expected by chance.[26,28] A value of +1 indicates perfect agreement, and some authorities consider a kappa value above 0.4 as evidence of useful agreement, but this threshold obviously depends on the clinical application and may need to be set at a level higher than 0.8 for the evaluation of retrieval performance.[27]

Concept	Site	Pathological process	Morphology	Histology	Causative agent	Function	Associated finding	Course
Acute left ventricular failure	Left ventricular structure	Pathological process	x	x	x	Cardiac	x	Acute
Aortic valve disease	Aortic valve structure	Pathological process	x	x	x	x	x	x
Bladder calculus	Urinary bladder structure	Pathological process	Calculus	x	x	x	x	x
Calculus of kidney	Kidney structure	Pathological process	Calculus	x	x	x	x	x
Clear cell carcinoma of kidney	Kidney structure	Malignant neoplastic	Mass - lesion	Clear cell carcinoma	x	x	x	x
Dermatitis herpetiformis	Skin of body region	Autoimmune	x	x	x	x	x	x
Ectopic pregnancy	Intrauterine conception structure	Pathological process	Malposition of	x	x	Pregnancy	x	x
Empyema	Pleural structure	Infection	Fluid collection	x	Microorganism	x	x	x
Enlarged tonsil	Tonsillar structure	x	Structural expansion	x	x	x	x	x
Fracture of vertebra	Bone structure of spine	Traumatic	Fracture - lesion	x	Mechanical force	x	x	x
Gangrene of foot	Foot structure	Pathological process	x	Gangrene	x	x	x	x
Ingrowing great toe nail	Nail of great toe	Pathological process	x	x	x	x	x	x
Medulloblastoma of	Cerebellar structure	Malignant neoplastic	Mass - lesion	Medulloblastoma	x	x	x	x
Myocardial infarction	Cardiac internal structure	Pathological process	x	Infarction	x	Blood flow	x	x
Otitis media	Middle ear structure	Inflammation	x	x	x	x	x	x
Paroxysmal atrial fibrillation	Cardiac conducting system	Pathological process	x	x	x	Cardiac	Heart irregularly	Paroxysmal
Pituitary-dependent Cushing's	Adrenal cortex	Metabolic	x	x	x	x	x	x
Pituitary-dependent Cushing's	Pars anterior of pituitary gland	Metabolic	x	x	x	x	x	x
Prepatellar bursitis	Prepatellar bursa	Inflammation	x	x	x	x	x	x
Proliferative diabetic	Retinal structure	Pathological process	x	x	x	x	Diabetes mellitus	x
Rectal abscess	Rectum structure	Infection	Abscess	x	Bacteria	x	x	x
Reiter's disease	Joint	Infection	x	x	Microorganism	x	x	x
Schizophrenia	x	Pathological process	x	x	x	Mental function	x	x
Tuberculosis of hip joint	Hip joint structure	Infection	x	x	Mycobacterium	x	x	x
Tumour of caecum	Caecum	Neoplastic	Mass - lesion	x	x	x	x	x
Viral meningitis	Meninges structure	Infection	x	x	Virus	x	x	x
Vulvovaginitis	Vulval structure	Inflammation	x	x	x	x	x	x
Vulvovaginitis	Vaginal structure	Inflammation	x	x	x	x	x	x

Figure 4 An extract of the semantic definition table from the experimental database, illustrating its use of a separate column for each attribute. The atoms for each concept are indicated by an entry of the appropriate value in the applicable attribute field. (Only a subset of attributes is shown.)

To express the collective results for all retrievals and produce a summary index of the overall performance of a terminology, means of the derived indexes from the 2 × 2 contingency were used. In addition, the Mantel-Haenszel chi-squared test was quoted, which also pools the results of the individual subsets using the following formula:

$$\chi^2_{MH} = \frac{(|\Sigma a - \Sigma E_a| - 0.5)^2}{\Sigma V_a}$$

where a is the observed value, E_a is the expected value of a, and V_a is the variance of a.

The Mann-Whitney test was used as a measure of the significance of association because it provides a more conservative estimate, as the assumption that the data always come from a normal distribution may not al-

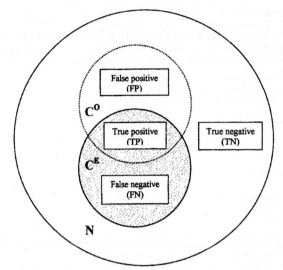

Figure 7 Venn diagram showing the relationship between the population of concepts observed by data retrieval (C^O), with respect to the actual (gold standard) expected population (C^E), and the total population (N); and the true positive, false positive, false negative and true negative populations forming the 2 × 2 contingency tables for each question in the experimental database.

ways be true. For example, the very fact that a question may (by design) retrieve concepts sharing one or more particular characteristics suggests that it is safer to assume that the data are nonparametric.

Results

A 2 × 2 contingency table was constructed for each of the 47 questions for all four methods relating to both concept and record retrieval (although free-text retrieval related only to records). These individual contingency tables related the actual numbers of concepts and records observed by each method compared with those expected (by the gold standard). The number of concepts expected to be retrieved ranged from 1 to 219 (from a total of 2,625 concepts); the number of records expected ranged from 0† to 4,231 (from a total of 106,000 records).

The mean detection rate of semantic differential retrieval was significantly better for both concept (0.86) and record (0.94) retrieval (Table 2). The use of the ICD-10 framework was slightly better than hierarchic retrieval, with free-text retrieval having the lowest de-

Query: All diseases affecting the limbs (and parts of)				
Concept	Site	Process	Morphology	Retrieved
Toe infection	**Toe structure**	Infection	-	✓
Rectal abscess	Rectum structure	Infection	Abscess	
Calculus of kidney	Kidney structure	-	Calculus	
Ulcer of foot	**Foot structure**	Inflammation	Ulcer	✓

Xa1Z8 **Limb structure**
 Xa1Z9 Lower limb structure
  XafX **Foot structure**
   Xa1tt **Toe structure**

Figure 5 The specification of a query to retrieve all disorders affecting the limb includes those disorder concepts having a semantic definition [Site]: Limb structure or part of limb structure. (An extract from the anatomy value limb structure hierarchy is illustrated.)

Query: All diseases affecting the limbs (and parts of) and due to infection				
Concept	Site	Process	Morphology	Retrieved
Toe infection	**Toe structure**	**Infection**	-	✓
Rectal abscess	Rectum structure	**Infection**	Abscess	
Calculus of kidney	Kidney structure	-	Calculus	
Ulcer of foot	**Foot structure**	Inflammation	Ulcer	

Xa1Z8 **Limb structure**
 Xa1Z9 Lower limb structure
  XafX **Foot structure**
   Xa1tt **Toe structure**

Figure 6 The specification of a query to retrieve all disorders caused by infection and affecting the limbs includes those concepts having *both* a semantic definition of [Pathological process]: Infection and [Site]: Limb structure or part of limb structure. (An extract from the anatomy value limb structure hierarchy is illustrated.)

---

†Zero records were retrieved for the question concerning the concept *Diabetes treated with diet alone* as the status of the patient whose record contained this entry changed during the interval between the original extraction of the Diabeta database and the subsequent retrieval experiments.

Table 2 ∎

Statistical Values for Free-text, ICD-10, Hierarchy, and Semantic Analysis for Concept and Record Retrieval in Response to the Battery of Clinical Questions

	Free Text	ICD	Hierarchy	Semantic
Concept retrieval (N = 2,625):				
Mean detection rate (SD)	NA	0.68 (0.35)**	0.66 (0.32)*	0.86 (0.26)
Mean positive predictive value (SD)	NA	0.79 (0.27)*	0.93 (0.19)	0.96 (0.08)
Mean Yates value (SD)	NA	955 (695)*	1034 (752)**	1537 (783)
Mantel-Haenszel chi-squared value	NA	11,467	10,013	19,302
Mean Cohen kappa value (SD)	NA	0.64 (0.30)*	0.73 (0.30)**	0.88 (0.21)
Record retrieval (N = 106,000)				
Mean detection rate (SD)	0.61 (0.34)*	0.81 (0.32)*	0.79 (0.32)*	0.94 (0.20)
Mean positive predictive value (SD)	0.82 (0.32)*	0.83 (0.29)*	0.95 (0.20)	0.99 (0.03)
Mean Yates value (SD)	57,969 (36,932)*	73,454 (33,154)*	79,520 (34,870)**	97,774 (23,962)
Mantel-Haenszel chi-squared value	987,190	1,243,364	1,277,119	1,550,356
Mean Cohen kappa value (SD)	0.65 (0.33)*	0.75 (0.32)*	0.83 (0.30)*	0.94 (0.19)

NOTE: Comparison of semantic differential retrieval is included with other methods. NA indicates not applicable. The performance of semantic retrieval with other methods is calculated using the Mann-Whitney test with P values expressed as $P < 0.001$ (indicated by a single asterisk) and $P < 0.01$ (indicated by a double asterisk).

tection rate (0.61). The detection rate is a useful indicator in assessing the ability of the retrieval method to identify all relevant concepts (avoiding false negatives), in contrast to the positive predictive value, which is a valuable indicator of the retrieval of false positives. This latter index again shows that semantic differential retrieval performs better than ICD-10, hierarchic, or free-text searching, although this does not reach significance in comparison with hierarchic retrieval.

The large mean Yates corrected chi-squared and Mantel-Haenszel chi-squared values confirm the expectation of a strong association between the focused set of concepts and records retrieved compared with the gold standard, in the context of a large total population. The strength of association indicated by the mean Yates chi-squared is significantly greater with semantic differential retrieval for both concepts and records, with ICD-10 and hierarchic retrieval being of intermediary status and free-text retrieval again fairing least well.

The calculated means of the Cohen kappa for all methods of retrieval were greater than 0.4 (empirically stated as evidence of useful agreement).[26,28] Cohen's kappa value for concept (0.88) and record (0.94) semantic retrieval were significantly better than for the other approaches and were above the benchmark of 0.81 (considered by some as almost perfect[29]), indicating that high levels of retrieval accuracy from clinical records are achievable.

Discussion

The evaluation of data retrieval can be tested against technical markers such as speed, but from the clinical perspective, although these usability issues are important, it is more vital to evaluate whether an information system can accurately answer the spectrum of questions that might be posed. The lack of reported work on the effect of different search methods on the efficacy of data retrieval from clinical records[1] is surprising, considering the large investment in terminology development in the United Kingdom and abroad[10-12] and the assumptions that data storage in computers will deliver sufficiently accurate information to underpin health service planning and decision support.[30] The effort required by terminology developers to semantically define concepts is considerable and has been quoted as varying between 4.6 and 20.5 minutes per concept.[22] The recent commencement of the cooperative development of SNOMED Clinical Terms (SNOMED CT)[31] heralds yet another massive effort embracing the principle of an underlying STM to provide reference functionality. This study provides the first practical evidence of the utility of such an approach in providing enhanced and accurate data retrieval from clinical records.

The clinical questions required retrieval of information from multiple perspectives. The multi-axial directed acyclic graph structure of CTV3[6] offered a moderately good mechanism for retrieval. This finding mirrors experiments using the cross-references of SNOMED International, which enabled the attainment of good detection rates and positive predictive values.[32] The performance of hierarchic retrieval in the study, however, was dependent on the expressed relationships between concepts in CTV3. Theoretically, if all possible relationships were expressed within the hierarchy, retrieval using this approach would be as good as any other method. The lack of some hierarchies representing a particular clinical perspective (e.g., "limb disorders") led to a number of false negatives, resulting in reduced performance (indicated by poor detection rates) in response to some clinical questions, e.g., retrieval of "limb complications." Creating an exhaustive list of all potential clinical perspectives could rectify hierarchy omissions, but these may be difficult to predict and would eventually cause an unwieldy "explosion" of large numbers of relationships. The performance measures indicate that, although the semantic method had significantly better detection rates compared with hierarchic retrieval rates, the positive predictive values were more comparable. This result reflects the formality of the pure subtype hierarchy and its success in providing a robust mechanism to avoid false positives.

While the disorder hierarchy present in CTV3 was unable to support retrieval of "limb disorders," the semantic method was able to exploit the more complete value hierarchy. The anatomy chapter of CTV3 utilizes the notion of "structure," which encompasses both the whole and "part of" descriptions of that site to ensure that the subtype structure is maintained.[33] This anatomy hierarchy contains the concept "limb structure" with applicable class members, allowing the creation of a semantic differential retrieval of all concepts having a definition [Site]: Limb structure or a type of limb structure (Figure 5). Thus, although the complete classification of "core" disorder concepts may not be possible (or desirable), the complete multiple classification of the underlying primitive values is essential. It is only with the exhaustive polyhierarchic arrangement (complete multiple classification) of primitive values that retrieval from the multiple perspectives that are clinically required is assured.

Evidence from examination of the raw free-text entries in Diabeta 1 suggests that clinicians may not always record the concepts they require with sufficient semantic pedantry. For example, the term "Paget's disease" may have a clear meaning in the context of a patient's record juxtaposed to an entry of *Mastectomy*, but following retrieval of the concept, outside this environment, it acquires ambiguity as to whether it is Paget's disease of the breast or Paget's disease of the bone. The study also revealed some discrepancy in the interpretation of the semantics of the question posed between the standard setter and the retrieval performer. This discrepancy was the main reason for the suboptimal performance of semantic differential retrieval in 13 of the 47 questions posed. For example, the meaning of the question "retrieve all cases of diabetic cataract" might be interpreted to include all cases of "cataract" (and its class) associated with di-

abetes; or only cases where the disorder of "diabetic cataract" was explicitly recorded. The rules of data entry can thus affect the result of the retrieval; e.g., if all cataracts in patients with diabetes mellitus are recorded as *Cataract* but retrieved as *Diabetic cataract*, no cases would be found. This experience identifies the important association between of the semantics of data entry and data retrieval and suggests that caution may be necessary before wholesale adoption of the principle of separation between the interface and reference features of terminologies that has been suggested.

The use of ICD-10 as a retrieval tool was comparatively effective as a method for retrieving data, a finding recently supported by an investigation of the coding and retrieval of stroke patients.[34] Retrieval with ICD-10 performed less well when questions fell outside its scope, e.g., levels of alcohol consumption, or required detail not present in the restricted number of categories available, e.g., absent foot pulses. Overall, the performance of ICD-10 as a retrieval tool was good when it was used within its scope. The method of free-text retrieval fared less well, despite this approach having previously been shown to be effective.[24] The performance may have been improved with the use of more sophisticated natural language processing tools,[35–37] and there have been reports of better detection rates in limited studies.[38]

The collected battery contained clinical questions from a diversity of perspectives, and the STM supported semantic differential retrieval from these various viewpoints significantly better than the other methods. The indications of the experiments on the Diabeta database are that good detection rates and Cohen's kappa values are achievable (despite the STM being incomplete), and the success supports further investment in exploring this approach. The success of the STM for retrieval was achieved by the flexibility of approach this afforded; however, this was at the expense of its being more complex to use. The method required the analyst to have a good understanding of relational databases and the resource tables (such as the hierarchy table) in CTV3. These operational issues could be improved by the fashioning of clinically intuitive human–computer interface designs.

Conclusion

The investigation has demonstrated a number of key points (see sidebar). It has shown that the use of an STM significantly improves information retrieval from a clinical database in response to physician-derived questions, in comparison with free-text, hierar-

Key Points

- The formal definition of concepts according to their meaning in a terminology (semantic terminological model) provides the potential for more accurate and flexible data retrieval.

- The International Classification of Diseases, 10th Revision, provides a useful framework for data retrieval when the question posed is within its scope.

- The recording of free text in computerized records, while useful for individual patient notes, is less amenable to information retrieval.

- High detection rates and levels of performance of information retrieval from electronic health care records in response to clinically relevant questions are attainable.

- The performance of semantic differential retrieval is dependent on complete formal sub-type classification of its constituent atoms.

- The complete semantic definition of health care concepts, while desirable, may not be possible; but this may not practically compromise data retrieval performance.

- The semantics of concept definition at data capture (interface functionality) needs to equate to that of data retrieval (reference functionality) to support accurate performance.

diabetes. These patients, with their diversity of complications and associated comorbidities, make the Diabeta database a valuable test bed for retrieval experiments. It is likely that the principles identified in this study are applicable to data represented by a terminology in other health care environments, but this will need confirmation.

The corpus of concepts in the disorder chapter of CTV3 is large, and the extent to which these have been completely semantically represented has been shown to be dependent on the specialist area.[20] For example, concepts describing mental health, neurologic, and dermatologic conditions are less amenable to complete characterization. Further effort is required to model these areas and to test whether such specialist extensions can be developed and be mutually compatible with a global STM for clinical findings. Finally, although the use of an STM as the basis for retrieval appears to be valuable technically, further investigation is required into the development of intuitive user-friendly interfaces and the practicability of its use by clinicians.

The authors thank Steve Carey at St. Thomas' Hospital for technical support in extracting data from the Diabeta database, the clinicians who contributed to the formulation of the battery of clinical questions, and Henri Brown for additional quality assurance. They are also indebted to Philip Young, Department of Mathematics, University of York, for statistical advice.

References ■

1. Hogan WR, Wagner MM. Accuracy of data in computer-based patient records. J Am Med Inform Assoc. 1997;4:342–55.
2. Johnson N, Mant D, Jones L, Randall T. Use of computerised general practice data for population surveillance: comparative study of influenza data. BMJ. 1991;302:763–5.
3. Rector AL, Nowlan WA, Kay S. Foundations for an electronic medical record. Methods Inf Med. 1991;30:179–86.
4. McDonald CJ. The barriers to electronic medical record systems and how to overcome them. J Am Med Inform Assoc. 1997;4:213–21.
5. Evans DA, Cimino JJ, Hersh WR, Huff SM, Bell DS, for the CANON Group. Toward a medical-concept representation language. J Am Med Inform Assoc. 1994;1:207–17.
6. O'Neil M, Payne C, Read JD. Read Codes version 3: a user-led terminology. Methods Inf Med. 1995;34:187–92.
7. Huff SM, Rocha RA, McDonald CJ, et al. Development of the Logical Observations Identifiers, Names, and Codes (LOINC) vocabulary. J Am Med Inform Assoc. 1998;5:276–92.
8. Côté RA, Rothwell DJ, Palotay JL, Beckett RS, Brochu L. The Systematized Nomenclature of Human and Veterinary Medicine: SNOMED International. Northfield, Ill: College of American Pathologists, 1993.
9. Rector AL, Glowinski AJ, Nowlan WA, Rossi-Mori A. Medical concept models and medical records: an approach

chic, and ICD-10 approaches. This indicates that an STM provides a useful framework for the representation of clinical findings and that there is merit in the current approach of defining health care concepts semantically. The study has also indicated that alternative methods of analysis will give different results, depending on the purpose for which they have been designed. Greater understanding of the design and scope of ICD may help with the appreciation of its merits as well as its restrictions as a statistical tool for data analysis.

The experiment used a clinical database that was oriented toward the collection of data from patients with

based on GALEN and PEN&PAD. J Am Med Inform Assoc. 1995;2:19–35.

10. Spackman KA, Campbell KE, Côté RA. SNOMED RT: a reference terminology for health care. Proc AMIA Fall Symp. 1997:640–4.

11. Stuart-Buttle CDG, Brown PJB, Price C, O'Neil MJ, Read JD. The Read Thesaurus: creation and beyond. In: Pappas C, et al. (eds). Proceedings of the 14th Medical Informatics Europe '97 Conference. Oxford, UK: IOS Press, 1997:416–20.

12. Rodgers JE, Rector AL. Terminology systems: bridging the generation gap. Proc AMIA Fall Symp. 1997:610–4.

13. Sönksen P, Williams C. Information technology in diabetes care "Diabeta": 23 years of development and use of a computer-based record for diabetes care. Int J Biomed Comput. 1996;42:67–77.

14. National Health Service Centre for Coding and Classification. Read Codes File Structure Version 3.0: Overview and Technical Description. Technical Report. Loughborough, UK: NHS: CCC, 1994.

15. World Health Organization. International Classification of Diseases and Related Health Problems (vol 1), 10th rev. Geneva, Switzerland: WHO, 1992.

16. Severs MP. The Clinical Terms Project. Bull R Coll Physicians. 1993;27(2):9–10.

17. Buckland R. The language of health. BMJ. 1993;306:287–8.

18. Office of Population Censuses and Surveys. Tabular list of the classification of surgical operations and procedures, 4th rev. London, UK: Her Majesty's Stationery Office, 1990.

19. National Health Service Centre for Coding and Classification. Read Codes File Structure Version 3.1: The Qualifier Extensions. Technical Report. Loughborough, UK: NHS CCC, 1994.

20. Brown PJB, O'Neil M, Price C. Semantic definition of disorders in version 3 of the Read Codes. Methods Inf Med. 1998;37:415–9.

21. Brown PJB. An examination of the conceptual components of disorders and their use in analysis of clinical records [MD thesis]. London, UK: University of London, 1999.

22. Brown PJB, Price C. Semantic-based concept differential retrieval and equivalence detection in Clinical Terms Version 3 (Read Codes). Proc AMIA Annu Symp. 1999:27–31.

23. Brown PJB, Price C, Sönksen P. Evaluating the terminology requirements to support multi-disciplinary diabetic care. Proc AMIA Fall Symp. 1997:645–9.

24. Steib SA, Reichley RM, McMullin ST, et al. Supporting ad-hoc queries in an integrated clinical database. Proc 19th Annu Symp Comput Appl Med Care. 1995:62–6.

25. National Health Service Centre for Coding and Classification. The Read Codes: Demonstrators, Oct 1997 [CD-ROM]. Loughborough, UK: NHSCCC, 1997.

26. Friedman CP, Wyatt JC. Evaluation Methods in Medical Informatics. New York, Springer, 1997:185–203.

27. Brown PJB, Sönksen P, Price C, Young P. A standard for evaluating the retrieval performance of clinical terminologies. Proc AMIA Fall Symp. 1999:1031.

28. Cohen J. Weighted kappa: nominal scale agreement with provision for scaled disagreement or partial credit. Psychol Bull. 1968;70:213–20.

29. Landis JR, Koch GG. The measurement of observer agreement for categorical data. Biometrics. 1977;33:159–74.

30. National Health Service Executive. Information for Health: An Information Strategy for the Modern NHS. London, UK: Her Majesty's Stationery Office, 1998.

31. National Health Service Information Authority and College of American Pathologists. SNOMED Clinical Terms: A Global Leader in Healthcare Terminology. 1999. Available from: http://www.coding.nhsia.nhs.uk. Accessed Jan 16, 2000.

32. Lussier YA, Bourque M. Comparing SNOMED and ICPC retrieval accuracies using relational database models. Proc AMIA Fall Symp. 1997:514–8.

33. Schulz EB, Price C, Brown PJB. Symbolic anatomical knowledge representation in the Read Codes version 3: structure and application. J Am Med Inform Assoc. 1997;4:38–48.

34. Mant J, Mant F, Winner S. How good is routine information? Validation of coding for acute stroke in Oxford hospitals. Health Trends. 1998;(4)29:96–9.

35. Friedman C. Toward a comprehensive medical language processing system: methods and issues. Proc AMIA Fall Symp. 1997:595–9.

36. Spyns P. Natural language processing in medicine: an overview. Methods Inf Med. 1996;35:285–301.

37. Haug PJ, Christensen L, Gundersen M, Clemons B, Koehler S, Bauer K. A natural language parsing system for admitting diagnoses. Proc AMIA Fall Symp. 1997:814–8.

38. Lin R, Lanert L, Middleton B, Shiffman S. A free-text processing system to capture physical findings: canonical phrase identification system (CAPIS). Proc 15th Annu Symp Comput Appl Med Care. 1992:843–7.

Patients with cancer holding their own records: a randomised controlled trial

MARK DRURY

PATRICIA YUDKIN

JEAN HARCOURT

RAY FITZPATRICK

LESLEY JONES

CHRIS ALCOCK

MICHAEL MINTON

SUMMARY

Background. The burden of cancer care in general practice is increasing. Patient-held records may facilitate effective, coordinated care, but no randomised controlled trials of their use in cancer care have been conducted, and concerns about possible negative effects remain.

Aim. To evaluate the use of a supplementary patient-held record in cancer care.

Method. Six hundred and fifty radiotherapy outpatients with any form of cancer were randomised either to hold a supplementary record or to receive normal care. It was explained to record holders that the supplementary record was intended to improve communication with health professionals and act as an aide memoire. After three months, patients' satisfaction with communication and with participation in their own care were assessed. Global health status, emotional functioning, and cognitive functioning were measured using the European Organization for Research and Treatment of Cancer QLQ-C30 questionnaire.

Results. There were no significant differences between groups in any of the outcome measures. Patients in both groups expressed a high level of satisfaction with communication and participation in their care. Mean (SD) scores in the intervention and control groups were: global health status, 66.8 (24.2) and 65.3 (23.7); emotional functioning, 75.0 (24.6) and 77.4 (22.8); cognitive functioning, 84.5 (21.0) and 84.0 (21.3).

Conclusion. A supplementary patient-held record for radiotherapy outpatients appears to have no effect on satisfaction with communication, participation in care, or quality of life.

Keywords: cancer patients; patient satisfaction; patient-held records; communication.

M Drury, MRCGP, general practitioner, Wantage, Oxfordshire. P Yudkin, MA, DPhil, university research lecturer; J Harcourt, BA, research nurse; and L Jones, BA, computer scientist, Imperial Cancer Research Fund General Practice Research Group, Department of Primary Health Care, University of Oxford. R Fitzpatrick, BA, MSc, PhD, professor, Division of Public Health and Primary Health Care, University of Oxford. C Alcock, FRCP, FRCR, clinical director of clinical oncology; and M Minton, FRCP, consultant in palliative medicine, Oxford Radcliffe Hospital, Headington, Oxford.

Submitted: 18 August 1998; final acceptance: 9 June 1999.

© British Journal of General Practice, 2000, **50**, 105-110.

Introduction

IN 1995, the report of the Expert Advisory Committee on Cancer Services (Calman–Hine Report[1]) proposed a three-tier service with specialised cancer centres at the top and primary care at the foundation. The effect will be to increase specialisation in hospital practice, which, with an already expanded primary care team, will tend to fragment care. Allying this with recommendations in the report — that cancer services should be patient-centred and give clear information about treatment options — will be difficult.

Cancer patients and their families crave information[2-6] but are often uncertain what to ask[4] and unhappy with the information they receive.[7,8] Communication is of central importance to patients[9] and carers[10] and is a common source of dissatisfaction.[11,12]

Patient-held records have been used successfully in obstetric and paediatric care to improve communication and promote patients' involvement in their own care.[13-15] Patients viewing their own general practitioner (GP) records reported a positive effect on communication, without increasing anxiety.[16] A review of the ethical and practical aspects of patient-held records[17] concluded that there were few drawbacks and considerable benefits. However, patient-held records have not been evaluated in cancer care.

In 1994, a pilot study of outpatients receiving palliative care[18] suggested a patient-held record was used and acceptable. In this study we investigated whether such a record for radiotherapy outpatients would affect their satisfaction with communication and with participation in their own care or their quality of life.

Method

Subjects

A total of 650 patients were recruited between April 1994 and April 1996 from consecutive attenders at radiotherapy clinics run by the Oxford Radcliffe National Health Service (NHS) Trust. All patients with cancer (except curable dermatological cancers) and aged 16 years or over were eligible.

Intervention

After randomisation in the clinic, patients in the intervention group were given the supplementary record. It consisted of an A4-size plastic wallet containing communication/diary sheets for use by the patient, their family, health professionals, and carers, as well as pages for appointments, medication, and addresses and telephone numbers. The study nurse explained the use of the record as a means of communication and as an *aide memoire*. Patients were encouraged to read and write in it and to show it to anyone concerned with their care. The record explicitly invited carers to use it as an aid to communication. Patients in both groups received an information sheet about the trial.

Six months after recruitment, all record-holding patients, if well enough, were asked to return the record.

Outcome measures

Psychometrically tested outcome measures directly relevant to the trial intervention are not available. We therefore used a validated instrument measuring quality of life that was specifically developed for cancer patients: the European Organization for Research and Treatment of Cancer QLQ-C30 questionnaire (EORTC QLQ C30).[19] The main outcomes were global health status, emotional functioning, and cognitive functioning at three months.

To examine outcomes more directly related to the trial intervention (i.e. patients' satisfaction with communication and with participation in their own care), a 19-item questionnaire (Box 1) was developed, based on evidence from the pilot study. Items were scored on a five-point scale: strongly agree to strongly disagree.

Sample size

To detect an effect size of 0.33 (considered a small but worthwhile effect)[20] in the mean EORTC QLQ C30 score between the two groups, with 90% power and at a significance level of 0.05, required 412 subjects (206 in each group). To allow for the high attrition rate expected in cancer patients, 650 were recruited.

Recruitment and randomisation

Clinic lists were reviewed and letters sent to eligible patients informing them about the study one week before their appointments. At the clinic, the study was explained to each patient by a study nurse who requested consent to take part. An explanatory letter and copy of the patient's consent was sent to their GP.

Participants were randomised by the study nurse, either to the record-holding group (RH) or to normal care (NC). The allocations, generated using random numbers and in blocks of 10, were in sealed, numbered, opaque envelopes, which were opened sequentially.

Data collected

Three months after recruitment, questionnaires relating to the

---

Identified in factor analysis:

Satisfaction with communication and with participation in care
 I have found it difficult to remember when to take my medicines and tablets
 Doctors and nurses keep me fully informed about my illness
 My doctors and nurses appear to be fully aware of all aspects of my illness and treatment
 I often forget what I want to say to my nurses and doctors
 I sometimes feel confused by the number of different doctors and nurses that I see
 I do not feel I have any control over the way my illness is treated
 My doctors and nurses often seem unaware of the problems I am facing
 I find it easy to remember everything my nurses and doctors say to me
 Those involved in my care do not seem to know what others are doing
 I feel I can take an active part in decisions about my treatment

Desire for information
 I would like to be fully informed about all matters that relate to my illness
 I would like to see all my medical records

Remaining statements
 I am unsure what my medicines and tablets are for
 I find it difficult to talk to my doctors
 I feel my family has not been told everything they would like to know about my illness
 I find it easy to ask for the help that I need from my doctors and nurses
 It has been easy to remember my appointments
 I find it easy to talk to my family about my illness
 I feel able to face all future aspects of my illness

Box 1. The 19 statements relating to communication and participation in care.

---

main outcomes of the trial, the use of the record, and contact with health professionals were sent to all patients (if well enough). Two reminders were sent to non-responders.

At the end of the study, a questionnaire about attitudes to patients holding their own records was sent to all GPs of RH patients ($n = 229$).

Statistical methods

The significance tests used were the *t*-test for comparing means, the chi-squared test for comparing proportions, and the Mann–Whitney test for comparing Likert scale scores.

To improve reliability of measurement and to reduce the number of statistical comparisons, the 19-item questionnaire was analysed using principal component analysis and a single varimax rotation of data. The raw scores were transposed, if necessary, so that higher scores always represented a greater sense of participation in care or a greater desire for information. Five factors with an Eigen value of greater than one were identified. On intuitive grounds and after examination of a scree plot, the two factors with the largest eigen values of 1.9 (desire for information) and 4.9 (satisfaction with communication and participation in care) were selected. They accounted for 35.9% of the variance. Items were selected that loaded on factors greater than 0.5. Clustering of items supported the use of two scales: satisfaction with communication and with participation in care (10 items), and desire for information (two items) (Box 1). Internal reliability for both scales was satisfactory (Cronbach's alpha = 0.81 and 0.74 respectively). The Central Oxford Research Ethics Committee granted approval for the study.

Results

Study population

The progress of patients through the study is shown in Figure 1. Of the 896 eligible patients presenting at the clinic, 246 (27.5%) refused to participate; 120 (13.4%) because the record would make them too anxious, 59 (6.6%) because they felt too well to need one, 40 (4.5 %) because they felt too ill, and 27 (3.0%) for other reasons. There was no difference in the pattern of diagnoses or in sex between refusers and participants, but the former were older ($P = 0.003$): mean (SD) ages were 65.0 (13.4) years and 62.1 (13.3) years respectively.

Of the 650 patients who entered the trial, 76 died or withdrew before three months. Thus, 574 patients were sent the three-month questionnaire, of whom 450 responded: 206/284 (72.5%) in the RH group and 244/290 (84.1%) in the NC group, a difference of 11.6% (95% confidence interval = 4.9 to 18.3; $P = 0.001$). Responses to individual questions were sometimes missing; details are given in the text.

Table 1 shows the age, sex, and diagnoses of patients enrolled in the study. Patients who died or withdrew before three months had a different pattern of diagnoses from those who remained ($P<0.001$): more had carcinoma of the bronchus (38.2% of those who died or withdrew compared with 14.1%) and fewer had carcinoma of the breast (18.4% compared with 35.2%). The remaining patients were similar in both groups. There were no statistically significant differences in age, sex, or diagnosis between those who responded to the questionnaire and those who did not, and these characteristics were comparable in the two groups of responders (Table 2).

Clinic attendance and contacts with professional carers

Very few patients (10/206, 4.9% in the RH group, and 13/244, 5.3% in the NC group) reported that they had not attended any

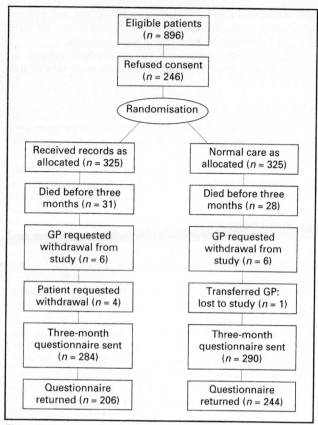

Figure 1. Progress of patients through the trial.

Table 1. Age, sex, and diagnoses of patients. Figures are % (*n*) except where otherwise stated.

	RH group (*n* = 325)	NC group (*n* = 325)
Mean (SD) age in years	61.9 (13.7)	62.2 (12.9)
Sex		
Female	60.6 (197	58.5 (190)
Male	39.4 (128)	41.5 (135)
Diagnosis of cancer		
Breast	32.9 (107)	33.5 (109)
Bronchus	16.9 (55)	16.9 (55)
Bowel	12.9 (42)	13.5 (44)
Gynaecological	9.5 (31)	7.4 (24)
Urogenital	7.1 (23)	5.5 (18)
Head and neck	4.0 (13)	4.6 (15)
Upper GI tract	4.0 (13)	4.3 (14)
Lymphoma	3.1 (10)	3.1 (10)
Unknown primary	0.6 (2)	3.4 (11)
Other	8.9 (29)	7.7 (25)

clinics in the three months since recruitment. The most commonly attended clinics were radiotherapy/oncology (82.7% of RH group and 84.6% of NC group), surgical (29.7% and 22.6% respectively), chest (8.5% and 10.0% respectively), and medical (8.1% and 10.9% respectively). Most patients (159/203, 78.3% in the RH group, and 156/183, 85.2% in the NC group) had visited their GP. Other carers most often seen were vicars/priests (16.7% and 10.6% respectively) and Macmillan nurses (13.1% and 11.5% respectively). There were no significant differences in attendance or contacts between the two groups.

Patients' reported use of the record

Three months after recruitment, 96.8% of those in the RH group who responded (184/190) still had their record. Of these, 91.8% (168/183) said that they understood how to use it, 88.9% (160/180) reported reading it, and 61.7% (113/183) said that they wrote in it themselves. A total of 82.2% (143/174) showed it to their hospital doctors when seen, and 66.7% (106/159) to their GP. Other people who patients commonly reported as reading or writing in the record included family members (33.5%; 59/176), radiotherapists (29.3%; 49/167), and hospital nurses (27.9%; 46/165).

Quality of life measured by EORTC QLQ C-30

There were no differences between groups in the study's main outcomes: global health status, emotional functioning, or cognitive functioning (Table 3). Overall, mean scores were similar in the two groups.

Patients' satisfaction with communication and with participation in their own care

Patients in both groups expressed a similarly high level of satisfaction. Mean (SD) scores for the 10 statements (each scored on a scale of 1 to 5) relating to satisfaction with communication and with participation in care were 3.83 (0.59) in the RH group and 3.80 (0.59) in the NC group (mean difference = 0.03; 95% CI = 0.09 to 0.15). Mean (SD) scores for the two statements relating to desire for information were 4.27 (0.79) and 4.14 (0.79) respectively (mean difference = 0.13; 95% CI = 0.02 to 0.28). There was little difference between groups in the responses to the seven statements not identified in the factor analysis (Table 4); however, patients in the RH group felt significantly less able to face all future aspects of their illness ($P = 0.05$).

GPs' views about the patient-held record

Of the 229 GPs of RH patients who received the questionnaire, 202 (88.2%) responded; only 27.3% (54/198) said they had seen the record. There were no significant differences between GPs who had and had not seen the record in views about patients with cancer having access to their medical records ($P = 0.90$) or being fully informed on all matters that relate to their illness ($P = 0.52$) (Table 5). Not all GPs who answered the questionnaire responded to these questions.

Discussion

In this large study, we did not find any significant benefit arising from cancer patients holding their own supplementary record, nor did we find any significant negative effect.

There were indications that record holding may have been a burden to some patients. Twenty-seven per cent of the eligible patients declined to participate; nearly half because they thought the record would generate anxiety. After three months, the response rate to the questionnaire was much lower among the record holders than the normal care group, and record holders more often failed to complete all the questions, particularly those concerning the record itself. Such discrepant response rates are unusual and suggest that something about the intervention itself affected the probability of response. It may be that patients felt a degree of guilt if they had failed to use the record, or that the record forced them to confront aspects of their illness that they did not wish to explore — a possibility supported by the finding that record holders appeared less able than non-record holders to face all future aspects of their illness. A sensitivity analysis suggested that the excess non-response among record holders might possibly have underestimated the negative effects of the records.

Table 2. Responders and non-responders to three-month questionnaire: age, sex, and diagnoses of patients. Figures are % (*n*) except where otherwise stated.

	Responders RH group (*n* = 206)	Non-responders NC group (*n* = 244)	*n* = 124
Mean (SD) age (years)	61.6 (13.2)	62.1 (12.8)	61.1(15.3)
Sex			
Female	64.6 (133)	59.0 (144)	58.9 (73)
Male	35.4 (73)	41.0 (100)	41.1 (51)
Diagnosis of cancer			
Breast	38.8 (80)	35.7 (87)	28.2 (35)
Bronchus	10.7 (22)	14.3 (35)	19.4 (24)
Bowel	12.1(25)	15.2 (37)	12.1 (15)
Gynaecological	9.2 (19)	8.2 (20)	8.1 (10)
Urogenital	7.3 (15)	5.3 (13)	10.5 (13)
Head and neck	4.9 (10)	4.5 (11)	4.0 (5)
Upper GI tract	3.4 (7)	2.5 (6)	7.3 (9)
Lymphoma	3.4 (7)	3.3 (8)	1.6 (2)
Unknown primary	-	3.7 (9)	0.8 (1)
Other	10.2 (21)	7.4 (18)	8.1 (10)

Note: There are no statistically significant differences in age, sex, or diagnosis between responders in the two groups, or between total responders and non-responders.

Table 3. Mean (SD) EORTC QLQ-C30 Quality of Life Scores.

	RH group (*n* = 206)	NC group (*n* = 244)	Difference (95% CI)
Functional Scales			
Physical	72.3 (26.7)	71.8 (27.1)	0.5 (-4.7 to 5.7)
Role	73.2 (34.4)	72.7 (35.2)	0.5 (-6.1 to 7.1)
Emotional	75.0 (24.6)	77.4 (22.8)	-2.4 (-6.9 to 2.1)
Cognitive	84.5 (21.0)	84.0 (21.3)	0.5 (-3.5 to 4.5)
Social	76.0 (28.9)	74.6 (29.9)	1.4 (-4.3 to 7.1)
Global health status	66.8 (24.2)	65.3 (23.7)	1.5 (-3.0 to 6.0)
Symptom Scales			
Fatigue	34.2 (27.9)	35.6 (27.3)	-1.4 (-6.6 to 3.8)
Nausea, vomiting	5.4 (11.6)	8.0 (15.9)	-2.6 (-5.2 to -0.1)
Pain	21.0 (26.3)	21.9 (26.6)	-0.9 (-6.0 to 4.2)
Dyspnoea	20.0 (26.5)	19.1 (24.7)	0.9 (-3.9 to 5.7)
Sleep disturbance	30.2 (33.0)	28.4 (31.0)	1.8 (-4.3 to 7.9)
Appetite loss	14.0 (27.2)	16.4 (27.0)	-2.4 (-7.5 to 2.7)
Constipation[a]	11.7 (21.8)	19.8 (29.9)	-8.1 (-13.1 to -3.1)
Diarrhoea	7.5 (18.8)	9.3 (20.8)	-1.8 (-5.6 to 2.0)
Financial impact	12.7 (25.9)	14.4 (28.3)	-1.7 (-6.9 to 3.5)

Note: scores range from 0 to 100, with higher scores representing better function or more symptomatology. [a]Difference between groups: $P = 0.002$

Only two-thirds of the record holders who had seen their GP said they had shown the GP their record. Recruitment in hospital outpatients may have led some patients to see it as belonging in secondary care. Even fewer (only a quarter) of the GPs of record-holding patients reported having seen it. This latter figure may be an underestimate, since we did not know which of these GPs had actually seen the patients. However, since questionnaires were sent to GPs at the end of the study, many may have forgotten seeing the record, and the low figure suggests that the record made relatively little impact on GPs.

The apparent lack of benefit of the record may reflect the particular circumstances of our study. The pilot study and other reports on the feasibility of patient-held records in cancer care[21,22] were limited to those receiving palliative care. Many of our study participants were in relatively good health and in infrequent contact with doctors and nurses. Patients in our study had a much better level of functioning and fewer symptoms, as measured by the EORTC QLQ C-30 questionnaire, than those with non-resectable lung cancer.[19] They also felt that communication with doctors and nurses was good, and had a real sense of participation in their care. Moreover, the majority of patients had access to a Cancer Information Centre onsite. In these circumstances it may be difficult to demonstrate that a supplementary record, even if valued, measurably improves outcome.

In two randomised trials comparing antenatal patients holding their own main records with those holding supplementary co-operation cards, patients holding the main record felt significantly more able to talk to their doctors and midwives, more in control of care,[13] and better informed.[14] One explanation for the null result in our study may be the difference between 'well' and 'sick' person care; although, in our pilot study in palliative care, patients reported that a supplementary record was valuable in promoting communication with carers and involvement with care. It may be that both obstetric and palliative care are areas in which the primary care team feels closely involved and therefore well motivated to use the record as a tool, whereas care for patients attending radiotherapy clinics is perceived as the province of the hospital.

Table 4. Statements[a] relating to communication and participation in care.

Statement	Group	Agree[b] (%)	Unsure (%)	Disagree[b] (%)	Total
I am unsure what my medicines and tablets are for	RH	6.1	2.8	91.1	179
	NC	5.6	6.1	88.3	213
I find it difficult to talk to my doctors	RH	11.4	6.5	82.1	184
	NC	8.5	6.7	84.8	224
I feel my family have not been told everything they would like to know about my illness	RH	14.6	10.3	75.1	185
	NC	15.0	11.4	73.6	220
I find it easy to ask for the help I need from doctors and nurses	RH	79.6	8.9	11.5	191
	NC	80.7	7.3	12.0	233
It has been easy to remember my appointments	RH	92.2	3.1	4.7	192
	NC	93.6	1.7	4.7	236
I find it easy to talk to my family about my illness	RH	76.9	6.5	16.7	186
	NC	84.1	5.6	10.3	233
I feel able to face all future aspects of my illness[c]	RH	61.9	28.6	9.5	189
	NC	71.4	21.8	6.7	238

[a]Statements not included in scales relating to satisfaction with communication and participation in care, and desire for information (see text). [b]Agree or strongly agree/disagree or strongly disagree. [c]Difference between groups: $P = 0.05$, Mann–Whitney test based on five-point scale.

Table 5. General practitioners' attitudes towards record holders and patient access to information (%).[a]

Q.1. Patients with potentially life-threatening cancer should have access to their medical records

	Strongly agree	Agree	Unsure	Disagree	Strongly disagree
GP had seen record ($n = 51$)	7.8	49.0	33.3	7.8	2.0
GP had not seen record ($n = 127$)	10.2	47.2	31.5	7.9	3.1
Total	9.6	47.8	32.0	7.9	2.8

Q.2. Patients should be fully informed about all matters that relate to their illness

	Strongly agree	Agree	Unsure	Disagree	Strongly disagree
GP had seen record ($n = 52$)	21.2	61.5	11.5	5.8	0.0
GP had not seen record ($n = 129$)	29.5	51.9	14.0	3.9	0.8
Total	27.1	54.7	13.3	4.4	0.6

[a]Not all GPs who answered the questionnaire responded to these questions; no significant difference between GPs who had seen and had not seen the record (Q.1: $P = 0.90$; Q.2: $P = 0.52$).

Selective use of supplementary patient-held records may be valuable in groups of patients at an active or critical stage in their disease, or in settings where there is an identified need for improved communication.

The momentum to develop tools that inform and empower patients with cancer is driven by an articulate voluntary sector, growing evidence of unmet need, and the search for mechanisms that facilitate shared care. Counter to this has been the concern that, indiscriminately used, such tools may have a negative effect on care. Our evidence shows that use of a supplementary patient-held record does not produce measurable benefit or harm.

References

1. Expert advisory Group on Cancer. *A policy framework for commissioning cancer services: Consultative Document.* London: EAGC, 1994.
2. Cassileth BR, Zupkis RV, Sutton-Smith K, March V. Information preferences among cancer patients. *Ann Intern Med* 1980; **92:** 832-836.
3. Derdiarian AK. Information needs of recently diagnosed cancer patients. *Nursing Res* 1986; **35:** 276-281.
4. National Cancer Alliance. *Patient centred cancer services: What patients say.* [Report of the National Cancer Alliance.] Oxford: National Cancer Alliance, 1996.
5. Blanchard CG, Labreque MS, Ruckdeschel JC, Balnchard EB. Information and decision making preferences of hospitalized adult cancer patients *Soc Sci Med* 1988; **27:** 1139-1145.
6. Meredith C, Symonds P, Webster L, *et al.* Information needs of cancer patients in west Scotland: cross sectional survey of patients' views. *BMJ* 1996; **313:** 724-726.
7. Fallowfield LJ. Giving sad and bad news. *Lancet* 1993; **341:** 476-470.
8. Seale C. Communication and awareness about death. A study of a random sample of dying people. *Soc Sci Med* 1991; **32:** 943-952.
9. Higginson I, Wade A, McCarthy M. Palliative care: Views of patients and their families. *BMJ* 1990; **301:** 277-281.
10. Robinson L, Stacy R. Palliative care in the community: setting guidelines for primary care teams. *Br J Gen Pract* 1994; **44:** 461-464.
11. Blythe A. Audit of terminal care in a general practice. *BMJ* 1990; **301:** 983-986.
12. Audit Comission. What seems to be the matter: communication between hospitals and patients. NHS Report 1993; no12 London. HMSO, 1993.
13. Elbourne D, Richardson M, Chalmers I, *et al.* The Newbury Maternity Care Study: a randomized controlled trial to assess a policy of women holding their own obstetric records. *Br J Obstet Gynaecol* 1987; **94:** 612-619.
14. Lovell A, Zander L, James C, *et al.* The St Thomas's Hospital maternity case notes study: a randomized controlled trial to assess the effects of giving expectant mothers their own maternity case notes. *Paediatr Perinat Epidemiol* 1987; **1:** 57-56.

15. Saffin K, Macfarlane A. How well are parent held records kept and completed? *Br J Gen Pract* 1991; **41:** 249-251.
16. Baldry M, Cheal C, Fisher B, *et al.* Giving patients their own records in general practice: experience of patients and staff. *BMJ* 1986; **292:** 596-598.
17. Gilhooly ML, McGhee SM. Medical records: practicalities and principles of patient posession. *J Med Ethics* 1991; **17(3):** 138-143.
18. Drury M, Harcourt J, Minton M. The acceptability of patients with cancer holding their own shared care record. *Psycho-oncology* 1996; **5:** 119-125.
19. Aaronson NK, Ahmedzi S, Bergman B, *et al.* The European Organization for the Treatment of Cancer QLQ-C30: A quality of life instrument for use in international clinical trials in oncology. *J Nat Cancer Inst* 1993; **85:** 365-376.
20. Wolf FM. Meta-analysis: *Quantitative Methods for Research Synthesis.* [Sage University Paper 59.] London: Sage Publications, 1986.
21. Latimer JL. A patient care travelling record for palliative care: A feasibility study. *J Palliat Care* 1991; **7:** 30-36.
22. Jones RVH. Dear Diary. *Nursing Times* 1990; **86:** 31-33.

Acknowledgements

We gratefully acknowledge the advice and support of Mrs Ella Barclay, Professor G Fowler, Dr Tim Lancaster, Professor D Mant, Dr Mike Murphy, and Dr Elaine Sugden.

Dedication

Mardy Bartlett died on 28 November 1995. Her work as a research nurse on the study continued even during her final illness. Her enthusiasm and commitment were invaluable. She is greatly missed.

Address for correspondence

Dr Mark Drury, Department of Primary Health Care, Institute of Health Sciences, Headington, Oxford OX3 7LF. E-mail: mdrury@server.dphpc.ox.ac.uk

Modelling nursing activities: electronic patient records and their discontents

Els Goorman and Marc Berg

Institute of Health Policy and Management, Erasmus University Rotterdam, Rotterdam, The Netherlands

Accepted for publication 22 September 1999

GOORMAN E and BERG M. *Nursing Inquiry* 2000; **7**: 3–9

Modelling nursing activities: electronic patient records and their discontents

A fully integrated and operating EPR in a clinical setting is hard to find: most applications can be found in outpatient or general practice settings or in isolated hospital wards. In clinical work practice problems with the electronic patient record (EPR) are frequent. These problems are at least partially due to the models of health care work embedded in EPRs. In this paper we will argue that these problems are at least partially due to the models of health care work embedded in current EPRs. We suggest that these models often contain projections of nurses' and doctors' work as it should be performed on the ward, rather than depicting how work is actually performed. We draw upon sociological insights to elucidate the fluid and pragmatic nature of healthcare work and give recommendations for the development of an empirically based EPR, which can support the work of nurses and other health care providers. We argue that these issues are of great importance to the nursing profession, since the EPR will help define the worksettings of the future. Since it is a tool that will impact the development of the nursing profession, nurses have and should have a stake in its development.

Key words: electronic patient record, nature of health-care work, nursing profession.

Electronic patient records (EPR) are expected to have a great impact on healthcare practice in the years to come. According to an influential report of the US Institute of Medicine, the EPR is 'an essential technology for health care today and in the future': the EPR will lead to a higher quality of health care, increase the scientific base of medicine and nursing, and reduce health care costs (Dick and Steen 1991). An immediate benefit of the use of EPRs, these authors argue, is the increased accessibility of the patient record. Healthcare providers who want information are no longer limited by the boundaries of wards and time because the record is always and from different places available. Moreover, an EPR is more structured and more readable than a paper record, which facilitates information retrieval.

In general, nurses seem to share these positive expectations (Goossen 1996). The majority of nurses expect that the computer will function as a nursing technology that

Correspondence: Els Goorman, Institute of Health Policy and Management, Erasmus University Rotterdam, PO Box 1738, 3000 DR Rotterdam, The Netherlands.

E-mail: <Goorman@bmg.eur.nl>; <M.Berg@bmg.eur.nl>

will make their work easier (Ngin et al. 1993). Similarly, nurses hope that the use of computerised technology will help improve their professional status (Axford and Carter 1996). More specifically, it is felt that computerization might help nurses make the high level of their skill and the complexity of their activities more visible, and attain a level of systematisation of nursing knowledge that makes it 'scientific' (based on theoretical models, empirically tested knowledge, scientific reasoning) (Wagner 1993).

Fully integrated and operating EPRs are rare, however, most applications can be found in outpatient or general practice settings, or in isolated hospital wards (Dick and Steen 1991; Collen 1995). Detailed research into the workings of EPRs in inpatient wards or emergency departments shows that problems are frequent (Harper et al. 1997; Berg 1998). Doctors often dislike working with the EPR, and nurses frequently complain about increased workloads due to a loss of overview, sluggish working routines and problems entering and locating information. Many different reasons for these problems are suggested, varying from shortcomings in present-day technology to psychological factors such as fear of change. Sociological studies suggest that problems with implementation and use of EPRs are partly related to the models that EPRs are based on (Nyce and Graves 1990; Forsythe et al. 1992; Berg et al. 1998). Technological applications that structure or guide work always require a model of that work to function. The sociological literature suggests that the model of the EPR contain a projection of medical and nursing activities, which does not match the activities of nurses and doctors as they actually take place at a ward.

The focus of this study is an investigation of the model of the EPR and its relationship to the nature of work performed by nurses. We investigated the practical functioning of an EPR on a neurological inpatients' ward in a Dutch regional hospital. To date, most studies of computer systems are based on methods that measure quantitative outcomes. Such studies often treat organizational features, user features, technological features, and information needs as static, independent, and objective rather than as dynamic, interacting constructs. Because such studies are often restricted to readily measurable static constructs, they tend to neglect aspects of cultural environment and processes of interaction and negotiation that could affect not only the outcomes, but also the constructs under study (Kaplan and Duchon 1988; Friedman and Wyatt 1997). For these reasons we decided to undertake a qualitative study and one of us (EG) spent several weeks at the ward, interviewing end-users and doing participatory observations. The interviews and participation notes were elaborated using grounded theory analysis methods (Strauss 1987). We shall briefly introduce the EPR used in the regional hospital.

The EPR is a system from a US vendor that is designed to support the primary care process. It is integrated with financial administration modules, resource management modules, and so forth. It is delivered as an assembly kit consisting of several basic screens that have to be expanded and tailored to adjust the system to the specific characteristics of the local hospital and its wards. Development of the system was a job for the automation team, which consisted of several nurses, doctors and laboratory workers who themselves had worked in this hospital for several years. Central to the system is the *order-communication* function that handles orders between different sub-information systems. This function allows orders entered by health care professionals in the nursing or doctors' room to be immediately communicated to the departments concerned (for example: the pharmacy, the X-ray department). The results of these tests are similarly made available on the system. Order-communication not only involves tests and examinations, doctors can also communicate new medication orders to nurses in this way. Patient

registration, management of waiting lists and planning of appointments is also included in the system of order-communication (Al et al. 1992).

In addition to the development of the order-communication functions, the replacement of the paper nursing and medical record keeping procedures by computer-based alternatives was also high on the agenda. By the summer of 1997, the system of order-communication was in use and the paper nursing record was largely replaced by the EPR. Due to doctors' resistance, attempts to automate medical records had not been successful, and these were therefore still in paper form. Implementation of the EPR in the regional hospital occurred step by step. At the moment of this research (summer 1997) the system was implemented in four wards. At these wards, terminals could be found in different locations: two terminals in the nursing room, two in the doctors' room, one in the investigation room and a last one in a so-called 'multifunctional' room (where meetings were held, health care professionals could speak to families, and so forth). As we will see, however, the system's functioning was far from smooth.

In the next paragraph, we will elucidate the model of work that is embedded in this EPR. We will show that this model corresponds with what we call the 'standard view' on healthcare activities as it can often be found, amongst others, in medical and nursing informatics literature.

THE EPR AND ITS MODEL OF HEALTH CARE WORK

The EPR used in the regional hospital consists of 27 000 different screens. On the neurological ward, where this investigation was undertaken, nurses have access to up to 10 000 screens. The screens are linked to each other in various ways and form several paths, consisting of up to 30 individual screens. When a nurse is working in a screen, the next screen is attainable by clicking with the mouse on a button on the screen. There is a path to order medication, a path to order an investigation and other paths for seeking information or reporting patient data. This EPR is highly structured — and it is in this structure that a model of nurses' and doctors' work can be found.

Any information technology application for workpractices relies upon, and reifies, some underlying conception of the activity that it is designed to support (Suchman 1987). This EPR is built in such a way, for example, that it can only accept data-entry in one, prefixed way. For each activity that is performed on the ward there is only one method (sometimes two) to enter the data produced by that activity. In this way the EPR contains a model of how people should handle the EPR, which implies a model of nursing and medical activities as they should be performed on the ward. As will be clear from the next three examples, this specific model derives from a 'standard', rationalist and non-empirical view of health care work.

The first example consists of the way in which medication was ordered on the ward before and after the implementation of the EPR. In theory, doctors are and were responsible for the prescription of medication and therefore should have written and signed the paper medication order forms. In daily practice, however, nurses often wrote the medication form and let doctors sign it. One management-derived goal of the implementation of the EPR was to obtain a better registration of the prescription and use of medication. So the EPR is built in such a way that it confirms the responsibility of the doctor in prescribing medication. Concurrently, the normal path to order medication via the EPR is a path for doctors. Only those users of the EPR who have an access code that is recognized by the system as a physician's code can use this specific path. In the case of an emergency, there is an alternative path, called the 'agent for' order which can be used by nurses. This 'agent for' order consists of a path that contains more screens, is more intricate and takes more time than the path designed for use by the physicians. Yet, although this path was designed as a detour, we noticed that when the EPR was implemented, nurses often ordered medication with an 'agent for' order. Why did this happen? Why did nurses order medication instead of the doctor?

Until the moment of the implementation of the EPR, doctors were used to working with the paper medication ordering system (Kardex), which is easy to handle and does not take much time. With the EPR it takes much more time for doctors to order medication, and time is a scarce resource for healthcare workers. Furthermore, experienced nurses often give patients medication when there is no doctor around to prescribe what is needed. They might consult the doctor by phone, or they might have been told what to do if a certain clinical situation would arise. Often, however, there is a whole repertoire of drugs (such as pain-relieving medication) which is informally agreed to be controlled by experienced nurses. For these practices, however, the 'agent for' order is too intricate and takes too much time. Our point is that the EPR is based upon an abstract conception in which medication is always ordered and prescribed by a doctor, who gives the order to the nurse, who, in turn, gives the medication to the patient. This standard model does not reckon with the fact that in daily practice there are many practical and good reasons for nurses to order medication.

The second example that shows the standard view of nursing and medical work embedded in the model of the EPR is closely related to the first one. It is about the paths of the EPR which consist of multiple, linked screens. To enter or retrieve information users must use the paths that are especially developed for these purposes. In practice, nurses and other users of the EPR complain about problems locating and seeking information. Nurses reporting on their care have to use a path that belongs to the 'main menu'. Often nurses need more information about a patient during this 'reporting' activity, so they want to search data in the EPR. Therefore they must go into the 'seek menu'. But before one can go into the 'seek menu' it is necessary to stop the activity in the 'main menu', leave this 'main menu' and start in the 'seek menu'. Switching between the menus is not possible. To work around this problem, nurses often work with two terminals at the same time: they report on one terminal and when they want to look for some information they log in on another terminal. In this way they overcome the EPR's limitation, and they do not have to leave the 'main menu' path they were working in.

Again, this example shows how the EPR embeds a standard view of nursing work that presumes that nurses first look for information, then take care of patients and after that report what they have been doing. The designers of this EPR conceptualize nursing and medical work as processes that can be split up in several steps with a logical sequence. But healthcare workers' need for information is not structured in the way presumed by this standard view of medical and nursing work. Rather, their need for information is fluid and diverse, and hard to predict at any given point. So, storing patient data in a rigid structure (in a long chain of screens, with prefixed entries) means that it is very difficult to retrieve information at the moment that health care providers need these patient data.

A third and last example is the way in which the screens of the EPR are built. By this we do not mean the construction of the paths, which we elucidated before, but the construction of the individual screens which make up the paths. The screens of the investigated EPR are filled with preprogrammed words and there is not much place to enter free text. To use the screens, a user must click with the mouse on the words in order to make a sentence. The construction of these screens is in line with the current tendency to thoroughly structure the EPR: to reduce the amount of free text as much as possible, to use prefixed options for input, to implement care maps and protocols and to build in workflows (Berg et al. 1998).

The use of the prefixed entries, combined with the fact that there is almost no space to enter free text, is another manifestation of the standard view of nursing work that is built into the EPR. According to the developers of this EPR, the reporting activities of healthcare professionals can or should be split up into several separated steps, using several screens with prefixed entries. Yet nurses often complain about how difficult it is to work with the prefixed words, especially if they want to report psychological, social or emotional information about patients. A screen with prefixed entries appears too limited to account for the richness of nurses' work tasks and the multiple dimensions of their work with patients.[1]

These three examples have shown aspects of a standard view of nurses' and doctors' work that is incorporated in the model of this EPR: diverse paths for different users, no possibility to switch between the paths, paths which are formed by numerous screens and prefixed entries that fill these screens. This system conceptualises health care activities as processes which can be split up in several steps with a logical sequence. It embeds, moreover, an individualised depiction of medical and nursing work (Berg 1997a). The EPR is set up in a step-by-step fashion, often directed at an individual 'user' and generally limited to medical data and interventions. Contextual aspects, the *process* of data gathering, and the interactions between healthcare workers are not taken to be important features for design. The structure of this EPR does not appear to be able to handle the fluidity and pragmatism that characterizes the daily practice of healthcare activities. It constantly generates clashes with the ongoing work, resulting in more work for nurses rather than less, and in less overview for healthcare workers rather than more. That, it seems, cannot be the goal of implementing high-tech IT applications in health-care.

It is important therefore to present an alternative, more empirically adequate perspective on healthcare activities. Only by starting from such a perspective can we hope to achieve systems that support rather than obstruct this practice.

SOCIOLOGICAL PERSPECTIVE ON HEALTHCARE ACTIVITIES

Typical of current inpatient care is the ongoing flow of activities with and around the patient, and the increasing number of health care professionals who have a function in this process. To conceptualize this stream of activities, and its unfolding over time, Strauss and his co-workers have coined the term 'patient trajectory' (Strauss et al. 1985). The term trajectory refers not only to the pathophysiological unfolding of patients' disease but to the total organization of work done over that course, plus the impact of these processes on those involved with that work and its organization. For different illnesses, the trajectory will involve different nursing and medical actions, different kinds of skills and other resources, a different parcelling out of tasks among the workers (including, perhaps, kin and the patient), and involving quite different relationships among the workers (Strauss et al. 1985). Patients' trajectories often involve several units and individuals within a hospital, which have to co-ordinate their efforts. This co-ordination is made difficult by the fact that work with patients is of an evolving and nonpredictable character, requiring continual readjustment and communication (Egger and Wagner 1993; Atkinson 1995). Depending on the physical condition of the patient, the results of the investigations and the observations of nurses and doctors, the management of the trajectory evolves. New medications are started, other medication is stopped, investigations are ordered and an operation is performed. Continuously readjusting the patients' management requires constant and intense communication between nurses, doctors and other healthcare providers (Timmermans et al. 1998).

Management of patient trajectories requires much *co-operative work:* the work of nurses and doctors is linked to the work of physiotherapists, dieticians, ward secretaries and lab technicians. At the core of this conception of co-operative work is the notion of *interdependence in work.* People engage in co-operative work when they are mutually dependent in their work and therefore are required to co-operate in order to get their work done (Schmidt and Bannon 1992). Being mutually dependent *in work* means that A relies positively on the quality and timeliness of B's work and vice versa. It should thus primarily be conceived of as a positive, though by no means necessarily harmonious, interdependence.

Yet at the same time, healthcare professionals are semi-autonomous in their work. Co-operative work is *distributed* in the sense that all people involved in the management of patients' trajectories have their own tasks and goals. They all work and make decisions in unique circumstances faced with different problems and confronted with varying contingencies. Different people react from differing points of view, and have different criteria, heuristics, interests and motives. This phenomenon can be witnessed in the

---

[1] One of the referees commented that the reason for the availability of pre-fixed texts is probably because 'outcomes' of practice are 'pre-figured' as being standard, and therefore amenable for costing calculations. Although this comment could be true for other EPRs with pre-fixed entries, the use of such entries in this case stems from the ideological belief in unifying and structuring reporting data throughout the organization. The data are not used for any other purpose.

constant transformations in the focus and content of the activities undertaken to manage a patient's trajectory (Bosk 1979; Frohock 1986; Berg 1992; Casper 1998).

Due to the very interdependence in work that gave rise to the co-operative work arrangement in the first place, the distributed nature of the arrangement must be managed. The distributed activities must be *articulated* with each other. Articulation work arises as an integral part of co-operation work, as a set of activities required to manage the distributed nature of co-operative work in order to ensure smooth co-ordination and co-operation (Schmidt and Bannon 1992). In the words of Strauss, articulation work is 'a kind of supra-type of work in any division of labour, done by various actors' (Strauss et al. 1985). Gerson and Star (1986) describe articulation work as follows:

> All tasks involved in assembling, scheduling, monitoring and co-ordinating all of the steps necessary to complete a production task (patient trajectory). This means carrying through a course of action despite local contingencies, unanticipated glitches, incommensurable opinions and beliefs or inadequate knowledge of local circumstances. Every real world system is an open system...No formal description of a system (or plan for its work) can thus be complete...every real world system thus requires articulation to deal with the unanticipated contingencies that arise. Articulation resolves these inconsistencies by packaging a compromise that 'gets the job done' that is, that closes the system locally and temporally so that the work can go on. (p. 166)

In healthcare work, articulation work is mostly done by nurses. It is mostly invisible: it is work that needs to be done but that is not often recognized by others as being an important aspect of the work (Star 1991). Yet the articulation work performed by nurses is essential in keeping healthcare practice operating smoothly (McCloskey 1995). Because of their proximity to the patient, nurses have a key role in co-ordinating patient care and protecting them from organizational turbulence (Allen 1997). Nurses are the 'glue' that holds complex healthcare practices together (Markussen 1995). In order to function as competent team members, then, nurses do not only have to be competent practitioners of their own profession: they need to have the skills to manage the turbulent intersection of *all* healthcare professionals' work tasks that constitute the work environment.

CONCLUSION AND CONSIDERATIONS FOR DESIGN

As we have elaborated above, the EPR studied embeds a model of nursing and medical activities that derives from a standard view on these activities. Although the study was conducted on an inpatient neurological ward, the theoretical points made here address medical work in general.[2] The examples discussed (the 'agent for' order, nurses working on two terminals, and the prefixed entries on the screens) illustrate the conflicts between the inbuilt structure of this EPR and the nature of nurses' and doctors' work. These are not isolated examples, specific to this single case: they reflect a recurrent set of issues that can be found in similar situations both within and outside medicine (Suchman 1987; Henderson 1991; Forsythe 1992; Star 1995; Wagner 1995; Berg 1997b). Although it was not the aim of this paper, it is worth noting that the use of an EPR also has consequences for other healthcare practitioners, such as laboratory, pharmacy and radiology staff.[3]

The reason for the conflicts described above is the gap between the model of work implemented in the structure of the EPR and the co-operative, pragmatically structured work of healthcare providers as it is actually performed on the ward. For developers to bridge this gap, several considerations are crucial.

First, developers of EPRs need to recognize that developing systems for healthcare practices should be based on empirical knowledge of the inner workings of such practices. In order to avoid building systems with built-in assumptions that clash with the realities of every day healthcare work, developers should acquire a more direct insight into the exigencies of this work before starting the design process. Such in-depth knowledge requires participatory observation and interviews with (future) end-users of an EPR. Only with such methods is it possible to recognize the pragmatically structured, complex functioning of medical work, and to build systems that encompass such awareness. Implementing information technologies necessarily transforms the healthcare practices at stake — this is unavoidable and, moreover, a central and legitimate reason to acquire IT technology. Yet some IT applications end

---

[2] On a neurological ward, turnover is low (patients are hospitalized for longer periods of time) and the amount and complexity of data captured is far less in comparison to highly specialized wards, such as intensive care. We assume that the problems addressed with the EPR on this specific neurological ward increase on wards where turnover and intensity of data capture and exchange are higher.

[3] Issues concerning the structure of an EPR and the organization of healthcare activities are not only relevant for nurses and doctors but apply also to all other health care professionals where organization of patient care is at stake. Likewise, not only positions of nurses and doctors could be transformed, but also those of other healthcare professionals. These comments stress the importance of involving future end-users in the development of EPRs, notwithstanding the fact that involvement of all end-users presumably hinders more than facilitates this development.

up fruitfully integrated with work practices (and enhance healthcare workers' responsibilities, enhance the quality of delivered care, and so forth) and others end up actually hindering the smooth flow of ongoing work. Ignoring the practical and often informal complexities of healthcare work is a certain way toward the latter option (Drazen 1995; Berg et al. 1998; Bowker et al. 1997).

Second, it is crucial that we start developing systems that acknowledge the fluid, pragmatic and practical nature of healthcare work. Only by avoiding the tendency to overly structure the EPR, and by allowing flexibility in roles and task sequences will it become possible to develop a record system that supports the work that is performed on the wards. We do not need to start from scratch here: there is a growing body of literature that takes the nature of work practices as described above as a starting point for adequate design (Nyce and Graves 1990; Schmidt and Bannon 1992; Schneider and Wagner 1993; Berg 1998; Bowker et al. 1997). Yet the issues are far from easy: how can an EPR facilitate the storage and retrieval of patient information in a way that matches doctors' and nurses' practical working routines and needs? How can an EPR truly facilitate the management of patients' trajectories without importing too much structure? Is it possible to support the invisible, articulation work that is mostly performed by nurses? These are some of the challenges that face us.

Third, it is important to draw the future end-users into the development and implementation of EPRs. They have hands-on experience about the tasks that have to be performed, and they can give suggestions and directions in order to develop an EPR in close co-operation with developers. An even more preferable situation would occur if nurses and other healthcare providers would be trained to function as nurse-developers. There are several specific tasks for these nurse-developers and doctor-developers. Analysis of nursing information needs by nurses and of doctors' information needs by doctors is one of these tasks. It is probable that these information needs will not always be the same for nurses and doctors. Another specific task for these nurse-developers is the marking out of the nursing profession. Since the model of the EPR is a representation of nursing activities, the development of EPRs is an opportunity for nurses to further define what the nursing profession consists of. The computerisation of health-care might be a forum to debate these questions and since these issues come to play anyway, it is more desirable to take up this challenge openly than to let others (often covertly) decide the matter for the profession.

Finally, it is important to realize that developing appropriate models for EPRs, and opting to embrace or oppose a standard view on medical and nursing activities, implies taking a political stand. As described above, an important part of nurses' work consists of the performance of mostly invisible work which contributes to the management of patient trajectories. This key role is not recognizable in the standard view of medical and nursing work that is conceptualized in the EPR. The development of appropriate models for EPR might help nurses to make the high level of their skill and the complexity of nursing activities more visible, and thereby attain a level of systematization of nursing knowledge that makes it 'scientific'. Along similar lines, the development of EPRs is an opportunity for nurses to further the struggle in professional autonomy. Computer-based documentation of nursing activities can be a political instrument in the demands for more adequate pay, better staffing and lower work loads (Wagner 1993). At the same time, however, this may turn out to be a risky strategy. The arguments described above can take another turn in the hands of managers, for example. With increasing visibility, then, nurses might find themselves becoming a target of social control and surveillance (Timmermans et al. 1998). In all these issues, the game is not yet fully played – but if the nursing profession wants to become a player in this game, we must not let the development of the EPR slip from our hands.

REFERENCES

Al CJ, J Driessen and J van Bokhoven. 1992. De Informatier-evolutie. Het Ziekenhuis 22: 234–59.

Allen D. 1997. The nursing-medical boundary: A negotiated order? *Sociology of Health and Illness* 19: 498–520.

Atkinson P. 1995. *Medical talk and medical work.* London: Sage.

Axford RI and BEL Carter. 1996. Impact of clinical information systems on nursing practice/nurses' perspectives. *Computers in Nursing* 14: 156–63.

Berg M. 1992. The construction of medical disposals: Medical sociology and medical problem solving in clinical practice. *Sociology of Health and Illness* 14: 151–80.

Berg M. 1997a. Problems and promises of the protocol. *Social Science of Medicine* 44: 1081–8.

Berg M. 1997b. *Rationalizing medical work: Decision support techniques and medical practices.* Cambridge: MIT Press.

Berg M. 1998. Medical work and the computer-based patient record: A sociological perspective. *Methods of Information in Medicine* 37: 294–301.

Berg M, C Langenberg, I van den Berg and J Kwakkernaat. 1998. Considerations for sociotechnical design: Experiences with an electronic patient record in a clinical context. *International Journal of Medical Informatics* 52: 243–51.

Bosk CL. 1979. *Forgive and remember: Managing medical failure.* Chicago: University of Chicago Press.

Bowker G, L Gasser, L Star and B Turner, eds. 1997. *Social science, technical systems, and cooperative work: Beyond the great divide.* Mahwah, NJ: Lawrence Erlbaum.

Casper MJ. 1998. *The making of the unborn patient: A social anatomy of fetal surgery.* New Brunswick, NJ, USA: Rutgers University Press.

Collen ME. 1995. *A history of medical informatics in the United States, 1950–90.* American Medical Informatics Association.

Dick RE and E Steen. 1991. *The computer based patient record: An essential technology for health care.* Washington D.C.: National Academy Press.

Drazen EL, ed. 1995. *Patient care information systems: Successful design and implementation.* New York: Springer.

Egger E and I Wagner. 1993. Negotiating temporal orders: The case of collaborative time management in a surgery clinic. *Computer Supported Cooperative Work* 1: 255–75.

Forsythe DE. 1992. *16th Symposium on computer applications in medical care,* ed. ME Frisse. New York: McGraw-Hill, 505–9.

Forsythe DE, BG Buchanan, JA Osheroff and RA Miller. 1992. Concept of medical information: An observational study of physicians' information needs. *Computers and Biomedical Research* 25: 181–200.

Friedman CP and JC Wyatt. 1997. *Evaluation methods in medical informatics.* New York: Springer.

Frohock FM. 1986. *Special care: Medical decisions at the beginning of life.* Chicago: University of Chicago Press.

Gerson E and SL Star. 1986. Analyzing due process in the workplace. *ACM Transactions on Office Information Systems* 4: 257–70.

Goossen WTF. 1996. Nursing information management and processing: A framework and definition for system analysis, design and evoluation. *International Journal of Bio-Medical Computing* 40: 187–95.

Harper R, KPA O'Hara, AJ Sellen and DJR Duthie. 1997. Towards the paperless hospital? *British Journal of Anaesthesia* 78: 762–7.

Henderson K. 1991. Flexible sketches and inflexible data bases: Visual communication, conscription devices,

and boundary objects in design engineering. 16: 448–73.

Kaplan B and D Duchon. 1988. Combining qualitative and quantitative methods in information systems research: A case study. *MIS Quarterly* 12: 570–86.

Markussen R. 1995. In *The cultures of computing,* ed. SL Star, 161–76. Oxford: Blackwell Publishers.

McCloskey JM. 1995. Recognizing the management role of all nurses. *N & HC: Perspectives on Community* 16: 307–8.

Ngin P, LM Simms and M Erbin-Roesemann. 1993. Work excitement among computer users in nursing. *Computers in Nursing* 11: 127–33.

Nyce JM and W Graves. III. 1990. The construction of knowledge in neurology: Implications for hypermedia system development. *Artificial Intelligence in Medicine* 2: 315–22.

Schmidt K and L Bannon. 1992. Taking CSCW seriously: Supporting articulation work. 1: 7–40.

Schneider K and I Wagner. 1993. Constructing the 'Dossier représentatif': Computer-based information-sharing in French hospitals. 1: 229–53.

Star SL. 1991. *Women, work and computerization: Understanding and overcoming bias in work and education,* eds I Erikson, B Kitchenham and K Tijdens, 81–92. North Holland: Elsevier Science Publishers BV.

Star SL, ed. 1995. *The cultures of computing.* Oxford: Blackwell Publishers.

Strauss A. 1987. *Qualitative analysis for social scientists.* Cambridge: Cambridge University Press.

Strauss A, S Fagerhaugh, B Suczek and C Wiener. 1985. *Social organization of medical work.* Chicago: University of Chicago Press.

Suchman L. 1987. *Plan and situated actions: The problem of human-machine communication.* Cambridge: Cambridge University Press.

Timmermans S, GC Bowker and SL Star. 1998. *Differences in medicine: Unraveling practices, techniques, and bodies,* eds M Berg and A Mol, 202–25. Durham, England: Duke University Press.

Wagner I. 1993. Women's voice: The case of nursing information systems. *AI and Society* 7: 295–310.

Wagner I. 1995. Hard times: The politics of women's work in computerized environments. *European Journal of Women's Studies* 2: 295–324.

UMLS Concept Indexing for Production Databases:

A Feasibility Study

PRAKASH NADKARNI, MD, ROLAND CHEN, MD, CYNTHIA BRANDT, MD, MPH

Abstract **Objectives:** To explore the feasibility of using the National Library of Medicine's Unified Medical Language System (UMLS) Metathesaurus as the basis for a computational strategy to identify concepts in medical narrative text preparatory to indexing. To quantitatively evaluate this strategy in terms of true positives, false positives (spuriously identified concepts) and false negatives (concepts missed by the identification process).

Methods: Using the 1999 UMLS Metathesaurus, the authors processed a training set of 100 documents (50 discharge summaries, 50 surgical notes) with a concept-identification program, whose output was manually analyzed. They flagged concepts that were erroneously identified and added new concepts that were not identified by the program, recording the reason for failure in such cases. After several refinements to both their algorithm and the UMLS subset on which it operated, they deployed the program on a test set of 24 documents (12 of each kind).

Results: Of 8,745 matches in the training set, 7,227 (82.6 percent) were true positives, whereas of 1,701 matches in the test set, 1,298 (76.3 percent) were true positives. Matches other than true positive indicated potential problems in production-mode concept indexing. Examples of causes of problems were redundant concepts in the UMLS, homonyms, acronyms, abbreviations and elisions, concepts that were missing from the UMLS, proper names, and spelling errors.

Conclusions: The error rate was too high for concept indexing to be the only production-mode means of preprocessing medical narrative. Considerable curation needs to be performed to define a UMLS subset that is suitable for concept matching.

■ **J Am Med Inform Assoc.** 2001;8:80–91.

Affiliation of authors: Yale University School of Medicine, New Haven, Connecticut.

This work was supported in part by National Institutes of Health grants R01 LM06843-01 from the National Library of Medicine and U01 CA78266-02 from the National Cancer Institute.

The authors will provide the relational UMLS schema used in this study (plus UMLS data from sources that have not imposed restrictions on distribution) and the Microsoft Access front end (which includes Concept Locator) to anyone who makes a written request.

Correspondence and reprints: Prakash M. Nadkarni, MD, Center for Medical Informatics, Yale University School of Medicine, P.O. Box 208009, New Haven, CT 06520-8009; e-mail: <Prakash.Nadkarni@yale.edu>.

Received for publication: 2/29/00; accepted for publication: 7/31/00.

Free text, like that found in discharge summaries and progress notes, is an important part of the electronic patient record, because it captures nuances of information that coded information cannot. *Information retrieval* is the field of informatics concerned with the processing of free text, typically by domain-independent methods.[1,2] With the ubiquity of the World Wide Web (where most information is textual), information retrieval technology is now mainstream. Several vendors of relational database management systems have integrated information retrieval with their technologies. We emphasize that information retrieval is ancillary to, and does not replace, conventional means of querying patient data through relational tables.

Information retrieval relies on preprocessing a collection of documents to speed up subsequent retrieval of documents that are relevant to a user's query, based on keywords of interest contained in them.* General-purpose Web retrieval engines, such as Yahoo or Excite, index the *words* in documents. For documents belonging to a single domain such as medicine, however, word indexing does not leverage domain knowledge; for example, synonymous phrases are not automatically recognized. Searches of medical free text that is indexed only by word would require a user to manually specify synonymous forms or risk missing relevant documents.

Using concepts in a domain-specific thesaurus can enhance retrieval; that is, we can index the *concepts* identified in a document. Concept-identification approaches are discussed in the next section. For medical records, detection of a concept in a document does not in itself make that document relevant for that concept. The concept may refer to a finding that was looked for but absent or ruled out, or that occurred in the remote past. The recording of "significant negatives" is important in medicine, and robust handling of negation in narrative is still an open problem in information retrieval.

The Unified Medical Language System (UMLS) Metathesaurus (the world's largest domain-specific thesaurus) of the National Library of Medicine (NLM)[3] has been the focus of much research. The present work explores the use of the UMLS for a high-specificity algorithm suitable for automated concept matching (and thereby, indexing) of medical free text.† We quantify the algorithm's success rate with sample data and quantify instances of failure. We use failure analysis to refine both the algorithm and the UMLS subset that it relies on, so that future efforts to improve the success rate may be directed appropriately and optimally.

Background

Approaches to Querying Medical Text Using Controlled Thesauri

One way to use a thesaurus in querying medical text is through close integration of the thesaurus with the query program. When a user specifies a query in terms of one or more keywords of interest, synonyms

of those keywords are located and added to the original query, thereby expanding (or broadening) it.

Studies using medical vocabularies for query broadening by intensive generation of lexical variants (including synonyms, abbreviations and acronyms, and morphological variants) have been carried out by the natural language processing group at the NLM and are described in Aronson et al.,[9] Aronson and Rindflesch,[10] Divita et al.,[11] and Rindflesch and Aronson.[12,13] An interesting approach described by Aronson et al.[9] uses a program called MetaMap. Metamap transforms the text in a document by limited syntactic analysis that recognizes simple noun phrases. After variant generation, the resulting phrases are matched to UMLS concepts, where possible, and then replaced with the preferred form of the matched concept (thereby reducing variability in the text). The transformed text, termed "surrogate text" by the authors, is then indexed with a retrieval system to allow query. The work described by Aronson et al.[9] used the well-known SMART retrieval system,[14] whereas the work described by Aronson and Rindflesch[10] used a more recent system, INQUERY.[15]

Srinivasan[16,17] has described an alternative approach that integrates thesaurus-derived document markup (though not the thesaurus itself). This method, termed *retrieval feedback* by the author, has been evaluated with a MEDLINE collection. It relies on the fact that two kinds of vocabularies are used to index MEDLINE documents. The first is the Medical Subject Headings (MeSH), a controlled vocabulary that is part of the UMLS; trained human indexers who carefully read the document's abstract have, historically, performed MeSH indexing. In addition, the documents are indexed by non-stop-words in the document title and abstract, which constitute a relatively uncontrolled vocabulary. In the retrieval feedback approach, documents that are returned with a high relevance rank in response to a user's query are selected, and the MeSH and non-MeSH keywords associated with them are used to expand the original query.

Concept Identification in Medical Narrative

We classify methods used to identify concepts in medical narrative into two categories, phrase-based and sentence-based. We discuss each in turn.

Phrase-based Methods

Phrase-based concept-identification methods use natural language processing to scan narrative and identify word and phrases of interest. These are then used to search the thesaurus. Most research has utilized noun phrases, as in the work of Elkin et al.[18] Aronson

---

* This process, termed *indexing*, is described in Appendix 1, which appears as supplemental material to this article in *JAMIA Online*, at www.jamia.org.
† An overview of the UMLS schema is provided in Appendix 2, which also appears as supplemental material to this article in *JAMIA Online*.

and Rindflesch's MetaMap program, summarized earlier, is an augmentation of the Elkin approach. A popular freeware natural language processing package for phrase recognition is the Xerox part-of-speech tagger[19]; this technology (used by Metamap, among others) has recently been commercialized as the LinguistX package.[20] Another commercial tagger is CLARIT, whose use has been described by Spackman and Hersh[21] and Evans et al.[22]

A criticism of the use of noun phrases alone is that, in medical narrative, many concepts can be identified correctly only through other parts of speech that are close to the noun phrase; for example, "blood pressure was *greatly elevated*" implies hypertension as opposed to blood pressure alone. Verb phrases such as "surgically resected" are intrinsically meaningful; the UMLS includes a large number of non-noun concepts. Furthermore, the same concept may be divided across two noun phrases, as in "hypertension is secondary to renal disease," which indicates renal hypertension.

Syntactic structure within a document determines the level of sophistication needed by a parser to successfully match concepts. Thus, in the above example, if the phrase "greatly elevated blood pressure" were encountered instead, it might be successfully matched because all four words constitute a single noun phrase with a terminal head ("pressure"). Aronson et al.[9] show that even a relatively simple parsing approach, "under-specified syntactic analysis" (identification of simple noun phrases with the head rightmost) is adequate in many cases.

In an attempt to overcome the limitations of single noun phrases, alternative approaches have attempted to use larger units of text; we will shortly illustrate, however, that these run against the limits of computational intractability. We believe that the phrase-based approach is fundamentally sound, and have used this approach for the work described in this paper.

Sentence-based Approaches

To address the problem of single concepts being split across multiple phrases, sentence-based approaches process a larger unit of text at a time. The approaches described to date rely on simple elimination of stop words and do not use part-of-speech tagging.

The SAPHIRE family of algorithms devised by Hersh and Greenes[23–25] exemplifies these approaches. The earliest SAPHIRE algorithm matched substrings of stemmed input text to stemmed concepts in a thesaurus,[23] making multiple passes across a block of text to identify all concepts. Its sensitivity was vulnerable

to the order of words in a phrase in the text, which needed to be the same as in the thesaurus to match. A newer, word-order-insensitive algorithm, first mentioned by Hersh et al.[24] and later described by Hersh and Hickman,[25] permuted the order of individual words in input text. It processed input documents a line at a time, up to each carriage return. To prevent concepts from being split by carriage returns, some carriage returns were first removed through a filtering program, so that the indexing process in effect processed the data a sentence at a time.

Some limitations of sentence-based approaches are as follows:

- In contrast to phrase-based approaches, sentence-based approaches err toward reduced specificity (i.e., more false positives). If a sentence contains multiple concepts, permuting words may spuriously generate valid concepts that were not implied in the original text. For example, the text segment "spleen rupture and normal stomach" (in an emergency surgery note) will match the concept of stomach rupture.

- While processing data a sentence at a time greatly improves recognition of concepts that are split across phrases, it cannot guarantee complete success. In the (admittedly artificial) example, "*Blood pressure* was recorded in the supine position. It was found to be *greatly elevated*," the concept of hypertension is split across two sentences.

- Finally, sentence-based approaches have the potential to be extremely machine-intensive.[‡]

Partial Matches in Concept Indexing

In 1995, Hersh and Leone[30] described a completely new SAPHIRE algorithm for interactive query of the UMLS. This algorithm allows partial matches and returns concepts in descending order of relevance; an elegant Web implementation can currently be accessed via http://www.ohsu.edu/cliniweb/saphint/. While it is appropriate for interactive UMLS query, however, we find this algorithm unsuitable for automated concept indexing of medical text, because there is no obvious computational strategy for eliminating false positive partial matches that pass the SAPHIRE threshold. If false positives are more numerous than true positives, then most entries in the concept index will be misleading.

---

‡ Sentence-based approaches are discussed in Appendix 3, which appears as supplemental material to this article in *JAMIA Online*, at www.jamia.org.

In a preliminary experiment, we implemented this algorithm and tested it with a surgery note containing the term "ligamentum flavum" (a ligament that connects adjacent vertebrae). Apart from the exact match "ligamentum flavum," we also got more than 30 partial matches for each pair of adjacent vertebrae—"C1/C2 ligamentum flavum," "C2/C3 ligamentum flavum," and so on, up to the coccyx. (The operation site, the lumbar spine, was noted two sentences previously in the narrative note.) This experience caused us to lean toward high specificity in our concept-matching approach, even at the cost of some sensitivity.

Thesaurus Issues: Composite vs. General Concepts

In the UMLS, which depends on its source vocabularies for comprehensiveness, *general* (primitive, atomic) concepts as well as relatively specific, *composite* concepts are formed by combining two or more general concepts. Thus, "carcinoma of pancreas" is a composite of "carcinoma" and "pancreas." The inclusion of composite terms depends on the source-vocabulary curators. Thus, "digitalis-induced atrial fibrillation" does not exist; if encountered in text, it can only match two separate concepts, "digitalis" and "atrial fibrillation." The most specific concept cannot always be matched. In the example "hypertension is secondary to renal disease," phrase-based approaches will miss "renal hypertension," instead matching "hypertension" and "renal disease" separately.

Sometimes, composite concepts exist, but the concepts from which they are derived are missing. For example, "seizure activity," an electroencephalographic finding, is missing, although "monitor for seizure activity" and "seizure activity not present" exist. When a particular general concept is missing from the thesaurus, false positive matches may result as an artifact of the concept-matching algorithm. A more specific concept (which is a child of the general concept) may be matched erroneously to a phrase in the text simply because it provides the closest (or a unique) match from all the concepts in the thesaurus.

Ambiguous Terms: Homonyms, Acronyms and Abbreviations

Homonyms are strings that map to multiple concepts. For example, "anesthesia" refers to loss of sensation as a clinical finding or to a procedure ancillary to surgery. Without contextual (i.e., domain plus syntactic) knowledge, it is difficult to match the phrase to the correct concept. To disambiguate the word "immunology"—which can refer to study of a bio-

logical function, a family of laboratory procedures, or a biomedical occupation—Rindflesch and Aronson[13] used a set of rules based on patterns in the enclosing sentence. Scaling up this approach is a daunting task, however; the 1999 UMLS lists 13,688 ambiguous term entries. Other methods, however, that are less labor intensive than manually devising rules (e.g., machine learning) have yet to be explored.

Much research in word-sense disambiguation tends to yield solutions that are highly domain-specific and nongeneralizable. However, Aronson et al.[9] describe a potentially powerful and generalizable approach, by which the contents of the UMLS Semantic Network (every concept has one or more semantic types) might be used to disambiguate homonymous concepts on the basis of the semantic types of adjacent, nonambiguous concepts.

Some acronyms and abbreviations in the UMLS are also words in their own right; e.g., "PEG" for polyethylene glycol and "cAMP" for cyclic adenosine monophosphate. While acronyms in published biomedical literature might be recognized by case, we found that case was too inconsistent to be relied on in medical notes. The UMLS's coverage of common abbreviations is not complete; missing, for example, is "VTach" for "ventricular tachycardia." There is currently no way to query the UMLS data for all instances of abbreviations or acronyms, because such terms are not explicitly flagged.

Methods

The experiment was divided into two phases. The first, *training* phase involved refinement of the concept-matching algorithm (and curation of the UMLS data on which it relied) by the first two authors, using a set of 50 discharge summaries and 50 surgery notes. These were obtained from the Veterans Administration Medical Center in West Haven, Connecticut, and were uploaded into a database table as text ("memo") fields. The notes spanned several specialties; for example, surgery notes spanned ophthalmology, neurosurgery, cardiac surgery, orthopedics, and general surgery.

The training phase was important in enabling us to identify the *range* of conditions under which concept matching could fail or be otherwise problematic. We used two different types of document to test our algorithm over a greater range of medical subdomains. The two documents types also differed significantly in structure. Surgery notes were typically very telegraphic, with sentences conveying the facts rather than possessing a fully formed grammatical structure. Discharge notes varied widely in structure. Some were terse, whereas others were highly verbose and contained enough explanatory text to be understood by a non-medical reader.[§]

In the second, *test* phase, we tested the algorithm with 24 new documents (12 discharge summaries, 12 surgery notes). An independent expert (the third author) first manually identified concepts in these notes, also recording negation of a concept where present. Subsequently, the third author inspected the output of the concept-identification program for these documents, and performed a failure analysis. The numbers obtained here provided a more realistic estimate of how the matching algorithm would perform in practice.

We first provide an overview of the steps performed in the training phase:

1. A list of stop-words was obtained from an electronic source[8] for use in other steps of our experiment. As will be described, we had to alter this list several times during the course of our experiment.

2. A Microsoft SQL Server database had been previously created to store a relational version of the UMLS 99 Metathesaurus. Only the English subset of UMLS was used. Extra tables were added to this database to store data and results for the present study, and a subset of the UMLS data was created for use in concept matching. We also created a Microsoft Access front end to access the database from our desktop machines over a local network.

3. The notes were preprocessed to remove standard headings (e.g., "diagnosis," "follow-up"). Each note was then written to a text file, which was then processed with a commercial phrase-identification program (described shortly). The program's output, which consists of delimited text fields, was imported programmatically into the database. The imported data were used for two different purposes.

   For the first, we created rich text format (RTF) equivalents of each note. (RTF is a machine-independent format originally defined by Microsoft.) We then programmatically color-coded different parts of the note text on the basis of phrases present in the parsed output. The purpose of the color-coding was to allow easy visual identification of possible problems with the phrase recognizer as

well as with our own concept-matching code. The color-coding scheme is described later in this section.

For the second, the phrases were processed with a concept-finding algorithm to identify matches from the UMLS subset, and matches were written to tables in the database.

4. Finally, the first two authors inspected each note visually along with the matches. Where our algorithm failed to recognize relevant concepts, these were manually added to the matches list and flagged as false negatives. (This study was not concerned with quantifying agreement between authors about which concepts were relevant. Therefore, the rule for resolving differences was that a concept was relevant if either author deemed it to be.) Each automatically matched concept was inspected manually for correctness in the context of its occurrence in the document, and problems were flagged with codes indicating the nature of failure.

We underwent several rounds of iteration. Thus, the output of an earlier stage of the experiment typically revealed shortcomings of the existing strategy and suggested obvious algorithmic or curation refinements.

For the test phase, the third author marked concepts of interest in each document through a macro that operated on the plain-ASCII document after it was imported into Microsoft Word. This macro (associated with a function key) allowed electronic highlighting of selected text by the addition of a yellow background. All the test documents were manually marked up this way and saved to disk. Then, a Microsoft Access program written by the third author opened each document in turn, identified phrases highlighted in yellow, and wrote each phrase, along with the document ID and the byte offset relative to the start of the document, to a database table. The test documents were then processed by the concept-recognition program, which also records byte offsets for matched concepts. The list of manually flagged concepts and automatically detected concepts were then visually compared side-by-side and sorted by document ID and byte offset, so that failure and problems in matching could be detected easily. The original documents were also inspected if the context of a particular phrase in a document had to be determined.[¶]

---

§ Part of a discharge summary is illustrated in Appendix 4, Figure 1, which appears as supplemental material to this article in *JAMIA Online*, at www.jamia.org.

¶ Details of each step, including the concept-matching algorithm, are also provided in Appendix 4, which appears online.

Table 1 ∎

The Results of Concept Matching

Match Type	Training Set (100 documents)			Test Set (24 documents)	
	No. of Matches	Percentage	Distinct Concepts	No. of Matches	Percentage
True positive	7,227	82.6%	2,268	1,298	76.3%
Redundant UMLS concept	490	5.6%	209	119	7.0%
Homonym	481	5.5%	127	45	2.6%
UMLS general concept missing	158	1.8%	86	38	2.2%
Concept not in UMLS	127	1.5%	31	42	2.5%
FP, acronym/abbrev	83	0.9%	51	15	0.9%
FN, variant not in UMLS	41	0.5%	16	44	2.6%
FN, inferable by ctx/expert	38	0.4%	12	31	1.8%
FN, acronym/abbreviation/elision	29	0.3%	6	37	2.2%
Concept not useful for indexing	25	0.3%	7	6	0.4%
Too many non-stop-words	25	0.3%	25	7	0.4%
FN, spelling/grammar error	8	0.1%	8	0	0.0%
FN/FP, proper name	10	0.1%	10	19	1.1%
FP, spelling/grammar error	3	0.0%	3	0	0.0%
TOTALS:	8,745		2,859	1,701	

NOTES: The three columns indicate category of match, the number of matches for each category, and the number of distinct concepts matched. FN indicates false negative; FP, false positive. The number of negated concepts in the test set was 110.

Results

The 100 notes used in the *training set* of documents contained 1.12 MB of text, with an average of 11,200 bytes and 1,800 words per note. Discharge notes were distinctly longer than surgery notes. It took an average of 55 seconds to process each note completely and recognize concepts. Much of this time involved database accesses over a local area network; the phrase recognition program, running locally, took less than a second per note. Time requirements might have been reduced somewhat if both the concept-indexing program and the database server had resided on the same machine. The characteristics of the test set are contrasted with those of the training set at the end of this section.

The results of the matching process for both training and test sets are summarized in Table 1. The columns in this table are as follows:

- *The category of match* ("Match Type"). The abbreviations FN and FP indicate false negative and false positive, respectively.

- *The number of matches for each category for both training and test sets, with percentages, after tallying matches for each note.* The total number of matches was 8,745 in the training set and 1,701 in the test set.

- *The number of distinct concepts matched across all notes for each category (training set only).* This is useful for analyzing failures without counting the same instance twice. Thus, the phrase "retrograde cold blood cardioplegia," a concept that probably should be in the UMLS but is currently missing, was seen in several open-heart surgery notes. The total number of distinct concepts matched was 2,859.

All categories other than "true positive" indicate problems either with vocabulary contents and curation or with the algorithm. Our definition of "true positive" was simply that the individual phrase matched to the correct concept, regardless of negation or tense. Therefore, "true positive" may or may not be the same as "relevant." For example, if a user were looking for patients presenting with alcoholism, a match to "alcoholism" would mean nothing per se. However, if the user were looking for all patients screened or interviewed for a history of alcoholism (whether it was actually present), every instance of "alcoholism" might well be relevant.

Match Failures

Failures to match unambiguously can be grouped into three categories:

- *Non-recognition due to the tagging / the noun-phrase method of targeting candidates.* Examples of these failures are spelling and grammatical errors in the text, and proper names. (As previously mentioned, grammatical errors cause subtle errors in the FET's phrase tagging process.) Although not discussed here, an artifact of the noun phrase method is that when a single concept is spread across two or more phrases, the matching process will match to two or more separate general concepts rather than one composite concept. Thus, as discussed previously, in the segment "hypertension is secondary to renal disease," the noun phrase approach would match the concepts "hypertension" and "renal disease" rather than the concept "renal hypertension." This is not necessarily bad, but it means that if a production system were to be consulted by a user searching for the concept of renal hypertension, it would need to consult the MRREL table of the UMLS, find the immediate "parent" concepts for renal hypertension, and expand the user's original query.

- *Problems due to UMLS content.* This category contains redundant UMLS concepts, term variants missing from the UMLS, missing general concepts (where a specific variant is present but the more general form is not), missing concepts, and concepts that are present in the UMLS but not useful for concept indexing.

- *Limitations of the matching algorithm.* Examples are homonyms, acronyms and abbreviations, phrases that are too long for the algorithm, and elided forms ("incomplete" phrases with one or more missing words). Some elided forms do not occur in the UMLS at all, whereas others need domain expertise to disambiguate in the context of their occurrence, as discussed shortly. Acronyms and abbreviations are partly a thesaurus problem; some are present in the UMLS, but others are not.

We discuss these categories in more details below; the numbers and percentages in parentheses refer to the training set. The numbers for the test set are not recapitulated in the text, but salient features are discussed toward the end of this section.

Redundant UMLS Concepts

Redundant UMLS concepts (5.6 percent, 490 matches) were cases in which a phrase or subphrase matched more than one concept even after disambiguation was attempted. Filtering on patterns like NOS (not otherwise specified) and NEC (not elsewhere classified) eliminated many but not all redundant concepts. For example, "spinal tap" and "spinal puncture" are two separate UMLS concepts even though they should be a single concept.

Another problem is noun-adjective variants. For example, "fibrosis" and "fibrotic" are two separate concepts, as are "necrotic" and "necrosis." From the concept-recognition viewpoint, the adjective is merely a variant of the noun form. Other instances include identical concepts with variations in spelling of the preferred term, e.g., "jaundice" and "Jaundice" (uppercase "J"). (The duplicate entries for "jaundice" appear to be due to a curation error; details of the two concepts are almost identical, except that "jaundice" has an associated definition, whereas "Jaundice" has none.) Only the last category is recorded in UMLS's ambiguous-terms list.

From the curation viewpoint, a genuine danger of recording two concepts instead of one is that the related concepts, recorded in the MRREL table of the UMLS, can be inconsistent with each other. Thus, the concept "necrosis" has the siblings "edema" and "gangrene," whereas "necrotic," the adjective form, has the child "gangrene," and "edema" is not associated with it. There is a continuing effort at the NLM to merge and eliminate duplicated concepts. The files merged.cui and deleted.cui, which record the changes made in this respect, are part of every annual UMLS release. This problem should, therefore, progressively abate with future releases.

Homonyms and Term Variants Not in the UMLS

Homonyms (5.5 percent, 481 matches) were described earlier in the Background section; we discuss term variants not found in the UMLS (0.47 percent, 41 matches) here.

In several cases, multiple matches for a phrase could not be disambiguated because the "default" concept that should match a word or phrase, if it stands by itself, was not recorded in the UMLS. For example, "xiphoid" in narrative typically refers to the "xiphoid bone" (a part of the sternum), whereas "flu vaccine" refers to "influenza vaccine." Some of these were abbreviations, such as IVP for "Intravenous Pyelography procedure" and CT for "X-Ray Tomography, Computed," respectively. (Currently UMLS records only "C.A.T." as a term for the procedure, even though "CT" is a more widely used abbreviation today.) Some verb forms of procedures are missing ("cardioverted," "cauterized"); the former verb is also missing from the SPECIALIST lexicon, which is part of the UMLS distribution.

Concepts Not in UMLS and Missing General Concepts

Concepts that are not in UMLS (1.45 percent, 127 matches) and missing general concepts (1.8 percent, 158 matches) were determined by manual inspection, either when a phrase did not match any concept or when it matched a wrong concept. The UMLS depends on its source vocabularies for comprehensiveness, and because vocabulary development has been driven by specific needs, such as publication indexing, diagnosis, and billing, some domains in medicine are under-represented. Thus, the concept of "relocation" as the opposite of "dislocation" (pertaining to a joint) is absent, although the UMLS records relocation of patients and of cardiac valves. Some missing concepts are compound words (e.g., "zygomaticofrontal"), verb forms of medication administration (e.g., heparinize/heparinization, coumadinize, digitalize), and adjective forms of procedures (e.g., Dopplerable). Most specialized surgical instruments are not recorded, nor are many descriptive psychiatry terms (e.g., "hyper-arousal"). Missing general concepts were discussed earlier.

Acronyms, Abbreviations, and Elided Forms

Acronyms resulted in false negatives (0.33 percent, 29 matches) when they were present in nonstandard forms that were not recorded in the UMLS. Abbreviations also caused false positives (0.95 percent, 83 matches) when they were identical to non-abbreviated words (e.g., "RAT," which refers to the animal or to recurrent acute tonsillitis). Elided forms led to false negatives (e.g., "white count" for "total white blood cell count," and "differential" for "differential white blood cell count"). Similarly, while the phrase "cocaine and alcohol dependence" implied the two concepts "cocaine dependence" and "alcohol dependence," the less specific concept, "cocaine," was identified instead. Disambiguation of some elided forms (e.g., "superior thyroid," which could refer either to the artery or to the vein) requires domain expertise. (In the context of carotid plaque-removal surgery, the phrase "superior thyroid" is more likely to refer to the artery.)

Concepts Not Useful for Indexing

Although we programmatically eliminated all suppressable synonyms as well as forms preceded by an acronym, several concepts of marginal utility (0.29 percent, 25 matches) were not removed. Examples were "In Blood" and "Stroke work right." These can be eliminated only through laborious manual curation.

Phrases Too Long for Algorithm (Too Many Non-stop-words)

Twenty-five phrases across all 100 notes were flagged as more than five non-stop-words long. In all cases but one ("chronic post traumatic stress disorder symptoms"), the phrases had conjunctions missing ("left hip open reduction [with] internal fixation") or were poorly phrased ("large left hemisphere MCA distribution stroke"). More important, the concepts embodied in the unprocessed phrase were present elsewhere in the note, where they were successfully matched. We regard this failure rate as acceptable, given efficiency considerations. In other words, the cut-off of five appears to provide reasonable computational efficiency with good coverage for the vast majority of phrases.

In production mode, rather than abandoning such phrases entirely, it might be desirable simply to attempt to match each individual word in the phrase to a concept. Although general matches are less useful than specific ones, they are better than no matches at all. For this study, however, we needed to determine the suitability of our arbitrarily chosen cut-off. (In an earlier stage of the experiment, we used a cut-off of four. This was found to be too low; among other concepts, "non-insulin dependent diabetes mellitus" was unprocessed.)

Spelling Errors and Proper Names

Spelling errors (0.12 percent, 11 matches) caused concepts to be missed as well as spuriously matched if the misspelling was a valid word in the thesaurus (e.g., "ilium" for "ileum"). Proper names (0.11 percent, 10 matches) posed a problem that we have not yet solved. For efficiency, it is desirable to filter out from a document most proper names—like that of the patient, which occurs repeatedly—prior to concept matching. In this way, the problem of trying to concept-match last names that are also words in the thesaurus (e.g., Black, Ward) is also bypassed.

The IBM FET program does a very good job of recognizing proper names. The problem, however, is that certain medically important names (e.g., Alzheimer, Romberg, Charcot) are also eliminated, and concepts containing them would never be matched. The only solution we can think of—manual creation of a list of such names, to be consulted in the preprocessing step—is significantly labor intensive but is probably necessary for production operation. Such an approach must also disambiguate such concept occurrences from instances in which a patient coincidentally has a medically important last name. (For example, when processing each note, a program can access the patient ID associated with it and use the ID to access patient demographic data, including name information.)

Salient Characteristics of the Test Document Set

Table 1 shows that the test set of documents differed somewhat from the training set in that the documents were shorter on average and each document contained fewer concepts. This was because they represented subdomains of medicine with a different frequency compared with the training set. Thus, cardiothoracic, vascular, and neurosurgical conditions were relatively over-represented in both discharge summaries and surgery notes.

The frequency distribution of the types of matches (discussed shortly) also differed significantly between the training and test sets ($P < 0.0001$ by the chi-square test). For example, missing variants of terms, elided forms, unrecognized acronyms, and unrecognized proper names were over-represented.

This is understandable; for example, documents in surgical specialties tend to contain proportionally more proper names that refer to instruments or surgical techniques. The difference in frequency distributions does not affect the validity of the results; the objective of the exercise is to see how the concept-matching algorithm performs when subjected to documents with different characteristics. The relative frequencies of different types of failures are less important than the fact that these failures must be systematically identified and categorized if we are to devise strategies that can address them.

Of the 1,298 "true positive" matches in the test set, 110 (8.5 percent) actually represented negation of a concept (with a condition being absent, denied by the patient, or ruled out). Although our test set of 24 documents is small, this relatively modest percentage seems to indicate that failure to handle negation robustly may not, by itself, make production concept indexing non-viable. This hypothesis needs to be tested with larger amounts of data; it may not apply universally and may well be false in the case of particular concepts that are routinely sought (but infrequently present) in a case.

In our test data, the words "lymphadenopathy" and "complications" were negated three times each; the former may be important for searching. If greater weight is given to documents in which a particular concept occurs more than once, as is likely if the concept is a significant theme of the document, then documents in which the concept is negated will get less weighting, because negation of a concept hardly ever needs to be stated more than once in a note.

Discussion

Although, in our results, the overall incidence of true positive matches (82.6 percent in the training set, 76.3 percent in the test set) appears superficially impressive, it also means that roughly one index entry in five had some problem that would manifest in production mode. In our opinion, accuracy needs to be much higher for concept indexing to be used in production mode. Certainly, a one-in-five error rate would be unacceptable for OCR (optical character recogition) software or for a human typist. Furthermore, concepts are rarely looked for in isolation; usually, a user is doing a Boolean search (e.g., show documents that contain concepts X and Y and Z) or a "vector-model" search (e.g., rank documents by relevance based on these three concepts). If a single concept has only a 0.8 chance of being a true positive, then the Boolean combination of three concepts has a chance of only 0.8^3, or 0.41, of being true positive. In addition, given the caveat that "true positive" is not necessarily the same as "relevant" (because of negation), the proportion of genuinely relevant documents for a given query may be somewhat lower still.

Concept indexing solves some problems but raises others. Previous experiments with it have not always yielded encouraging results. On the basis of experiments conducted with the SMART system, Salton et al.[33] have asserted that indexing with words is superior to indexing on phrases in a controlled vocabulary. Several experiments conducted by Hersh et al.,[24,25,34,35] have indicated that concept indexing with the earlier versions of SAPHIRE was somewhat less effective, with respect to retrieval, than indexing with traditional word-based methods. Although traditional word indexing, as performed with off-the-shelf software, also has its limitations (chiefly with synonyms), word indexing does not make any claims to intelligence. On the other hand, concept indexing, which aims to partly address the problem of the *meaning* of text, implicitly does make such claims. Therefore, users may well react to perceived lapses in concept indexing much more negatively. Our experience also indicates that concept indexing alone is not sufficiently viable to support robust querying of medical record data.

However, approaches that combine concepts in the UMLS (or the MeSH, one of its major components) with word-indexing approaches have been more encouraging. Thus, the work of Aronson et al.[9] reported a modest improvement with the combined approach than with word indexing or concept indexing alone. Srinivasan's work on retrieval feedback using MeSH terms[16] reported a significant improvement with a combined strategy. In a subsequent paper, Aronson and Rindflesch,[10] while reviewing and validating Srinivasan's work with further experiments, concluded that an optimal strategy would be to combine their own approach (MetaMap) with a retrieval feedback approach.

We envisage a somewhat different approach to integration of concept indexing with word indexing. We propose a user interface that allows query explicitly by words, concepts, or both. If by both, a query would be a two-step process. The UMLS concepts would be matched to the keywords in the user's query and displayed to the user, who could then select the concepts of interest. The retrieval engine would then do both a word search and a concept search, giving greater weight to documents that matched both words and concepts. We have not yet created such an interface or retrieval engine; the task should prove to be an interesting software challenge, and many issues (such as the weighting scheme) need to be resolved.

MetaMap's intensive variant-generation phase yields more sensitivity but less specificity than our own algorithm. In their 1993 paper, Rindflesch and Aronson[12] describe false positives due to variant generation artifacts; thus, "base" (a variant of "foundation") maps to "inorganic chemical" because of the homonym phenomenon. As previously stated, our algorithm is biased toward high specificity for the concept match because of our hypothesis (to be tested in future work) that the accompanying word index might provide the requisite sensitivity.

Conclusions and Future Directions

The present work is concerned with the important prerequisite of highly specific concept matching, without which a concept index is of little use. Our algorithm is, of course, tailored to the UMLS, and some of the problems encountered might not apply to the much smaller controlled vocabularies of other domains.

Many of the categories of false negative, false positive, and ambiguous matches with concept indexing need to be addressed through curation of the UMLS subset used for matching. In 1992, Hersh and Hickam[25] expressed the hope that future editions of

the UMLS would be enhanced to be useful for concept indexing. However, because the UMLS has to support varied audiences, enhancements for one audience might be deleterious for another. Two UMLS enhancements—creation of the ambiguous terms/strings tables and the flagging of suppressable synonyms—are aimed specifically at the concept-matching audience, but clearly much more needs to be done. Some issues are highlighted below.

First, for now, ambiguous terms are the Achilles heel of concept indexing. The ambiguous-entries tables in the UMLS do not currently list acronyms and abbreviations. As stated earlier, we have generated a table of terms with non-unique stemmed forms. Although many entries in this list are of the "NOS/NEC" variety, the list also includes abbreviations that are identical to non-abbreviated words. However, this list is so large (49,800 stemmed forms from 132,300 terms, incorporating 111,300 unique concepts) that we have currently been able to access it only programmatically—to look for similar forms, for example, with and without "NEC." We will eventually need to process the list manually or devise clever ways of processing it algorithmically.

One admittedly ad hoc strategy to deal with ambiguous terms is to treat them as "pseudo-concepts," assigning them IDs beyond the range of UMLS concepts proper, and index them with these IDs. (The method of assigning IDs beyond the UMLS range is widely used to maintain local vocabularies, as described in Rocha et al.,[36] for example) The table of ambiguous terms must be available to the query process, so that if the user specifies such terms in the query expression, the program can warn the user that the matches might lack specificity. The alternative approach of Aronson et al.,[9] which seeks to use the UMLS Semantic Network for disambiguation, was cited earlier in the Background section.

Second, to make the existing term list more useful for concept matching, it might be necessary to store the "default concept" against a term if the term is encountered as an isolated noun phrase. For example, CT and IVP by themselves would imply X-Ray Computed Tomography and Intravenous Pyelography, respectively.

Third, in addition to incorporating more concepts for medical subdomains that are currently under-represented in the UMLS (e.g., orthopedics), the vocabulary may need to be expanded by the incorporation of more high-level, general concepts that are currently missing from the UMLS, even though they form parts of composite concepts. The creation of algorithms to identify potential higher-level concepts from the existing contents of the UMLS is an open problem.

Concurrently, the suitability for concept indexing of many highly composite concepts present in the UMLS needs to be carefully assessed. This applies especially to concepts derived from sources such as ICD-9 and ICD-10. For example, several concepts are very similar, being distinguished from each other by the presence of one or more negations. Thus, we have "acute gastrojejunal ulcer with hemorrhage, without mention of obstruction" vs. "acute gastrojejunal ulcer with hemorrhage and obstruction," and so on. These are formed from the general concepts "acute," "gastrojejunal ulcer," "hemorrhage,"and "obstruction."

The question is whether the general concepts are useful enough by themselves. In medical narrative, the clinical condition codified by the composite concepts would be described over multiple phrases and possibly over multiple sentences, and would hardly ever be matched by a phrase-based approach. One way to curate ICD codes is to go to the original source and use the decimal nomenclature (there are fewer decimals for higher-level, general concepts) as the basis for creation of subsets.

Finally, it would be very useful if future editions of the UMLS explicitly recorded, against each string for a term, whether the term was an abbreviated form (e.g., an acronym) or not. This would greatly reduce the incidence of false positive and false negative matches. Currently, it requires a human curator to perform this interpretation. Unfortunately, the SPE-CIALIST lexicon, a component of the UMLS distribution that records abbreviations explicitly, is currently too limited in this matter. Many of the problematic abbreviations (e.g., PEG for polyethylene glycol) are not recorded in SPECIALIST.

The authors thank Dr. Michael Hehenberger of IBM Corporation for providing the Intelligent Miner for Text software at no cost. Dr. Betsy Humphreys of the National Library of Medicine provided valuable information about the UMLS, as well as pointers to previous work. The test data was made available through Dr. H. David Stein, Forrest W. Levin and Dr. Joseph Erdos of the VAMC, West Haven, Connecticut. Finally, they thank the National Library of Medicine for making a valuable resource like the UMLS freely available, and making this research possible.

References ■

1. Salton G. Automatic text processing: the transformation, analysis, and retrieval of information by computer. Reading, Mass: Addison-Wesley, 1989.
2. Hersh WR. Information Retrieval: A Health Care Perspective. New York: Springer-Verlag, 1996.
3. Lindberg DAB, Humphreys BL, McCray AT. The Unified Medical Language System. Methods Inf Med. 1993;32:281–91.
4. Salton G, Wu H, Yu CT. Measurement of Term Importance in Automatic Indexing. J Am Soc Inf Sci. 1981;32(3):175–86.
5. Wilbur WJ, Yang Y. An analysis of statistical term strength and its use in the indexing and retrieval of molecular biology texts. Comput Biol Med. 1996;26(3):209–22.
6. National Library of Medicine. UMLS Knowledge Sources. 9th ed. Bethesda, Md: NLM, 1999.
7. Porter MF. An algorithm for suffix stripping. Program. 1980;14(3):130–7.
8. Baeza-Yates R, Frakes WB. Information Retrieval: Data Structures and Algorithms. Englewood Cliffs, NJ: Prentice Hall, 1993.
9. Aronson A, Rindflesch T, Browne A. Exploiting a large thesaurus for information retrieval. Proc RIAO '94. 1994:197–216.
10. Aronson AR, Rindflesch TC. Query expansion using the UMLS Metathesaurus. Proc AMIA Annu Fall Symp. 1997:485–9.
11. Divita G, Browne AC, Rindflesch TC. Evaluating lexical variant generation to improve information retrieval. In: Proc AMIA Annu Symp. 1998:775–9.
12. Rindflesch TC, Aronson AR. Semantic processing in information retrieval. Proc 17th Annu Symp Comput Appl Med Care. 1993:611–5.
13. Rindflesch TC, Aronson AR. Ambiguity resolution while mapping free text to the UMLS Metathesaurus. Proc Annu Symp Comput Appl Med Care. 1994:240–4.
14. Salton G. The SMART Retrieval System: Experiments in Automatic Document Processing. Englewood Cliffs, NJ: Prentice Hall, 1971.
15. Callan J, Croft W, Harding S. The INQUERY retrieval system. Proc Int Conf Database Expert Syst Appl. 1992:347–56.
16. Srinivasan P. Retrieval feedback in MEDLINE. J Am Med Inform Assoc. 1996;3(2):157–67.
17. Srinivasan P. Query Expansion and MEDLINE. Inf Proc Manage. 1996;32(4): 431–43.
18. Elkin PL, Cimino JJ, Lowe HJ, et al. Mapping to MeSH: the art of trapping MeSH equivalence from within narrative text. Proc 12th Symp Comput Appl Med Care. 1988:185–190.
19. Cutting D, Pedersen J. The Xerox Part-of-Speech Tagger. Palo Alto, Calif: Xerox Corporation, 1994. Available freely online for downloading as LISP code from: ftp://parcftp.xerox.com/pub/tagger/tagger-1-0.tar.Z:.
20. Inxight Corporation. LinguistX Platform [product summary]. Palo Alto, Calif: Inxight Corp., 1999. Available at: http://www.inxight.com/Products/Developer/Platform.
21. Spackman K, Hersh W. Recognizing noun phrases in medical discharge summaries: an evaluation of two natural language parsers. ProcAMIA Annu Fall Symp. 1996:155–8.
22. Evans D, Brownlow N, Hersh W, Campbell E. Automating concept identification in the electronic medical record: an experiment in extracting dosage information. Proc AMIA Annu Fall Symp. 1996:388–92.
23. Hersh W, Greenes R. SAPHIRE—an information retrieval system featuring concept matching, automatic indexing, probabilistic retrieval, and hierarchical relationships. Comput Biomed Res. 1990; 23(5): 410–25.
24. Hersh W, Hickam D, Leone T. Words, concepts, or both: optimal indexing units for automated information retrieval. Proc 16th Annu Symp Comput Appl Med Care. 1992:644–8.
25. Hersh W, Hickam D. A comparison of retrieval effectiveness for three methods of indexing medical literature. Am J Med Sci. 1992;303(5):292–300.

26. Gordon H. Discrete Probability. (Undergraduate Texts in Mathematics.) New York: Springer-Verlag, 1997.

27. Aho A, Ullman J. Foundations of Computer Science. "C" ed. New York: WH Freeman, 1995.

28. Hersh W, Leen T, Rehfuss P, Malveau S. Automatic prediction of trauma registry procedure codes from emergency room dictations. MedInfo '98. 1998:665–9.

29. Miller R, Myers JD. Quick medical reference (QMR) for diagnostic assistance. MD Comput. 1986;3(5):34–48.

30. Hersh WR, Leone TJ. The SAPHIRE server: a new algorithm and implementation. Proc 19th Annu Symp Comput Appl Med Care. 1995:858–62.

31. Huff S, Rocha R, McDonald C, et al. Development of the Logical Observations Identifiers, Names, and Codes (LOINC) vocabulary. J Am Med Inform Assoc. 1998;5(3):276–92.

32. Nadkarni PM. Concept Locator: a client-server application for retrieval of UMLS Metathesaurus concepts through complex Boolean query. Comput Biomed Res. 1997;30: 323–36.

33. Salton GB, Buckley C, Smith M. On the application of syntactic methodologies in automatic text analysis. Inf Proc Manage. 1990;26(1):73–92.

34. Hersh W, Hickam D. A comparison of two methods for indexing and retrieval from a full-text medical database. Med Decis Making. 1993;13(3):220–6.

35. Hersh W, Hickam D. Information retrieval in medicine: the SAPHIRE experience. MedInfo '95. 1995:1433–7.

36. Rocha RA, Huff SM, Haug P, Warner HR. Designing a controlled medical vocabulary server: the VOSER project. Comput Biomed Res. 1994;27(6):472–507.

G. Nilsson[1], H. Petersson[2], H. Åhlfeldt[2], L.-E. Strender[1]

[1]Family Medicine Stockholm, Karolinska Institute, Sweden
[2]Medical Informatics, Linköping University, Sweden

Evaluation of Three Swedish ICD-10 Primary Care Versions: Reliability and Ease of Use in Diagnostic Coding

Abstract: If computer-stored information is to be useful for purposes other than patient care, reliability of the data is of utmost importance. In primary healthcare settings, however, it has been found to be poor. This paper presents a study on the influence of coding tools on reliability and user acceptance. Six general practitioners coded 152 medical problems each by means of three versions of ICD-10, one with a compositional structure. At code level the reliability was poor and was almost identical when the three versions were compared. At aggregated level the reliability was good and somewhat better in the compositional structure. Ideas for improved user acceptance arose, and the study explored the need for several different tools to retrieve diagnostic codes.

Keywords: Coding, ICD, Reliability, Family Medicine, Medical Modeling

1. Introduction

Primary healthcare in Sweden is provided at about 1,000 health centers by more than 4000 general practitioners (GP). The use of electronic patient records (EPR) is increasing, and in 1995 approximately 85% of patient records were computerized [1].

Swedish GPs have a tradition of using a primary healthcare version of the International Classification of Diseases (ICD) [2] for diagnostic labeling in the EPR. The general practitioner is responsible for the diagnostic coding. A Swedish primary healthcare version of ICD-10 (KSH97P) has been put to use [3]. It was developed by a working group within the Swedish Association of General Practice on behalf of the Swedish National Board of Health and Welfare, and is based on experiences from the widespread use of the primary healthcare version of ICD-9.

Identifying problems and diagnoses is vital in the medical problem-solving process, is a basis for decision-making, and strongly influences the outcome of medical care. Proper coding of these clinical data is essential for diagnosis-related data retrieval, which is mainly used to support quality assessment and research.

A correct diagnosis is important for patient care, and the validity (the extent to which an instrument measures what it is intended to measure, e.g. the extent to which a physician codes the correct diagnosis for a patient) of physicians' diagnoses has been documented previously. In a recent study Ridderikhoff et al. found a completely correct diagnosis in only 43% of consultations in primary health care [4]. This is not surprising, as primary healthcare deals with a blend of widely varying problems, which are often in an early stage. Furthermore, the diagnosis is based on patient data such as symptoms and findings that also have limited validity, as reported by de Dombal et al. [5]. The same range of diagnostic validity has been found in hospital settings [6, 7].

If computer-stored information is to be useful for data retrieval, then the reliability (the extent to which the same measure will provide the same results under the same conditions, e.g. the extent to which two physicians code for the same diagnosis for a patient's problem) of the patient data is of utmost importance [8]. This is due to the fact that information coded by different GPs is compared. Consequently, consistent use of the same code for the same clinical entity becomes important in order to facilitate data retrieval. The reliability of coded diagnoses, however, is poor both in primary healthcare [9-11] and in hospital settings [12].

Possible ways of improving the reliability of diagnostic coding are to improve coding routines, coding tools, and coding schemes. For example, computerized coding tools have been found by Hohnloser et al. [13] to save time and result in higher quality codes when medical concepts are extracted from narrative text from clinical cases. Natural language analysis methods have been found suitable for suggesting potentially correct codes from free text pathology reports [14]. In addition, physicians' motivation and the purpose of diagnostic coding are important factors to stress in order to improve the reliability.

The relevance of the structure of KSH97P to diagnostic coding and to data retrieval is reduced by a number of compromises among classifications based on etiology, anatomical site, circumstances of onset, etc. For example,

Table 1 Compositional structure of state of health as a systematic list in alphabetic order.

Location	Etiology
Blood	Circumstances
Circulatory organs	Deficiency
Digestive organs	Endogenous
Ear	Infection
Eye	Injury
Inner secretory organs	Mixed etiology
Mammary gland	Poisoning
Multiple organs/functions	
Musculoskeletal system	**Type**
Nervous system	Disease
Psychological functions	Healthy
Respiratory organs	Risk
Sexual organs	Symptom
Skin	
Urinary tract organs	

clinical problems related to an upper respiratory tract infection can be found in Chapter 1 where they are based on etiology, in Chapter 10 where they are based on exclusion criteria and location, and in Chapter 18 where they are based on exclusion criteria and symptoms. Users may wish to be able to access diagnoses based on location or on etiology in a poly-hierarchic system [15]. In the KSH97P and other ICD-based coding schemes, this flexibility is hindered by the mono-hierarchic structure.

A model for evaluation of computerized coding systems has been proposed by Bolton et al. [16]. This model includes evaluation of the structure of the coding system, the reliability of coding, the ease of use of the codes, the infra-structure supporting the coding system, and the overall usefulness. In the present study, evaluation is focused on reliability and ease of use. The structure of the coding system is discussed, but the infrastructure and overall usefulness are not analyzed in this study.

The major objective of this study was to see if the reliability of diagnostic coding and ease of use can be improved by attaching a new structure to the official book version of KSH97P. As the new structure is computerized, the comparison was done in two steps, a comparison of the two media, and a comparison of the two structures. The reliability of diagnostic coding and the ease of use were thus studied by means of three versions of the coding scheme. To evaluate the new structure as an aggregation scheme, the reliability of diagnostic code aggregation was compared with the traditional ICD-structure.

---

2. Material and Methods

2.1 Coding Tools

Three versions of the KSH97P were used in the coding trial:
1. The Book – the official book version
2. The Chapter Browser – a computerized version with the traditional ICD-structure
3. The Cube Browser – a computerized version with a new compositional structure

Altogether there are 972 codes with preferred terms and 1,566 alternative terms, collected from the vocabulary of Swedish GPs, in KSH97P. The chapters are the same as in ICD-10 except that Chapter 20 is excluded in KSH97P.

The compositional structure is based on a conceptual model of primary healthcare and state of health developed by GPs in a terminology working group in the Stockholm County Council [17]. The basic concepts in this model are patient, care contact, care provider, intervention, and state of health. The concept model of state of health has three dimensions: location, etiology, and type (Table 1). It is possible to combine the elements from one, two or three dimensions to retrieve a group of diagnoses from different ICD-chapters.

The computerized versions were modifications of the web-based Classification Browser described earlier [17]. Two almost identical browsers, the Chapter Browser and the Cube Browser, were produced. The string matching function was excluded in order to focus on the differences between the structures. The only differences between them were the browsing functions effected by the structure.

This study was approved by the local ethics committee.

2.2 Encounters

Records from 89 encounters were used for the coding trial. They concerned 152 medical problems, and were randomly selected from a two-year period at a healthcare center with an EPR system within the Stockholm County Council. The cases were considered fairly representative of Swedish general practice regarding distribution of age, sex and other population factors.

The records were problem-oriented, i.e. all notes were recorded in the context of a specific problem [18]. The cases were presented on paper and concerned one, two or three problems arranged according to the SOAP-structure (Subjective, Objective, Assessment, and Plan). The records averaged 164 words per encounter and 105 words per problem. The complete record of the encounter was presented, thus including prescriptions, laboratory tests and referrals. Original diagnostic codes, assigned according to the Swedish primary healthcare version of ICD-9, were excluded.

2.3 Subjects

Six GPs from different healthcare centers, three in each of two Swedish

Subjects	The Book		The Chapter Browser		The Cube Browser	
	Agreements	K	Agreements	K	Agreements	K
1 and 2	32/51	0.62	27/50	0.53	29/51	0.58
3 and 4	27/50	0.53	31/51	0.60	30/51	0.58
5 and 6	31/51	0.60	24/51	0.46	27/50	0.53
Total	90/152		82/152		86/152	
Percent	(59)		(54)		(57)	
Mean Kappa		0.58		0.53		0.56

Table 2 Inter-coder reliability. The number of agreements per set of codes in different subject pairs in relation to the total number of codes, the Kappa statistics (K) values, and the percentage level of agreement (%) (N = 152).

cities, were selected for the study. All subjects had previous experience with EPRs ranging from 3–10 years. Three different EPR systems were in use in their health-care settings, one with graphical interface and two that were text-oriented. The subjects were familiar with computers and word processing. On the other hand, they were not especially skilled Web surfers, which is the primary skill required for this application. Three out of six subjects routinely used the official KSH97P.

In their day-to-day practice the subjects apply a variety of methods to retrieve the codes. Their EPR systems provide convenient string matching functions, but the book (KSH97P or the previous version) as well as crib sheets were used. As reported by the participants, in about 95% of their encounters one or more diagnostic codes or rubrics from a coding scheme were recorded.

The subjects were considered representative of GPs in Sweden in terms of computer experience. Some GPs had more knowledge of the KSH97P than the average GP.

2.4 Experimental Setup

Prior to the experiment day, each GP was briefly introduced to the coding scheme, the model of state of health, and the computer applications, and they each had the opportunity to practice using training cases.

The encounters were divided into three sets of 50 or 51 problems. Each GP was asked to code one set of problems by means of each method (the Book, the Chapter Browser, and the Cube Browser) in an order established by random. They were instructed to select one code for each problem in the record. The GPs were divided randomly into three pairs in order to measure agreement, i.e. inter-rater reliability. One GP repeated the coding trial after four weeks to make it possible to measure intra-rater reliability.

Sessions were held at two locations with the client and server computers connected over the Internet. Diagnostic codes for each case were recorded manually by the GPs and handed in for compilation at the end of each session.

Table 3 Inter-coder reliability measured with percentage level of agreement (%) and the Kappa statistics (K) at code level and aggregated levels (N = 152).

Abstraction level	The Book		The Chapter Browser		The Cube Browser	
	%	K	%	K	%	K
Code level	59	0.58	54	0.53	57	0.56
Aggregated level						
ICD-10 chapter	84	0.82	80	0.76	81	0.79
location	89	0.87	84	0.81	88	0.86
etiology	84	0.75	80	0.69	84	0.76
type	82	0.62	82	0.64	82	0.64

2.5 Evaluation

The inter- and intra-rater *reliability of diagnostic coding* was measured on code level and on aggregated levels. The *reliability of diagnostic code aggregation* was measured on aggregated levels in the traditional ICD-chapter structure, as well as in the new compositional structure, thereby comparing the two methods with respect to the structuring of categorical data. In the coding trial each physician generated 152 codes, and they accordingly generated 912 codes in all. This whole set of codes was used to compare the reliability of the two alternative structures as aggregation schemes.

The ease of use was measured by the time used, the number of queries sent to the database in which the computerized versions were represented (for example, the content of an ICD-chapter, or alternative terms for a diagnosis), and subjective opinions. The time used was

Table 4 Comparison of aggregation based on the two structures. The number of classes and inter-coder reliability measured by the Generalized Kappa statistic (K_G).

Categorization scheme	Number of classes	K_G
The chapter structure	18	0.81
The compositional structure		
location	16	0.86
etiology	8	0.74
type	4	0.66
location and etiology	38	0.76
location and type	29	0.76
etiology and type	15	0.71

measured for each set of problems, and the number of queries was extracted from the log files of the web server. Information about subjective opinions on the three versions, aspects of the subjects' previous experiences, and the experimental setup was obtained through a survey and an individual interview. In the survey, a total of 44 questions were used, 18 of which were answered with 100-mm visual analogue scales (VAS) [19], where the answer was pointed to on a line. For example, 0 corresponded to worst possible and 100 to best possible. Multiple-choice items and comments comprised the remaining 26 questions.

2.6 Statistical Analysis

The number of agreements, the percentage level of agreement, and Cohen's Kappa (K) were used to measure reliability. The Kappa statistics can range from –1 to 1, but values for K will usually lie between 0 and 1, where 0 indicates only chance agreement and 1 indicates perfect chance corrected agreement. Suggested interpretations of agreement for different scores are <0.20 poor, 0.21–0.40 fair, 0.41–0.60 moderate, 0.61–0.80 good, and 0.81–1.00 very good [20]. However, a sound interpretation of K must take into account the prevalence of each category, the number of categories, as well as the number of agreements [21, 22]. The confidence intervals of K were not calculated, as that would require a much larger sample size than in this study [23].

The three pairs of physicians yielded one set of codes for each method, respectively. Thus three different K values for each method were calculated

Requested information	Median	Range
The Chapter Browser:		
Content of a chapter	55	45-68
Information about a diagnosis	12	2-59
Total	66	53-116
The Cube Browser:		
Content of a Cube category	62	59-67
Combination of two Cube categories	24	5-72
Combination of three Cube categories	3	0-27
Information about a diagnosis	20	2-62
Categories on a Cube axis	69	49-71
Total	176	128-299

Table 5 Number of queries, per set of codes, sent to the database using the two computerized versions, measured at different levels of abstraction.

and merged into a K value for the method by means of the arithmetic mean value (as seen in Table 2). When measuring agreement among more than two examiners, such as when comparing the reliability of the two aggregation schemes, Generalized Kappa (K_G) [23] was used.

Since the VAS data were considered as an ordinal scale and not normally distributed, medians and range are presented. Data were analyzed with non-parametric statistical methods. Friedman's ANOVA was used for comparing related samples with respect to the three versions, such as for evaluating the physicians' ranking of ease of use. The Wilcoxon matched-pairs signed-ranks test was used for comparing the versions two by two.

A p-value <0.05 was considered to be statistically significant.

3. Results

3.1 Reliability of Diagnostic Coding

The number of agreements at code level showed only a small variation, from 24/51 to 32/51 per set of codes, and from 82/152 to 90/152 per version (Table 2). The inter-coder reliability at code level was moderate (54–59%, K = 0.53–0.58), and was almost the same using the three versions. The inter-coder reliability at aggregated levels was good or very good (80–89%, K = 0.62–0.87) (Table 3).

The intra-coder reliability at code level was good, with a percentage level of agreement of 73–76% (N = 51) and K = 0.72–0.76. At aggregated levels the percentage level of agreement was 86–98% (N = 51) and K = 0.72–0.96. The highest scores for intra-coder reliability were achieved with the Cube Browser, but the differences among the three versions were small.

3.2 Reliability of Diagnostic Code Aggregation

The Kappa scores for the whole set of 912 codes at aggregated levels were good or very good (0.66–0.86). The highest score was measured using the dimension of location in the compositional structure. The number of classes ranged from 4–38, and was highest in

Table 6 Usability in VAS scores where 0 indicates completely impossible and 100 indicates easiest possible.

Question	Median	Range
Ease of use in practice :		
The Book	64	40-91
The Chapter Browser	64	25-90
The Cube Browser	66	46-80
Ease of getting overview :		
The Book	68	16-80
The Chapter Browser	45	27-89
The Cube Browser	67	40-73

the compositional structure in the combinations of location and etiology (38) and location and type (29), respectively (Table 4). In both these groups the reliability was good. This part of the study was based on the assumption that with respect to coding, the three versions are equal. This was supported by the finding that when the three versions were compared, the reliability of diagnostic coding was almost identical.

3.3 Used Time

Differences were found in the time required for solving cases with the alternative versions, and the overall differences were significant (p <0.05). Most time was used with the Cube Browser, with a median time of 62 (range 40–104) minutes per set of 50-51 codes. The Chapter Browser required 58 (range 35–79) minutes, and the Book 51 (range 35–70) minutes per set, respectively. There was a statistically significant difference only between the Book and the Chapter Browser. The time required for solving different case sets also varied, but the differences were not statistically significant. In the trial for intra-rater reliability it was found that the required time for solving cases with the two browsers decreased by 16% using the Chapter Browser, and by 18% using the Cube Browser. The time for solving cases with the Book was reduced by 28%.

3.4 Number of Queries

To code a specific problem, the median number of queries to the database was lower using the Chapter Browser, as compared to the Cube Browser, per set of codes, and this difference was statistically significant (p <0.05) (Table 5). There were no statistically significant differences between the number of queries to the database for further information about diagnoses, i.e. alternative terms, chapter and category assignments, and inclusion and exclusion criteria. In the trial for intra-rater reliability it was found that the number of queries was reduced in the second session by 10% using the Chapter Browser, and by 32% using the Cube Browser.

The number of queries to the database was commented on in the interviews. The subjects preferred to use only a few combinations in the compositional structure and go through a longer list of codes. It was thought that there was a risk of missing potentially useful diagnoses when using many combining criteria.

3.5 Subjective Opinions

In the survey, the scores for ease of use in practice did not vary much for the different methods. The scores for ease of getting an overview did vary, but the differences were not significant (Table 6).

The subjects also ranked the methods according to the overall criterion "best". Both the Chapter Browser and the Cube Browser, but not the Book, were ranked as number one by single GPs. The rank sums were higher for the two computerized versions compared to the Book, but this difference was not statistically significant.

Regarding the Book, the comment was made that the overview would benefit from having the chapter structure printed on the inside of the cover. The Book provided a better overview of terms than the list of diagnoses in the browsers, where only the preferred terms are presented by default.

The Chapter Browser was discussed and comments were made concerning how all synonyms and other information about a diagnosis can be seen. In order to see the inclusion and exclusion criteria, for example, the user has to request that information explicitly by clicking a link. In the Book, this information is presented close to the code.

It was suggested that the Cube Browser should also be available in paper form, which is possible in part. This would make it easier to choose a particular method depending on the diagnostic problem of the specific patient. The overview provided by the Cube Browser was to some extent disrupted by the fact that the logic of the combining function was not sufficiently obvious.

The Cube Browser was thought of as a feasible tool for finding uncertain diagnoses or when the GP does not really know what diagnosis he/she is looking for. Interpretation of some categories, for example the Healthy and Mixed etiology, was found to be difficult or uncertain. It was mentioned that there is a risk of missing diagnoses because of misinterpretation when combinations are used.

The physicians found that three dimensions in the compositional structure were sufficient for retrieving diagnoses. Some subjects suggested that a number of compositional categories should be further subdivided in order to reduce the number of diagnoses in each class, but others had the opposite opinion.

Most GPs commented on the lack of a string matching function, which was present in their own EPRs. String matching functions, specifically excluded in this study, were thought to function well for certain types of diagnoses, and two examples, spinal stenosis and tonsillitis, were pointed out. Some wanted to be able to have the diagnoses presented alphabetically instead of being ordered according to code. Another comment concerned sorting out diagnoses by means of a string matching function, for example fractures. Yet another wish was to have a personalized list of 'favorites' or of the most common diagnoses.

---

4. Discussion

4.1 Limitations of the Study

The number of practitioners and encounters in the study was limited, but is considered adequate for the objectives of this study. It is difficult to draw conclusions reflecting primary healthcare in Sweden in general, even if the subjects were considered to be representative, the encounters were randomly selected, and the patient mix, when evaluated in the survey, was found to conform to everyday practice.

As noted by some of the subjects, the coding results might have been different under normal circumstances, when actually seeing the patient. Furthermore, the subjects did not always agree with the course of the examination as it was presented (i.e. the information taken from the history, physical examination, and tests), and in some cases more information was sought. In the survey, however, the subjects found that it was reasonable to use cases described on paper and that it was fairly easy to assign diagnoses to the cases.

The interviews indicated that the introduction to the trial resulted in the GPs feeling confident in using the systems, but some physicians nevertheless thought they needed more time to really compare the versions. Also, the decreased amount of time required at the repeated trial, along with statements from the interviews regarding the experience gained by the physicians during the trial, indicate that they had not reached the plateau of the learning curve. However, the effects of any such improved learning on the results of the experiment were minimized by means of the experimental design.

4.2 Follow-up of Clinical Encounters

4.2.1 Quality of Clinical Information

There is a need for high quality data retrieval from the EPR, and ideally all clinically relevant information should be of high quality. For a number of reasons this is not possible, however, and this part of the discussion is focused on the amount of clinically relevant information that can be retrieved with high reliability. The fact that information about many day-to-day activities in general practice is of low quality is due in part to characteristics of the information itself, i.e. some clinically relevant information has poor reliability. One example of clinically relevant but not reliable data is found in the distinction between the concepts of symptom and disease. But to some extent this poor reliability is also due to limitations in coding and classification of information, which can be improved.

Trying to improve the reliability of diagnostic data is complex and problematic. Many factors, such as the purpose of recording the data, the recorders themselves, the number of diagnoses, diagnostic criteria, and the coding methods, all have the potential to influence the reliability [24]. The reliability can consequently be affected, although perhaps to only a very limited extent, by coding tool development such as attaching a new structure to a traditional classification as was done in this study. Improvements suggested by the subjects in the interview, such as several different tools to retrieve diagnostic codes, could also improve the reliability, but they need further evaluation.

The compositional structure used in this study was created to cover all clinical concepts of state of health that are relevant to data retrieval, i.e. the information from the encounters that general practitioners in the terminology working group, which developed the conceptual model of state of health, want to follow-up. This structure does not take into account whether it is possible to follow-up that information. However, since concept systems, regarded as abstract and static systems consisting of several components (concepts) and their relationships, are fundamental to the ability to structure experience and knowledge [25], we believe that they are useful for producing meaningful classes for data retrieval.

The main aim of this study was to see if the new structure attached to the KSH97P increased the reliability of coding, i.e. if it resulted in a better correlation between clinically relevant and reliable information. Contrary to our expectation, the Cube Browser did not improve the reliability at code level as compared to the traditional structure, but some aspects of the reliability were improved and guidance for further studies was obtained. The lack of improvement could be due to the absence of an actual difference, but it is possible that the data sample was too small to show a minor difference. Also, the limited training with, and limitations of, the compositional structure may have affected the reliability negatively.

4.2.2 Level of Granularity

The moderate level of inter-rater reliability at code level indicates its limitations with respect to diagnosis-related data retrieval in Swedish primary health-care settings. The reliability that can be achieved at code level is however, a matter for discussion. The study explored the need for research on the reliability at code level for different types of diagnostic codes, e.g. codes for well-defined diagnoses such as diabetes that may be more reliable than codes for diagnoses that include vague descriptions such as hyperplasia. The intra-rater reliability results, based here on one subject, indicate that data re-

trieval at code level is not useful for retrieval of high quality. In both structures the reliability at aggregated levels indicates that these are more useful for data retrieval. It may be that due to the nature of general practice, it is only possible to follow-up the aggregated levels of diagnostic data with high reliability.

On aggregated levels the low reliability at the dimension of type (disease/symptom/risk/healthy) indicates that these concepts could be less useful, or not useful at all, for follow-up with data retrieval. Distinguishing between diagnoses and symptoms in clinical practice is difficult, since in many cases they are present at the same time, and most diagnoses are associated with one or more symptoms. The results indicate that the dimensions of both location and etiology may be more reliable, and that these concepts probably could be more useful for data retrieval. As the interviews indicate that the three-dimensional view might be difficult, it could be beneficial to use only these two axes for most cases.

4.2.3 Categorization of Data

From one point of view the compositional structure did improve the reliability of the clinically relevant information wanted for follow-up. Used as an aggregation scheme, it seemed to have advantages over the traditional ICD-chapter structure, and it seemed to be more suitable for diagnosis-related data retrieval. These results are indicative of the difference between the coding system as a *coding tool* for code generation, and as a *categorization scheme* for code aggregation. The structure can affect the reliability in the choice of a code as well as when codes are aggregated. In this study the effect on the latter was greater. The reliability on code level is generally found to be moderate, and it may not be possible to improve it very much. Consequently, improvement of the structure and any possible effect on reliability at aggregated levels becomes important for diagnosis-related data retrieval.

Further development of the compositional structure should focus on improvement in the reliability of diagnostic data, but the extent to which this is possible is uncertain. Subdivision of a

number of compositional categories, as suggested by the subjects, could improve the structure by reducing the number of diagnoses in large classes. For example, the most frequently used categories in this study, circulatory organs, mixed etiology, and disease, contain 21.7, 49.6, and 65.2% of the diagnoses, respectively (N = 972). Feasible subdivisions of the circulatory organ system, musculoskeletal system, and respiratory organ system were suggested, but there are also other categories that could be split into subclasses.

The basic problem involved in high reliability in diagnostic coding is to make clear which set of states of health can be denoted by each code, and to make that information explicit and easily accessible. Extending the compositional structure by means of the kind of multiple classification mentioned in the interview where, for example, each state of health can be associated with several locations in the compositional structure, could possibly improve the reliability. One example is Sjögren's syndrome, which has manifestations in both the musculoskeletal system and the eye, and which should be possible to access both ways in the compositional structure.

Extending the description of diagnoses, however, requires a thorough approach in order to be reliable. For example, for a state of health with two locations it is necessary to specify the quantity as well as the quality of the way in which the locations are affected, i.e. to state whether it concerns both locations at the same time, or only one of them, and in what way each location is influenced. In terms of Rossi Mori's meta-classification [26], this corresponds to transforming the classification into a third generation terminology, i.e. a formally represented system with an inference engine. The two structures tested in our study, the traditional and the compositional, are to some extent first generation (an enumerated term list) and second generation (a predefined categorical structure of descriptors) structures, respectively. The essence of the transformation would be the defining information built into the formalization, and it is possible that the proper use of that information could improve the reliability of coding.

4.3 Ease of Use

User acceptance should have high priority in the development of EPR facilities [27]. As the time for coding activities in day-to-day practice is limited, user acceptance of coding tools is dependent on time effectiveness. High reliability in diagnostic coding without automatic coding tools is time consuming. Time could be saved, however, by diagnostic coding support and terminology development.

A shorter time for coding was expected for the two browsers as compared to the Book. The time did correlate to the version, but the Book was faster. In the repeated trial performed by one subject, both the time and number of queries were reduced. This indicates that coding performance could improve after longer implementation. The time savings reported by Hohnloser et al. [13], which was due to the linking of the users' vocabulary to the target term, could probably have been demonstrated by using the string matching function and the alternative terms in KSH97P.

Additional information about the diagnoses, however, such as alternative terms and exclusion criteria, was not often sought. This could be due to the lack of different kinds of diagnostic coding support suggested by the subjects, such as explanations of a text book type, rule-based representations of diagnostic criteria, and annotations like "have you thought of … ", although exclusion and inclusion criteria are definitional information.

The subjects expressed the need for several different tools to retrieve diagnosis codes, and they thought it was important to study these. Depending on personal preferences and the type of encounter, different methods were preferred. These included an alphabetic list, a personalized or local short list, the string matching function, the three versions in this study, parts of the Cube Browser in paper form, as well as others. The user acceptance of coding tools is, however, limited to some extent by the variety of personal preferences. Personal preferences often favor alphabetic or short lists, which need to be evaluated, as these probably affect the reliability negatively.

5. Conclusions

The reliability of diagnostic coding was not improved by the new compositional structure of the KSH97P as compared to the traditional ICD-structure. It seems that the reliability of diagnostic code aggregation was improved by the new structure, which would make it suitable for diagnosis-related data retrieval. Compared to the traditional book, the computerized version of the KSH97P with the traditional structure required a longer time for coding. Coding tools in general practice require high functionality in order to be accepted by the users.

Acknowledgment

This study was supported by grants from the Stockholm County Council.

REFERENCES

1. Patientjournaler med datorstöd (Computer-supported patient records). Stockholm: SPRI, 1995.
2. Klassifikation av sjukdomar 1987. Primärvård (Classification of Diseases 1987. Primary Care). Stockholm: Socialstyrelsen, 1987.
3. Klassifikation av sjukdomar och hälsoproblem 1997. Primärvård (Classification of Diseases and Health Problems 1997. Primary Care). Stockholm: Socialstyrelsen, 1997.
4. Ridderikhoff J, van Herk E. A diagnostic support system in general practice: is it feasible? Int J Med Inform 1997; 45: 133-43.
5. Gill PW, Leaper DJ, Guillou PJ, Staniland JR, Horrocks JC, de Dombal FT. Observer variation in clinical diagnosis. A computer-aided assessment of its magnitude and importance in 552 patients with abdominal pain. Method Inform Med 1973; 12: 108-13.
6. Zarling EJ, Sexton H, Milnor P. Failure to diagnose acute myocardial infarction. The clinicopathologic experience at a large community hospital. JAMA 1983; 250: 1177-81.
7. de Dombal FT, Dallos V, McAdam WA. Can computer aided teaching packages improve clinical care in patients with acute abdominal pain? Br Med J 1991; 302: 1495-7.
8. James NK, Reid CD. Plastic surgery audit codes: are the results reproducible? Br J Plast Surg 1991; 44: 62-4.
9. Bentsen BG. The accuracy of recording patient problems in family practice. J Med Educ 1976; 51: 311-6.
10. Bridges-Webb C. Classifying and coding morbidity in general practice: validity and reliability in an international trial. J Fam Pract 1986; 23: 147-50.
11. Britt H, Angelis M, Harris E. The reliability and validity of doctor-recorded morbidity data in active data collection systems. Scand J Prim Health Care 1998; 16: 50-5.
12. Dixon J, Sanderson C, Elliot P, Walls P, Jones J, Petticrew M. Assessment of the reproducibility of clinical coding in routinely collected hospital activity data: a study in two hospitals. J Public Health Med 1998; 20: 63-9.
13. Hohnloser JH, Kadle P, Peurner F. Coding Clinical Information: Analysis of Clinicians Using Computerized Coding. Method Inform Med 1996; 35: 104-7.
14. De Bruijn LM, Hasman A, Arends JW. Automatic coding of diagnostic reports. Method Inform Med 1998; 37: 260-5.
15. Rector AL, Faithfulness or comparability [editorial; comment]. Method Inform Med 1996; 35: 218-9.
16. Bolton P, Mira M, Usher H, Prior G. A model for the evaluation of computerized codes. The Gabrieli Medical Nomenclature as an example. Aust Fam Physician 1997; 26 Suppl 2: S76-8.
17. Petersson H, Nilsson G, Åhlfeldt H, Malmberg B-G, Wigertz O. Design and implementation of a World Wide Web accessible database for the Swedish ICD-10 primary care version using a concept system approach. In: Masys DR, editor. Proceedings of the 1997 AMIA Annual Fall Symposium; 1997 Oct 25-29; Nashville, USA. Philadelphia: Hanley & Belfus, 1997: 885.
18. Weed LL. Medical records, patient care, and medical education. Chicago: Year Book Medical Publishers, 1969.
19. Gaston-Johansson F. Measurement of pain: the psychometric properties of the Pain-O-Meter, a simple, inexpensive pain assessment tool that could change health care. J Pain Symptom Manage 1996; 12: 172-81.
20. Altman DG. Practical Statistics for Medical Research. London: Chapman and Hall, 1991.
21. Gjorup T. The Kappa coefficient and the prevalence of a diagnosis. Method Inform Med 1988; 27: 184-6.
22. Brennan P, Silman A. Statistical methods for assessing observer variability in clinical measures. Br Med J 1992; 304: 1491-4.
23. Haas M. Statistical methodology for reliability studies. J Manipulative Physiol Ther 1991; 14: 119-32.
24. Anderson JE. Reliability of morbidity data in family practice. J Fam Pract 1980; 4: 677-83.
25. Nuopponen A. Begreppssystem för terminologisk analys (Concept Systems for Terminological Analysis) [dissertation]. English summary. Vaasa: University of Vaasa 1994.
26. Rossi Mori A, Consorti F, Galeazzi E. Standards to support development of terminological systems for healthcare telematics. Method Inform Med 1998; 37: 551-63.
27. Van Ginneken AM. The Structure of Data in Medical Records. In: Van Bemmel JH, McCray AT. editors. Yearbook of Medical Informatics 1995. Stuttgart, New York: Schattauer, 1995: 61-70.

Address of the authors:
G. Nilsson, M.D.,
Family Medicine Stockholm,
Department of Clinical Science,
Karolinska Institutet,
Novum,
Blickagången 6
SE-141 57 Huddinge,
Sweden
E-mail: gunnar.nilsson@nvso.sll-se

Section 3:

<table>
<tr>
<td>

Health Information Systems

Reprinted by kind permission of:
American Academy of Pediatrics (399)
American Medical Informatics Association (389)
BMJ Publishing Group (406)
College of American Pathologists (410)
Lippincott Williams & Wilkins (414)

</td>
</tr>
</table>

387 Isaacs S.
   Some Evaluations of Informatics Applications in Health Care.
   Synopsis.

389 Coiera E.
   When conversation is better than computation.
   J Am Med Inform Assoc 2000 May-Jun;7(3):277-86.

399 Gray JE, Safran C, Davis RB, Pompilio-Weitzner G, Stewart JE, Zaccagnini L, Pursley D.
   Baby CareLink: using the internet and telemedicine to improve care for high-risk infants.
   Pediatrics 2000 Dec;106(6):1318-24.

406 Mair F, Whitten P.
   Systematic review of studies of patient satisfaction with telemedicine.
   BMJ 2000 Jun 3;320(7248):1517-20.

410 Marcelo A, Fontelo P, Farolan M, Cualing H.
   Effect of image compression on telepathology. A randomized clinical trial.
   Arch Pathol Lab Med 2000 Nov;124(11):1653-6.

414 Nahm R, Poston I.
   Measurement of the effects of an integrated, point-of-care computer system on quality of nursing documentation and patient satisfaction.
   Comput Nurs 2000 Sep-Oct;18(5):220-9.

S. Isaacs

Department of Medical Informatics,
Groote Schuur Hospital
Observatory, South Africa

Synopsis

Some Evaluations of Informatics Applications in Health Care

The papers selected for this section address the issues of effectiveness and utility of a selection of informatics applications in health care from diverse perspectives.

Telemedicine and informatics are sometimes regarded as technology looking for a use. When any new device is introduced into an area where resources are scarce it is therefore necessary to prove from the onset that the new techniques are effective as well as cost effective and acceptable by all parties involved in its usage. Much of the usefulness of applications in medical informatics as well as in medicine are often based on 'good feel' on the part of the experts and also of the sales people. In a world where medical devices and materials are big business research is often directed to the sale of medical cures and devices with the profit motive as the main factor. About 90% of research is directed to the treatment of the ailments of the richest 10% of the population. In the area dealing with the application of informatics and telematics we need to prove that the methods used or proposed are cost effective and useful. The papers in this section deal specifically with these issues.

The first paper in this section is a thoughtful presentation by Coiera on the limitations of the computerization of human communication that occurs in the medical care process. This paper should be of particular interest to those who are concerned about the 'over computerization' of human activity and of the Medical Care Process. The writer points to the evidence for the relation between communication breakdown and morbidity and mortality in the clinical settings thereby emphasizing the need for this process to be efficient. This is therefore an area which requires serious attention by informaticians. The author discusses what he calls the communication space and appeals for a better understanding of the health care communication process in a complex organization such as a health care facility so that better systems can be designed. He also discusses the possible non technical interventions such as the change in the communication process as well as the teaching of cost and benefits of other communication channels. The author points out the need of the Informatician to understand the process of communication and the resources constraints when building an information model for an organization.

The paper by Gray et al. looks for evidence that the internet and telemedicine is 'personal' enough to be amenable and useful for the co-operative care and management of low birth weight babies and their families. The authors believe that their result shows that the emotional and educational needs of the very low birth weight infants and their families can me met through the telemedicine methods they investigated. The overall length of stay in the care facility of these infants also improved. Whether these methods are applicable in a community with less resource needs to be investigated.

The question posed in the paper by Francis Mair and Pamela Whitten is fundamental to telematics and many experts are of the opinion that satisfaction with telematics care has been proven if not experimentally at least by consensus of expert opinion. The author reviews carefully selected papers from a number of databases and examined patient reported satisfaction with the telematics service. The authors discuss shortcoming of the reported studies and generalisabilities of the studies. They suggest that the evidence of the effectiveness of the teleconsultation is inconclusive. A useful addition to this study would be to follow up reports of successful implementations of systems and telematics applications in order to see if there is a sustained benefit.

The paper by Marcello and others deals with the practical issues of clarity of image transmitted in telepathology, size of files and the means of handling file size by compression. The concern most people have is whether file compression has an effect of image quality when the file is decompressed for use. The authors approach the problem using the method of the randomized double blind controlled trial which has been proven so successfully in Clinical Research [1]. The evidence produce will assure areas which do not have many resources at their disposal that image quality is not compromised with the more economical forms of file compression.

The paper by Nahm and Poston is another paper which deals with what is fundamental in Medical Informatics application. They investigated the effectiveness of a point of care system on the nursing process and concluded that their data shows that a point of care computer system does improve nursing documentation as measured by compliance to the Joint Commission on Accreditation of Health Care Organisation. An additional value in the paper is the care with which the analysis was done.

References

1. NHS Centre for Reviews and Dissemination. Report number 4. York: York University; 1996.

Address of the author:
Dr. Sedick Isaacs
Department of Medical Informatics
M51 OMB Groote Schuur Hospital
Observatory 7925,
Republic of South Africa
E-mail: Seisaacs@pawc.wcape.gov.za

When Conversation Is Better Than Computation

ENRICO COIERA, MB, BS, PHD

Abstract   While largely ignored in informatics thinking, the clinical communication space accounts for the major part of the information flow in health care. Growing evidence indicates that errors in communication give rise to substantial clinical morbidity and mortality. This paper explores the implications of acknowledging the primacy of the communication space in informatics and explores some solutions to communication difficulties. It also examines whether understanding the dynamics of communication between human beings can also improve the way we design information systems in health care. Using the concept of common ground in conversation, proposals are suggested for modeling the common ground between a system and human users. Such models provide insights into when communication or computational systems are better suited to solving information problems.

■ **J Am Med Inform Assoc.** 2000;7:277–286.

The current decision-support paradigm in health informatics is a computational one. The computer sits at the center of information systems that acquire, manipulate, store, and present data to clinicians. Computational models of clinical problems allow computers to make inferences and create views on data or perhaps prompt, critique, or actually make clinical decisions.

In this computational paradigm, human information processes are shaped into a form dictated by techno-

Affiliation of the author: University of New South Wales, Sydney, Australia.

This paper is based on a presentation by Dr. Coiera that was part of the Cornerstone on Acquiring and Presenting Data, one of four Cornerstone sessions included in the program of the AMIA Annual Fall Symposium, Washington, D.C., November 6–8, 1999.

Correspondence and reprints: Enrico Coiera, MB, BS, PhD, Professor, Office of the Dean, Faculty of Medicine, University of New South Wales, Sydney 2052, Australia; e-mail: ⟨ewc@pobox.com⟩.

Received for publication: 11/24/99; accepted for publication: 1/19/00.

The papers in this section continue the Cornerstones focus begun in the Mar/Apr issue of the Journal.

logic structure. Yet we know empirically that the development of technology is actually socially shaped.[1] The value of any particular information technology can be determined only with reference to the social context in which it is used and, more precisely, with reference to those who use it.[2,3] For example, in one study the strongest predictor of e-mail adoption in an organization had nothing to do with system design or function, but with whether the e-mail user's manager also used e-mail.[4] Furthermore, a highly structured view of human processes sits uneasily with the clinical workplace. It is not just that people have difficulty accepting information technology in a social setting because their interactions are loosely structured. We know that people will treat computers and media as if they *were* people.[5] Consequently, they superimpose social expectations on technologic interactions.

So, should we recast the tasks of acquiring and presenting clinical information socially? In the computational paradigm, clinicians faced with a decision problem turn to computer-based systems for support. However, if we examine what actually happens clinically, it is clear that people preferentially turn to each other for information and decision support. It is through the multitude of conversations that pepper the clinical day that clinicians examine, present, and interpret clinical data and ultimately decide on clinical actions. In contrast to the computational view of decision support, this conversational view emphasizes social interaction in health care and sees the sharing and interpretation of information as an interactive process that emerges out of communication. Rather than "acquiring" and "presenting" data in some mechanistic way, conversations are better characterized by the fluid and interactive notions of asking and telling, inquiring and explaining.

Although few studies have attempted to quantify directly the size of the communication space that contains the direct interactions between clinicians, those that have all paint a similar picture. Covell et al.[6] reported that colleagues, rather than document sources, met about 50 percent of information requests by clinicians in clinic. In a similar study, Tang et al.[7] found that about 60 percent of clinician time in clinic is devoted to talk. Safran et al.,[8] reviewing the information transactions in a hospital with a mature computer-based record system, still found that about 50 percent of information transactions occurred face-to-face between colleagues, with e-mail and voicemail accounting for about another quarter of the total. Only about 10 percent of the information transactions occurred through the electronic medical record.

Not only is the communication space huge in terms of the total information transactions and clinician time, it is also a source of significant morbidity and mortality. Communication failures are a large contributor to adverse clinical events and outcomes. In a retrospective review of 14,000 in-hospital deaths, communication errors were found to be the lead cause, twice as frequent as errors due to inadequate clinical skill.[9] Furthermore, about 50 percent of all adverse events detected in a study of primary care physicians were associated with communication difficulties.[10] If we look beyond the raw numbers, the clinical communication space is interruption-driven and has poor communication systems and poor practices.[11]

In summary, the communication space is apparently the largest part of the health system's information space. It contains a substantial proportion of the health system information "pathology" but is usually ignored in our informatics thinking. Yet it seems to be where most of the information in the clinical workplace is acquired and presented. The biggest information repository in health care lies in the people working in it, and the biggest information system is the web of conversations that link the actions of these individuals.

Possible Responses to the Communication Paradigm

How do we respond to the idea that information exchanges in the social communication space are primary and, therefore, that this is where substantial informatics efforts need to be focused? There seem to be four plausible responses, depending on how one views communication tasks and what technical interventions are considered to support those tasks:

■ *Identity: Communication tasks are replaceable with information tasks.* In this view, the problem is the size and behavior of the communication space, and the solution is to transform communication interactions into information transactions. For example, we replace information-seeking questions that currently occur in conversation with queries to databases. The identity response implies a 1:1 correspondence hypothesis, that all communication tasks can be replaced by computational tasks. It is similar to the so-called strong hypothesis in artificial intelligence, which states that human intelligence can be directly simulated in a computational system. The strong hypothesis is a matter of ongoing debate in the artificial intelligence community. For our purposes, it should be sufficient to say that pragmatically we do not currently have the technology capable of transforming any arbitrary conversation between humans into identical human–computer interactions. Consequently, we must for now dismiss the identity response.

■ *Exclusivity: Communication tasks are necessary and not replaceable.* This view emphasizes the necessity for communication and considers the size of the communication space to be natural and appropriate. Communication tasks are essentially "different" from the ones we currently support with information systems and, consequently, accomplish different things and need to be supported in different ways. For example, the informal and interactive nature of most conversations is essential, since the types of questions we seek to answer might be poorly structured and become clear only through the act of conversation. The idea that a query to a database could replace a conversation is meaningless, because the query only comes into existence as a result of the discussion. The exclusivity of communication response suggests that problems in the communication space arise because of the way we support these tasks, either ignoring them completely or shoe-horning them into formal information technology solutions that misunderstand the nature and role of communicative interaction.

- *Mixed: Some but not all tasks can be satisfied in either the information or the communication space.* Attempting to find common ground between the previous identity and exclusivity responses, the mixed hypothesis suggests that some communication tasks should be replaced by information systems. For example, information requests that occur frequently in the communication space, such as requests for laboratory results or drug information, could be gainfully replaced by information systems. The regularity of these requests permits them to be modeled accurately and serviced by a formal information system. The mixed response is probably the status quo viewpoint in informatics thinking, albeit an implicit one, since active consideration of tasks in the communication space is rare.

- *Continuum: Communication and information tasks are related but drawn from different parts of a task space.* This view holds that, while there are essential differences between what happens in an informal conversation and what happens in a formal information system transaction, these differences are simply those we find at different ends of the same continuum. Unlike the previous responses, the continuum view sees the whole information-communication task problem as a false dichotomy, perpetrated in part by technology. We see information and communication interactions as different only because we support them with different tools. While the telephone and the computer might rightly be seen as supporting one or the other type of task, a complex system like the Web begs classification and can support both communication and information tasks. As a result, the continuum view aims to understand which specific task characteristics would indicate where along the technologic continuum we look for solutions. However, to build tools tuned to the specific needs of information and communication tasks, we need to more precisely characterize this continuum. For example, is there some parameter in a clinical process that we could measure to help us decide when communication is better than computation? Without such precision, we are left to rely on rules of thumb or case lore and have progressed only little beyond the mixed hypothesis.

Two implications arise from the above analysis. First, and pragmatically, on the basis of either the exclusivity (necessity-of-communication) response or the mixed hypothesis, we need to recognize the importance of the informal transactions that occur in the communication space. Direct support of the communication between clinicians should substantially improve how our organizations acquire, present, and use information. By recognizing the communication space as an essential part of any organization's information systems, we avoid depending solely on the computational paradigm, which can end up shaping our view of how clinical decisions are made and cause us to ignore features of clinical practice that sit outside it. Thinking only in computational terms, we run the risk of becoming focused exclusively on re-engineering all clinical work into formal behaviors that are suitable for computational treatment.

Second, the continuum view suggests that developing a richer understanding of communication tasks should help us more appropriately craft and target information and communication technologies for our organizational information needs. Both of these implications will now be examined in turn.

Supporting Clinical Communication

To create processes and technologies that support the communication space, we first need to characterize the activities that occur within it and understand where improvement is needed. While much has been written about the dynamics of patient–clinician communication, very little is known about the way clinicians communicate with each other. More pertinently, the studies of communication processes from the wider perspective of the clinical organization are almost nonexistent. Perhaps the only shining exception here is the development of the structured clinical interview and problem-oriented medical record. These are communication innovations as much as information ones. They ensure that messages between clinicians are well formed and maximize the likelihood that critical information is "sent" and "received" via the reliable communication channel that we call the medical record.

What we do know about clinical communication systems in an organization like a hospital is that they carry a heavy burden of traffic and create an interrupt-driven workplace.[12] Clinical tasks generate many communication requests, and inefficiencies in communication system design, technology, and clinical behavior lead to an apparently much higher level of interaction than is necessary.

It is only by delving into the details of the specific conversations that we can start to understand who is responsible for the high level of traffic across communication systems and what the reasons for it are. In one analysis of a U.K. hospital, doctors were found to be the highest generator of communication traffic, sending almost twice as many messages as they received.[11] Furthermore, doctor–doctor interactions made up more than 40 percent of the calls made by the doctors in the study, denying the truism that medical staff suffer constant interruption because of the actions of other clinical staff in the hospital.

Of concern is that the high level of interruption, whatever its source or reason, may lead to errors by clinical staff. Well-known cognitive costs are associated with interruption, leading to diversion of attention, forgetfulness, and errors.[13-15] Furthermore, interruption often requires rescheduling of work plans. The interrupt-driven nature of the hospital work environment thus has the potential to generate extra costs in staff time and efficiency.

There are many potential reasons for the high level of call traffic in an organization. Many are specific to the systems in place in particular organizations, but others are general characteristics of clinical work and human interaction. Some potential causes of the high level of call traffic in hospitals include[11]:

- *Synchronous bias.* People seem to favor interruptive communication mechanisms, such as face-to-face discussion, paging, and the telephone, over less interruptive methods that are available to them. This may be because, in busy environments, tasks need to be "ticked off the list" once completed, to reduce cognitive load. For example, asking someone directly to complete a task produces immediate acknowledgment that the hand-over has occurred, but asynchronous channels like e-mail, voicemail, or notes are usually not designed to deliver the appropriate acknowledgment of message receipt and task acceptance.

- *Information seeking from humans.* The reliance of clinicians on discussion to resolve information needs has suggested to some that this is in response to poor printed or computer-based information sources.[6] Another hypothesis is that communication is actually the preferred mechanism for information gathering. Clinical problems are often poorly defined, and clarification can be obtained through conversation. Thus, clinical staff may opportunistically interrupt each other because face-to-face discussion is highly valued but difficult to schedule, and any opportunity is avidly seized.

- *Poor directory information about roles and responsibilities.* Up to a quarter of calls in hospital may be associated with identifying the name of an individual occupying a specific role. This suggests that poor support for identifying role occupants contributes significantly to overall call traffic.

- *Failure to reason about the impact of individual behavior.* Most clinicians seek to maximize their personal efficiency in serving their patients but do not seem to consider the consequences of their behavior on the overall operational efficiency of their organizations. However, the consequence of interrupting colleagues to satisfy individual needs may be a far more inefficient organization overall. This is analogous to a situation in which everyone elects to drive a car rather than take public transport, because the car is more convenient personally, but the overall impact is congested roads and slower transport times for all on the road.

While it is clear that much more research is needed into the nature of clinical communication processes, we can begin to outline the types of intervention that should lead to improved communications.

Nontechnical Interventions

Although it is tempting to immediately suggest new technical solutions, a variety of powerful nontechnical interventions can profoundly alter the communication dynamics of an organization. First, communication behaviors can be altered. Individuals can be encouraged to regard communication behaviors not as a personal style choice but as a professional skill. Educational programs can emphasize the individual and organizational costs of interruption, and staff can be trained to consider the costs and benefits of different communication channels and services. Second, communication policies can be altered. Beyond educational interventions, organizations have some power to institute mandatory policies that constrain professional behavior involving poor communication practice. For example, it might be reasonable to prohibit the sending of e-mail organizationwide unless strict criteria are met.

Technical Interventions

With the merging of information and communication technologies into new classes of communication networks and devices, the opportunity to innovate technically to improve communication is enormous. When faced with a communication task, system designers have the opportunity to introduce a variety of different interventions:

- *Channels.* One of the simplest interventions is to improve organizational infrastructure by introducing new channels for staff. For example, the introduction of pagers, mobile phones, or e-mail offers new options for interaction among staff who might otherwise have difficulty contacting each other. When faced with apparent difficulties in information flows in an organization, one should remember that communication channels are prime bearers of information and are a part of the solution to information problems—the telephone is an information system, too! For example, members of a clinical team may spend much of their days geographically separated. Providing team members with an asynchronous channel like a shared "to-do" list on a wireless palmtop device would allow team members to track one anothers' activities and prevent duplication of tasks as well as provide a check to ensure that all team tasks are completed.

- *Communication services.* Communication channels can bear a variety of different services or applications on top of them.[16] The telephone channel, for example, can bear voice, fax, and e-mail services. Thus, if analysis of organization call traffic reveals that many calls are attempting to identify who occupies a specific role or that errors occur because of a failure to contact an individual in a role, then a role-based call-forwarding service might help.[12,17] Teams of individuals can also be coordinated using complex role-based calling services. For example, calls to a medical emergency team can be managed by a system that uses knowledge of team roles to ensure that someone in each designated role is called and acknowledges receipt of a call.[12] Such information-enhanced communication systems use specific knowledge about communication patterns and users to optimize the routing and management of messages.

- *Types of message.* Fine-grained analysis of communication traffic may reveal that certain classes of message may benefit from automation. For example, computer-generated alerts can be sent to physicians to notify them of significant clinical events, with substantial clinical benefit.[18] Computer-based notification systems thus integrate with the communication infrastructure of an organization and offer a mechanism to extend the level of interaction between traditional information systems and clinicians.[19] Sometimes, even simpler methods of sending messages can help. For example, individuals in specific roles can be routinely interrupted with the same request from different individuals. The number of calls they receive could be reduced by providing a page of information on a Web-based local directory with answers to these frequent questions.

- *Agents.* The notion that some computational services can act as semi-autonomous proxies for their owners is now well established. Agents responsible for creating, receiving, or filtering messages can be created. As with human beings, interesting conflicts arise between the needs of individuals and the needs of organizations. For example, clinicians may wish to instruct an agent to filter certain classes of message they consider annoying, but organizational policy may wish to override such individual preferences when wider concerns are taken into account.

Typically, a communication system will introduce a bundle of new interventions into an organization, each with different effects. For example, introducing a computer-based notification system for alerts will have channel, service, and message effects. The channel effect may be positive, by permitting a shift of existing events from the synchronous to the asynchronous domain, reducing the number of interruptions. Thus, rather than receiving pages from laboratories or the pharmacy, a clinician will instead receive e-mail that can be read at the time of the clinician's choosing. However, the message effect of introducing a new communication system may be to generate new types of events in the asynchronous domain. This could increase the overall message load, with consequent increases in demand on user time and effort. Such systems thus have the potential to either harm or help, depending on which of the effects dominates and the state of the local environment.

The Continuum View

The continuum view suggests that developing a richer understanding of the connection between communication and information tasks should help in the design and blending of information and communication technologies. It is easy to construct specific examples, in which a solution to a problem can be engineered using different mixes of computational or communication technologies. For example, to minimize the efforts of clinical staff in learning to use an electronic record system, one might use speech recognition and synthesis technologies. Alternatively, using a communication channel like the phone, and alternative structuring of processes and roles, staff can dictate notes and send orders via trained computer operators[20] (Figure 1).

The challenge is to develop a set of principles that permit choices between such alternatives to be made rationally and to guide the design and implementation of systems along different points of the continuum. From an informatics viewpoint, we can take a first-principle approach, which regards all informatics tasks as model construction and application.[16] It makes sense, therefore, to look at how models are handled in information and communication technologies.

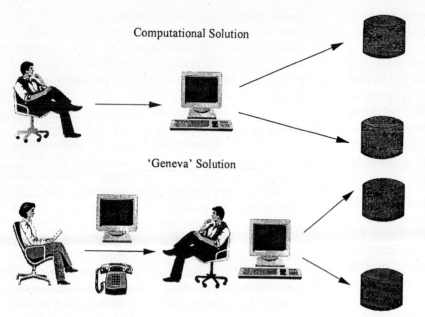

Computational Solution

'Geneva' Solution

Figure 1 A voice-driven interface to an electronic medical record system can use a computational solution relying on speech technologies or a hybrid approach using communication and information technology. One design solution developed at the University Hospital in Geneva allowed clinical staff to interact with the medical record via a telephone pool of trained operators.

In simple terms, we can say that information technologies require explicit formalizations of information processes for them to operate, whereas communication systems remain relatively informal to process models.[21] A telephone, for example, needs no model of the conversation that occurs across it to operate. In contrast, a computer system would need to explicitly model any dialog that occurs across it. From this point of view, we can say that a continuum of possible model formalization is available to us. For a given task, system designers make an explicit choice to model some or all of a process, based on their perception of costs and benefits. When the choice is to formalize the process substantially, computational solutions are sometimes used. When the task is left informal, we find instead that communication solutions are required.

Searching for a similar characterization of the continuum, one can turn to the literature in psychology and linguistics. While much communication research is focused on the specifics of conversational structure, some work does step back and look at the underlying notions of how much of a conversation has been explicitly modeled. In particular, the psychological notion of *common ground* is a strong match with the notion of relative formality of model construction.

Common ground refers to the knowledge shared by two communicating agents.[22] For a conversation to occur, agents have to share knowledge about language as well as knowledge about the subject under discussion. We know intuitively, for example, that discussing a medical problem with a clinical colleague or with a patient results in very different conversations. While messages can be concise and much mutual knowledge can be assumed between colleagues, explaining an issue to a nonexpert requires the main message to be sent along with the background knowledge needed to make the message understandable.

Unsurprisingly then, human agents communicate more easily with others of similar occupation and educational background, since they have similar experiences, beliefs, and knowledge.[23] Furthermore, the more individuals communicate, the more similar they become.[24] We can recognize the sharing of common ground as a key reason that similar agents find it easy to converse with each other. In addition, two separate streams of dialogue actually occur during any given conversation. The first is concerned with the specifics of the conversation, while the second is devoted to checking that messages have been understood, and may result in the sharing of common ground when it is clear that assumptions about shared knowledge do not hold.[25] Thus, building common ground requires mutual effort and consent between participating agents.

The notion of common ground holds whether we are discussing a conversational interaction between human beings or a human–computer interaction. For a computationally rendered information system, the system designer must create a model of what the user will want to do with the application. For their part, users have to learn a model of how to operate the computer application. When both computer and user share this common ground, the interaction should be succinct and effective. When the user and system do not share mutual knowledge, we run into difficulty. If the user lacks knowledge of the system's operation, the human–computer dialogue will be ineffective. On the other hand, a system that does not model its context of use will be regarded as an inappropriate intrusion into the workplace.

Building common ground incurs costs for the participating agents. For example, a computer user spends some time up front learning the functions of a system in anticipation of having to use them for future interactions. Inevitably, not everything that can be "said" to the computer is learned in this way, and users also typically learn new features of a system as they interact with it for particular tasks. This means that agents have two broad classes of grounding choice:

- *Pre-emptive grounding.* Agents can share knowledge prior to a specific conversational task, assuming that it will be needed in the future. They elect to bear the grounding cost ahead of time and risk the effort being wasted if it is never used. This is a good strategy when task time is limited. For example, if a rare event is nonetheless an urgent one, preparation is essential. Thus, pilots, nuclear power plant operators, and clinicians all train rigorously for rare but mission-critical events, since failure to prepare has potentially catastrophic consequences. Training a medical emergency team on how to interact with each other makes sense because at the time of a real clinical emergency, there is no time for individuals to question each other to understand the meaning of any specific orders or requests. Pre-emptive grounding is a bad strategy when the shared knowledge is never used and the time and effort in grounding becomes wasted. For example, training students with knowledge that is unlikely to be used when they face a task in the workplace is usually a poor allocation of resources. From first principles, the cost of pre-emptive grounding is proportionate to the amount of common ground an agent has to learn. For example, the length of messages increases, as does the cost of checking and maintaining the currency of the knowledge once received (Figure 2)

- *Just-in-time grounding.* Agents can choose to share only specific task knowledge at the time they have a discussion. This is a good strategy when there are no other reasons to talk to an agent. For example, if the task or encounter is rare, it probably does not make sense to expend resources in the anticipation of an unlikely event. Conversely, it is a bad strategy when there is limited task time for grounding at the time of the conversation. Just-in-time grounding is also a poor strategy if one of the agents involved in the dialogue is reluctant to expend energy learning. Thus, computer system designers might face difficulties if they assume that users are willing to

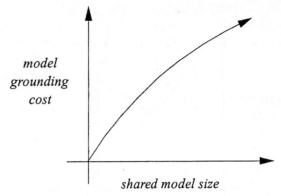

Figure 2 The cost of pre-emptive grounding increases with the amount of knowledge agents share: The more we share, the greater the cost of telling and maintaining.

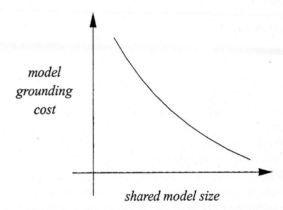

Figure 3 The cost of "just-in-time" grounding decreases with the amount of prior knowledge agents already share about a task: The less we share, the more I have to share now.

spend time during the routine course of their day learning new features of their system, when the users are already overcommitted to other tasks. The cost of just-in-time grounding is inversely proportional to the amount of prior shared knowledge between agents. For example, a message between agents with a high degree of common ground will be very terse, but the length (and thus cost) of transmitting a message to an agent with little common ground will be greater (Figure 3).

Any given interaction between two agents usually involves costs borne at the time of the conversation, as well as costs borne previously in pre-emptive groundings (Figure 4). Information system designers thus have choices about the amount of grounding they expect of the agents who will participate in organizational interactions. At the "solid-ground" end of the spectrum, the effective or efficient completion of tasks requires agents to share knowledge ahead of time. At the other end of the spectrum, on "shifting ground,"

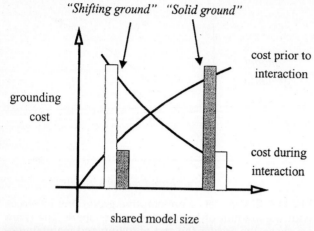

Figure 4 For any given interaction, some of the grounding costs are borne at the time of the interaction and some have been borne earlier. This means that an information system designer has a spectrum of options for designing the interaction between computer and user.

it is hard or uneconomic to decide what ground should be pre-emptively shared.

Thus, with solid-ground interactions, a user is expected to have learned most of the formalities of an information system or, conversely, the system is expected to have adapted to the needs of the users. On shifting ground, the information system is designed to handle interactions that require new knowledge to be exchanged at the time of interaction. This may be in the form of online help to the user or the acquisition of data from the user.

When Is Conversation Better than Computation?

Common ground is a candidate for the continuum parameter, which links information and communication system design. It offers us an operational measurement that can be used to define the characteristics of specific interactions between agents, whether they are human or computational. Using it, we should be able to analyze the specifics of a particular set of interactions and make broad choices about whether they would be better served by communication or computational systems. It should also allow us to make finer-grained distinctions about the dynamics of such interactions as, for example with regard to the amount of grounding that needs to be supported in a specific human–machine conversation.

With this in mind, we can now simply regard information models as part of the common ground of an organization and its members. We can choose to model any interaction across a spectrum from zero to a "complete" formal description (Figure 5). Further-

more, the models of our organizational systems have value only when we interact with them through our information or communication systems. In other words, for computational tools to be of value, they have to share ground with human beings. Users need to know how to use the system, and the system needs to be fashioned to users' needs. If an information system is perfectly crafted to model the processes of an organization but not the resource constraints of those who will need to learn to use it, the logic that predicts its failure is inevitable. Consequently, we should no longer consider information models in isolation but rather include the models that users will need to carry with them. Simply building an information model without regard to how it will be shared with those who interact with it ignores the complex realities of the workplace and does not factor in the costs and benefits of using the model for individuals.

"Pure" communication tools such as the telephone can now be seen to be neutral in any particular conversation that occurs over them, and they need no common ground with the agents using them. As such, they are well suited to support poorly grounded conversations, when it is hard to predict ahead of time what knowledge needs to be shared. We thus favor the use of communication tools across shifting ground with a high just-in-time grounding component. This may be because the interacting agents do not share sufficient ground, or it may be because it simply is not economic to do the modeling. The transacted information is thus often personal, local, informal, or rare. It is up to the agents having the discussion to share knowledge. The channel simple provides basic

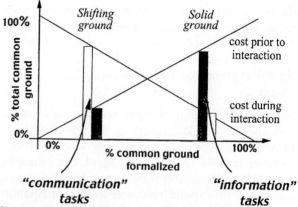

Figure 5 A continuum of common ground between agents defines how much of the interaction can be modeled formally ahead of time and how much needs to be left informal until the time of the interaction. Computational systems work well when substantial modeling can occur ahead of time, while communication systems can be used when agents are unable to reliably model their interactions ahead of time.

support to ensure that the conversation takes place. Communication channels are thus used de facto when no computational tools exist to support the interaction.

Furthermore, for highly grounded conversations, we know that the agents will be able to have succinct conversations. One can predict that they will need lower bandwidth channels than if the message exchange were poorly grounded. Poorly grounded conversations, in contrast, need a higher bandwidth, since more information has to be exchanged between the conversing agents. Building such common ground between agents may require the sharing of information objects such as images and designs.[26]

In contrast, we favor computational tools when it is appropriate to formalize interactions ahead of time and when the users of the system are willing, able, and resourced to build common ground with the tool. Such interactions occur over solid ground, having a high pre-emptive grounding component. The information exchanged in such situations is worth formalizing, perhaps because it is stable, repetitive, archival, or critical but rare. The computational system moves from being a passive channel to the interaction to either modifying what is said or becoming a conversational agent itself.

An information system designer also needs to take into account the common ground that is expected of the system users. For example, the voice-driven electronic record system illustrated in Figure 1 requires users to understand both their clinical task ground and the operation of the electronic tool. For complicated systems, the resource implications of mastering both clinical task and tool ground can be unacceptable to users. In contrast, using operators to drive the computer system allows the clinical users to master only their clinical tasks, leaving mastery of the computational system to the operators. Thus, clinicians can devote most of their pre-emptive efforts to clinical tasks and learn most about the specifics of the computational tool on a needs-only basis during interactions.

For computational tools, choices also need to be made between the traditional process of information modeling prior to system construction and a more interactive approach to building models. Thus, a system designer may try to model all the user needs prior to the construction of a system or engineer some flexibility into the architecture that will allow personalization of the interaction for specific users. For example, a system may gather data about the frequency of different requests from a specific user and customize its behavior to optimize for the most frequent requests of the individual, rather than the population as a whole. Such computational systems build common

ground with their users in a just-in-time fashion, as well as having pre-emptive modeling to cover the most common features users will need.

Conclusion

The communication space is the largest part of the health information space and seems to contain a substantial proportion of the health system's information "pathology." Nevertheless, it has been largely ignored in our informatics thinking. In this paper, two implications of acknowledging the primacy of communication have been explored. First, there is an immediate need to support communication in our health care organizations, since this should lead to substantial improvements in organizational efficiency and effectiveness as well as offering a genuine opportunity to improve patient care. To do this we need to develop a richer understanding of the specific communication systems in our health care organizations. With such an understanding, a variety of technical and nontechnical interventions can be brought into play to improve poor communication processes.

Communication research is also important for developing our understanding of the basic principles of informatics. Understanding the interrelationship between communication and information tasks may help us re-evaluate the role of technologic support. Common ground is a powerful candidate concept that may help unify our understanding of information and communication in just such a way.

References ■

1. Coiera E. The impact of culture on technology. Med J Aust. 1999;171:508–9.
2. Berg M. Rationalizing Medical Work: Decision Support Techniques and Medical Practice. Cambridge, Mass: MIT Press, 1997.
3. Lorenzi NM, Riley RT, Blyth JC, Southon G, Dixon BJ. Antecedents of the people and organizational aspects of medical informatics: review of the literature. Journal of the American Medical Informatics Association. 1997;4:79–101.
4. Markus ML. Electronic mail as the medium of managerial choice. Organisation Sci. 1994;5(4):502–27.
5. Reeves B, Nass C. The Media Equation. Cambridge, UK: Cambridge University Press, 1996.
6. Covell DG, Uman GC, Manning PR. Information needs in office practice: are they being met? Ann Intern Med. 1985; 103:596–9.
7. Tang P, Jaworski MA, Fellencer CA, Kreider N, LaRosa MP, Marquardt WC. Clinical information activities in diverse ambulatory care practices. Proc AMIA Annu Fall Symp. 1996:12–6.
8. Safran C, Sands DZ, Rind DM. Online medical records: a decade of experience. Methods Inf Med. 1999;38:308–12.
9. Wilson RM, Runciman WB, Gibberd RW, et al. The Quality

in Australian Health Care Study. Med J Aust. 1995;163:458–71.

10. Bhasale AL, Miller GC, Reid SE, et al. Analysing potential harm in Australian general practice: an incident-monitoring study. Med J Aust. 1998;169:73–6.

11. Coiera E, Tombs V. Communication behaviours in a hospital setting: an observational study. BMJ. 1998;316:673–6.

12. Coiera E. Clinical communication: a new informatics paradigm. Proc AMIA Annu Fall Symp. 1996:17–21.

13. Reitman JS. Without surreptitious rehearsal, information in short-term memory decays. J Verbal Learning Behav. 1974; 13:365–77.

14. Baddeley AD. Working Memory. Oxford, UK: Oxford University Press, 1986.

15. Reason J. Human Error. Cambridge, UK: Cambridge University Press, 1990.

16. Coiera E. Guide to Medical Informatics, the Internet and Telemedicine. London, UK: Arnold, 1997.

17. Coiera E, Gupta A. A communication system for organizations incorporating task and role identification, and personal and organizational communication policy management. U.S. patent 5,949,866; granted Sep 7, 1999.

18. Sullivan F, Mitchell E. Has general practitioner computing made a difference to patient care? A systematic review of published reports. BMJ. 1995;311:848–52.

19. Wagner MM, Tsui F, Pike J, Pike L. Design of a clinical notification system. Proc AMIA Annu Symp. 1999:989–93.

20. Scherrer JR, Baud RH, Hochstrasser D, Ratib O. An integrated hospital information system in Geneva. MD Comput. 1990;7(2):81–9.

21. Coiera E. Informality. Bristol, UK: Hewlett Packard Laboratories, Bristol, Feb 1997. Technical report HPL-97-37 970212. Also available at: http://www.coiera.com/publica.htm

22. Clarke H, Brennan S. Grounding in communication. In: Resnick LB. Levine J, Behreno SD (eds). Perspectives on Socially Shared Cognition. Washington, DC: American Psychological Association, 1991.

23. Lazarsfeld PF, Merton RK. Friendship as social process: a substantive and methodological analysis. In Berger M, et al. (eds.). Freedom and Control in Modern Society. New York: Octagon, 1964.

24. Rogers EM. Diffusion of Innovations. 4th ed. New York: Free Press, 1995.

25. Clark HH. Using Language. Cambridge, UK: Cambridge University Press, 1996.

26. Ramsay J, Barabesi A, Preece J. Informal communication is about sharing objects and media. Interact Comput. 1996; 8(3):277–83.

Baby CareLink: Using the Internet and Telemedicine to Improve Care for High-Risk Infants

James E. Gray, MD, MS*‡; Charles Safran, MD, MS‡; Roger B. Davis, ScD‡;
Grace Pompilio-Weitzner, RN*‡; Jane E. Stewart, MD, MS*; Linda Zaccagnini, RN, NNP*; and
DeWayne Pursley, MD, MPH*

GLOSSARY

Broadband: A high-speed Internet connection

ISDN: Integrated Services Digital Network provides high-speed digital phone service that can be delivered through standard phone lines and facilitates videoconferencing

Mb, Gb: Megabyte and gigabyte, respectively. A measure of the amount of memory contained in a computer

RAM: Random access memory

Shockwave Applet: A computer application used within a World Wide Web (WWW) browser to display animated and interactive content

Virtual house calls: The use of videoconferencing technology to allow clinicians to check on a patient without the need for a home visit

WWW browser: A program such as Microsoft Internet Explorer or Netscape Navigator that allows a computer user to view information contained on the World Wide Web

Secure Sockets Layer: A standard method for encrypting data during transit across the Internet

---

ABBREVIATIONS. NICU, neonatal intensive care unit; VLBW, very low birth weight; WWW, World Wide Web; PIN, personal identification number; ICU, intensive care unit.

ABSTRACT. *Objective.* To evaluate an Internet-based telemedicine program designed to reduce the costs of care, to provide enhanced medical, informational, and emotional support to families of very low birth weight (VLBW) infants during and after their neonatal intensive care unit (NICU) stay.

Background. Baby CareLink is a multifaceted telemedicine program that incorporates videoconferencing and World Wide Web (WWW) technologies to enhance interactions between families, staff, and community providers. The videoconferencing module allows virtual visits and distance learning from a family's home during an infant's hospitalization as well as virtual house calls and remote monitoring after discharge. Baby CareLink's WWW site contains information on issues that confront these families. In addition, its security architecture allows efficient and confidential sharing of patient-based data and communications among authorized hospital and community users.

Design/Methods. A randomized trial of Baby CareLink was conducted in a cohort of VLBW infants born between November 1997 and April 1999. Eligible infants were randomized within 10 days of birth. Families of intervention group infants were given access to the Baby CareLink telemedicine application. A multimedia computer with WWW browser and videoconferencing equipment was installed in their home within 3 weeks of birth. The control group received care as usually practiced in this NICU. Quality of care was assessed using a standardized family satisfaction survey administered after discharge. In addition, the effect of Baby CareLink on hospital length of stay as well as family visitation and interactions with infant and staff were measured.

Results. Of the 176 VLBW infants admitted during the study period, 30 control and 26 study patients were enrolled. The groups were similar in patient and family characteristics as well as rates of inpatient morbidity. The CareLink group reported higher overall quality of care. Families in the CareLink group reported significantly fewer problems with the overall quality of care received by their family (mean problem score: 3% vs 13%). In addition, CareLink families also reported greater satisfaction with the unit's physical environment and visitation policies (mean problem score: 13% vs 50%). The frequency of family visits, telephone calls to the NICU, and holding of the infant did not differ between groups. The duration of hospitalization until ultimate discharge home was similar in the 2 groups (68.5 ± 28.3 vs 70.6 ± 35.6 days). Among infants born weighing <1000 g ($n = 31$) there was a tendency toward shorter lengths of stay (77.4 ± 26.2 vs 93.1 ± 35.6 days). All infants in the CareLink group were discharged directly to home whereas 6/30 (20%) of control infants were transferred to community hospitals before ultimate discharge home.

Conclusions. CareLink significantly improves family satisfaction with inpatient VLBW care and definitively lowers costs associated with hospital to hospital transfer. Our data suggest the use of telemedicine and the Internet support the educational and emotional needs of families facilitating earlier discharge to home of VLBW infants. We believe that further extension of the Baby CareLink model to the postdischarge period will significantly improve the coordination and efficiency of care. *Pediatrics* 2000;106:1318–1324; *neonatal intensive care unit, very low birth weight (infant), telemedicine, Internet, videoconferencing, randomized controlled trial, medical informatics.*

From the *Department of Neonatology, Beth Israel Deaconess Medical Center; and the ‡Center for Clinical Computing, Beth Israel Deaconess Medical Center, Harvard Medical School, Boston Massachusetts.

Disclosure: Dr Safran is Chief Executive Officer of Clinician Support Technology (CST). Ms Pompilio-Weitzner is currently clinical content specialist to CST. Dr Gray holds equity in and serves as a consultant to CST. CST is a developer and distributor of CareLink applications.

The Baby CareLink Clinical and Technical Team consists of the following individuals: Sheleagh Alsop-Somers, MSW; Hollis Caswell, RN; Peter Jones; Alison Levy, MS; Glen Low, RRT, PhD; Alfredo Morales, MS; Michele Phillips, RN, PhD; Mary Quinn, RN, NNP; Annette Roberts, RN; David Veroff; Qiang Wang, MD; and Gail Wolfsdorf, MSW.

Received for publication May 26, 2000; accepted Jul 3, 2000.

Reprint requests to (J.E.G.) Beth Israel Deaconess Medical Center, Department of Neonatology, 330 Brookline Ave, Boston, MA 02115. E-mail: jgray@bidmc.harvard.edu

---

The original paper contained coloured figures.

The admission of a newborn child to the neonatal intensive care unit (NICU) is among the most emotionally distressing situations that a family can face. Young families with little experience with critical care medicine are thrown into a high-tech environment that is bewildering and foreign to most parents.[1] A sick child may pose emotional, educational, and logistic problems for a parent. During a family's stay in the NICU and after discharge, they need not only top-quality medical care, but also effective and creative information sharing. We hypothesized that Internet and telemedicine technologies could influence these family needs and lower health care costs. In this report we will describe our efforts to design, implement, and test a high-tech approach to provide individualized support to the families of very low birth weight (VLBW) infants.

Telemedicine broadly defined means care at a distance. Early telemedicine approaches could almost be characterized as medicine with 2-way television.[2] The convergence of voice, data, and video on the broadband Internet lends support to the notion that telemedicine can and should use this new medium for transmitting and obtaining clinically relevant information. Almost 120 million Americans have accessed the Internet from home and office. The use of the World Wide Web (WWW) to gather medical information has also skyrocketed with over 45 million Americans using the WWW to gather health information.[3] Fast access to the Internet within the home is happening more rapidly then any other technological introduction in modern history. Despite the ubiquitous availability of the Internet in the home, the use of the Internet to evolve new models of care is unexplored. Here we report the first randomized, controlled clinical trial of this technology to change the delivery of care.

METHODS

Baby CareLink

Baby CareLink was created by a team of neonatologists, nurse practitioners, nurses and respiratory therapists, social workers, child life specialists, medical informatitions, and software engineers. Baby CareLink provides information to families using both a specially designed WWW-based system and a system of videoconferencing from the NICU. The CareLink system is programmed using Microsoft BackOffice (Microsoft Corporation, Redmond, WA) components including Internet Information Server 4.0, Active Server Pages and SQL Server 6.5. Security Services were provided using ACE Server (RSA Security Incorporated, Bedford, MA). Baby CareLink dynamically generates WWW pages that can be accessed from a standard web browser. Educational content is enhanced with video, audio, and ShockWave applets (Macromedia Company, San Francisco, CA).

Six major areas of clinical content and resources are present within Baby CareLink Web including a daily clinical report, a message center, a see your infant section, a family room, a clinical information section, and a section focused on preparation for discharge to home (Fig 1). The daily report is a web-page that provides clinical updates about an infant's clinical care and status. This report relies on dynamic links to the NICU's electronic medical record system (HP CareVue, Hewlett Packard Company, Andover, MA) to avoid the need for clinicians to enter information into 2 separate systems. The message center is a WWW-based messaging system through which parents can share confidential communications with members of the NICU staff. Baby CareLink also contains a context sensitive messaging throughout the CareLink site to allow parents to easily compose messages related

to the content they are viewing. The see your infant section is a pictorial daily journal comprised of images captured by the staff with a consumer grade digital camera. Baby CareLink also provides a mechanism for allowing families to share these photographs outside of the confines of the CareLink security architecture. By changing a picture's status through the WWW-based interface, parents can post pictures to a password protected WWW where their families and friends can see their infant. This approach maintains the locus of control for making these photographs public with the parents. The family room provides a potpourri of supports including answers to common questions, information about services available to families, links to WWW-based resources, an on-line library for browsing available print and video resources. "The Kid's Corner" provides a collection of information and support materials specifically geared for older siblings of our patients. "The Emotional Side of the NICU" allows parents to both read about the issues that confront families of high-risk newborns and view high-quality digital video of NICU families discussing how they coped with their NICU experience. The clinical information and care section describes the issues present at various stages in an infant's NICU stay including when an infant is first admitted, as an infant stabilizes and family members becomes more active participants in their infant's care, and the period before discharge when families prepare to take over all of their infant's care at home. The "NICU-Pedia" provides an on-line encyclopedia of clinical conditions, tests, treatments, and medications relevant to the care of high-risk newborns. The preparing for discharge section is an on-line discharge teaching module where parents can view multimedia modules describing the knowledge and competencies they must acquire before discharge. This module is constructed so that NICU clinicians can individualize the content for each infant's needs using a simple WWW interface. It also allows parents and clinicians to track acquisition of knowledge.

Patients enrolled in the evaluation study intervention group received a standard Hewlett Packard Vectra 233 MHz Pentium II processor computer with 32 MB of RAM, a 3.1 GB hard disk, a 12X CD-ROM drive, a 33.6 baud full duplex fax modem with a speakerphone, a 16-bit sound card, and a 17-inch SVGA color monitor with integrated speaker. The homestation, which has Windows 95, was equipped with PictureTel (Andover, MA) Live 200 desktop videoconferencing equipment. Families could access the WWW-based information from any computer equipped with a standard web browser. Connections to CareLink were made through standard phone lines for WWW access, while videoconferencing used 128Kb ISDN lines. Both the computer equipment and communication lines were provided to families at no cost to them. Arrangements for installation of home units were made at the time of randomization. Units were left in the families' home for 4 to 6 months after discharge. An outside company installed the equipment in each family's home and retrieved it at the end of the study period. Clinicians in the NICU had Internet access through hospital clinical workstations. Three mobile videoconferencing carts with a PictureTel group conferencing system allowed conferencing from each of the NICU's 33 bedspaces.

The identity of users is verified using RSA SecurID hardware tokens (RSA Security Inc, Bedford, MA). These tokens are small, handheld devices containing microprocessors that calculate and display unpredictable, one-time-only codes. The codes automatically change every 60 seconds. To access patient-specific data, the CareLink site requires that a user begin a session by entering a username and a password. The password is the combination of a memorized personal identification number (PIN) and the currently displayed 6-digit code on the RSA SecurID device. This information is transmitted to a security server that authenticates the user and verifies that the correct password was entered. The security server compares the user-entered password with its knowledge of the correct password for that 60-second period. If the password does not match, it also checks the password from the previous minute to account for delays in typing and transmission. Once a password is verified, the user is authenticated for the entire CareLink site for the duration of the web session or 15 minutes, whichever is less. Each user is assigned to a group (parent, NICU staff, community provider, or administrator) and is linked to 1 or more patients. This information is initialized at the beginning of a session and then used for the entire session. CareLink dynamically generates web pages based on the group identifier and patient links of the user. CareLink uses the group identifier to provide

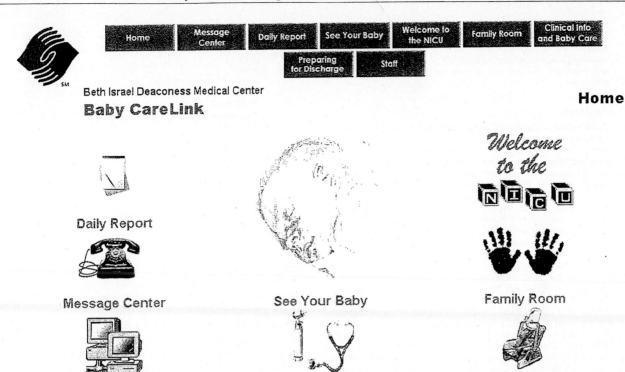

Fig 1. The home page of Baby CareLink.

different features on the web pages and uses patient links to limit patient data access to patients linked to that user. The RSA SecurID username, password, and all patient data are transmitted through the standard Secure Sockets encryption Layer to protect confidentiality. Extensive audit logs are kept for each session.

Study Design

Project participants were selected from VLBW infants born at Beth Israel Deaconess Medical Center, Boston Massachusetts, between November 1, 1997, and March 30, 1999 and cared for in its NICU. Infants were excluded if ISDN access was not available at their family's primary residence or if the infants expected length of stay in the study NICU was expected to be <14 days (eg, because of need for transfer for surgical care at the nearby Children's Hospital, or because of planned transfer back to a referring community hospital for infants born weighing >1250 g). In addition, infants were excluded if their family lacked a permanent residence, did not speak English, or if discharge to other than the biological family was expected. Lack of basic telephone service in the family residence was not used as an exclusion criterion. For such families, basic telephone service was arranged for the duration of the study period. Attending physicians could exclude a family from the study if they felt enrolling the family in a study would be clinically inappropriate. The families of eligible study infants were approached for consent to participate between the infant's third and tenth hospital day.

After informed consent was obtained, infants were randomized to the intervention or control group using a birth weight-stratified permuted block design. Infants in the control group received information and support as usually provided in the NICU, while those in the intervention group were given access to the Baby CareLink system as described above. In cases of multiple deliveries (ie, twins/triplets etc), 1 infant was randomly selected for random assignment to either the intervention or the control group. Treatment status of the remaining siblings was yoked to that of the selected sibling (ie, if the infant was assigned to the intervention arm, his or her siblings also received the intervention). Only data about the randomized infant is included in analyses. The clinical team made all decisions regarding clinical care including those regarding the timing of discharge.

Sociodemographic and clinical information was collected from the medical record and from family interviews. Recorded elements included birth weight, gestational age, sex, plurality, maternal race, mode of delivery, and Apgar scores as well as maternal characteristics including maternal educational level, gravidity, parity, and marital status. Disposition from the study NICU was recorded as 1) alive and discharged from the hospital, 2) alive and transferred to another facility (eg, level II, III or rehabilitation facility), or 3) died. Discharge date from the study hospital was recorded, as was the date of ultimate discharge home for those transferred to other facilities. Information on the frequency of family visits and telephone calls to the NICU as well as episodes of kangaroo care and other types of holding by the family was abstracted from the medical record. Information on a family's previous experience with the use of computer technologies was recorded at the time of family training using a structured written survey instrument.

Each family in the Baby CareLink group was given a single training session that focused on the hardware and software to be used in their home. These sessions lasted between 45 and 120 minutes with most lasting <75 minutes. The local phone company installed ISDN lines in the family residence and computer hardware was placed and tested by a local hardware service provider. Hardware and ISDN lines were placed in most homes within 12 days of randomization. In only 1 case, installation required more than 3 weeks.

The Picker Institute's Neonatal Intensive Care Unit Family Satisfaction survey[4] was used to assess family perceptions of the quality of care provided to them and their infant by the NICU. This 80-item written questionnaire was administered to families between 1 and 4 months after their child's discharge from the NICU. Surveys were not sent to families of infants who died in the NICU or whose child was discharged to chronic care facilities. The Picker instrument is designed to assess family experiences within the following 8 dimensions of care: 1) information and education to parents, 2) environment and visitation policies, 3) family and infant support by the NICU, 4) confidence and trust in the NICU, 5) continuity and transition, 6) family participation in care, 7) overall impressions, and 8) coordination of care. Responses to each question and within each dimension are tabulated to form a problem score, representing the percentage of questions within a dimension that elicited a problem response. For example, Item 67 asks, "How would you rate the way the NICU staff worked together? Possible responses included poor, fair, good, very good, and excellent. The first two of these are characterized as problem responses.

Analyses

Statistical analysis was performed using the SAS Statistical Software version 6.12 for Windows (SAS Institute, Cary, NC). Simple comparisons were done using χ^2 testing or Wilcoxon rank sum tests where appropriate. Length of stay was compared with the Wilcoxon rank sum test. Additionally, proportional hazards models were fit, allowing adjustment for birth weight and the ability to treat in-hospital deaths as incomplete (ie, censored) observations. Because the more complicated model did not change the conclusions, only the Wilcoxon test results are reported.

Comparison of problem scores for both individual questions and dimensions was done using Fisher's exact test.

Descriptive analysis of web utilization was performed using 2 methods. Family and staff sessions were identified and tabulated using the CareLink Security logs. Utilization of individual sections and pages within CareLink was identified from the web server logs maintained by Internet Information Server. Because the breadth of WWW content changed during the course of the study, we analyzed a 6-month period during which all content was present and was unchanging (November 7, 1998, through April 7, 1999). This tabulation was done using Web Trends Log Analyzer Version 5.0 (WebTrends Corporation, Portland, OR). Utilization of videoconferencing was assessed by review of the ISDN line billing records.

The Beth Israel Deaconess Medical Center's Committee on Clinical Investigation approved the study.

RESULTS

One hundred seventy-six VLBW infants were admitted to the NICU during the study period. Eighty-eight infants (50%) were excluded from the trial because of the presence of 1 or more exclusion criteria (Table 1). Eighty-eight infants were eligible for randomization. The families of 9 infants declined to participate and 4 were unavailable to provide consent during the enrollment period. Of the 75 remaining infants, 26 were randomized to the Baby CareLink arm and 30 were randomized to receive usual care. The 7 siblings of infants in the Baby CareLink group and 12 siblings of control infants were placed in the same study group as their randomized sibling.

The 120 excluded infants were of slightly higher birth weight (1087 ± 286 vs 995 ± 290 g; $P < .05$) and higher gestational age (28.8 ± 2.7 vs 27.7 ± 2.3 weeks; $P < .05$) than the 56 study infants. The excluded infants and 56 study infants did not differ in gender distribution, plurality, maternal race, or insurance status.

Demographic and clinical characteristics of the 2 study groups are presented in Table 2. The 2 groups were similar in birth weight, gestational age, plurality, maternal race, and educational level, as well as insurance status. Infants in the Baby CareLink group were more likely to have been delivered by cesarean section (92.3% vs 63.3%; $P < .05$) and to be born to a single mother (38.5% vs 13.3%; $P < .05$). Similar percentages of parents of each group lived together in the same home (88.5% vs 90.0%; $P \geq .85$).

Infants in the CareLink group remained hospitalized for a shorter time than those in the usual care group although this difference was not significant

TABLE 1. Reasons for Exclusion

Admitted to NICU During Study Period		176
Ineligible		88
Reasons*		
Expected length of stay		39
ISDN service not available		29
Early death		12
Non-English speaking family		7
Attending exclusion		5
No permanent residence		3
Consent not obtained	13	
Parents unavailable for consent		4
Parents did not consent		9
Eligible for randomization	75	
Randomized		56
Sibling of randomized infant		19

* Not mutually exclusive.

(68.5 ± 28.3 vs 70.6 ± 35.6 days; $P \geq .05$). Interestingly, posthoc subgroup analysis showed the difference among infants born weighing <1000 g to be even greater (77.4 ± 26.2 vs 93.1 ± 35.6 days; $P \geq .05$). The difference in lengths of stay among infants of higher birth weight was smaller (54.4 ± 26.9 vs 48.2 ± 16.8 days; $P \geq .05$) Of note, control infants were significantly more likely to be back-transported to level II facilities (20% vs 0%; $P < .05$).

During the study period, 1033 CareLink WWW sessions were initiated by NICU and project staff members (1.8 sessions/day). During the same period, the 26 CareLink families initiated 1744 sessions. This represents 67 sessions per family and an average of 0.98 sessions per inpatient day. The average duration of WWW sessions for all users was 5.4 minutes. Most family sessions were initiated from the home. The mother's security token was used to initiate 64% of the WWW sessions. Table 3 shows that the patient-specific areas within the CareLink WWW were the most commonly visited. During the study period, families initiated 328 videoconferencing sessions. These sessions lasted on average 6 minutes.

Postdischarge surveys were administered to 51 families. Five families were not surveyed because of NICU death (1 family) or transfer to and discharge from another level III or rehabilitative facility (4 families). Responses were received from 31 families (61% response rate). The response rate was similar in both groups. There was no difference between responders and nonresponders when compared on birth weight, gestational age, Apgar scores, length of stay, and maternal age or educational level.

As can be seen in Fig 2, CareLink usage was associated with significant improvements in family satisfaction in the overall quality of care and environment and visitation dimensions. CareLink families also reported higher scores in all other dimensions except in coordination of care. Within the dimension of overall quality, (Fig 3A) CareLink families were 85% less likely to report problems with the duration of their child's hospitalization (6.7% vs 43.8%; $P = .04$). Of those reporting problems most noted that their NICU stay was shorter than they felt necessary. Interestingly, even though the same visitation policies applied to both groups, CareLink families were

TABLE 2. Characteristics of Study Participants

	CareLink Group	Usual Care Group	
Birth weight (mean ± SD)	960 ± 278	1026 ± 302	$P = .38$
<750 g (n)	8	8	
750–999 g	8	7	
1000–1500 g	10	15	
Gestational age (wk) (± SD)	27.8 ± 2.4	27.5 ± 2.3	$P = .73$
Gender (% female)	35%	30%	$P = .80$
5-minute Apgar ≤7 n (%)	9 (35%)	9 (30%)	$P = .78$
Plurality			
Singleton n (%)	19 (73%)	19 (63%)	
Twin n (%)	6 (23%)	10 (33%)	
Triplet n (%)	1 (48%)	1 (3%)	
C-section n (%)	2 (8%)	11 (37%)	$P = .01$
Maternal race (% African-American)	19%	23%	
Maternal age (y ± SD)	31.3 ± 7.3	31.4 ± 6.4	$P = .69$
<21 n (%)	1 (4%)	2 (7%)	
>35 n (%)	6 (23%)	9 (30%)	
Insurance status			$P = .052$
Commercial (n)	21	19	
Health Maintenance Organization (HMO) (n)	0	6	
Self-pay or government program (n)	5	5	
High-risk maternal antenatal transfer (%)	30%	19%	$P = .35$

also less likely to report problems when asked if the unit's visitation policy met the needs of their other family members (13.3% vs 50%; $P = .02$; Fig 3B). CareLink families also showed a trend toward fewer problems related to receiving practical support from the NICU (33.3% vs 68.7%; $P = .08$).

DISCUSSION

We have demonstrated that emerging communication technologies such as the WWW and videoconferencing can be successfully integrated into practice within a busy NICU and that they significantly improve family perceptions of care quality and lower costs associated with transfers. NICUs and the care of VLBW children are costly, constituting the single largest segment of hospitalized care for children. Previous studies have shown that improved home care lowers costs for VLBW infants.[5] Yet home care by appropriately trained nurses is expensive and logistically difficult in many settings. We believe extension of Baby CareLink into the postdischarge period can provide this type of support to families and the clinical staff and will significantly improve the coordination and efficiency of care.

Families and staff alike enthusiastically embrace the use of the Baby CareLink system. Parents used

TABLE 3. WWW Utilization: CareLink Sessions Initiated by Families During Five-Month Period Beginning November 1998

Area	Sessions	Percentage of Total Sessions
Picture gallery	452	91%
Daily report	281	57%
Message center	230	46%
Growth chart	134	27%
Staff photos and roster	84	17%
Discharge teaching	70	14%
Family room	58	12%
NICU-Pedia	53	11%

Total sessions during this period were 496.

the system daily mostly looking at their infant's WWW home page and the photograph gallery. Some content in Baby CareLink such as the NICU-Pedia's section on retinopathy of prematurity were less frequently accessed. However, given the small number of families in our study ($n = 26$) and the rarity of the condition, this finding is not surprising. Moreover, the total number of accesses to a section should not be equated to the potential impact even a single reading might have for the family. From the staff perspective, they now have adopted Baby CareLink as part of the care for each child in the NICU. Children routinely have postdischarge virtual visits, and families have experimenting with virtual support groups.

The ability and willingness of families in the NICU to use the Baby CareLink WWW to gather information about their child's care in the NICU parallels the experience of Bass et al.[6] In their study of elderly patients with Alzheimer's disease they found a computer support network to be heavily used by the patient's family caretakers. In addition, they found that the system significantly reduced stress among caregivers. Although our project facilitated access to the WWW by providing computer hardware and access to the Internet, our surveys show that 70% of families by the end of our study already have home-based WWW access. These figures are similar to that found by other Boston-based research,[7,8] but is higher than the 38% found nationally in 1999.

Others have also demonstrated the ability of telemedicine technologies to be valuable in the care of pediatrics patients. Karp et al[9] in their study of a population of children with special health care needs found a telemedicine system to be both well-received and well-utilized in providing distance consultation within the state of Georgia. The use of telemedicine to provide post-intensive care unit (ICU) home monitoring and care has been described by Miyasaka et

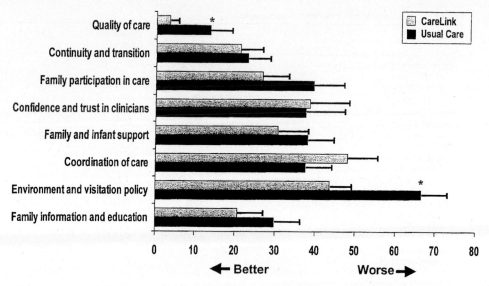

Fig 2. Family satisfaction survey results. Mean problem scores (± SE) are presented for each of 8 Picker survey dimensions. (*P < .05 for group comparison).

al.[10] Using a system of videophones in the patient's home and the pediatric ICU, they were able to demonstrate reduced need for physician home visits, unscheduled hospital visits, and days hospitalized. Despite these successes, obstacles do exist to the routine implementation of systems such as these. These issues include the ability of providers to recoup costs associated with providing telemedicine consultations,[11] medicolegal issues,[12] as well as issues related to access.[8]

Almost all families can learn to use CareLink, which is designed for a 6th grade reading level. The lack of access to the Internet by many families poses logistic problems for the NICU wishing to adopt this kind of approach. In our study, we had governmental support that provided equipment and telecommunications into the home. Work by Gustafson (personal communication, April 2000) has shown that patients without traditional access to health care derive greater benefit from computer-assisted decision support. Homes with televisions and telephones can be made Internet-ready for as little as $200. Learning centers at the hospital can help provide access when there is none at home. Local libraries can also provide needed access for families as well.

The small size of our study group limits the power of our analyses to detect differences. Our analyses do suggest that Baby CareLink improved the transition from NICU to home. Although their NICU stays were shorter, parents in the Baby CareLink group expressed greater comfort with the timing of their infant's discharge. We believe that Baby's CareLink allows families to attain the skills, knowledge, comfort, and confidence necessary to become the primary caretaker for their child(ren) earlier in their NICU stay. Furthermore, extension of the Baby CareLink model and technologies into the postdischarge period and enhancing communication be-

tween families, community, and tertiary providers may further improve care.

Families in the CareLink group reported greater satisfaction with care across multiple dimensions. In addition to the improvements documented by the results of our Picker surveys, we believe the decreased rates of retrotransfer among CareLink families was the result of improved satisfaction with the care received in the study NICU. In this NICU, it is a part of standard procedures to retrotransfer infants back to their referring level II facility when they no longer require level III care. This process occurs unless families actively decline this transfer.

To our surprise, families in the Baby CareLink group expressed greater satisfaction with the NICU's physical environment and visitation policies despite the fact that both groups were cared for in the same NICU and experienced the same set of clinical policies. Although not immediately self-evident, it appears that this results in part from Baby CareLink's ability to facilitate alternative methods of visiting for extended family members. For example, families often used videoconferencing to allow daily visiting of young children with their hospitalized siblings. Our experience suggests that such "real world" visiting is often limited by the need for parents to divide their attention between their hospitalized and older child.

The ability to support low birth weight infants (<1000 g) is a marvel of modern medicine, but extracts an emotional toll on the family. Our study suggests that our intervention designed to support the emotional and educational needs of families actually improved care and supported families who felt comfortable taking their children home sooner. Families without CareLink technology tended to stay longer but felt that their stay was too short. Technologies such as the ones we have evaluated can offer

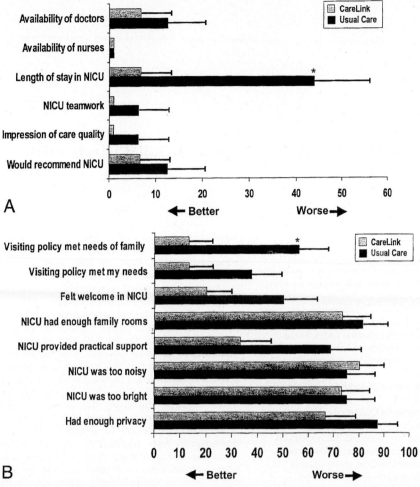

Fig 3. A, Proportion of families (± SE) reporting problems for each component question from overall quality of care dimension (*P < .05 for group comparison). B, Proportion of families (± SE) reporting problems for each component question from physical environment and visitation policy dimension (*P < .05 for group comparison).

every family better communication with their physicians, better coordination of care with their nurses, and better collaboration with other members of their community. Paradoxically, we have used a high-tech approach in a high-tech environment to provide a more humane high-touch.

ACKNOWLEDGMENTS

This study was funded by the National Library of Medicine's Telemedicine Initiative (NO1-LM-6-3535).

We would like to thank the members of the Baby CareLink Study Advisory Panel for their guidance during the course of this project. Panel members included Heidelise Als, PhD, Mary Ellen Avery, MD, Patricia Flatley Brennan, RN, PhD, Jerold Lucey, MD, and Marie McCormick, MD, ScD.

We would also like to thank Ms Beth Hinton for her help with manuscript preparation.

REFERENCES

1. Wasserman W. Complications. *New Yorker.* February 28, 2000:87–109
2. Field MJ, ed. *Telemedicine: A Guide to Assessing Telecommunications for Health Care.* Institute of Medicine; 1996
3. Peterson A. Lost in the maze: the web's explosive growth poses a challenge for users: making the most of it. *Wall Street Journal.* December 6, 1999, Section R:6 (column 1)
4. The Picker Institute. Improving the quality of health care though the eyes of patients: Surveys. 2000. Available at URL: http://www.picker.org/surveys/default.htm
5. Brooten D, Kumar S, Brown LP, et al. A randomized clinical trial of early hospital discharge and home follow-up of very-low-birth-weight infants. *N Engl J Med.* 1986;15:934–939
6. Bass DM, McClendon MJ, Brennan PF, McCarthy C. The buffering effect of a computer support network on caregiver strain. *J Aging Health.* 1998;10:20–43
7. Goldsmith D, Safran C. Using the web to reduce postoperative pain following ambulatory surgery. *Proc AMIA Symp.* 1999;780–784
8. Mandl KD, Katz SB, Kohane IS. Social equity and access to the World Wide Web and E-mail: implications for design and implementation of medical applications. *Proc AMIA Symp.* 1998;215–219
9. Karp WB, Grigsby K, McSwiggan-Hardin M, et al. Use of telemedicine for children with special health care needs. *Pediatrics.* 2000;105:843–847
10. Miyasaka K, Suzuki Y, Sakai H, Kondo Y. Interactive communication in high-technology home care: videophones for pediatric ventilatory care. *Pediatrics.* 1997;99(1). URL: http://www.pediatrics.org/cgi/content/full/99/1/e1
11. Sorum PC, Mallick R. Physicians' opinions on compensation for telephone calls. *Pediatrics.* 1997;99(4). URL: http://www.pediatrics.org/cgi/content/full/99/4/e3

Systematic review of studies of patient satisfaction with telemedicine

Frances Mair, Pamela Whitten

Abstract

Objective To review research into patient satisfaction with teleconsultation, specifically clinical consultations between healthcare providers and patients involving real time interactive video.

Design Systematic review of telemedicine satisfaction studies. Electronic databases searched include Medline, Embase, Science Citation Index, Social Sciences Citation Index, Arts and Humanities Citation Index, and the TIE (Telemedicine Information Exchange) database.

Subjects Studies conducted worldwide and published between 1966 and 1998.

Main outcome measures Quality of evidence about patient satisfaction.

Results 32 studies were identified. Study methods used were simple survey instruments (26 studies), exact methods not specified (5), and qualitative methods (1). Study designs were randomised controlled trial (1 trial); random patient selection (2); case-control (1); and selection criteria not specified or participants represented consecutive referrals, convenience samples, or volunteers (28). Sample sizes were ≤ 20 (10 trials), ≤ 100 (14), > 100 (7), and not specified (1). All studies reported good levels of patient satisfaction. Qualitative analysis revealed methodological problems with all the published work. Even so, important issues were highlighted that merit further investigation. There is a paucity of data examining patients' perceptions or the effects of this mode of healthcare delivery on the interaction between providers and clients.

Conclusions Methodological deficiencies (low sample sizes, context, and study designs) of the published research limit the generalisability of the findings. The studies suggest that teleconsultation is acceptable to patients in a variety of circumstances, but issues relating to patient satisfaction require further exploration from the perspective of both clients and providers.

Introduction

Telemedicine can be defined as the use of telecommunications technologies to provide medical information and services.[1] There is increasing interest in the use of telemedicine as a means of healthcare delivery. This is partly because technological advances have made the equipment less expensive and simpler to use and partly because increasing healthcare costs and patient expectations have increased the need to find alternative modes of healthcare delivery.

A wide variety of studies concerning telemedicine, interactive video consultations, have been performed in different settings throughout the world. Commentators on telemedicine frequently highlight the need for research into safety, efficacy, and cost effectiveness. Telemedicine literature abounds with publications about patient satisfaction, which are generally positive, and as a result there is a tendency to assume that the need for further research into this is less of a priority.

We argue in this paper that (a) the available research fails both to provide satisfactory explanations of the underlying reasons for patient satisfaction or dissatisfaction with telemedicine and to explore communication issues in any depth and (b) generalisations about satisfaction with telemedical care are difficult because of methodological deficiencies of the current evidence. To support this perspective, we provide the results of a systematic literature review of research into telemedicine satisfaction, in the context of interactive video.

Methods

Search strategy

To identify telemedicine satisfaction studies the following electronic databases were searched: Medline 1966 to 1998, Embase 1988-98, Science Citation Index 1981-98, Social Sciences Citation Index 1981-98, Arts and Humanities Citation Index 1981-98, and the TIE (Telemedicine Information Exchange) database. Searches were restricted to English language papers, and the keywords used were: "patient satisfaction," "consumer satisfaction," "telecommunications," and "telemedicine." The reference lists of papers identified were hand searched for other relevant references.

We included only clinical trials that explored patient satisfaction with teleconsultation, specifically those clinical consultations between healthcare providers from any discipline and patients that involve the use of real time interactive video. We excluded review or discussion papers, studies in which the use of telecommunications technologies was primarily for educational or administrative purposes and not linked to direct patient care, and studies in which the patient was not physically present at either point of care. In

Department of Primary Care, Whelan Building, Quadrangle, University of Liverpool, Liverpool L69 3GB
Frances Mair
senior lecturer in general practice

Department of Telecommunication, Michigan State University, 409 Communication Arts and Sciences Building, East Lansing, MI 48824-1212, USA
Pamela Whitten
assistant professor

Correspondence to:
F Mair
f.s.mair@liv.ac.uk

BMJ 2000;320:1517-20

addition, if any single study resulted in multiple publications, we reviewed only the principal paper focusing on patient satisfaction. The studies we reviewed had evaluation of patient satisfaction either as the main outcome measure or at least as a prominent feature of their overall assessment of the project. We did not include telemedicine projects that did not directly measure patient satisfaction but reported "unsolicited feedback" that suggests a reasonable degree of satisfaction with telemedicine services.[2]

Selection criteria

It is acknowledged that well designed and executed trials, particularly randomised controlled trials, provide the most reliable evidence for inclusion in any systematic review.[3] However, in view of the limited number of patient satisfaction studies that met the search criteria outlined above, we analysed data from all clinical trials identified irrespective of sample size or methodologies used. Titles and abstracts of the studies identified by the outlined search strategy were read to determine their potential eligibility for the review. The full articles were then assessed for relevance.

Outcome measures and data extraction

The outcome measures we examined included patients' satisfaction (principally overall satisfaction with the telemedicine service but also including levels of satisfaction with communication via this medium,

telemedicine consultations compared with traditional face to face consultations, and technical performance) and patients' willingness to use telemedicine in the future.

We recorded the studies' bibliographic details; descriptions of study setting and study population; subject selection criteria; details of form and delivery of the intervention; and outcome measures. We also noted patient numbers, response rates, study methodologies, and other factors affecting the validity of results, including effect modifiers.

Qualitative analysis

In view of the heterogeneous nature of the studies identified, the dearth of randomised controlled trials, and the preponderance of demonstration and feasibility studies, the data available did not permit the use of formal statistical techniques such as meta-analysis. Instead, we conducted a broad qualitative overview of the data, including a critical review of the strength of the findings. We judged the reliability and validity of data by the methodologies used in each study and judged their generalisability from the study context. We did not use a formal scoring method as no well validated instrument for qualitative review yet exists.[3] [4] However, as the basis for our critical appraisal of the studies, we used a checklist designed for assessing the methodological quality of both randomised and non-randomised studies of healthcare interventions.[4]

Results

Thirty two studies met our selection criteria. The studies examined the use of interactive video in diverse contexts ranging from specialist consultations to home nursing. Many of these represented demonstration and feasibility studies rather than full scale trials. This is reflected in their sample sizes often being small and selection criteria for study participants rarely being random in nature. Only seven studies had more than 100 participants,[5–11] 14 were small pilot studies with less than 100 patients,[12–25] and 10 were simple feasibility studies with 20 or fewer patients.[26–35] One paper, which presented an overview of an Australian regional telepsychiatry project, did not provide patient numbers.[36]

The table lists the studies by type of consultation. (An extra table on the *BMJ*'s website provides further detail of studies in which patient numbers were over 20 and methods of measuring patient satisfaction were explicitly described. None of these studies declared any conflicts of interest.)

In terms of methodologies used, 26 studies used simple survey instruments, five did not specify the exact methods, and one used qualitative methods. Only one study was a randomised controlled trial,[10] in two others patients were randomly selected,[19] [23] and one was a case-control study.[20] In the remaining 28 studies selection criteria were not specified or participants represented consecutive referrals, convenience samples, or volunteers.

Measures of patient satisfaction

The studies mainly used simple survey instruments to ascertain patient satisfaction. Firm conclusions are limited by methodological difficulties, but it would seem that the patients found teleconsultations acceptable;

Studies of patient satisfaction with teleconsultations

Study	Type of teleconsultation	No of participants	Location
Callahan et al[13]	Psychiatry	93	USA
Blackmon et al[16]	Psychiatry (child)	43	USA
Baigent et al[19]	Psychiatry	63	Australia
Dongier et al[20]	Psychiatry (adult and child)	50	Canada
Clarke[22]	Psychiatry	32	Australia
Graham[25]	Psychiatry	39	USA
Baer et al[30]	Psychiatry (obsessive compulsive disorder)	10	USA
Ball et al[33]	Psychiatry	6	UK
McLaren et al[35]	Psychiatry	3	UK
Trott[36]	Psychiatry	Not specified	Australia
Loane et al[6]*	Dermatology	334	UK
Lowitt et al[7]	Dermatology	139	USA
Gilmour et al[8]*	Dermatology	126	UK
Oakley et al[9]	Dermatology	104	Australia
Jones et al[18]	Dermatology	51	UK
Brecht et al[5]	Multispecialty consultations	585	USA
Huston et al[12]	Multispecialty consultation	96	USA
Harrison et al[17]	Multispecialty consultation	54	UK
Brennan et al[10]	Emergency medicine	104	USA
Allen et al[21]	Oncology	39	USA
Kunkler et al[32]	Oncology	6	UK
Doolittle et al[31]	Hospice	6	USA
Conrath et al[14]	Family practice consultations	32	Canada
Itzak et al[29]	Primary care consultations	11	Israel
Pedersen et al[23]	Otolaryngology	26	Norway
Blakeslee et al[15]	Otolaryngology	36	USA
Duffy et al[11]	Diagnosis of speech and language disorders	150 in group A, 8 in group B	USA
Takano et al[27]	Home health care (including medical consultations, physiotherapy, health and welfare services)	20	Japan
Whitten et al[24]	Home nursing	22	USA
Allen et al[34]	Home nursing	3	USA
Couturier et al[28]	Orthopaedic consultation	15	France
Hubble et al[26]	Patients with Parkinson's disease	9	USA

*Study by Gilmour et al[8] used some of same subjects as study by Loane et al.[6]

noted definite advantages, particularly increased accessibility of specialist expertise, less travel required, and reduced waiting times; but also had some disquiet about this mode of healthcare delivery, particularly relating to communication between provider and client via this medium.

Shortcomings of studies

We identified several problems with the studies that affect their reliability and validity. Many studies had small sample sizes, almost a third having 20 or fewer participants, and low response rates, as low as 50%.[22] Patient selection criteria were often not clearly specified, or there were no formal selection criteria. Most of the studies (28) used volunteers or physician referrals and provided no information about refusal rates at point of initial referral. Thus, it is not possible to discount selection bias in favour of those likely to be positive about teleconsultation.

Methodologies used for assessing satisfaction were not clearly specified in many studies, making interpretation and comparison of results problematic. Most studies sought to measure whether patients would use the systems again or were "satisfied" with the service. However, few studies defined what satisfaction meant. Therefore, we are unable to discern whether the participants said they were satisfied because telemedicine didn't kill them, or that it was "OK," or that it was a wonderful experience. The available evidence does not help us to understand the reasons underlying satisfaction or dissatisfaction. In addition, most of the studies presented only initial impressions and failed to explore what happened to patient satisfaction over time, thereby making it possible that the novelty value of the technology resulted in a positive bias.

The cost of teleconsultations compared with routine consultations was not addressed. This is particularly pertinent to the US studies, which account for over 45% of the studies found. The US system of healthcare delivery is a fee for service system, yet the US studies do not mention whether patients attending for teleconsultation paid for the service in the usual way or whether they received this service free of charge. As many US telemedicine projects are primarily grant funded, it is possible that in some studies participants received free teleconsultations, which could affect their satisfaction with the service provided.

Because of the survey nature of most of the studies, there are often inconsistencies in responses that remain unexplained. One possible explanation lies in the survey design. Many surveys have questions with multiple constructs (such as: "I felt the physician was easy to talk to and understood everything I said"). When a single question contains two constructs it is not possible to know which actual construct the participant is responding to, making the data difficult to interpret.

The effects, if any, of telemedicine on communicative behaviours and the interaction between provider and patient during the consultation remained virtually unexplored. There was a lack of data examining patients' perceptions.

Generalisability of results

The generalisability of much of the published research is limited because of effect modifiers such as study setting. One of the largest studies examined teleconsulta-

tion in a prison in the United States.[5] Clearly, there are several reasons why satisfaction in prisoners may be different from that in the general population. Thus, the peculiarities of the setting mean that this study's results cannot be applied reliably to the general population of that country or more widely.

Furthermore, the delivery of health care was somewhat artificial in many studies. Participants often received a teleconsultation in addition to a routine consultation, and so were really being asked to make a hypothetical judgment as to its value. In many studies participants also received "special" treatment, with every effort being made to minimise inconvenience. Satisfaction in these somewhat artificial contexts may not be readily translatable to satisfaction with telemedicine when it is being used in routine practice.

Discussion

The published research suggests that healthcare delivery via telemedicine is acceptable to patients in a variety of circumstances, but, by addressing this issue in a rather superficial manner, most studies have produced more questions than answers. Thus far, most telemedicine research has had a technological focus. We know a great deal about bandwidths and resolution, but little about the human dimensions that make the practice possible. Pragmatic information that can benefit future delivery of health care via telemedicine is needed.

The following issues need to be addressed:

- What types of consultation are suitable for teleconsulting? Is it suitable for initial consultations, or do patients find it more acceptable to use telemedicine technology just for follow up appointments?
- What are the effects of this mode of healthcare delivery on the doctor-patient relationship? Examining patient perceptions would help to address the reasons why patients liked or disliked a service and help healthcare providers to better understand patients' subjective definitions of acceptability and utility.
- How do communicative issues affect the delivery of health care via telemedicine? We need to better understand the effects of telemedicine on consultations in order to improve the services we provide through this medium.
- What are the possible limitations of telemedicine in clinical practice?

In addition, we need to use research tools that have been shown to be reliable and valid. Questionnaires have advantages and disadvantages, but if they are to be used in future research we need to use instruments that have undergone rigorous testing and have been shown to produce repeatable results and to measure what they are intended to measure. Future evaluations need to start with a set of clear hypotheses and objectives and to use clearly defined methodologies that will increase the likelihood of meeting the initial aims. Although randomised controlled trials may not always be practical, representative patient samples are necessary in order to improve the usefulness of results obtained.

This review serves to highlight methodological deficiencies in the published research. Although there are practical obstacles to evaluating telemedicine,[37] there remains a need for further exploration of this field in order to facilitate an evidence based approach

What is already known on this topic

Telemedicine is currently advocated as a mode of healthcare delivery because of its potential to diminish inequalities in service provision and to improve access to care

Studies of interactive teleconsultations have been performed in a diversity of settings throughout the world, and most suggest that patients are satisfied with this mode of healthcare delivery

However, preliminary review of this literature indicates there are still many gaps in knowledge in relation to patient satisfaction with telemedicine

What this study adds

This systematic review of the telemedicine literature demonstrates that methodological deficiencies in the published research affect the validity and generalisability of the results and that communication issues, the quality of interpersonal relationships with this medium, and subsequent effects, if any, on the outcome of consultations have yet to be fully explored

Future research in this subject needs to be more scientifically robust in order to assist policymakers in reaching informed decisions about the appropriate use of this technology

to the wider introduction of this new technology. It is an oversimplification to suggest that this aspect of telemedicine has undergone sufficient scrutiny.

We thank Dr Mark Gabbay, senior lecturer, Department of Primary Care, University of Liverpool, and Dr Maria Leitner, Health and Community Care Research Unit, University of Liverpool, for advice and comments.

Contributors: FM contributed to initiation of the research, discussed core ideas, designed the protocol, participated in data collection, analysed and interpreted the data, and participated in writing the paper. PW initiated the primary study hypothesis and the research, discussed core ideas, and participated in study design, data collection, and writing of the paper. FM is guarantor of this paper.

Funding: None.

Competing interests: None.

1 Perednia DA, Allen A. Telemedicine technology and clinical applications. *JAMA* 1995;273:483-8.
2 Mahmud K, Lenz J. The personal telemedicine system. A new tool for the delivery of health care. *J Telemed Telecare* 1995;1:173-7.
3 NHS Centre for Reviews and Dissemination. *Report Number 4*. York: University of York, 1996.
4 Downs SH, Black N. The feasibility of creating a checklist for the assessment of the methodological quality both of randomised and non-randomised studies of health care interventions. *J Epidemiol Community Health* 1998;52:377-84.
5 Brecht RM, Gray CL, Peterson C, Youngblood B. The University of Texas Medical Branch-Texas Department of Criminal Justice telemedicine project: findings from the first year of operation. *Telemed J* 1996;2:25-35.
6 Loane MA, Bloomer SE, Corbett R, Eedy DJ, Gore HE, Mathews C, et al. Patient satisfaction with realtime teledermatology in Northern Ireland. *J Telemed Telecare* 1998;4:36-40.
7 Lowitt MH, Kessler II, Kauffman CL, Hooper FJ, Siegel E, Burnett JW. Teledermatology and in-person examinations: a comparison of patient and physician perceptions and diagnostic agreement. *Arch Dermatol* 1998;134:471-6.
8 Gilmour E, Campbell SM, Loane MA, Esmail A, Griffiths CE, Roland MO, et al. Comparison of teleconsultations and face-to-face consultations: preliminary results of a United Kingdom multicentre teledermatology study. *Br J Dermatol* 1998;139:81-7.
9 Oakley AMM, Astwood DR, Loane M, Duffill MB, Rademaker M, Wootton R. Diagnostic accuracy of teledermatology: results of a preliminary study in New Zealand. *NZ Med J* 1997;110:51-3.
10 Brennan JA, Kealy JA, Gerardi L, Shih R, Allegra J, Sannipoli L, et al. A randomized controlled trial of telemedicine in an emergency department. *J Telemed Telecare* 1998;4(suppl 1):18-20.
11 Duffy JR, Werven GW, Aronson AE. Telemedicine and the diagnosis of speech and language disorders. *Mayo Clin Proc* 1997;72:1116-22.
12 Huston JL, Burton DC. Patient satisfaction with multispecialty interactive teleconsultations. *J Telemed Telecare* 1997;3:205-8.
13 Callahan EJ, Hilty DM, Nesbitt TS. Patient satisfaction with telemedicine consultation in primary care: comparison of ratings of medical and mental health applications. *Telemed J* 1998;4:363-9.
14 Conrath DW, Buckingham P, Dunn EV, Swanson JN. An experimental evaluation of alternative communication systems as used for medical diagnosis. *Behav Sci* 1975;20:296-305.
15 Blakeslee DB, Grist WJ, Stachura ME, Blakeslee BS. Practice of otolaryngology via telemedicine. *Laryngoscope* 1998;108:1-7.
16 Blackmon LA, Kaak HO, Ranseen J. Consumer satisfaction with telemedicine child psychiatry consultation in rural Kentucky. *Psychiatr Serv* 1997;48:14644-66.
17 Harrison R, Clayton W, Wallace P. Can telemedicine be used to improve communication between primary and secondary care? *BMJ* 1997;313:1377-81.
18 Jones DH, Crichton C, Macdonald A, Potts S, Sime D, Toms J, et al. Teledermatology in the highlands of Scotland. *J Telemed Telecare* 1996;2(suppl 1):7-9.
19 Baigent MF, Lloyd C, Kavanagh SJ, Ben-Tovim DI, Yellowlees PM, Kalucy RS, et al. Telepsychiatry: 'tele' yes, but what about the 'psychiatry'? *J Telemed Telecare* 1997;3(suppl 1):3-5.
20 Dongier M, Tempier R, Lalinec-Michaud M, Meunier D. Telepsychiatry: psychiatric consultation through two-way television. A controlled study. *Can J Psychiatry* 1986;31:32-4.
21 Allen A, Hayes MPA. Patient satisfaction with teleoncology: a pilot study. *Telemed J* 1995;1:41-6.
22 Clarke PHJ. A referrer and patient evaluation of a telepsychiatry consultation-liaison service in South Australia. *J Telemed Telecare* 1997;3(suppl 1):12-4.
23 Pedersen S, Holand U. Tele-endoscopic otorhinolaryngoligical examination: preliminary study of patient satisfaction. *Telemed J* 1995;1:47-52.
24 Whitten P, Mair FS, Collins B. Home tele-nursing care in Kansas: patients' perceptions of uses and benefits. *J Telemed Telecare* 1997;3:67-9
25 Graham M. Telepsychiatry in Appalachia. *Am Behav Sci* 1996;39:602-15.
26 Hubble JP, Pahwa R, Michalek DK, Thomas C, Koller WC. Interactive video conferencing: a means of providing interim care to Parkinson's disease patients. *Mov Disord* 1993;8:380-2.
27 Takano T, Nakamura K, Akao C. Assessment of the value of videophones in home healthcare. *Telecom Policy* 1995;19:241-8.
28 Couturier P, Tyrrell J, Tonetti J, Rhul C, Franco A. Feasibility of orthopaedic teleconsulting in a geriatric rehabilitation service. *J Telemed Telecare* 1998;4(suppl 1):85-7.
29 Itzak B, Weinberger T, Berkovitch E, Reis S. Telemedicine in primary care in Israel. *J Telemed Telecare* 1998;4(suppl 1):11-4.
30 Baer L, Cukor P, Jenike MA, Leahy L, O'Laughlen J, Coyle JT. Pilot studies of telemedicine for patients with obsessive-compulsive disorder. *Am J Psychiatry* 1995;152:1383-5.
31 Doolittle GC, Yaezel A, Otto F, Clemens C. Hospice care using home-based telemedicine systems. *J Telemed Telecare* 1998;4(suppl 1):58-9.
32 Kunkler IH, Rafferty P, Hill D, Henry M, Foreman D. A pilot study of teleoncology in Scotland. *J Telemed Telecare* 1998;4:113-9.
33 Ball CJ, McLaren PM, Summerfield AB, Lipsedge MS, Watson JP. A comparison of communication modes in adult psychiatry. *J Telemed Telecare* 1995;1:22-6.
34 Allen A, Roman L, Cox R, Cardwell B. Home health visits using a cable television network: user satisfaction. *J Telemed Telecare* 1996;2(suppl 1):92-4.
35 McLaren PM, Blunden J, Lipsedge ML, Summerfield AB. Telepsychiatry in an inner-city community psychiatric service. *J Telemed Telecare* 1996;2:57-9.
36 Trott P. The Queensland Northern Regional Health Authority telemental health project. *J Telemed Telecare* 1996;2(suppl 1):98-104.
37 Wootton R. Telemedicine in the National Health Service. *J R Soc Med* 1998;91:614-21.

(Accepted 5 April 2000)

Corrections and clarifications

Letter
In the issue of 15 April in the first letter on p 1074, headed "Further research is needed on why rates of caesarean section are increasing," we inadvertently omitted the second author's first initial: his name is S W Lindow.

ABC of arterial and venous disease: acute stroke
In this article by Philip M W Bath and colleagues (1 April, pp 920-3), an error persisted to the final published version. The second paragraph in the section "Acute intervention" (p 922), gives the impression that alteplase is currently licensed in New Zealand; it is not.

Guidelines for managing acute bacterial meningitis
In this editorial by Kirsten Møller and Peter Skinhøj (13 May, p 1290), a manuscript note was misread, which led to a redundant "t" and a missing "l" in Møller's email address. The correct address is kirsten.moller@dadlnet.dk.

Effect of Image Compression on Telepathology

A Randomized Clinical Trial

Alvin Marcelo, MD; Paul Fontelo, MD, MPH; Miguel Farolan, MD; Hernani Cualing, MD

● **Context.**—For practitioners deploying store-and-forward telepathology systems, optimization methods such as image compression need to be studied.

Objective.—To determine if Joint Photographic Expert Group (JPG or JPEG) compression, a lossy image compression algorithm, negatively affects the accuracy of diagnosis in telepathology.

Design.—Double-blind, randomized, controlled trial.

Setting.—University-based pathology departments.

Participants.—Resident and staff pathologists at the University of Illinois, Chicago, and University of Cincinnati, Cincinnati, Ohio.

Intervention.—Compression of raw images using the JPEG algorithm.

Main Outcome Measures.—Image acceptability, accuracy of diagnosis, confidence level of pathologist, image quality.

Results.—There was no statistically significant difference in the diagnostic accuracy between noncompressed (bit map) and compressed (JPG) images. There were also no differences in the acceptability, confidence level, and perception of image quality. Additionally, rater experience did not significantly correlate with degree of accuracy.

Conclusions.—For providers practicing telepathology, JPG image compression does not negatively affect the accuracy and confidence level of diagnosis. The acceptability and quality of images were also not affected.

(*Arch Pathol Lab Med.* 2000;124:1653–1656)

Medical specialties that rely on images to formulate a diagnosis lend themselves to the store-and-forward method of telemedicine. With this method, images are captured and then forwarded, often through the Internet, to a remote expert for asynchronous review at a later time. Pathology (telepathology), radiology (teleradiology), and dermatology (teledermatology) are among the most advanced areas of telemedicine because of their image-intensive nature and minimal requirement for patient interaction.[1–3]

Telepathology in particular requires the evaluation of microscopic images to formulate a diagnosis. Store-and-forward telepathology allows a pathologist in a remote location to digitize images of a challenging case for second opinion consultation. These images are usually transmitted through the Internet, which is now widely used as an exchange medium for scientific data. Efficient methods of image transmission, especially by compression, are of great interest to the scientific community, since high-quality digital images may attain sizes of 1 megabyte or greater. While larger files generally produce better images, they also take longer to send through the Internet. Depending on the type of Internet connection and the amount of "traffic," a 1-megabyte file may take 5 minutes or more to download. Its compressed version, on the other hand, may be received in less than 30 seconds.

Joint Photographic Experts Group (JPG) is a widely accepted image compression algorithm. Any Internet-connected computer today will have a web browser, such as Netscape or Internet Explorer, which is capable of displaying JPG files.[4–7] This algorithm accomplishes compression by exploiting known limitations of the human eye, particularly its inability to detect minute color and shades-of-gray details.[8] During the compression process, these small details are removed without noticeable difference if viewed with the naked eye. The final compressed image, therefore, will contain less data than the original. It is this loss of data, its possible effect on the quality of the image, and ultimately its effect on diagnosis that generates a cause for concern.

Many studies have been published on telepathology,[9–14] but only a few researchers[15,16] have actually compared noncompressed with compressed images using a structured study design. The aim of this study was not to compare the diagnostic accuracy of telepathology with that of glass slide diagnosis, but rather to determine whether the loss of data in JPG compression adversely affects the quality of images and the accuracy of diagnosis.

METHODS

Ten previously diagnosed cases were chosen from the teaching files of the Department of Pathology, University of Illinois University Hospital Chicago (UIC). Six representative snapshots from each case (magnifications ×2.5, ×10, and ×40) were captured using a Polaroid DMC 1 digital camera (Polaroid Corp,

Accepted for publication June 16, 2000.

From High Performance Computing and Communications, National Library of Medicine (Drs Marcelo and Fontelo), Bethesda, Md; Department of Pathology, University of Illinois, Chicago (Dr Farolan); and Department of Pathology, University of Cincinnati, Cincinnati, Ohio (Dr Cualing).

Presented as an electronic poster at Advancing Pathology Informatics, Imaging, and the Internet (APIII 99), sponsored by University of Pittsburgh School of Medicine, Marriott City Center, Pittsburgh, Pa, October 14–16, 1999.

Reprints: Alvin B. Marcelo, MD, National Library of Medicine, 8600 Rockville Pike, 38A, B1N30, Bethesda, MD 20894.

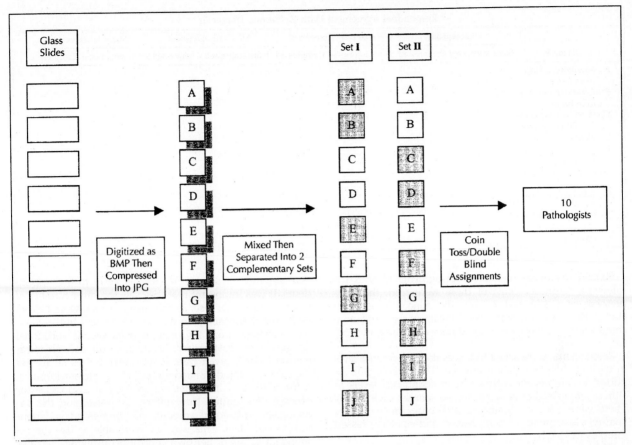

Schema for assignment of cases to pathologists.

Cambridge, Mass) mounted on a Leica DMLB (Leica Microsystems, Heidelberg, Germany). All initial images were saved in the Windows bit-map (BMP), noncompressed format (average size ~1000 kilobytes, at 667 × 500 pixel resolution). Bit-map images were then compressed using Adobe PhotoShop 5.0 (Adobe Systems, San Jose, Calif). The resulting compressed files were about 100 kilobytes at 90% compression. Images were archived on Macintosh 8100 computer (Apple Computers, Cupertino, Calif) and served on the World Wide Web using Quid Pro Quo 2.1.2 (Social Engineering, Berkeley, Calif) on a T-3 (45 megabits/s) line. The Web site was password protected and was accessible only after proper authentication. File extensions were masked server-side using randomly selected letters.

Two test sets were prepared (Figure). Set 1 had 5 cases in noncompressed (BMP) and 5 in compressed (JPG) format, and set 2 was its complement. Participants were assigned randomly to a set by coin toss.

Using Internet Explorer 5.0 (Microsoft Corporation, Redmond, Wash), 5 pathologists each from UIC and the University of Cincinnati (Cincinnati, Ohio) viewed the randomly assigned sets on the Internet at their convenience and assessed the images according to protocol. Server-side and client-side caching was allowed to minimize the effect of variable Internet transmission. Parameters measured were acceptability of a case for diagnosis, accuracy of diagnosis, confidence in diagnosis, and image quality (if found acceptable for diagnosis). Each rater's level of experience was also recorded.

The final diagnosis based on the glass slides from UIC was used as the reference diagnosis. Three of the authors (PAF, MF, and HC) independently compared the respondents' diagnoses with the reference diagnosis (blinded). By consensus, they classified the responses into 4 categories: no diagnosis (n = 0), no

difference (n = 1), minor difference (n = 2), and major difference (n = 3). A response was labeled "no difference" if it agreed completely with the reference diagnosis, "minor difference" if it signified a minor disagreement in terminology with no alteration in management, and "major difference" if the disagreement required a major change in management, usually benign to malignant or vice versa.

Categories for confidence level were no response (n = 0), very confident (n = 1), quite confident (n = 2), and not confident (n = 3). Categories for image quality were: no response (n = 0), excellent (n = 1), very good (n = 2), fair (n = 3), and poor (n = 4). Comparison of proportions was used to analyze results.

RESULTS

Ten pathologists examined 10 cases each for a total of 100 samples (50 compressed, 50 noncompressed). Seven of the 100 samples were labeled unacceptable (poor and unfit for diagnosis). Of these 7, 4 were from the compressed set (8%) and 3 from the noncompressed (6%). The acceptability rates for compressed and noncompressed samples were not statistically different (at 95% confidence interval [CI]). Reasons given for unacceptability were "too dark," "too few images," and "no intermediate power." From the 93 samples judged acceptable, respondents concurred with the reference diagnosis in 71 cases (Table). The accuracy rates for compressed and noncompressed samples were not statistically different (at 95% CI).

Six responses had minor disagreements with the reference diagnosis. An equal number of compressed and noncompressed samples were classified as such (6% each).

	Unacceptable		Complete Agreement		Minor Disagreement		Major Disagreement	
Diagnosis	Noncompressed	Compressed	Noncompressed	Compressed	Noncompressed	Compressed	Noncompressed	Compressed
A. Mucinous adeno-carcinoma	2	. . .	2	2	1	1	1	1
B. Complete hydatidi-form mole	. . .	. . .	4	2	2	2	. . .	. . .
C. Pheochromocytoma	1	2	1	4	. . .	. . .	2	. . .
D. Carotid body tumor	. . .	1	4	4	. . .	. . .	. . .	1
E. Nephroblastoma	. . .	. . .	6	4	. . .	. . .	. . .	. . .
F. Endometrial carci-noma	. . .	. . .	4	6	. . .	. . .	. . .	. . .
G. Medullary carcino-ma	. . .	. . .	6	4	. . .	. . .	. . .	. . .
H. Tubulovillous ade-noma	. . .	. . .	. . .	. . .	. . .	. . .	4	6
I. Prostate adenocar-cinoma	. . .	1	4	5	. . .	. . .	. . .	. . .
J. Crohn disease	. . .	. . .	6	3	. . .	. . .	. . .	1

Respondent Agreement With Reference Diagnosis

Sixteen responses had major disagreements with the reference diagnosis. Nine of these were from the compressed set (18%) and 7 from the noncompressed set (14%). The disagreement rates for compressed and noncompressed samples were not statistically different (95% CI).

Respondents were asked to assess their confidence level in each of the cases they examined. The pathologists reported no significant differences in confidence levels in either compressed or noncompressed samples (at 95% CI). There were also no significant differences in the image quality assessments of compressed and noncompressed samples (95% CI).

Of the 16 responses with major disagreements with the reference diagnosis, 10 were made by pathologists with less than 7 years of experience and 6 by those with more experience. This difference was not statistically significant (95% CI).

COMMENT

We compared the effect of compression on a pathologist's ability to diagnose using static telepathology techniques. It should be emphasized that the "diagnostic" aspect of the study was only one of the parameters used for comparison and was not the end in itself. Therefore, our results are best viewed within their relations to each other (compressed vs noncompressed) rather than by their absolute relation to the reference diagnosis. An important caveat, therefore, is that the results obtained in this study are applicable to telepathology only. They cannot be extrapolated to a comparison between telepathology and glass slide diagnosis, since the respondents did not evaluate the original glass slides.

Several technical limitations were observed while conducting this study. The cases chosen had varying degrees of diagnostic difficulty. As pathologists well know, some cases may only require one slide or one area to formulate a diagnosis, whereas others may need more. For example, some cases may be so challenging that even 20 images may not be sufficient, or special stains might be required to arrive at a diagnosis. This variability between amount of data presented (the images) and the amount of information that can be extracted from them (for diagnosis) is a known limitation of static telepathology. The best way to control this variable in this study was to provide iden-

tical amounts of data (6 images per case) to the respondents. It was important that they saw the same number of images from each case, as this ensured they were able to make the diagnosis from the same data and not because they received more information from seeing additional images. If the respondents could not cull enough information from a given case, it was recorded as such, and the case was rated "unacceptable" in its current form.

Interrater and intrarater variability was also cause for concern. We limited these effects by presenting the pathologists with equal amounts of compressed and noncompressed data. This way, we were able to use the respondent as his or her own control by applying the rater variable across both experimental and control populations.

There was also the limitation imposed by carry-over errors. Carry-over errors occur when compressed images are derived from flawed originals. A defective original noncompressed image would necessarily give poor compressed counterparts. This may explain why all respondents missed case H (tubulovillous adenoma). It is important to identify such errors, since these may detract from the value of a good telepathology system when the actual flaw may be due to poor technique or human error.

The level of resolution chosen was the best achievable using commercially available off-the-shelf software and currently standard monitor resolutions. To emphasize the ease of use of the Internet, the study employed a Web browser interface for presentation. By doing so, minimal training (point-and-click), if any, was required from the respondents. This is consistent with our goal of reproducing conditions in a typical pathologist's workstation.

The respondents included 4 attending pathologists, 2 sixth-year fellows, 1 fifth-year fellow, and 3 chief residents. Although it was expected that experience would be a significant factor in telepathology, the results showed that this may not be the case. A possible explanation is the familiarity of the younger respondents with computer-based displays. This premise is consistent with the findings of Krupinski et al,[17] who noted a negative correlation between years of clinical experience with performance when viewing images from a monitor display.

In summary, image compression using commonly available software can reduce image files to approximately one-tenth their original size. Such compression may be beneficial in reducing transmission time over the Internet. User acceptance of JPG-compressed images for diagnosis is not significantly different from that with noncompressed formats. Other factors, such as poor selection of fields, poor lighting, and insufficient number of image samples, can influence acceptability by causing carry-over errors. It should be stressed that these factors are independent of the compression algorithm and are related more to technique and methodology. Once deemed acceptable, however, compressed images are diagnosed correctly and incorrectly with the same frequency as noncompressed images. Lastly, no difference in performance was observed between young and experienced pathologists for both image formats.

Store-and-forward telepathology is useful for second-opinion consultation for pathologists and physicians with access to the Internet in locations where rapid courier services are not available. We believe that this study provides evidence to support the use of JPG compression in telepathology. These findings may also apply to other image-dependent telemedicine applications in dermatology and radiology.

References

1. Jukic DM. Telepathology and pathology at distance: an overview. *Croat Med J.* 1999;40:421–424.

2. Fontelo PA. Telepathology and the Internet. *Adv Clin Pathol.* 1997;1:95–96.

3. Szymas J, Wolf G. Remote microscopy through the internet. *Pol J Pathol.* 1999;50:37–42.

4. Nagata H, Mizushima H. World wide microscope: new concept of internet telepathology microscope and implementation of the prototype. *Medinfo.* 1998; 9(pt 1):286–289.

5. Szymas J, Wolf G. Telepathology by the internet. *Adv Clin Pathol.* 1998;2: 133–135.

6. Singson RP, Natarajan S, Greenson JK, et al. Virtual microscopy and the Internet as telepathology consultation tools: a study of gastrointestinal biopsy specimens. *Am J Clin Pathol.* 1999;111:792–795.

7. Kim CY. Compression of color medical images in gastrointestinal endoscopy: a review. *Medinfo.* 1998;9(pt 2):1046–1050.

8. Lane T. Frequently asked questions about JPEG image compression. Available at: http://www.faqs.org/faqs/jpeg-faq/part1. Accessed March 15, 1999.

9. Danilovic Z, Seiwerth S, Kayser K, et al. Experience based approach to interactive versus "store and forward" telepathology. *Adv Clin Pathol.* 1998;2: 149–150.

10. Felten CL, Strauss JS, Okada DH, et al. Virtual microscopy: high resolution digital photomicrography as a tool for light microscopy simulation. *Hum Pathol.* 1999;30:477–483.

11. Dunn BE, Almagro UA, Choi H, Recla DL, Weinstein RS. Use of telepathology for routine surgical pathology review in a test bed in the Department of Veterans Affairs. *Telemed J.* 1997;3:1–10.

12. Berman B, Elgart GW, Burdick AE. Dermatopathology via a still-image telemedicine system: diagnostic concordance with direct microscopy. *Telemed J.* 1997;3:27–32.

13. Kuakpaetoon T, Stauch G, Visalsawadi P. Image quality and acceptance of telepathology. *Adv Clin Pathol.* 1998;2:305–312.

14. Versteeg CH, Sanderink GC, Lobach SR, et al. Reduction in size of digital images: does it lead to less detectability or loss of diagnostic information? *Dentomaxillofac Radiol.* 1998;27:93–96.

15. Sneiderman C, Schosser R, Pearson TG. A comparison of JPEG and FIF compression of color medical images for dermatology. *Comput Med Imaging Graph.* 1994;18:339–342.

16. Yamamoto LG. Using JPEG image compression to facilitate telemedicine. *Am J Emerg Med.* 1995;13:55–57.

17. Krupinski EA, Weinstein RS, Rozek LS. Experience-related differences in diagnosis from medical images displayed on monitors. *Telemed J.* 1996;2:101–108.

Measurement of the Effects of an Integrated, Point-of-Care Computer System on Quality of Nursing Documentation and Patient Satisfaction

Rosemary Nahm, MSN, RN, and Iona Poston, PhD, RN

This quasi-experimental, modified time series study measured the effects of the nursing module of a point of care clinical information system on nursing documentation and patient satisfaction. Measurements were taken before implementation of the module and at 6-, 12-, and 18-month intervals postimplementation. Quality of nursing documentation was measured by compliance to items applicable to nursing documentation selected from the Joint Commission on Accreditation of Healthcare Organizations (JCAHO) Closed Medical Review Tool. Patient satisfaction was measured by using the Risser Patient Satisfaction Scale. The study data showed a statistically significant increase in the quality of nursing documentation after implementation of the computerized nursing documentation system, as well as a decrease in variability in charting, as evidenced by a decrease in standard deviations. A significant increase in charting compliance was still occurring between the 12- and the 18-month time points after initiation of automated documentation. The point of care computer system did not seem to affect patient satisfaction with the nurse–patient relationship.

Key words: Nursing documentation, Quality, Hospital information systems, Patient satisfaction, Evaluation studies

In today's healthcare environment, documentation requirements of nurses are growing because of issues of risk management, state and nursing organizations' standards of practice, and requirements of external regulatory agencies such as the Joint Commission on Accreditation of Healthcare Organization (JCAHO) and the Health Care Financing Agency (HCFA). Computer systems are providing nurses an alternative to time-consuming and ineffective methods of manual documentation. Does this technology increase the quality of nursing documentation? Do newer integrated, bedside (ie, point of care) computer systems further affect the quality of information recorded about the patient and the documentation of nursing care delivered to the patient at the bedside? How much time is needed after implementation to realize the benefits of the system on documentation? The purpose of this study was to evaluate the effects of an integrated point of care computer system on the quality of nursing documentation and patient satisfaction over time.

The Staggers and Parks Nurse–Computer Interaction Framework was used as the conceptual framework for this research because it portrays the nurse–computer dyad interaction as a developmental process that occurs over time, moving along a nursing informatics developmental trajectory.[1] As the relationship between the nurse and the computer unfolds, the interaction changes, and the outcome is influenced by the length of time the two have been interacting. For this reason, as well as for reasons related to resources, the study was performed over an 18-month period after implementation of the point of care computer system. According to the Staggers and Parks model, the interaction between the nurse and the computer also occurs within the nursing context. Therefore, this study was also designed to explore the effect of the presence of bedside computers on patients' perceptions of changes in nurses' behaviors that influence nurse–patient relationships.

REVIEW OF THE LITERATURE

Studies measuring the effects of computerization on the quality of nursing documentation have found mixed results, with most reporting a positive relationship between automation and quality. Dennis and colleagues[2] used a combination of external standards from JCAHO and internal standards established by the hospital's nursing department to measure quality of computerized nursing documentation. They reported a 34% increase in compliance with 11 standards and a 10% decrease in three other standards for which the computer software did not provide word cues. They also reported a significant increase in the frequency of charting when bedside terminals were used. Investigating charting in a burn unit, Hammond and colleagues[3] found that errors occurred in 25% of handwritten flow sheets. Installation of a Patient Data Management System virtually eliminated these errors and significantly increased the number of progress notes documented. Miller and Sheridan[4] reported an increase in compliance with documentation audit criteria of 25% and 27%, respectively, in two nursing units piloting a bedside computer system. Minda and Brundage[5] also reported an increase in the number of nursing observations recorded with automated versus handwritten documentation. Measuring compliance scores with internal documentation policies and external regulatory standards, White and Hemby[6] observed an increase from 62% to 95% for the eight indicators monitored before and after installation of a computer system. Other researchers have shown more comprehensive or more accurate documentation when patient records were compared before and after computerization.[7-9]

Some studies, however, have not found a positive relationship between computerization and the quality of nursing documentation. In a study evaluating the effectiveness of a computerized nursing information system on one nursing unit, there were mixed results in the completeness of nursing documentation.[10] Whereas an increase was shown in the documentation of nursing interventions, there was little change in the evaluation of the effects of the interventions, and there was no significant change in the percentage of patient problems charted. Marr et al.[11] were unable to support their hypotheses of positive relationships between the presence of bedside terminals and the completeness of nursing documentation of medication administration, admission notes, or of daily charting. Most charting was being done at places other than the bedside, such as the nursing circle and in empty patient rooms.[11] Pabst and colleagues[12] reported mixed results regarding quality of documentation when evaluating an automated documentation system. They found that care plans were updated more frequently on the unit that was automated; however, no significant differences were shown in the quality of charting.

Using the Health Care Technology Assessment framework, Happ[13] investigated the effectiveness of point of care technology on several aspects of the quality of patient care. She compared a convenience sample of patients from five nursing units in three hospitals. Half of the patients selected had computers at their bedsides, and half did not. She found the charts of patients with point of care technology (PCT) to be less compliant to JCAHO Chart Audit scores and concluded that the quality of patient care, as measured by patient satisfaction and documentation of nursing care given, did not improve with the implementation of PCT. This study has limitations because (1) there was no randomization of patients or units, (2) documentation of nursing care may not be reflective of the quality of patient care delivered, and (3) the control group was at a different hospital from the experimental groups.

In summary, the findings regarding the impact of computer systems on documentation were mixed. Furthermore, few studies reported the type of computer systems, for example, whether it was a stand-alone system or a integrated system, functions used, and placement of computer terminals, thus making comparison of results difficult. Data must be accumulated on various types of computer systems to judge which characteristics are most successful in providing an automated structure for nursing documentation. Other limitations exist. Many studies measured nursing units on-line against those nursing units that were not, instead of looking at the same unit before and after implementation. There was no standardized tool for data collection across studies. Few measured the impact at several time points after implementation. Measurements made too soon after implementation may underestimate the benefits derived from the system. For these reasons, this study, using JCAHO standards to measure quality of documentation, investigated the effects of time on the same nursing units before and after implementation of an integrated point of care system.

Fewer studies were available that investigated the effects of computerization on patient satisfaction. Happ[11] reported high patient satisfaction with nursing care and that patients were positive about bedside computer technology. However, when time and the presence of a computer were controlled for, Happ found that patients on nursing units without computers were more satisfied with nursing care than patients with computers in their rooms. No significant changes in patient satisfaction secondary to computerization were found in a study by Bernard and colleagues.[14] These findings are consistent with studies investigating the effects of computerization on the patient–physician relationship.[15-17] However, Siders and Peterson[18] found that implementing an automated nursing discharge summary increases patient satisfaction.

COMPUTER SYSTEM

The computer system implemented, on the units under study, is ULTICARE (Health Data Sciences, San Bernardino, CA), a UNIX-based, fully integrated, menu-driven hospital information system that provides an electronic medical record that includes a longitudinal clinical database repository. The computer is designed to allow real-time documentation at the point of care and provides clinicians access to the most recent patient information from anywhere in the hospital. All members of the healthcare team use the computer, enter orders, document patient care, and retrieve information based on their security level. At the time the study was conducted, the bedside terminal workstations, which are located at the head of the bed, ran Windows 3.1 or Windows 95, using TCP/IP connecting them to the 10–Base T Ethernet.

The nursing module of this clinical information system contains five elements of the nursing process; the sixth element, Outcomes Identification, was not added as a component of the nursing process until after this study was conducted. Because the vendor's software is flexible, a team of nurses representing each nursing unit was able to customize on-screen content. The nursing module of this clinical information system was implemented in stages by bringing up various aspects of nursing documentation at different time intervals. Six months after automation, nurses on all inpatient units were documenting admission, shift, and focused assessments as well as the plan of care on-line. Nursing assistants were also documenting their patient care on the computer system. By the 12-month time interval, screening assessments had been added to the admission database. By the 18-month time interval, tubes, drains, additional interventions, intake, and output had been added to on-line documentation procedures. Documentation of medication administration was not automated.

METHODS

The purpose of this study was to evaluate the effects of an integrated point of care computer system on the quality of nursing documentation and patient satisfaction.

The three research hypotheses were:

1. There will be a difference in the quality of nursing documentation before and after implementation of an integrated, point of care, computerized nursing documentation system, as measured by the percent compliance to the modified 35-item JCAHO Closed Medical Record Review Tool.
2. The quality of computerized nursing documentation will improve over each of the three postimplementation measurements of preimplementation to 6-month, 6- to 12-month, and 12- to 18-month pairwise comparisons.
3. There will be a difference in patient satisfaction before and after implementation of an integrated point of care system.

A quasi-experimental, modified time series research design was used to test the hypotheses that quality of nursing documentation and patient satisfaction will be improved by the implementation of an integrated, point of care, nursing documentation system. This study was conducted on four nursing units at a 282–licensed bed, not for profit, community hospital in North Carolina. Because implementation of the nursing module of the computer system was staggered over a 2-month period, data were collected with respect to each unit's implementation date, maintaining a 6-, 12-, and 18-month interval after implementation data collection for each unit. A limitation of the study is that only one preimplementation data collection was done because of the extensive resources necessary for manual data extraction from paper/microfiche charts. Quality of nursing documentation was operationally defined as compliance to JCAHO standards. Approval for the study was sought and obtained from the hospital's Institutional Review Board (IRB) committee.

Sample

The sample was selected by use of a simple random technique, using a proportion of each unit's patient admissions at each time interval (3 months before and 6, 12, and 18 months after implementation). At onset of the study, 11 of the hospital's 13 nursing units were scheduled for a point of care computer system within the time limits of this study. Four study nursing units were randomly picked: a 10-bed intensive care unit (study unit I), a 20-bed progressive care telemetry unit (study unit II), a 20-bed general surgery unit (study unit III), and a 12-bed gynecologic surgery unit (study unit IV). Because the computer system was implemented at different times over a 2-month period for the study nursing units, data were collected at 6-, 12-, and 18-month time points with respect to each unit's implementation date, at 6-month intervals.

The sample size of 288 charts used in the quality of documentation part of the study was calculated to detect a 6% increase in documentation compliance. The calculation was based on the known variance from previous chart reviews for a level $\alpha = .05$ one-sided test with a power of 95% for all units combined. The sample population for the quality of documentation segment of the study was derived by obtaining a list of all admissions to each unit during a 30-day period, for each of the four measurement time intervals. Charts were coded, and then a random number table was used to select a proportional, random sampling that consisted of 32% to 35% of the patients admitted to those respective nursing units during the 30-day period, at each time interval.

For the patient satisfaction segment, a convenience sample of patients from the four randomly selected nursing units was used. The only criterion for inclusion was that the patient was alert and oriented. Participation was voluntary, and participants remained anonymous. Informed consent was obtained before data collection. A total of 108 patients agreed to participate.

Instrumentation

Quality of Documentation

Each chart from the total sample of 288 charts was reviewed for compliance to the 35 nursing documentation items from the 96 "General Items" on the 1995 JCAHO Closed Medical Record Review tool. JCAHO does not report reliability and validity for the Closed Medical Record Review tool. This study found the reliability of the selected 35 items to be 0.71. The study tool measured nursing documentation in five categories: General, Assessment, Reassessment, Education, and Discharge. The tool was scored as a percent compliance to the 35 items. Possible responses were *Y, N,* and *N/A. Y* represented compliance to the standard. *N* represented noncompliance with the standard. *N/A* represented "not applicable to the patient whose chart was being reviewed." The percent compliance (PC) was calculated from the number of positive responses (Y) divided by the number of possible positive responses (Total answers − N/A).

Patient Satisfaction

Patient satisfaction was measured by using the Risser Patient Satisfaction Scale,[19] as revised by Hinshaw and Atwood[20] for use with inpatient hospital subjects. This tool was chosen because it was the only published patient satisfaction tool available with high reliability. The Risser Patient Satisfaction Scale (PSI) is a 25-item self-reporting attitude scale. It is subdivided into three subscales: I. technical professional behavior, for example, nursing knowledge and physical care; II. interpersonal–educational relationship, for example, social aspects as well as information exchange between nurse and patient; and III. interpersonal trusting relationship, for example, sensitivity to people and their feelings as well as listening to patient problems. Reliability coefficients (alpha) for the tool were reported by Risser as follows: Subscale I was 0.64, subscale II was 0.83, subscale III was 0.82, and the total was 0.91. Hinshaw and Atwood[20] found subscale I to be 0.79, subscale II to be 0.78, and subscale III to be 0.88. They did not report the total score. This study found subscale I to be 0.63, subscale II to be 0.70, subscale III to be 0.68, with the total being 0.87. Risser determined content validity through the method of item selection and revision. The distribution of scores was found to be positively skewed. Risser considered this fact to be

indicative of content validity, because other estimates of patient satisfaction show similar skewness. Hinshaw and Atwood[20] established construct validity by use of convergent and discriminant validity analysis, as well as predictive modeling. They concluded that the numerous validity estimates used across successive samples indicated moderate to strong validity for the PSI in general.

Data Collection Procedures

Data for the quality of documentation portion of the study were collected by two healthcare professionals. To determine interrater reliability, the two data collectors examined the same three charts, using the 35-item quality of documentation tool. Their interrater reliability averaged 92% for these three charts. Data were collected at 3 months before implementation of the computer system and again at 6, 12, and 18 months after implementation. The data collectors were blinded as to unit and data collection time interval.

Data for the patient satisfaction portion of the study were collected by distributing the Risser Patient Satisfaction Scale to the subjects. The instruments were collected approximately 30 minutes after distribution. Data were collected before implementation of the computer system and again at 6 and 18 months after implementation. Only three time periods (pre, 6, and 18 months postimplementation) were used for data collection because of the limited time between the decision to do the study and bringing the units on-line, as well as limits on data collection resources.

RESULTS

The analysis for the first and second hypotheses was performed by using SAS General Linear Models (GLM) procedure, Least Squares Means (LS) with a Step-down Bonferroni adjustment for five multiple comparisons, to test both hypotheses 1 and 2.

Hypothesis 1

There will be a difference in the quality of nursing documentation before and after implementation of an integrated, point of care, computerized nursing documentation system, as measured by the percent compliance to the modified 35-item JCAHO Closed Medical Record Review Tool.

A total of 288 charts were audited from the study nursing units, 61 at 3 months before implementation, 67 at 6 months after implementation, 82 at 12 months after implementation, and 78 at 18 months after implementation. Mean percent compliance was calculated, at each time interval, for each of

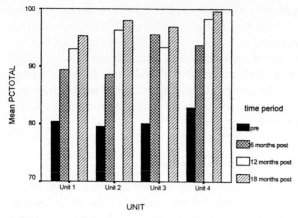

FIGURE 1
Mean percent documentation compliance over time by individual unit.

the four study nursing units (Fig. 1) and for all of the units combined. For all units combined, there was a 13% increase in compliance to JCAHO standards from a mean prescore of 85% to an 18-month postimplementation score mean of 98%, with a highly significant P-value, $t(135) = 4.01$, $P = 0.0003$. Hypothesis 1 was, therefore, accepted.

Hypothesis 2

The quality of computerized nursing documentation will improve over each of the three postimplementation measurements of: preimplementation to 6-month, 6- to 12-month, and 12- to 18-month pairwise comparisons.

The pairwise comparisons from LS Means indicate the differences between each of the three time periods to be statistically significant with P-values, $t(124) = 4.02$, $P = 0.0003$ for the comparison be-

tween the preimplementation and 6-month time points, $t(147) = 2.50$, $P = 0.0134$ for the comparison between the 6- and 12-month time points, and $t(158) = 2.40$, $P = 0.0134$ for the comparison between the 12- and 18-month time points. Hypothesis 2 was, therefore, accepted.

Post hoc analyses were performed by Nursing Unit and Sub Category on the modified JCAHO Review Tool:

By Unit

Because of the highly significant results for hypotheses 1 and 2, the effect of time on quality of nursing documentation was analyzed for each nursing unit. Modified Step-Down Bonferroni was used to adjust for the 30 comparisons shown in Table 1, for hypothesis 1 subgroup analysis. These post hoc tests showed that each of the four study units had a statistically significant increase in percent compliance for the preimplementation to 18-month comparison. The P-values, t-values and corresponding degrees of freedom for each unit are given in Table 1. For hypothesis 2, the subgroup analysis showed that, by themselves, only two units showed statistically significant increases in percent compliance. Unit III showed the only significant increase from the preimplementation to 6-month time period; unit II showed the only significant increase from the 6- to 12-month time period. When evaluated individually, no unit showed significance at the 12- to 18-month time period. The lack of significance for individual units over preimplementation to 6-month, 6- to 12-month, and 12- to 18-month comparisons is attributed to the lower power to detect a significant difference, given that there is one, for the single unit in the situation where the sample size is approximately one fourth of all four units combined,

TABLE 1
Subgroup Analysis for Hypothesis One T-Test* (3 Months Preimplementation to 18 Months Postimplementation)

Unit	General	Assessment	Reassessment	Education	Discharge	Total
I	$t(18) = 4.97$	$t(18) = 4.97$	$t(18) = 1.47$	$t(18) = 1.74$	$t(18) = 0.73$	$t(18) = 4.65$
	p = 0.0015	p = 0.0015	p = 0.6408	p = 0.5253	p = 0.9448	p = 0.0017
II	$t(46) = 4.26$	$t(46) = 1.95$	$t(46) = 0.49$	$t(46) = 4.26$	$t(46) = 1.09$	$t(46) = 4.26$
	p = 0.0015	p = 0.3426	p = 0.9448	p = 0.0015	p = 0.8508	p = 0.0015
III	$t(41) = 4.31$	$t(41) = 3.05$	$t(41) = 1.26$	$t(41) = 3.34$	$t(41) = 0.31$	$t(41) = 4.31$
	p = 0.0015	p = 0.0280	p = 0.7550	p = 0.0144	p = 0.9448	p = 0.0015
IV	$t(26) = 4.59$	$t(26) = 0.47$	$t(26) = 1.69$	$t(26) = 3.36$	$t(26) = 2.72$	$t(26) = 4.59$
	p = 0.0015	p = 0.9448	p = 0.5253	p = 0.0180	p = 0.0754	p = 0.0015
Total	$t(135) = 4.01$	$t(135) = 4.01$	$t(135) = 1.68$	$t(135) = 4.01$	$t(135) = 1.02$	$t(135) = 4.01$
	p = 0.0015	p = 0.0015	p = 0.5253	p = 0.0015	p = 0.8508	p = 0.0015

*Boldface values indicate significant p-values.

and where we are looking at incremental percent increases. The study was sampled and powered to detect a 6% increase for all units combined; thus, for individual units with smaller sample sizes, statistically significant results would not be expected unless the gain in percent compliance was greater than 6%. The *P*-values, *t*-values, and corresponding degrees of freedom for each unit are given in Table 2.

By Subcategory

Because of the highly significant results for hypotheses 1 and 2, the effect of time on quality of nursing documentation was also analyzed for each of the five categories on the modified JCAHO Closed Medical Record Review Tool. For hypothesis 1, post hoc tests for the General, Assessment, and Education categories indicated a statistically significant increase in the preimplementation to 18-month comparison. No significant differences were found in the preimplementation to 18-month comparison for either the Reassessment or the Discharge category. The *P*-values, *t*-values, and corresponding degrees of freedom for each category are given in Table 1.

For hypothesis 2, post hoc tests for the General and Assessment categories indicated a statistically significant difference for the preimplementation to 6 month comparison. The General category also showed a statistically significant increase between the 12- and 18-month time points. The Education category indicated a statistically significant increase between the 6- and 12-month time points. Post hoc tests for the Reassessment and Discharge categories showed no statistical significance between any of the four time points. The *P*-values, *t*-values, and corresponding degrees of freedom for each category are given in Table 2.

Hypothesis 3

There will be a difference in patient satisfaction before and after implementation of an integrated point of care system.

A total of 108 inpatients agreed to complete the Risser Patient Satisfaction tool, 49 in the preimplementation group, 30 in the 6-month postimplementation group, and 29 in the 18-month postimplementation group. A one-way analysis of variance (ANOVA) was computed to compare preimplementation and postimplementation data. There was no statistical significance at the 0.05 level for any subgroup, nor for the total score. Therefore, the hypothesis was rejected.

DISCUSSION

The computer system in this study has several attributes that encourage quality charting. One attribute is the prompts provided within the assessments and interventions, which remind nurses of the specific data that need to be documented for each type of assessment and intervention. Another attribute is the ability to collect and chart data real time, at the bedside. The standardization of assessment and other charting is also an attribute as the nurse is guided through the screens by menus and templates. Also, some information is required and must be entered before the nurse can continue; other information is historical and pulls forward from past visits or previous shifts. Finally, the system contains electronic work tools that consolidate, sequence, and constantly update patient care tasks and provide notification when interventions are missed. Hypotheses 1 and 2 were designed to confirm that, collectively, these attributes had the desired effect on quality of nursing documentation. This was achieved as evidenced by the significance test results for the two hypotheses and by the decreasing trend in standard deviation of the percent compliance. The decrease in standard deviation across time indicated decreased variability in charting across nursing units. The values for the standard deviation, for all nursing units, at each of the four successive measurement time points from preimplementation to 18 months were: 9.7%, 8.2%, 6.8%, and 3.8%, respectively.

The preimplementation to 18-month comparison for hypothesis 1 showed a significant increase in the quality of nursing documentation after implementation of the computerized nursing system. The combined scores on the JCAHO Closed Medical Record Review increased from a mean of 85% before computerization to 98% at 18 months after implementation of computerization. Hypothesis 2 was designed to capture the maturation as people learn over time and become comfortable with a computer system. The between time-point comparisons for hypothesis 2 showed significance between all time points, thus, when the units were evaluated collectively, increase in compliance was continuing to take place throughout the entire 18-month postimplementation phase.

The subgroup analyses for both hypotheses give further insight into which components of nursing documentation, as operationalized in this computer system, are contributing to the increased compliance. As shown in Figure 2, the compliance across JCAHO subcategories varied by category at the preimplementation time point. The compliance to the *Reassessment* and *Discharge* components of nursing documentation was already high at 95% and 94%, respectively, before implementation of the computer system. The 18-month compliance scores for reassessment and discharge were 97% and 98%; although not increased enough to be statistically significant, both show an upward trend, as shown in

TABLE 2
Subgroup Analysis for Hypothesis Two T-Test (Time Comparison by JCAHO Subcategory and by Unit)

Time Comparison	JCAHO Subcategory		
	Pre to 6	6 to 12	12 to 18
General	t(124) = 4.02 p = 0.0014	t(147) = 1.85 p = 0.6289	t(158) = 3.55 p = 0.0058
Assessment	t(124) = 3.14 p = 0.0231	t(147) = 0.82 p = 1.000	t(158) = 0.06 p = 1.000
Reassessment	t(124) = 0.07 p = 1.000	t(147) = 1.51 p = 0.9373	t(158) = 0.32 p = 1.000
Education	t(124) = 0.48 p = 1.0000	t(147) = 4.00 p = 0.0014	t(158) = 0.45 p = 1.0000
Discharge	t(124) = 0.73 p = 1.0000	t(147) = 1.35 p = 1.0000	t(158) = 1.68 p = 0.7110
Total	t(124) = 4.02 p = 0.0003	t(147) = 2.50 p = 0.0134	t(158) = 2.40 p = 0.0134
Unit	**Unit**		
	Pre to 6	6 to 12	12 to 18
I	t(16) = 2.20 p = 0.4515	t(17) = 1.19 p = 1.000	t(19) = 0.75 p = 1.000
II	t(41) = 1.87 p = 0.6289	t(41) = 3.86 p = 0.0048	t(46) = 0.86 p = 1.000
III	t(40) = 4.32 p = 0.0014	t(56) = 1.13 p = 1.000	t(57) = 1.87 p = 0.6289
IV	t(23) = 2.01 p = 0.5620	t(27) = 1.88 p = 0.6289	t(30) = 5.28 p = 1.000
Total	t(124) = 4.02 p = 0.0003	t(147) = 2.50 p = 0.0134	t(158) = 2.40 p = 0.0134

Boldface values indicate significant *p*-values.

Figure 2. The subgroup analysis investigating the incremental increases in compliance between time points for these two subcategories showed no statistical significance between any two time points as expected (Table 2). The subcategories *General, Assessment,* and *Education,* with more improvement opportunity, attributable to lower compliance before implementation, showed statistically significant increases in percent compliance between one or more of the various time points as well as significance for the preimplementation to 18-month comparison. Thus, the model of nursing documentation components, in this computer system, that were contributing most to the increased compliance is:

Assessment + General + Education

This model is heavily dependent on the strengths, weaknesses, and adherence to the prior documentation system. These results illustrate the sensitivity of system evaluation to the preimplemen-tation charting methods and compliance profile. For example, an institution with a different compliance profile or charting method may have unique tools for charting assessment in place before implementation, and thus have a high percent compliance in this JCAHO subcategory. Therefore, the preimplementation compliance must be thoroughly characterized before interpreting postimplementation evaluative measures.

The increase in charting compliance was not achieved by every nursing unit, for all categories combined until 12 months after initiation of automated documentation. For example, unit II showed a statistically significant increase during the 6- to 12-month time period, when no other unit showed a statistically significant increase. Unit III showed a statistically significant increase in the preimplementation to 6-month time period, during which no other unit showed a statistically significant increase. One possible reason for this may be the differences in

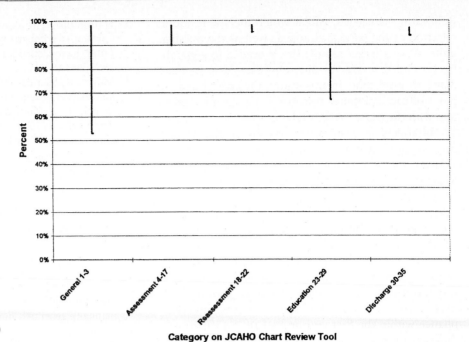

FIGURE 2
Change in percent compliance from pre- to
18 months by category.

Category on JCAHO Chart Review Tool

learning curve among the various staff nurses as they worked with the new system. Additionally, as the nursing staff adjusted to the new system, some also may have been adapting their nursing care by making process changes accordingly. This has implications for others who are evaluating computer systems. Because the relationship between the nurse and the computer is dynamic and evolves over time, adequate time should be allowed to see the benefits. Evaluation should be repeated at set intervals until the desired target level of documentation compliance is reached or until no further gains are being made. In this study, measurements were terminated at 18 months because documentation compliance had reached the 98th percentile. Chief Financial Officers of healthcare institutions want, and expect to see, immediate benefits that will justify the high expense of a computer system; however, the true extent of these benefits may not be evident until 18 months postimplementation. An additional implication is that longitudinal research designs extending to 18 months are needed to provide insight into the time needed to reap expected benefits.

The nursing context, in which nurse–computer interactions occur, includes many variables. Although unable to control for these extraneous variables in an active clinical environment, there was an awareness of these variables and their possible effects on the findings. For example, the nursing unit census fluctuated in the preimplementation data collection from 75% to 100% on the sample nursing units. Perhaps a lower census would decrease the nurse–patient ratio and allow the nurse more time for

charting. However, by flexing staff up and down according to patient census, the nurse–patient ratio remained essentially constant on each unit during the course of the study. Other variables that could affect the quality of documentation or patient satisfaction, that were not controlled for, included patient acuity, unit management changes on two of the four study units, attitude of management and staff toward the computer system, and where the nurses chose to do their charting (bedside vs. hallway).

A limitation of the study is that only one preimplementation data collection was done because of the extensive resources necessary for manual data extraction from paper/microfiche charts. Any future research should equalize preimplementation and postimplementation data collection time points. This will strengthen the experimental design and conclusions by controlling or quantifying documentation process stability both before and after implementation.

Because the patient satisfaction mean scores did not significantly change from before to after implementation in this study, the third hypothesis was rejected. Although consistent with some of the previous literature, there are limitations to this finding. Because the self-reporting patient satisfaction tool was used on a convenience sample of patients who voluntarily participated in the study, this finding may not be indicative of the total patient population even though the nursing units from which the convenience sample was obtained were randomly selected. The confirmed lower reliability scores for subscale I and our finding of low score for subscale III of the Risser Patient Satisfaction Tool is also a limitation.

Replication is needed, which would include random selection of the patient sample as well as the nursing units. Also, a larger sample size is needed to generalize beyond this research site. However, it is encouraging to note that, in this study, the use of a new point of care computer system did not seem to interfere with the nurse–patient relationship.

In conclusion, this study has shown that documenting with a point of care, integrated computer system can increase compliance to JCAHO Standards without negatively affecting patient satisfaction. Based on the increases in percent compliance achieved in this study, each of the four nursing units had a percent increase ranging from a 9.4% to 11.6% increase within 18 months of implementation of computerized charting. Therefore, this research suggests that implementation of similar systems, in institutions with a similar compliance profile, and nursing context, may expect similar increases in compliance within the first year and a half. Furthermore, different nursing units can be expected to attain the expected compliance gains at different time points within 1 year of implementation.

The authors conclude that the evaluation of the implementation of a computerized nursing documentation system should include more than the evaluation of the change in percent compliance. One should also consider the initial level of compliance and what factors, for example, JCAHO subcategories, were contributing to the initial level of compliance. In addition, it is important to know the length of time required for nurses to achieve the gains sought and the effect on the nurse–patient relationship.

Further research remains to be done to refine the practice of nursing by using the rich data accumulated from information systems, to establish links between nursing interventions and patient outcomes. The first step is to establish that computer systems can lead to an increase in the quality of documentation. Next, whether better organization and display of data can assist the nurse to assimilate information needs to be determined. Then, research is needed on how that information is being used. Does better information lead to more knowledgeable and better clinical decision making? Finally, exploration is needed to determine whether these elements affect the quality of care and the outcomes for the patient.

REFERENCES

1. Staggers N, Parks PL. Description and initial applications of the Staggers & Parks nurse-computer interaction framework. *Comput Nurs.* 1993;11:282–290.
2. Dennis KE, Sweeney PM, MacDonald LP, Morse NA. Point of care technology: Impact on people and paperwork. *Nurs Econ.* 1993;11:229–237, 248.
3. Hammond J, Johnson HM, Varas R, Ward CG. Qualitative comparison of paper flowsheets vs a computer based clinical information system. *Chest.* 1991;99:155–157.
4. Miller ER, Sheridan EA. Integrating a bedside nursing information system into a professional nursing practice model. In: Arnold JM, Pearson GA, eds. *Computer Applications in Education and Practice.* New York: National League for Nursing; 1992;60–72.
5. Minda S, Brundage DJ. Time differences in handwritten and computer documentation of nursing assessment. *Comput Nurs.* 1994;12:277–279.
6. White C, Hemby C. Automating the bedside. *Heath Informatics.* 1997;February:68–74.
7. Belcher AJ, Cunningham LS. Implementation of bedside computers in critical care. In: Arnold JM, Pearson GA, eds. *Computer Applications in Education and Practice.* New York, NY: National League for Nursing; 1992:53–61.
8. Holzemer WL, Henry SG. Computer supported vs manually generated nursing care plans: A comparison of patient problems, nursing interventions, and AIDS patient outcomes. *Comput Nurs.* 1992;10:19–24.
9. Hendrickson G, Kovner CT, Knickman JR, Finkler SA. Implementation of a variety of computerized bedside nursing information systems in 17 New Jersey hospitals. *Comput Nurs.* 1995;13:96–102.
10. Hinson DK, Huether SE, Blaufuss JA, et al. Measuring the impact of a clinical nursing information system on a nursing unit. *Proceedings of the Seventeenth Annual Symposium on Computer Applications in Medical Care;* 1993:203–210.
11. Marr PB, Duthie E, Flassman KS, et al. Bedside terminals and quality of nursing documentation: Part 1. *Comput Nurs.* 1993;11:176–182.
12. Pabst MK, Scherubel JC, Minnick AF. The impact of computerized documentation on nurses' use of time. *Comput Nurs.* 1996;14:25–30.
13. Happ MA. The effect of point of care technology on the quality of patient care. *Proceedings of the Seventeenth Annual Symposium on Computer Applications in Medical Care,* 1993:183–187.
14. Bernard AM, Hayward RA, Anderson JE, Rosevear JS, McMahon LF Jr. The integrated inpatient management model: Lessons for managed care. *Med Care.* 1995:663–675.
15. Aydin CE, Rosen PN, Jewell SM, Felitti VJ. Computers in the examining room: The patient's perspective. *Proceedings of the Annual Symposium on Computer Applications in Medical Care.* 1995:824–828.
16. Legler JD, Oates R. Patients' reactions to physician use of a computerized medical record system during clinical encounters. *J Fam Pract.* 1993;37:241–244.
17. Solomon GL, Dechter M. Are patients pleased with computer use in the examination room? *J Fam Pract.* 1995;41:241–244.
18. Siders AM, Peterson M. Increasing patient satisfaction and nursing productivity through implementation of an automated nursing discharge summary. *Proceedings of the the Annual Symposium on Computer Applications in Medical Care.* 1991:136–140.

19. Risser NL. Development of an instrument to measure patient satisfaction with nurses and nursing care in primary care settings. *Nurs Res*. 1975;24:45–52.

20. Hinshaw AS, Atwood JR. A patient satisfaction instrument: Precision by replication. *Nurs Res*. 1982;31:170–175, 191.

Rosemary Nahm, MSN, RN, is a Clinical Research Associate with Duke Clinical Research Institute, Durham, North Carolina.

Iona Poston, PhD, RN, is an Associate Professor, School of Nursing, East Carolina University. Her research focus is utilization of computers, in both education and practice.

This collaborative study was conducted as part of an evaluation project of the nursing component of the new hospital information system installed at Nash General Hospital, a part of Nash Health Care Systems, Rocky Mount, North Carolina. Portions of this study have been presented as a paper at the Rutgers State College Fifteenth Annual International Nursing Informatics Conference, March 1997, Atlantic City, New Jersey; and as a poster at the North Carolina Nurses Association annual meeting, September 1997, Greensboro, North Carolina.

The authors gratefully acknowledge the statistical help of Meredith Nahm, MS, Duke Clinical Research Institute, and Dr. Melvin Swanson, School of Medicine, East Carolina University.

Address for correspondence: Rosemary Nahm, MSN, RN, 617 Edinborough Drive, Durham, NC 27703.

Section 4:

Reprinted by kind permission of:
John Wiley & Sons, Inc. (431)
International Federation for Medical
& Biological Engineering (443)
The Institute of Electrical and
Electronical Engineers, Inc. (455, 465)
Elsevier Science (449)

P. Laguna

Synopsis

Dept. of Electronic Engineering and
Communications
University of Zaragoza, Spain

Signal Processing

Signal processing is generally referred to as the technique to analyze time domain series acquired from a physical phenomenon, representing some physical time-varying magnitude. Signals can be of different nature: one-dimensional continuous signals (e.g. bioelectric signals, speech, etc); two-dimensional signals (images, etc); three-dimensional signals (video, etc). However, when we use the term signal we will tacitly refer here (and in many references) to one-dimensional signals. One-dimensional signals can also be continuous or discrete in time. The latest are such either by nature or by discretization of a continuous signal, as is usually the case in biomedical signal analysis. These time-discrete one-dimensional signals have been subjected to the huge development of the information processing techniques of the last decades, particularly to signal processing techniques focusing on obtaining the information of interest carried by the signal.

In the biomedical system field, Electrocardiogram (ECG), Electroencephalogram (EEG), and to a lower extent Electromyogram (EMG) bioelectric signals possess a broader history in signal processing development. The aim has always been to obtain relevant information to diagnose, evaluate, monitor, and/or follow-up the physiological system under study. Special and separate atten-tion has been given to the voice signal. This pressure signal, converted to electrical signal by a microphone transducer and of biological origin, has been the subject of many signal processing developments in the context of communication (speech recognition, synthesis, enhancement, etc). In the particular use of biomedical application synthesis is playing a major role in helping the speech impaired. Also the transient evoked otoacoustic emissions (TEOAE), generated by the cochlea as response to acoustic stimuli, are of interest for hearing impaired identification. The five selected papers for the signal processing section of the 2002 Yearbook deal with EEG, ECG and TEOAE.

Signal processing is a very useful technique in many biomedical applications. Therefore, it should be restated that most biological system diagnosis involving biomedical signals can be done, and in most cases largely outperformed, by more elaborate techniques, such as imaging, invasive test, etc.. These techniques, even with their better sensitivity and specificity, present two major drawbacks: the price paid by the patient or the public health system, which has made them prohib-itive for massive screening, and the invasive aspect, resulting in highly uncomfortable procedures for the patient with collateral risks in some cases. These two reasons still make it very challenging to push signal process-ing techniques developments that improve actual levels of sensitivity/specificity in the related domain diagnosis. Both low cost and non-invasive techniques are important aspects of signal processing. Recording equipment today is within very acceptable price ranges, and processing has been implemented in computers today. Limitations of the computers are often procedural rather than computational. These two properties are very valuable in screening large populations and in pathologies associated with large prevalence, such as cardiac disorders in western countries.

In the last decades, signal processing researchers have developed well-established linear time-discrete signal processing techniques. Linear processing allows accounting for most of the phenomena that can be modeled as linear, or whose real behavior is not far from being linear. Thus the signal can be filtered to separate undesired components, or those originated in a biological subsystem other than the one under study. The system parameters that generate the signal can, in many cases, be estimated based on linear system identification techniques. From these system parameters, clinically valuable indices can be inferred. Examples are spectral analysis in EEG for sleep analysis, ECG filtering (to remove the EMG and baseline wander that essentially lies on different frequency bands), heart rate variability (HRV) analysis to identify the influence the central nervous system has on rhythm by evaluating the relative frequency band power content, etc..

In many cases, linear techniques alone are not enough to extract clinically relevant information. Therefore, other ad hoc rules are introduced to the linear analysis, depending on its purpose. Examples of these structures are: threshold based QRS detectors to combine linear and non-linear techniques (such as squaring with threshold decision rules), fiducial point identification in ECG wave analysis with threshold based rules, arrhythmia analysis and beat type identification systems (requiring feature extraction from linearly processed signals plus some classification criteria), high frequency indices extraction to stratify post myocardial infarction patients at risk of sudden cardiac death (late potentials or intra-QRS potentials), ischemia detection and monitoring, otoacoustic emission detection. Many of these ad hoc techniques can be studied using detection or estimation theory, after which the optimum rules can be estimated from the statistics of the problem.

Beside measuring particular signal parameters, the problem of identifying hidden parameters has also been addressed. These parameters give relevant information for some diagnostic objective that is not apparent in signal visual inspection or its automated, measured descriptive parameters. This is often addressed by statistical signal processing in reference to data from documented patient databases and should be investigated further by prospective studies. The classification rules, typically used to separate patient groups, can be linear (MANOVA) or non-linear, such as higher order classifiers or neural networks. In terms of patient screening

and decision rules based on signal-extracted parameters, neural network non-linear classifiers have developed greatly. They possess better classification properties than linear rules and often involve simpler algorithmic implications. These nonlinear interpolators are always based on the availability of an appropriate training set with which the network can be trained and further studies conducted.

In addition to the ad hoc non-linear rules introduced in many parts of signal processing, linear approximations are often far from the reality of biological systems, in which very complex cross-systems influences take part. This implies that linear analysis of the signals generated by the system gets lost within the system. Frequently, if we were able to study the non-linear relationships within the signal in a way related to the non-linearity inherent in the system, we will be able to gain better insight into the physiological processes than by just using linear strategies. Non-linear signal processing is under development and some indices based on chaos studies, fractal dimension of signal etc. are being considered to extract useful information from signals that usually remains hidden in linear analysis. These indices will add strength to signal analysis if they are able to relate closely to the underlying physiological mechanisms of the system. Since these mechanisms are often unknown, and non-linear signal analysis can be performed in many ways with a less well-established framework than linear analysis, in my opinion, more fundamental work is still required to assess the real impact of these techniques and to obtain the most suitable non-linear representation in each case. Examples of these non-linear approaches are the studies on heart rate variability carried out in the past decade, and the similarity index to predict seizures [4] in EEG analysis.

The phenomenon behind biomedical signals is typically spatial and requires at least three orthogonal dimensions (signals) to describe it. Analysis recordings are well established in cardiac and brain multi-channel (leads). Time-space signal processing techniques have also recently been explored to diagnose brain and cardiac dysfunction. These techniques, within the scope of the author, still have room to grow, since they have not achieved maximum possible information extraction.

The five selected papers for this section on signal processing deal with three types of biomedical signals: Electrocardiogram [1], otoacoustic emissions [2], and Electroencephalogram [3, 4, 5]. The paper by Zigel et al. [1], proposes very important ECG data compression evaluation strategies. One of the main evaluation strategies of signal data compression is the use of mathematical distortion measures as percentile root mean square difference (PRD) which is a quadratic norm of the differences between original and reconstructed signal. Other alternatives have introduced linear norms. In any case, this gives a general idea of the shape distance (measured sample by sample) between the signals. However, interest in the biomedical signal is not in the overall waveshape, but in the clinical information carried by the signal. A reduced PRD, or its variations, does not guaranty the preservation of the clinical information. The introduced Weighted Diagnostic Distortion (WDD) index evaluates the difference between the clinical parameters measured in the original and the reconstructed signals (waves amplitudes, intervals duration, etc.) and is much more suitable for the purpose of clinical diagnoses. It will be desirable in the future for data compression techniques to measure their performance with these or related alternative indices rather than mathematical ones. A mean opinion score (MOS) given by expert cardiologists in terms of diagnosticability has been used to compare the WDD and the classical PRD. Not surprisingly, the WDD correlated much better with the expert MOS, corroborating the convenience of using this kind of WDD index to evaluate data compression algorithms. This approach is parallel to coders evaluations in speech processing. Here, the overall waveshape is not of interest, but the perception of the listener when listening to the reconstructed signal.

The approach presented by Janušaukas et al. in [2] deals with the pass/fail separation problem for hearing impairment screening. The otoacoustic emissions are carefully analyzed both in time and frequency to design ad hoc linear processing detection strategies. Different time windows are taken from the elicited stimulus as functions of the frequency bands under analysis, according to the different lags of the three different bands reported for these emissions. The very poor signal to noise ratio of this signal is treated in the wavelet transform domain by clipping (time-varying linear operation) the coefficients under some selected threshold and thus just keeping those components of dominant energy at the averaged TEOAE. This operation is performed on two subaverage sets of TEOAE. If the obtained signal is not noise, it should present correlation between the two subaverages. This correlation at three different wavelet scales is used to decide the pass/fail strategy using a threshold based rule. For a sensitivity of 90%, the received operating curves (ROC) evaluated on a very large subject database allow an increase in specificity from 68% (classical detection methods) to 90%, which is a remarkable improvement. This paper corroborates that fine knowledge of the signal under study and its underlying mechanisms allow

ad hoc signal processing refinement which results in further improvement. More elaborated decision rules or similarity measures from the two subaverages TEOAE will probably be the direction to pursue in these kind of studies.

The remaining three papers [3, 4, 5] deal with the EEG problem. This signal is more random in nature than ECG or TEOAE. The mechanisms of brain behavior are more complex and make the inference of valuable clinical decisions from the EEG more difficult. The EEG represents a spatio-temporal summation of the total brain activity. The difficulty in obtaining information from the EEG is reduced when the objective is to locate areas of particularly intense activation as in epileptic patients, or in evoked responses to a particular stimuli.

The paper by Zhukov et al. [3] presents a very interesting strategy to integrate most of the available developments in identifying source location (if a single source is assumed) and extends this technique to multifocal source location. The work assumes that the different focuses are not correlated. By using Independent Component Analysis (ICA), it separates the EEG component related to each focus. Single focus techniques are then applied. The computational load is greatly reduced and more effective results in this simpler case of the single-focus inverse problem in Electroencephalography are achieved. First, it achieves noise reduction by applying principal component analysis. After using the ICA techniques, it isolates every focus-related EEG component. Since the inverse EEG source location is an ill-posed problem, there is no guarantee that the solution is correct, due to the solution's multiplicity. In simulations, the work reports precision in locating the focuses between 2 and 5 mm.

The work presented by le van Quyen et al. [4] deals with well in advance prediction of epileptic seizure. This will be especially useful in uncontrolled epilepsy patients, allowing application of preventive measures and improvement of quality of life. The rational behind the work is to compare, from the non-linear point of view, scalp-EEG signals time windows from a reference period and a running window recording. Since the recordings are highly noisy, many non-linear techniques fail due to the noise influence. In this work, a similarity index based on zero crossing of the signal which makes the noise influence very limited, is used. A threshold based rule is then used to decide when the time window under analysis is different from the reference one. In a set of 23 patients with temporal-lobe epilepsy (TLE), the anticipation of the seizures was 416 s (SD 356), suggesting that the preictal state is a process which largely varies within individual patients. Details about the non-linear technique are referred to the appendix in www.thelancet.com. The finding that similar results can be obtained from the scalp-EEG and from intracranial recordings is both surprising and challenging. Surprising, because the scalp-EEG is an attenuated and blurred version of the intracranial activity and challenging, because of the convenience in practical clinical implications.

The work by Gonzalez Andino et al. [5] also deals with EEG signal analysis. They try to infer neurophysiological activation with measures of signal complexity. They assume that signals of low complexity belong to organized sources, and signals of high complexity belong to unorganized sources and represent noise or unstructured activation. In this work, the time-frequency representation of the signal is performed, and, in the time-frequency plane, the Renyi entropy throughout the Renyi number is computed. This number gives an estimate of the degree of ordering in the signal. If the signal is organized with well defined elementary function in the time frequency plane, the degree of complexity will be low. If no elementary function can be identified at the frequency plane, the Renyi number will be low representing a higher degree of complexity and no relation with synchronized activity. This technique allows cerebral maps of activation areas according to the Renyi number at each lead. This approach, in addition, does not require strong assumptions about noise statistics and is less restricted than other techniques with the same objective.

Acknowledgements

Thanks to S. Olmos, J. García, R. Bailón, R. Jané and L. Sörnmo for reading and commenting on the synopsis.

References

1. Zigel Y, Cohen A, Katz A. The weighted diagnostic distortion (WDD) measure for ECG signal compression. IEEE Trans Biomed Eng 2000;47:1422-30.
2. Janušaukas A, Marozas V, Engdahl B, Hoffman HJ, Svensson O, Sörnmo L. Otoacoustic emissions and improved pass/fail separation using wavelet analysis and time windowing. Med Biol Eng Comput 2001;39:134-9.
3. Zhukov L, Weinstein D, Johnson C. Independent component analysis for EEG source localization. IEEE Eng Med Biol 2000;357:87-96.
4. le van Quyen M, Martinerie J, Navarro V, Boon P, D'Havé M, Adam C, et al.. Anticipation of epileptic seizures from standard EEG recordings. Lancet 2001;357:183-8.
5. Gonzalez Andino SL, de Peralta Menendez RG, Thuut G, Spinelli L, Blanke O, Michel CM et al.. Measuring the complexity of time series: An application to neurophysiological signals. Hum Brain Mapp 2000;11:46-57.

Address of the author:
Pablo Laguna Lasaosa
Dept. of Electronic Eng. and Communications
Centro Politécnico Superior
University of Zaragoza
María de Luna 3
50015 Zaragoza, Spain
E-mail: laguna@posta.unizar.es

Measuring the Complexity of Time Series: An Application to Neurophysiological Signals

S.L. Gonzalez Andino,[*] **R. Grave de Peralta Menendez, G. Thut,
L. Spinelli, O. Blanke, C.M. Michel, M. Seeck, and T. Landis**

[1]*Functional Human Brain Mapping Laboratory and Presurgical Epilepsy Laboratory, Neurology
Department, University Hospital Geneva, Geneva, Switzerland*
[2]*Plurifaculty Program of Cognitive Neuroscience, University of Geneva, Geneva, Switzerland*

Abstract: Measures of signal complexity can be used to distinguish neurophysiological activation from noise in those neuroimaging techniques where we record variations of brain activity with time, e.g., fMRI, EEG, ERP. In this paper we explore a recently developed approach to calculate a quantitative measure of deterministic signal complexity and information content: The Renyi number. The Renyi number is by definition an entropy, i.e., a classically used measure of disorder in physical systems, and is calculated in this paper over the basis of the time frequency representation (TFRs) of the measured signals. When calculated in this form, the Renyi entropy (RE) indirectly characterizes the complexity of a signal by providing an approximate counting of the number of separated elementary atoms that compose the time series in the time frequency plane. In this sense, this measure conforms closely to our visual notion of complexity since low complexity values are obtained for signals formed by a small number of "components". The most remarkable properties of this measure are twofold: 1) It does not rely on assumptions about the time series such as stationarity or gaussianity and 2) No model of the neural process under study is required, e.g., no hemodynamic response model for fMRI. The method is illustrated in this paper using fMRI, intracranial ERPs and intracranial potentials estimated from scalp recorded ERPs through an inverse solution (ELECTRA). The main theoretical and practical drawbacks of this measure, especially its dependence of the selected TFR, are discussed. Also the capability of this approach to produce, with less restrictive hypothesis, results comparable to those obtained with more standard methods but is emphasized. *Hum. Brain Mapping 11:46–57, 2000.* © 2000 **Wiley-Liss, Inc.**

Key words: Renyi entropy; ERPs; Evoked potentials; EEG; Complexity

Contract grant sponsor: Swiss National Foundation; grant numbers: 2053-059341.99 and 31-57112.99. Contract grant sponsor: Programme commun de recherche en genie biomedical 1999–2002.

Correspondence to: S.L. Gonzalez Andino, Functional Brain Mapping Lab., Neurology Dept., University Hospital Geneva, 24 Rue Micheli du Crest, 1211 Geneva, Switzerland.
E-mail: slgandino@hotmail.com

Received for publicaton 25 April 2000; accepted 2 June 2000.

INTRODUCTION

Functional neuroimaging aims to study the dynamic functioning of the human brain while subjects are at rest or performing controlled perceptual or cognitive tasks. Electroencephalography (EEG), Magnetoencephalography (MEG), Event related potentials (ERPs) or functional magnetic resonance imaging (fMRI) are some of the techniques currently in use to quantify and localize in space and/or in time some correlates of neuronal activity related to a task. While fMRI has direct localizing value, i.e., it provides images of functional activation within the brain, EEG, MEG, or ERP provide maps over the scalp surface and one has to solve an inverse problem to obtain estimates of the electrical activity within the brain. In any case, these techniques usually lead to a large number of signals (time series) which are a function of space and time and which have to be further analyzed in order to detect the brain or scalp sites in which consistent patterns of activation arise. Concretely we have to differentiate signal from noise on the basis of the time series measured or from those estimated by an inverse solution.

The intuitive rationale behind the visual identification of a signal is the presence of an organized response, that is, the emergence of a typical pattern that a trained observer can often differentiate from a "non signal" (noise). Although this pattern usually differs from one technique to another, the common rule that differentiate signal from noise on visual basis is that signals seem to be composed of a few elementary waveshapes sometimes referred to as components.

In this paper we explore a recently developed approach to calculate a quantitative measure of deterministic signals complexity and information content: The Renyi number [Renyi, 1961]. The Renyi number is by definition an entropy, i.e., a quantitative measure of the level of disorder in a physical system. Entropy has been used in statistics and information theory to develop measures of the information content of signals [Shannon, 1948]. The novelty of the approach presented in this paper resides in that the Renyi entropy (RE) is calculated over the basis of the time frequency representation (TFR) of the measured signals as suggested by Willians et al. [1991]; Flandrin et al. [1994] and Baraniuk et al. [submitted]. This measure relies on the "counting" of the number of components (energy spots) that appear in the time frequency representation of a signal. In this sense, this measure closely conforms with our visual notion of complexity and assumes nearly nothing about the properties of the process generating the signal or about the signal itself. For these reasons, the Renyi entropy calculated over the basis of TFRs is a measure particularly suitable to analyze the complexity of a large range of neurophysiological signals.

Like many other methods in use nowadays the methodology described in this paper aims to detect activation in functional neuroimaging data on the basis of the measured time series. However, in contrast with many of the currently used methods it requires nearly no assumptions about the signals itself or the neural process generating it. By using the natural association between organization of the signal over time and activation there is no need to model the underlying neural process, e.g., the hemodynamic response for fMRI. Besides, the estimation of the RE based on the TFR allows for the analysis of signals which are non stationary or non gaussian. It relies only on the assumption that the properties of signals and noise differ in the time-frequency plane.

In the initial part of the paper the concept of Renyi entropy and the basis for its calculation using TFRs are presented. An initial section discusses the concept of complexity and its relationship to disorder and noise and illustrates how these aspects are reflected by a time frequency representation. Synthetic data are used to reveal the capabilities of the time frequency representation to separate independent signals in the time frequency plane and to clarify how the RE indirectly counts them. It is shown that the estimate of the number of components is stable for a fixed TFR once an adequate separation between the elementary signals is reached. The applicability of the Renyi number to differentiate signals from noise are then exemplified using data from different neuroimaging modalities, namely, fMRI time series, intracranial event related potentials and the time series obtained from applying a distributed inverse solution termed ELECTRA [Grave et al., 2000] to scalp recorded event related potentials. Some theoretical limitations associated with the analogy probability density and TFRs used to calculate the RE are discussed. These aspects are confronted to the practical merits of the measure to reflect our visual perception of complexity for many different types of neurophysiological signals.

Basic theory

This section first describes the concept of time frequency representations and shows the applicability of them to differentiate elementary signal components in the time frequency plane. It follows the definition of complexity and the basis to calculate it using TFRs. A third section discusses the selection of the TFR. Finally the concrete steps to be followed in the analysis are itemized. Basic concepts are marked in italics.

Signals, complexity, elementary components and time frequency representations

Many neurophysiological signals are obtained by receivers recording variations of brain activity over time. Brain signals are in general non-stationary, that is, their frequency content is varying with time [Gersch, 1987; Unser and Aldroubi, 1996]. Therefore the

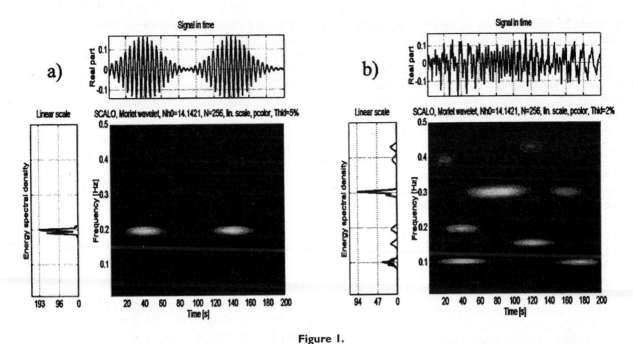

Figure I.

Time, frequency and time-frequency representations of two signals. At the top of each inset is the time course of the signals depicted. The power spectrum is shown at the left of each inset.

The big square shows the time frequency representation (Morlet scalogram) for two signals composed by two (**a**) and eight (**b**) elementary gaussian atoms.

most informative description of such signals is achieved by directly represent their frequency content while still keeping the time description parameter. This is precisely the aim of time frequency representations [Boudreaux-Barte, 1996; Lin and Chen, 1996]. Time frequency representations (TFRs) generalize the concept of the time and frequency domains to a joint time-frequency function $C_s(t, f)$ that indicates how the frequency content of a signal s changes over time, i.e., they tell us which frequencies are contained in a signal and when these frequencies appear.

There are a multitude of time frequency representations that range from the well known spectrogram to the more recently developed scalogram based on wavelet transform. All TFR have in common that they transform a one dimensional signal to a two dimensional representation in the time frequency plane where the spectral properties are tracked over time. Thus, spots or energy concentrations in the time frequency plane identify the elementary signals, sometimes referred as components or atoms, that superimpose to form the original signal. This is the key point in the relationship between our visual notion of complexity and the estimates provided by the method discussed in this paper. It is intuitively reasonable to assume that signals of high complexity (noise) must be constructed from large numbers of elementary com-

ponents while signals of low complexity should be composed of a few elementary components. Activation is in this sense associated to organization of the signals (few components in the time frequency plane) while noise is associated to disorder (a multiplicity of components). It is important to note that this intuitive idea of complexity does not rely upon the locations in time of these elementary components but instead in their number. Independently of the neuroimaging modality, a signal reflecting activation arises directly or indirectly from the "synchronized" activity of groups of neurons and such synchronization leads to less complex signals than the chaotic firing of the same group.

In Figure 1a and b we illustrate the characteristics of the time (uppermost insets), the frequency (leftmost insets) and the time-frequency representations of two signals. They are composed by two (a) and eight (b) elementary gaussian atoms, i.e., concentrations (spots) of energy in the time frequency plane. It is clear from the figure that the signal composed by the largest number of components visually resembles more a disorganized or noisy process than the one formed by only two components. Note also how the TFR (Morlet scalogram) adequately identifies the number and frequencies of these atoms while the power spectrum does not.

Measures of the complexity of signals: the renyi's numbers or renyi's entropies

The concept of complexity is far too diffuse to expect any quantitative measure of it to apply universally. So far, two main basic approaches have been used to evaluate complexity of time series: a) Entropy measures derived in the framework of information theory and calculated on the basis of probabilistic models [Willians et al., 1991; Flandrin et al., 1994; Barniuk et al., submitted] and 2) Entropy measures derived in the context of non linear analysis or chaos theory [Wackermann et al., 1993; Weber et al., 1998; Cerutti et al., 1996]. One common element between both is the underlying association between highly complex signals and noise.

Here we relate the term complexity to the idea described in the previous section, i.e., to the amount of elementary atoms or components constituting the signal. The concept of complexity will be quantified by means of the most classical measure of disorder in a physical system: the entropy. Besides its initial application in the field of molecular physics, entropy has been used in statistics and information theory to develop measures of the information content of signals [Shannon, 1948]. Shannon entropy is the classical measure of information content and is defined for an n-dimensional probability density (PD) distribution $P(x)$ as:

$$H(P) = \int_{-\infty}^{\infty} P(x) \log P(x) dx \qquad (1)$$

An efficient estimator for the probability density distribution usually requires either several samples of the process or strong assumptions about the properties of the studied process. Thus, here we explore a novel approach to measure complexity trough entropy suggested by Willians et al., [1991] and further developed by Flandrin et al., 1994 and Baraniuk et al., [submitted] in the field of signal processing. In this approach the probability density function is replaced by the coefficients $C_s(t, f)$ of a given time frequency representation of the signal $s(t)$ which leads for the Shannon entropy to:

$$H(C) = \int_{-\infty}^{\infty} \int_{-\infty}^{\infty} C(t, f) \log C(t, f) dt df \qquad (2)$$

This approach exploits the apparent analogy between time frequency representations and probability densities described in Willians et al. [1991]. In such an approach, TFRs are interpreted as bidimensional energy densities in the time-frequency domain. This analogy relies partially upon the parallelism that exists for the marginal properties of some TFRs and those of the probability densities, namely:

a) time marginal preservation: $\int C_s(t, f) df = |s(t)|^2$
b) frequency marginal preservation: $\int C_s(t, f) dt = |S(f)|^2$
c) energy preservation: $\int C_s(t, f) dt df = \int |s(t)|^2 dt = \|s\|_2^2$

where $|.|$ stands for the modulus and $\|.\|$ for the signal norm. Since several time frequency representations can achieve negative values the use of the more classical Shannon information as a measure of complexity is prohibited (due to the presence of the logarithm within the integral in (3)) and some authors [Willians et al., 1991; Flandrin et al., 1994, Baraniuk et al., submitted] have proposed the use of a relaxed measure of entropy known as the Renyi entropy of order α:

$$H_\alpha^R(P) = \frac{1}{1-\alpha} \log_2 \frac{\int P^\alpha(x) dx}{\int P(x) dx} \qquad (3)$$

$$H_\alpha(C_s) = \frac{1}{1-\alpha} \log_2 \int\int \left(\frac{C_s(t, f) dt df}{\int\int C_s(t, f) dt df} \right)^\alpha \qquad (4)$$

Following Baraniuk, the passage from the Shannon entropy H to the class of Renyi entropies H_α^R involves only the relaxation of the mean value property from an arithmetic to an exponential mean and thus in practice H_α^R behaves much like H. The Shannon entropy can be recovered as $\lim_{a \to 1} H_\alpha^R(P) = H(P)$.

The rationale behind substituting the probability density function P by the coefficients $C_s(t, f)$ of the time frequency representation of the time series s is appealing: the peaky TFRs of signals comprised of a small numbers of elementary components (organized signals) would yield small entropy values, while the diffuse TFRs of more complicated or noisy signals would yield large entropy values. Based on this idea and several empirical studies, Willians et al., [1991] proposed the use of the 3rd order Renyi entropy ($\alpha = $

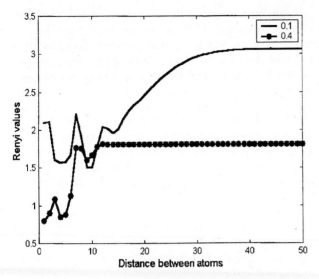

Figure 2.

Saturation values of the RE vs. atoms separation: The curves reflect the RE value estimated for different distances between the gaussian atoms when the Morlet scalogram is used. Two normalized frequencies are shown (0.01 and 0.04).

3 in equation 4) as a measure of the complexity of the signal. Note that that (3) and (4) not only differ in the substitution of the probability density by the TFR coefficients but also that (4) is a prenormalized version, equivalent to normalizing the signal energy before raising the TFR coefficients to the α power. Thus we will use definition (4) for the rest of the paper.

Selecting the time frequency representation

The complexity value estimated through the analogy probability density and TFR depends upon the TFR employed. While this element certainly play havoc with a uniquely defined measure of complexity, the results of the numerical experiment carried out by Willians et al. [1991], as described below shed light on how the RE behaves. In practice and in agreement with these authors we have found that the RE value tends to stabilize for a fixed number of components or atoms once the atoms are clearly resolved in the time frequency plane. This stabilization occurs for all time frequency representations even if they differ in the value at which the RE saturates.

To test the counting behavior of $H_3(C_s)$, Willians et al. [1991] selected two gaussian atoms and plotted the values of the RE vs. the separation in time of the atoms. They observed that the H_3 value stabilized once the two atoms became disjoint in the time frequency plane. In Figure 2, we present the results of a

similar simulation that we carried out for the Morlet scalogram (the square of the wavelet transform) instead of the Wigner Ville originally used in Willian's paper (Willians et al., 1991]. The results for the scalogram are similar, i.e., the Renyi value stabilizes for adequate separation between atoms.

This analysis reflects the well known trade-off between time and frequency (or scale) resolution. High frequency regions of the wavelet transform have very good time resolution whereas low frequency regions have very good spectral resolution. The two atoms are better resolved in time for the higher frequencies than for the lower ones which explains why the counting of elementary components reaches a stable value for smaller distance when the frequencies of the components are higher.

These elements lead to an important question: which is the more suitable TFR to obtain the most accurate estimates of complexity for a given data set? In practice, the best estimates are obtained with the TFR which is better in separating the elementary atoms that conform our signal. While quasi-stationary signals could be adequately analyzed with the simple spectrogram its low resolution at high frequencies affects the differentiation between signals and noise when noise is concentrated in the high frequency band. As shown below an adequate tuning of the scalogram reached by changing the length of the Morlet analyzing wavelet at coarsest scale is sufficient to separate the components for signals of different nature. In summary, because there is no ideal TFR that fulfills all desirable properties, we recommend to explore the kind of signals to be analyzed with at least one member of each class (i.e., Cohen's class, the hyperbolic class, the affine class, etc., see Boudreaux-Bartel, 1996) to check for auto term preservation and cross term removal in the particular application.

Algorithm

In summary, the concrete steps that we propose to detect activation in neurophysiological signals are:

1) Choose a time frequency representation and tune its parameter with a few signals to achieve adequate discrimination of the basic elementary components. Note that this step is not needed for each individual data set but for a given experimental design.

2) Compute the preselected time frequency representation for each signal.

3) Compute the Renyi entropies of order three us-

ing equation (3) for each of the TFRs of the processed signals.

A Matlab toolbox developed by the Digital Signal Processing group from the Rice University comprising a large number of TFRs as well as a subroutine to compute the Renyi entropy is freely available on the Web (www-isis.enst.fr/Applications/tftb/iutsn.univ-nantes.fr/auger/tftb.html).

Measuring the complexity of neurophysiological signals

In this section we describe the results obtained in the classification of signals from noise using the RE in three types of neurophysiological signals. This analysis has two goals: 1) Demonstrate that this method provides results comparable to those obtained by means of more standard techniques that require stronger a priori assumptions about the signals and 2) Illustrate that the same analysis procedure leads to reasonable results for signals arising from the diverse neuroimaging techniques commonly used nowadays.

The whole analysis was carried out using the MAT-LAB time frequency toolbox [Auger et al., 1996] and all the signals were analyzed using the Morlet scalogram. After some numerical simulations we decided for the default parameters reported in the toolbox in the computation of the scalogram. The RE of order three was subsequently calculated using the same toolbox.

Analyzing fMRI signals

A variety of methods for analyzing fMRI signals in the time or the frequency domain have been proposed in the last few year [see e.g. Bandettini et al., 1993; Baker et al., 1994; Worsley and Friston, 1995; Xiong et al., 1996; Lange and Zeger, 1997; Ruttimann et al., 1998 among others]. Some of these methods rely upon some model and/or assumption about the fMRI acquisition, e.g. concerning the stimulus (binary baseline-activation conditions), or the haemodynamic response.

The blood oxigenation level dependent (BOLD) images were obtained with a 1.5T Edge system (Picker Int. Cleveland OH) using single shot echo planar imaging (EPI) with the following parameters: echo time (TE) = 40 ms, repetition time (TR) −2s, number of averages = 1, field of view (FOV) = 25∗16 cm^2, matrix size 128 × 82, number of slices = 11, slice thickness = 5 mm with no gap. The acquisition time was 1.1 s. The experimental task consisted in a sequential right thumb to right digit opposition.

After motion correction and linear detrend of the signals we computed the Morlet scalogram for each of the fMRI time series. Typical patterns found in this data set for this time frequency representation are shown in Figure 3. Left panels (a and b) correspond to regions of no activation and show a more diffuse or widespread pattern with atoms dispersed over the whole time frequency plane. In contrast, the TFR of the time series associated to activated regions shown in the right panels (c and d) show a consistent regular pattern at the low frequency band. In the TFR of organized signals the regular pattern dominates over the components of the noise. Note also that since the temporal position of the atoms has no influence on the RE computation this measure will be robust to different haemodynamic delays at different sites or to non periodic fMRI signals likely to arise in event related fMRI paradigms.

In figure 4 we represent eight fMRI signals with their corresponding RE values at the top of each signal. The four signals at the left column are signals with low linear correlation coefficient (CC < 0.5) with a preselected reference vector [Bandettinni, 1993] while the ones in the right were classified as signals reflecting activation (CC > 0.7) on the same basis. Exact values for the CC for each signal are given at the figure legend. Signals on the right also correspond to brain sites known to be activated by the functional motor task, i.e., they are located on the left primary motor cortex.

For this data set, the Renyi entropy values showed a clear gap between activation and no activation independently of the amplitude of the responses. The appealing aspects in this analysis which contrast with the comparison with a preselected reference vector are twofold: 1) There is no need to guess or model such a reference vector since the classification is based on the counting of the number of elementary components and 2) The method can be applied to experiments where sequences of on-off conditions are not available.

Still, in the whole analysis of a fMRI (not discussed here) statistical methods will probably be needed to set the threshold between signals and noise (as done in correlation analysis) if a clear gap as the one observed in this example does not appear.

Analyzing intracranial ERPs

Intracranial ERPs were obtained from 94–100 recording sites of two epileptic patients (A.M. and N.B.). The patients had subdural grids or strips implanted on their left hemispheres as part of presurgical diagnostic investigations including electrical cortical stimulation

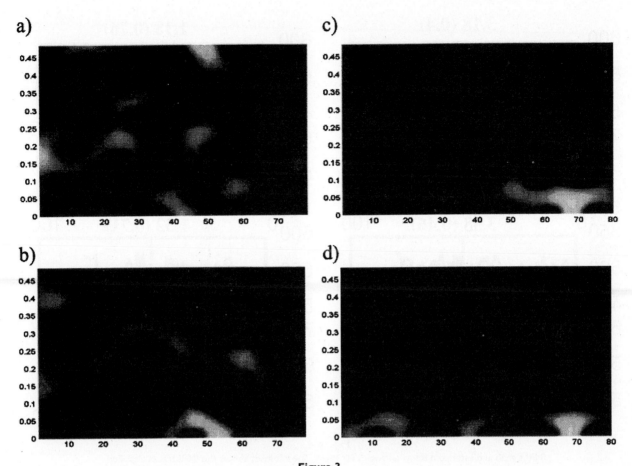

Figure 3.
Morlet scalogram (a TFR) for fMRI traces arising at non activated brain areas (3a and 3b) and activated areas (3c and 3d). Note the diffuse pattern in the non activated areas which contrast with the regular one found in the right panel.

to map brain functions. After informed consent had been obtained, both patients participated in a study on visuomotor integration. As a part of this study patients performed simple unimanual index finger responses to black dots, which were presented every 5–6 sec for 60 msec in random order either to the left or to the right of a central fixation cross on a gray computer screen. Here two conditions were further evaluated: 1) Right visual field stimulation, right hand response (RR) 2) Left visual field stimulation, right hand response (LR). After having performed a training session, NB was tested in 80 trials per condition and AM in 60.

The EEG was recorded continuously with a sampling rate of 190 Hz (AM) or 200 Hz (NB) in a bipolar montage, bandpass 0.1–100 Hz. EEG was analyzed off-line and EEG epochs (100 ms before and 500 ms after stimulus onset) were computed and averaged after artifact rejection. Averages were later bandpass

filtered (Butterworth) between 1 and 50 Hz. The motor responses recorded with a response key device were situated within the time window of analysis. Mean reaction times were 352.4 ± 76 ms for NB and 257 ± 47 ms for AM.

For each averaged signal, we computed first the scalogram and then the Renyi entropy of order three [Auger et al., 1996]. Figure 5 shows the plot of the values of the Renyi's number superimposed over the grid or stripes in the individual MRIs of the two patients. The darker the region the lower the RE. The regions with the lowest REs were encircled to outline the sites where the most organized responses appeared. For surgical reasons the grid had to be oriented horizontally in NB and vertically in AM. In Figure 4b we display the results of the electrical cortical stimulation. The different symbols represent the brain sites from which visual illusions, right hand

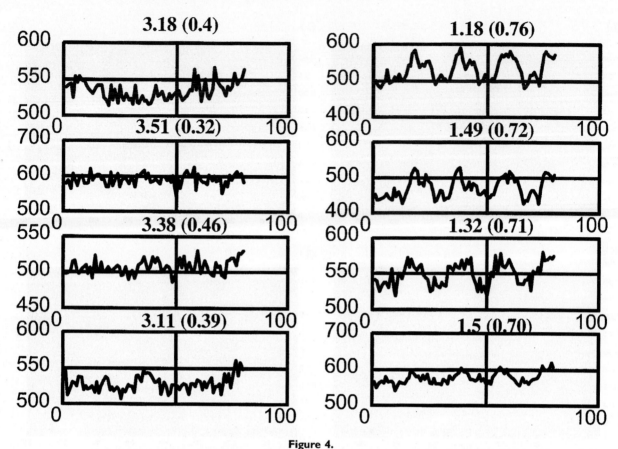

Figure 4.
fMRI signals and estimated Renyi entropies for them. The left inset shows the fMRI traces classified as noise by classical correlation coefficient analysis (CC values from top to bottom are 0.04, 0.32, 0.46 and 0.39 respectively). On the right, signals classified as reflecting activation (CC are 0.76, 0.72, 0.76, 0.72), are shown.

somato-sensory phenomena or right hand movements were elicited. These areas were expected to be activated during the performance of the simple visuomotor reaction time task.

In line with these expectations we found that the regions with highest organized signals in terms of RE correspond for both patients to the contacts over motor and sensory motor areas, and for one patient (NB) to contacts over visual areas. No highly organized signals are observed over the visual areas of AM. However, these contacts lie more anterior than the visual ones in NB, and are thus likely to cover higher order visual cortex not necessarily engaged in visual information processing in this simple task.

Analyzing time series estimated by ELECTRA

While fMRI is able to detect functional activation with excellent spatial resolution, this technique lacks the capability to track neural events at the milliseconds level. Temporal evolution of such events can be traced by electrophysiological techniques such as EEG, ERP or MEG which are nonetheless unable to provide accurate spatial localization. Therefore, there is an increasing tendency to combine both neuroimaging techniques. Such combination generally requires the solution of the electromagnetic inverse problem either using spatio temporal source models or distributed inverse solutions.

One aspect that has somehow limited the combination of fMRI and EEG/MEG inverse solutions is that the relationship between hemodynamic responses and underlying electrophysiological events is not yet clearly established. It is however reasonable to assume that fMRI images provide a coarse temporal average of electrophysiological events. One manner to further assess this hypothesis is to compare for similar experiments fMRI images with temporal averages of intra-

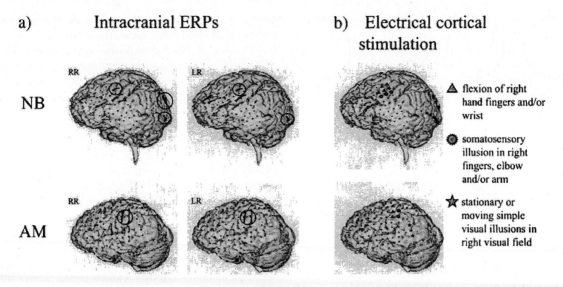

Figure 5.

Estimated response complexity in a visuo motor task in two epileptic patients. (**a**) Calculated Renyi's entropies superimposed on the individual MRIs of the two epileptic patients. The regions with the lowest NNREs (darkest values) are encircled to outline the sites where the most organized and strongest responses appeared. (**b**) Results of the electrical cortical stimulation. The different symbols represent the brain sites from which visual or right hand somato-sensory illusions or right hand movements were elicited.

cranial recordings or distributed inverse solutions. While intracranial recordings are usually restricted to a few brain sites in pathological brains, the results of inverse solutions are not always reliable especially in terms of the estimated amplitudes of the deeper sources. Recent simulations have suggested that the temporal courses of the generators tend to be more reliably estimated (except for an amplitude factor) than the instantaneous amplitude map [Grave de Peralta et al., 2000]. This reason speaks in favor of searching for methods to analyze the estimated signals in terms of their temporal organization rather than relying on the instantaneous maps. Obviously the methods to analyze these time series should not depend upon a scale factor which is insured here by the use of equation (3).

We concretely propose to compare fMRI results with the images obtained by determining the traces of the estimated inverse solution which show a consistent activation over time. Activation will be measured trough the Renyi entropy. For simplicity we use a recently developed distributed inverse solution coined ELECTRA [Grave de Peralta and Gonzalez, 1999; Grave de Peralta et al., 2000] which restricts the source model to the kind of currents that can be actually detected by scalp electrodes. Besides it's mathematical properties, ELECTRA is particularly appealing for the analysis described here because it is the first inverse

solution that attempts to estimate the three dimensional potential distribution inside the human brain such as the one provided by implanted intracranial electrodes. In this sense ELECTRA's results can be compared with those measured experimentally and all procedures employed to analyze these traces, as the one proposed in this paper, can be applied.

In Figure 6 we present an example of application of the RE to the detection of signals in the potentials estimated by ELECTRA in a simple visual task. In the experimental protocol, 41 channel evoked potentials (EP) were recorded in 25 healthy subjects. Checkerboard reversal stimuli (500 ms) were presented to the left, the center or the right visual field. The mean average response over subjects was computed and ELECTRA solution was obtained for this grand mean data using an spherical volume conductor model of the head.

Figure 6a and b show the 3-dimensional RE maps for the right and central visual field stimulation, respectively. The sites with the most organized responses (lower RE) are shown. Consistent with the basic anatomical, electrophysiological and clinical knowledge [Regan, 1989], the lateralized stimuli (right) mainly led to activation of the occipital areas contralateral to the stimulated field, while full-field stimulation induced symmetrical activation of the occipital areas of both hemispheres.

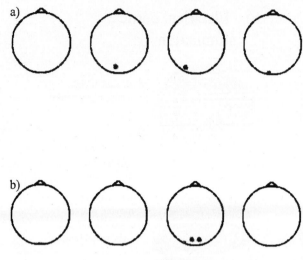

Figure 6.
The lowest RE values for the time series estimated by ELECTRA in a simple visual task. Top: Right visual field stimulation and Bottom: Central visual field stimulation. Only the four lower slices of the solution space are shown.

DISCUSSION

We have described and illustrated here an approach to differentiate activation from noise in neurophysiological signals of diverse origins with minimal assumptions. This approach uses as a measure of activation the RE calculated over the basis of the time frequency representation of the measured signals. Although many additional theoretical properties of the RE are discussed in Baraniuk et al, (submitted), we prefer to discuss here those merits, pitfalls and caveats of more practical relevance. It should not be neglected that the lack of uniqueness in this definition of complexity given its dependence of the selected TFR is an obvious theoretical flaw of this method. More relevant on practical grounds are the presence of cross-components or interference terms in the TFR which affect the counting property of the RE. Also amplitude and phase differences between the components of the signal alter the asymptotic saturation levels as illustrated in Figure 2. This is why the selection of an adequate TFR, able to extract the relevant features of the signal to be processed with a minimum of interference terms, is a crucial aspect in the analysis proposed. Probably even more important than the selection of the TFR itself is the adequate tuning of its parameters taking into account the unavoidable trade off between time and frequency resolution. On one hand, a good time resolution requires a short temporal analysis window; on the other hand a good frequency resolution re-

quires a long time window. Unfortunately both wishes cannot be simultaneously granted. In the particular case of ERPs and fMRI signals it can be assumed that their frequency changes over time are not very fast and thus the time resolution is not as important as the frequency resolution [McGillem and Aunon, 1987]. Consequently, in this case a long temporal window can be chosen which might not be adequate for other types of data.

It is also relevant that this measure of complexity is closely related to our intuitive notion of organization of the signals. If the TFR adequately separates the elementary components of the signals in the time frequency plane, then this measure reflects more or less adequately the number of components. Usually, the more peaky time frequency representation of signals comprised of small numbers of elementary components yield small entropy values (small Renyi numbers), while the diffuse TFRs of more complicated signals yield large entropy values (large Renyi numbers).

One could also wonder if other measures derived from the TFR of a signal such as moment-based measures, e.g., time-bandwidth and its generalizations to second order time frequency moments could replace the RE as measures of complexity. A simple example described by Baraniuk (submitted) shows that this is not the case. Let's consider a signal comprised of two components of compact support, i.e., which are zero outside a certain region of the time frequency plane. While the time-bandwidth product increases without bound with separation, the complexity does not increase once the components become disjoint as illustrated in the basic theory section.

Alternative measures of complexity have already been applied to the analysis of electrophysiological signals [Wackermann et al., 1993; Tononi et al., 1996; Aftanas et al., 1998; Micheloyannis et al., 1998; Weber et al., 1998 among others]. Most of these measures are derived in the context of non linear analysis and chaos [Cerutti et al., 1996] and are difficult to apply to general neurophysiological signals. The main reason is that an adequate estimate of the complexity requires a large number of samples, i.e., either signals sampled at a very high sampling frequency or very long periods. These conditions are not always fulfilled in practice. Additional difficulties of using non linear analysis techniques are described in Nunes [1995].

The applications described and illustrated here merely scratch the surface of potential applications of TFRs or RE for the analysis of brain signals. An interesting potential application is to exploit the "analogy" TFR and probability density for the calculation of the average amount of mutual information, a measure of the interdependence between time series applicable to the study of information transmission between brain areas [Mars and Da Silva, 1987]. A generalization of the Shannon measure known as the Gelfand and Yaglom measure have been already used in the EEG/ERP literature to study the structure of brain interdependencies [Mars and Da Silva, 1987, for a review]. An understanding of the principles governing the behavior of epileptiform activity, where the complexity is reported to decrease preceding the seizure [Lehnertz et al., 1997; Weber et al., 1998] or the analysis of changes and transitions of the brain electric activity before and after drugs intake can be obtained from the application of the methods described here.

CONCLUSIONS

In this paper we describe a measure of the complexity of neurophysiological signals: the Renyi entropy. This measure is conceptually simple to understand and as illustrated in the analysis of several types of neurophysiological signals, it corresponds well with our visual notion of complexity. In contrast with measures derived in the framework of non linear analysis this measure does not require long time series. Worthy to note is that this method implies nearly no assumptions about the underlying processes or the recorded signals, which makes this measure of complexity robust and generally applicable. All these properties are essential for the analysis of the diverse signals arising from different modalities of brain imaging which describe very different neurophysiological processes.

Our goal with this paper is not to describe an approach able to access information invisible to other methods. We aim instead to describe a tool to extract the same information with less assumptions. It is important to realize that most of the standard methods available to distinguish signals from noise imply requirements such as gaussianity or stationarity, demand lengthy time series or presuppose some a priori knowledge about the underlying neurophysiological process. Many of these hypothesis do not necessarily hold for each neuroimaging modality or for each experimental paradigm, and their validity is hardly ever tested in practice. Therefore, a method like the one proposed here, general enough to handle a multiplicity of neurophysiological signals without needing assumptions about them, should not be disregarded.

ACKNOWLEDGMENTS

Work supported by the Swiss National Foundation Grants 4038-044081, and 21-45699.95

REFERENCES

Aftanas LI, Lotova NV, Koshkarov VI, Makhnev VP, Mordvintsev YN, Popov SA (1998): Non-linear dynamic complexity of the human EEG during evoked emotions. Int J Psychophysiol 28(1): 63–76.

Auger F, Flandrin A, Goncalves P, Lemoine O (1996): Time Frequency Toolbox for use with Matlab.

Baker J, Weisskoff R, Stem C, Kennedy D, Jiang A, Kwong K, Kolodny L, Davis T, Boxerman J, Buchwinder B, Wedeen B, Bellivau J, Rosen B (1994): Statistical assessment of functional MRI signal change. In: Proceedings of the second annual meeting of the society of magnetic resonance, p 626.

Bandettini PA, Jesmanowicz A, Wong EC, Hyde JS (1993): Processing strategies for time-course data sets in functional MRI of the human brain. Magn Res Med 30:161–173.

Baraniuk RG, Flandrin P, Hansen AJEM, Michel O (submitted): Measuring time frequency information content using the Renyi entropies. Postscript version available at www-dsp. rice.edu/publications.

Bodreaux-Bartel GF (1996): Mixed time-frequency signal transformations. In: The transforms and applications handbook (Poularikas, Ed.) pp. 887–963. Boca Raton-CRC Press.

Cerutti S, Carrault G, Cluitmans OJ, Kinie A, Lipping T, Nikolaidis N, Pitas I, Signorini MG (1996): Non-linear algorithms for processing biological signals. Comput Methods Programs Biomed 51:51–73.

Flandrin P, Baraniuk RG, Michel O (1994): Time frequency complexity and information. Proc IEEE Int Conf Acoust, Speech, Signal Processing-ICASSP'94. III: 329–332.

Grave de Peralta Menendez R, Gonzalez Andino SL (1999): Distributed source models: Standard solutions and new developments. In: Uhl C, ed. Analysis of Neurophysiological Brain Functioning. Heidelberg: Springer Verlag.

Grave de Peralta Menendez R, Gonzalez Andino SL, Morand S, Michel CM, Landis TM (2000): Imaging the electrical activity of the brain: ELECTRA. Hum Brain Mapp 9(1)1–12.

Gersch W (1987): Non-stationary multichannel time series analysis. In: Handbook of Electroencephalography and Clinical Neurophysiology. (Gevins AS, Remond A, eds) Vol. 1., Methods of Analysis of Brain Electrical and Magnetic Signals. Amsterdam-New York-Oxford: Elsevier. p 261–296.

Lange N, Zeger SL (1997): Non linear Fourier time series analysis for human brain mapping by functional magnetic resonance imaging. Journal of the Royal Statistical Society. Series C, Applied Statistics, 46(1) p 1–30.

Lehnertz K, Elger CE, Weber B, Wieser HG (1997): Neuronal complexity loss in temporal lobe epilepsy: effects of carbamazepine on the dynamics of the epileptogenic focus. Electroencephalogr Clin Neurophysiol 103(3):376–380.

Lin Z, Chen JD (1996): Advances in time-frequency analysis of biomedical signals. Crit Rev Biomed Eng 24(1):1–72.

Mars NJ, Lopes da Silva FH (1987): EEG analysis methods based on information theory. In: Handbook of Electroencephalography and Clinical Neurophysiology. (Gevins AS, Remond A, eds) Vol. 1., Methods of analysis of Brain Electrical and Magnetic Signals. Amsterdam-New York-Oxford: Elsevier. p 297–307.

McGillem CD, Aunon JI (1987): Analysis of event-related potentials. In: Handbook of Electroencephalography and Clinical Neurophysiology. (Gevins AS, Remond A, eds) Vol. 1., Methods of analysis of Brain Electrical and Magnetic Signals. Amsterdam-New York-Oxford: Elsevier. p 131–170.

Micheloyannis S, Flitzanis N, Papanikolau E, Bourkas M, Terzakis D, Arvanitis S, Stam CJ (1998): Usefulness of non-linear EEG analysis. Acta Neurol Scand. 97 (1):13–9.

Nunes PL (1995): Non linear analysis and chaos. In: Neocortical dynamics and human EEG rhytms. (Nunes PL, ed). New York-Oxford: Oxford University Press. p 417–474.

Regan D (1989): Human Brain Electrophysiology. Elsevier.

Renyi A (1961): On measures of entropy and information. In: Proc. 4th Berkeley Symp. Math. Stat. and Prob. Vol. 1, p 547–561.

Ruttimann UE, Unser M, Rawlings RR, Rio D, Ramsey NF, Mattay VS, Hommer DW (1998): Statistical analysis of functional MRI data in the wavelet domain. IEEE Trans. Medical Imaging, 17(9) p 2555–2558.

Shannon CE (1948): A mathematical theory of communication. Part I, Bell Sys Tech J 27:379–423.

Tononi G, Sporns O, Edelman GM (1996): A complexity measure for selective matching of signals by the brain. Proc Natl Acad Sci USA. 93(8):3422–7.

Unser M, Aldroubi A (1996): A review of wavelets in biomedical applications. Proc IEEE, vol. 84, p 626–638.

Wackermann J, Lehmann D, Michel CM (1993): Global dimensional complexity of multichannel EEG indicates change of human brain functional state after single dose of a nootropic drug. Electroenceph Clin Neurophysiol 86:193198.

Weber B, Lehnertz K, Elger CE, Wieser HG (1998): Neuronal complexity loss in interictal EEG recorded with foramen ovale electrodes predicts side of primary epileptogenic area in temporal lobe epilepsy: a replication study. Epilepsy, 39(9):922–7.

Willians WJ, Brown ML, Hero AO (1991): Uncertainty, information and time-frequency distributions. In: Proc SPIE Int Soc Opt Eng, vol. 1566, p 144–156.

Worsley K, Friston K (1995): Analysis of fMRI time series revisited-again. Neuroimage 2:173–181.

Xiong J, Gao JH, Lancaster JL, Fox PT (1996): Assessment and optimization of fMRI analysis. Hum Brain Mapp 4:153–167.

Otoacoustic emissions and improved pass/fail separation using wavelet analysis and time windowing

A. Janušauskas[1,2]   V. Marozas[1,2]   B. Engdahl[3]   H. J. Hoffman[4]
O. Svensson[1]   L. Sörnmo[1]

[1]Signal Processing Group, Department of Applied Electronics, Lund University, Lund, Sweden
[2]Department of Biomedical Engineering, Kaunas University of Technology, Kaunas, Lithuania
[3]Department of Environmental Medicine, National Institute of Public Health, Oslo, Norway
[4]Epidemiology, Statistics & Data System Branch, National Institute on Deafness and Other Communication Disorders, NIH, Bethesda, Maryland, USA

Abstract—*A new method is presented for the purpose of improving pass/fail separation during transient evoked otoacoustic emission (TEOAE) hearing screening. The method combines signal decomposition in scales using the discrete wavelet transform, non-linear denoising and scale-dependent time windowing. The cross-correlation coefficient between two subaveraged, processed TEOAE signals is used as a pass/fail criterion and assessed in relation to the pure-tone, mean hearing level. The performance is presented in terms of receiver operating characteristics for a database of 5214 individuals. The results show that the specificity improves from 68% to 83% at a sensitivity of 90% when compared with the conventional wave reproducibility parameter.*

Keywords—*Transiently evoked otoacoustic emissions, Hearing screening, Wavelets, Denoising, Time windowing*

Med. Biol. Eng. Comput., 2001, **39**, 134–139

1 Introduction

TRANSIENTLY EVOKED otoacoustic emissions (TEOAEs) are low-level sounds produced by the cochlea in response to short acoustic stimuli and recorded in the external ear canal. The TEOAE signal has been found useful in clinical practice, as it is usually present in the normal hearing ear but absent, or attenuated, in the dysfunctional cochlea (KEMP, 1978; GRANDORI *et al.*, 1990; BRAY, 1989). Tests for identification of moderate hearing loss based on TEOAE detection have become very popular, for example in large hearing screening programs, because the test can be completed in a few minutes using non-invasive, inexpensive equipment.

Several studies have shown that the signal-to-noise ratio (SNR) is critical for achieving an acceptable performance of the TEOAE test (GORGA *et al.*, 1993; BRASS *et al.*, 1994; PRIEVE *et al.*, 1993; LUTMAN, 1993). For example, an increase in SNR of 0.6 dB was found to improve specificity (the 'pass' percentage) from 83 to 86% when sensitivity was held constant (BRAY, 1989). Reduction of the noise level in recorded data can be achieved by various approaches, e.g. careful fitting of the probe in the ear canal, adding more sweeps to the synchronous signal average, and enhancement of emission-specific features relying on the fact that signal components exhibit a frequency-dependent latency (KEMP, 1978; NEELY *et al.*, 1988).

In this study, the last of the above approaches is further pursued for noise reduction. This approach has recently been investigated in other studies of, for example, time windowing of the TEOAE signal (WHITEHEAD *et al.*, 1995), highpass filtering removing frequencies below 800 Hz (RAVAZZANI *et al.*, 1998), signal splitting into bandpass components (GORGA *et al.*, 1993) or time-frequency analysis (TOGNOLA *et al.*, 1998). Here, a wavelet-based approach for signal decomposition and denoising is presented, evaluated and compared with other approaches.

2 Wavelet method

The present method is based on the discrete wavelet transform (DWT) for the decomposition of subaveraged TEOAEs into scales. The decomposed signal is subjected to non-linear denoising and time windowing of each scale. Crosscorrelation coefficients are then computed for the subaveraged and processed signals in three different scales. Finally, the cross-correlation coefficients are averaged and used as a decision parameter for pass/fail separation. The method is summarised by the block diagram in Fig. 1.

2.1 *Mapping subaverages onto time-scale plane*

For signal decomposition in the time-scale plane, we have used the orthogonal DWT (DAUBECHIES, 1992; STRANG and NGUYEN, 1996), which represents the signal $s(n)$ by

$$s(n) = \sum_{j=1}^{K} \sum_{k=-\infty}^{\infty} w_j(k) \psi(2^j n - k) \tag{1}$$

Correspondence should be addressed to Prof. L. Sörnmo;
e-mail: leif.sornmo@tde.lth.se

First received 3 February 2000 and in final form 16 October 2000

MBEC online number: 20003534

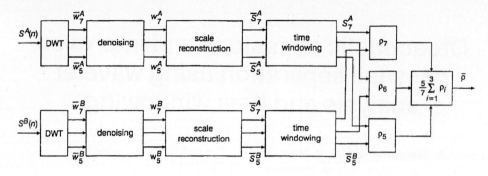

Fig. 1 *Block diagram of wavelet method*

where the function $\psi(n)$ is a discrete analysis wavelet, and the coefficients $w_j(k)$ represent the signal at scale j. In the present paper, the DWT is performed using lowpass filters for the 'approximate' signal and highpass filters for the 'detailed' signal, followed by downsampling (Mallat's pyramid algorithm (MALLAT, 1989)).

Each TEOAE signal was acquired during 20 ms at a sampling rate of 25 600 Hz, resulting in a recording of 512 samples. Using the Mallat algorithm with dyadic time-scale tiling, the 512 samples covered 8 octaves in frequency (DAUBECHIES, 1992); however, most of the energy of the TEOAE signal can be represented by three different scales (numbered 5, 6 and 7). The Coiflet5 wavelets were used for decomposition, as these are the most symmetrical among finite-in-time wavelets (DAUBECHIES, 1992) and resemble the shape of a TEOAE (see Fig. 2).

2.2 Denoising

The motivation behind studying wavelet-based denoising is that the DWT concentrates the signal energy in a few wavelet coefficients, while spreading out the energy of the noise over a large number of coefficients. The original signal can then be estimated by processing of the coefficients in the wavelet domain. Denoising procedures in orthogonal wavelet bases can be considered as non-linear signal-dependent filtering. An early approach to such filtering was presented by WEAVER *et al.* (1991) and was based on the thresholding of wavelet coefficients. Donoho and Johnstone introduced the concept of denoising by 'wavelet shrinkage' (DONOHO and JOHNSTONE, 1995) and proposed various strategies for threshold selection (DONOHO and JOHNSTONE, 1992).

In the present study, the denoising process uses a hard thresholding technique, defined by

$$\tilde{w}_j(k) = \begin{cases} 0 & |w_j(k)| < \lambda_j \\ w_j(k) & |w_j(k)| > \lambda_j \end{cases} \qquad (2)$$

where λ_j is a threshold at scale j. The thresholds are chosen individually for each scale j

$$\lambda_j = \lambda_0 \cdot \max_k(|w_j^A(k)|, |w_j^B(k)|) \qquad (3)$$

where $w_j^A(n)$ and $w_j^B(n)$ are wavelet coefficients of the sub-averaged signals $s^A(k)$ and $s^B(k)$, respectively. The parameter λ_0 was set to 0.2.

We suggest the use of 'percentile-related' thresholds when analysing TEOAE signals. The maximum percentage of zeroed coefficients in eqn 2 is set to 60% of the total number of coefficients in the two subaverages. This percentage is selected to avoid poor statistics for the crosscorrelation computation. If more than 60% of the coefficients are zeroed, the parameter λ_0 is successively decreased until this percentage is reached. Fig. 3 illustrates how the denoising procedure improves the TEOAE signal quality.

2.3 Scale reconstruction and time windowing

The signals in different scales are reconstructed by taking the corresponding subset of wavelet coefficients at scale j

$$\hat{s}_j(n) = \sum_k \tilde{w}_j(k)\psi(2^j n - k) \qquad (4)$$

where the reconstructed signal $\hat{s}_j(n)$ refers to the jth scale.

It is well known from clinical practice that the latency of TEOAE components depends on frequency, i.e. higher-frequency components occur earlier in the emission signal. To account for this feature, different time windows were

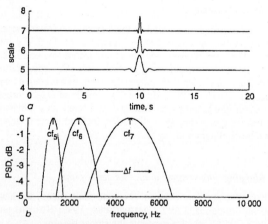

Fig. 2 *Splitting of spectrum into octave bands by Coiflet5 wavelets. (a) Coiflet5 wavelets at scales 5, 6 and 7. (b) $cf_5 = 1150\,Hz$; $\Delta f_5(-3\,dB) = 817\,Hz$; $cf_6 = 2200\,Hz$; $\Delta f_6(-3\,dB) = 1585\,Hz$; $cf_7 = 4400\,Hz$; $\Delta f_7(-3\,dB) = 3121\,Hz$*

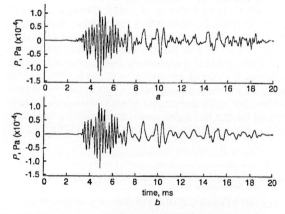

Fig. 3 *Denoising of TEOAE signal: (a) original signal, and (b) signal after denoising*

introduced. In the high-frequency scale, the signal was windowed from 2.5 to 7.5 ms, and the middle- and low-frequency scales were windowed from 2.5 to 9.0 ms and from 3.5 to 14.0 ms, respectively (see Fig. 4). In all cases, a window of rectangular shape (with raised cosines attached to the onset and end) was applied.

2.4 Crosscorrelation coefficient of two subaverages

The processed subaveraged signals $\hat{s}_j^A(k)$ and $\hat{s}_j^B(k)$, obtained from the inverse DWT in eqn 4, are used for calculation of the crosscorrelation coefficient ρ_j in each scale. The average of the crosscorrelation coefficients $\bar{\rho}$ for the three specified scales is then used as the final pass/fail separation parameter.

3 Existing methods for the signal-to-noise ratio improvement

The predominant OAE recording device in clinical routine is the so-called ILO*. Its analysis software computes a set of parameters that can be used for detection of hearing impairment. The crosscorrelation coefficient between two subaverages ('wave reproducibility') is the most frequently used parameter for such detection (PRIEVE *et al.*, 1993; DIRCKX *et al.*, 1996). As the SNR is essential for the final screening result, a number of methods have been included for improving the performance of the wave reproducibility parameter, e.g. time windowing or bandpass filtering (WHITEHEAD *et al.*, 1995; GORGA *et al.*, 1993).

The performance of the wavelet method was compared with the wave reproducibility parameter obtained either directly from the ILO device or after the TEOAE response had been subjected to bandpass filtering or time windowing (see Section 5). The main specifications of these three techniques are given below:

Wave reproducibility: The ILO analysis software calculates the wave reproducibility parameter from the bandpass filtered (0.6–6.0 kHz) input signal in an interval ranging from 2.5 to 20 ms after click stimulus (DIRCKX *et al.*, 1996). The ILO software also offers a 'Quick screen' operating mode using a shorter interval (2.5–12.5 ms).

Time windowing: Four different window lengths and locations were considered when the crosscorrelation coefficient was computed: 2.5–7.5 ms, 2.5–9.0 ms, 7.75–14.25 ms and 13.0–19.5 ms (WHITEHEAD *et al.*, 1995) and 2.5–12.5 ms (as in Quick screen).

Bandpass filtering: This approach was designed to extract signal components with a high SNR by calculating the crosscorrelation from the bandpass-filtered OAE responses (GORGA *et al.*, 1993). Four different octave bandpass filters were considered with the following centre frequencies: 500 Hz, 1000 Hz, 2000 Hz and 4000 Hz.

4 Database of TEOAE records

The database consists of 5214 TEOAE records that were collected during the health screens of 65 604 subjects in the Norwegian county of Nord-Tröndelag (HUNT); a more detailed description of the subsample has been given in ENGDAHL (1998). Transient evoked OAEs were recorded in an attenuation booth or in a relatively quiet, but not sound-proof, room. The ILO92 analyser[†] was used for data acquisition. The rejection criterion for the averaging process on the analyser was set to a fixed level (4 mPa) throughout the acquisition.

Air conduction pure-tone audiograms were recorded using Interacoustics AD25 automatic audiometers during the same screening test. The audiometric criterion used to separate normal hearing ears from impaired ears was defined by a pure-tone mean hearing threshold (MHL) above 30 dB HL obtained at the frequencies 0.5, 1, 2 and 4 kHz. The MHL distribution for the database is shown in Fig. 5. It is obvious from this Figure that the majority of the subjects had normal hearing. A total of 4404 subjects were classified as normal, whereas 810 exhibited impaired hearing. The age ranged from 20 to 96 years, and the average age was 49 years.

5 Results

5.1 Comparison of TEOAE detection methods

The receiver operating characteristic (ROC) was computed to assess the pass/fail separation capability of the methods mentioned above. This type of curve quantifies the diagnostic accuracy in terms of sensitivity and specificity: sensitivity indicates the percentage of correctly detected subjects with hearing impairment, and specificity indicates the percentage of correctly detected subjects with normal hearing. Each point in the ROC corresponds to a certain value of the decision threshold. Here, the threshold is applied to the average crosscorrelation coefficient. Although an ROC presents the performance for a wide range of values of the decision threshold, special attention is given below to the case when the sensitivity is held fixed at 90%; this case is considered to be of particular interest for the screening application.

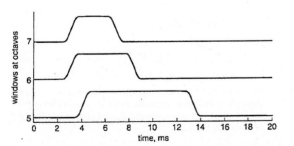

Fig. 4 *Time windows for subaveraged TEOAE signals containing high-frequency (j = 7), middle-frequency (j = 6) and low-frequency (j = 5) components*

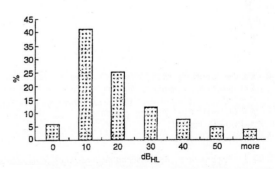

Fig. 5 *Distribution of mean hearing level in database*

---

* Manufactured by Otodynamics Ltd

† Otodynamics Ltd

The results are first presented for time windowing and bandpass filtering using different sets of parameter values on our TEOAE database. The values yielding the best result are then used for comparison with wave reproducibility and the wavelet method.

Time windowing: The results obtained using different window definitions showed that the time window extracting the initial signal part (2.5–7.5 ms and 2.5–9.0 ms) produces the largest specificity (72%) at a sensitivity of 90%, whereas the windows including the later parts yield significantly worse results (56% and 38%); the Quick screen window produced a specificity of 71%. Obviously, the initial part, containing high-frequency components, appears to be more important for TEOAE detection purposes than the later parts, which primarily contain lower-frequency components.

Bandpass filtering: The results obtained using bandpass filtering in four octave bands confirm the observation made in the preceding paragraph. The signal components of the high-frequency bands, centred at 2 and 4 kHz, produce the largest specificity (73% and 78% respectively), whereas the components of the low-frequency bands, centred at 500 Hz and 1 kHz, produce very poor specificity (29% and 52%, respectively).

The wavelet method: A performance comparison of the wavelet method and the other methods is found in Fig. 6. It can be seen that the wavelet method outperforms the other methods by achieving a better specificity at all investigated sensitivity values. At a sensitivity of 90%, the specificity of wave reproducibility was 68%, that of time windowing was 72%, that of bandpass filtering was 78%, and that of the wavelet method was 83%. The improvement is illustrated by an example with a considerable change in crosscorrelation coefficient after wavelet processing (see Appendix).

To provide further insight into the above results, the sensitivity and specificity are presented as functions of the decision threshold in Fig. 7. (A sensitivity curve that is less steep indicates that, for a certain value of the separation parameter, a larger number of cases are mistaken as true OAEs as a consequence of residual stimuli or correlated noise artefacts. A specificity curve that is less steep indicates a larger number of cases where noise is insufficiently reduced or where an OAE was not present because of methodological problems.) Again, it is evident that time windowing corresponds to a less favourable sensitivity and specificity than does the wavelet method. Bandpass filtering has a better sensitivity but a poorer specificity than the other methods; the sensitivity characteristic is explained by lower noise contamination in the higher-frequency region, which reduces the likelihood of high crosscorrelation values due to correlated noise artefacts.

5.2 *Influence of different wavelet method components*

The wavelet method can be divided into four components: scale decomposition, denoising, time windowing and averaging of crosscorrelation coefficients. The relative importance of each of these components is studied in this Section.

First, the performances resulting from scale decomposition and the other techniques are presented in Table 1; the best performance is obtained for the wavelet method, as described in Section 2. The effects of using no time windowing, scale-independent windowing (with length according to the 'Quick screen' mode; see Section 3) and scale-dependent windowing are presented in Table 2. The results show that the use of scale-dependent time windows gives an increase in specificity from 79% to 82% at a sensitivity level of 90%. This result can be explained by an improvement in the SNR when only the time interval containing the highest TEOAE energy is used in each scale. The Quick screen window did not improve the results.

We also studied the effect of averaging ρ_j for different scale combinations; see Table 3. The results indicate that averaging of all three scales yields the best performance, and therefore this type of averaging was chosen for the wavelet method.

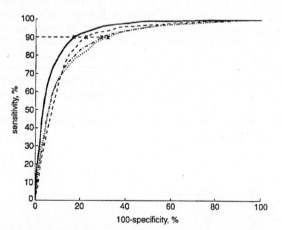

Fig. 6 *Receiver operating characteristics for wave reproducibility, time windowing, bandpass filtering and wavelet analysis. (···) ILO wave reproducibility; (-·-·) windowing (interval 2.5–12.5 ms); (---) filtering (fourth octave $f_c = 4000$ Hz); (—) wavelet method*

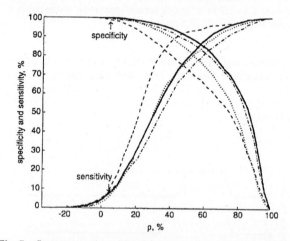

Fig. 7 *Sensitivity and specificity against crosscorrelation coefficient value. (···) ILO wave reproducibility; (-·-·) windowing (interval 2.5–12.5 ms); (---) filtering (fourth octave $f_c = 4000$ Hz); (—) wavelet method*

Table 1 *Performance using subband decomposition in combination with various techniques (CC denotes crosscorrelation)*

Additional technique	CC averaging	Denoising and CC averaging	Time windowing and denoising	Wavelet method
Specificity (sensitivity = 90%)	79%	80%	82%	83%

Table 2   Influence of time windowing (no denoising)

Technique	No windowing	Scale-independent windowing (Quick screen)	Scale-dependent windowing
Specificity (sensitivity = 90%)	79%	78%	82%

Table 3   Influence of averaging (time windowing and denoising included)

Parameter	Scales 5 and 6	Scales 5 and 7	Scales 6 and 7	Scales 5, 6 and 7
Specificity (sensitivity = 90%)	71%	79%	81%	83%

Finally, the influence of wavelet denoising was found to increase specificity from 82% to 83%, compared with the case without denoising (Tables 1 and 2). Thus, we conclude that the main improvement obtained by the wavelet method can be attributed to subband decomposition and scale-dependent time windowing.

6 Discussion

Several parameters were considered in the development of the wavelet method. The bandwidth in the time-scale decomposition was selected as one octave, which is in agreement with earlier results (GORGA *et al.*, 1993). In that study, it was found that OAE signals decomposed by octave filters provided a better separation between normal subjects and hearing-impaired subjects than did the one-third octave filter.

In certain studies, the continuous wavelet transform has been chosen for TEOAE frequency decomposition, for example TOGNOLA *et al.* (1998). In the present study, the DWT was employed because it results in an octave frequency band decomposition and is computationally much faster. The speed can be further increased by omitting the IDWT and, instead, calculating the separation parameter $\bar{p}$ in the wavelet domain (MAROZAS *et al.*, 1999). However, the IDWT can be preferable to use, as sampling in the wavelet domain is sparse at scales with lower resolution. Accordingly, it is difficult to construct a window in the wavelet domain that has an exact counterpart in the time domain (JANUŠAUSKAS *et al.*, 1999).

Another important consideration is the selection of length and the position of the scale-dependent windows. Here, these quantities were selected based on the results from a pilot study with 70 subjects with normal hearing. The TEOAE signals were decomposed into the scales chosen by the wavelet method, and the window lengths and positions were decided according to where the main OAE signal energy was found. Further investigations on a larger population are needed to obtain a better statistical description of the distribution of OAE signal energy in different frequency bands.

The separation parameter was defined as a simple average of the crosscorrelation coefficients over three frequency bands. In a pilot study, we investigated more complex relationships in terms of an artificial neural network. However, preliminary results showed that only a marginal increase in specificity could be obtained, and therefore averaging of crosscorrelation coefficients was used.

It is highly desirable for the audiologist to have an objective method that can determine the hearing threshold at different frequencies. Although many have hoped that the OAE test would be such a method, no strong evidence has so far been presented in the literature. In our study, we could observe that, in terms of specificity (measured at 90% sensitivity in one scale), the separation of hearing threshold above and below 30 dB$_{HL}$ for closest audiometric frequency was inferior to the separation of

the MHL (60% for closest audiometric and 75% for MHL). This observation was valid for scales 6 and 7, whereas scale 5 showed better separation for the closest audiometric frequency (70%) compared with the MHL (54%). A possible explanation for this can be predominant high-frequency hearing loss among the subjects in our database. The higher-frequency hearing loss leads to a decrease of the MHL, whereas OAE at low frequencies is still present. This results in a poor pass/fail separation in low-frequency scale when 30 dB$_{HL}$ MHL is used as an audiological criterion.

The European Consensus Statement on Neonatal Hearing Screening, taken in Milan, 1998, (DAVIS *et al.*, 1998), states that the audiological criterion for neonatal screening should be the MHL of 40 dB$_{HL}$ over the frequencies of 0.5, 1, 2 and 4 kHz. In the present study, different screening levels were investigated, and it was found that the wavelet method exhibited a worse specificity for 20 dB$_{HL}$ than for 30 dB$_{HL}$, i.e. 65% and 83%, respectively, at 90% sensitivity. This result supports the observation that fragmented OAE activity exists in signals from persons with mean hearing levels between 20 and 30 dB$_{HL}$ (ROBINETTE and GLATTKE, 1997). For 40 dB$_{HL}$, the corresponding specificity was found to be 85%.

No data records were excluded from the database owing to noise, possible retrocochlear hearing loss or middle-ear dysfunctionality. It is likely that a better performance would have resulted with additional quality criteria. The fact that such criteria were not applied may explain that the performance figures were lower than those presented in other studies (GORGA *et al.*, 1993; PRIEVE *et al.*, 1993).

Bandpass filtering with centre frequency at 4000 Hz yielded good performance in terms of sensitivity (Fig. 7). This result can be explained by the fact that the correlation of low-frequency signals in a short window causes a larger variance of the results and can therefore cause undesirable high correlation values leading to false OAE detections. Another, perhaps more important, reason is that patient-related noise is primarily characterised by low-frequency components that increase the likelihood of false detections; this likelihood is reduced by bandpass filtering. The cost in terms of specificity for the bandpass filter with centre frequency at 4000 Hz is, however, substantial, and the results from the ROC analysis in Fig. 6 are still inferior to those for the wavelet method.

In conclusion, the performance comparison of the wavelet method with the existing techniques indicates that the diagnostic accuracy can be increased by enhancement of both time and frequency TEOAE features, compared with the case when either time or frequency properties are considered.

Acknowledgments—We are grateful to Professor Arūnas Lukoševičius from Kaunas Technology University, Lithuania, for valuable comments. Thanks are also due to the National Health Screening Services in Norway for assistance with data collection.

This work was supported in part by grants from the Swedish Institute and the US National Institute on Deafness and Other Communication Disorders, National Institutes of Health (contract number NO1-DC-6-2104).

Appendix

We present here an example of a TEOAE signal before (Fig. 8) and after (Fig. 9) processing and the corresponding crosscorrelation ρ between subaverages for both cases. As the MHL for this particular subject was 14 dB, it is expected that otoacoustic emissions are present. To determine the performance of the wavelet method, we added signals from the three scales processed by this method. The wave reproducibility was then used for the detection of TEOAE. Fig. 8 shows that no emission is present in the unprocessed signal ($\rho = 35\%$); however, it is obvious from Fig. 9 that TEOAEs are detected from the processed signal ($\rho = 81\%$).

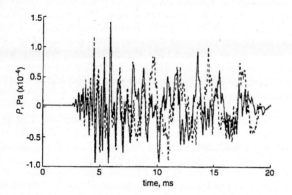

Fig. 8 *Subaveraged TEOAE signals before processing. $\rho = 35\%$; noise $= 2.2\,dB$*

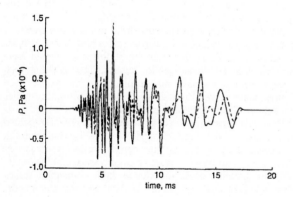

Fig. 9 *Subaveraged TEOAE signals after processing with wavelet method. $\rho = 81\%$; noise $= -5\,dB$*

References

BRASS, D., WATKINS, P., and KEMP, D. T. (1994): 'Assessment of an implementation of a narrow band, neonatal otoacoustic emission screening method', *Ear Hearing*, **15**, pp. 467–475

BRAY, P. (1989): 'Click evoked otoacoustic emissions and the development of a clinical otoacoustic hearing test instrument'. PhD thesis, University of London

DAUBECHIES, I. (1992): 'Ten lectures on wavelets' (SIAM)

DAVIS, A., LUTMAN, M., GRANDORI, F., and PROBST, R. (1998): 'European consensus statement on neonatal hearing screening', *ENT News*, **7** (http://ent-news.com/)

DIRCKX, J. J. J., DAEMERS, K., SOMERS, T., OFFECIERS, F. E., and GOVAERTS, P. J. (1996): 'Numerical assessment of TEOAE screening results: currently used criteria and their effect on TEOAE prevalence figures', *Acta Otolaryng.*, **116**, pp. 672–679

DONOHO, D. L., and JOHNSTONE, I. M. (1992): 'Minimax estimation via wavelet shrinkage'. Technical Report 402, Stanford University, Department of Statistics

DONOHO, D. L., and JOHNSTONE, I. M. (1995): 'Adapting to unknown smoothness via wavelet shrinkage', *J. Am. Stat. Ass.*, **90**, p. 432

ENGDAHL, B. (1998): 'Otoacoustic emissions as a function of age, gender and hearing loss in a large general adult population'. Proc. AHEAD Eur. Meeting: Psychoacoust. and OAEs, Basel, 1998

GORGA, M. P., NEELY, S. T., BERGMAN, B. M., BEAUCHAINE, K. L., KAMINSKI, J. R., PETERS, J., SCHULTA, L., and JESTEADT, W. (1993): 'A comparison of transient-evoked and distortion product otoacoustic emissions in normal-hearing and hearing-impaired subjects', *J. Acoust. Soc. Am.*, **94**, pp. 2639–2648

GRANDORI, F., CIANFRONE, G., and KEMP, D. (1990): 'Cochlear mechanisms and otoacoustic emissions', *Adv. Audiol.*, **7**, pp. 99–109

JANUŠAUSKAS, A., ENGDAHL, B., SVENSSON, and O., SÖRNMO, L. (1999): 'Latency of otoacoustic emission frequency components', *Med. Biol. Eng. Comput.*, **37**, (Suppl. 1), pp. 332–333

KEMP, D. T. (1978): 'Stimulated acoustic emissions from within the human auditory system', *J. Acoust. Soc. Am.*, **64**, pp. 1386–1391

LUTMAN, M. E. (1993): 'Reliable identification of click-evoked otoacoustic emissions using signal processing techniques', *Brit. J. Audiol.*, **27**, pp. 103–108

MALLAT, S. (1989): 'Multiresolution approximation and wavelets', *Trans. Am. Math. Soc.*, **315**, pp. 69–88

MAROZAS, V., JANUŠAUSKAS, A., ENGDAHL, B., SVENSSON, O., and SÖRNMO, L. (1999): 'Detection of otoacoustic emission in wavelet domain', *Med. Biol. Eng. Comput.*, **37**, (Suppl. 1), pp. 334–335

NEELY, S. T., NORTON, S. J., GORGA, M. P., and JESTEADT, W. (1988): 'Latency of auditory brain stem responses and acoustic emissions using tone-burst stimul.', *J. Acoust. Soc. Am.*, **83**, pp. 652–656

PRIEVE, B. A., GORGA, M. P., SCHMIDT, A., NEELY, S., PETERS, J., SCHULTES, L., and JESTEADT, W. (1993): 'Analysis of transient-evoked otoacoustic emissions in normal-hearing and hearing-impaired ears', *J. Acoust. Soc. Am.*, **93**, pp. 3308–3319

RAVAZZANI, P., TOGNOLA, G., GRANDORI, F., and RUHONEN, J. (1998): 'Two-dimensional filter to facilitate detection of transient-evoked otoacoustic emissions', *IEEE Trans.*, **BME-45**, pp. 1089–1096

ROBINETTE, M., and GLATTKE, T. (1997): 'Otoacoustic emissions: clinical applications' (Thieme, New York)

STRANG, G., and NGUYEN, T. (1996): 'Wavelets and filter banks' (Wellesley-Cambridge Press)

TOGNOLA, G., RAVAZZANI, P., and GRANDORI, F. (1998): 'Wavelet analysis of transient-evoked otoacoustic emissions', *IEEE Trans.*, **BME-45**, pp. 686–697

WEAVER, J. B., HANSUN, X., HEALY, D. M., and CROMWELL, L. D. (1991): 'Filtering noise from images with wavelet transforms', *Magnet. Res. Med.*, **21**, pp. 288–295

WHITEHEAD, M. L., JIMENEZ, A. M., STAGNER, B. B., MCCOY, M. J., LONSBURY-MARTIN, B. L., and MARTIN, G. K. (1995): 'Time windowing of click evoked otoacoustic emissions to increase signal-to-noise ratio', *Ear Hearing*, **16**, pp. 599–611

Author's biography

VAIDOTAS MAROZAS received his BS in Engineering Electronics in 1993, MS in Metrology and Measurements in 1995, and PhD in Electrical and Electronics Engineering from Kaunas University of Technology in 2000. Since August 2000 he has been employed as a research scientist at the Institute of Biomedical Engineering, Kaunas University of Technology. He is a member of the Lithuanian Society of Biomedical Engineering. His research interests include biomedical signal processing, time-frequency analysis, wavelet analysis and neural networks.

Anticipation of epileptic seizures from standard EEG recordings

Michel Le Van Quyen, Jacques Martinerie, Vincent Navarro, Paul Boon, Michel D'Havé, Claude Adam, Bernard Renault, Francisco Varela, Michel Baulac

Summary

Background New methods derived from non-linear analysis of intracranial recordings permit the anticipation of an epileptic seizure several minutes before the seizure. Nevertheless, anticipation of seizures based on standard scalp-electroencephalographical (EEG) signals has not been reported yet. The accessibility to preictal changes from standard EEGs is essential for expanding the clinical applicability of these methods.

Methods We analysed 26 scalp-EEG/video recordings, from 60 min before a seizure, in 23 patients with temporal-lobe epilepsy. For five patients, simultaneous scalp and intracranial EEG recordings were assessed. Long-term changes before seizure onset were identified by a measure of non-linear similarity, which is very robust in spite of large artifacts and runs in real-time.

Findings In 25 of 26 recordings, measurement of non-linear changes in EEG signals allowed the anticipation of a seizure several minutes before it occurred (mean 7 min). These preictal changes in the scalp EEG correspond well with concurrent changes in depth recordings.

Interpretation Scalp-EEG recordings retain sufficient dynamical information which can be used for the analysis of preictal changes leading to seizures. Seizure anticipation strategies in real-time can now be envisaged for diverse clinical applications, such as devices for patient warning, for efficacy of ictal-single photon emission computed tomography procedures, and eventual treatment interventions for preventing seizures.

Lancet 2001; **357**: 183–88
See Commentary page 160

Introduction

In most patients with epilepsy, seizures occur suddenly and without identifiable external precipitants. The unpredictability of seizure onset is a major threat for people with uncontrolled epilepsy and a cause of disability[1] and mortality.[2] Prediction of seizure onset, even in the short-term, would provide time for the application of preventive measures to keep the risk of seizure to a minimum and, ultimately, improve quality of life.

Intracranial recordings of patients who are candidates for surgical treatment offers the most precise access to the emergence of a seizure.[3] Ways to anticipate seizure onset before the first intracranial electrical changes have been

---

The original paper contained coloured figures.

Laboratoire de Neurosciences Cognitives et Imagerie Cérébrale
(M Le Van Quyen PhD, J Martinerie PhD, V Navarro MD, C Adam PhD,
B Renault PhD, F Varela PhD, Prof M Baulac MD) **and Unité
d'Epileptologie** (V Navarro, C Adam, Prof M Baulac), **CNRS UPR
640, Hôpital de la Pitié-Salpêtrière, 75651 Paris, Cedex 13,
France; and Department of Neurology, Epilepsy Monitoring Unit and
Laboratory of Clinical Neurophysiology, University of Gent, 185 De
Pintelaan, B-9000 Gent, Belgium** (Prof P Boon PhD, M D'Havé MS)

Correspondence to: Dr Francisco Varela
(e-mail: fv@ccr.jussieu.fr)

intensively investigated by conventional linear (ie, frequency) analyses.[4-6] Nevertheless, prediction does not exceed more than a few seconds before visual detection of the seizure. Non-linear analysis is an alternative way to characterise qualitative changes in the dynamics of complex systems[7] and could be important in clinical practice.[8] Applied to intracranial recordings of patients with temporal-lobe epilepsy (TLE), these methods have shown that the evolution toward a seizure involves not just two states—interictal and ictal—but also a preictal transitional phase of several minutes that is not detected by linear methods.[9-11] This preictal transitional phase could become the basis to anticipate seizures in clinical applications.

To make seizure anticipation practical in real life conditions, and to study types of epilepsy that do not warrant intracranial implantation, we analysed scalp-electroencephalographical (ECG) recordings. Scalp EEG, however, is well known to be subject to signal attenuation, poor spatial resolution, and noise or artifacts,[12] which may render delicate[13] and even questionable[14] the detection of changes with current non-linear measures, originally designed to analyse systems with little noise.

To improve non-linear analysis we have proposed a strategy well suited to track dynamical changes in complex brain signals,[11,15] which measures similarity of EEG dynamics between recordings taken at distant moments in time. This relative measure indicates changes in brain electrical activity with greater accuracy than other non-linear techniques.[16-17] Furthermore, it has the advantage of being very robust against noise and artifacts, and is fast enough to be carried out in real-time.

In the present study, we have applied this non-linear strategy to analyse scalp-EEG recordings from patients with TLE to assess whether changes in brain dynamics can be detected early enough to anticipate the onset of the clinical seizure. In a subgroup of patients, we validated our results on simultaneous surface and intracranial recordings.

Methods

Scalp EEG recordings

We studied a sample of 18 patients with refractory TLE who required continuous EEG recording and video monitoring to localise seizure onsets. Hippocampal sclerosis as defined by magnetic resonance imaging was the most frequent pathological condition associated with TLE (table). Patients were free to move in the recording room.

To avoid changes induced by variation of arousal states,[5] only seizures in which the patients were awake (14 seizures) or asleep (four seizures) for the entire preictal hour were studied. This selection was done with a minimum of a priori knowledge about the quality of the signal. Recordings were obtained from a 32 channel Biomedical Monitoring Systems Inc system (Nicolet-BMSI, Madison, Wisconsin, USA) with 21 or 27 electrodes, placed according to the extended International 10–20 System.[18] The scalp potentials were passed to a channel amplifier system with band-pass filter settings of 0·5–99 Hz by an external reference over linked ears, and were digitised at 200 Hz. We obtained 18 long-term scalp recordings of 60–90 min duration including the 30–60 min before the clinical seizure, as defined by either the time of the first symptoms (including aura sensation) or the first electrographical

---

Patient number	Brain magnetic resonance imaging	Epileptic focus (EEG-video)
1 to 8	Left hippocampal sclerosis	Left temporal
9 to 13	Right hippocampal sclerosis	Right temporal
14	Right hippocampal sclerosis and right external temporo-occipital scar	Right temporal
15	Right internal temporo-occipital tumour	Right temporal
16	Normal	Right hemisphere (right medial temporal*)
17	Normal	Left temporal
18	Right external temporo-occipital scar	Right temporo-occipital or right anterior temporal
19 to 21	Left hippocampal sclerosis	Left hippocampus*
22	Bilateral hippocampal sclerosis	Right hippocampus*
23	Right hippocampal sclerosis	Right hippocampus*

*Intracranial recording.

Electroradiological features of the patients

changes (burst of spikes, electrodecremental events, or sinusoidal waves) noted by the epileptologist electroencephalographer. None of the recordings were rejected.

Simultaneous scalp and intracranial recordings
We also studied seizures of five patients with TLE using both scalp and intracranial electrodes. The patients were implanted with mediotemporal intracerebral electrodes by use of a posteroanterior trajectory. These electrodes recorded the medial structures of the temporal lobe (amygdala and hippocampus) and the temporo-occipital cortical junction. In addition, subdural strips inserted through burr holes sampled the lateral or inferior-temporal cortex. Postimplantation location of the electrodes was verified by magnetic resonance imaging. The EEG-video recordings were made with a 64-channel Telefactor system (Conshohocken, PA, USA). The raw data were filtered with a band-pass of 0·1–70 Hz and digitised at 200 Hz using an external passive reference. We analysed 8 epochs of 60 min duration 50 min before the seizure. The patients were awake (six seizures) or asleep (two seizures) for the entire preictal hour. Seizure onset was defined by electrographical criteria as localised, sustained rhythmic discharges greater than 2 Hz in frequency (burst of spikes, low voltage, fast, &c) and associated with subsequent clinical seizure activity.[3]

Data analysis
The anticipation method, which has been described in detail previously,[15] includes four main steps, which are done independently on each EEG channel to obtain the spatial distribution of dynamical changes (figure 1).

Reconstruction of EEG dynamics by time intervals
The recording was segmented into consecutive non-overlapping windows of 30 s duration. For each window, the signal was transformed to pure-phase information by taking the sequence of time intervals between positive-going crossings of a fixed threshold (set here to the zero of the signal; figure 1A). An important advantage of this zero-crossing approach is that the time intervals are robust to noise components of the signal amplitude. Furthermore, the approach achieves a substantial decrease (by ten orders of magnitude) in the volume of data, providing the computational speed for real-time procedures. Finally, the sequence of time intervals contains the pertinent dynamical information. Following standard techniques,[19] we converted time-serial data to a geometric representation (figure 1B) which describes the EEG dynamics in a high-dimensional state space (see mathematical appendix on *The Lancet*'s website www.thelancet.com)

Calculation of a similarity index between EEG time windows
The dynamical similarity between any pairs of EEG windows is quantified by the crosscorrelation integral between the two dynamics (see mathematical appendix). If the EEG is stationary, the similarity index yields a value close to 1. By contrast, if changes in the dynamical state occur, the similarity index decreases below 1.

Detection of preictal changes by comparison with a reference state
To give the most general picture of the preseizure changes, we chose a long reference window (300 s) during a stationary sequence and distant in time from the seizure. This reference window contained common features of interictal activity, including isolated spikes, and was chosen at the same time for all channels. We computed the similarity index between this reference window and consecutive test windows moved over the whole recording epoch. The timecourse of the similarities, the similarity profile, provides information about long-term changes before seizure onset. Figure 1C illustrates a representative example of this step of our analysis applied to a single scalp EEG channel (left frontotemporal channel FT9, same seizure as figure 2) and covering 50 min before a left medial-lobe seizure. Seizure onset was identified by localised periodic low-frequency spikes in the left hippocampus (window 97). The similarity profile, during the first part of the recording (1–60 windows), shows a segment of windows with high similarity, suggesting fairly uniform dynamical properties. After this first dynamical state, and before the seizure, there is a transitional preictal state that begins around 18 min before seizure onset (windows 60–96) and differs dynamically from the interictal and ictal states. We also did a spectral analysis over the same period, to see if preictal changes could also be detected by this linear method. As seen in figure 1C, this was not the case, supporting the view that non-linear analysis is essential.

Statistical analysis
We assessed the significance of the preictal changes by quantifying the deviation of the test window from the reference state. Let μ and σ be the mean and SD of similarity variations (γ) during the baseline. We define here the significance Σ of the deviation by the ratio $\Sigma=(\gamma-\mu)/\delta$ whose p-value is given by the Chebyshev's inequality (for any statistical distribution of γ: $P[|\Sigma|\geqslant k] \leqslant 1/k^2$ where k is the chosen statistical threshold). The temporal evolution of the statistical significance Σ is used to detect when the similarity index reaches a critical value. We define the anticipation time as when the ratio Σ reaches a critical value of $k=5$ (p=0·04), and remains at or above this fixed deviation threshold up to the time when the seizure occurs.

Results
Figure 2 shows a representative example of the results for simultaneous intracranial and scalp recording 50 min before a spontaneous seizure of left-temporal origin. The similarity profiles, relative to a reference state taken at the beginning of the recording, are depicted for selected scalp and depth channels in the left-temporal region (figure 2A). A persistent deviation from the reference state is recorded around 18 min before the seizure in both the scalp and intracranial similarity profiles. No consistent changes in preictal spiking nor other electroencephalographical features correlated with these dynamical changes. After this preictal state, the electrographic seizure was accompanied by a second drop to the lowest similarity. Postictally, the

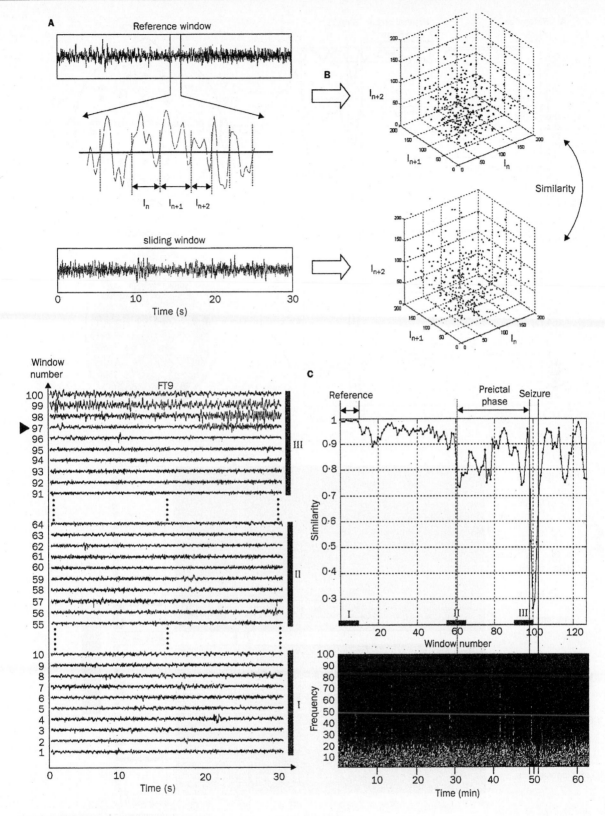

Figure 1: Quantification of preictal changes

A: The first step is to transform the recording into sequences of time intervals I_n between successive zero-crossings for pairs of windows that are not necessarily adjacent in time.

B: The second step is to define a multidimensional reconstruction of the dynamics by a time delay embedding of the intervals, shown here with $m=3$ for a schematic representation. The third step consists of the comparison of the two reconstructed dynamics by a measure of similarity.

C: Analysis of 50 min of a scalp EEG channel before a spontaneous temporal lobe seizure; left, examples of consecutive windows of 30 s duration in the recording, the seizure onset occurs at window 97; right, the similarity profile (upper panel) from a long "reference phase" chosen here from windows 1 to 10. A sustained preictal state is identified 18 min before seizure onset. The spectrogram (lower panel) display over the same epoch shows no relation to the similarity profile.

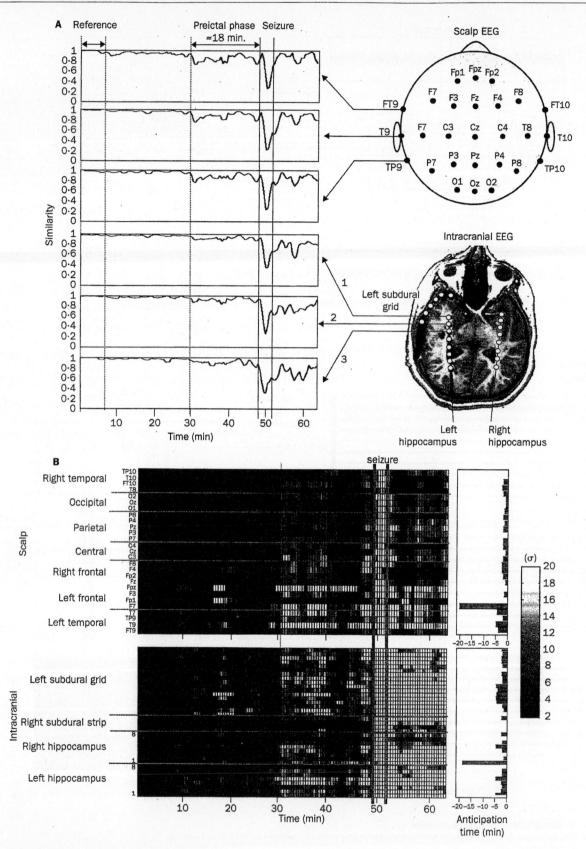

Figure 2: Representative example of our analysis

A: left, for several scalp and intracranial channels in the left temporal region, the timecourse of the similarities from a reference state taken at the beginning of the recording; right, schematic location of the scalp and intracranial electrodes.

B: Spatiotemporal deviation map of preseizure changes. The deviations from the reference state of each contact are depicted as a function of time in SDs by a colour scale. The corresponding anticipation times are indicated on the right of each contact. Long lasting decreases around 18 min before seizure were found at a large number of the recording sites.

similarity index increased again and tended to reach the interictal level. There was a large correlation between the intercranial and the scalp similarity profiles (ρ=78·8% at lag zero between T9 and LH1).

To obtain a complete spatiotemporal picture of preictal dynamics, this analysis was applied to all recorded channels (figure 2B). Significant decreases in similarity were uniformly recorded several minutes before the seizure. These changes were present at almost all recording sites in both scalp (25 of 27) and intracranial recordings (29 of 32). For many channels, state transitions before the seizure seem to wax and wane and are occasionally disrupted, in particular, shortly before seizure onset. Nevertheless, some channels (scalp: F7; intracranial: left hippocampus 5, right hippocampus 1) show sustained deviations above the statistical threshold up to the onset of the electrographic seizure. In the example shown, the preictal changes are more pronounced and sustained in the left-temporal lobe (scalp: FT9 to F7, intracranial: left hippocampus) but can also be seen in contralateral contacts (scalp: T8 to TP10, intracranial: right hippocampus). The spatial distribution of preseizure changes is widespread and projects beyond the epileptogenic focus.

Figure 3 shows the seizure anticipation times we recorded from the 23 patients with TLE. Definition of the dynamical properties of the scalp EEG allowed, in 25 of 26 cases, anticipation of a seizure several minutes before it occurred (mean 416 s [SD 356]). When multiple seizures were recorded in single patients, the corresponding anticipation times were highly variable. This finding is consistent with our previous results[9,11] and suggests that the preictal state is a complex process which varies within individual patients. For the group of patients with both scalp and intracranial recordings, there was a significant

correlation between the timecourse of scalp and intracranial preictal changes (figure 3). In most cases, anticipation times from scalp and intracranial recordings were similar.

Preictal state changes were in the temporal lobe ipsilateral to the epileptic focus in most cases. The contralateral temporal lobe was often the site of changes, although these changes were less precocious and pronounced. In some patients the changes appeared in parasagittal and frontal areas and were not spatially congruent with the epileptic area. The detected changes frequently showed a widespread topography that projected beyond the limits of the epileptogenic temporal lobe.

Discussion

Our results indicate that preseizure changes in brain dynamics can be detected from recordings of scalp-EEG activity. These changes were characterised with a reference state taken 1 h before the ictus, and were detected several minutes before the earliest clinical or overt EEG manifestations of the seizure. We chose this reference state to analyse only preictal epochs recorded during stable states of wakefulness or during sleep, to avoid changes in the interictal dynamics induced by major changes in the physiological state of the brain.[5]

Our finding that the changes in scalp electrical activity were similar to those detected from intracranial recordings is surprising, given that the scalp EEG is an attenuated and blurred vision of direct intracranial recording because of the distance between the brain and scalp, with the skull as an interposing medium. However, the relations between activity recorded with intracranial and extracranial electrodes is more complex than a simple decrease in the signal-to-noise ratio because of cortical convolutions, anatomical anisotropies, and the orientation, shape, and extension of the underlying generators.[20] Also, potentials produced by neocortical changes and recorded from scalp electrodes might also be driven by events in deeper cerebral structures. For instance, changes in the hippocampal activity could cause secondary activation of several neocortical areas, producing synchronised local field potentials. Further studies are required to identify the extent of generators giving rise to the global dynamics ultimately detected on the scalp, particularly the use of more extensive intracranial sampling or source localisation methods.

Keeping in mind these uncertainties, we have nevertheless shown that scalp recordings retain sufficient information for use as a preictal marker. A remarkable property of the similarity estimation is the robustness against noise compared with other non-linear methods.[9,10] Furthermore, our anticipation times determined from scalp electrodes, even for data with poor signal-to-noise ratios, indicate an extensive spatial distribution of the preictal condition, necessarily involving multiple sources from both the epileptogenic region and distant non-epileptogenic regions. This finding is confirmed by our analysis of simultaneous intracranial recordings and consistent with our previous results.[11] These findings are further concordant with the notion that TLE is not a perfect model of a purely focal process, but often exhibits widespread functional, cognitive, electrical, and structural abnormalities, with frequent contralateral temporal-lobe involvement.[21]

It could be argued that our findings cannot be explained by ictal discharges present at depth but not recognised at the scalp, which is unlikely for two reasons: the time difference between intracranial seizure onset and the first clinical or scalp-EEG signs should have been of several minutes; simultaneous surface and intracranial recordings

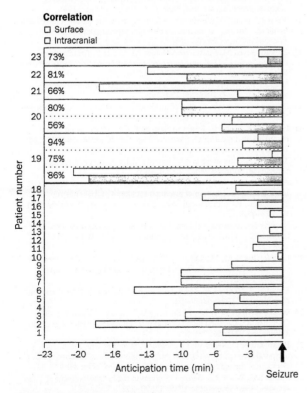

Figure 3: Anticipation times for all the patients and seizures under investigation

Defined as the earliest anticipation recorded across all the channels. Correlation coefficients are expressed as percentages.

show that the timecourses of preictal change occur in parallel—scalp preictal changes takes place before the intracranial-seizure onset.

The presence of widespread preictal changes raises the question of their relation to the process of seizure generation. As previously suggested,[9,10] one hypothesis is that preictal changes are due to subthreshold epileptic recruitment. Large scale drivings starting from the epileptogenic region can be involved in this process, as recorded during interictal activity.[22] A second hypothesis is that the preictal state might not be part of the ictal process itself, but reflects a facilitating state of the brain, which allows a susceptible region to generate sustained epileptic discharges. From this perspective, two interrelated processes with different timescales can be distinguished: long-lasting and non-specific generalised changes that could create favourable conditions for the appearance of seizures; and focal epileptogenic processes in regions prone to hypersynchronous behaviour in response to these generalised changes. A possible candidate for this long-term facilitation process could be a decrease in remote inhibitory control of the epileptogenic zone.[23]

To further understand the pathophysiological basis of preictal changes, it would be of interest to know if other physiological indices also show preictal modification. Invasive techniques to measure regional cerebral blood flow in a continuous fashion[24] or fortuitous non-invasive single photon emission computed tomography observations[25] have shown preictal modifications around 10 min before temporal-lobe seizures. Interestingly, large alterations in regional cerebral blood flow have been reported in both epileptogenic and contralateral non-epileptogenic neocortices, consistent with a widespread perturbation of brain perfusion before medial-temporal-lobe seizure onset.

From a clinical point of view, the ability to anticipate seizure with the scalp EEG may have considerable practical implications for the large population of patients with uncontrolled epilepsy. The computational cost of our method is quite small and it can be implemented in real-time with a personal computer, facilitating ambulatory application. Our method holds the potential for clinical application, warning patients at home or in a hospital setting. A careful study of the specificity and sensitivity of this method over long recording periods and larger patient populations needs to be done. If proven reliable, such an application would lower the medical consequences of seizures and improve the quality of life of people with epilepsy by decreasing the risk of injury, and the sense of helplessness fostered by the unpredictability of the disease. The scalp EEG could also facilitate EEG/video monitoring of surgery candidates by allowing early injection of the peri-ictal single photon computed tomography emission tracer, which would lower the cost of the procedure. In addition, identifying preictal changes would also allow treatment intervention such as administration of a short-acting anticonvulsant drug,[26] electrical stimulation,[27] or cognitive intervention with neurophysiological or behavioural countermeasures.

Contributors

Michel Le Van Quyen, Jacques Martinerie, and Francisco Varela initiated the study and did the signal analysis. Vincent Navarro collected the data with the assistance of Claude Adam and provided substantial input into the interpretation of the results. Bernard Renault provided assistance during the early stages of the project. Paul Boon and Michel D'Havé provided the data of simultaneous scalp and intracranial recordings. Michel Baulac supervised the clinical part of the study. Michel Le Van Quyen and Francisco Varela wrote the paper, with input from Vincent Navarro and Michel Baulac.

Acknowledgments

This work was supported by the Fondation Française pour la Recherche sur l'Epilepsie, Fondation pour la Recherche Médicale, the Institut National de la Santé et de la Recherche Médicale (INSERM), Institut Electricité Santé de France, Laboratoire Sanofi-Synthelabo.

We are grateful to Robert B Duckrow for his help in the preparation of the manuscript.

References

1   Devinsky O, Vickrey BG, Cramer J, et al. Development of the quality of life in epilepsy inventory. *Epilepsia* 1995; **36**: 1089–104.

2   Cockerell OC, Johnson AL, Sander JW, Hart YM, Goodridge DMG, Shorvon SD. Mortality from epilepsy: results from a prospective population-based study. *Lancet* 1994; **344**: 918–21.

3   Engel J Jr. Seizure and epilepsy. Philadelphia, USA: F A Davis Company, 1989.

4   Rogowski Z, Gath I, Bental E. On the prediction of epileptic seizures. *Biol Cybern* 1981; **42**: 9–15.

5   Katz A, Marks DA, McCarthy G, Spencer SS. Does interictal spiking rate change prior to seizure? *Electroencephalogr Clin Neurophysiol* 1991; **79**: 153–56.

6   Osorio I, Frei M-G, Wilkinson SB. Real-time automated detection and quantitative analysis of seizures and short-term prediction of clinical onset. *Epilepsia* 1998; **39**: 615–27.

7   Kantz H, Schreiber T. Nonlinear time series analysis. Cambridge, UK: Cambridge University Press, 1997.

8   Goldberger AL. Nonlinear dynamics for clinicians: chaos theory, fractals and complexity at the bedside. *Lancet* 1996; **347**: 1312–14.

9   Martinerie J, Adam C, Le Van Quyen M, et al. Epileptic seizures can be anticipated by non-linear analysis. *Nat Med* 1998; **4**: 1173–76.

10 Lehnertz K, Elger CE. Can epileptic seizures be predicted? Evidence from nonlinear time series analysis of brain electrical activity. *Phys Rev Lett* 1998; **80**: 5019–22.

11 Le Van Quyen M, Adam C, Martinerie J, Baulac M, Clémenceau S, Varela F. Spatio-temporal characterizations of nonlinear changes in intracranial activities prior to human temporal lobe seizures. *Eur J Neurosci* 2000; **12**: 1224–34.

12 Quesney L. Extracranial EEG evaluation. In: Engel J Jr, ed. Surgical treatment of the epilepsies. New York: Raven Press, 1987: 129–66.

13 Schreiber T, Kantz H. Observing and predicting chaotic signals: is 2% noise too much? In Kravtsov YA, Kadtke JB, eds. Predictability of complex dynamical systems. New York, USA: Springer, 1996.

14 Theiler J, Rapp PE. Re-examination of the evidence for low-dimensional nonlinear structure in the human electroencephalogram. *Electroencephalogr Clin Neurophysiol* 1996; **98**: 213–23.

15 Le Van Quyen M, Martinerie J, Baulac M, Varela F. Anticipating epileptic seizure in real time by a nonlinear analysis of similarity between EEG recordings. *Neuroreport* 1999; **10**: 2149–55.

16 Manuca R, Savit R. Stationarity and nonstationarity in time series analysis. *Physica D* 1996; **99**: 134–61.

17 Schreiber T, Schmitz A. Classification of time series data with nonlinear similarity measures. *Phys Rev Lett* 1997; **79**: 1475–78.

18 Nuwer MR, Comi G, Emerson R, et al. IFCN standards for digital recording of clinical EEG. *Electroencephalogr Clin Neurophysiol* 1998; **106**: 259–61.

19 Taken F. Lecture notes in mathematics: dynamical systems and turbulence. Springer Verlag: Berlin, 1981.

20 Alarcon G, Guy CN, Binnie CD, Walker SR, Elwes RDC, Polkey CE. Intracerebral propagation of interictal activity in partial epilepsy: implications for source localization. *J Neurol Neurosurg Psychiatry* 1994; **57**: 233–43.

21 Spencer SS. Substrates of localization-related epilepsies: biologic implications of localizing findings in humans. *Epilepsia* 1998; **39**: 114–23.

22 Le Van Quyen M, Martinerie J, Adam C, Varela F. Nonlinear analyses of interictal EEG map the brain interdependences in human focal epilepsy. *Physica D* 1999; **127**: 250–67.

23 Depaulis A, Vergnes M, Marescaux C. Endogenous control of epilepsy. *Prog Neurobiol* 1994; **42**: 33–52.

24 Weinand ME, Carter LP, El-Saadany WF, Sioutos PJ, Labiner DM, Oommen KJ. Cerebral blood flow and temporal lobe epileptogenicity. *J Neurosurg* 1997; **86**: 226–32.

25 Baumgartner C, Serles W, Leutmezer F, et al. Pre-ictal SPECT in temporal lobe epilepsy: regional cerebral blood flow is increased prior to electroencephalography-seizure onset. *J Nucl Med* 1998; **39**: 978–82.

26 Akinbi MS, Welty TE. Benzodiazepines in the home treatment of acute seizures. *Ann Pharmacother* 1999; **33**: 99–102.

27 Schiff S, Jerger K, Chang T, Sauer T, Spano M, Ditto W. Controlling chaos in the brain. *Nature* 1994; **370**: 615–20.

Independent Component Analysis for EEG Source Localization

An Algorithm that Reduces the Complexity of Localizing Multiple Neural Sources

A pervasive problem in neuroscience is determining which regions of the brain are active, given voltage measurements at the scalp. If accurate solutions to such problems could be obtained, neurologists would gain noninvasive access to patient-specific cortical activity. Access to such data would ultimately increase the number of patients who could be effectively treated for neural pathologies such as multifocal epilepsy [5, 6].

However, estimating the location and distribution of electric current source within the brain from electroencephalographic (EEG) recordings is an ill-posed problem. Specifically, there is no unique solution, and possible solutions do not depend continuously on the data. The ill-posedness of the problem makes finding the correct solution a challenging analytic and computational problem.

In this article, we consider a spatiotemporal method for sources localization, taking advantage of the entire EEG time series to reduce the configuration space we must evaluate. The EEG data are first decomposed into signal and noise subspaces using a principal component analysis (PCA) decomposition. This partitioning allows us to easily discard the noise subspace, which has two primary benefits: the remaining signal is less noisy, and it has lower dimensionality. After PCA, we apply independent component analysis (ICA) on the signal subspace. The ICA algorithm separates multichannel data into activation maps due to temporally independent stationary sources. For each activation map we perform an EEG source-localization procedure, looking only for a single dipole per map. By localizing multiple dipoles independently, we substantially reduce our search complexity and increase the likelihood of efficiently converging on the correct solution.

Leonid Zhukov, David Weinstein, Chris Johnson
Scientific Computing and Imaging Institute, University of Utah

Measuring Brain Activity

Electroencephalography is a technique for the noninvasive characterization of brain function. Scalp electric potential distributions are a direct consequence of internal electric currents associated with the firing of neurons. These potentials can be measured over a period of time at discrete recording sites on the scalp surface.

Most measured nonbackground brain activity is generated within the cerebral cortex, the outer surface (1.5-4.5 mm thick) of the brain, which is comprised of approximately 10 billion neurons. The active regions within the cortex are generally fairly well localized, or *focal*. Their activity is the result of synchronous synaptic stimulation of a very large number (10^5-10^6) of neurons. Cortical neurons align themselves in columns oriented orthogonally to the cortical surface [1]. When a large group of such neurons all depolarize or hyperpolarize in concert, the result is a dipolar current source oriented orthogonal to the cortical surface. It is the propagation of this current that we measure as the EEG.

The Source-Localization Problem

Estimation of the location and distribution of current sources within the brain, based on potential recordings from the scalp (source localization), is one of the fundamental problems in electroencephalography. It requires the solution of an inverse problem; i.e., given a subset of electrostatic potentials measured on the surface of the scalp, and the geometric and

conductivity properties within the head, calculate the current sources and potential fields within the cerebrum. This problem is challenging because solutions do not depend continuously on the data, and because it lacks a unique solution. (Mathematically, problems fitting such a profile are termed ill-posed [2].) The lack of continuity implies that small errors in the measurement of the voltages on the scalp can yield unbounded errors in the recovered solution. The nonuniqueness is a consequence of the linear superposition of the electric field: different internal source configurations can produce identical external electromagnetic fields, especially when only measured at a finite number of electrode positions [1, 3, 4].

Advances in Source Localization

There exist several different approaches to solving the source-localization problem. Initially, many of these methods were implemented on spherical models of the head [7, 8], and those that proved promising were then extended to work on realistic geometry [9]. One of the most general methods for inverse source localization is source imaging. Source imaging involves starting from some initial distributed estimate of the source and then recursively enhancing the strength of some of the solution elements, while decreasing the strength of the remainder of the elements until they become zero. In the end, only a small number of elements will remain nonzero, yielding a localized solution. This method is implemented, for example, in the FOCUSS algorithm [10]. Another example of an iterative reweighting technique is the LORETA algorithm [11].

A second source-localization approach incorporates a priori assumptions about the sources and their locations in the model. Electric current dipoles are usually used as sources, provided that the re-

---

The original paper contained coloured figures.

Access to such data would ultimately increase the number of patients who could be effectively treated for neural pathologies.

gions of activations are relatively focused [3]. Although a single dipole is the most widely used model, it has been demonstrated that a multiple-dipole model is required to account for the complex field distribution on the surface of the head [12]. If the distance between the dipoles is large, or if the dipoles have entirely different temporal behavior, the field patterns may exhibit only minor overlap and can be fitted individually using the single-dipole model. However, more often than not, examination of spatial surface topographies can be misleading, as the time series of multiple dipoles overlap and potentials cancel each other out [4, 13]. In such cases, one must employ a third approach: a spatio-temporal model.

The main assumption of the spatio-temporal model is that there are several dipolar sources that maintain their position and orientation but vary just their strength (amplitude) as a function of time. Now, rather than fit dipoles to measurements from one instant in time, dipoles are fit by minimizing the least-square error residual over the entire evoked potential epoch [14].

A more advanced version of this spatio-temporal approach is developed in the multiple signal classification algorithm, MUSIC [15], and in its extension, RAP-MUSIC [16]. A signal subspace is first estimated from the data, and the algorithm then scans a single-dipole model through the three-dimensional (3-D) head volume and computes projections onto this subspace. To locate the source, the user must search the head volume for local

peaks in the projection metric. The RAP-MUSIC extension of this algorithm automates this search, extracting the location of the sources through a recursive use of subspace projection.

Independent Sources

While the above methods represent significant advances in source localization, they fail to address the problem most recently identified by Cuffin in [17]: "Solutions to multiple dipole ... sources are much less reliable than solutions for single-dipole sources. These solutions can be very sensitive to ... noise. At present, this sensitivity limits the usefulness of these solutions as clinical and research tools." We introduce a novel approach for spatio-temporal source localization of *independent* sources. In our method, we first separate the raw EEG data into independent sources. We then perform a separate localization procedure on each independent source. Because we localize sources independently, our method is just as reliable as single-dipole source-localization methods.

The steps of our method are depicted in Fig. 1. We begin by extracting the signal subspace of the EEG data using a PCA algorithm. This step removes much of the noise from the data and reduces its dimensionality by truncating lower-order terms of the decomposition (i.e., discarding the noise subspace). We then divide the PCA signal subspace into individual components, using the recently developed ICA signal processing technique [18-20]. The result of this preprocessing is a set of time-series signals (which sum to the original signal) at each electrode, where each time series corresponds to an independent source in the model. The number of different maps created by ICA is equal to the number of temporally independent stationary sources in the problem. To localize each of these independent sources, we solve a separate source-localization problem. Specifically, for each independent component, we employ a downhill simplex search method [21] to determine the dipole that best accounts for that particular component's contribution of the signal.

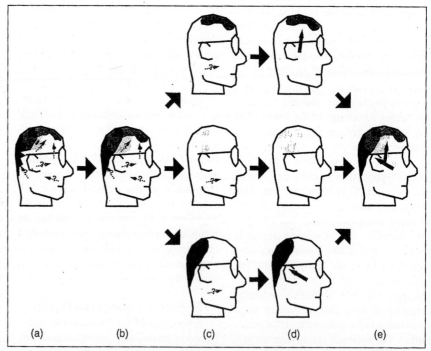

1. A depiction of the steps of our algorithm. (a) Measured signals are recorded at the scalp surface through EEG electrodes; the underlying neural sources (which we will model as dipoles) are unknown. (b) With PCA decomposition, truncation, and reconstruction, much of the noise is removed from the EEG data. (c) Using the ICA algorithm, the time signals can be decomposed into statistically independent activation maps (summing these activation maps returns the signal subspace). (d) For each independent activation map, the single-dipole source that best accounts for the map's voltages is localized. (e) Integrated together, these independent dipole sources reproduce the signal from (b).

In our method we first separate the raw EEG data into independent sources. We then perform a separate localization procedure on each source.

In our study, we use simulated data obtained by placing dipoles in a computational model at positions corresponding to observed epileptic sources in children with Landau-Kleffner syndrome [6]. We chose to simulate three tangential epileptogenic right-hemisphere sources, as shown in Fig. 2: the temporal lobe, the occipital lobe, and the Sylvian fissure. This distributed configuration is typical of multifocal epilepsy, where each source has an independent time course [6]. For each of these sources, we use a time signal from a clinical study to vary its magnitude over time. That is, we place the three current dipoles inside our finite element model, and for each instant in time we project the activation signals onto 32 clinically measured scalp electrode positions and add 2% noise to the signals. The electrode positions are shown in Fig. 3. Projecting the sources onto the electrodes requires the solution of a so-called forward problem.

Forward Problem

The EEG forward problem can be stated as follows: given the positions, orientations, and magnitudes of dipole current sources, as well as the geometry and electrical conductivity of the head volume Ω, calculate the distribution of the electric potential on the surface of the head (scalp) Γ_Ω. Mathematically, this problem can be described by Poisson's equation for electrical conduction in the head [22]:

$$\nabla \cdot (\sigma \nabla \Phi) = \sum I_s(\mathbf{r}), \text{ in } \Omega \quad (1)$$

and Neumann boundary conditions on the scalp:

$$\sigma(\nabla \Phi) \cdot \mathbf{n} = 0, \text{ on } \Gamma_\Omega \quad (2)$$

where σ is a conductivity tensor and I_s are the volume current's density due to current dipoles placed within the head. The unknown Φ is the electric potential created in the head by the distribution of current from the dipole sources. An ideal current dipole source can be described as two point sources of opposite polarity, with infinitely large current density I_0 and infinitely small separation d:

$$I_s(r) = \lim_{d \to 0} I_0 \left[\delta \left(\mathbf{r} - \mathbf{r}_s - \frac{d}{2} \right) - \delta \left(\mathbf{r} - \mathbf{r}_s + \frac{d}{2} \right) \right] \quad (3)$$

and $d \cdot I_0 = P$, the dipole strength.

To solve Poisson's equation numerically, we began with the construction of a computational model. The realistic head geometry was obtained from MRI data, where the volume was segmented and each tissue material was labeled in the underlying voxels [23]. The segmented head volume was then tetrahedralized via a mesh generator that preserved the classification when mapping from voxels to elements [24]. For each tissue classification, we assigned a conductivity tensor as obtained from the literature [25]. A cut-through of the classified mesh is shown in Fig. 4.

We then used the finite-element method (FEM) to compute a solution within the entire volume domain [26]. The FEM allows us to capture the anisotropy of conductivity and accurate boundaries of the volume. The main idea behind the FEM is to reduce a continuous problem that has an infinite number of unknown field values, with a finite number of unknowns, by discretizing the solution region. Then the values of the field at any point can be approximated by interpolation functions within every element in terms of the field values at specified points, called nodes. Nodes are located at the element vertices where adjacent elements are connected. Details of the FEM method can be found in [26-28].

In our study, we use tetrahedral elements and linear interpolation functions within each tetrahedron. Our head model consists of approximately 768,000 elements and $N = 164,000$ nodes. Once we

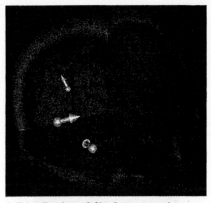

2. Distribution of dipole sources (arrows) visualized with orthogonal MRI slices (background).

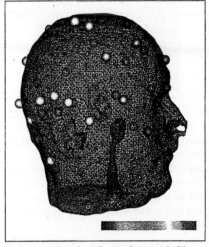

3. Triangulated scalp surface with 32 electrodes. The electrodes have been color-mapped to indicate order: they are colored from blue to red as the channel number increases.

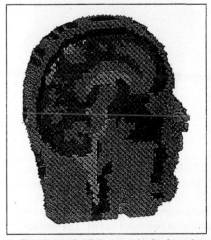

4. Cut-through of the tetrahedral mesh, with elements colored according to conductivity classification. Green elements correspond to skin, blue to skull, yellow to cerebro-spinal fluid, purple to gray matter, and light blue to white matter.

have a geometric model, we can assemble the matrix equations (build the matrix **A**) for relating field values at different nodes. This can be done by using, for example, a Rayleigh-Ritz or Galerkin method [28]. Finally, we impose boundary conditions and apply source currents. These boundary and source conditions are incorporated within the right-hand side (RHS) of

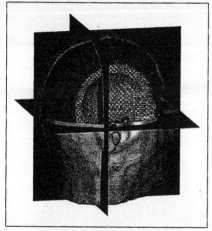

5. Solution to a single-dipole source forward problem. The underlying model is shown in the MRI planes, the dipole source is indicated with the red and blue spheres, and the electric field is visualized by a cropped scalp potential mapping and a wire-frame equipotential isosurface.

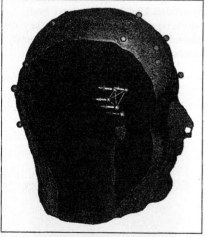

6. Visualization of the downhill simplex algorithm converging to a dipole source. The simplex is indicated by the gray vectors joined by yellow lines. The true source is indicated in red. The surface potential map on the scalp is due to the forward solution of one of the simplex vertices, whereas the potentials at the electrodes (shown as small spheres) are the "measured" EEG values (potentials due to the true source).

the system (vector **b**). As a result, when we move sources we do not have to re-build the mesh or matrix **A**. We note that for linear-interpolation functions, the RHS vector is not sensitive to the position of a source within an element; that is, for any position (though not orientation) within a particular tetrahedron, the contribution to the RHS vector is the same. This ambiguity is relevant because it will restrict the accuracy of our inverse solution when we attempt to recover the exact source positions.

Using the FEM, we obtain the linear system of equations:

$$\mathbf{A}_{ij}\Phi_j = \mathbf{b}_i \qquad (4)$$

where $\mathbf{A}_{ij}$ is an $N \times N$ stiffness matrix, $\mathbf{b}_i$ is a source vector, and Φ is the vector of unknown potentials at the nodes within the head volume. The **A** matrix is sparse (containing approximately 2 million nonzero entries), symmetric, and positive definite.

The solution of this linear system was computed using a parallel conjugate gradient (CG) method and required approximately 12 sec of wall-clock time on a 14 processor SGI Power Onyx with 195 MHz MIPS R10000 processors. The solution to a radially oriented, single-dipole source, forward problem is visualized in Fig. 5. In this image, we display an equipotential surface in wire frame, indicating the dipole location with red and blue spheres, cut-through the initial MRI data with orthogonal planes, and render the surface potential map of the bioelectric field on the cropped scalp surface.

In order to simulate time-dependent recordings, we first computed a forward solution due to each epileptic source, assuming dipoles of unit strength. Each source produced a map of values at the simulated electrode sites. Running forward simulations for each of several dipoles resulted in a collection of several maps. To extend the single-instant values at the electrodes into time-dependent signals, we scaled the values of each map by prerecorded clinical activation signals. Finally, we added noise to the projected data to better simulate physical EEG measurements.

The above method for solving the forward problem is needed not only to derive the simulated electrode recordings but also as the iterative engine for solving the inverse source-localization problem.

One of the challenges of solving the inverse EEG source-localization problem is choosing the initial configuration of sources.

Inverse Problem

The general EEG inverse problem can be stated as follows: given a set of electric potentials from discrete sites on the surface of the head, and the associated positions of those measurements, as well as the geometry and conductivity of the different regions within the head, calculate the locations and magnitudes of the electric current sources within the brain.

Mathematically, it is an inverse source problem in terms of the primary electric current sources within the brain, which can be described by the same Poisson's equation as the forward problem, Eq. (1), but with a different set of boundary conditions on the scalp:

$$\sigma(\nabla\Phi)\cdot\mathbf{n} = 0, \text{ and } \Phi_j = \phi_j \text{ on } \Gamma_\Omega$$

$$(5)$$

where ϕ_j is the electrostatic potential on the surface of the head known at discrete points (electrode locations), and I_s in Eq. (1) are now unknown current sources.

The solution to the inverse problem can be formulated as the nonlinear optimization problem of finding a least-squares fit of a potential due to a set of current dipoles to the observed data over the entire time series, or as minimization with respect to the model parameters of the following cost function:

$$\left\| \phi - \hat{\phi} \right\| = \sum_{k} \sum_{j=1}^{32} \left(\phi_j(t_k) - \hat{\phi}_j(t_k) \right)^2 \quad (6)$$

where $\phi_j(t_k)$ is the value of the measured electric potential on the jth electrode at time instant t_k, and $\hat{\phi}_j(t_k)$ is the result of the forward model computation for a particular source configuration; the sum extends over all channels and time frames.

A brute-force implementation of the above method would require solving the forward problem for every possible configuration of dipoles in order to find the configuration that minimizes Eq. (6). Each dipole in the model has six parameters: location coordinates (x, y, z), orientation (θ, ϕ), and time-dependent dipole strength $P(t)$. The number of dipoles is usually determined by iteratively adding one dipole at a time until a "reasonable" fit to the data has been found. Even when restricting the location of the dipole to a lattice of sites, the configuration space is factorially large. This is a bottleneck of many localization procedures [12, 29].

Assume now that we could decompose the signals on the electrodes, such that we know electrode potentials due to each dipole *separately*. Then, for every set of electrode potentials, we would need to search for only one dipole, thus dramatically reducing our search space. We will discuss this useful filtering technique below.

Statistical Preprocessing of the Data

In EEG experiments, electric potential is measured with an array of electrodes (typically 32, 64, or 128) positioned primarily on the top half of the head, as shown in Fig. 3. The data are typically sampled every millisecond during an interval of interest.

For a given electrode configuration, the time-dependent data can be arranged as a matrix, where every column corresponds to the sampled time frame and every row corresponds to a channel (electrode). For example, the data obtained by 32 electrodes in 180 msec can be sampled in 180 frames and represented as a matrix (32×180). Below, we will refer to this matrix as $\phi(t_k)$, where instead of a continuous variable t, we have sampled time frames t_k.

Before performing source localization, we will preprocess the EEG activation maps in order to decompose them into several *independent* activation maps. The source for each activation map will then be localized independently. This is accomplished as follows:

- First, we will process the raw signals $\phi(t_k)$ in order to reduce the dimensionality of the data and to remove some of its noise. The projection of the data on the signal subspace will be referred to as $\phi_s(t_k)$.
- The signal subspace $\phi_s(t_k)$ will then be decomposed into statistically independent components $\phi_s^i(t_k)$.
- Each independent activation $\phi_s^i(t_k)$ will be assumed to be due to a single stationary dipole, which we will then localize using a parameterized search algorithm.

As outlined above, the first step in processing the raw EEG data, $\phi(t_k)$ is to decompose it into signal and noise subspaces by applying the PCA method [30] (in the signal processing literature it is also known as the Karhunen-Loeve transform). The decomposition is achieved by finding the Eigen decomposition of the data covariance matrix

$$\mathbf{R} = E\left\{ \phi(t_k)\phi^T(t_k) \right\} \approx \frac{1}{n} \sum_k \phi_s(t_k) \cdot \phi_s(t_k)^T \quad (7)$$

and constructing signal and noise subspaces [15]. The noise subspace will constitute the singular vectors with singular values less than a chosen noise threshold:

$$\mathbf{R} = \mathbf{U} \cdot \Lambda \cdot \mathbf{U}^T$$
$$= \mathbf{U}_s \cdot \Lambda_s \cdot \mathbf{U}_s^T + \mathbf{U}_n \cdot \Lambda_n \cdot \mathbf{U}_n^T. \quad (8)$$

Having constructed the subspaces, we can project the original data onto the signal subspace by

$$\phi_s(t_k) = \sqrt{\Lambda_s}^{(-1)} \cdot \mathbf{U}_s^T \cdot \phi(t_k) \quad (9)$$

where Λ_s and $\mathbf{U}_s$ are the signal subspace singular values and singular vectors.

Though PCA allows us to estimate the number of dipoles, in the presence of noise it does not necessarily give an accurate result [15]. In order to separate out any remaining noise, as well as each statistically independent term, we will use the recently derived *infomax* technique, ICA. (It is worth noting that PCA not only filters out noise from the data but also makes a preliminary step of ICA decomposition by decorrelating the channels, or removing linear dependence; i.e., $E\{\mathbf{s}_i \cdot \mathbf{s}_j\} = 0$. ICA then makes the chan-

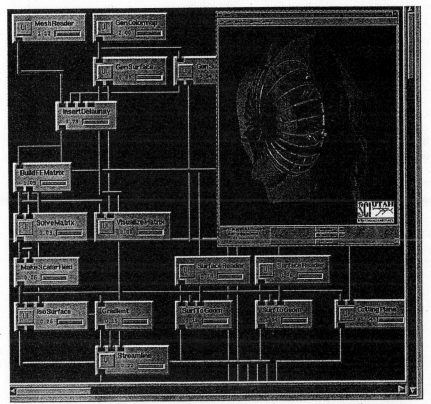

7. The SCIRun problem-solving environment. The user can select physiologically plausible regions of the model in which to seed the downhill simplex algorithm, thereby steering the algorithm to a more rapid convergence.

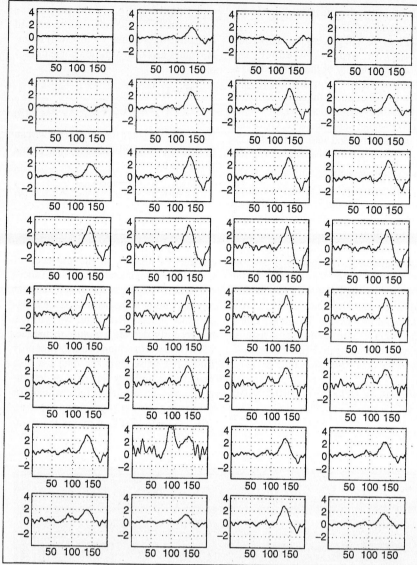

8. Simulated scalp potentials due to three dipole sources mapped onto 32 channels (electrodes). Channels are numbered left to right, top to bottom. The first channel is the reference electrode. These signals are the input data for the ICA algorithm. The locations of these 32 electrodes are shown in Fig. 3.

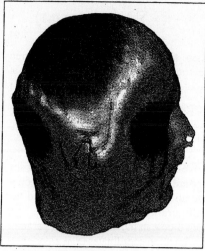

9. Scalp surface potential map due to several dipoles, corresponding to time T = 160 msec from the signals shown in Fig. 8.

$$\mathbf{W} \cdot \phi_s(t_k) = \mathbf{W} \cdot \mathbf{M} \cdot \mathbf{s}(t_k) = \mathbf{s}(t_k)$$

$$(11)$$

or, in other words, $\mathbf{W} = \mathbf{M}^{-1}$; but we do not know $\mathbf{M}$: the only data we have is the $\phi_s(t_k)$ matrix.

Under the assumption of *independent* sources, ICA allows us to construct such a matrix; however, since neither the $\mathbf{W}$ matrix or the sources are known, $\mathbf{W}$ can be restored only up to scaling and permutations (i.e., $\mathbf{W} \cdot \mathbf{M}$ is not an identity matrix but rather is equal to $\mathbf{S} \cdot \mathbf{P}$, where $\mathbf{S}$ is a diagonal scaling matrix and $\mathbf{P}$ is a permutation matrix). This problem is often referred to as blind-source separation (BSS) [18, 31-33].

The ICA process consists of two phases: learning and processing. During the learning phase, the ICA algorithm finds a weighting matrix $\mathbf{W}$, which minimizes the mutual information among channels (variables); i.e., it makes output signals that are statistically independent in the sense that the multivariate probability density function of the input signals becomes equal to the product of $f_{\mathbf{u}} = \prod_i f_{u_i}(\mathbf{u_i})$ probability density functions of every independent variable. This is equivalent to maximizing the entropy of a nonlinearly transformed vector $\mathbf{u} = \mathbf{g}(\mathbf{W}\phi_s)$:

$$H(\mathbf{u}) = -E\{\log f_u(\mathbf{u})\}$$
$$= -\int f_u(\mathbf{u}) \log f_u(\mathbf{u}) d\mathbf{u} \quad (12)$$

where $\mathbf{g}$ is some nonlinear function.

nels *independent*; i.e., $E\{\mathbf{s}_i^n \cdot \mathbf{s}_j^m\} = 0$ for any powers n and m.)

There are several assumptions one needs to make about the sources in order to apply the ICA algorithm in electroencephalography [19]:

- The sources must be independent (signals come from statistically independent brain processes). We note that this assumption is thought to be valid for our multifocal epilepsy source-localization problem; however, it may not be valid for other neural events.
- There is no delay in signal propagation from the sources to the detectors (conducting media without delays at source frequencies).

- The mixture is linear (Poisson's equation is linear).
- The number of independent signal sources does not exceed the number of electrodes (we expect to have fewer strong sources than our 32 electrodes).

It follows then that since the PCA-processed EEG recordings $\phi_s(t_k)$ are the result of linear combinations of the source signals $\mathbf{s}(t_k)$, they can therefore be expressed as:

$$\phi_s(t_k) = \mathbf{M} \cdot \mathbf{s}(t_k) \quad (10)$$

where $\mathbf{M}$ is the so-called "mixing" matrix and each row of $\mathbf{s}(t_k)$ is a source's time activation. What we would like to find is an "unmixing" matrix $\mathbf{W}$ such that:

There exist several different ways to estimate the **W** matrix. For example, the Bell-Sejnowski infomax algorithm [18] uses weights that are changed according to the entropy gradient. Below, we use a modification of this rule as proposed by Amari, Cichocki, and Yang [20], which uses the natural gradient rather than the absolute gradient of $H(\mathbf{u})$. This allows us to avoid computing matrix inverses and to speed up solution convergence. Weighting matrix **W** is constructed iteratively by:

$$\mathbf{W}_{k+1} = \mathbf{W}_k + \mu_k \cdot \left[\mathbf{I} + 2g(\mathbf{y}_k) \cdot \mathbf{y}_k^T \right] \cdot \mathbf{W}_k$$

(13)

where the vector **y** is defined as:

$$\mathbf{y}_k = \mathbf{W}_k \cdot \phi_s(t_k) \qquad (14)$$

and for the nonlinear function g we used:

$$g(\mathbf{y}_k) = \tanh(\mathbf{y}_k). \qquad (15)$$

In the above equation, μ_k is a learning rate and **I** is the identity matrix [33]. The learning rate decreases during the iterations, and we stop when μ_k becomes smaller than a predefined tolerance (e.g., 10^{-6}).

The second phase of the ICA algorithm is the actual source separation. Independent components (activations) can be computed by applying the unmixing matrix **W** to the signal subspace data:

$$\mathbf{s}(t_k) = \mathbf{W} \cdot \phi_s(t_k). \qquad (16)$$

Projection of independent activation maps $\mathbf{s}(t_k)$ back onto the electrodes, one at a time, can be done by:

$$\phi^i(t_k) = \mathbf{U}_s \cdot \sqrt{\Lambda} \cdot \mathbf{W}^{(-1)} \cdot \mathbf{s}_i(t_k) \quad (17)$$

where $\phi^i(t_k)$ is the set of scalp potentials due to just the ith source. For $\mathbf{s}_i(t_k)$, we zero out all rows but the ith; that is, all but the ith source are "turned off." In practice, we will not need the full time sequence $\phi^i(t_k)$ in order to localize source $\mathbf{s}_i$ but rather simply a single instant of activation. For this purpose, we set the $\mathbf{s}_i$ terms to be unit sources (i.e., $\mathbf{s} = \mathbf{I}$), resulting in ϕ^i row elements that are simply the corresponding columns of $\mathbf{U}_s \cdot \sqrt{\Lambda} \cdot \mathbf{W}^{(-1)}$.

Source Localization

For each electrode potential map ϕ^i, we can now localize a single dipole using a search method to minimize Eq. (6). We have chosen to use the straightforward downhill simplex search. Since we know we are only searching for one dipole source that produced each activation map,

ϕ^i, we will only need to optimize six degrees of freedom: the position (x, y, z), orientation (θ, ϕ) and strength P of a single dipole. The last three variables can be thought of as components (p_x, p_y, p_z), the dipole strength in the x, y, and z direction.

Since the potential is a linear function of dipole moment, we can further reduce our search space by using the analytic optimization from [34, 35]. Specifically, for each location to be evaluated for the simplex, we separately compute the solutions

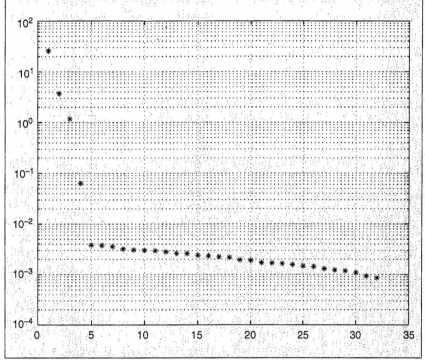

10. Singular values of the covariance matrix. It appears that only the first four singular values contribute to the signal subspace, with the rest constituting the noise subspace.

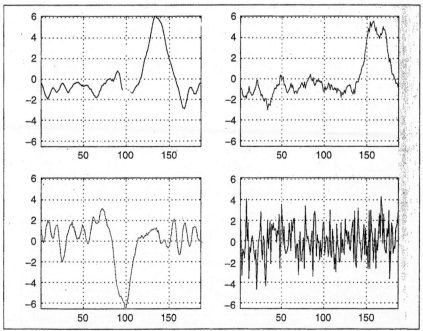

11. ICA activation maps obtained by unmixing the signals from the signal subspace. We observe that there are only three independent patterns, indicating the presence of only three separate signals in the original data; the fourth component is noise.

due to dipoles oriented in the x, y and z directions and solve a 3×3 system to determine the optimal strength and orientation for that position [37]. The minimization cost function now explicitly depends on only the coordinates of the dipole:

$$R(x, y, z) = \left\| \phi^i - \overline{p}_x \hat{\phi}_x - \overline{p}_y \hat{\phi}_y - \overline{p}_z \hat{\phi}_z \right\|.$$

(18)

To perform nonlinear minimization of $R(x, y, z)$, we applied the multistart downhill simplex method [21, 36], as implemented in [38]. In an N-dimensional space, the simplex is a geometric figure that consists of $N + 1$ fully interconnected vertices. In our case, we are searching a 3-D coordinate space, so the simplex is just a tetrahedron with four vertices. The downhill simplex method searches for the minimum of the 3-D function by taking a series of steps, each moving a point in the simplex (a dipole) away from where the function is largest (see Fig. 6).

The single-dipole solution to the source-localization problem is unique [39]. This follows from the fundamental physical properties of the model and can be illustrated by considering the cost function, Eq. (6), over its entire 3-D domain. A computationally efficient method for evaluating the cost function using lead-field theory is discussed in [37]. However, despite the uniqueness of the solution, in the case of linear finite elements the downhill simplex search method may fail to reach the global minimum. This can happen when the nodes of the simplex (and its attempted extensions) are all contained within a single element of the finite element model. In such situations, the simplex must be restarted several times in order to find the true global minimum.

After all of the dipoles have been localized, the only step that remains is to determine their absolute strengths. This can be accomplished by solving a small, $m \times m$, linear minimization problem, where m is the number of dipoles. For this study, we recovered three dipoles, so we solved a 3×3 system, where the RHS is formed by the inner products of optimized single-dipole solutions and EEG recordings ϕ.

An Inverse EEG Problem-Solving Environment

One of the challenges of solving the inverse EEG source-localization problem is choosing initial configurations for the downhill simplex solver. A good choice can result in rapid convergence, whereas a bad choice can cause the algorithm to search somewhat randomly for a very long time before closing in on the solution. Furthermore, because the solution space has many plateaus as a result of the linear finite element model used, it is generally necessary to re-seed the algorithm multiple times in order to find the global minimum.

We have brought the user into the loop by enabling seed-point selection within the model. The user can seed specifically within physiologically plausible regions. This focus enables the algorithm to converge much more quickly, rather than repeatedly wandering through non-interesting regions.

To steer our algorithm, we utilized the SCIRun problem-solving environment [40]. SCIRun is a scientific programming environment that allows the interactive construction, debugging, and steering of large-scale scientific computations. SCIRun can be envisioned as a "computational workbench" in which a scientist can design and modify simulations interactively via a dataflow programming model. As opposed to the typical "off-line" simulation mode (in which the scientist manually sets input parameters, computes results, visualizes the results via a separate visualization package, and then starts again at the beginning), SCIRun "closes

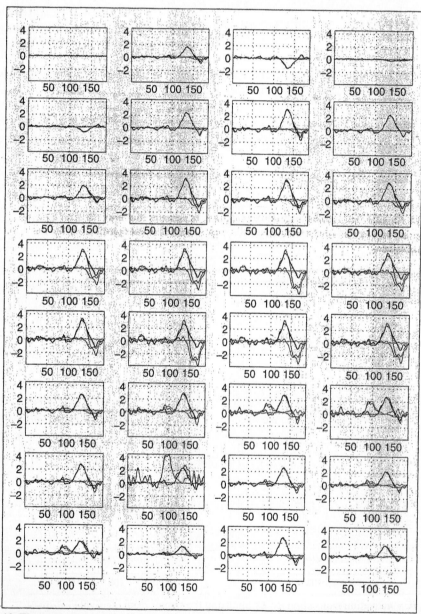

12. The projection of the first three activation maps from Fig. 11 (as well as the original signals from Fig. 10) onto the 32 electrodes.

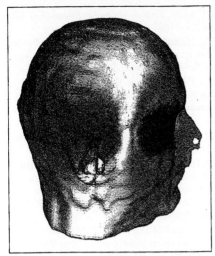

13. Projection of the first ICA component onto the 32 channels at the time of *T* = 160 msec.

the loop" and allows interactive steering of the design, computation, and visualization phases of a simulation. The images of our algorithm running within the SCIRun environment are shown in Figs. 6 and 7.

Numerical Simulations

We prepared the simulated data as described above. The time-dependent course of 180 msec for all 32 channels is shown in Fig. 8. We also provide a color mapped plot of the potentials on the surface of the head for the time step at 160 msec (maximum variance), as seen in Fig. 9. As shown there, the distribution of potentials on the scalp can hardly be attributed to a single dipole but rather to a configuration of several dipoles. We perform PCA on the original EEG time-dependent data, and the singular values are shown in Fig. 10. Analyzing the singular values, we can deduce that the signal subspace consists of the first four singular vectors. Working with just the contribution of these four components, ϕ, s, t, k, and using Eq. (16), we perform the ICA procedure, resulting in the activation maps shown in Fig. 11. Notice that there are only three different activation patterns presented; the fourth component is actually just noise.

Projecting the first activation back onto all 32 channels, we get the signals shown in Fig. 12, which are the potentials due to a single temporal lobe dipole. Plotting the potentials again for the time step at 160 msec in Fig. 13, one can recognize the surface potential map as resulting from the activation of a single dipole source. This is evidenced by the

well-defined foci near the right eye and ear, as well as the symmetric potential fall-off about the dipole plane.

We can check the accuracy of the ICA decomposition by comparing the above results to the results of the forward simulation run with the two other dipoles "turned off." Because ICA does not preserve scale, we use time-space correlation coefficients as our metric for comparing the potentials at the electrodes. The sets of electrode potentials are viewed as vectors in time-space, and the cosine of the "angle" between them is calculated by taking the dot-product of the two vectors after they have been normalized. Evaluated this way, our three activation projections restored the original (unmixed) potential distribution with RMS errors of 2%, 3%, and 5%.

We now turn our attention to the last step of the procedure: source localization. For our head model, on average, the downhill simplex algorithm required only two or three interactive restarts in order to converge to the correct solution, with an average run of 30 or 50 iterations. This is a substantial speed-up compared to the batch-mode multistart multiple-dipole localization methods reported in [36]. The localized temporal lobe dipole was found to be accurate within 4 mm of the actual source. We repeated this localization procedure for the occipital lobe and Sylvian fissure dipoles and were able to determine their positions with errors of 5 and 2 mm, respectively.

Conclusions

We have presented an algorithm that reduces the complexity of localizing multiple neural sources by exploiting the time dependence of the data. We have shown that, on a realistic head model with simulated EEG data, our algorithm is capable of correctly predicting the number of independent sources in the model and of reconstructing potentials due to each source separately. These potential maps can be successfully used by source-localization methods to localize sources independently.

By integrating our algorithm within the SCIRun problem-solving environment, we were able to computationally steer the multistart downhill simplex algorithm toward probable regions of activation. Interactive control of the simulation coupled with statistical data preprocessing of the data enable us to increase dramatically the efficiency and ac-

curacy of recovering multiple sources from EEG data.

Acknowledgments

This work was supported in part by the National Science Foundation, the Department of Energy, the National Institutes of Health, and the Utah State Centers of Excellence Program.

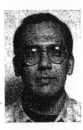

Leonid Zhukov received his B.S and M.S. in physics from Moscow Engineering and Physics Institute in 1991 and 1993, and his Ph.D. from the University of Utah in 1998. His research interests are in the field of scientific computing, modeling, and simulation. Specific interests include inverse problems, multiresolution methods for large-scale computational problems, scientific visualization, and statistical signal and image processing. He is currently a research scientist in the Scientific Computing and Imaging Institute within the Department of Computer Science at the University of Utah.

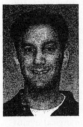

David Weinstein received his B.A. in applied mathematics and computer science from the University of California at Berkeley in 1993. He was a National Science Foundation Graduate Research Fellow from 1995-1998 and a University of Utah Graduate Research Fellow from 1997-1998. His research interests include scientific computing, scientific visualization, neuroscience, and computer graphics. He is currently the technical manager for the NIH NCRR Center for Bioelectric Field Problems within the Department of Computer Science at the University of Utah.

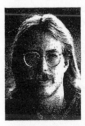

Chris Johnson holds faculty positions in the departments of Computer Science, Bioengineering, Mathematics, and Physics at the University of Utah, where he directs the Scientific Computing and Imaging Institute. His research interests are in the area of scientific computing. Particular interests include inverse and imaging problems, adaptive methods for partial differential equations, large-scale computational problems in medicine, problem-solving environments, and scientific visualization. Prof. Johnson was awarded a FIRST Award from the NIH in 1992, a National Young Investigator (NYI) Award from the NSF in 1994, and the Presidential Faculty Fellow (PFF) Award in 1995. This past year, Prof. Johnson was Awarded the Governor's Medal for Science and Technology from the State of Utah Governor.

Address for Correspondence: Chris R. Johnson, Center for Scientific Computing and Imaging, Department of Computer Science, Merill Engineering Building, 50 South Campus Central Dr., Room 3490, University of Utah, Salt Lake City, UT 84112. Tel: +1 801 581 7705. Fax: +1 801 585-6513. E-mail: crj@cs.utah.edu.

References

1. **Gulrajani RM:** *Bioelectricity and Biomagnetism.* New York: Wiley, 1998.

2. **Hadamard J:** Sur les problemes aux derivees parielies et leur signification physique. *Bull Univ of Princeton* pp. 49-52, 1902.

3. **Nunez PL:** *Electric Fields of The Brain.* New York: Oxford, 1981.

4. **Koles ZJ:** Trends in EEG source localization. *Electroenceph and Clin Neurophysiol* 106: 127-137, 1998.

5. **Huiskamp GGM, Maintz JBA, Wieneke GH, Viergever VA, and van Huffelen AC:** The influence of the use of realistic head geometry in the dipole localization of interictal spike activity in MTLE patients. *NFSI* 97: 84-87, 1997.

6. **Paetau R, Granstrom M, Blomstedt G, Jousmaki V, Korkman M, et al.:** Magnetoencephalography in presurgical evaluation of children with Landau-Kleffner syndrome. *Epilepcia* 40: 326-335, 1999.

7. **Rush S and Driscoll DA:** EEG electrode sensitivity - An application of reciprocity. *IEEE Trans Biomed Eng* 16: 15-22, 1969.

8. **Smith DB, Sidman RD, Flanigin H, Henke J, and Labiner D:** A reliable method for localizing deep intracranial sources of the EEG. *Neurology* 35: 1702-1707, 1985.

9. **Roth BJ, Balish M, Gorbach A, and Sato S:** How well does a three-sphere model predict positions of dipoles in a realistically shaped head? *Electroenceph and Clin Neurophysiol* 87: 175-184, 1993.

10. **Gorodnitsky IF, George JS, and Rao BD:** Neuromagnetic source imaging with FOCUSS: A recursive weighted minimum norm algorithm. *Electroenceph and Clin Neurophysiol* 95: 231-251, 1995.

11. **Pascual-Marqui RD, Michel CM, and Lehnam D:** Low resolution electromagnetic tomography: A new method for localizing electrical activity in the brain. *Int J Psychophysiol* 18: 49-65, 1994.

12. **Supek S and Aine CJ:** Simulation studies of multiple dipole neuromagnetic source localization: Model order and limits of source resolution. *IEEE Trans Biomed Eng* 40: 354-361, 1993.

13. **Achim A, Richer F, and Saint-Hilaire:** Methods for separating temporally overlapping sources of neuroelectric data. *Brain Topography* 1: 22-28, 1988.

14. **Scherg M and von Cramon D:** Two bilateral sources of the late AEP as identified by a spatio-temporal dipole model. *Electroenceph Clin Neurophysiol* 62: 290-299, 1985.

15. **Mosher JC, Lewis PS, and Leahy RM:** Multiple dipole modeling and localization from spatio-temporal MEG data. *IEEE Trans Biomed Eng* 39: 541-57, 1992.

16. **Mosher JC and Leahy RM:** Source localization using recursively applied (RAP) MUSIC. *IEEE Trans Signal Processing* 47(2): 332-340, 1999.

17. **Cuffin BN:** EEG dipole source localization. *IEEE Eng Med Biol Mag* 17(5): 118-122, 1998.

18. **Bell AJ and Sejnowski TJ:** An information-maximization approach to blind separation and blind deconvolution. *Neural Computation* 7: 1129-1159, 1995.

19. **Makeig S, Bell AJ, Jung T-P, and Sejnowski TJ:** Independent component analysis of electroencephalographic data. *Advances in Neural Information Processing Systems* 8: 145-151, 1996.

20. **Amari S, Cichocki A, and Yang HH:** A new learning algorithm for blind signal separation.In: Touretsky D et al. (Eds): *Advances in Neural Information Processing Systems*. Vol. 8, pp. 757-763, 1996.

21 **Nedler JA, Mead R:** A simplex method for function minimization. *Compt J* 7: 308-313, 1965.

22. **Plonsey R:** Volume conductor theory. In: Bronzino JD (Ed): *The Biomedical Engineering Handbook*. Boca Raton, FL: CRC Press, pp. 119-125, 1995.

23. **Wells WM, Grimson WEL, Kikinis R, and Jolesz FA:** Statistical intensity correction and segmentation of MRI data. In Proc 3rd Conf Visualization in Biomedical Computing, Rochester, NY, pp. 13-24, 1994.

24. **Schmidt JA, Johnson CR, Eason JC, and MacLeod RS:** Applications of automatic mesh generation and adaptive methods in computational medicine. In: Babuska I et al. (Eds): *Modeling, Mesh Generation, and Adaptive Methods for Partial Differential Equations*. Berlin: Springer-Verlag, pp. 367-390, 1995.

25. **Foster KR and Schwan HP:** Dielectric properties of tissues and biological materials: A critical review. *Critical Reviews in Biomed Eng* 17: 25-104, 1989.

26. **Miller CE and Henriquez CS:** Finite element analysis of bioelectric phenomena. *Critical Reviews in Biomed Eng* 18: 181-205, 1990.

27. **Yan Y, Nunez PL, and Hart RT:** Finite-element model of the human head: Scalp potentials due to dipole sources. *Med Biol Eng Comp* 29: 475-481, 1991.

28. **Jin J:** *The Finite Element Method in Electromagnetics*. New York: Wiley, 1993.

29. **Harrison RR, Aine CJ, Chen H-W, Flynn ER, and Huang M:** Investigation of methods for spatiotemporal neuromagnetic source localization. Los Alamos National Laboratory, Report LA-UR-96-2042.

30. **Glaser EM and Ruchkin DS:** *Principles of Neurobiological Signal Analysis*, New York: Academic, pp. 233-285, 1976.

31. **Jutten C and Herald J:** Blind separation of sources, part I: An adaptive algorithm based on neurometric architecture. *Signal Processing* 24: 1-10, 1991.

32. **Comon P:** Independent component analysis, a new concept? *Signal Processing* 36: 287-314, 1994.

33. **Makeig S, Jung T-P, Bell AJ, Ghahremani D, and Sejnowski TJ:** Blind separation of event-related brain responses into independent components. In *Proc Natl Acad Sci USA*, 1997.

34. **Awada KA, Jackson DR, Williams JT, Wilton DR, Baumann SB, and Papanicolaou AC:** Computational aspects of finite element modeling in EEG source localization. *IEEE Trans Biomed Eng* 44: 736-752, 1997.

35. **Salu Y, Cohen LG, Rose D, Sato S, Kufta C, and Hallett M:** An improved method for localizing electric brain dipoles. *IEEE Trans Biomed Eng* 37: 699-705, 1990.

36. **Huang M, Aine CJ, and Flynn ER:** Multi-start downhill simplex method for spatio-temporal source localization in magnetoencephalography. *Electroenceph and Clin Neurophysiol* 108: 32, 1998.

37. **Zhukov LE and Weinstein DW:** Lead field basis for FEM source localization. University of Utah, Technical Report UUCS-99-014, Oct 1999.

38. **Press WH, Teukolsky SA, Vetterling WT, and Flannery BP:** *Numerical Recipes in C*. Cambridge: Cambridge Univ. Press, 1992.

39. **Amir A:** Uniqueness of the generators of brain evoked potential maps *IEEE Trans Biomed Eng* 41: 1-11, 1994.

40. **Parker SG, Weinstein DM, and Johnson CR:** The SCIRun computational steering software system. In Arge E, Bruaset AM, and Langtangen HP (Eds): *Modern Software Tools in Scientific Computing*. Boston: Birkhauser Press, pp. 1-44, 1997.

The Weighted Diagnostic Distortion (WDD) Measure for ECG Signal Compression

Yaniv Zigel*, Arnon Cohen, and Amos Katz

Abstract—In this paper, a new distortion measure for electrocardiogram (ECG) signal compression, called weighted diagnostic distortion (WDD) is introduced. The WDD measure is designed for comparing the distortion between original ECG signal and reconstructed ECG signal (after compression). The WDD is based on PQRST complex diagnostic features (such as P wave duration, QT interval, T shape, ST elevation) of the original ECG signal and the reconstructed one. Unlike other conventional distortion measures [e.g. percentage root mean square (rms) difference, or PRD], the WDD contains direct diagnostic information and thus is more meaningful and useful.

Four compression algorithms were implemented (AZTEC, SAPA2, LTP, ASEC) in order to evaluate the WDD. A mean opinion score (MOS) test was applied to test the quality of the reconstructed signals and to compare the quality measure (MOS_{error}) with the proposed WDD measure and the popular PRD measure. The evaluators in the MOS test were three independent expert cardiologists, who studied the reconstructed ECG signals in a blind and a semiblind tests.

The correlation between the proposed WDD measure and the MOS test measure (MOS_{error}) was found superior to the correlation between the popular PRD measure and the MOS_{error}.

Index Terms—Electrocardiogram, ECG compression, distortion measures, PRD, PQRST complex, weighted diagnostic distortion.

I. INTRODUCTION

MANY algorithms for electrocardiogram (ECG) compression have been proposed in the last 30 years [1]–[17]. Until recently, all ECG compression algorithms have used simple mathematical distortion measures such as the percentage root mean square (rms) difference (PRD) for evaluating the reconstructed signal. Such measures are almost irrelevant from the point of view of diagnosis.

In this paper, a new distortion measure for ECG signal compression called weighted diagnostic distortion (WDD), based on diagnostic features is introduced.

One of the important problems in ECG compression is the definition of the error criterion. The purpose of the compression system is to remove redundancy, the irrelevant information (which does not contain diagnostic information—in the ECG case). Consequently, the error criterion has to be defined such that it will measure the ability of the reconstructed signal to preserve the relevant diagnostic information. The main problem here is that such information is subjective and is determined by the expert cardiologists perception. The problem has been defined in the past as "diagnostability" [18]. The problem of objective evaluation criteria arises in many applications where the resultant processed signal is to be presented to a human operator, such as in the case of speech and image processing [19].

Today the accepted way to examine diagnostability is to get cardiologists' evaluations of the system's performance. This solution is expensive and may be applied only for research or offline evaluation of coder's performance. Its advantage, of course, lies in the fact that it yields direct information on experts' impression. As yet, there is no mathematical measure which is correlated with diagnostic information. Such a measure is described in this paper. It has been successfully used in an ECG compression system [20], [31].

II. CONVENTIONAL DISTORTION MEASURES

In most ECG compression algorithms, the PRD measure is employed

$$PRD = \sqrt{\frac{\sum_{n=1}^{N}(x(n) - \tilde{x}(n))^2}{\sum_{n=1}^{N} x^2(n)}} \times 100 \qquad (1)$$

where $x(n)$ is the original signal, $\tilde{x}(n)$ is the reconstructed signal, and N is the length of the window over which the PRD is calculated. Some papers use a version of PRD with different normalization

$$PRD' = \sqrt{\frac{\sum_{n=1}^{N}(x(n) - \tilde{x}(n))^2}{\sum_{n=1}^{N}(x(n) - \bar{x})^2}} \times 100 \qquad (2)$$

where $\bar{x}$ is the signal's mean. Definition (2) is independent of the dc level of the original signal. Definitions (1) and (2) are of course the same, for a signal with zero mean.

In the literature, there are some other error measures for comparing original and reconstructed ECG signals [21], such as the root mean square error (rms):

$$rms = \sqrt{\frac{\sum_{n=1}^{N}(x(n) - \tilde{x}(n))^2}{N}} \qquad (3)$$

or the signal-to-noise ratio (SNR), which is expressed as

$$SNR = 10\log\left(\frac{\sum_{n=1}^{N}(x(n) - \bar{x})^2}{\sum_{n=1}^{N}(x(n) - \tilde{x}(n))^2}\right). \qquad (4)$$

Manuscript received October 27, 1999; revised June 30, 2000. *Asterisk indicates corresponding author.*

*Y. Zigel is with the Electrical and Computer Engineering Department, Ben-Gurion University, P.O. Box 653, Beer-Sheva 84105, Israel (e-mail: yaniv@ee.bgu.ac.il).

A. Cohen is with the Electrical and Computer Engineering Department, Ben-Gurion University, Beer-Sheva 84105, Israel.

A. Katz is with the Cardiology Department Faculty of Health Sciences, Ben-Gurion University, Beer-Sheva 84105, Israel.

Publisher Item Identifier S 0018-9294(00)08809-1.

The relation between the SNR and the PRD (2) is: $\text{SNR} = -20 \log(0.01 \text{PRD})$.

A maximum amplitude error [21], or peak error (MAX or PE), is also an error measure, which may be used in ECG compression; it is expressed as

$$\text{MAX} = \max_n \{|x(n) - \tilde{x}(n)|\}. \qquad (5)$$

All these error measures have many disadvantages, which all result in poor diagnostic relevance. For example, if the signal has baseline fluctuations, the variance of the signal will be higher, the PRD will be artificially lower, and the SNR will be artificially higher. Furthermore, every segment in the PQRST complex has a different diagnostic meaning and significance. A given distortion in one segment does not necessarily have the same weight as the same distortion in another segment. For example, in many patients' ECGs, the ST segment is much more diagnostically significant than the TP segment.

III. THE WDD MEASURE

The proposed WDD measure was first introduced in [22]. This measure is based on comparing the PQRST complex features of the two ECG signals, the original ECG signal and the reconstructed one (the signal recovered from the compressed signal). The WDD measures the relative preservation of the diagnostic information in the reconstructed signal. The relevant diagnostic information in the ECG signals exists in the form of PQRST complex features. The PQRST complex features (diagnostic features) are the location, duration, amplitudes, and shapes of the waves and complexes that exist in every beat (PQRST complex). These were chosen with the help of an experienced cardiologist.

A. The Diagnostic Features

The diagnostic features can be divided into three groups: **duration** features (of waves, segments, and intervals), **amplitude** features, and **shape** features. The duration features are the most significant features in most of the applications. Fig. 1 shows some amplitude and duration of the diagnostic features.

The WDD requires the extraction of the location, the amplitudes and the shapes of the PQRST waves and segments.

B. Diagnostic Feature Extraction

The main effort in the PQRST feature extraction is the segmentation, namely the determination of the exact location of the waves (Fig. 2 shows an example of PQRST waves and the location points). After segmentation, the determination of the waves amplitudes and shapes is much simpler. The strategy for finding the waves' locations is to first recognize the QRS complex, which has the highest frequency components. The T wave is recognized next, and, finally, the P wave, which is usually the smallest wave. The baseline and the ST features are relatively easily estimated later [22], [29]. Several algorithms for ECG segmentation have been suggested. Most are based on time and frequency domain recognition of the waves [23]–[26], but other methods such as for example HMM segmentation [27] have also been published.

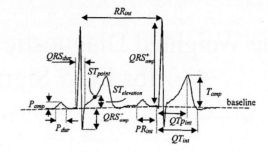

Fig. 1. Some of the amplitude and duration diagnostic features.

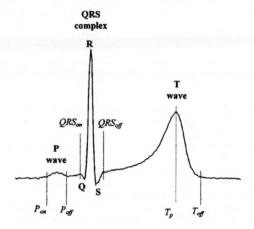

Fig. 2. PQRST waves and location points of one beat.

C. The WDD Measure

For every beat of the original signal and for the reconstructed signal, a vector of diagnostic features is defined

$$\boldsymbol{\beta}^T = [\beta_1, \beta_2, \dots, \beta_p]; \quad \text{original signal} \qquad (6)$$
$$\hat{\boldsymbol{\beta}}^T = [\hat{\beta}_1, \hat{\beta}_2, \dots, \hat{\beta}_p]; \quad \text{reconstructed signal} \qquad (7)$$

where p is the number of features in the vector, $p = 18$ is used in this work. The diagnostic parameters (β_i, $i = 1, 2, \dots, p$) were chosen to be: $RR_{\text{int}}, QRS_{\text{dur}}, QT_{\text{int}}, QTp_{\text{int}}, P_{\text{dur}}, PR_{\text{int}}, QRS_{\text{peaks}}, QRS_{\text{sign}}, \Delta_{\text{wave}}, T_{\text{shape}}, P_{\text{shape}}, ST_{\text{shape}}, QRS^+_{\text{amp}}, QRS^-_{\text{amp}}, P_{\text{amp}}, T_{\text{amp}}, ST_{\text{elevation}},$ and ST_{slope}. Table I describes these features.

The WDD between these two vectors is

$$\text{WDD}(\boldsymbol{\beta}, \hat{\boldsymbol{\beta}}) = \Delta\boldsymbol{\beta}^T \cdot \frac{\boldsymbol{\Lambda}}{\text{tr}[\boldsymbol{\Lambda}]} \cdot \Delta\boldsymbol{\beta} \times 100 \qquad (8)$$

where $\Delta\boldsymbol{\beta}$ is the normalized difference vector

$$\Delta\boldsymbol{\beta}^T = [\Delta\beta_1, \Delta\beta_2, \dots, \Delta\beta_p] \qquad (9)$$

and $\boldsymbol{\Lambda}$ is a diagonal matrix of weights, defined in (16) below.

Every scalar in this vector gives the distance between the original signal feature and the reconstructed signal feature. For the

TABLE I
DESCRIPTION OF THE DIAGNOSTIC FEATURES. (* 10 mm = 1 mV)

Feature's serial number	Feature symbol	Feature description	Units
1	RR_{int}	The time duration between the current and the previous location of the R waves	msec
2	QRS_{dur}	The time duration between the onset and the offset of the QRS complex	msec
3	QT_{int}	The time duration between QRS_{on} and T_{off}	msec
4	QTp_{int}	The time duration between QRS_{on} and T_p	msec
5	P_{dur}	The time duration between P_{on} and P_{off}	msec
6	PR_{int}	The time duration between P_{on} and QRS_{on}	msec
7	QRS_{peaks}	The number of peaks and notches in the QRS complex	(>= 1)
8	QRS_{sign}	The sign of the first peak in the QRS complex	(1 or −1)
9	$\Delta_{wave?}$	The existence of delta wave [28]	(0 or 1)
10	T_{shape}	The shape of T wave (see table 2)	
11	P_{shape}	The shape of P wave (see table 2)	
12	ST_{shape}	The shape of ST segment (see table 2)	
13	QRS_{amp}^+	The maximum positive amplitude of the QRS complex	mm
14	QRS_{amp}^-	The minimum negative amplitude of the QRS complex	mm
15	P_{amp}	The amplitude of P wave	mm
16	T_{amp}	The amplitude of T wave	mm
17	$ST_{elevation}$	The ST elevation [29]	mm
18	ST_{slope}	The ST slope [29]	mm/sec

duration features and the amplitude features, the distance is defined as

$$\Delta\beta_i = \frac{|\beta_i - \hat{\beta}_i|}{\max\{|\beta_i|, |\hat{\beta}_i|\}}. \qquad (10)$$

For the shape features (T_{shape}, P_{shape}, and ST_{shape}), the distance is determined by fixed penalty matrices $\mathbf{W}^i = \{w^i_{\beta_i, \hat{\beta}_i}\}$ $i \in (T_{shape}, P_{shape}, ST_{shape})$(one matrix for each shape feature)

$$\mathbf{W}^i = \begin{bmatrix} w^i_{11} & w^i_{12} & \cdots & w^i_{1Z_i} \\ w^i_{21} & w^i_{22} & \cdots & w^i_{2Z_i} \\ \vdots & \vdots & \ddots & \vdots \\ w^i_{Z_i 1} & w^i_{Z_i 2} & \cdots & w^i_{Z_i, Z_i} \end{bmatrix} \qquad (11)$$

where Z_i is the number of shapes for the relevant feature ($Z_P = 9$ for P_{shape}, $Z_{ST} = 5$ for ST_{shape}, and $Z_T = 3$ for T_{shape}). Each element of the penalty matrices $w^i_{\beta_i \hat{\beta}_i}$ is the cost measure or the distance between the shape code β_i and the shape code $\hat{\beta}_i$ of the original shape feature and the reconstructed one, respectively ($\beta_i, \hat{\beta}_i \in 1, 2, \ldots, Z_i$). $w^i_{\beta_i \hat{\beta}_i}$ is determined such that its value is between 0 to 1, $w^i_{\beta_i \hat{\beta}_i} = 0$ for $\beta_i = \hat{\beta}_i$, and $w^i_{\beta_i \hat{\beta}_i} = w^i_{\hat{\beta}_i \beta_i}$. For the shape features, the distance $\Delta\beta_i$ is given as:

$$\Delta\beta_i = w^i_{\beta_i \hat{\beta}_i}. \qquad (12)$$

Table II describes the shape features and their codes.

The values of the matrices $\mathbf{W}^i$ $i \in (T_{shape}, P_{shape}, ST_{shape})$ that were used in this work were

$$\mathbf{W}^T = \begin{bmatrix} 0 & .2 & .4 \\ .2 & 0 & .2 \\ .4 & .2 & 0 \end{bmatrix} \qquad (13)$$

$$\mathbf{W}^P = \begin{bmatrix} 0 & .2 & .2 & .2 & .3 & .2 & .2 & .2 & .4 \\ .2 & 0 & .1 & .1 & .3 & .4 & .4 & .4 & .2 \\ .2 & .1 & 0 & .1 & .3 & .4 & .4 & .4 & .2 \\ .2 & .1 & .1 & 0 & .3 & .4 & .4 & .4 & .2 \\ .3 & .3 & .3 & .3 & 0 & .3 & .3 & .3 & .3 \\ .2 & .4 & .4 & .4 & .3 & 0 & .1 & .1 & .2 \\ .2 & .4 & .4 & .4 & .3 & .1 & 0 & .1 & .2 \\ .2 & .4 & .4 & .4 & .3 & .1 & .1 & 0 & .2 \\ .4 & .2 & .2 & .2 & .3 & .2 & .2 & .2 & 0 \end{bmatrix} \qquad (14)$$

$$\mathbf{W}^{ST} = \begin{bmatrix} 0 & .1 & .2 & .1 & .4 \\ .1 & 0 & .2 & .4 & .1 \\ .2 & .2 & 0 & .2 & .2 \\ .1 & .4 & .2 & 0 & .1 \\ .4 & .1 & .2 & .1 & 0 \end{bmatrix} \qquad (15)$$

where the shapes are numbered as Table II shows.

The types of shapes were determined using an experienced cardiologist, and the penalty matrices were determined arbitrarily using the subjective logic of noncardiologist.

The algorithm for the estimation of shape features may be found in [29].

TABLE II
THE CODING OF THE WDD SHAPE FEATURES

Code / Shape feature	1	2	3	4	5	6	7	8	9
P_{shape}	biphasic II	notched negative	pulmonale negative	negative	flat	positive	pulmonale positive	notched positive	biphasic I
T_{shape}	positive	flat	negative						
ST_{shape}	straight positive	concave	flat	convex	straight negative				

Λ [in (8)] is a diagonal weighting matrix

$$\Lambda = \mathrm{diag}[\lambda_i]; \quad \lambda_i > 0; \quad (i = 1, 2, \ldots, p). \quad (16)$$

This matrix provides a way to emphasize certain parameters or regions in the ECG complex. When compressing the ECG of a certain subject, the matrix Λ may be adjusted to match the effects of the specific pathology (for example emphasizing the ST segment). Note that in (8) the WDD is normalized to the sum of the weights. The values of the weights: $\lambda_i, i = 1, \ldots, p$ which were determined for checking the algorithm, are determined to be as shown in (17) at the bottom of the page.

For the sake of this work, the weights were determined arbitrarily using the subjective logic of a noncardiologist. In practice, the weights should reflect the relevant clinical importance of the features. The extraction of the diagnostic features used for the WDD is described in [29]. Some other feature extraction algorithms may be used. Of course, lack of precision in the extraction is a source of error and can affect the WDD score of a reconstructed signal.

IV. THE MEAN OPINION SCORE (MOS) TEST

In order to analyze the proposed WDD measure, a reference qualitatively based distortion measure is needed, which represents the "true" quality of every reconstructed signal ("gold" standard). Therefore, MOS test was performed, which contained a blind test and a semiblind test (these two tests, in medical terms, are **single**-blind tests, because the tested signals are known to the test manager but not to the test evaluators—the cardiologists). The evaluators for this test were three experienced cardiologists. The results of this MOS test are combined in a distortion measure, called: MOS_{error}. Every tested signal (reconstructed ECG signal), was printed on paper, in the form and the scale that a cardiologist is used to seeing.

The aim of the **blind-test** was to get the cardiologists' evaluation of reconstructed signals from different compression algo-

TABLE III
THE BLIND MOS TEST QUESTIONNAIRE

analysis of ECG signal No. ###

1. Details of tester

Name: _____

Date: _____

2. General quality score for the signal (circle one number)

1 – very bad , 2 – almost tolerable , 3 – tolerable , 4 - good , 5 – excellent

3. Interpretation (circle one interpretation for each parameter)

Parameter	Interpretation							
	1	2	3	4	5	6	7	8
1 P	normal	pulmonale	mitrale	abnormal	non-specific	unable to decode	____	abnormal
2 QRS	normal	IVCD	LBBB	RBBB	delta wave	pace maker	unable to decode	abnormal
3 T	normal	positive	negative	biphasic	symmetric	a-symmetric	unable to decode	abnormal
4 ST	normal	depressed	elevated	flat	unable to decode	other	____	abnormal
5 abnormal beats	none	PVC's	VF	bradycardia	pace maker	AV-block	other	____

4. Comments:

rithms without knowing the source of each tested signal (original, reconstructed and the compression method). In every test, the cardiologist was given one strip of signal (marked by a serial number), which contained the unknown signal and some mean estimated features (see example in Fig. 3). The signal was one channel, 27 seconds in duration [29]. For every tested signal, the cardiologist was asked to fill a questionnaire, which is shown in Table III.

The aim of the **semiblind test** was to get cardiologists' evaluation of reconstructed signals from different compression algorithms by comparing each of the reconstructed signals (without knowing the compression method) to the original signal. In every test, the cardiologist was given one strip of signal, which contained the original signal (marked as "original") and the reconstructed signal (marked as "reconstructed"). 13.5 seconds were allocated for each signal (see example in

$$\Lambda = \mathrm{diag}[2 \quad 1 \quad 1 \quad 1 \quad 1 \quad 1 \quad 1 \quad 0.25 \quad 0.25 \quad 1 \quad 1 \quad 1 \quad 2 \quad 2 \quad 1 \quad 1 \quad 1 \quad 1] \quad (17)$$

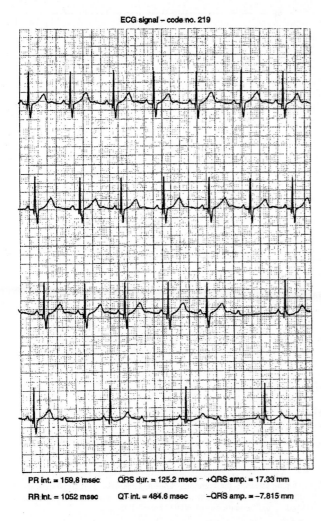

ECG signal – code no. 219

| PR int. = 159.8 msec | QRS dur. = 125.2 msec | +QRS amp. = 17.33 mm |
| RR int. = 1052 msec | QT int. = 484.6 msec | –QRS amp. = –7.815 mm |

Fig. 3. One of the strips used for the blind test. Each line is the continuation of the previous line (total duration is 27 seconds). The vertical grid lines are 0.2 second (5 mm) apart. The horizontal grid lines are 0.5 mV (5 mm) apart. The feature values on the bottom are the mean values.

Fig. 4). The evaluator was aware of which strip is original and which is reconstructed, however he was not aware of the compression algorithm and its parameters. For every tested signal, the cardiologist was asked to fill a questionnaire, which is shown in Table IV.

A **weighted MOS error** was calculated from the results of the blind and semiblind tests of three independent cardiologists for every tested signal.

For the blind test, the MOS error (MOS_k^B) of one tested signal is the relative error (in percentage) between the evaluation of the reconstructed signal and the evaluation of the suitable original signal. The MOS error of one tested signal from the kth cardiologist is given by

$$\mathrm{MOS}_k^B = factor \times \max\left\{\frac{S_o - S_t}{S_o}, 0\right\} \times 100$$
$$+ (1 - factor)\frac{\sum_{i=1}^{5} |\mathrm{sgn}(I_{ti} - I_{oi})|}{5} \times 100 \quad (18)$$

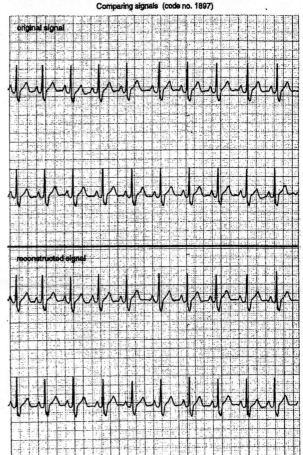

Comparing signals (code no. 1897)

original signal

reconstructed signal

Fig. 4. One of the strips used for the semiblind test.

TABLE IV
THE SEMI-BLIND MOS TEST QUESTIONNAIRE

Comparison of ECG signal No. ### with its original signal

1. Details of tester
   Name: _____
   Date: _____

2. The measure of similarity between the original signal and the reconstructed one (circle one number):

1	2	3	4	5
completely different				identical

3. Would you give a different diagnosis with the tested signal if you had not seen the original signal? (circle YES or NO),

YES	NO

4. Comments:

where

S_t general quality score of the reconstructed signal (1–5);

S_o general quality score of the original signal (1–5);

I_{ti} interpretation of the ith parameter of the reconstructed signal (1–8);

I_{oi} interpretation of the ith parameter of the original signal (1–8);

factor   weighting coefficient between the general quality score and the interpretation (in the experiments performed here: $factor = 0.5$);

k number of the testing cardiologist.

The MOS error for the blind-test of one tested signal from all N cardiologists ($N = 3$) was then calculated by

$$\text{MOS}^B = \frac{\sum_{k=1}^{N} \text{MOS}_k^B}{N} \qquad (19)$$

For the semiblind test, the MOS error (by percentage) of one tested signal from the k_{th} cardiologist is given by:

$$\text{MOS}_k^{SB} = factor \times \frac{5-C}{5} \times 100 + (1 - factor)$$
$$\times (1 - D) \times 100 \qquad (20)$$

where

C measure of similarity between the original signal and the reconstructed one (1–5);

D answer to the Boolean question about the diagnosis (0—YES, 1—NO);

factor   weighting coefficient between the measure of similarity and the Boolean question ($factor = 0.5$).

For the semiblind test, the MOS error of one tested signal from all N cardiologists ($N = 3$) is given by

$$\text{MOS}^{SB} = \frac{\sum_{k=1}^{N} \text{MOS}_k^{SB}}{N}. \qquad (21)$$

The **MOS error** of one tested signal is given by

$$\text{MOS}_{\text{error}} = \frac{\text{MOS}^B + \text{MOS}^{SB}}{2}. \qquad (22)$$

The lower the value of the $\text{MOS}_{\text{error}}$ the better the quality evaluation of the reconstructed signal. This is perhaps different from other applications (such as the speech MOS test), where the higher the value of the MOS the better the signal quality. The $\text{MOS}_{\text{error}}$ in this work was defined as such in order to be similar to the PRD/WDD measures.

V. RESULTS AND DISCUSSION

Four compression algorithms were implemented in order to yield reconstructed signals with different qualities. The reconstructed signals were used for analysis and comparison between the WDD and the PRD measure. The ECG signals were taken from the MIT-BIH Arrhythmia database [30] and the compression algorithms were chosen to be: analysis by synthesis ECG compressor (ASEC) with WDD minimization and with PRD minimization [20], [31], LTP [13], SAPA2 [8], and AZTEC [3]. These compressors were chosen, because AZTEC and SAPA2 are often referred for comparison in the literature, and ASEC and LTP are two of the best ECG compressors available today. ECG records from the MIT-BIH database (records: 104, 107, 111, 112, 115, 116, 118, 119, 201, 207, 208, 209, 212, 213, 214, 228, 231, and 232) were used in the evaluation. These signals were chosen by an experienced cardiologist and they consist of a large variety of pathological cases. Every original signal was

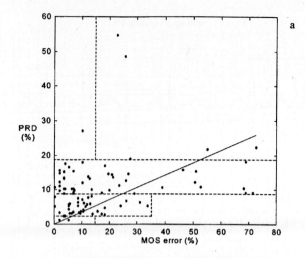

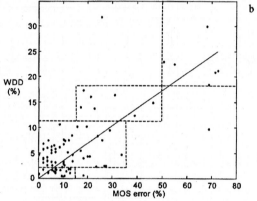

Fig. 5. The scattering of the distortion measures for the reconstructed signals. (the sloping lines are the regression lines and the dashed rectangles are the quality areas of reconstructed signals. (a) The scattering of PRD versus $\text{MOS}_{\text{error}}$, (b) The scattering of WDD versus $\text{MOS}_{\text{error}}$.

preprocessed to have zero mean and flat baseline. From these 18 original signals, 92 reconstructed records were produced. For every reconstructed signal, three distortion measures were calculated: WDD, PRD, and $\text{MOS}_{\text{error}}$ (from the MOS test described before). The $\text{MOS}_{\text{error}}$ was used as the "gold standard".

Fig. 5 shows the scattering of the distortion measures for the reconstructed signals. Each point represents the distortion values of one reconstructed record. Fig. 5(a) shows the scattering of PRD versus $\text{MOS}_{\text{error}}$, and Fig. 5(b) shows the scattering of WDD versus $\text{MOS}_{\text{error}}$.

The results were analyzed in two ways:

1) A measure of deviation from the regression line between two distortion measures was defined. It is given as the variance of the points' vertical deviation from the regression line

$$\text{VAR} = \frac{\sum_{i=1}^{n}(r_i - \mu_r)^2}{n} \qquad (23)$$

where

r_i vertical deviation of the ith point from the regression line;

n total number of points (signals);

μ_r mean value of r_i; ($i = 1, \ldots, n$).

TABLE V
QUALITY GROUPS DEFINED BY MOS_{error}

MOS error:	0		15		35		50	
Quality of tested signal	very good		good		not good		bad	

The regression line (the linear lines in Fig. 5) and the variance were calculated with the MATLAB function *regress.m*, which was programmed using equations from [32].

The deviation variance between the PRD and the MOS error [Fig. 5(a)] is 80.91, and the deviation variance between the WDD and the MOS error [Fig. 5(b)] is 22.04, four times better than the PRD case.

2) A rough classification of signal quality was defined by dividing the MOS_{error} into four quality groups [33]. These are shown in Table V.

The ability of the distortion measure (PRD or WDD) to predict the quality of the ECG record was then examined. For every tested measure (PRD and WDD), four prediction ranges were determined. Fig. 6 shows the PRD and WDD values of each quality group of signals and these ranges.

The boundaries (thresholds) of each prediction range were manually determined, such that all the signals in the prediction range (except 3% outliers) would be included in a minimum number of quality groups. For example, Th_L in the PRD was determined to be 2. For this value, all the signals in the first prediction range (PRD: 0–2) belong to the "very good" quality group. Th_M in the same case was determined to be 9, because for this value, all the signals in the second prediction range (PRD: 2–9) belong to the "very good" and "good" quality groups—the minimum number of quality groups.

Table VI shows the prediction ranges of the tested measures and their quality group connection (confusion matrix). Every number (p_{ij}) inside the 4 × 4 matrix, is the percentage of signals from the ith prediction range, which belong to the jth quality group (including outliers).

Table VI demonstrates the prediction ability of the two distortion measures. For example, if some signal has a PRD between 9%–19%, one can not determine its quality group, while the range of WDD between 12–18 predicts a quality group of "good" or "not good". The percentage numbers on the main diagonal represent the correct prediction. The mean correct prediction of the WDD is 59% while that of the PRD is only 40.5%. Furthermore, let us define normalized prediction error as follows:

$$\varepsilon_p = \frac{1}{4}\sum_{i=1}^{4}\frac{\sum_{j=1}^{4}\rho_{ij}p_{ij}}{\sum_{k=1}^{4}\rho_{ik}} \qquad (24)$$

where ρ_{ij} is the weight of the ith row and the jth column, defined as follows:

$$\rho_{ij} = |i - j|. \qquad (25)$$

The normalized prediction error of the WDD is 10.25% while that of the PRD is 20.4%.

The superiority of the WDD over the PRD is clearly demonstrated by these results.

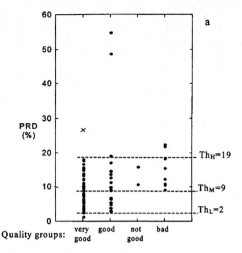

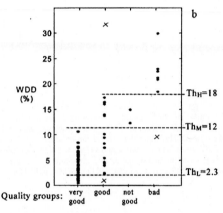

Fig. 6. The scattering and thresholds of the prediction ranges for each quality group of reconstructed signals (outliers are marked with x). (a) For the PRD measure, (b) for the WDD measure.

TABLE VI
MEASURES' RANGES AND QUALITIES CONNECTION

PRD Range	Quality Groups					WDD Range	Quality Groups			
	very good	good	not good	bad			very good	good	not good	bad
0 - 2	100	0	0	0		0 – 2.3	95	5	0	0
2 - 9	76	24	0	0		2.3 - 12	71	27	0	2
9 - 19	55	23	5	17		12 - 18	0	71	29	0
19 - 60	17	50	0	33		18 - 40	0	14	0	86

Fig. 7 shows an example of original ECG signal (from MIT-BIH record 214) and two extremely "bad" quality reconstructed signals. Observing these signals and the MOS_{error} values, one can say that these reconstructed signals are definitely "bad" quality signals.

Fig. 8 shows an example of two "very good" quality reconstructed signals. Observing these signals and the MOS_{error} values, one can say that these reconstructed signals are "very good" quality signals.

Note that the PRD value for the "bad" SAPA2 reconstructed signal [Fig. 7(c)] is 9.2%, which is less than the PRD value (15.41%) for the "very good" ASEC reconstructed signal

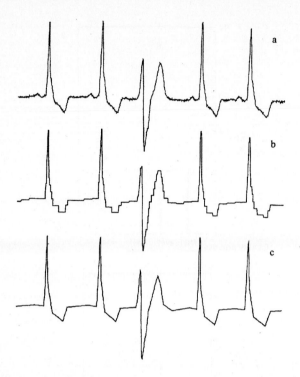

Fig. 7. Example of bad quality reconstructed signals. (a) Original ECG signal (MIT-BIH record 214), (b) reconstructed signal, which was compressed by the AZTEC algorithm. The distortion values for this signal are: $MOS_{error} = 67.9\%$, $PRD = 10.6\%$, and $WDD = 30.1\%$, (c) reconstructed signal, which was compressed by the SAPA2 algorithm. The distortion values for this signal are: $MOS_{error} = 71.2\%$, $PRD = 9.2\%$, and $WDD = 21\%$.

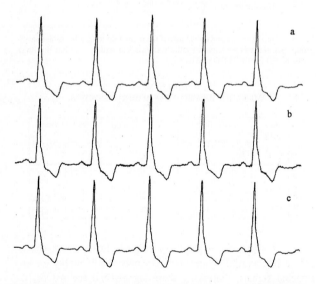

Fig. 8. Example of very good quality reconstructed signals. (a) Original ECG signal (MIT-BIH record 214), (b) reconstructed signal, which was compressed by the LTP algorithm. The distortion values for this signal are: $MOS_{error} = 12.1\%$, $PRD = 7.88\%$, and $WDD = 7.55\%$ (note the addition of high frequency low amplitude noise), (c) reconstructed signal, which was compressed by the ASEC algorithm (with WDD minimization). The distortion values for this signal are: $MOS_{error} = 3.33\%$, $PRD = 15.41\%$, and $WDD = 3.52\%$.

[Fig. 8(c)]. This is a clear example of the diagnostic irrelevance of the PRD measure.

The ASEC consists of WDD minimization, and it is superior to most available compression algorithms. A detailed information and results of this compression algorithm can be found in [20], [29], and [31].

The PRD measure has the advantage of low complexity. It is very inexpensive to calculate the PRD. We emphasize again that when using the PRD, care must be taken to remove the baseline (to have zero and flat baseline), or, at least, to eliminate the dc component of the signal.

The WDD measure is well correlated with cardiologists' perception. Its disadvantage is the fact that it is expensive to calculate. In cases where the automatic diagnostic features are required for other purposes than compression (screening, monitoring, alarms), this may not be a disadvantage. The WDD may be calculated in real time by a digital signal coprocessor, or by a sufficiently powerful CPU.

Based on the results reported here, it is concluded that the proposed WDD measure is much more suitable for evaluating ECG reconstructed signals than the popular PRD measure.

REFERENCES

[1] J. P. Abenstein and W. J. Tompkins, "A new data reduction algorithm for real time ECG analysis," *IEEE Trans. Biomed. Eng.*, vol. BME-29, pp. 43–48, Jan. 1982.

[2] G. D. Barlas and E. S. Skordalakis, "A novel family of compression algorithms for ECG and other semiperiodical, one dimensional, biomedical signals," *IEEE Trans. Biomed. Eng.*, vol. 43, Aug. 1996.

[3] J. R. Cox, F. M. Nolle, H. A. Fozzard, and C. G. Oliver, "AZTEC, a preprocessing program for real time ECG rhythm analysis," *IEEE Trans. Biomed. Eng.*, vol. 15, pp. 128–129, Apr. 1968.

[4] B. Furht and A. Perez, "An adaptive real-time ECG compression algorithm with variable threshold," *IEEE Trans. Biomed. Eng.*, vol. 35, pp. 489–494, June 1988.

[5] D. J. Hamilton, D. C. Thomson, and W. A. Sandham, "ANN compression of morphologically similar ECG complexes," *Med. Biol. Eng. Comput.*, vol. 33, pp. 841–843, Nov. 1995.

[6] P. S. Hamilton and W. J. Tompkins, "Compression of the ambulatory ECG by average beat subtraction and residual differencing," *IEEE Trans. Biomed. Eng.*, vol. 38, pp. 253–259, Mar. 1991.

[7] M. L. Hilton, "Wavelet and wavelet packet compression of electrocardiograms," *IEEE Trans. Biomed. Eng.*, vol. 44, May 1997.

[8] M. Ishijima, S. B. Shin, G. H. Hostetter, and J. Sklansky, "Scan along polygon approximation for data compression of electrocardiograms," *IEEE Trans. Biomed. Eng.*, vol. BME-30, pp. 723–729, Nov. 1983.

[9] S. M. Jalaleddine and C. G. Hutchens, "SAIES—A new ECG data compression algorithm," *J. Clin. Eng.*, vol. 15, no. 1, pp. 45–51, Jan./Feb. 1990.

[10] S. M. Jalaleddine, C. G. Hutchens, R. D. Strattan, and W. A. Coberly, "ECG data compression techniques—A unified approach," *IEEE Trans. Biomed. Eng.*, vol. 37, pp. 329–343, Apr. 1990.

[11] G. B. Moody, K. Soroushian, and R. G. Mark, "ECG data compression for tapeless ambulatory monitors," *Comput. Cardiol. 1988*, pp. 467–470, 1988.

[12] T. Uchiyama, K. Akazawa, and A. Sasamori, "Data compression of ambulatory ECG by using multi-template matching and residual coding," *IEICE Trans. Inform. Syst.*, vol. E76-D, no. 12, pp. 1419–1424, Dec. 1993.

[13] G. Nave and A. Cohen, "ECG compression using long term prediction," *IEEE Trans. Biomed. Eng.*, vol. 40, pp. 877–885, Sept. 1993.

[14] C. Paggetti, M. Lusini, M. Varanini, A. Taddei, and C. Marchesi, "A multichannel template based data compression algorithm," *Comput. Cardiol. 1994*, pp. 629–632, 1994.

[15] A. G. Ramakrishnan and S. Supratim, "ECG coding by wavelet-based linear prediction," *IEEE Trans. Biomed. Eng.*, vol. 44, Dec. 1997.

[16] U. E. Ruttiman and H. V. Pipberger, "Compression of the ECG by prediction or interpolation and entropy encoding," *IEEE Trans. Biomed. Eng.*, vol. 26, pp. 613–623, Nov. 1979.

[17] S. C. Tai, "ECG data compression by corner detection," *Med. and Biol. Eng. and Comp.*, vol. 30, pp. 584–590, Nov. 1992.

[18] A. Cohen, P. M. Poluta, and R. Scott-Millar, "Compression of ECG signals using vector quantization," in *Proc. IEEE-90 S. A. Symp. Communications and Signal Proc., COMSIG-90*, 1990, pp. 45–54.

[19] W. B. Kleijn and K. K. Paliwal, *Speech Coding and Synthesis*, Amsterdam, The Netherlands: Elsevier, 1995.

[20] Y. Zigel, A. Cohen, and A. Katz, "ECG signal compression using analysis by synthesis coding," *IEEE Trans. Biomed. Eng.*, vol. 47, pp. 1308–1316, Oct. 2000.

[21] M. Ishijima, "Fundamentals of the decision of optimum factors in the ECG data compression," *IEICE Trans. Inf. and Sys.*, vol. E76-D, no. 12, Dec. 1993.

[22] Y. Zigel, A. Cohen, and A. Katz, "A diagnostic meaningful distortion measure for ECG compression," in *Proc. 19th Conf. IEEE in Israel*, 1996, pp. 117–120.

[23] F. Gritzali, G. Frangakis, and G. Papaconstantinou, "Detection of P and T waves in ECG," *Comput. Biomed. Res.*, vol. 22, pp. 83–91, 1989.

[24] P. S. Hamilton and W. J. Tompkins, "Quantitative investigation of QRS detection rules using the MIT/BIH arrhythmia database," *IEEE Trans. Biomed. Eng.*, vol. 33, Dec. 1986.

[25] P. Laguna, N. V. Thakor, P. Caminal, R. Jane, and H.-R. Yoon, "New algorithm for QT interval analysis in 24-hour Holter ECG: Performance and applications," *Med. Biol. Eng. Comput.*, vol. 28, pp. 67–73, Jan. 1990.

[26] O. Pahlm and L. Sornmo, "Software QRS detection in ambulatory monitoring—A review," *Med. Biol. Eng. Comput.*, pp. 289–297, July 1984.

[27] A. Koski, "Modeling ECG signals with HMM," *A.I. in Med.*, vol. 8, pp. 453–471, 1996.

[28] R. J. Huszar, *Basic Dysrhythmias: Interpretation & Management*, 2nd ed. St. Louis, MO: Mosby Lifeline, 1994.

[29] Y. Zigel, "ECG Signal Compression," M.Sc. Thesis, Ben-Gurion University, Beer-Sheva, Israel, Aug. 1998. [Online]. Available: http://www.ee.bgu.ac.il/~spl/publication.

[30] G. B. Moody, *The MIT-BIH Arrhythmia Database CD-ROM*, 2nd ed: Harvard-MIT Division of Health Sciences and Technology, Aug. 1992.

[31] Y. Zigel, A. Cohen, A. Abu-Ful, A. Wagshal, and A. Katz, "Analysis by synthesis ECG signal compression," *Comput. Cardiol. 1997*, vol. 24, pp. 279–282, 1997.

[32] N. R. Draper and H. Smith, *Applied Regression Analysis*, 2nd ed. New York: Wiley, 1981.

[33] Y. Zigel and A. Cohen, "On the optimal distortion measure for ECG compression," *Proc. Eur. Medical & Biological Eng. Conf., EMBEC 99*, vol. 37, pp. 1618–1619, Nov. 1999.

[34] A. Cohen and Y. Zigel, "Compression of multichannel ECG through multichannel long-term prediction," *IEEE Eng. Med. Biol. Mag*, vol. 17, no. 1, pp. 109–115, Jan./Feb. 1998.

[35] A. Cohen, *Biomedical Signal Processing*. Boca Raton, FL: CRC, 1986.

[36] A. Gersho and R. M. Gray, *Vector Quantization and Signal Compression*. Norwell, MA: Kluwer Academic Publishers, 1992.

[37] N. S. Jayant and P. Noll, *Digital Coding of Waveforms*. Englewood Cliffs, NJ: Prentice-Hall, 1984.

[38] A. M. Kondoz, *Digital Speech*. New York: Wiley, 1994.

[39] G. B. Moody and R. G. Mark, "The MIT-BIH arrhythmia database in CD-ROM and software for use with it," *Comput. Cardiol.*, vol. 17, pp. 185–188, 1990.

[40] J. G. Proakis, *Digital Communications*, 3rd ed. New York: McGraw-Hill, 1995.

[41] K. Sayood, *Introduction to Data Compression*. San Mateo, CA: Morgan Kaufmann, 1996.

[42] W. J. Tompkins, *Biomedical Digital Signal Processing*. Englewood Cliffs, NJ: Prentice-Hall, 1993.

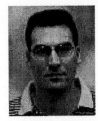

Yaniv Zigel was born in Tel-Aviv, Israel, in 1970. He received the B.Sc. and M.Sc. degrees in electrical and computer engineering from the Ben-Gurion University, Beer-Sheva, Israel, in 1992 and in 1998, respectively. He is working toward the Ph.D. degree at the Department of Electrical and Computer Engineering of the same university.

From 1992–1995, he was a Technical Officer at the communication and computer corps in the Israeli Defense Forces (IDF). Currently, he is working as a Teaching and Research Assistant at the Department of Electrical and Computer Engineering of the Ben-Gurion University. His research interests include one-dimensional signal processing, signal compression, and speech and speaker recognition.

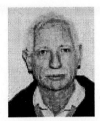

Arnon Cohen was born in Haifa, Israel, in 1938. He received the B.Sc. and M.Sc. degrees in electrical engineering from the Technion-Israel Institute of Technology, Haifa, Israel, in 1964 and 1966, respectively, and the Ph.D. degree in electrical and biomedical engineering, from Carnegie-Mellon University, Pittsburgh, PA, in 1970.

Since 1972, he has been with the Department of Electrical and Computer Engineering, and the Biomedical Engineering Program, Ben-Gurion University, Beer-Sheva, Israel, where he is a Professor of Electrical and Biomedical Engineering. His research interests are in signal processing, mainly with biomedical and speech applications. He is the author of *Biomedical Signal Processing*, (Boca Raton, Fl: CRC, 1986).

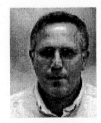

Amos Katz was born in Ramat Gan, Israel, in 1952. He received the M.D. degree from the Faculty of Health Sciences at Ben Gurion University of the Negev, Beer Sheva, Israel. He was trained in cardiology at the Soroka Medical Center, Beer Sheva, and in electrophysiology at the St. Vincent Hospital, Indianapolis, IN.

He is currently the Director of the Electrophysiology Laboratory at the Soroka Medical Center. He is a Senior Lecturer in Cardiology in the Faculty of Health Sciences and Vice Dean for Student Affairs at Ben Gurion University. His research interests are in cardiac electrophysiology, sudden death, pacemakers, implantable defibrillators, and heart rate variability.

Section 5:

G.F. Cooper

Center for Biomedical Informatics
University of Pittsburgh
Pittsburgh, Pennsylvania, USA

Synopsis

Knowledge Processing and Decision Support Systems

The section on knowledge processing and decision support systems contains four papers. One paper highlights methodological issues in developing and evaluating predictive clinical models. Although the emphasis is on artificial neural networks, most of the points apply to all types of predictive models. The remaining three papers in the section are about guidelines. Two evaluate guidelines that are integrated into the physicians' workflow; they show increased physician compliance with the use of computer-based guidelines. The other describes a novel method for converting decision models into guidelines; this paper describes a pilot study that shows relatively high user subjective satisfaction with the generated guidelines. The remainder of this synopsis discusses each paper in turn.

A clinical decision support system for prevention of venous thromboembolism

The first paper, which is by Durieux et al. [1], describes the evaluation of physician compliance with a guideline-based clinical decision-support system. The system recommends anticoagulant therapy for surgical patients as a prophylactic measure to prevent venous thromboembolism.

The clinical guideline for thromboembolism prophylaxis was developed locally. Clinicians complied with the guideline about 95% of the time in the intervention period, during which the decision-support system presented the guideline. When the system was removed, clinician practice reverted back to near a pre-intervention level of about 84%. On the whole, this pattern is consistent with the results of previously published studies of reminder systems. It further shows that even *locally* developed guidelines are not heeded automatically, but rather, require continual reminding to be highly effective.

The decision-support system improved the clinical practice of all clinicians except one, whose guideline compliance was close to 100% during the non-intervention (control) period. The greatest improvement in guideline compliance was observed among the five surgeons who operated on fewer than 40 patients.

The greatest effect of the decision-support system was for patients at moderate risk for venous thromboembolism. It is understandable that a decision-support system might have the most influence on decision making for those patients in the "gray area" (e.g., moderate risk patients). For those patients at low or at high risk, the best decision may be more obvious.

On the misuses of artificial neural networks for prognostic and diagnostic classification in oncology

The second paper, which is by Schwarzer et al.[2], discusses problems with how artificial neural networks (ANN) are derived and evaluated. Although the paper focuses on ANN models, the caveats are applicable for most predictive modeling techniques. Indeed, it is not clear that more traditional statistical models (e.g., logistic regression models) are being derived and evaluated in a manner that is any better than for ANNs.

The paper describes how feedforward neural network models are a generalization of logistic regression models. As pointed out, a more expressive modeling methodology may in theory be able to generate better (i.e., more predictive) models, but any given application of the methodology may not actually result in a better model. Models that are highly expressive (and therefore highly "tunable") are particularly subject to overfitting, which can inhibit predictive performance. Overfitting occurs when the model is tuned too closely to the training (derivation) data in ways that do not correspond well to the process that is generating the data. The paper illustrates the problem and describes how penalty terms can attenuate it. Although not mentioned, Bayesian approaches to learning neural networks intrinsically include such penalty terms [3]. These and other advanced approaches for deriving ANNs are described in papers at [4]. On the whole, current ANN researchers are aware of the problems that were reviewed by Schwarzer et al. and are avoiding those problems. As this paper indicates, however, recent application of those methods by clinical researchers is lagging behind.

Schwarzer et al. describe problems in evaluating ANNs. It is worth noting that the evaluation of most predictive models is subject to these same problems. For example, validating a model only on the dataset that was used to derive the model is usually a bad idea, regardless of the type of model being validated. The paper mentions the use of cross-validation methods as a way of efficiently using the data, while avoiding a biased evaluation. The computer-intensive nature of these methods is rarely a problem nowadays, and these methods are being used routinely in machine-learning research.

Beyond ANNs, other statistical and machine-learning methodologies continue to be explored. For example, in recent years, increasing attention has been focused on Support Vector Machines (SVM) and related methodologies [5,6]. Hopefully the current paper by Schwarzer et al. [2] will lessen the chance that a similar paper will need to be written in ten years about the misuses of SVMs for prognostic and diagnostic classification.

Assessment of decision support for blood test ordering in primary care

The paper by van Wijk et al. [7] studies physician compliance with a computer-based guideline for blood-test ordering, which was integrated into the physicians' workflow. The physician control group received an electronically displayed list of possible blood tests, which were organized to highlight 15 tests that cover most of the clinical situations in primary care.

Seventy four percent of the eligible practices participated in the study. Among the physicians receiving the guideline, 71% of their orders were generated by using the decision-support system.

Overall, there was 20% more reduction in test ordering for those physicians who used the guideline versus those in the control group. Interestingly, the reduction was due primarily to a decrease in the ordering of some specific tests. For example, there was a marked reduction in the number of tests for creatinine, but little reduction in the number of tests for sodium. Like the Durieux et al. [1] study discussed above, this investigation by van Wijk et al. indicates that the impact of a guideline on clinician behavior can be selective in interesting and at times non-obvious ways.

Design and pilot evaluation of a system to develop computer-based site-specific practice guidelines from decision models

The paper by Sanders et al. [8] introduces a method for converting a decision model (e.g., a decision tree) into a clinical guideline that is made available on the web. By modifying the parameters in the decision model, the guideline can be tailored to a clinical site or even a particular patient. Doing so may make decision support more accessible, relevant, and helpful.

The paper describes a pilot study that involved participants from the authors' department and program who used the decision-model-generated guideline versus a control guideline from the literature. The domain area was the treatment of non-small cell lung cancer.

Results show that the decision-model-generated guideline was rated relatively highly by the participants. As the paper points out, however, the participants were not blinded to the source of the guideline they used, and thus the possibility of a rating bias is a concern. Therefore, the results are quite preliminary. Nonetheless, the approach seems sound and promising.

Discussion

The four papers in this section provide solid contributions in the area of knowledge processing and decision support systems. Several trends are suggested, which this author believes will continue for many years to come.

Traditionally, a clinical guideline or model has been developed from knowledge and data at one or a few study sites and then applied (perhaps with ad hoc modification) at many local clinical sites. Increasingly, these guidelines and models are likely to be automatically or semi-automatically tailored based on local knowledge and data. Taken to its logical conclusion, this trend leads to patient-specific computer-based guidelines and models.

A closely related issue is the use of experimental and observational data in the development of guidelines and models. Experimental studies, such as randomized controlled trials, often provide the most trustworthy methods we have for establishing causal relationships from clinical data. Such studies, while potentially highly informative, may not always be safe, ethical, logistically feasible, or financially worthwhile. Observational data are passively observed. Such data are more readily available than experimental data and, indeed, most clinical databases are observational. As clinical data become more and more routinely recorded electronically, the opportunities for using such local observational data increase. Interestingly, recent analyses of the literature indicate that experimental and observational studies often yield similar predictions about the direction and magnitude of causal relationships in clinical medicine [9, 10]. These results suggest that both experimental and observational data have powerful roles to play in deriving clinical knowledge of cause and effect. Increasingly, it is likely that the data from (typically) *non-local* experimental studies will be tailored using data from *local* observational databases in order to develop clinical guidelines and models that are applied locally. Such approaches will leverage the power of both experimental and observational data [11].

Finding a bridge between the development of sophisticated diagnostic, predictive, and therapeutic models and the presentation of such models to clinical users is likely to remain an important issue. Although at the present time the targeted users are usually clinicians, increasingly there are likely to be other users (particularly patients) of the underlying computer-based clinical models. Each user will

be able to provide their own input into the models and receive tailored output. As one example, direct computer-based assessment of patient symptoms, preferences and subjective outcomes is likely to grow significantly in the years ahead [12].

The evaluation of computer-based clinical guidelines and models will continue to be critically important. Such studies are usually expensive in terms of time and money. As our understanding of such evaluations develops, it seems likely we will see sophisticated computer-based tools that assist in designing, performing, and analyzing such experiments in a manner that is both efficient and sound.

References

1. Durieux P, Nizard R, Ravaud P, Mounier N, Lepage E. A clinical decision support system for prevention of venous thromboembolism: Effect on physician behavior. JAMA 2000;283:2816-21.
2. Schwarzer G, Vach W, Schumacher M. On the misuses of artificial neural networks for prognostic and diagnostic classification in oncology. Stat Med 2000;19:541-61.
3. MacKay DJC. Bayesian methods for supervised neural networks. In: Arbib MA, editor. The Handbook of Brain Theory and Neural Networks. Cambridge, MA: M.I.T. Press; 1995. p. 144-9.
4. NIPS Online website at http://nips.djvuzone.org/
5. Cristianini N, Shawe-Taylor J. An Introduction to Support Vector Machines. Cambridge, U.K.: Cambridge University Press; 2000.
6. Herbrich R, Graepel T, Campbell C. Bayes point machines. Journal of Machine Learning Research 2001;1:245-279 (Available at http://www.ai.mit.edu/projects/jmlr/papers/volume1/herbrich01a/herbrich01a.pdf).
7. van Wijk MAM, van der Lei J, Mosseveld M, Bohnen AM, Van Bemmel JH. Assessment of decision support for blood test ordering in primary care: A randomized trial. Ann Intern Med 2001;134:274-81.
8. Sanders GD, Nease RF, Owens DK. Design and pilot evaluation of a system to develop computer-based site-specific practice guidelines from decision models. Med Decis Making 2000;20:145-59.
9. Benson K, Hartz AJ. A comparison of observational studies and randomized, controlled trials. N Engl J Med 2000;342: 1878-86.
10. Ioannidis JPA, Haidich AB, Pappa M, Pantazis N, Kokori SI, Tektonidou MG, et al. Comparison of evidence of treatment effects in randomized and nonrandomized studies. JAMA 2001;286:821-30.
11. Cooper GF, Yoo C. Causal discovery from a mixture of experimental and observational data. In: Proceedings of the Conference on Uncertainty in Artificial Intelligence; Morgan Kaufmann; 1999. p. 116-25.
12. Treadwell JR, Soetikno RM, Lenert LA. Feasibility of quality-of-life research on the Internet: A follow-up study. Qual Life Res 1999;8:743-7.

Address of the author
Gregory F. Cooper, M.D., Ph.D.
Center for Biomedical Informatics
University of Pittsburgh
Suite 8084 Forbes Tower
200 Lothrop Street
Pittsburgh, PA 15213-2582
U.S.A.
E-mail: gfc@cbmi.upmc.edu

A Clinical Decision Support System for Prevention of Venous Thromboembolism

Effect on Physician Behavior

Pierre Durieux, MD, MPH

Rémy Nizard, MD

Philippe Ravaud, MD, PhD

Nicolas Mounier, MD

Eric Lepage, MD, PhD

COMPUTER-BASED CLINICAL DEcision support systems (CDSSs) are defined as "any software designed to directly aid in clinical decision making in which characteristics of individual patients are matched to a computerized knowledge base for the purpose of generating patient-specific assessments or recommendations that are then presented to clinicians for consideration."[1] Clinical decision support systems have been promoted for their potential to improve the quality of health care by supporting clinical decision making. In particular, it has been suggested that physicians have difficulties processing complex information[2] and will improve their prescription practices in response to electronically delivered recommendations.[3] However, given their rapid rate of development and the limited range of clinical settings in which they have been tested to date, it has been stressed that CDSSs should be rigorously evaluated before widespread introduction into clinical practice.[1,4]

In clinical hospital practice, venous thromboembolism remains a serious problem and pulmonary embolism is a major cause of death.[5] Fatal pulmo-

Context Computer-based clinical decision support systems (CDSSs) have been promoted for their potential to improve quality of health care. However, given the limited range of clinical settings in which they have been tested, such systems must be evaluated rigorously before widespread introduction into clinical practice.

Objective To determine whether presentation of venous thromboembolism prophylaxis guidelines using a CDSS increases the proportion of appropriate clinical practice decisions made.

Design Time-series study conducted between December 1997 and July 1999.

Setting Orthopedic surgery department of a teaching hospital in Paris, France.

Participants A total of 1971 patients who underwent orthopedic surgery.

Intervention A CDSS designed to provide immediate information pertaining to venous thromboembolism prevention among surgical patients was integrated into daily medical practice during three 10-week intervention periods, alternated with four 10-week control periods, with a 4-week washout between each period.

Main Outcome Measure Proportion of appropriate prescriptions ordered for anticoagulation, according to preestablished clinical guidelines, during intervention vs control periods.

Results Physicians complied with guidelines in 82.8% (95% confidence interval [CI], 77.6%-87.1%) of cases during control periods and in 94.9% (95% CI, 92.5%-96.6%) of cases during intervention periods. During each intervention period, the appropriateness of prescription increased significantly ($P<.001$). Each time the CDSS was removed, physician practice reverted to that observed before initiation of the intervention. The relative risk of inappropriate practice decisions during control periods vs intervention periods was 3.8 (95% CI, 2.7-5.4).

Conclusions In our study, implementation of clinical guidelines for venous thromboembolism prophylaxis through a CDSS used routinely in an orthopedic surgery department and integrated into the hospital information system changed physician behavior and improved compliance with guidelines.

JAMA. 2000;283:2816-2821   www.jama.com

nary embolism may occur in up to 1% of general surgery patients and 3% of orthopedic surgical patients who do not receive prophylaxis.[6] The most efficient way to prevent both fatal and nonfatal venous thromboembolism is to use

Author Affiliations: Department of Public Health, Faculté de Médecine Broussais Hôtel Dieu (Dr Durieux), Department of Orthopedics, Lariboisière Hospital, Assistance Publique–Hôpitaux de Paris (Dr Nizard), Epidemiology Unit, Bichat Hospital, Assistance Publique–Hôpitaux de Paris (Dr Ravaud), Paris, France; and the Department of Biostatistics and Medical Informatics, Henri Mondor Hospital, Assistance Publique–Hôpitaux de Paris, Créteil, France (Drs Mounier and Lepage).
Corresponding Author: Pierre Durieux, MD, MPH, Santé Publique, Faculté de Médecine Broussais Hôtel Dieu, 15 rue de l'Ecole de Médecine, 75006 Paris, France (e-mail: pierre.durieux@egp.ap-hop-paris.fr).
Reprints not available from the author.

routine prophylaxis for moderate- to high-risk patients. Despite the publication of several clinical guidelines for venous thomboembolism prophylaxis in both Europe and North America[6-9] as well as studies suggesting that prophylaxis remains underused, few studies aimed at improving prophylaxis practices have been performed.[10,11] One probable reason is that optimal decisions about the use of anticoagulants in prevention of venous thromboembolism require access to a large amount of complex information to evaluate the degree of risk of hospitalized patients. We have developed a CDSS to implement clinical guidelines on venous thromboembolism prophylaxis in an orthopedic surgery department. In this study, we evaluated the effect of this system on physician behavior. We aimed to determine whether real-time presentation of venous thromboembolism prophylaxis guidelines through a CDSS increases the proportion of appropriate anticoagulant prescriptions ordered and whether this behavior change was extinguished after discontinuing use of the CDSS.

METHODS
Study Site and Population

The study was conducted in the orthopedic surgery department of Lariboisière Hospital, a 1000-acute-bed teaching hospital of the Assistance Publique–Hôpitaux de Paris group (the Paris, France, metropolitan area public hospital network). About 2400 patients are hospitalized annually in this department. All surgeons (7 full-time, 7 part-time) working in the orthopedic surgery department were involved in the study. All orthopedic patients who underwent surgery in the department (from December 1997 to July 1999) were included in the study.

The Assistance Publique–Hôpitaux de Paris Institutional Review Board determined that, according to French policy, the study was exempt from review requirement and could be conducted without informed consent from patients.

Table 1. Guidelines for Venous Thromboembolism Prophylaxis*

Surgical Risk Level	Patient Risk Level	Venous Thromboembolism Risk Level
1	1	Low (No treatment recommended)
	2	
2	3	Moderate (Low dosage of low-molecular-weight heparin recommended)
	1	
	2	
3	3	High (High dosage of low-molecular-weight heparin recommended)
	1	
	2	
	3	

*See "Methods" section of text for details. See Table 2 for explanation of patient and surgical risk levels.

Guideline and Software Development

Clinical guidelines for venous thromboembolism prophylaxis were developed at Assistance Publique–Hôpitaux de Paris.[12,13] These local guidelines for general surgery, urologic surgery, gynecologic surgery, and orthopedic surgery were created by local hospital experts. In this study, assessment of guideline use with and without the CDSS was restricted to orthopedic surgery patients.

The risk of thromboembolism in a hospital patient depends on the planned surgical procedure (or the reason for admission) and on preexisting patient-related variables. Each of these factors has been classified in existing guidelines as low, moderate, or high risk.[6-9] There is no published classification of risk that combines patient risk factors and surgical risk factors to obtain an overall risk of venous thromboembolism. However, taking into account both types of risk for a given patient is crucial in clinical practice. Thus, the local hospital expert group proposed a classification system in which, for each patient, the presence of patient risk factors and surgical risk factors are combined to classify patients as having a low, moderate, or high risk for venous thromboembolism. A prophylactic strategy is recommended for each level of risk. When the risk level is low, no medication is recommended; when the risk level is moderate, prescription of a low dosage of low-molecular-weight heparin is recommended; and when the risk level is high, prescription of a high

dosage of low-molecular-weight heparin is recommended (TABLE 1).

Our CDSS is an online computer application designed as a tool to provide clinicians with relevant, real-time information pertaining to venous thromboembolism prevention among surgical patients. This application is linked to the diagnosis related group–based information system that is implemented in all French hospitals. Patients' administrative and clinical data are collected by direct entry in admitting, operating room, and medical care units. These data are stored in a coded and integrated clinical patient database and are available for computer-assisted decision making.

The CDSS can be accessed through computer terminals available just outside each operating room. Following each surgical procedure, after entering an identification code, the physician enters data related to the clinical situation of the patient (age, sex, disease, surgical procedure, and preexisting patient and surgical risk factors of venous thromboembolism). The physician orders all treatments necessary for patient follow-up (eg, antibiotic therapy, pain management, immobilization), including venous thromboembolism prophylaxis, through the computer system. The computer system critiques the orders using data contained in the patient's database and guideline-based criteria stored in the system's knowledge base. If the computer detects a discrepancy between the prescription and the corresponding information in the database, the physician is immediately notified via a message on the computer screen suggesting the appropriate prescription and explaining the reasons. The physician can choose to maintain or change his/her order. At the end of the process, the patient follow-up and prescription information, including venous thromboembolism prophylaxis, is printed out and included in the patient's file.

Study Design

The study had an alternating time-series design, with three 10-week intervention periods, four 10-week control periods, and a 4-week washout between each period.

During intervention periods, physicians received a message from the CDSS if their prescriptions were not appropriate according to the guidelines. During control periods, physicians ordered all treatment related to thromboembolism prophylaxis through the computer system but received no critiquing messages from the CDSS.

Outcome Measures

To evaluate the effects of the CDSS, the proportion of venous prophylaxis prescriptions that was appropriate according to clinical guidelines was considered to be the main end point. This proportion was estimated based on the final prescription order for each patient compared with treatment designated by algorithms established prior to the study and derived from the guidelines. Each prescription could be classified as appropriate or not appropriate. A prescription was classified as not appropriate when no medication was ordered by the physician when the CDSS recommended prescription of low-molecular-weight heparin (type 1 error), when the wrong dosage of low-molecular-weight heparin was prescribed (type 2 error), or when a prescription of low-molecular-weight heparin was made when the CDSS proposed no medication (type 3 error).

The percentage of inappropriate initial prescriptions that were changed after advice was given by the CDSS during intervention periods was also calculated according to each level of risk of venous thromboembolism. We also recorded the number of pulmonary embolisms and deep vein thromboses diagnosed in the orthopedic department during the study period.

Statistical Analysis

Analysis included all eligible patients. Comparisons of clinical characteristics of patients during intervention and control periods were tested using the χ^2 test and the *t* test where appropriate. The nominal significance level for the end points was .05 (2-sided formulation).

Table 2. Characteristics of Patients Enrolled During Control and Intervention Periods

Characteristics	Control Periods	Intervention Periods
No. of patients	1112	859
Mean age, y	51.1	52.2
Length of intervention, min	77.2	80.4
Male, No. (%)	484 (47.1)	430 (50.8)
Patient Risk		
No. (%) of patients		
Level 1 (no risk factors)	411 (37.0)	270 (31.4)
Level 2	658 (59.2)	551 (64.1)
Age >40 y	654 (58.8)	559 (65.1)
Combined oral contraceptive	15 (1.3)	19 (2.2)
Heart failure	13 (1.2)	14 (1.6)
Preoperative bed rest >4 d	34 (3.1)	39 (4.5)
Venous insufficiency	24 (2.2)	29 (3.4)
Presurgery acute infection	15 (1.3)	9 (1.1)
Postpartum (1 mo)	81 (7.3)	74 (8.7)
Obesity	18 (1.6)	21 (2.4)
Level 3	43 (3.9)	38 (4.4)
Recent or metastatic malignancy	23 (2.1)	23 (2.7)
Previous deep vein thrombosis or pulmonary embolism	3 (0.3)	0 (0)
Lower limb paralysis	8 (0.7)	6 (0.7)
Myeloproliferative disease	9 (0.8)	8 (0.9)
Thrombophilia	2 (0.2)	6 (0.7)
Surgical Risk		
No. (%) of patients		
Level 1	402 (36.1)	302 (35.2)
Upper limb surgery	363 (32.7)	286 (33.3)
Diagnostic arthroscopy	3 (0.2)	6 (0.7)
Foot surgery	35 (3.1)	22 (2.6)
Device removal	16 (1.4)	9 (1.1)
Herniated disk surgery	2 (0.2)	0 (0)
Level 2	53 (4.8)	40 (4.6)
Lower limb immobilization	2 (0.2)	3 (0.4)
Spine surgery (without neurological impairment)	36 (3.2)	26 (3.0)
Therapeutic arthroscopy	20 (1.8)	13 (1.5)
Level 3	657 (59.1)	517 (60.2)
Spine surgery (with neurological impairment)	4 (0.4)	9 (1.1)
Hip surgery and surgery of the pelvis	633 (56.9)	509 (59.3)
Lower limb trauma	22 (2.0)	0 (0)
Multiple trauma	0 (0)	0 (0)
Venous Thromboembolism Risk		
No. (%) of patients		
Low risk	397 (35.7)	299 (34.8)
Moderate risk	58 (5.2)	40 (4.6)
High risk	657 (59.1)	520 (60.6)

To evaluate the effect of the decision-making application on appropriateness of prescription, we first chose the patient as the unit of analysis because the patient experiences the care and generates the original data. Then we took into account as a unit of analysis the physician (eg, the sequence of prescriptions of 1 physician). We accounted for the potential nonindependence of patient observations of a physician resulting from clustering by using a logistic regression model for binary data with random effect. We assumed that only the intercept, not the decision-making application effect, varies among physicians. The decision-making application effect was tested using the logit of the probability of appropriateness as response, while the period (control vs intervention) was considered the explicative covariate. The intercept was regarded as a random effect and the period as a fixed effect. Model parameters were estimated using the iteratively reweighted restricted likelihood method and fixed effects were tested with the Fisher exact test (SAS GLIMIX macro).[14] Mean probability of appropriateness of prescription according to study period was then generated by taking the exponential transformation of the logit.

All statistical analyses were performed using SAS version 6.12 computer software (SAS Institute Inc, Cary, NC).

RESULTS

A total of 1971 patients were included in the study; 1112 during control periods and 859 during intervention periods. The computer system was used in 100% of patients who underwent surgery during the study period. Patient characteristics were comparable in the intervention and control periods, except for patient risk factors. There were more patients with no preexisting risk factors during the control periods than in the intervention periods (36.9% vs 31.5%; $P=.04$). However, distribution of venous thromboembolism risks were comparable in the 2 groups (TABLE 2). A total of 696 patients (35.3%) were at low risk of venous thromboembolism,

98 patients (5.0%) were at moderate risk, and 1177 patients (59.7%) were at high risk. During the study period, the mean number of patients per surgeon was 141 (range, 4-370). Five surgeons operated on fewer than 40 patients each and 8 surgeons operated on more than 100 patients.

Physicians complied with guidelines in 82.8% (95% confidence interval [CI], 77.6%-87.1%) of cases during control periods and in 94.9% (95% CI, 92.5%-96.6%) of cases during intervention periods. Logistic regression analysis, performed using the physician as the unit of analysis, demonstrated a significant physician effect ($P<.001$) and a significant difference between the 2 study periods on appropriateness of prescription ($P<.001$). The relative risk of inappropriateness was 3.8 (95% CI, 2.7-5.4) for control periods vs intervention periods, equivalent to a 73% reduction in risk of inappropriate prescription.

Results according to period are shown in the FIGURE. During each intervention period, the proportion of appropriate prescriptions ordered increased significantly. Each time the CDSS was removed, physician compliance with guidelines reverted to that observed before initiation of the intervention.

Results according to venous thromboembolism risk are shown in TABLE 3. A total of 191 prescriptions (17.2%) were judged inappropriate by the CDSS during control periods and 113 prescriptions (13.2%) were judged inappropriate during intervention periods. Among these 113 prescriptions, 69 (61.1%) were modified by the physician according to the recommendation of the CDSS and 44 (38.9%) remained unchanged. Overall, the effect of the CDSS was greatest for patients at moderate risk of venous thromboembolism. In this group, 18 (81.8%) of 22 inappropriate prescriptions were changed after advice given by the CDSS. The CDSS appeared to have less effect for patients at high risk of venous thromboembolism. In this group, 24 (51.1%) of 47 inappropriate prescriptions were changed.

TABLE 4 presents the number of errors by type for the 191 inappropriate

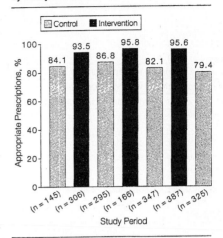

Figure. Appropriateness of Prescription by Study Period

For intervention periods, data are percentages of appropriate prescriptions ordered after opportunity to correct initial decision. See "Study Design" for a description of the study periods.

prescriptions ordered during the control periods and the 44 inappropriate prescriptions that were not changed during the intervention periods. The system did not allow for analysis of the 69 initial prescriptions that were changed according to the recommendation. During intervention periods, the error rate decreased by 86% for type 1 errors, by 59% for type 2 errors, and by 66% for type 3 errors.

The CDSS improved the clinical practice of all physicians except 1 whose proportion of appropriate prescriptions was close to 100% during control periods. The greatest improvement was observed among the 5 surgeons who operated on fewer than 40 patients.

One pulmonary embolism and 2 deep vein thromboses were diagnosed during control periods. No pulmonary embolisms and 2 deep vein thromboses were diagnosed during intervention periods.

COMMENT

Our study showed that implementation of clinical guidelines for venous thromboembolism prophylaxis through a CDSS in an orthopedic surgery department significantly changed physician behavior and improved compliance with guidelines. The improvement was

Table 3. Appropriate and Inappropriate Prescriptions According to Venous Thromboembolism Risk During Intervention and Control Periods*

| | Venous Thromboembolism Risk | | | | | | | |
| | Low | | Moderate | | High | | Total | |
	C (n = 397)	I (n = 299)	C (n = 58)	I (n = 40)	C (n = 657)	I (n = 520)	C (n = 1112)	I (n = 859)
Initial prescription was appropriate	344 (86.7)	255 (85.3)	3 (5.7)	18 (45.0)	574 (87.4)	473 (91)	921 (82.8)	746 (86.8)
Initial prescription was not appropriate	53 (13.3)	44 (14.7)	55 (94.3)	22 (55.0)	83 (12.6)	47 (9.0)	191 (17.2)	113 (13.2)
And was changed after advice given by the CDSS	...	27 (9.0)	...	18 (45.0)	...	24 (4.6)	...	69 (8.0)
And remained inappropriate after advice given by the CDSS	...	17 (5.7)	...	4 (10.0)	...	23 (4.4)	...	44 (5.1)
Total appropriate prescriptions	344 (86.7)	282 (94.3)	3 (5.7)	36 (90)	574 (87.4)	497 (95.6)	921 (82.8)	815 (94.9)

*Data are number (percentage) of prescriptions. C indicates control period; I, intervention period; CDSS, clinical decision support system; and ellipses, data not applicable.

Table 4. Inappropriate Prescriptions by Type of Error*

	Control Periods (n = 1112)	Intervention Periods (n = 859)†
Total No. of errors	191 (17.2)	44 (5.1)
Error type		
1	65 (5.8)	7 (0.8)
2	73 (6.6)	23 (2.7)
3	53 (4.8)	14 (1.6)

*Data are number (percentage) of total prescriptions. Type 1 errors indicate no medication was ordered by the physician when prophylaxis was recommended; type 2 errors, wrong dosage of medication was prescribed; and type 3 errors, medication was ordered by the physician when prophylaxis was not recommended.
†Data are not available for prescriptions changed according to the guidelines.

greater for patients at moderate risk of venous thromboembolism than for patients at high risk of venous thromboembolism where practices were already appropriate for more than 90% of patients before any intervention. In patients with elective hip surgery and hip fractures, drug regimens including subcutaneous heparin and low-molecular-weight heparin have been proven effective in prevention of deep vein thrombosis[6-8] and this strategy is well accepted by French surgeons. However, the moderate risk constitutes a gray zone of uncertainties and is more difficult to define. Physicians may also have difficulty remembering the guidelines for this category involving relatively few patients (5% of the total). This explains the dramatic effect of the CDSS on physician behavior concerning this subgroup of patients during intervention periods. For the same group, the percentage of appropriate initial prescriptions (before advice was given by the CDSS) was much more important

during intervention periods (45%) than during control periods (5.7%). Due to a Hawthorne effect, the physicians involved in the study were probably more watchful when the CDSS was in use than when it was not in use. This was an indirect effect of the CDSS.

The CDSS reduced all types of errors but its input seemed to be particularly important for type 1 errors (failure to order a medication when prophylaxis was recommended).

Our study contributes several important considerations to the understanding of the potential role of CDSSs in clinical guideline implementation. First, this study confirms that use of a CDSS at the time of prescription constitutes an effective guideline implementation strategy.[15-18] A significant effect on physician behavior was observed despite a high baseline compliance to guidelines (84.1%) before intervention. In 2 recent studies performed in surgical and medical-surgical patients, 86% and 85%, respectively, received venous thromboembolism prophylaxis before any intervention.[10,19]

The CDSS was able to maintain a sustained effect of guidelines for a relatively long period. Failure to do so constitutes a major weakness of most guideline implementation strategies, including paper reminders.[20,21] The guidelines can also be easily updated on the CDSS, which facilitates the implementation over time of up-to-date guidelines.[15,16]

The CDSS was integrated into the daily practice of physicians. Thus, all consecutive patients who underwent

surgery during the study period were included in the study. Since the computer system was used as a data collection tool, it was easy to evaluate the effect of the system.

Second, when we designed the CDSS, we chose to establish a critiquing system rather than a reminding system. Such critiquing systems, which advise clinicians about what should be done after a prescription contrary to guidelines has been ordered, have been commonly applied.[22] A simple reminder system that notifies clinicians before prescription of tasks that should be done probably can be disregarded more easily by the clinician. A critiquing system can also be used on a routine basis to calculate physician deviation rates before intervention, thus facilitating efforts toward continuous quality improvement.[23]

Third, some investigators have considered that reminding or alerting clinicians about what constitutes appropriate practice is a continuing medical education strategy.[24] The rate of reversion of compliance to guidelines to baseline values during each control period, even after 15 months, showed that a CDSS cannot be considered an educational tool or that education alone is unable to sustain substantial changes in physician practice as has been suggested previously.[25,26]

Our study had several limitations. The clinical guidelines, particularly the combination of patient- and surgery-related risk factors used to generate venous thromboembolism risk, were developed locally and may not be acceptable to other groups of physicians. The CDSS was implemented in 1 department of 1 hospital and, therefore, the applicability of our results to other settings is unknown. Another limitation is that we evaluated the effect of implementing a CDSS on process, not on patient outcomes. The number of pulmonary embolisms and deep vein thromboses diagnosed among patients during their hospital stay is insufficient to evaluate patient outcomes since a thromboembolism event can occur after discharge. However, the aim of the CDSS was to increase the appropriateness of prophylaxis, not to demonstrate a relationship between prophylaxis and thromboembolism. In addition, there is no noninvasive, accurate, and inexpensive diagnostic test to identify patients with deep vein thrombosis.[27] The difficulties in interpreting outcomes are widely recognized.[28] Numerous authors now consider it better to evaluate process rather than outcomes when assessing quality of care.[29-31] Outcomes have multiple determinants and it is impossible to know what proportion of a given health outcome is determined by quality factors (ie, processes and structure of care) and what proportion is due to patient-related risk factors.[32] Interpretation of health outcomes is hampered by the problem of case-mix.[28] Statistical analyses require an adequate number of outcomes for the results to be meaningful.[29,32] Conversely, the use of process measures can identify specific shortcomings (eg, proportion of inappropriate prescriptions) and point toward what needs to be changed.[28]

Clinical decision support systems have been successfully implemented for preventive care, drug dosing, and management of diseases.[1] Our study shows that implementation of clinical guidelines for venous thromboembolism prophylaxis through a CDSS used routinely in an orthopedic surgery ward and integrated into a computerized hospital information system significantly changed physician behavior and improved compliance with guidelines. This system, integrated in the daily practice of physicians, appeared to constitute a way to obtain a sustained effect of clinical guidelines. Given the limited range of clinical settings and health systems in which CDSSs have been tested, it is important to evaluate such systems on physician behavior.

Funding/Support: This study was supported by the Direction des Hôpitaux, Ministère de l'Emploi et de la Solidarité (Projets Hospitaliers de Recherche Clinique, Délégation à la Recherche Clinique d'Ile de France grant AOM 95-239).

Acknowledgment: We thank Cédric Belliot for data management, the physicians at the Department of Orthopedics of Lariboisière Hospital, and Laurent Sedel, MD, head of the department. We especially thank Michael Fine, MD, University of Pittsburgh, Pittsburgh, Pa, for comments during preparation of the manuscript. We also acknowledge the contribution of the physicians who participated in the development of the clinical guidelines, particularly Yves Chapuis, MD (Cochin Hospital, Paris, France), president of the expert group, Meyer Samama, MD (Hôtel Dieu, Paris, France), and Marc Samama, MD (Pitié-Salpétrière Hospital, Paris, France).

REFERENCES

1. Hunt DL, Haynes RB, Hanna SE, Smith K. Effects of computer-based clinical decision support systems on physician performance and patient outcome: a systematic review. *JAMA.* 1998;280:1339-1346.
2. Weed LL, Weed L. Opening the black box of clinical judgment—an overview. *BMJ.* 1999;319:1279.
3. Schiff GD, Rucker D. Computerized prescribing: building the electronic infrastructure for better medication usage. *JAMA.* 1998;279:1024-1029.
4. Evans RS, Pestotnik SL, Classen DC, et al. A computer-assisted management program for antibiotics and other anti-infective agents. *N Engl J Med.* 1998;338:232-238.
5. Anderson FA, Wheeler HB, Goldberg RJ, et al. A population-based perspective of the hospital incidence and case-fatality rates of deep vein thrombosis and pulmonary embolism. *Arch Intern Med.* 1991;151:933-938.
6. Clagett GP, Anderson FA, Heit J, Levine MN. Prevention of thromboembolism. *Chest.* 1995;108:312S-334S.
7. Prophylaxie des thromboses veineuses profondes et des embolies pulmonaires post-opératoires (chirurgie générale, gynécologique et orthopédique). *Ann Fr Anesth Reanim.* 1991;10:417-421.
8. Nicolaides AN, Arcelus J, Belcaro G, et al. Prevention of venous thromboembolism: European Consensus Statement. *Int Angiol.* 1992;1:151-159.
9. Thromboembolic Risk Factors (THRIFT) Consensus Group. Risk of and prophylaxis for venous thromboembolism in hospital patients. *BMJ.* 1992;305:567-574.
10. Anderson FA, Wheeler HB, Goldberg RJ, Hosmer DW, Forcier A, Patwardhan NA. Changing clinical practice: prospective study of the impact of continuing medical education and quality assurance programs on use of prophylaxis for venous thromboembolism. *Arch Intern Med.* 1994;154:669-677.
11. Patterson R. A computerized reminder for prophylaxis of deep vein thrombosis in surgical patients. *Proc AMIA Symp.* 1998:573-576.

12. Durieux P, Ravaud P. From clinical guidelines to quality assurance: the experience of Assistance Publique–Hôpitaux de Paris. *Int J Qual Health Care.* 1997;9:215-219.
13. Ravaud P, Durieux P, Fourcade A, and the Comité Scientifique Thrombose AP-HP. Prophylaxie des thromboses veineuses post-opératoires: recommendations de l'Assistance Publique–Hôpitaux de Paris. *Sang Thromb Vaisseaux.* 1995;7:119-129.
14. Wolfinger R, O'Connell M. Generalized linear mixed models: a pseudo-likelihood approach. *J Stat Comput Simulation.* 1993;48:233-243.
15. NHS Centre for Reviews and Dissemination. Implementing clinical practice guidelines: can guidelines be used to improve medical practice? *Effective Health Care.* 1994;8:1-12.
16. Oxman AD, Thomson MA, Davis DA, Haynes RB. No magic bullets: a systematic review of 102 trials of interventions to improve professional practice. *CMAJ.* 1995;153:1423-1431.
17. Shea S, DuMouchel W, Bahamonde L. A meta-analysis of 16 randomized controlled trials to evaluate computer-based clinical reminder systems for preventive care in the ambulatory setting. *J Am Med Inform Assoc.* 1996;3:399-409.
18. Balas EA, Austin SM, Mitchell JA, Ewigman BG, Bopp KD, Brown GD. The clinical value of computerized information services: a review of 98 randomized clinical trials. *Arch Fam Med.* 1996;5:271-278.
19. Ryskamp RP, Trottier SJ. Utilization of venous thromboembolism prophylaxis in a medical-surgical ICU. *Chest.* 1998;113:162-164.
20. McNally E, de Lacey G, Lowell P, Welch T. Posters for accident departments: simple method of sustaining reduction in x-ray examinations. *BMJ.* 1995;310:640-642.
21. Auleley G-R, Ravaud P, Giraudeau B, et al. Implementation of the Ottawa ankle rules in France. *JAMA.* 1997;277:1935-1939.
22. Randolph AG, Haynes RB, Wyatt JC, Cook DJ,

Guyatt GH. Users' guides to the medical literature, XVIII: how to use an article evaluating the clinical impact of a computer-based clinical decision support system. *JAMA.* 1999;282:67-74.
23. Schriger DL, Baraff LJ, Rogers WH, Cretin S. Implementation of clinical guidelines using a computer charting system: effect on the initial care of health care workers exposed to body fluids. *JAMA.* 1997;278:1585-1590.
24. Davis DA, Thomson MA, Oxman AD, Haynes B. Changing physician performance: a systematic review of the effect of continuing medical education strategies. *JAMA.* 1995;274:700-705.
25. Soumerai SB, McLaughlin TJ, Avorn J. Improving drug prescribing in primary care: a critical analysis of the experimental literature. *Milbank Q.* 1989;67:268-317.
26. Weingarten SR, Riedinger MS, Conner L, et al. Practice guidelines and reminders to reduce duration of hospital stay for patients with chest pain. *Ann Intern Med.* 1994;120:257-263.
27. Goldhaber SZ, Morpurgo M, for the WHO/International Society and Federation of Cardiology Task Force. Diagnosis, treatment, and prevention of pulmonary embolism. *JAMA.* 1992;268:1727-1733.
28. Davies HT, Crombie IK. Assessing the quality of care. *BMJ.* 1995;311:766.
29. Mant J, Hicks N. Detecting differences in quality of care: the sensitivity of measures of process and outcomes in treating acute myocardial infarction. *BMJ.* 1995;311:793-796.
30. Brook RH, McGlynn EA, Cleary PD. Quality of health care: measuring quality of care. *N Engl J Med.* 1996;335:966-970.
31. McKee M. Indicators of clinical performance: problematic, but poor standards of care must be tackled. *BMJ.* 1997;315:142.
32. Hammermeister KE. Participatory continuous improvement. *Ann Thorac Surg.* 1994;58:1815-1821.

Design and Pilot Evaluation of a System to Develop Computer-based Site-specific Practice Guidelines from Decision Models

GILLIAN D. SANDERS, PhD, ROBERT F. NEASE, JR., PhD,
DOUGLAS K. OWENS, MD, MSc

Background. Local tailoring of clinical practice guidelines (CPGs) requires experts in medicine and evidence synthesis unavailable in many practice settings. The authors' computer-based system enables developers and users to create, disseminate, and tailor CPGs, using normative decision models (DMs). *Methods.* ALCHEMIST, a web-based system, analyzes a DM, creates a CPG in the form of an annotated algorithm, and displays for the guideline user the optimal strategy. ALCHEMIST's interface enables remote users to tailor the guideline by changing underlying input variables and observing the new annotated algorithm that is developed automatically. In a pilot evaluation of the system, a DM was used to evaluate strategies for staging non–small-cell lung cancer. Subjects ($n = 15$) compared the automatically created CPG with published guidelines for this staging and critiqued both using a previously developed instrument to rate the CPGs' usability, accountability, and accuracy on a scale of 0 (worst) to 2 (best), with higher scores reflecting higher quality. *Results.* The mean overall score for the ALCHEMIST CPG was 1.502, compared with the published-CPG score of 0.987 ($p = 0.002$). The ALCHEMIST CPG scores for usability, accountability, and accuracy were 1.683, 1.393, and 1.430, respectively; the published CPG scores were 1.192, 0.941, and 0.830 (each comparison $p < 0.05$). On a scale of 1 (worst) to 5 (best), users' mean ratings of ALCHEMIST's ease of use, usefulness of content, and presentation format were 4.76, 3.98, and 4.64, respectively. *Conclusions.* The results demonstrate the feasibility of a web-based system that automatically analyzes a DM and creates a CPG as an annotated algorithm, enabling remote users to develop site-specific CPGs. In the pilot evaluation, the ALCHEMIST guidelines met established criteria for quality and compared favorably with national CPGs. The high usability and usefulness ratings suggest that such systems can be a good tool for guideline development. *Key words*: clinical practice guidelines; computer-based systems; normative decision models; guideline development. **(Med Decis Making 2000;20:145–159)**

Rising health care costs, combined with documented variation in practice patterns,[1-8] have pro-

Received February 10, 1999, from the Center for Primary Care and Outcomes Research, Department of Medicine, Stanford University, Stanford, California (GDS, DKO); the Division of General Medical Sciences, Washington University School of Medicine Washington University, St. Louis, Missouri (RFN); the VA Palo Alto Health Care System, Palo Alto, California (DKO); and Stanford Medical Informatics, Department of Medicine, Stanford University (GDS, DKO). Revision accepted for publication October 13, 1999. Presented at the 20th annual meeting of the Society for Medical Decision Making. Boston, Massachusetts, October 25–28, 1998. Dr. Owens is supported by a Career Development Award from the VA Health Services Research and Development Service.

Address correspondence and reprint requests to Dr. Sanders: Center for Primary Care and Outcomes Research, 179 Encina Commons, Room 182, Stanford, CA 94305-6019; telephone: (650) 723-0407; fax: (650) 723-1919; e-mail: ⟨sanders@stanford.edu⟩.

duced widespread interest in methods for improving quality of care, and in dissemination of guidelines for clinical practice.[9] The Institute of Medicine (IOM) defines clinical practice guidelines (CPGs) as "systematically developed statements to assist physician and patient decisions about appropriate health care for specific clinical circumstances."[10] CPGs provide a systematic means to review patient management and a formal description of appropriate levels of care. Their use can enhance the quality, appropriateness, and effectiveness of health care, and may also contain costs.[11]

Development of CPGs, however, requires input from experts in clinical medicine, meta-analyses, decision analyses, clinical epidemiology, cost–effectiveness analyses, and evidence synthesis. Such experts often are not available, or are prohibitively costly, on a local level.[12-14] Therefore, CPGs often are developed by national organizations[15,16] for populations that have "average" characteristics. These CPGs may need to be adapted to local settings in which the characteristics of the patient populations or practices are different.[17–19] In addition, traditional guidelines are normally static and thus may become out-of-date as new information about the interventions under consideration emerges.[20]

To offer potential solutions to obstacles to CPG success, we use decision models (DMs) as an aid for developing CPGs. We define DMs as abstract representations of decision problems that take into account the uncertain, dynamic, and complex consequences of a decision, and that assign values to those consequences.[21,22] Our approach allows developers and users to create, disseminate, and tailor CPGs, using normative DMs. Our approach is designed to improve CPG applicability, relevance, and acceptance by local clinicians and guideline developers, and thus to promote high-quality and cost-effective health care.

Our objective, therefore, was to develop a web-based system, ALCHEMIST, that creates high-quality guidelines automatically from decision models. In this work, we describe the ALCHEMIST system and a pilot evaluation of guidelines that it generated. We first frame the problem.

CLINICAL PRACTICE GUIDELINES

Current CPGs encompass numerous formats and levels of complexity. Each CPG has its own methods of development and dissemination, and therefore its own strengths and limitations. CPGs can be represented in several different formats, including text, protocol charts or lists, flowcharts, or any combination thereof. We concentrate on CPGs that are represented as clinical algorithms as defined by the Society for Medical Decision Making Committee on Standardization of Clinical Algorithms,[23] and that allow the guideline developer to communicate a complex series of conditional statements in a structured manner. The flowchart representation (figure 1) is integrated with textual output that follows a published structure for CPGs developed by Hayward and colleagues.[24] This organization and content promote a consistent structure for reporting CPGs and enhance a user's ability to determine the applicability, importance, and validity of a CPG for his or her specific population.[24]

After a CPG is created, problems with dissemination and maintenance often impede its success.[25–27] Local users who were not involved in the CPG-development process may feel removed from the policy-making process or may not believe that the CPG is applicable to their specific site or patients.[28] This lack of local involvement and validation de-

creases the likelihood of CPG dissemination and implementation.

DECISION MODELS

Decision models provide a normative analytic framework for representing the evidence, outcomes, and preferences involved in a clinical decision. Basing CPG creation on DMs enriches the CPGs.[19,29,30] DMs define clearly the available alternatives and events of interest, and combine these elements in an objective and predictable way to produce a recommendation that is consistent with underlying data and assumptions. In addition, sensitivity analyses of DMs allow a guideline user to identify critical variables to focus refinement of that guideline. We assume that guideline developers and clinicians desire such a normative model of a decision, and create CPGs based on such models. A growing number of guidelines have been developed with the aid of DMs.[31–44] Some clinical problems, however, particularly those with many sequential decisions, are difficult to represent with DMs. In addition, current CPGs are not often based on DMs; even when a DM representation exists for the same clinical problem, its advice or logic may not correlate with that of a published CPG.[45] Our research addresses this lack of correlation and provides a method for mapping between DMs and CPGs.

There are several DM representations, including decision trees, influence diagrams,[46,47] spreadsheet models, and state-transition models. We concentrate on the decision-tree representation, because the medical decision-making community commonly uses it as a model representation for simple decision analyses, Markov models, and cost–effectiveness studies. Several software packages are available for building such decision trees on the computer, including Decision Maker,[48] SMLtree,[49] and Data by TreeAge. In this research, we used decision trees modeled with the Decision Maker software.

Methods

SYSTEM DEVELOPMENT AND DESCRIPTION

ALCHEMIST is a web-based system that evaluates a DM and automatically generates an annotated guideline. We defined conceptual models—descriptions of a part of the world, the concepts about that part of the world, and the relationships among these concepts—of the knowledge represented by DMs and CPGs and formalized a method for mapping between these two representations.[50,51] Referring to these models, ALCHEMIST analyzes a DM and deter-

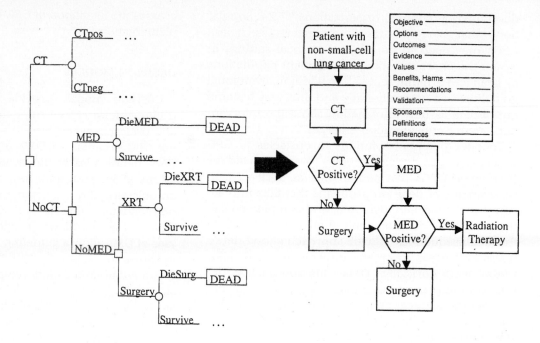

FIGURE 1. Decision-tree (left) and flowchart (right) representations for staging of non–small-cell lung cancer. The decision-tree schematic represents the alternatives, outcomes, and preferences in the clinical decision; the annotated flowchart (right) represents the optimal strategy for a specific instantiation of the underlying decision model.

mines what information it can extract automatically from the DM representation and what knowledge it needs to obtain from the decision analyst. ALCHEMIST uses this combined information to create a global CPG that represents the recommended strategy for the base-case patient population. This guideline comprises a flowchart algorithm showing the optimal recommended strategy and additional information, such as the guideline's options, outcomes, evidence, values, benefits, harms and costs, recommendations, methods of validation, sponsors, and sources. ALCHEMIST also creates a balance sheet of the benefits, harms, and costs[52]; a tornado diagram of the changes in expected utility (a graphic representation of the change in the expected utility of a given strategy as each variable value is varied along its sensitivity-analysis range); and a list of the variables to which the guideline is sensitive. This guideline is then made available over the web and can be custom-tailored by a user to specific clinical settings or can be modified automatically over time as the underlying DM or evidence evolves. We now describe the functionality of the ALCHEMIST system and step through how the various users would interact with ALCHEMIST.

We envision two main user groups for ALCHEMIST: decision analysts and guideline developers. The decision analyst identifies a clinical problem and builds a clinically valid DM that he or she loads into ALCHEMIST. Sufficient knowledge for producing a CPG usually is not contained in the DM representation. For example, the DM representation normally does not include a description of the target health problem or population. The ALCHEMIST implementation uses a web-based interface and common-gateway interface (CGI) scripts, so it can be run on any computer platform, and the decision analyst can load any decision tree in his or her personal-computing environment. ALCHEMIST reviews the DM to determine what additional knowledge is needed for it to create a CPG. Based on this review, ALCHEMIST creates the DM annotation editor to query the decision analyst for additional information and evidence pertaining to the DM.[51] Because this step requires the decision analyst to state explicitly the evidence used for the DM, the underlying assumptions, and the other key elements of a high-quality guideline that are normally not available in a DM, it represents additional work. This work, however, provides structure to the modeling and evidence-gathering process and helps the analyst to create a DM that has no inconsistencies, and that therefore can be transformed into a CPG. This additional information may also increase the transparency of the model to other users. The analyst can update the information that he or she enters into the DM annotation editor if new evidence becomes available or if he or she wants to reflect different patient populations. Implementation of the annotation editor on the web gives decision analysts access to the editor from different institutions, and allows decision-analysis teams to share decision-modeling tasks among members who are located at geographically disparate institutions and are using different computing platforms.[20,50]

As part of the DM annotation process, the decision analyst may indicate a clinically valid range for the input variable values. After the decision-analytic

Table 1 • Endorsing Societies and Locations of Comparison Clinical Practice Guidelines (CPGs)

Endorsing Society	Title of CPG	URL
American Society of Clinical Oncology	Clinical Practice Guidelines for the Treatment of Unresectable Non–Small-cell Lung Cancer	https://asco.infostreet.com/prof/pp/html/m_lung.htm
National Cancer Institute	Non–Small Cell Lung Cancer	http://imsdd.meb.unibonn.de/cancernet/100039.html
Canadian Medical Association	Cancer Management: Lung Tumor Group	http://www.bccancer.bc.ca/cmm/08-1.html
American Thoracic Society	Pretreatment Evaluation of Non–Small-cell Lung Cancer	http://www.ajrccm.org/cgi/content/full/156/1/320#T6

team has entered all the requisite information in the annotation editor, ALCHEMIST runs an additional analysis of the information and creates the global CPG. For each variable for which the decision-analytic team has defined a sensitivity-analysis range, ALCHEMIST calculates the expected outcome across this range—to be incorporated into the tornado diagram—and determines whether varying the variable within the given range changes the optimal guideline. Those variables in which such variance results in a changed guideline are flagged and noted for the end user. The guideline developer who implements the resulting CPG has access to the structured DM and to that model's various input variables. He or she therefore can tailor and update the clinical guideline based on patient- and site-specific information, or on new clinical information. The assumptions in the DM are explicit, so that the guideline developer can determine the model's applicability to a specific patient population.

TAILORING OF CPGs

ALCHEMIST's initial CPG reflects the DM base-case values. To make this CPG applicable to the specific site or patient, the local user must tailor the input variables. Tailoring abilities are beneficial when clinical circumstances vary substantially such that the user can't know whether the guideline recommendations will differ before tailoring.[18,19,53] The user of the CPG is able to change the base-case variable values to reflect his or her specific patient population. After determining that none of the DM modeling assumptions is violated, ALCHEMIST updates the results and recommended CPG flowchart algorithm. To help maintain the validity of the resulting CPG, ALCHEMIST represents and makes explicit to the CPG user information indicating to which variables the CPG is sensitive within the predetermined clinically valid range, plausible ranges for given variables, and modeling assumptions. ALCHEMIST does not allow structural updating or custom-tailoring of the underlying DM. Although it is possible to implement changes to the DM from a web interface, the re-

quirements for ensuring that the structurally changed model is complete and that the resulting CPG is valid are complex and are not part of this research. In short, the current implementation of ALCHEMIST allows CPGs to be tailored by changing the values of variables in the underlying DM, and seeks to ensure that such tailoring is consistent with the assumptions inherent in the DM.

PILOT EVALUATION

After completing the design and implementation of the ALCHEMIST system, we performed a pilot evaluation of the quality and usability of the ALCHEMIST guidelines.

Our objective was to evaluate the quality of an ALCHEMIST CPG, and to assess the usability of the ALCHEMIST browser and custom-tailoring editor. After we determined ALCHEMIST's implementation to be sufficiently complete, we created—using the DM annotation editor—the global CPG for a decision model for staging of lung cancer. We then solicited to serve as subjects 15 experienced guideline users affiliated with Stanford's Department of Health Research and Policy or Stanford Medical Informatics. None of the subjects had worked on constructing or testing ALCHEMIST's representation of DMs or CPGs, although one subject had worked extensively on the underlying lung-cancer DM. Ten of the 15 users were physicians, and 12 reported that they had had exposure to current clinical guidelines. Although the test subjects were affiliated with the Health Policy and Informatics departments at Stanford, they were not all familiar with decision analysis.

The subjects were asked to compare two guidelines—the lung-cancer CPG produced by ALCHEMIST and a current CPG available over the web for the same clinical domain—in terms of quality. The subjects chose one comparison CPG from a set of four current CPGs for the treatment of non–small-cell lung cancer.

We determined the set of comparison guidelines by performing a 1998 Medline search of publication type "Practice Guideline" and using the keyword term "non small cell." This search returned three guidelines,[54-56] two of which were available in full text over the web.[54,55] Using the Medical Matrix index of medical resources ⟨http://www.medmatrix.org/SPages/Practice_Guidelines.asp⟩, we then performed a search of the World Wide Web. This search yielded two additional CPGs. Table 1 lists the endorsing societies and URLs for the four comparison guidelines available on the web. Each subject was presented with the list of these endorsing societies and was asked to choose one society's guideline for the comparison. We allowed the subjects this choice of current CPGs to mimic the choice that practitioners would have available and to allow the users to choose the CPGs in which they had the greatest faith.

GUIDELINE CRITERIA USED

In 1992, the IOM published an instrument for critiquing CPGs.[10] Several investigators have developed guideline evaluations based on the IOM criteria.[57-61] To develop an operationalized rating procedure, Sonnad and colleagues combined the IOM criteria with Eddy's objectives of accuracy, accountability, predictability, defensibility, and usability.[61,62] Unlike the others available, this rating procedure allows the guideline user to calculate a numeric score for a CPG, thereby allowing quantitative comparison of two or more CPGs. We therefore used the criteria developed by Sonnad and colleagues to assess the quality of the CPGs in our evaluation. Note that we were assessing the *quality* of the CPG, rather than the *effectiveness* of the CPG in changing physician behavior or in improving patient care. Underlying this approach is the implicit assumption that the quality of the CPG will correlate with the clinical effectiveness of the CPG.[13,52,62-67]

We asked the subjects to complete the 15-item

guideline-rating questionnaire for both the ALCHEMIST CPG and the comparison CPG. The questionnaire included a guideline-rating key that provided additional information for each question in the questionnaire. We randomized the order in which the subjects rated the two CPGs. Using the guideline-rating key, we calculated a quality score for a CPG as the weighted average of the individual sections. Each guideline was assigned a score between 0 and 2, with greater scores reflecting higher quality.

After the 15 subjects completed the guideline-rating questionnaire for both guidelines, we asked them to change input variables of the ALCHEMIST CPG to reflect different clinical scenarios. To help the subjects determine which variables to change, we allowed them to use the listed sensitive variables and the tornado diagram. For this evaluation, the subjects were able to change any combination of the values listed in the input-variables table. Each subject then recorded whether the algorithm was sensitive to these changes and what effect the changes had on the (quality-adjusted) expected utility. ALCHEMIST generated a new CPG, and we compared the expected health benefit and flowchart algorithm produced by ALCHEMIST with that produced through manual computation. This component of our evaluation demonstrated the feasibility and accuracy of ALCHEMIST in producing tailored CPGs. The subjects then completed an end-user computing-satisfaction questionnaire (adapted from Doll and Torkzadeh, 1988[68]). In addition, we solicited from each subject answers to five open-ended questions. The duration of the evaluation was unconstrained; the total participation time for each subject was approximately 60 minutes.

The three outcomes of the user-evaluation study were 1) the difference between the quality score of the ALCHEMIST CPG and that of the comparison CPG; 2) the degree of user satisfaction with the CPG

FIGURE 2. Schematic representation of the staging lung-cancer effectiveness model. Square nodes represent decision nodes, circles represent chance nodes. The first decision is whether to perform a CT, followed by the decision whether to perform mediastinoscopy. Mediastinoscopy includes a small (but not insignificant) risk of death. Survival of mediastinoscopy—or the absence of mediastinoscopy—is followed by the treatment decision (thoracotomy versus radiation therapy). Both treatments incur a risk of death and each has a specified life expectancy based on the presence or absence of mediastinal metastases. CT = computed tomography, MED = mediastinoscopy, XRT = radiation therapy, Surgery = thoracotomy, MedMets = mediastinal metastases.

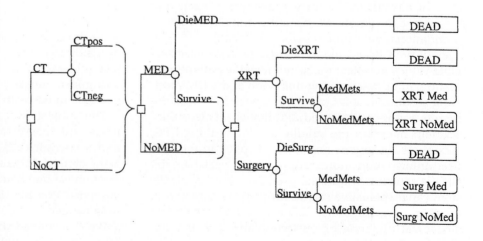

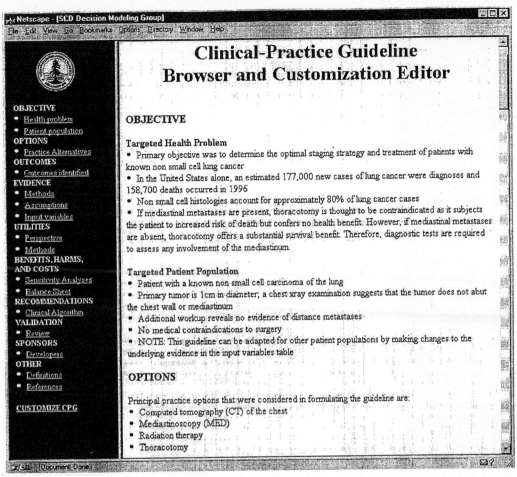

FIGURE 3. Clinical practice guideline (CPG) that ALCHEMIST produces using information from the annotation editor. The menu on the left side of the screen outlines the structure of the CPG and allows the user to move through the elements of the CPG.

browser and custom-tailoring editor; and 3) the responses to the structured interview.

Results

INTERACTION WITH ALCHEMIST: AN EXAMPLE

To demonstrate the abilities of ALCHEMIST, we step through how a user interacts with the system. In our scenario, a guideline-developing organization builds a standard DM that represents the alternatives, outcomes, evidence, assumptions, and knowledge for a decision problem. The example decision is what mediastinal-staging strategy to use in managing patients who have non–small-cell lung cancer. The outcomes modeled were life expectancy and quality-adjusted life expectancy; there are also sequential decisions representing the numerous tests that can be used.[47,69,70] Although we do not provide details in this paper, ALCHEMIST is also able to represent and generate guidelines from DMs that have dual utili-

ties (e.g., cost–effectiveness models) or that use Markov processes (e.g., time-dependent models).

In the example DM, a chest x-ray examination reveals that the tumor does not abut the chest wall or the mediastinum. If mediastinal metastases are found to be present, then thoracotomy is contraindicated, and the preferred treatment is radiation therapy. However, if mediastinal metastases are absent, then thoracotomy offers a substantial survival advantage. There are several diagnostic tests available to assess any involvement of the mediastinum.[47] In this example DM, we consider the use of only computed tomography (CT) of the chest and mediastinoscopy. Figure 2 is a schematic representation of the decision tree for the staging of lung cancer.

The first decision is whether to perform CT, followed by the decision whether to perform mediastinoscopy (note that, if CT is performed, the results of this test are available before the decision to perform mediastinoscopy is made). Mediastinoscopy includes a small (but not insignificant) risk of death.

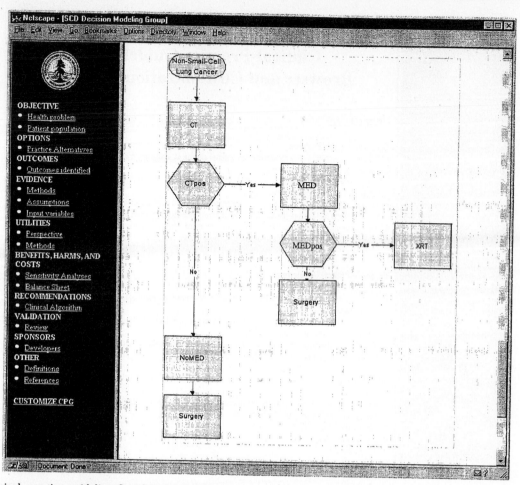

FIGURE 4. Clinical practice guideline flowchart representation generated by ALCHEMIST. Clinical-state boxes are rounded rectangles, action boxes are rectangles, and decision boxes are hexagons. This flowchart shows that, for the best-estimate values of the decision model for lung-cancer staging, the optimal strategy is to perform a CT examination. If the CT is negative, then surgery should be performed. If the CT is positive, then the physician should order mediastinoscopy. If this second diagnostic test is positive, then radiation therapy should be administered; otherwise, surgery is the treatment of choice.

Survival of mediastinoscopy—or the absence of mediastinoscopy—is followed by the treatment decision (thoracotomy versus radiation therapy). The results of both CT and mediastinoscopy, if performed, are known before the treatment decision is made. Both treatments incur a risk of death and each has a specified quality-adjusted life expectancy based on the presence or absence of mediastinal metastases, and on utilities for the various health states.

The DM is loaded into the ALCHEMIST system, which analyzes it and maps the information obtained explicitly from it onto the global CPG. ALCHEMIST then creates a web-based DM annotation editor that queries the decision analyst for additional information where needed. The information that the decision analyst is required to enter should be readily available: it comprises the data and knowledge that the analytic team used in creating the DM. The decision analyst enters it and submits it to ALCHEMIST, which then produces the global CPG, as well

as creating an editor for browsing and customtailoring the guideline (figures 3 and 4). The DM annotation editor website and the website that includes a catalog, browser, and editor of the available global guidelines are located on two separate websites in the ALCHEMIST system.

After the global guideline is made available over the web, local guideline implementers can explore it; can examine its evidence and recommendations, results of sensitivity analyses, balance sheet of benefits, harms, and costs; and can specify site- or patient-specific input values to produce an updated tailored CPG. Figure 5 shows a guideline user changing the prior probability of mediastinal metastases from the base-case value of 0.46 to a new value of 0.80. ALCHEMIST takes this new value, and—after checking that none of the underlying assumptions in the DM is violated—produces a new CPG. Using a base-case value for the prior probability of mediastinal metastases of 0.46, the generated CPG (figure

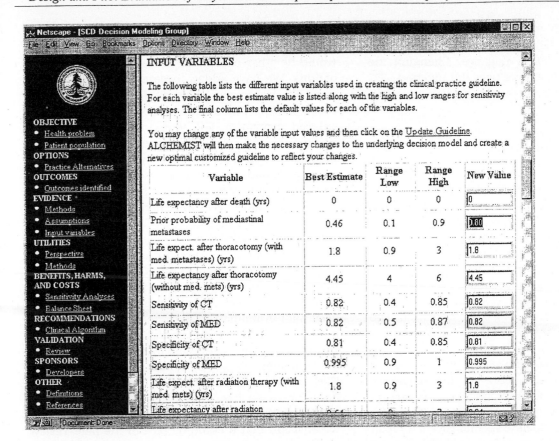

INPUT VARIABLES

The following table lists the different input variables used in creating the clinical practice guideline. For each variable the best estimate value is listed along with the high and low ranges for sensitivity analyses. The final column lists the default values for each of the variables.

You may change any of the variable input values and then click on the Update Guideline. ALCHEMIST will then make the necessary changes to the underlying decision model and create a new optimal customized guideline to reflect your changes.

Variable	Best Estimate	Range Low	Range High	New Value
Life expectancy after death (yrs)	0	0	0	0
Prior probability of mediastinal metastases	0.46	0.1	0.9	0.80
Life expect. after thoracotomy (with med. metastases) (yrs)	1.8	0.9	3	1.8
Life expectancy after thoracotomy (without med. mets) (yrs)	4.45	4	6	4.45
Sensitivity of CT	0.82	0.4	0.85	0.82
Sensitivity of MED	0.82	0.5	0.87	0.82
Specificity of CT	0.81	0.4	0.85	0.81
Specificity of MED	0.995	0.9	1	0.995
Life expect. after radiation therapy (with med. mets) (yrs)	1.8	0.9	3	1.8
Life expectancy after radiation				

FIGURE 5. Tailoring of the clinical practice guideline (CPG). The user here has entered 0.80 for the prior probability of mediastinal metastases.

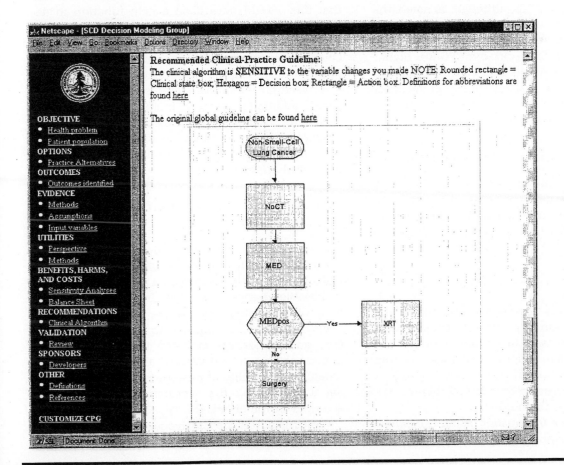

Recommended Clinical-Practice Guideline:
The clinical algorithm is SENSITIVE to the variable changes you made NOTE: Rounded rectangle = Clinical state box; Hexagon = Decision box; Rectangle = Action box. Definitions for abbreviations are found here

The original global guideline can be found here

FIGURE 6. Tailored CPG. The flowchart representation has been updated to reflect the 80% prior probability of mediastinal metastases that the user entered in figure 5.

4) recommends a CT examination followed by mediastinoscopy if the CT is positive, and followed by thoracotomy if the CT is negative. Changing the prior probability to 0.80 produces the updated CPG (figure 6), which recommends immediate mediastinoscopy.

QUALITY SCORE OF THE CPGs

Table 2 summarizes the results of the user evaluation. On a scale from 0 (worst) to 2 (best), the mean score for ALCHEMIST CPG was 1.502, compared with the comparison-CPG score of 0.987. The difference of 0.515 between these two scores was statistically significant (p = 0.002). Considering only the subscores of the questionnaire, the ALCHEMIST CPG scores for usability, accountability, and accuracy were 1.683, 1.393, and 1.430, respectively; the comparison CPG scores were 1.192, 0.941, and 0.830. The differences between these means were statistically significant (p < 0.05) in all cases.

Among the subjects who rated the ALCHEMIST guideline first, the mean score for the ALCHEMIST guideline was 1.550 and that for the comparison guideline was 0.939 (p = 0.006). Those subjects who rated the ALCHEMIST guideline second gave it a mean score of 1.460 and the comparison guideline a score of 1.029 (p = 0.067). The orders in which the users rated the guidelines did not change significantly the scores on either of the CPGs, although, as noted, the difference between the guidelines' scores was greater when ALCHEMIST was rated first.

The mean score for the ALCHEMIST CPG was higher than that of the comparison CPG for every question in the guideline-criteria instrument except the question asking whether the guideline had been submitted to any formal peer review (table 2).

USER SATISFACTION WITH THE ALCHEMIST CPG

Using an ordinal scale of 1 to 5, where 5 is ideal, the subjects rated ALCHEMIST's ease of use as 4.76, the usefulness of the content as 3.98, and the format of the presentation as 4.64. Table 3 details these results.

RESPONSES TO THE STRUCTURED INTERVIEW

Overall, the subjects' experience with the ALCHEMIST system was extremely positive. All subjects who held medical degrees said they would consider using a guideline system such as ALCHEMIST to help them in clinical practice. The free-form comments from the subjects revealed four broad themes. We list and explore these themes here.

1. Need for clearer information about exceptions to the CPG. Several subjects expressed a desire for more information about when the CPG would *not* apply to their patient population or when there would be other exceptions to treatment recommendations. We have added these exclusion criteria to our CPG framework. One subject noted that, because an expert panel does not review each custom-tailored algorithm, she would question the algorithm's accuracy. Although ALCHEMIST does check to make sure that the sensitivity-analysis ranges of the underlying decision model are not violated, we must develop methods to ensure the validity of tailored guidelines before systems such as ALCHEMIST are used in clinical practice.

2. Need for additional evidence for best-estimate values. The subjects expressed a desire to view the evidence tables on which the CPG was based. Although the evidence tables are now part of ALCHEMIST, this capability was not implemented when the user pilot evaluation took place. It is likely that the inclusion of these evidence tables would have strengthened the accountability scores of the ALCHEMIST guideline. One subject said that approval of the CPG by a recognized clinical organization would have increased her faith in the CPG. Although we did not solicit such approval for the example DM, we envision that it could be part of the peer-review process and would be required before a CPG was implemented into a clinical setting.

3. Need for help functionality. Many subjects said that they would have liked a help function to describe decision-analytic terms such as QALY, societal perspective, tornado diagram, and time tradeoff. One subject also wanted a more detailed introduction to the site and its functionality.

4. Need for additional features. The subjects suggested additional features, including a method for indicating visually in the flowchart algorithm the strength of the recommendations (e.g., by the thickness of the line), links to the relevant Medline citations, and an explanation facility.

EVALUATION OF THE CPG CUSTOM-TAILORING AND UPDATING EDITOR

In the final part of our evaluation, we assessed ALCHEMIST's ability to custom-tailor and update clinical guidelines. We restricted all changes to the CPG to variable changes (e.g., updating the prior probability of mediastinal metastases in the lung-cancer decision model), as opposed to structural changes (e.g., adding positron-emission tomography examinations as a possible diagnostic alternative). We evaluated the feasibility of custom-tailoring and updating a CPG using the ALCHEMIST system, and the accuracy of the changed CPG.

We considered the CPG accurate if the new CPG produced the same expected outcomes and flow-

Table 2 • Responses to Guideline-rating Questionnaire

Question	Mean*	Median	Standard Deviation	Difference between Means	p Value†
Usability					
U1. Is the intervention clearly defined?					
ALCHEMIST CPG	1.867	2	0.3519		
Comparison CPG	1.467	1	0.516	0.400	0.014
U2. Is the desired goal of the intervention clearly stated?					
ALCHEMIST CPG	1.867	2	0.3519		
Comparison CPG	1.267	1	0.704	0.600	0.004
U3. Does the guideline state explicitly the population to which the statements apply?					
ALCHEMIST CPG	2.000	2	0		
Comparison CPG	1.333	1	0.724	0.667	0.002
U4. Does the guideline identify the specifically known or generally expected exceptions to this recommendation?					
ALCHEMIST CPG	1.400	2	0.828		
Comparison CPG	1.200	1	0.775	0.200	0.266
U5. Is guidance offered about how to modify the guideline for differing clinical circumstances?					
ALCHEMIST CPG	1.467	2	0.743		
Comparison CPG	0.867	1	0.743	0.600	0.017
Usability total					
ALCHEMIST CPG	*1.683*	*1.750*	*0.403*		
Comparison CPG	*1.192*	*1.125*	*0.506*	*0.492*	*0.006*
Accountability					
A1. Was the guideline developed in a multidisciplinary process?					
ALCHEMIST CPG	1.600	2	0.632		
Comparison CPG	1.400	2	0.737	0.200	0.192
A2. Is the evidence used in drawing conclusions included?					
ALCHEMIST CPG	1.267	1	0.704		
Comparison CPG	1.133	1	0.915	0.133	0.335
A3. Can you determine the process used to synthesize evidence and develop the guideline?					
ALCHEMIST CPG	1.133	1	0.743		
Comparison CPG	0.733	1	0.799	0.400	0.116
A4. Are the assumptions used in guideline development clearly stated?					
ALCHEMIST CPG	1.933	2	0.258		
Comparison CPG	0.600	0	0.737	1.333	<0.001
A5. Is there a procedure for scheduled reviews included in this guideline?					
ALCHEMIST CPG	1.133	1	0.516		
Comparison CPG	0.600	0	0.828	0.533	0.036
Accountability total					
ALCHEMIST CPG	*1.393*	*1.444*	*0.409*		
Comparison CPG	*0.941*	*0.778*	*0.618*	*0.452*	*0.02*
Accuracy					
B1. Are intermediate events and their relationships to final outcomes clearly stated, including intermediate events?					
ALCHEMIST CPG	1.333	2	0.816		
Comparison CPG	1.000	1	0.655	0.333	0.087
B2. Are the methods of measurement for the intervention and the outcomes clearly stated?					
ALCHEMIST CPG	1.600	2	0.632		
Comparison CPG	1.133	1	0.743	0.467	0.065

Table 2 • Continued

Question	Mean*	Median	Standard Deviation	Difference between Means	p Value†
B3. Is the method used in linking the intervention and guideline clearly stated?					
ALCHEMIST CPG	1.733	2	0.704		
Comparison CPG	0.733	1	0.799	1.00	0.002
B4. Has the guideline been through some form of formal peer review?					
ALCHEMIST CPG	0.933	1	0.884		
Comparison CPG	1.133	1	0.915	−0.200	0.745
B5. Are patient preferences explicitly considered in development of the guideline?					
ALCHEMIST CPG	1.800	2	0.561		
Comparison CPG	0.400	0	0.632	1.400	<0.001
Accuracy total					
ALCHEMIST CPG	*1.430*	*1.333*	*0.314*		
Comparison CPG	*0.830*	*0.667*	*0.524*	*0.600*	*0.002*
TOTAL					
ALCHEMIST CPG	**1.502**	**1.519**	**0.274**		
Comparison CPG	**0.987**	**0.986**	**0.461**	**0.515**	**0.002**

*To calculate a guideline's score, we used the following scoring system: usability = {[(U1 + U2)/2] + U3 + U4 + U5}/4, accountability = {A1 + [(A2 + A3 + A4)/3] + A5}/3, accuracy = {[(B1 + B2 + B3)/3] + B4 + B5}/3. The guideline's overall quality score is the average of these three scores.
†We calculated p values using a paired t-test.

chart algorithm as those obtained directly by the DM and through manual computation. The clinical validity of the new CPG was not assessed. The 15 subjects completed 38 such scenarios, all of which corresponded to the expected utility and algorithm calculated through manual derivation. All the subjects said that they were pleased with the custom-tailoring abilities of the ALCHEMIST system.

Discussion

We developed a web-based system, ALCHEMIST, that creates an annotated flowchart algorithm automatically by analyzing an underlying decision model. The ALCHEMIST system thus constructs CPGs that represent the optimum policy as determined by the evidence and values reflected in the decision model. Users can view the evidence on which the guideline is based, review model inputs, or interrogate and rerun the model using a web-based interface. Thus, users can determine the degree to which the resulting CPG is pertinent to their patient population, and can explore whether a guideline should be tailored to their clinical population. ALCHEMIST demonstrates that it is possible to transform DMs into CPGs automatically in a computer-based system, and to tailor and update the CPGs by modifying the inputs to the decision model.

In a pilot evaluation, our users rated the ALCHEMIST guidelines comparable to or better than current published CPGs in quality and usability, and

Table 3 • Responses to the User-satisfaction Section of the Guideline-rating Questionnaire

Statement about ALCHEMIST	Subject Agreement with Statement	Agreement* (%)
The information is clear	4.333	93
ALCHEMIST provides the precise information you need	3.733	73
ALCHEMIST is user-friendly	4.200	87
The information content meets your needs	3.933	73
The output is presented in a useful format	4.600	100
ALCHEMIST is easy to use	4.800	100
ALCHEMIST provides sufficient information	3.467	67
ALCHEMIST provides reports that seem to be just about exactly what you need	3.733	73

*Assignment of a score of 4 or 5 to the question.

they preferred the ALCHEMIST guideline for lung-cancer staging to guidelines published by nationally recognized organizations. The subjects were pleased with the system's presentation of information, with the usefulness of that information, and with the system's ease of use. Although our study was small and evaluated only the lung-cancer CPGs, this preliminary evaluation is encouraging, and suggests that a larger and more broad-based evaluation is warranted.

Current CPGs, although promoted by policymakers and health-care institutions, have been hindered in effectiveness because they are difficult to keep up to date[71]; the methods by which they are created may not be rigorous,[72] their development requires extensive resources,[71] and they may not adequately account for legitimate variation in clinical settings and populations.[19,73] Use of DMs can overcome several of these limitations: DMs provide a systematic means for integrating and updating evidence,[47] for understanding the importance of uncertainty, for representing values explicitly,[18,74] and for evaluating differences across patient populations.[19] Despite the advantages of these models, users have hitherto had to be familiar with highly specialized, often difficult-to-use software, as well as to have direct access to the models. With the ALCHEMIST system, guideline developers or end users can perform limited analyses without knowing how to build decision models, and the web-based system provides near-universal access by allowing remote users to perform analyses.[20] Thus, systems such as ALCHEMIST may help us to resolve the tension between performing comprehensive high-quality analyses, which require extensive resources and expertise, and accommodating legitimate variations in circumstances and practice settings.

Our evaluation has several limitations. First, as noted, our study was small, and we compared only the lung-cancer guidelines. Second, users were not blinded to the origin or development method of the CPGs, and all subjects were from Stanford University. To blind the users, we would have had to eliminate the ability of the ALCHEMIST to tailor CPGs—and thus to eliminate a core element of the system's design. To provide the greatest advantage to the published guidelines, we allowed each subject to choose for the comparison the guideline that he or she preferred. Although all subjects were affiliated with Stanford University, they were not all familiar with decision analysis. We do realize, however, the limit of the generalizability of our pilot evaluation, and therefore plan to evaluate the use of ALCHEMIST within a diverse set of clinicians as detailed below. Third, we did not formally train our subjects to use the CPG-assessment tool. Although there were several instances in which the subjects had questions about how to apply the assessment tool to the specific guideline that they were assessing, we had no indication of any systematic problems that would explain the differences in ratings between the ALCHEMIST and comparison CPGs. Fourth, we did not evaluate the efficacy of any implementations of the ALCHEMIST or published CPGs. To affect patient outcomes, guidelines must be disseminated and understood by physicians[75]; in addition, the physicians must agree with the guideline recommendations,[76] and must translate those recommendations into changes in their clinical practice.[75,77–79] Such an eval-

uation was beyond the scope of our study.

As a next step, we have designed a larger evaluation to address several of these limitations. In this planned study, we will use the ALCHEMIST system to create an evidence-based customizable guideline for the prevention of sudden cardiac death based on decision models developed as part of the Cardiac Arrhythmia Patient Outcomes Research Team.[20,80–82] We will then evaluate, in a randomized clinical trial, the use by members of the American College of Cardiology (ACC) of our web-based guideline system and their satisfaction with it compared with traditional guidelines. The large ACC membership (more than 21,000 in 1999) will give us ample power and a diverse set of subjects for our analyses. Our long-term goal is to evaluate ALCHEMIST in routine clinical practice. Specifically, we would like to perform a randomized clinical trial that compares the ALCHEMIST guideline system with current practice. We would like the measure the adherence of clinicians to the ALCHEMIST guidelines, the effects of the ALCHEMIST system on both the process of care and patients' outcomes, and the costs of disseminating and implementing guidelines generated by ALCHEMIST. We believe that this pilot evaluation and our planned evaluation with the ACC will lay a firm foundation for a future clinical trial. Another important step in our evaluation of the ALCHEMIST system is to evaluate the DM annotation process by remote decision-analytic teams using diverse decision models and clinical domains.

Various extensions to our system would be useful, and their incorporation into the ALCHEMIST system would increase the potential effectiveness of ALCHEMIST in a future clinical trial. Such extensions include expansion to other decision-modeling software and representations, including influence diagrams; allowing users to explore the structure of the underlying decision model; incorporation of a controlled clinical vocabulary into the DM modeling process and into the DM annotation editor, to simplify integration of ALCHEMIST guidelines with a computer-based patient record; and combination of our generated CPGs with an explanation module.[83–85]

Although we envision the primary users of the ALCHEMIST system to be decision analysts and local guideline developers, clinicians could also use the generated CPG. ALCHEMIST would provide these clinicians with access to the CPG recommendations, evidence, and modeling assumptions, and to ALCHEMIST's custom-tailoring capabilities on a patient-specific level. To facilitate such patient-specific tailoring, we plan to incorporate a utility-assessment module—such as the U-titer utility-assessment tool[86]—to help the guideline user to determine his or her patient's preferences.[87,88] Although use of ALCHEMIST for patient-specific decision support raises questions about how to represent a specific patient's decision problem with sufficient fidelity, there is no technical barrier that prevents this use of ALCHEMIST. Determination of how to make such features useful in a clinical setting requires careful evaluation.

We believe that systems such as the one that we developed have the potential to increase the usefulness of both DMs and CPGs. Such systems may enable a broad audience to incorporate systematic analyses into both policy and clinical decisions. In an era in which great importance is placed on defending clinical practice with rigorous supporting evidence, our approach suggests a powerful method for mapping from such evidence to familiar guidelines suitable for clinical adoption.

The non–small-cell lung cancer guideline can be viewed at ⟨http://alchemist.stanford.edu/guidelines/index.html⟩. Please contact the authors at ⟨sanders@stanford.edu⟩ for access.

The authors thank Dr. Frank Sonnenberg and Greg Hagerty for use of the Decision Maker software, Dr. Edward Shortliffe for comments on earlier versions of this manuscript, and Lyn Dupré for editorial assistance.

References

1. Chassin MR, Brook RH, Keesey J, et al. Variations in the use of medical and surgical services by the Medicare population. N Engl J Med. 1986;314:285–90.

2. Conway AC, Keller RB, Wennberg DE. Partnering with physicians to achieve quality improvement. Joint Commission Journal on Quality Improvement. 1995;21:619–26.

3. Fisher ES, Welch HG, Wennberg JE. Prioritizing Oregon's hospital resources. An example based on variations in discretionary medical utilization [see comments]. JAMA. 1992; 267:1925–31.

4. Health Services Research Group. Standards, guidelines, and clinical policies. Can Med Assoc J. 1992;146:833–7.

5. Iscoe NA, Goel V, Wu K, Fehringer G, Holowaty EJ, Naylor CD. Variation in breast cancer surgery in Ontario. Canad Med Assoc J. 1994;150:345–52.

6. Keller RB, Soule DN, Wennberg JE, Hanley DF. Dealing with geographic variations in the use of hospitals. The experience of the Maine Medical Assessment Foundation Orthopaedic Study Group. J Bone Joint Surg. 1990;72:1286–93.

7. Welch WP, Miller ME, Welch HG, Fisher ES, Wennberg JE. Geographic variation in expenditures for physicians' services in the United States [see comments]. N Engl J Med. 1993;328: 621–7.

8. Wennberg J, Gittelsohn A. Small area variations in health care delivery. Science. 1973;182:1102–8.

9. Woolf SH. Practice guidelines: a new reality in medicine. I. Recent developments. Arch Intern Med. 1990;150:1811–8.

10. Institute of Medicine. Guidelines for Clinical Practice: From Development to Use. Washington, DC: National Academy Press, 1992.

11. U.S. Department of Health and Human Service. Using Clinical Practice Guidelines to Evaluate Quality of Care. Volume 1: Issues. Rockville, MD: U.S. Department of Health and Human Services, 1995.

12. Brook R. Practice guidelines and practicing medicine. JAMA. 1989;262:3027–30.

13. Eddy DM. Anatomy of a decision. JAMA. 1990;263:441–3.

14. Fletcher RH, Fletcher SW. Clinical practice guidelines. Ann Intern Med. 1990;113:645–6.

15. American College of Physicians. Clinical Practice Guidelines. 1995 ed. Philadelphia, PA: American College of Physicians, 1995.

16. U.S. Preventive Services Task Force. Guide to Clinical Preventive Services. 2nd ed. Baltimore, MD: Williams & Wilkins, 1996.

17. Carter AO, Battista RN, Hodge MJ, et al. Proceedings of the 1994 Canadian Clinical Practice Guidelines Network Workshop. Can Med Assoc J. 1995;153.

18. Nease RF, Owens DK. A method for estimating the cost-effectiveness of incorporating patient preferences into practice guidelines. Med Decis Making. 1994;14:382–92.

19. Owens DK, Nease RF. A normative analytic framework for development of practice guidelines for specific clinical populations. Med Decis Making. 1997;17:409–26.

20. Sanders GD, Hagerty CG, Sonnenberg FA, Hlatky MA, Owens DK. Distributed decision support using a web-based interface: prevention of sudden cardiac death. Med Decis Making. 1999;19:157–66.

21. Owens DK, Sox HCJ. Medical decision making: probabilistic medical reasoning. In: Shortliffe E, Perreault L, Fagan L, Widerhold G (eds). Medical Informatics: Computer Applications in Health Care. Reading, MA: Addison–Wesley; 1990:70–116.

22. Owens DK, Nease RF. Development of outcome-based practice guidelines: a method for structuring problems and synthesizing evidence. Joint Commission Journal on Quality Improvement. 1993;19:248–63.

23. Society for Medical Decision Making (SMDM) Committee on Standardization of Clinical Algorithms (CSCA). Proposal for clinical algorithm standards. Med Decis Making. 1992;12: 149–54.

24. Hayward RSA, Wilson MD, Tunis SR. More informative abstracts of articles on clinical practice guidelines. Ann Intern Med. 1993;118:731–7.

25. Grimshaw JM, Russell IT. Achieving health gain through clinical guidelines: II. Ensuring the guidelines change medical practice. Quality in Health Care. 1994;March.

26. Danila RN, MacDonald KL, Rhame FS, et al. A look-back investigation of patients of an HIV-infected physician. Public health implications. N Engl J Med. 1991;325:1406–11.

27. Davis DA, Taylor-Vaisey A. Translating guidelines into practice. A systematic review of theoretic concepts, practical experience and research evidence in the adoption of clinical practice guidelines. Can Med Assoc J. 1997;157:408–16.

28. Carter AO, Battista RN, Hodge MJ, et al. Report on activities and attitudes of organizations active in the clinical practice guidelines field. Can Med Assoc J. 1995;153:901–7.

29. Nease RF, Owens DK. Decision models as an aid to short-term evaluation of clinical guidelines [abstr]. Med Decis Making. 1991;11:325.

30. Oddone EZ, Samsa G, Matchar DB. Global judgments versus decision-model–facilitated judgments: are experts internally consistent? Med Decis Making. 1994;14:19–26.

31. American College of Physicians. Guidelines for counseling postmenopausal women about preventive hormone therapy. Ann Intern Med. 1992;117:1038–41.

32. American College of Physicians. Screening for ovarian cancer: recommendations and rationale. Ann Intern Med. 1994; 121:141–2.

33. Carlson KJ, Skates SJ, Singer DE. Screening for ovarian cancer. Ann Intern Med. 1994;121:124–32.

34. Eddy DM. Screening for breast cancer. In: Eddy DM (ed). Common Screening Tests. Philadelphia, PA: American College of Physicians, 1991:229–54.

35. Eddy DM. Screening for lung cancer. In: Eddy DM (ed). Common Screening Tests. Philadelphia, PA: American College of Physicians, 1991:312–25.

36. Eddy DM. Screening for cervical cancer. In: Eddy DM (ed). Common Screening Tests. Philadelphia, PA: American College of Physicians, 1991:255–85.

37. Eddy DM. Screening for colorectal cancer. In: Eddy DM (ed). Common Screening Tests. Philadelphia, PA: American College of Physicians, 1991:286–311.

38. Fahs MC, Mandelblatt J, Schechter C, Muller C. Cost effectiveness of cervical cancer screening for the elderly. Ann Intern Med. 1992;117:520–7.

39. Grady D, Rubin SM, Petitti DB, et al. Hormone therapy to prevent disease and prolong life in postmenopausal women. Ann Intern Med. 1992;117:1016–37.

40. Littenberg B, Garber AM, Sox HC Jr. Screening for hypertension. In: Eddy DM (ed). Common Screening Tests. Philadelphia, PA: American College of Physicians, 1991:22–46.

41. Melton JL III, Eddy DM, Johnston CC. Screening for osteoporosis. In: Eddy DM (ed). Common Screening Tests. Philadelphia, PA: American College of Physicians, 1991:202–28.

42. Schapira MM, Matchar DB, Young MJ. The effectiveness of ovarian cancer screening. A decision analysis model. Ann Intern Med. 1993;118:838–43.

43. Singer DE, Samet JH, Coley CM, Nathan DM. Screening for diabetes mellitus. In: Eddy DM (ed). Common Screening Tests. Philadelphia, PA: American College of Physicians, 1991: 154–178.

44. Sox HC Jr, Garber AM, Littenberg B. The resting electrocardiogram as a screening test: a clinical analysis. In: Eddy DM (ed). Common Screening Tests. Philadelphia, PA: American College of Physicians, 1991:47–80.

45. Wears RL, Stenklyft PH, Luten RC. Using decision tables to verify the logical consistency and completeness of clinical practice guidelines: fever without source in children under three. Acad Emerg Med. 1994;1:A35.

46. Owens DK, Schacter RD, Nease RF. Representation and analysis of medical decision problems with influence diagrams. Med Decis Making. 1997;17:241–62.

47. Nease RF, Owens DK. Use of influence diagrams to structure medical decisions. Med Decis Making. 1997;17:263–75.

48. Sonnenberg FA, Pauker SG. Decision maker: an advanced personal computer tool for clinical decision analysis. Proceedings of the Eleventh Annual Symposium Computer Applications in Medical Care. Washington, DC: IEEE Computer Society, 1987.

49. Hollenberg JP. The decision tree builder: an expert system to simulate medical prognosis and management. Med Decis Making. 1984;4:531.

50. Sanders GD. Automated creation of clinical-practice guidelines from decision models. Stanford Medical Informatics. Stanford, CT: Stanford University, 1998.

51. Sanders GD, Nease RF, Owens DK. Design and implementation of a computer-based system to annotate decision models for use in guideline development [abstr]. Med Decis Making. 1998;18:469.

52. Eddy DM. Comparing benefits and harms: the balance sheet. JAMA. 1990;263:2493–505.

53. Owens DK, Nease RF. A model-based approach for prioritizing information acquisition during guideline development [abstr]. Med Decis Making. 1991;11:330.

54. American Society of Clinical Oncology. Clinical practice guideline for the treatment of resectable non–small-cell lung cancer. J Clin Oncol. 1997;15:2996–3018.

55. American Thoracic Society, European Respiratory Society. Pretreatment evaluation of non–small-cell lung cancer. Am J Respir Crit Care Med. 1997;156:320–32.

56. Ettinger DS, Cox JD, Ginsberg RJ, et al. NCCN Non–small-cell lung cancer practice guidelines. The National Comprehensive Cancer Network Oncology. 1996;10:81–111.

57. Cluzeau F, Littlejohns P. Towards valid clinical guidelines: development of a critical appraisal instrument. Health Care Risk Report. 1996;2:16–8.

58. Cluzeau F, Littlejohns P, Grimshaw J, Feder G. Appraisal instrument for clinical guidelines. Version 1 ed. London, U.K.: St. George's Hospital Medical School, 1997.

59. Cluzeau F, Littlejohns P, Grimshaw J, Hopkins A. Appraising clinical guidelines and the development of criteria—a pilot study. J Interprofessional Care. 1995;9:227–35.

60. Scottish Intercollegiate Guidelines Network (SIGN). Draft criteria for appraisal of clinical guidelines for national use. Web document, 1995.

61. Sonnad S, McDonald TW, Nease RF, Oleske J, Owens DK. An evaluation of the methodology of guidelines for zidovudine therapy in HIV disease. Med Decis Making. 1993;13:398.

62. Eddy DM. Guideline for policy statements: the explicit approach. JAMA. 1990;263:2239–43.

63. Eddy DM. Clinical policies and the quality of clinical practice. N Engl J Med. 1982;307:343–7.

64. Eddy DM. Designing a practice policy. Standards, guidelines, and options. JAMA. 1990;263:3077–84.

65. Eddy DM. Practice policies: guidelines for methods. JAMA. 1990;263:1839–41.

66. Eddy DM. Practice policies: what are they? JAMA. 1990;263: 877–80.

67. Basinski ASH. Evaluation of clinical practice guidelines. Can Med Assoc J. 1995;153:1575–81.

68. Doll WJ, Torkzadeh G. The measurement of end-user computing satisfaction. MIS Quarterly. 1988;12:259–74.

69. Gould MK, Nease RF, Sox HC, Owens DK. A decision model for mediastinal staging in non–small cell lung cancer. J Gen Intern Med. 1997;12:61.

70. Owens DK, Sox HCJ, Inouye SK. Strategies for test selection in the staging of lung neoplasms. Seminars in Respiratory Medicine. 1989;10:195–202.

71. U.S. Congress Office of Technology Assessment. Identifying Health Technologies That Work: Searching for Evidence. Washington, DC: U.S. Government Printing Office, 1994.

72. Eddy DM. A Manual for Assessment of Health Practices and Designing Practice Policies: The Explicit Approach. Philadelphia, PA: American College of Physicians, 1992.

73. Owens DK. The use of medical informatics to implement and develop clinical-practice guidelines. West J Med. 1998;168: 166–75.

74. Owens DK. Spine update. Patient preferences and the development of practice guidelines. Spine. 1998;23:1073–9.

75. Pierre KD, Vayda E, Lomas J, Enkin MW, Anderson GM. Obstetrical attitudes and practices before and after the Canadian Consensus Conference Statement on Cesarean Birth. Soc Sci Med. 1991;32:1283–9.

76. Burack RC, Liang J. The early detection of cancer in the primary care setting: factors associated with the acceptance and completion of recommended procedures. Prev Med. 1987;16:739–51.

77. Grilli R, Apolone G, Marsoni S, Nicolucci A, Zola P, Liberati A. The impact of patient management guidelines on the care of breast, colorectal, and ovarian cancer patients in Italy. Med Care. 1991;29:50–63.

78. Kosecoff J, Kanouse DE, Rogers WH, McCloskey L, Winslow CM, Brook RH. Effects of the National Institutes of Health Consensus Development Program on physician practice. JAMA. 1987;258:2708–13.

79. Lomas J, Anderson GM, Domnick-Pierre K, et al. Do practice guidelines guide practice? The effect of a consensus statement on the practice of physicians. N Engl J Med. 1989;321: 1306–11.

80. O'Campo PO, De Boer MA, Faden RR, Gielen AC, Kass N,

Chaisson R. Discrepancies between women's personal interview data and medical record documentation of illicit drug use, sexually transmitted diseases, and HIV infection. Med Care. 1992;30:965–71.

81. Owens DK, Sanders GD, Harris RA, et al. Cost effectiveness of implantable cardioverter defibrillators relative to amiodarone for prevention of sudden cardiac death. An Intern Med. 1997;126:1–12.

82. Sanders GD, Harris RA, Hlatky MA, Owens DK. Prevention of sudden cardiac death: a probabilistic model for decision support. Proceedings of the Nineteenth Annual Symposium on Computer Applications in Medical Care. Philadelphia, PA: Hanley & Belfus, 1995:258–62.

83. Jimison HB. A representation for gaining insight into clinical decision models. Proceedings of the Twelfth Annual Symposium on Computer Applications in Medical Care. Los Angeles, CA: IEEE Computer Society Press, 1988:110–3.

84. Langlotz CP, Shortliffe EH, Fagan LM. A methodology for generating computer-based explanations of decision-theoretic advice. Med Decis Making. 1988;8:290–303.

85. Suermondt HJ, Cooper GF. An evaluation of explanations of probabilistic inference. Proceedings of the Sixteenth Annual Symposium on Computer Applications in Medical Care. New York: McGraw–Hill, 1992:579–85.

86. Sumner W, Nease R, Littenberg B. U-titer: a utility assessment tool. Proceedings of the Fifteenth Annual Symposium on Computer Applications in Medical Care. New York: McGraw–Hill, 1991:701–5.

87. Lenert LA, Michelson D, Flowers C, Bergen MR. IMPACT: an object-oriented graphical environment for construction of multimedia patient interviewing software. Proceedings of the Nineteenth Annual Symposium on Computer Applications in Medical Care. Philadelphia, PA: Hanley & Belfus, 1995:319–23.

88. Sanders GD, Owens DK, Padian N, Cardinalli AB, Sullivan AN, Nease RF. A computer-based interview to identify HIV risk behaviors and to assess patient preferences for HIV-related health states. Proceedings of the Eighteenth Annual Symposium on Computer Applications in Medical Care. Philadelphia, PA: Hanley & Belfus, 1994:20–24.

On the misuses of artificial neural networks for prognostic and diagnostic classification in oncology

Guido Schwarzer[1,*,†], Werner Vach[2] and Martin Schumacher[1]

[1] *University of Freiburg, Institute of Medical Biometry and Medical Informatics, Stefan-Meier-Straße 26, D-79104 Freiburg, Germany*
[2] *University of Southern Denmark/Odense University, Department of Statistics and Demography, Campusvej 55, DK-5230 Odense M, Denmark*

SUMMARY

The application of artificial neural networks (ANNs) for prognostic and diagnostic classification in clinical medicine has become very popular. In particular, feed-forward neural networks have been used extensively, often accompanied by exaggerated statements of their potential. In this paper, the essentials of feed-forward neural networks and their statistical counterparts (that is, logistic regression models) are reviewed. We point out that the uncritical use of ANNs may lead to serious problems, such as the fitting of implausible functions to describe the probability of class membership and the underestimation of misclassification probabilities. In applications of ANNs to survival data, further difficulties arise. Finally, the results of a search in the medical literature from 1991 to 1995 on applications of ANNs in oncology and some important common mistakes are reported. It is concluded that there is no evidence so far that application of ANNs represents real progress in the field of diagnosis and prognosis in oncology. Copyright © 2000 John Wiley & Sons, Ltd.

1. INTRODUCTION

During the last years, the application of artificial neural networks (ANNs) for prognostic and diagnostic classification in clinical medicine has attracted growing interest in the medical literature. For example, a 'mini-series' on neural networks that appeared in the *Lancet* contained three more or less enthusiastic review articles [1–3] and an additional commentary expressing some scepticism [4]. In this commentary as well as in other, more balanced reviews [5], the comparison with competing statistical methods is emphasized.

The relationship between ANNs and statistical methods, especially logistic regression models, has been described in several articles [6–10]. We start with a brief summary of feed-forward neural networks and logistic regression models and their extensions. We then illustrate by means

---

* Correspondence to: Guido Schwarzer, University of Freiburg, Institute of Medical Biometry and Medical Informatics, Stefan-Meier-Straße 26, D-79104 Freiburg, Germany
† E-mail: sc@imbi.uni-freiburg.de

of a simple example that uncritical use of ANNs can lead to functions describing the probability of class membership that are far from plausible. This is due to the flexibility of ANNs which is often cited as an advantage [2]; we argue that it must be seen as a major concern. Problems associated with the estimation of misclassification probabilities and the application of ANNs to survival data that often occur in oncology are outlined. In addition to these general methodological considerations we report the results of a literature search on the application of ANNs in oncology; the most frequently occurring mistakes are identified and commented on. Finally, an attempt is made to summarize our findings in the conclusions section.

2. ESSENTIALS OF LOGISTIC REGRESSION AND NEURAL NETWORKS

The common principle of diagnosis and prognosis in oncology or other areas is to decide to which class k, $k \in \{0, \dots, K\}$, an individual belongs by using information on a set of p covariate values $x = (x_1, \dots, x_p)'$. The simplest but most common case is to consider only two possible classes. Examples are the diagnosis of a tumour as 'benign' or 'malignant' or the prediction of the recurrence of a disease up to a specified point in time. We restrict our attention to the special case of two classes and call the class indicator $Y \in \{0, 1\}$.

The aim is to construct a decision rule for individuals with known covariate values but unknown class level. Many approaches to constructing such a decision rule are based on estimating the conditional probability of observing an individual with class level 1 given the covariates $x = (x_1, \dots, x_p)'$. Such an estimation is often based on a parametric model

$$P(Y = 1 \mid X = x) = f(x, \beta) \tag{1}$$

for the conditional probabilities, where β is a vector of unknown parameters. The parameters are called 'regression coefficients' in statistics and 'weights' by the neural net community. Estimation of these parameters is done by using information from a sample of individuals with known class levels and known covariate values. Based on an estimate $\hat{\beta}$ of the parameters, we can estimate for each future individual with covariate values x the conditional probability of belonging to class 1 by $f(x, \hat{\beta})$. The classification rule is given as: class 1, if $f(x, \hat{\beta})$ is greater than some cut-off level, for example, 0.5; class 0, otherwise.

Logistic regression and feed-forward neural networks differ in the functional form $f(x, \beta)$ assumed for the conditional probability $P(Y = 1 \mid X = x)$.

2.1. Logistic regression

The linear logistic regression model [11] assumes that

$$f(x, \beta) = \frac{1}{1 + \exp(-\beta_0 - \sum_{i=1}^{p} \beta_i x_i))} = \Lambda\left(\beta_0 + \sum_{i=1}^{p} \beta_i x_i\right) \tag{2}$$

with $\Lambda(.)$ denoting the logistic function. The model can be re-expressed in terms of the odds of observing an individual with class level 1 given the covariates x in the following way:

$$\text{Odds}(x) = \frac{P(Y = 1 \mid X = x)}{P(Y = 0 \mid X = x)} = \exp\left(\beta_0 + \sum_{i=1}^{p} \beta_i x_i\right).$$

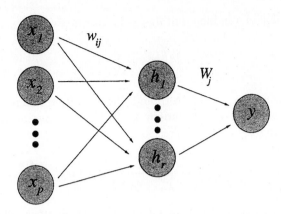

Figure 1. Graphical representation of a feed-forward neural network with p input units, r hidden units and one output unit.

Thus the essential assumption of the linear logistic regression model is that the logarithm of the odds is linear in x. The odds ratio of two individuals, showing a difference of Δ for the ith covariate and no difference for the others, is equal to $\exp(\beta_i \Delta)$. Hence, the regression coefficients β_i are directly interpretable as log-odds ratios or, in terms of $\exp(\beta_i)$, as odds ratios. This property of the logistic regression model enables one to assess the effect of a single covariate and is one major reason for the widespread use of this method in the biomedical sciences.

A natural extension of the linear logistic regression model is to include quadratic terms and multiplicative interaction terms:

$$f(x, \beta) = \Lambda \left(\beta_0 + \sum_{i=1}^{p} \beta_i x_i + \sum_{i=1}^{p} \gamma_i x_i^2 + \sum_{i < i'} \delta_{ii'} x_i x_{i'} \right). \tag{3}$$

These more general logistic regression models are usually considered as the first step to overcome the stringent assumption of additive and purely linear effects of the covariates. Other approaches to model the conditional probability $P(Y = 1 \mid X = x)$ in a more flexible manner include generalized additive models [12], fractional polynomials [13] and feed-forward neural networks.

2.2. Feed-forward neural networks

In articles published in biomedical journals, ANNs are typically introduced as a computer-based procedure functioning in a manner analogous to the human brain. The description is often accompanied by a graphical representation like that in Figure 1. This figure illustrates a feed-forward neural network with one hidden layer. The number of hidden layers may vary but is almost always chosen to be one. The network consists of p input units, r hidden units and one output unit. The flow of information is indicated by the arrows.

The units in the input layer $x = (x_1, \ldots, x_p)'$ correspond to the covariates in a logistic regression model. The hidden units $h_1, \ldots, h_r$ are the result of applying a so-called 'activation function' to a weighted sum of the input units plus a constant which is called 'bias' in the neural net framework. The value of a hidden unit h_j, $j = 1, \ldots, r$ is given by

$$h_j = \phi_j^h \left(w_{0j} + \sum_{i=1}^{p} w_{ij} x_i \right)$$

with unknown parameters $w_{0j}, \ldots, w_{pj}$. Although the activation functions $\phi_j^h(.)$ could be mutually different they are almost always chosen as the logistic function $\Lambda(.)$. Thus the value of a hidden unit appears to be

$$h_j = \frac{1}{1 + \exp(-w_{0j} - \sum_{i=1}^{p} w_{ij} x_i)} = \Lambda \left(w_{0j} + \sum_{i=1}^{p} w_{ij} x_i \right).$$

The value of the output unit y is calculated by applying another activation function $\phi^o(.)$ to the weighted sum of the values of the hidden units plus bias. The output activation function must not coincide with any $\phi_j^h(.)$ but in most applications it is also chosen as the logistic function. Hence

$$y = f(x, w) = \Lambda \left(W_0 + \sum_{j=1}^{r} W_j h_j \right) = \Lambda \left(W_0 + \sum_{j=1}^{r} W_j \Lambda \left(w_{0j} + \sum_{i=1}^{p} w_{ij} x_i \right) \right) \qquad (4)$$

with unknown weights $w = (W_0, \ldots, W_r, w_{01}, \ldots, w_{pr})$, which have to be estimated in a 'learning' or 'training' process. This representation of a feed-forward neural network may not have the appeal of Figure 1, but is the basis for analytical comparisons of feed-forward neural nets and logistic regression models.

One drawback of feed-forward neural networks is that the weights w have no clear interpretation. Except for a neural net without a hidden layer and with a logistic activation function, the weights lack the interpretation as log-odds ratios. In this special case formula (4) reduces to formula (2) which is a linear logistic regression model. This specific network type is called 'logistic perceptron' in the neural network literature. An extension of model (4) for $K > 2$ unordered categories is a feed-forward neural network with K output units and a softmax activation function [14,15] in the output layer. Such a network without a hidden layer is equivalent to use of a polytomous logistic regression model [16,17] for the conditional probabilities $P(Y = k \mid X = x)$, $k = 1, \ldots, K$. A feed-forward neural network with p input units, r hidden units and K output units is denoted by p-r-K in the following.

2.3. Estimation

A sample of N individuals with known covariate values $x^{(n)} = (x_1^{(n)}, \ldots, x_p^{(n)})'$ and known class level $y^{(n)} \in \{0, 1\}$ is used to estimate regression coefficients β or weights w, respectively. 'Training a network' is equivalent to estimation.

In neural net science, estimation is usually based on the minimization of a distance measure called 'energy function' or 'learning function'. In most applications the distance measure chosen is the least squares criterion:

$$D_{\mathrm{LS}}(w) = \sum_{n=1}^{N} (y^{(n)} - f(x^{(n)}, w))^2. \qquad (5)$$

Especially for classification problems, the Kullback–Leibler distance [18] has been proposed in the neural net literature [19,20] as an alternative:

$$D_{\mathrm{KL}}(w) = \sum_{n=1}^{N} \left[y^{(n)} \log \frac{y^{(n)}}{f(x^{(n)}, w)} + (1 - y^{(n)}) \log \frac{1 - y^{(n)}}{1 - f(x^{(n)}, w)} \right]. \qquad (6)$$

In statistical science, estimation is usually based on the maximum likelihood principle [21]. It is well-known that fitting neural networks or logistic regression models by the maximum likelihood principle is equivalent to minimization of the Kullback–Leibler distance [8].

Standard numerical optimization algorithms, like quasi-Newton or Levenberg–Marquardt algorithms, can be used to minimize the chosen distance measure. However, for the training of neural networks other algorithms are preferred. In particular, the back-propagation algorithm or one of its variants is implemented in most commercial neural net programs and thus utilized by the (biomedical) users of this software. The algorithm is known to suffer from convergence problems and difficulties in choosing values for the tuning-parameters embedded in this algorithm ('learning rate', 'momentum' etc.) [22,23]. The literature on numerical optimization provides many simple alternatives like Newton–Raphson methods allowing maximization of (5) or (6) within a few steps and the automatic choice of the tuning parameters.

3. IMPLAUSIBLE FUNCTIONS FITTED BY NEURAL NETWORKS

Feed-forward neural networks with one hidden layer are universal approximators [24–26] and thus can approximate any function defined by the conditional probability (1) with arbitrary precision by increasing the number of hidden units. However, the question in practice is whether we can expect valid approximations to the true function f by solving (5) or (6) based on the limited data available in biomedical applications. To examine this question we consider a simple example that was first presented by Finney [27] and has extensively been used for illustrative purposes [28–30].

The data set consists of a class indicator $Y \in \{0, 1\}$ and two covariates X_1 and X_2 measured on 39 individuals. A scatter plot of the data displayed in Figure 2 indicates that, when considering both covariates, the two classes are well separated, except for two individuals marked in Figure 2. However, for each single covariate the separation is not as obvious.

In the single plots of Figure 3 we included the pairs (Y, X_2), and we observe that the ranges of values of X_2 for $Y = 0$ and $Y = 1$, respectively, clearly overlap. For small values of X_2 the probability of $Y = 1$ is small but it increases with increasing X_2. We first fit a linear logistic regression model to this data, using the maximum-likelihood principle as provided by PROC LOGISTIC in SAS 6.11 [31]. The resulting estimated function $x \mapsto f(x, \hat{\beta})$ is shown in the first plot; it is a smooth and hence plausible proposal for the true f.

Next we fit feed-forward neural networks with logistic activation functions by minimizing the Kullback–Leibler distance (6), using the back-propagation algorithm provided by the public domain software package Stuttgart Neural Network Simulator (SNNS) [32], version 4.1, with a self-written extension for the Kullback–Leibler criterion. Using a simple logistic perceptron, we achieve of course the same function $x \mapsto f(x, \hat{w})$ as in the case of linear logistic regression. Using neural networks with a hidden layer, we find ourselves confronted with functions becoming more and more warped with increasing numbers of hidden units. Such functions are increasingly

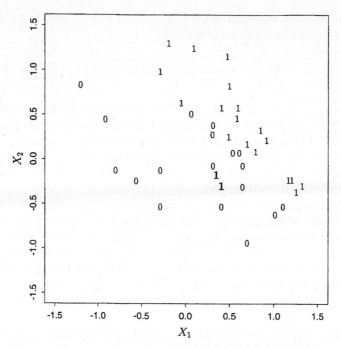

Figure 2. Scatter plot of the Finney data [27]; class membership is indicated by the plotting symbol; two influential observations are printed in bold font.

implausible, because the true function f should reflect some biological or medical relationship that can assumed to be smooth, not warped.

Mathematically, the extreme fluttering of the functions shown in Figure 3 is due to some very large weights. This undesirable feature is well recognized in the literature on neural nets, and there exists the suggestion of introducing some weight decay [7] to overcome this problem, that is, to add the sum of squared weights to the distance measure $D(w)$ as penalty term

$$D^*(w) = D(w) + \lambda \left(\sum_{j=1}^{r} W_j^2 + \sum_{j=1}^{r} \sum_{i=1}^{p} w_{ij}^2 \right)$$

with $D(w)$ according to (5) or (6). The smoothness of the resulting function is controlled by the decay parameter λ. The effect of using weight decay is illustrated in the lower part of Figure 3. A neural network with 15 hidden units and $\lambda = 0.005$ results in a fit comparable to that of to the logistic regression model. However, weight decay seems to have rarely been used in biomedical applications.

The tendency of neural nets to fit implausible functions can also be illustrated by considering both covariates. Fitting a linear logistic model results in a function (Figure 4) which is still smooth, but clearly indicates the difference between the lower left and upper right part of Figure 2. The two observations printed in bold font in Figure 2 are here regarded as indicators that the change from the upper right part to the lower left part is not a change from a region with definite membership of class 1 to a region with definite membership of class 0, but that there is an

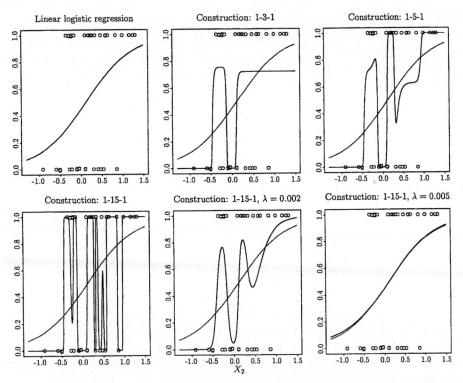

Figure 3. Estimated functions $x \mapsto f(x, \hat{\beta})$ for the probability of belonging to class 1 from the linear logistic regression model and from feed-forward neural networks with different number r of hidden units and logistic activation function for covariate X_2 of the Finney data represented in Figure 2.

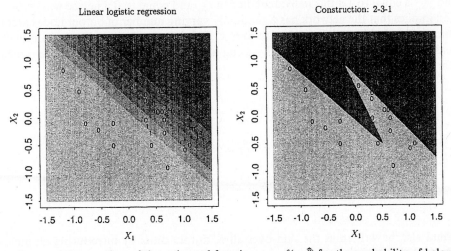

Figure 4. Grey scale image plots of the estimated function $x \mapsto f(x, \hat{\beta})$ for the probability of belonging to class 1 of linear logistic regression and neural networks analyses for both covariates of the Finney data represented in Figure 2. Darker grey scale levels represent higher probabilities of membership in class 1; displayed grey scale levels range from 0 to 1.

intermediate region where both memberships are possible. Feed-forward neural networks with one to five hidden units were fitted to the data. A feed-forward neural network with three hidden units fits almost perfectly but fails to recognize the intermediate region. Instead, a strict frontier between class 1 and class 0 membership is postulated, but this frontier is not smooth and hence barely plausible.

4. SURVIVAL DATA AND NEURAL NETWORKS

The application of feed-forward neural nets to survival data has recently been discussed [33–39]. It is fairly straightforward [37] to consider a 'grouped' version of the Cox regression model [40] in the framework of this paper. Denoting by T the survival time random variable and by I_k the time interval $t_{k-1} \leqslant t < t_k$, $k = 1, \ldots, K$, where $0 = t_0 < t_1 < \cdots < t_K < \infty$, the model can be specified through the conditional probabilities

$$P(T \in I_k \,|\, T \geqslant t_{k-1}, x) = \Lambda \left(\beta_{0k} + \sum_{i=1}^{p} \beta_{ik} x_i \right) \qquad (7)$$

for $k = 1, \ldots, K$. This is the original proposal by Cox [40]; other models for grouped survival data can be obtained using other link functions [41,42]. The neural network corresponding to (7) is an extension of model (4) without a hidden unit to K output units $y_1, \ldots, y_K$. The output y_k at the kth output unit corresponds to the conditional probability of dying in the kth time interval I_k, $k = 1, \ldots, K$.

Data for the nth individual consists of a vector $x^{(n)} = (x_1^{(n)}, \ldots, x_p^{(n)})'$ of regressor variables and a vector $y^{(n)} = (y_1^{(n)}, \ldots, y_{K_n}^{(n)})'$ where $y_k^{(n)}$ is an indicator for individual n dying in the interval I_k and $K_n \leqslant K$ is the number of intervals in which individual n is observed. Thus $y_1^{(n)}, \ldots, y_{K_n-1}^{(n)}$ are all zero and $y_{K_n}^{(n)}$ is equal to 1 if this individual died in I_{K_n} and equal to 0 if he/she was censored. This situation implies that the network has a randomly varying number of output nodes according to those time intervals where an individual is 'at risk'. This is a standard problem of survival analysis [43] and can easily be accommodated by using a slight modification of distance measure (6).

In particular, setting

$$y_k = f(x, w) = \Lambda \left(\beta_{0k} + \sum_{i=1}^{p} \beta_{ik} x_i \right)$$

where w summarizes $\beta_{01}, \ldots, \beta_{0K}, \beta_{11}, \ldots, \beta_{pK}$, we obtain

$$D_{\mathrm{KL}}^{*}(w) = \sum_{n=1}^{N} \sum_{k=1}^{K_n} \left[y_k^{(n)} \log \frac{y_k^{(n)}}{f(x^{(n)}, w)} + (1 - y_k^{(n)}) \log \frac{1 - y_k^{(n)}}{1 - f(x^{(n)}, \omega)} \right].$$

This could also be written as the sum over all K output units by introducing an indicator for individual n being at risk at the kth time interval I_k, $k = 1, \ldots, K$, as it is usually done in survival analysis [44]. The proportional hazards assumption can then be implemented in (7) through the constraints $\beta_{ik} = \beta_i$ for $i = 1, \ldots, p$ and $k = 1, \ldots, K$ whereas the parameters β_{0k} are allowed to differ for $k = 1, \ldots, K$.

There have been some other unsound proposals for analysing grouped survival data by means of a feed-forward neural net. In order to predict outcome (death or recurrence) of individual breast cancer patients, Ravdin and Clark [38] and Ravdin *et al.* [39] use a network with only one output unit but using the number k of the time interval as additional input. Moreover, they consider the unconditional survival probability of dying before t_k rather than the conditional one as output. Their underlying model then reads

$$P(T < t_k \,|\, x) = \Lambda \left(\beta_0 + \sum_{i=1}^{p} \beta_i x_i + \beta_{p+1} k \right) \tag{8}$$

for $k = 1, \ldots, K$. This parameterization ensures monotonicity of the survival probabilities but also implies a rather stringent and unusual shape of the survival distribution, since in the case that no covariates are considered (8) reduces to

$$P(T < t_k) = \Lambda (\beta_0 + \beta_{p+1} k)$$

for $k = 1, \ldots, K$. Obviously, the survival probabilities do not depend on the length of time intervals I_k, which is a rather strange and undesirable feature. Including a hidden layer in (8) is a straightforward extension retaining all the features summarized above. De Laurentiis and Ravdin [34] call such type of neural networks 'time-coded models'.

Another form of neural networks that has been applied to survival data are the so-called 'single time-point models' [34]. Since they are identical to a logistic perceptron or a feed-forward neural network with a hidden layer (4) they correspond to fitting of logistic regression models (2) or their generalizations (3) to survival data. In practice, a single time-point t is fixed and the network is trained to predict the t-year survival probabilities. The corresponding model is given by

$$P(T < t \,|\, x) = \Lambda \left(\beta_0 + \sum_{i=1}^{p} \beta_i x_i \right)$$

or its generalization when introducing a hidden layer. This approach is used by Burke [33] to predict 10-year survival of breast cancer patients based on various patient and tumour characteristics at time of primary diagnosis. McGuire *et al.* [45] utilized this approach to predict 5-year disease-free survival of patients with axillary node-negative breast cancer based on seven potentially prognostic variables. Kappen and Neijt [36] used it to predict 2-year survival of patients with advanced ovarian cancer [46] obtained from 17 pre-treatment characteristics. The neural network they actually used reduced to a logistic perceptron.

Of course, such a procedure can be repeatedly applied for the prediction of survival probabilities at fixed time-points $t_1 < t_2 < \cdots < t_K$. For example, Kappen and Neijt [36] trained several ($K = 6$) neural networks to predict survival of patients with ovarian cancer after $1, 2, \ldots, 6$ years. The corresponding model reads

$$P(T < t_k \,|\, x) = \Lambda \left(\beta_{0k} + \sum_{i=1}^{p} \beta_{ik} x_i \right)$$

in the case that no hidden layer is introduced.

Note that without restriction on the parameters such an approach does not guarantee that the probabilities $P(T < t_k \,|\, x)$ increase with k, and hence may result in life-table estimators suggesting non-monotone survival functions. Closely related to such an approach are the so-called 'multiple time-point models' [34] where one neural network with K output units with or without a hidden layer is used.

The common drawback of these naive approaches is that they do not allow one to incorporate censored observations in a straightforward manner, which is closely related to the fact that they are based on unconditional survival probabilities instead of conditional survival probabilities as the Cox model. Neither omission of the censored observations – as suggested by Burke [33] – nor treating censored observations as uncensored are valid approaches, but a serious source of bias, which is well-known in the statistical literature. De Laurentiis and Ravdin [34] propose to impute estimated survival probabilities for the censored cases from a Cox regression model, that is, they use a well established statistical procedure just to make an artificial neural network work. Future developments should be based on the considerations given by Liestøl et al. [37] where the standard requirements for the analysis of survival data are incorporated. Biganzoli et al. [47], for example, use a similar approach. Faraggi and Simon [35] use the regression model arising from a neural network with a hidden layer to define an extension of Cox's proportional hazards regression model that is applied to the well-known prostate cancer data [48].

5. ESTIMATION OF MISCLASSIFICATION PROBABILITIES

In constructing a new rule for prognosis or diagnosis, it is necessary not only to know the new rule, but also to know its accuracy. A simple, meaningful and popular measure to describe the accuracy of a rule is its misclassification probability, that is, the probability of classifying future objects incorrectly. An obvious estimate of the misclassification probability is the apparent error rate defined as the relative frequency of incorrect classifications if the new rule is applied in the current sample, that is, in that sample we have used to construct the rule. However, this rate tends seriously to underestimate the true misclassification probability, because the rule is made as similar as possible to the current data, not to future data. This is especially true for classification rules developed by neural networks where the tendency to overfitting constitutes a major problem. To avoid this underestimation of the true misclassification probability, a widespread technique is to split the sample randomly into a learning set and a test set. The learning set is used to construct the new rule, and the test set is used to estimate the misclassification probability by applying the new rule and counting the incorrect classifications. This test set based error rate is unbiased.

We illustrate the difference between the apparent error rate and the test set based error rate by a small artificial example. We consider a constellation with five covariates, which are independently and identically distributed as standard Gaussian. The probability of an object belonging to one of the classes $Y = 0$ or $Y = 1$ depends only on the first two covariates, and is given by

$$P(Y = 1 \mid X = x) = \begin{cases} 0.85 & \text{if } x_1 > 0 \quad \text{and} \quad x_2 > 0 \\ 0.15 & \text{otherwise.} \end{cases}$$

This reflects a possible situation in medical applications: if two specific variables both exceed a given threshold, we have a high probability that the object belongs to class $Y = 1$, otherwise this probability is small. We draw a sample of size 400 according to this law and split it randomly into a learning set and a test set. Figure 5 shows the distribution of the first two covariates and the

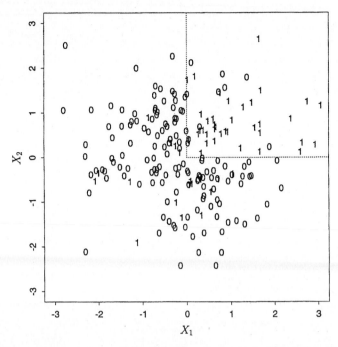

Figure 5. Scatter plot of an artificial example; class membership is indicated by the plotted symbol; region with a high probability for $Y = 1$ in the upper right corner is demarcated by the dotted line.

class membership indicator in the learning set. To the data of the learning set we fit feed-forward neural nets with a logistic activation function and one hidden layer with the number of hidden units r varying between 0 and 15. Figure 6 illustrates the apparent error rates observed in the learning sample and the test set based error rates. We observe that the apparent error rate decreases with increasing number of hidden units and hence suggests (incorrectly) that a neural net with many hidden units should be chosen, whereas the unbiased test set based error rate suggests a neural net with two or three hidden units and indicates that neural nets with a large number of hidden units have a higher misclassification probability. This is expected from the results of Section 3. With increasing number of hidden units we fit more and more implausible functions which move away from the true law f, and hence the misclassification probability increases. On the other hand, the fitted functions resemble more and more closely the data of the learning set, and the apparent error rate decreases. In this artificial example we known the true law generating the data, thus we can compute the true misclassification probability of each rule, which is also shown in Figure 6. The test set based error rates vary around the true probabilities, which illustrates their unbiasedness.

Although such a splitting into a learning set and a test set is widely recommended, it is in general wasteful of information. One should be aware that accurate estimation of misclassification probabilities requires large samples. For example, in order to estimate a true misclassification probability of 20 per cent with an absolute standard error of 1 per cent requires a sample size of 1600. Hence it is usually desirable to use the complete sample both for construction of a rule and for estimation of misclassification probabilities. There exist several techniques for this task,

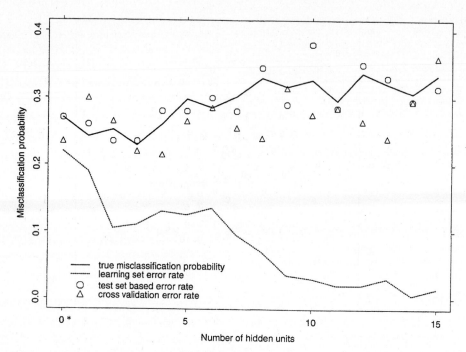

Figure 6. Error rates and true misclassification probabilities of rules based on fitting feed-forward neural networks with one hidden layer with different number *r* of hidden units and logistic activation function. (* The feed-forward neural network with no hidden units is the simple logistic perceptron and equivalent to a simple linear logistic regression model.)

the most well-known being cross-validation. The idea of cross-validation is to split the complete data set several times into a learning set and a test set, to perform estimation of the model parameters in each learning set, and estimation of the misclassification probability in the corresponding test set, and finally to use the average of the test set based error rates as an estimate of the misclassification probability of the rule derived from estimation of the model parameters in the complete sample. Often, the sample is split *k* times with *k* disjoint test sets, and is referred to as *k*-fold cross-validation. If each test set contains only one data point, we speak of leave-one-out cross-validation. To illustrate the power of this approach we have used it in the above example to estimate the misclassification probabilities using only the learning set. The resulting error rates based on leave-one-out cross-validation are also shown in Figure 6. We can observe that these estimates vary around the true misclassification probability in a similar manner as the test set based estimates, so that they are of comparable quality.

In developing rules based on neural nets, the computation of test set based error rates is often an intermediate step in the process of finding the optimal number of hidden units. Then the neural net with the smallest test set based error rate is selected as the new rule. A common mistake is to report the minimal test set based error rate, that is, the rate observed for the selected rule, as an estimate for the misclassification probability in classifying future objects using the selected rule. However, this is a biased estimate which tends to underestimate the true misclassification probability. A closer look at Figure 6 may illustrate the reason; the test set based error rates vary around the true misclassification probabilities and by selecting the rule with the minimal rate – here the rule based on a 5-2-1 or 5-3-1 network – we have a high probability of selecting a rate smaller than the corresponding true rate. Because a single example may not be convincing, we performed a small simulation study where we generated 500 pairs of learning and test sets of size 200 according to the above law. We always fitted as above the 16 different neural nets and selected that with minimal test set based error rate. On average we observe a true misclassification probability of 0.233, but a test set based error rate of only 0.211, that is, an average difference of 0.022. Looking at the ratio between the test set based error rate of the selected rule and the true misclassification probability of the selected rule, we observe on average an underestimation of 9 per cent. Moreover, in 75 per cent of the repetitions the test set based error rate of the selected rule was smaller than the true misclassification probability. If we consider the same problem with a smaller sample size of 100 for learning and test set (and many examples of the use of neural nets in medical applications are even smaller, see the next section), then the results are even worse; we observe an average difference of 0.036 and an average relative underestimation of 13 per cent.

A general strategy to avoid this underestimation is to split the available sample into three subsamples: learning, validation, and test set [5,22]. The learning set is used to estimate the parameters in models with a varying number of hidden units. The validation set is used for an unbiased estimation of the misclassification probability of the rule based on the parameter estimates obtained in the learning set for each model. Then the rule with the smallest error rate is selected, and finally, the test set is used to obtain an unbiased estimate of the misclassification probability of the selected rule. This is a nice paradigm, but even more wasteful of information. Again cross-validation allows to make use of all data. However, it requires a very computer time intensive nested loop. In each subset with one observation left out we have to repeat the complete process of selecting a rule, that is, for each considered model we have to estimate first the parameters and then the error rate by cross-validation. From this point of view alternative methods to allow a direct selection among different models are helpful. This can be done by adding some penalty to the minimal Kullback–Leibler distance achieved in fitting the single models, where the penalty depends on the number of parameters of each model. The most prominent measures following this idea are Akaike's information criterion [49], and its analogue, the network information criterion [50]. Using such criteria, we need cross-validation only to assess the misclassification probability of the resulting rule.

In addition to the misclassification probability, other measures for the accuracy are possible. Especially in diagnostic studies one should report additionally the sensitivity and specificity of a new rule or the whole receiver operating characteristic (ROC) curve [51]. If – as it is often the case in diagnostic studies – the sample is not drawn from one population, but separately from two populations of diseased and healthy subjects, these are the only meaningful measures, as the misclassification probability depends on the prevalence, that is, a chance of selecting a diseased or healthy subject which is arbitrary.

6. FREQUENTLY MADE MISTAKES IN APPLICATIONS OF ANNS

We reviewed the medical literature between 1991 and 1995 to examine applications of feed-forward neural networks for prognostic and diagnostic classification in oncological studies.

A Medline search conducted in May 1996 yielded 173 articles in English or German concerning the use of artificial neural networks and artificial intelligence in oncology. After reading the available abstracts, 43 articles, summarized in Table I, remained in which feed-forward neural nets were used for classification, some of which considered statistical methods as alternatives. The topics of these articles were diagnosis of cancer (23 articles), automatic tumour grading (6 articles) and prognosis (10 articles), and a further 3 reviews and 2 commentaries. Most of the excluded articles dealt with the application of artificial intelligence in image analysis and the use of expert systems for classification. We reviewed the methodological quality of these publications and identified some common mistakes which are indicated in Table I and are now described in detail.

6.1. Mistakes in estimation of misclassification probabilities

6.1.1. Biased estimation. The dramatic underestimation of the apparent error rate seems to be well-known. In none of the articles was the apparent error rate used as an estimate of the misclassification probability. For estimation, either an independent test set or cross-validation or another resampling method was always used. However, in most cases, the network with the smallest test set based error rate or the smallest cross-validation error rate was selected and this minimal error rate was regarded as a valid estimate of the true misclassification probability, which is not true, as shown in the last section. There are only a few articles following the paradigm of a split into learning, validation and test sets ensuring unbiased error rates.

6.1.2. Inefficient estimation. In many articles the size of the test set was very small; in six articles it contains less than 20 observations. Consequently, the estimates of the misclassification probabilities are highly unstable, but this problem is totally ignored. In general, all applications using a split sample approach could have been improved by using cross-validation techniques.

6.2. Fitting of implausible functions

In Section 3 we have demonstrated that due to overfitting the available data fitting neural nets with many hidden units results in implausible functions to describe the probability of class membership; there exists no generally valid limit where overfitting begins, but a key number is the ratio between the number of observations and the number of parameters in a model. In the example of Figure 3 with 39 observations we can observe that we have distinct overfitting for a 1-5-1 network with 16 parameters, and already some overfitting for a 1-3-1 network with 10 parameters. This agrees with traditional rules of thumb in the statistical literature, requiring 5 or 10 observations for each parameter to be estimated, which are also considered in the literature on neural networks [52]. If we assume that overfitting occurs at least if the ratio between the number of observations and the number of parameters is smaller than two, then in 23 of the 43 articles we are concerned that the resulting rule suffers from overfitting, that is, it is based on a highly implausible function. The use of weight decay was not mentioned in any of these articles.

6.3. Incorrectly describing the complexity of a network

The above rules of thumb are also used in the literature on neural networks. In the selected applications several authors tried to overcome a possible criticism with respect to overfitting by reporting the ratio between the number of observations and the complexity of the network. However, to measure the complexity they only use the number of input units, which is usually

Table I. Applications of feed-forward neural networks for diagnostic and prognostic classification in oncological studies.

Year	First author	Study type*	Number of individuals Training	Validation	Test	Network	Number of weights	Common mistakes†
1991	Dawson [53]	g	12	31		17-4-4	92	2, 5
	Maclin [54]	d	52	leave-one-out		21-10-3	253	2
	Ostrem [55]	g	87	31		6-12-9-3	231	2
	Piraino [56]	d	110	44		20-40-55	3095	2
1992	Astion [57]	d	57	20		9-15-2	182	1, 2, 3, 5, 6
	Cicchetti [58]	r		*Commentary*				3
	Goldberg [59]	d	200	leave-one-out		3-2-1	11	—
	McGuire [45]	p	133	66		7-6-2	62	1
						8-7-2	79	
	Nafe [60]	d	58	leave-one-out		⋮	⋮	2, 5, 6
						40-14-5	649	
	O'Leary [61]	d	36	19		2-4-1	17	1
	Ravdin [38]	p	500	420	453	8-6-1	61	7
	Ravdin [39]	p	508	500	960	8-4-1	41	7
1993	Kappen [36]	p	269	10% of the data		17-0-1	18	6, 7
						1-5-2	22	
	Schweiger [62]	d	90	16		⋮	⋮	1, 2, 3, 4, 5, 6
						7-15-5	200	
1994	Becker [63]	d	36	19		2-4-1	17	1, 3, 5
	Bugliosi [64]	p	153	19		19-?-?	?	1, 4
	Burke [33]	p	3500	3500	3500	3-9-1	46	7
	Burke [65]	r		*Review*				4
	Clark [66]	r		*Review*				—
	Ercal [67]		240	40%, 60%, 80%		14-7-1	113	2
		d	216	of the data		8-4-1	41	
						5-3-1	22	
	Erler [68]	d	45	45		or	or	2, 5, 6
						5-5-2	42	
	Floyd [69]	d	260	leave-one-out		8-16-1	161	1, 2
	Giger [70]	d	53	leave-one-out		2-4-1	17	—
	Kolles [71]	g	?	?	?	?-?-?	?	4
	Maclin [72]	d	72	leave-four-out		35-35-35-5	2700	1, 2
	Reinus [73]	d	709	4-fold crossval.		95-0-45	4320	1, 2
1994	Rogers [74]	r		*Review*				—
	Snow [75]	d	1578	209		14-50-1	801	1, 2
		p	938	5% of the data		12-5-1	71	
	Wilding [76]	d	104	5-fold crossval.		3-6-2	38	2
			98			⋮	⋮	
						10-10-2	132	
	Wu [77]	d	727	leave-one-out		9-8-1	89	1, 5
1995			78	258				
	Attikiouzel [78]	p	65	248		6-18-1	145	1, 2
			477	952		4-12-1	73	
	Baker [79]	d	206	leave-one-out		18-10-1	201	1, 2
	Christy [80]	g	52	29		10-10-2	132	2, 5
	Doyle [81]	p	528	5-fold crossval.		33-48-30-1	3133	1, 2
	Fogel [82]	d	400	283		9-2-1	23	—
	Gurney [83]	d	318	271 bootstrap.		7-3-1	28	—
	Hamamoto [84]	p	54	11		9-14-1	155	1, 2
	Kolles [85]	g	226	679		4-30-10-3	493	1, 2, 5
						4-1-1	7	
	Moul [86]	g	93	9-fold crossval.		⋮	⋮	1, 2
						7-14-1	127	
	Niederberger [87]	r		*Commentary*				—
	Simpson [88]	d	64	27		?-?-?	?	1, 4, 5, 6
	Strotzer [89]	d	115	115		28-?-1	?	2, 4
			45			28-?-23	?	
	Truong [90]	d	56	56		7-10-1	91	1, 2

* d, diagnosis/differential diagnosis; g, automatic grading/cytology; p, prognosis/survival; r, review/commentary

† 1, mistakes in estimation of misclassification proabilities; 2, fitting of implausible functions; 3, incorrectly describing the complexity of a network; 4, no information on complexity of the network; 5, use of inadequate statistical competitors; 6, insufficient comparison with statistical method; 7, naive application of artifical neural networks to survival data.

much smaller than the number of parameters to describe the network. Hence the reported ratios are much too large and the danger of overfitting is underestimated.

6.4. No information on complexity of the network

In order to enable the reader to judge the danger of an overfitted rule using some rule of thumb, it is necessary to know the number of hidden layers and hidden units to calculate the number of fitted weights. However, some publications even omit this basic information.

6.5. Use of inadequate statistical competitors

Some authors compared the performance of a feed-forward neural network with that of a statistical competitor, in all but one of these applications linear or quadratic discriminant analysis. All results reported were in favour of the artificial neural network. This is not surprising since feed-forward neural networks are highly flexible classification tools and 'may yield better classification results than DFs (discriminant functions) since they form complex, non-linear associations between input data and output results' [68]. An adequate and fair comparison of the performance of feed-forward neural networks and statistical methods must be based on statistical tools of similar flexibility like nearest-neighbour methods [91], generalized additive models [12], CART [92] or logistic regression models with quadratic terms and multiplicative interaction terms. Such comparisons were made by Ripley [7] and Vach *et al.* [93], for example, and demonstrated that the discriminative power of neural networks and flexible statistical methods are similar.

6.6. Insufficient comparison with statistical method

Astion and Wilding [57] concluded that 'results from neural networks compare favorably with those obtained for the same sets of patients as analyzed by QDFA (quadratic discriminant function analysis)'. This conclusion was solely based on four (feed-forward neural network) and five (quadratic discriminant analysis) misclassified observations for a test set of 20 observations, that is, highly unstable estimates of the misclassification probabilities. No attempt was made to prove the significance of the difference between the observed misclassification rates, which is necessary to conclude that one rule outperforms the other. This testing can be done by use of the McNemar test, for example. The performance of a feed-forward neural network and a statistical competitor was evaluated by simply inspecting the estimates of the misclassification probability in several applications.

6.7. Naive application of artificial neural networks to survival data

All applications of feed-forward neural networks to survival data [33,36,38,39] suffer from the deficiencies mentioned in Section 4. The approach used in Kappen and Neijt [36] does not guarantee monotonicity of the estimated survival curves. Burke [33] omitted the censored cases, which is a serious source of bias. Ravdin and Clark [38] and Ravdin *et al.* [39] used the number of the time interval as additional input unit, hence the estimated survival probabilities do not depend on the length of the time intervals. These obvious deficiencies show that there is some danger that the fruitful development of statistical methodology for survival data during the last three decades may be wasted with these naive applications of neural networks to such data.

7. CONCLUSIONS

We have seen that most applications of artificial neural networks for prognosis and diagnosis in oncology during the last years suffer from methodological deficiencies. In many applications some overfitting probably occurs, resulting in biologically implausible functions to describe the class membership probability. In many applications the reported error rate for the selected neural network underestimates the true misclassification probability. Moreover, we often observed a fundamental misunderstanding of the mathematics of neural networks and basic statistical principles. Examples are the use of two output units in the case of two classes, which gives the same result as using only one output unit, the fitting of non-monotone survival curves, misunderstanding of sensitivity and specificity measures or error rates based on very small samples, ignoring the instability of such estimates. One might hope that review papers and textbooks on artificial neural networks available for any potential user (for example, Cheng and Titterington [6], Hecht-Nielsen [94] and Ripley [7]), which include warnings against the common mistakes we mentioned, may lead to a better understanding and use of artificial neural networks. However, we could not observe any improvement in the quality of applications of artificial neural networks in oncological studies over time (see Table I). In revising this paper, we picked out two recent articles on the application of artificial neural networks in oncology that appeared in prominent journals [95, 96]. In these two articles several of the commonly made mistakes appeared again, giving rise to the conjecture that the situation has not improved substantially after our literature review.

Incidentally, we came across a paper by Peter Lachenbruch entitled 'Some misuses of discriminant analysis' [97] where he identified frequently made mistakes of similar type. This paper was written in 1977, at a time where statistical packages like BMDP, SAS, or SPSS became widely available to non-specialists. This seems to have been a similar situation to today where numerous user-friendly neural network packages are available which can in principle be used by everyone who is able to click the mouse button on a personal computer.

The application of artificial neural networks in biomedical applications is often accompanied by grossly overstated claims, praising neural networks as the ultimate solution to the problem of diagnosis and prognosis. For example, neural networks 'ability to learn … make them formidable tools in the fight against cancer' [33] and 'neural computation may be as beneficial to medicine and urology in the twenty-first century as molecular biology has been in the twentieth' [87].

In our opinion, there is no evidence that artificial neural networks have provided real progress in the field of diagnosis and prognosis in oncology. We have tried to demonstrate that feedforward neural networks are nothing more than regression models like logistic regression models, the only differences being that feed-forward neural networks (with hidden layers) provide a larger class of regression functions. This is often referred to as the greater flexibility of neural networks. However, greater flexibility is only of value if the true regression function is far away from that of a linear logistic model. Small deviations from a linear logistic model do not matter, because due to the small sample sizes of a few hundred typical in oncological applications, such a difference may be small relative to random errors. Large deviations, especially functions with many jumps, are not very plausible, because biological relationships tend to be smooth. Hence one cannot expect that the greater flexibility of neural networks helps them to outperform logistic models, especially if the latter are combined with careful model building, allowing use of quadratic or higher interaction terms, for example. In a recent publication, Ennis *et al.* [98] compared the results of a logistic regression approach [99] with that of artificial neural networks and several flexible statistical modelling approaches using data from a large clinical trial in cardiology [100].

They concluded that 'with such a large data set none of the adaptive non-linear methods that we tried could outperform the logistic regression model of Lee *et al.*'. Similar experiences have been encountered in other applications in cardiology [101, 102]. Additionally, in contrast to neural network such logistic models still allow one to describe and evaluate the influence of the single covariates. This information is often of equal importance as the decision rule, as it may allow a better understanding of the underlying process.

Nevertheless, how can we explain that the comparison with statistical procedures reported in some of the selected articles almost always favour neural networks? In our opinion, this may at least partially be due to some methodological deficiencies. Usually many different neural networks are fitted on the same data set. Without using an independent test set, the minimal error rate observed within the class of neural nets underestimates the true misclassification probability. If, on the other hand, only one or two statistical procedures are used for such a comparison, corresponding error rates will not be biased to such an extent. Moreover, it seems absolutely unfair to allow an intensive model selection procedure for neural networks but not for their statistical competitors. Indeed, investigations comparing neural networks with flexible statistical methods which also allow some model building do not indicate great differences.

One should also be aware that the results favouring neural nets are based on a comparison with statistical procedures. To prove the significance of neural nets to oncology, one should at least find one application where neural nets succeed in finding a new rule proven to be better than an existing one in the literature, depending on the same covariates, which cannot be developed by statistical procedures. All applications listed in Table I avoid a comparison with an existing prognostic index or a diagnostic rule, and hence are inadequate to demonstrate the value of neural networks for medical research in oncology.

REFERENCES

1. Baxt WG. Application of artifical neural networks to clinical medicine. *Lancet* 1995; **346**:1135–1138.
2. Cross SS, Harrison RF, Kennedy RL. Introduction to neural networks. *Lancet* 1995; **346**:1075–1079.
3. Dybowski R, Gant V. Artificial neural networks in pathology and medical laboratories. *Lancet* 1995; **346**:1203–1207.
4. Wyatt J. Nervous about artificial neural networks? *Lancet* 1995; **346**:1175–1177.
5. Penny W, Frost D. Neural networks in clinical medicine. *Medical Decision Making* 1996; **16**:386–398.
6. Cheng B, Titterington DM. Neural networks: a review from a statistical perspective (with discussion). *Statistical Science* 1994; **9**:2–54.
7. Ripley BD. Statistical aspects of neural networks. In *Networks and Chaos – Statistical and Probabilistic Aspects*, Barndorff-Nielsen OE, Jensen JL (eds). Chapman and Hall: London, 1993.
8. Schumacher M, Roßner, R, Vach W. Neural networks and logistic regression: Part I. *Computational Statistics and Data Analysis* 1996; **21**:661–682.
9. Stern HS. Neural networks in applied statistics (with discussion). *Technometrics* 1996; **38**:205–220.
10. Warner B, Misra M. Understanding neural networks at statistical tools. *American Statistician* 1996; **50**:284–293.
11. Cox DR, Snell EJ. *Analysis of Binary Data*, 2nd edn. Chapman and Hall: London, 1992.
12. Hastie TJ, Tibshirani RJ. *Generalized Additive Models*. Chapman and Hall: London, 1990.
13. Royston P, Altman DG. Regression using fractional polynomials of continuous covariates: parsimonious parametric modelling (with discussion). *Applied Statistics* 1994; **43**:429–467.
14. Bridle JS. Probabilistic interpretation of feedforward classification network outputs with relationships to statistical pattern recognition. In *Neuro-Computing: Algorithms, Architectures and Applications*, Fogleman SF, Hérault J (eds), Springer-Verlag: New York, 1990.
15. Bridle JS. Training stochastic model recognition algorithms as networks can leads to maximum mutual information estimation of parameters. In *Advances in Neural Information Processing Systems 2*, Touretzky DS (ed.), Morgan Kaufmann: San Mateo, CA, 1990.
16. Engel J. Polytomous logistic regression. *Statistica Neerlandica* 1988; **42**:233–252.
17. McCullagh P, Nelder JA. *Generalized Linear Models*, 2nd edn. Chapman and Hall: London, 1989.
18. Kullback S, Leibler RA. On information and sufficiency. *Annals of Mathematical Statistics* 1995; **22**:79–86.

19. Barron AR, Barron RL. Statistical learning networks: a unifying view. In *Computing Science and Statistics: Proceedings 20th Symposium Interface*, Wegman E (ed.) American Statistical Association: Washington, 1988.
20. Hinton GE. Connectionist learning procedures. *Artificial Intelligence* 1989; **40**:185–234.
21. Mood AM, Graybill FA, Boes DC. *Introduction to the Theory of Statistics*, 3rd edn. McGraw-Hill: Singapore, 1974.
22. Ripley BD. *Pattern Recognition and Neural Networks*. University Press: Cambridge, 1996.
23. Sarle WS. Neural networks and statistical models. In Proceedings of the 19th Annual SAS Users Group International Conference, 1994.
24. Cybenko G. Approximation by superpositions of a sigmoidal function. *Mathematics of Controls, Signals, and Systems* 1989; **2**:303–314.
25. Funahashi K. On the approximate realization of continuous mappings by neural networks. *Neural Networks* 1989; **2**:183–192.
26. Hornik K, Stinchcombe M, White H. Multilayer feedforward networks are universal approximators *Neural Networks* 1989; **2**:359–366.
27. Finney DJ. The estimation from individual records of the relationship between dose and quantal response. *Biometrika* 1947; **34**:320–334.
28. Fahrmeir L, Tutz G. *Multivariate Statistical Modelling Based on Generalized Linear Models*. Springer-Verlag: New York, 1994.
29. Morgenthaler S. Least-absolute-deviations fits for generalized linear models. *Biometrika* 1992; **79**:747–754.
30. Pregibon D. Resistant fits for some commonly used logistic models with medical applications. *Biometrics* 1982; **38**:485–498.
31. SAS-Institute Inc. *SAS/STAT User's Guide, Version 6*, 4th edn. SAS-Institute Inc: Cary NC, 1990.
32. Zell A, Mamier G, Vogt M, Mache N, Hübner R, Döring S, Herrmann KU, Soyez T, Schmalzl M, Sommer T, Hatzigeorgiou A, Posselt D, Schreiner T, Kett B, Clemente G, Wieland J. *Stuttgart Neural Network Simulator, User Manual, Version 4.1, Report no 6/95*. Institute for Parallel and Distributed High Performance Systems, 1995.
33. Burke HB. Artificial neural networks for cancer research: outcome prediction. *Seminars in Surgical Oncology* 1994; **10**:73–79.
34. De Laurentiis M, Ravdin PM. Survival analysis of censored data: neural network analysis detection of complex interactions between variables. *Breast Cancer Research and Treatment* 1994; **32**:113–118.
35. Faraggi D, Simon R. A neural network model for survival data. *Statistics in Medicine* 1995; **14**:73–82.
36. Kappen HJ, Neijt JP. Neural network analysis to predict treatment outcome. *Annals of Oncology* 1993; **4**:Supplement S31–34.
37. Liestøl K, Andersen PK, Andersen U. Survival analysis and neural nets. *Statistics in Medicine* 1994; **13**:1189–1200.
38. Ravdin PM, Clark GM. A practical application of neural network analysis for predicting outcome of individual breast cancer patients. *Breast Cancer Research and Treatement* 1992; **22**:285–293.
39. Ravdin PM, Clark GM, Hilsenbeck SG, Owens MA, Vendely P, Pandian MR, McGuire WL. A demonstration that breast cancer recurrence can be predicted by neural network analysis. *Breast Cancer Research and Treatment* 1992; **21**:47–53.
40. Cox DR. Regression models and life tables (with discussion). *Journal of the Royal Statistical Society, Series B* 1972; **34**:187–220.
41. Doksum KA, Gasko M. On a correspondence between models in binary regression analysis and in survival analysis. *International Statistical Review* 1990; **58**:243–252.
42. Prentice RL, Gloeckler LA. Regression analysis of grouped survival data with application to breast cancer data. *Biometrics* 1978; **34**:57–67.
43. Kalbfleisch JD, Prentice RL. *The Statistical Analysis of Failure Time Data*. Wiley:New York, 1980
44. Andersen PK, Borgan Ø, Gill RD, Keiding N. *Statistical Models Based on Counting Processes*. Springer-Verlag: New York, 1993.
45. McGuire WL, Tandon AK, Allred DC, Chamness GC, Ravdin PM, Clark GM. Treatment decisions in axillary node-negative breast cancer patients. *Monographs – National Cancer Institute* 1992; **11**:173–180.
46. Van Houwelingen JC, ten Bokkel Huinink WW, van der Burg ME, van Oosterom AT, Neijt JP. Predictability of the survival of patients with advanced ovarian cancer. *Journal of Clinical Oncology* 1989; **7**:769–773.
47. Biganzoli E, Boracchi P, Mariani L, Marubini E. Feed forward neural networks for the analysis of censored survival data: a partial logistic regression approach. *Statistics in Medicine* 1998; **17**:1169–1186.
48. Andrews DF, Herzberg AM. *Data – a Collection of Problems from many Fields for the Student and Research Worker*. Springer-Verlag: New York, 1985.
49. Akaike H. Fitting autoregressive models for prediction. *Annals of the Institute of Statistical Mathematics* 1969; **21**:243–247.
50. Murata N, Yoshizawa S, Amari SI. Network information criterion — determining the number of hidden units for artificial neural network models. *IEEE Transactions on Neural Networks*, 1994; **5**:865–872.
51. De Leo JM, Campbell G. Receiver operating characteristic (ROC) methodology in artificial neural networks with biomedical applications. In *Proceedings of the World Congress on Neural Networks*, 1995.

52. Livingstone DJ, Manallack DT. Statistics using neural networks: chance effects. *Journal of Medicinal Chemistry* 1993; **36**:1295–1297.
53. Dawson AE, Austin RE, Weinberg DS. Nuclear grading of breast carcinoma by image analysis classification by multivariate and neural network analysis. *American Journal of Clinical Pathology* 1991; **95**:Supplement S29–37.
54. Maclin PS, Dempsey J, Brooks J, Rand J. Using neural networks to diagnose cancer. *Journal of Medical Systems* 1991; **15**:11–19.
55. Ostrem JS, Valdes AD, Edmonds PD. Application of neural nets to ultrasound tissue characterization. *Ultrasonic Imaging* 1991; **13**:298–299.
56. Piraino DW, Amartur SC, Richmond BJ, Schils JP, Thome JM, Belhobek GH, Schlucter MD. Application of an artifical neural network in radiographic diagnosis. *Journal of Digital Imaging* 1991; **4**:226–232.
57. Astion ML, Wilding P. Application of neural networks to the interpretation of laboratory data in cancer diagnosis. *Clinical Chemistry* 1992; **38**:34–38.
58. Cicchetti DV. Neural networks and diagnosis in the clinical laboratory: state of the art. *Clinical Chemistry* 1991; **38**:9–10.
59. Goldberg V, Manduca A, Ewert DL, Gisvold JJ, Greenleaf JF. Improvement in specificity of ultrasonography for diagnosis of breast tumors by means of artificial intelligence. *Medical Physics* 1992; **19**:1475–1481.
60. Nafe R, Chortiz H. Introduction of a neuronal network as a tool for diagnostic analysis and classification based on experimental pathologic data. *Experimental and Toxicologic Pathology* 1992; **44**:17–24.
61. O'Leary TJ, Mikel UV, Becker RL. Computer-assisted image interpretation: use of a neural network to differentiate tubular carcinoma from sclerosing adenosis. *Modern Pathology* 1992; **5**:402–405.
62. Schweiger CR, Soeregi G, Spitzauer S, Maenner G, Pohl AL. Evaluation of laboratory data by conventional statistics and by three types of neural networks. *Clinical Chemistry* 1993; **39**:1966–1971.
63. Becker RL. Computer-assisted image classification: use of neural networks in anatomic pathology. *Cancer Letters* 1994; **77**:111–117.
64. Bugliosi R, Tribalto M, Avvisati G, Boccadoro M, De Martinis C, Friera R, Mandelli F, Pileri A, Papa G. Classification of patients affected by multiple myeloma using a neural network software. *European Journal of Haematology* 1994; **52**:182–183.
65. Burke HB. Increasing the power of surrogate endpoint biomarkers: the aggregation of predictive factors. *Journal of Cellular Biochemistry* 1994; **19**:Supplement 278–282.
66. Clark GM, Hilsenbeck SG, Ravdin PM, De Laurentiis M, Osborne CK. Prognostic factors: rationale and methods of analysis and integration. *Breast Cancer Research and Treatement* 1994; **32**:105–112.
67. Ercal F, Chawla A, Stoecker WV, Lee H, Moss RH. Neural network diagnosis of malignant melanoma from color images. *IEEE Transations on Biomedical Engineering* 1994; **41**:837–845.
68. Erler BS, Hsu L, Truong HM, Petrovic LM, Kim SS, Huh MH, Ferrell LD, Thung SN, Geller SA, Marchevsky AM. Image analysis and diagnostic classification of hepatocellular carcinoma using neural networks and multivariate discriminant functions. *Laboratory Investigation* 1994; **71**:446–451.
69. Floyd Jr CE, JYL, Yun AJ, Sullivan DC, Kornguth PJ. Prediction of breast cancer malignancy using an artificial neural network. *Cancer* 1994; **74**:2944–2948.
70. Giger ML, Vyborny CJ, Schmidt RA. Computerized characterization of mammorgraphic masses: analysis of spiculation. *Cancer Letters* 1994; **77**:201–211.
71. Kolles H, von Wangenheim A, Niedermayer I, Vince GH, Feiden W. Computer assisted grading of astrocytoma. *Verhandlungen der Deutschen Gesellschaft für Pathologie* 1994; **78**:427–431.
72. Maclin PS, Dempsey J. How to improve a neural network for early detection of hepatic cancer. *Cancer Letters* 1994; **77**:95–101.
73. Reinus WR, Wilson AJ, Kalman B, Kwasny S. Diagnosis of focal bone lesions using neural networks. *Investigative Radiology* 1994; **29**:606–611.
74. Rogers SK, Ruck DW, Kabrisky M. Artificial neural networks for early detection and diagnosis of cancer. *Cancer Letters* 1994; **77**:79–83.
75. Snow PB, Smith DS, Catalona WJ. Artificial neural networks in the diagnosis and prognosis of prostate cancer: a pilot study. *Journal of Urology* 1994; **152**:1923–1926.
76. Wilding P, Morgan MA, Grygotis AE, Shoffner MA, Rosato EF. Application of backpropagation neural networks to diagnosis of breast and ovarian cancer. *Cancer Letters* 1994; **77**:145–153.
77. Wu YC, Doi K, Giger ML, Metz CE, Zhang W. Reduction of false positives in computerized detection of lung nodules in chest radiographs using artificial neural networks, discriminant analysis, and a rule-based scheme. *Journal of Digital Imaging* 1994; **7**:196–207.
78. Attikiouzel Y, de Silva CJ. Applications of neural networks in medicine. *Australasian Physical & Engineering Sciences in Medicine* 1995; **18**:158–164.
79. Baker JA, Kornguth PJ, Lo JY, Williford ME, Floyd CE. Breast cancer: prediction with artificial neural network based on bi-rads standardized lexicon. *Radiology* 1995; **196**:817–822.
80. Christy PS, Tervonen O, Scheithauer BW, Forbes GS. Use of a neural network and a multiple regression model to predict histologic grade of astrocytoma from mri appearances. *Neuroradiology* 1995; **37**:89–93.

81. Doyle HR, Parmanto B, Munro PW, Marino IR, Aldrighetti L, Doria C, McMichael J, Fung JJ. Building clinical classifiers using incomplete observations – a neural network ensemble for hepatoma detection in patients with cirrhosis. *Methods of Information in Medicine* 1995; **34**:253–258.
82. Fogel DB, Wasson 3rd EC, Boughton EM. Evolving neural networks for detecting breast cancer. *Cancer Letters* 1995; **96**:49–53.
83. Gurney JW, Swensen ST. Solitary pulmonary nodules: determining the likelihood of malignancy with neural network analysis. *Radiology* 1995: **196**:823–829.
84. Hamamoto I, Okada S, Hashimoto T, Wakabayashi H, Maeba T, Maeta H. Prediction of the early prognosis of the hepatectomized patient with hepatocellular carcinoma with a neural network. *Computers in Biology and Medicine* 1995; **25**:49–59.
85. Kolles H, von Wangenheim A, Vince GH, Niedermayer I, Feiden W. Automated grading of astrocytomas based on histomorphometric analysis of Ki-67 and Feulgen stained paraffin sections. classification results of neuronal networks and discriminant analysis. *Annals Cellular Pathology* 1995; **8**:101–116.
86. Moul JW, Snow PB, Fernandez EB, Maher PD, Sesterhenn IA. Neural network analysis of quantitative histological factors to predict pathological stage in clinical stage i nonseminomatous testicular cancer. *Journal of Urology* 1995; **153**:1674–1677.
87. Niederberger CS. Commentary on the use of neural networks in clinical urology. *Journal of Urology* 1995; **153**:1362.
88. Simpson HW, McArdle C, Pauson AW, Hume P, Turkes A, Griffiths K. A non-invasive test for the pre-cancerous breast. *European Journal of Cancer* 1995; **31A**:1768–1772.
89. Strotzer M, Krös P, Held P, Feuerbach S. Die Treffsicherheit künstlicher neuronaler Netze in der radiologischen Differentialdiagnose solitärer Knochenläsionen. *Fortschritte auf dem Gebiete der Röntgenstrahlen und der Neuen Bildgebenden Verfahren* 1995; **163**:245–249.
90. Truong H, Morimoto R, Walts AE, Erler B, Marchevsky A. Neural networks as an aid in the diagnosis of lymphocyte-rich effusions. *Analytical and Quantitative Cytology and Histology* 1995; **17**:48–54.
91. Hand DJ. *Discrimination and Classification.* Wiley: New York, 1981.
92. Breiman L, Friedman JH. Olshen RA, Stone CJ. *Classification and Regression Trees.* Wadsworth and Brooks: Monterey, California, 1984.
93. Vach W, Roßner R, Schumacher M. Neural networks and logistic regression: Part II. *Computational Statistics and Data Analysis* 1996; **21**:683–701.
94. Hecht-Nielsen R. *Neurocomputing.* Addison-Wesley: New York, 1990.
95. Bottaci L, Drew PJ, Hartley JE, Hadfield MB, Farouk R, Lee PWR, Macintyre IMC, Duthie GS, Monson JRT. Artificial neural networks applied to outcome prediction for colorectal cancer patients in separate institutions. *Lancet* 1997; **350**:469–472.
96. Burke HB, Goodman PH, Rosen DB, Henson DE, Weinstein JN, Harrell FE, Marks JR, Winchester DP, Bostwick DG. Artificial neural networks improve the accuracy of cancer survival prediction. *Cancer* 1997; **79**:857–862.
97. Lachenbruch PA. Some misuses of discriminant analysis. *Methods of Information in Medicine* 1977; **16**:255–258.
98. Ennis M, Hinton G, Naylor D, Revow M, Tibshirani R. A comparison of statistical learning methods on the GUSTO database. *Statistics in Medicine* 1998; **17**:2501–2508.
99. Lee KL, Woodlief LH, Topol EJ, Weaver WD, Betriu A, Col J, Simoons M, Aylward P, Van de Werf F, Califf RM. Predictors of 30-day mortality in the era of reperfusion for acute myocardial infarction. results from an international trial of 41 021 patients. *Circulation* 1995; **91**:1659–1668.
100. GUSTO-1 Investigators. An international randomized trial comparing four thrombolytic strategies for acute myocardial infarction. *New England Journal of Medicine* 1993; **329**:673–682.
101. Tu JV. Advantages and disadvantages of using artificial neural networks versus logistic regression for predicting medical outcomes. *Journal of Clinical Epidemiology*, 1996; **49**:1225–1231.
102. Tu JV, Weinstein MC, McNeill BJ, Naylor CD and the Steering Committee of the Cardiac Care Network of Ontario. Predicting mortality after coronary artery bypass surgery: what do artifical neural networks learn? *Medical Decision Making* 1998; **18**:229–235.

Assessment of Decision Support for Blood Test Ordering in Primary Care
A Randomized Trial

Marc A.M. van Wijk, MD, PhD; Johan van der Lei, MD, PhD; Mees Mosseveld, MSc; Arthur M. Bohnen, MD, PhD; and Jan H. van Bemmel, PhD

Background: Different methods for changing blood test–ordering behavior in primary care have been proven effective. However, randomized trials comparing these methods are lacking.

Objective: To compare the effect of two versions of BloodLink, a computer-based clinical decision support system, on blood test ordering among general practitioners.

Design: Randomized trial.

Setting: 44 practices of general practitioners in the region of Delft, the Netherlands.

Participants: 60 general practitioners in 44 practices who used computer-based patient records in their practices.

Intervention: After stratification by solo practices and group practices, practices were randomly assigned to use BloodLink-Restricted, which initially displays a reduced list of tests, or Blood-Link-Guideline, which is based on the guidelines of the Dutch College of General Practitioners.

Measurements: Average number of blood tests ordered per order form per practice.

Results: General practitioners who used BloodLink-Guideline requested 20% fewer tests on average than did practitioners who used BloodLink-Restricted (mean [±SD], $5.5 ± 0.9$ tests vs. $6.9 ± 1.6$ tests, respectively; $P = 0.003$, Mann–Whitney test).

Conclusions: Decision support based on guidelines is more effective in changing blood test–ordering behavior than is decision support based on initially displaying a limited number of tests. Guideline-driven decision support systems can be effective in reducing the number of laboratory tests ordered by primary care practitioners.

Ann Intern Med. 2001;134:274-281.   www.annals.org

For author affiliations, current addresses, and contributions, see end of text.

The majority of general practitioners in the Netherlands have replaced traditional paper-based patient records with computer-based records; physicians enter patient data themselves in the computer during patient encounters (1). The use of electronic patient records creates new opportunities to influence physician behavior through implementation of decision support systems (2–7). In recent years, researchers have documented various computer-based decision support systems that have influenced physician behavior (8–17). Other investigators, however, have reported that computer-based decision support has not affected patient care (18). To resolve the issue, investigators have compared the results of studies that were conducted in different settings, used different methods, and involved different populations (19). Studies comparing different methods of providing computer-based decision support in randomized trials are not available.

In the Netherlands, 3% to 4% of patient encounters with general practitioners in primary care result in the ordering of blood tests (20). However, ordering of blood tests is not always appropriate (21–29). Researchers argue that excessive ordering of tests causes physicians to pursue evaluation of false-positive results, which in turn leads to additional unnecessary diagnostic examinations (30–35). Two methods have proven effective in reducing the number of tests ordered by Dutch general practitioners. The first method is based on restricting the number of tests that are listed on an order form. Zaat and colleagues (36, 37) developed a restricted paper order form that replaced the existing form. The second method involves introduction of indication-oriented order forms that are based on clinical practice guidelines (38–40).

We hypothesized that an indication-oriented order form based on guidelines, which would provide an optimally "restricted" list of tests that are relevant for a specific indication, would be more effective in decreasing the number of tests ordered compared with an order form that provides an initially limited list of tests. We therefore conducted a randomized trial to compare the effect of two versions of BloodLink, a computer-based clinical decision support system, on blood test ordering among Dutch general practitioners.

METHODS
Participants

In August and September 1995, all 64 practices (94 general practitioners) in the region of Delft, the Netherlands, were invited to participate in the study. Only practices that had replaced their paper-based patient records with electronic records and were using the computer during patient encounters were eligible. A total of 46 practices (62 general practitioners) agreed to participate.

Randomization

To avoid contamination, we performed random allocation at the level of the practice (41, 42). The practices were first stratified by type: solo practices or group practices (two or more general practitioners in the same practice). Each practice was subsequently assigned by simple random allocation to use BloodLink-Restricted or BloodLink-Guideline for the full study period. A researcher who was not involved in the study and was blinded to the identity of the practices performed the randomization by using a random-numbers table. After randomization, 22 practices involving 30 general practitioners were assigned to use BloodLink-Restricted and 24 practices involving 32 general practitioners were assigned to use BloodLink-Guideline.

Intervention

We developed two versions of BloodLink, a computer-based decision support system. BloodLink-Restricted initially displays a reduced list of tests, whereas BloodLink-Guideline is based on the guidelines of the Dutch College of General Practitioners. Both versions of BloodLink are integrated with the computer-based patient record (43).

The option to use BloodLink was added to the screen that the general practitioner uses when entering data in the electronic patient record during patient encounters. The general practitioner can activate Blood-Link to order blood tests as an alternative to using paper order forms. Because the total number of tests that can be ordered is too large to display on a computer screen, a set of tests is presented for selection. If the physician

requires additional tests that are not currently displayed, he or she can type the first few letters of the names of the required tests, and the system will present all possible matches (including those corresponding to possible typing errors of the general practitioner) for selection. The number of tests that the general practitioners had at their disposal was the same both before and during the intervention (52 clinical chemistry tests and 46 microbiological tests). Options for specific instructions to the laboratory (for example, "urgent processing" or "fasting values") are available. Once the physician has made his or her selections, BloodLink prints a patient-specific test order form and instructions for the laboratory and updates the patient record with the tests that have been ordered. The only difference between the two versions of BloodLink is the method used to present the initial set of tests to the general practitioner.

BloodLink-Restricted is based on the idea of a restricted order form. It offers the general practitioner an initial set of 15 tests that have been shown to cover most of the clinical situations seen in primary care (36). BloodLink-Restricted can be viewed as a general electronic order form that presents only 15 tests on the screen, together with a field labeled "other tests" that allows the physician to request any other blood test (43). The 15 tests are alanine aminotransferase, aspartate aminotransferase, total bilirubin, cholesterol, creatinine, erythrocyte sedimentation rate, free thyroxine, γ-glutamyl-transferase, glucose (and fasting glucose), glycosylated hemoglobin, hemoglobin, mean corpuscular volume, Paul–Bunnell, potassium, and thyroid-stimulating hormone. At any time, the physician can customize tests for individual patients by adding or deleting tests.

BloodLink-Guideline is based on the guidelines of the Dutch College of General Practitioners. By January 1996, the Dutch College of General Practitioners had published 54 guidelines. Some guidelines focus on symptoms that are frequently seen in the primary care setting, such as acute diarrhea, acute sore throat, low back pain, alcohol abuse, fever in children, and sleeping disorders. Other guidelines focus on common diseases in primary care, such as diabetes, asthma, depression, dementia, and eczema. Finally, a set of guidelines covers preventive medicine. We reviewed the most recent version of each guideline, available in January 1996, and noted whether it contained a reference to a blood test (44). We determined the clinical situation in which the test should be performed (indication) and the tests that should be performed in that situation (advised tests).

When general practitioners activate the system, BloodLink-Guideline first provides an overview of the available guidelines. The names of these guidelines are familiar to Dutch general practitioners. The general practitioner selects the appropriate guideline. A guideline may describe several different indications for requesting blood tests; for example, the guideline for blood tests and liver disease mentions 10 different indications. After the indication has been identified, the system proposes the relevant tests. The general practitioner then decides whether to adhere to the protocol. At any time, the physician can customize tests for individual patients by adding or removing tests from the proposed list. Although new guidelines are published at regular intervals, the currently available guidelines cover only a limited set of indications for blood tests (44). In the absence of national guidelines, local or regional guidelines may be used.

The version of BloodLink-Guideline used during the clinical trial in the Delft region included three regional guidelines for anemia, AIDS, and clotting disorders, in addition to all national guidelines. Even with these additional guidelines, BloodLink-Guideline does not cover all possible indications for blood tests in primary care. To deal with these situations, the general practitioner can select the heading "other indication" and order any test.

Protocol

Before the study, the general practitioners were using two paper order forms: one for clinical chemistry and one for microbiology. After BloodLink was installed, one of the authors gave a brief orientation presentation to the participating practitioners. During a 3-month phase-in period, the general practitioners were allowed to use BloodLink in their practices to become acquainted with the system. After this period, the general practitioners were asked whether they were willing to participate in the trial. The study period was March 1996 through February 1997.

Physicians always had the choice to use either the BloodLink software or the paper forms to order clinical chemistry and microbiology tests; thus, paper order forms were still available during the entire intervention

period. When the general practitioner ordered blood tests during a patient encounter, only one order form was generated regardless of whether the general practitioner used paper forms or BloodLink. The electronic patient record monitored use of BloodLink by the practitioners. To include the requests for blood tests that were made by using traditional paper forms, we retrieved from the regional laboratory all requests for blood tests.

Outcomes

We counted the number of order forms that the laboratory received from the general practitioners and the number of tests on each form. The main outcome measure was the average number of tests per order form (including paper forms) per practice (summary variable). We defined the most frequently ordered tests as the tests that accounted for 80% of the total number of tests ordered. For these tests, we computed per practice the percentage of order forms that included the test.

Statistical Analysis

We used t-tests to compare the distribution of baseline characteristics of practices and general practitioners. The differences in the number of tests per order form were analyzed by using the Mann–Whitney test, with practice as the unit of analysis. We conducted a multivariate Poisson regression analysis to estimate the difference in number of tests per order form between the two intervention groups while controlling for historic (1 July 1994 through 30 June 1995) test-ordering behavior of the general practitioners, size of the practice, and composition of the practice (sex of the patients, average patient age, and type of insurance). For all analyses, we used the number of tests as a count variable and the number of forms as an offset variable. Since the number of tests does not follow a Poisson distribution, we adjusted the standard errors for overdispersion (scale parameter estimated by using the square root of the Pearson chi-square value divided by the degrees of freedom). For frequently ordered tests, we computed per practice the percentage of order forms that included that test and then applied the Student t-test; equal variance was not assumed, and the unit of analysis was the practice. All analyses were performed by using SAS statistical soft-

Table 1. **Baseline Characteristics of Practices**

Characteristic	BloodLink-Restricted Group (n = 21)		BloodLink-Guideline Group (n = 23)		P Value*
	Mean	Median (25th, 75th percentiles)	Mean	Median (25th, 75th percentiles)	
Enrolled patients, n	3683	3399 (2930, 4400)	3411	3205 (2917, 3796)	>0.2
Patient age, y	36.3	36.3 (35.1, 37.8)	37.1	37.6 (35.0, 39.4)	>0.2
Female patients, %	48.3	49.4 (48.2, 50.0)	49.5	49.9 (49.0, 50.3)	>0.2
Patients insured through government insurance, %	53.2	53.5 (50.9, 56.4)	52.9	53.7 (50.7, 58.9)	>0.2
Tests per order form from 1 July 1994 through 30 June 1995, n†	7.7	7.8 (5.8, 9.3)	7.2	7.3 (6.1, 8.1)	>0.2

* By *t*-test on means.
† Two practices missing in each group.

ware, version 6.12 (SAS Institute, Inc., Cary, North Carolina).

Role of the Funding Source

Our funding source, the European Commission, had no influence on the collection, analysis, or interpretation of the data or in the decision to submit the study for publication.

RESULTS

BloodLink software was installed in 46 practices. During the 3-month phase-in period, two solo practitioners did not want to proceed with the experiment; one practitioner assigned to BloodLink-Restricted stated that the response time of his computer had deteriorated with use of the software, and one practitioner assigned to BloodLink-Guideline did not like the software. Thus, 44 practices consisting of 60 general practitioners completed the study (21 practices involving 29 general practitioners were assigned to BloodLink-Restricted and 23 practices involving 31 general practitioners were assigned to BloodLink-Guideline).

Baseline Data

As of 1 March 1996, 77 336 patients were enrolled in the practices assigned to BloodLink-Restricted. Of these patients, 41 174 (53.2%) were insured through government insurance, 37 397 (48.4%) were female, and the average age was 36.2 years (median, 33.7 years [25th and 75th percentiles, 21.0 and 50.6 years]). A total of 78 461 patients were enrolled in the practices assigned to BloodLink-Guideline as of 1 March 1996; 41 198 (52.5%) patients were insured through government insurance, 38 743 (49.9%) were female, and the

average age was 37.1 years (median, 34.7 years [25th and 75th percentiles, 21.5 and 51.9 years]). **Table 1** shows the baseline characteristics of the practices involved in the study. **Table 2** shows the baseline characteristics of the general practitioners.

Tests per Order Form per Practice

The general practitioner had the choice of using BloodLink or a paper form to order tests. Of the 12 742 order forms that the laboratory received from practices using BloodLink-Restricted, 11 151 orders (88%) were made by using the software; the remaining 1591 orders were placed by using traditional paper order forms. Of the 12 668 orders placed by the practices using Blood-Link-Guideline, 9091 (71%) were generated by using the decision support system. We calculated as a summary variable the average number of tests ordered per order form per practice. General practitioners who had access to BloodLink-Guideline ordered 20% fewer tests per form than did general practitioners who had access to BloodLink-Restricted (mean [±SD], 5.5 ± 0.9 tests vs. 6.9 ± 1.6 tests [median, 6.6 vs. 4.6], respectively; $P = 0.003$, Mann–Whitney test).

Table 3 shows the results of multivariate Poisson regression analysis comparing the number of tests per order form with use of BloodLink-Restricted or Blood-Link-Guideline, adjusted for practice characteristics and historic test-ordering behavior. These results are similar to those found in univariate comparisons. The group that used BloodLink-Restricted ordered 19% more tests per order form than did the group that used BloodLink Guideline. No demographic practice variable was independently associated with the number of tests per order form. Practices that ordered more tests before the inter-

Table 2. Baseline Characteristics of General Practitioners*

Characteristic	BloodLink-Restricted Group (n = 29)		BloodLink-Guideline Group (n = 31)		P Value†
	Mean	Median (25th, 75th percentiles)	Mean	Median (25th, 75th percentiles)	
Age at start of study, y	43.7	42.0 (38.7, 48.2)	43.2	43.0 (39.0, 47.0)	>0.2
Experience at start of study, y	16.5	15.0 (12.5, 22.2)	15.6	16.0 (12.0, 20.0)	>0.2
CME credits in 1996	44.3	42.0 (33.7, 56.5)	43.1	42.0 (31.0, 50.0)	>0.2
CME credits in 1997	51.7	47.0 (38.0, 56.5)	43.7	43.0 (31.0, 60.0)	0.126

* CME = continuing medical education.
† By *t*-test on means.

vention continued to order more tests per form, independent of the type of form.

The general practitioners ordered 157 360 tests in total during the study period. Although the practitioners requested 351 different laboratory tests, the 20 most frequently ordered tests accounted for 80% of the total number of ordered tests (**Table 4**). **Table 4** also shows the percentage of order forms per practice that included that test. In the BloodLink-Restricted group, for example, 61.2% of the order forms included an erythrocyte sedimentation rate test, compared with 44.1% in the BloodLink-Guideline group ($P < 0.001$, Student *t*-test).

DISCUSSION

Physicians who used BloodLink-Guideline, an indication-oriented test-ordering system, ordered fewer tests per form compared with those who used BloodLink-Restricted, which initially presented a limited list of tests (5.5 tests vs. 6.9 tests). For some frequently ordered tests, the difference between the BloodLink-Guideline and BloodLink-Restricted groups was large; we observed differences of 28% for erythrocyte sedimentation rate,

Table 3. Association between the Number of Tests per Form and Type of Form*

Factor	Relative Risk (95% CI)†
Use of BloodLink-Guideline order form	1.0 (referent)
Use of BloodLink-Restricted order form	1.19 (1.10–1.29)
Average number of tests per form in the year before the start of the study (per 1% increase)	1.12 (1.10–1.15)
Percentage of women (per 1% increase)	2.15 (0.23–20.6)
Percentage of patients with government insurance	0.63 (0.23–20.6)

* Two practices are missing from each group because data on historic ordering behavior are lacking.
† Based on multivariate Poisson regression model and adjusted for the factors listed in the table and practice size.

32% for creatinine concentration, 46% for γ-glutamyl-transferase level, and 49% for aspartate aminotransferase level (**Table 4**). For other tests, however, there were no significant differences (for example, glucose, cholesterol, thyroid-stimulating hormone, and high-density lipoprotein cholesterol levels; erythrocyte count; and sodium and alkaline phosphatase levels). We conclude that the overall reduction of ordered tests in the BloodLink-Guideline group was caused predominantly by a decrease in the ordering of some specific tests. BloodLink-Guideline does not reduce all test ordering to the same degree, but instead singles out various tests.

Increasingly, the literature shows that provision of decision support can change health care delivery (8–13, 15). BloodLink-Guideline, which is based on five categories of indications and involves 68 different indications (44), manages the ordering of 37 different tests; in contrast, BloodLink-Restricted initially lists 15 tests in alphabetical order. Use of BloodLink-Guideline resulted in a much larger reduction in ordered tests.

A limitation of our study is the absence of a gold standard to judge whether the reduction in the number of ordered tests translates into more appropriate ordering patterns. Our results, however, indicate that with regard to blood test ordering, providing more options that are embedded in a system driven by guidelines leads to a larger reduction in the number of tests ordered than does merely reducing the form to a limited set of tests. This larger reduction can be explained by the fact that BloodLink-Guideline shows an "optimal" restricted list of tests relevant for a specific indication. BloodLink-Guideline can be regarded as an attempt to limit the number of choices available on the basis of medical knowledge about a specific indication. BloodLink-Guideline enables physicians to apply the medical

Table 4. **Order Forms per Practice That Included the 20 Most Frequently Ordered Tests***

Test	Order Forms		P Value†
	BloodLink-Restricted Group	BloodLink-Guideline Group	
	%		
Erythrocyte sedimentation rate	61.2 ± 12.0	44.1 ± 10.9	<0.001
Hemoglobin	58.5 ± 11.9	47.8 ± 11.7	0.004
Glucose	47.1 ± 17.4	41.4 ± 12.3	>0.2
Leukocyte count	38.6 ± 15.3	29.7 ± 8.9	0.03
Hematocrit	36.0 ± 21.1	26.6 ± 2.3	0.08
Creatinine	40.0 ± 11.2	27.4 ± 10.8	<0.001
Erythrocyte count	34.7 ± 21.5	24.3 ± 11.6	0.06
Mean corpuscular volume	34.4 ± 21.5	23.0 ± 12.0	0.04
Leukocyte count (differential analysis)	31.3 ± 16.2	23.3 ± 7.2	0.05
Cholesterol	28.7 ± 12.1	25.7 ± 9.0	>0.2
Thyroid-stimulating hormone	26.9 ± 14.3	25.3 ± 5.3	>0.2
γ-Glutamyltransferase	31.3 ± 15.4	16.9 ± 9.2	<0.001
Alanine aminotransferase	24.7 ± 13.6	15.2 ± 6.8	0.008
Potassium	17.7 ± 11.3	8.8 ± 5.4	0.003
Aspartate aminotransferase	16.7 ± 10.8	8.5 ± 6.5	0.005
Triglycerides	11.4 ± 9.9	9.9 ± 6.5	>0.2
High-density lipoprotein cholesterol	11.7 ± 11.1	9.5 ± 6.8	>0.2
Sodium	6.9 ± 7.4	6.2 ± 3.5	>0.2
Free thyroxine	8.4 ± 6.2	4.8 ± 3.7	0.03
Alkaline phosphatase	5.4 ± 4.9	7.0 ± 5.4	>0.2

* Data are presented as the mean ± SD.
† By *t*-test.

knowledge of guidelines, whereas BloodLink-Restricted applies the notion of an initially limited set of tests that should fit most circumstances.

Many investigators have lamented the fact that the availability of guidelines is no guarantee that physicians actually will use them (45–47). Although physicians did not receive formal training in use of the BloodLink software (only brief instruction was given) and the usual paper forms were still available during the intervention period, physicians used BloodLink to place the majority of their orders. Our study provides additional evidence that computer-based decision support systems can be an effective method for incorporating guidelines into daily practice.

Paper forms have been used to change physician behavior in blood test ordering (28, 36, 38–40, 48). Paper forms, however, do not allow expression of the detailed information available in current guidelines. Studies conducted with paper forms, therefore, have been limited to only a few guidelines. Paper forms based on a limited set of guidelines do not solve the fundamental problem of introducing guidelines into clinical

practice. BloodLink-Guideline is based on the complete set of recommendations for test ordering provided by the Dutch College of General Practitioners. Although BloodLink could have been used as a stand-alone application, the introduction of BloodLink into daily practice was facilitated by the fact that the general practitioners were already using computer-based patient records.

In conclusion, our study highlights the potential advantage of computer-based patient records as a vehicle for changing physician behavior (49). The results should encourage the adoption of computer-based patient records to enhance test ordering during patient encounters.

From Institute of Medical Informatics and Institute of Primary Care Medicine, Faculty of Medicine and Health Sciences, Erasmus University Rotterdam, Rotterdam, the Netherlands.

Acknowledgments: The authors thank the general practitioners who participated in the study: J.M. Baks, R.D.W. van Bentveld, Y.J. Bezuijen, J.P. Bijl, P. de Blooy, C.M.J. Bonekamp, G.O. Boonstra, H. Breedveldt Boer, J. Breugem, J.A. Brienen, P.J.A. Bucx, H.B.F. Derksen, W. van Donselaar, E. Driever, R.H. Dupuis, P. van der Endt, J.A.J. Garretsen, R. Glotzbach, R.J. de Haan, H. Harmans, M. Human-Breedveld, C. Jansen, C.H.F. Jonker, M. Jonquiere, P.E. Kalsbeek, W. Kamermans, L.E.M. Kleipool, A.M.A. van der Knaap, S.J. Kool, M.I.Th. Koopmans, P.C.J.M. Kop, E.H.M. Lange, S. Laverman, S.J. Lindenhout, M. Luitse, D. Maring, S. van der Meer, P.J.Th.M. Meijs, J.E.G. Nieuwkamer, J.B.M. Nijkamp, J. Oosthoek, M.A. Plasmans, L. Redel, A.R.N. van Rijckevorsel, F.J.N. Rijkee, W.F. Sandhövel, P.P.M. Schijen, F. Schreuder, H.S. Spijker, M. Steentjes, R. van Stijn, E.P.L.A. Timmermans, F.C.M. Touw, P.S.W. Verheyden, P.D. Visser, H.W. Visser, H.J.P. Vos, C. van der Weg, W. Wierema.

Grant Support: By Ziektekostenverzekering Delft Schieland Westland, Institüt Ziektekostenverzekering Ambtenaren, and the European Commission Fourth Framework Health Telematics Programme (project PROMPT [Protocols for Medical Procedures and Therapies]).

Requests for Single Reprints: Marc A.M. van Wijk, MD, PhD, Institute of Medical Informatics, Faculty of Medicine and Health Sciences, Erasmus University Rotterdam, PO Box 1738, 3000 DR Rotterdam, the Netherlands; e-mail, wijk@mi.fgg.eur.nl.

Current Author Addresses: Drs. van Wijk, van der Lei, and van Bemmel and Mr. Mosseveld: Department of Medical Informatics, Faculty of Medicine and Health Sciences, Erasmus University Rotterdam, PO Box 1738, 3000 DR Rotterdam, the Netherlands.
Dr. Bohnen: Department of Primary Care Medicine, Faculty of Medicine and Health Sciences, Erasmus University Rotterdam, PO Box 1738, 3000 DR Rotterdam, the Netherlands.

Author Contributions: Conception and design: M.A.M. van Wijk, A.M. Bohnen, J.H. van Bemmel.

Analysis and interpretation of the data: M.A.M. van Wijk, J. van der Lei, A.M. Bohnen.

Drafting of the article: M.A.M. van Wijk, J. van der Lei.

Critical revision of the article for important intellectual content: M.A.M. van Wijk, J. van der Lei, A.M. Bohnen.

Final approval of the article: J. van der Lei, A.M. Bohnen.

Statistical expertise: J. van der Lei.

Administrative, technical, or logistic support: M. Mosseveld.

Collection and assembly of data: M.A.M. van Wijk, M. Mosseveld.

References

1. van der Lei J, Duisterhout JS, Westerhof HP, van der Does E, Cromme PV, Boon WM, et al. The introduction of computer-based patient records in The Netherlands. Ann Intern Med. 1993;119:1036-41. [PMID: 0008214981]

2. Baily GG, Hammer MR, Hanley SP, Pattrick MG, De Kretser DM. Implementing clinical guidelines. Computers allow instant access [Letter]. BMJ. 1993; 307:679. [PMID: 0008401062]

3. Tierney WM, Overhage JM, Takesue BY, Harris LE, Murray MD, Vargo DL, et al. Computerizing guidelines to improve care and patient outcomes: the example of heart failure. J Am Med Inform Assoc. 1995;2:316-22. [PMID: 0007496881]

4. Elson RB, Connelly DP. Computerized patient records in primary care. Their role in mediating guideline-driven physician behavior change. Arch Fam Med. 1995;4:698-705. [PMID: 0007620600]

5. Connelly DP, Willard KE, Hallgren JH, Sielaff BH. Closing the clinical laboratory testing loop with information technology. Am J Clin Pathol. 1996; 105:S40-7. [PMID: 0008607461]

6. Henry SB, Douglas K, Galzagorry G, Lahey A, Holzemer WL. A template-based approach to support utilization of clinical practice guidelines within an electronic health record. J Am Med Inform Assoc. 1998;5:237-44. [PMID: 0009609493]

7. Chin HL, Wallace P. Embedding guidelines into direct physician order entry: simple methods, powerful results. Proc AMIA Symp. 1999:221-5. [PMID: 0010566353]

8. Johnston ME, Langton KB, Haynes RB, Mathieu A. Effects of computer-based clinical decision support systems on clinician performance and patient outcome. A critical appraisal of research. Ann Intern Med. 1994;120:135-42. [PMID: 0008256973]

9. Margolis A, Bray BE, Gilbert EM, Warner HR. Computerized practice guidelines for heart failure management: the HeartMan system. Proc Annu Symp Comput Appl Med Care. 1995:228-32. [PMID: 0008563274]

10. Hollingworth GR, Bernstein RM, Viner GS, Remington JS, Wood WE. Prompting for cost-effective test ordering: a randomized controlled trial. Proc Annu Symp Comput Appl Med Care. 1995:635-9. [PMID: 0008563364]

11. Zielstorff RD. Online practice guidelines: issues, obstacles, and future prospects. J Am Med Inform Assoc. 1998;5:227-36. [PMID: 0009609492]

12. Ohno-Machado L, Gennari JH, Murphy SN, Jain NL, Tu SW, Oliver DE, et al. The guideline interchange format: a model for representing guidelines. J Am Med Inform Assoc. 1998;5:357-72. [PMID: 0009670133]

13. Jenders RA, Hripcsak G, Sideli RV, DuMouchel W, Zhang H, Cimino JJ, et al. Medical decision support: experience with implementing the Arden Syntax at the Columbia-Presbyterian Medical Center. Proc Annu Symp Comput Appl Med Care. 1995:169-73. [PMID: 0008563259]

14. Hunt DL, Haynes RB, Hanna SE, Smith K. Effects of computer-based clinical decision support systems on physician performance and patient outcomes: a systematic review. JAMA. 1998;280:1339-46. [PMID: 0009794315]

15. Smith BJ, McNeely MD. The influence of an expert system for test ordering and interpretation on laboratory investigations. Clin Chem. 1999;45:1168-75. [PMID: 0010430781]

16. Shiffman RN, Liaw Y, Brandt CA, Corb GJ. Computer-based guideline implementation systems: a systematic review of functionality and effectiveness. J Am Med Inform Assoc. 1999;6:104-14. [PMID: 0010094063]

17. Cannon DS, Allen SN. A comparison of the effects of computer and manual reminders on compliance with a mental health clinical practice guideline. J Am Med Inform Assoc. 2000;7:196-203. [PMID: 0010730603]

18. Montgomery AA, Fahey T, Peters TJ, MacIntosh C, Sharp DJ. Evaluation of computer based clinical decision support system and risk chart for management of hypertension in primary care: randomised controlled trial. BMJ. 2000; 320:686-90. [PMID: 0010710578]

19. Cook DJ, Greengold NL, Ellrodt AG, Weingarten SR. The relation between systematic reviews and practice guidelines. Ann Intern Med. 1997;127: 210-6. [PMID: 0009245227]

20. Kluijt I, Zaat JO, Van der Velden J, van Eijk JT, Schellevis FG. Voor een prikje: huisarts en bloedonderzoek [The general practitioner and blood tests]. Huisarts en Wetenschap. 1991;34:67-71.

21. Ornstein SM, Markert GP, Johnson AH, Rust PF, Afrin LB. The effect of physician personality on laboratory test ordering for hypertensive patients. Med Care. 1988;26:536-43. [PMID: 0003379985]

22. Kassirer JP. Our stubborn quest for diagnostic certainty. A cause of excessive testing. N Engl J Med. 1989;320:1489-91. [PMID: 0002497349]

23. Kassirer JP. Diagnostic reasoning. Ann Intern Med. 1989;110:893-900. [PMID: 0002655522]

24. Axt-Adam P, van der Wouden JC, van der Does E. Influencing behavior of physicians ordering laboratory tests: a literature study. Med Care. 1993;31:784-94. [PMID: 0008366680]

25. Eisenberg JM, Nicklin D. Use of diagnostic services by physicians in community practice. Med Care. 1981;19:297-309. [PMID: 0007218895]

26. Wong ET, Lincoln TL. Ready! Fire! . . . Aim! An inquiry into laboratory test ordering. JAMA. 1983;250:2510-3. [PMID: 0006632145]

27. van Walraven C, Naylor CD. Do we know what inappropriate laboratory utilization is? A systematic review of laboratory clinical audits. JAMA. 1998;280: 550-8. [PMID: 0009707147]

28. van Walraven C, Goel V, Chan B. Effect of population-based interventions on laboratory utilization: a time-series analysis. JAMA. 1998;280:2028-33. [PMID: 0009863855]

29. Solomon DH, Hashimoto H, Daltroy L, Liang MH. Techniques to improve physicians' use of diagnostic tests: a new conceptual framework. JAMA. 1998;280:2020-7. [PMID: 0009863854]

30. Boohaker EA, Ward RE, Uman JE, McCarthy BD. Patient notification and follow-up of abnormal test results. A physician survey. Arch Intern Med. 1996; 12:327-31. [PMID: 0008572844]

31. DeKay ML, Asch DA. Is the defensive use of diagnostic tests good for patients, or bad? Med Decis Making. 1998;18:19-28. [PMID: 0009456202]

32. Epstein AM, Begg CB, McNeil BJ. The effects of physicians' training and personality on test ordering for ambulatory patients. Am J Public Health. 1984; 74:1271-3. [PMID: 0006496824]

33. Rosser WW. Approach to diagnosis by primary care clinicians and specialists: is there a difference? J Fam Pract. 1996;42:139-44. [PMID: 0008606303]

34. Sox HC. Decision-making: a comparison of referral practice and primary care. J Fam Pract. 1996;42:155-60. [PMID: 0008606305]

35. Kristiansen IS, Hjortdahl P. The general practitioner and laboratory utilization: why does it vary? Fam Pract. 1992;9:22-7. [PMID: 0001634022]

36. Zaat JO, van Eijk JT, Bonte HA. Laboratory test form design influences test

ordering by general practitioners in The Netherlands. Med Care. 1992;30:189-98. [PMID: 0001538607]

37. Zaat JO, van Eijk JT. General practitioners' uncertainty, risk preference, and use of laboratory tests. Med Care. 1992;30:846-54. [PMID: 0001518316]

38. Smithuis LO, Van Geldrop WJ, Lucassen PL. Beperking van het laboratoriumonderzoek door een probleemgeorienteerd aanvraagformulier. Een partiele implementatie van NHG-standaarden [Reducing test ordering by introducing a problem oriented order form. Partial implementation of the guidelines of the Dutch College of General Practitioners]. Huisarts en Wetenschap. 1994;37:464-66.

39. van Gend JM, van Pelt J, Cleef TH, Mangnus TM, Muris JW. [Quality improvement project "laboratory diagnosis by family physicians" leads to considerable decrease in number of laboratory tests]. Ned Tijdschr Geneeskd. 1996; 140:495-500. [PMID: 0008628438]

40. Van Geldrop WJ, Lucassen PLBJ, Smithuis LO. Een probleemgeorienteerd aanvraagformulier voor laboratoriumonderzoek. Effecten op het aanvraaggedrag van huisartsen [A problem oriented test order form. Impact on test ordering behavior of general practitioners]. Huisarts Wet. 1992;35:192-6

41. Eccles M, Grimshaw J, Steen N, Parkin D, Purves I, McColl E, et al. The design and analysis of a randomized controlled trial to evaluate computerized decision support in primary care: the COGENT study. Fam Pract. 2000;17:180-6. [PMID: 0010758083]

42. Kerry SM, Bland JM. Trials which randomize practices I: how should they be analysed? Fam Pract. 1998;15:80-3. [PMID: 0009527302]

43. van Wijk M, Mosseveld M, van der Lei J. Design of a decision support system for test ordering in general practice: choices and decisions to make. Methods Inf Med. 1999;38:355-61. [PMID: 0010805028]

44. van Wijk MA, Bohnen AM, van der Lei J. Analysis of the practice guidelines of the Dutch College of General Practitioners with respect to the use of blood tests. J Am Med Inform Assoc. 1999;6:322-31. [PMID: 0010428005]

45. Lomas J, Anderson GM, Domnick-Pierre K, Vayda E, Enkin MW, Hannah WJ. Do practice guidelines guide practice? The effect of a consensus statement on the practice of physicians. N Engl J Med. 1989;321:1306-11. [PMID: 0002677732]

46. McColl A, Smith H, White P, Field J. General practitioner's perceptions of the route to evidence based medicine: a questionnaire survey. BMJ. 1998;316:361-5. [PMID: 0009487174]

47. Grol R, Dalhuijsen J, Thomas S, Veld C, Rutten G, Mokkink H. Attributes of clinical guidelines that influence use of guidelines in general practice: observational study. BMJ. 1998;317:858-61. [PMID: 0009748183]

48. Durand-Zaleski I, Rymer JC, Roudot-Thoraval F, Revuz J, Rosa J. Reducing unnecessary laboratory use with new test request form: example of tumour markers. Lancet. 1993;342:150-3.

49. van Bemmel JH, Van Ginneken AM, Van der Lei J. A progress report on computer-based patient records in Europe. In: Dick RS, Steen EB, Detmer DE, eds. The Computer-Based Patient Record: An Essential Technology for Health Care. Washington, DC: National Academy Pr; 1997:21-43.

I killed them because I felt a little fatigued and suffered from a slight, persistent cough. Thinking I was overworked and hadn't been getting enough sleep, I went home for a short visit, just a few days to relax in the country while the sweet corn and the raspberries were ripe. From the city I brought fancy ribbon, two boxes of Ambrosia chocolate, and a deadly gift . . . I gave the influenza to my mother, who gave it to my father, or maybe it was the other way around.

Christina Schwarz
Drowning Ruth
New York: Doubleday; 2000

Submitted by:
Fred Campbell, MD
San Antonio, TX 78260

Submissions from readers are welcomed. If the quotation is published, the sender's name will be acknowledged. Please include a complete citation (along with page number on which the quotation was found), as done for any reference.—*The Editor*

Section 6:

J. Dørup

Section for Health Informatics
University of Aarhus, Denmark

Synopsis

Educational technology as a scientific discipline

Teaching and learning are integral parts of all clinical activity. Yet medical education is only slowly finding its place among other scientific medical specialities. Why is this? And why is computer-based learning software putting conscious pedagogy on the agenda?

Doctors have been teaching and learning at least since Aristotle. However, it is still unusual for many physicians to consider education a scientific discipline. How can we conduct double blinded, placebo controlled educational trials? And if we can't, how can we justify any change in approach towards education? The question may, however, be reversed: How can we justify status quo with no other evidence than the existence of present day doctors and patients with present day status of knowledge and skills? In other words: How do we know if what we do is the best? Educational research has progressed dramatically over the past 100 years (see a timeline at http://www.ittheory.com/timelin2.htm, refer to (1) and (2) for recent perspectives from the medical domain). Still, implementation of research from the area of education seems to be lagging behind. The situation resembles that faced by Archibald L. Cochrane (http://www.cochrane.org/cochrane/archieco.htm) in the 1960's and 70's. Available evidence from clinical trials did not induce changes in clinical practice. Patients who could have been cured with new evidence-based treatments may have lost their lives. Considering the importance of well educated physicians and patients, ineffective education may be equally fatal.

The need to increase the efficiency of education worldwide is urgent. Lecturing, tutoring and traditional classroom teaching is time consuming and expensive, and there is a limit to its spread. As more knowledge must be disseminated to an increasing number of patients suffering from the major non-communicable diseases, educational technology will no longer be optional. In spite of improvements in the health care systems of most countries, we have not seen successes in limiting the number of patients with these conditions. On the contrary, failure of effective primary prophylaxis has shifted the focus of much research towards limiting complications and the impact on living conditions. Important results of such research are waiting to be incorporated in clinical praxis around the world. Changing practice, however, is also about changing culture. In some areas, this can be done rapidly, but progress is slow in others. Decision makers in medical faculties and hospitals are often recruited from the basic scientific community and good scientific evidence from well-conducted studies is particularly important for pushing a cultural shift in medical education. The outstanding papers presented in the following section may well serve not only their own purposes. Rather, promotion of well-conducted educational research serves as evidence that educational research also works without placebo control and double blinding and that this field of research is both possible and necessary.

The learning patient

In the first years of computer-assisted learning, much focus was placed on educating medical students, less on patients and doctors. This may be a logical consequence of a more formal approach towards teaching medical students. The primary goal of medical students is learning. Also, they may take structured teaching from professional teachers for granted. Postgraduate students and patients must emphasize other important activities. Learning takes place when time can be found, and often with little or no instruction. Here computer-based materials come in handy.

Patients as learners, especially those suffering from chronic diseases, have some benefits compared to physicians:
1) Motivation: The chronic disease provides the learning patient with constant motivation. Any new relevant knowledge may be immediately put to use.
2) Time: Disease, to some extent, prevents normal working activities, but leaves the patient with more time to establish networks within patient groups for self-paced learning and

in-depth study of specific areas of current importance.

3) Control: In conditions requiring tight control of medication, like diabetes and asthma, the well-educated patient may be able to obtain a better regulation when sharing part of the responsibility with medical professionals. As an example, it has recently been shown that, among specific groups of patients, self-management of oral anticoagulant therapy may be more efficient than conventional control (3). As the availability of computers and the Internet among patients increases, dissemination of clinical information and use of interactive medical learning software via the web may solve many key patient problems.

Four research papers on educational technology

The papers selected for the Computer Supported Education section of the 2002 IMIA Yearbook illustrate that medical education is a scientific discipline and that valid conclusions can be drawn from such studies.

Web-based clinical guidelines are finding increased use for many reasons. First, they can be updated easily and inexpensively. Second, users can find the materials on any computer connected to the web. Third, publishing the guidelines on the web enables easy comparison and stimulates collaboration between clinical departments. The study by Douglas Bell and colleagues from University of California, Los Angeles, compares web-based and printed guidelines for care after acute myocardial infarction. Residents were randomized to either web-based or written guides. It was concluded that learning was more efficient in the group receiving web-based study materials. Higher knowledge scores in the web group were not statistically significant, but less time was spent, and the learner

satisfaction scale was significantly higher. As such, the study adds educational scientific evidence to the practical advantages mentioned above.

The study by Emma-Jane Berridge and colleagues from London, UK, was aimed both at patients and family practitioners, since the general practitioner will always play a crucial role as a consultant for a well-educated patient. In this project, programming was preceded by a thorough analysis, including identification of objectives, design principles, domain and more. The strategy is known among computer scientists as Object Oriented Analysis and Design, usually deploying the Unified Modeling Language. It has been described, among others, by Martin Fowler in his book UML Distilled: A Brief Guide to the Standard Object Modeling Language (4). Briefly, modeling of real-world objects is conducted as a first step in developing an object-oriented design methodology. Numerous programs, which were developed without going through the modelling phases failed to reach their goal simply because the programmers' aims differed from those of users, programming strategy was not selected in the most effective way, or human factors and user perspectives were not sufficiently taken into consideration. The process is iterative, as described in Figure 1 of the paper, with special focus on the returning arrows: Should problems arise at one level, development will need to take one or more steps back to assure a sound further development. This study is not only a valuable important educational resource for patients and their doctors. The description of how the program was developed may be directly re-used as inspiration for others planning similar projects. In addition to the design principles mentioned above, the study also contains a valuable description of how various media elements were included and deployed, as well as a discussion of the pros and cons of each element.

Ross Shegog and colleagues from Houston, Texas, present another perspective to patient education in an approach directed at asthma patients aged 9-13 years. As realized by most parents and school teachers, at this age, many children want excitement and entertainment as they often find in computer games. Developing educational software for this group of patients by using principles of computer games corresponds to meeting the children on their own playground, which may probably be the only way to maintain their attention. The study showed that this was indeed possible and that learning took place in such important areas as knowledge on self-regulation, prevention and treatment.

The study by Viorel G. Popescu and co-workers from New Jersey and California, presents an orthopaedic tele-rehabilitation system, connecting the patient at home with the orthopaedic clinic via the Internet and a web-based teleconferencing system. Considering the large number of patients in need for rehabilitation, a number that may well increase as the percentage of elderly citizens increases, the possibility for in-home tele-rehabilitation opens new perspectives for more effective rehabilitation in the future. As with other new technologies, it may be that the advanced hardware and software used in the present study will be too complicated for some patients, but the study shows important and promising results upon which further progress may rest.

Success or failure with medical learning software

Not all learning software will result in learning. The road from idea to final product is paved with challenges and many projects fail to reach their goal. Unsuccessful projects may be as expensive and demanding as successful ones, but software that end up not being used may influence decision makers negatively when new projects are judged. Several initiatives have tried to analyze and describe success criteria for learning software. I will mention a few here. In the present context, medical learning software is a subset of academic learning software, and much of what is true for academic software also applies to medical learning software.

A comprehensive study, which deals with success criteria for academic educational software, was conducted by the CUTSD, Committee for University Teaching and Staff Development in Australia (5), (executive summary can be found at http://www.iim.uts.edu.au/about/sa_pubs/cautexec.html). The study reviewed 104 projects, which received funding from the Committee for the Advancement of University Teaching (CAUT) in 1994 or 1995, and which made significant use of a range of information technologies to develop student learning materials. The study made a series of useful conclusions directly suited for consideration by others. Without going into detail here, many conclusions coincide with what was previously established by Laurillard (6): the importance of an organizational infrastructure and collaboration between a number of people or groups with responsibilities for separate segments of the software design. Other important criteria were the use of a conscious learning design strategy; the reassurance of the integration of the software in the curriculum, including its acceptance by all teachers, and its usability (7) for both teachers and students.

It is not easy to prove the impact of standards, guides and guidelines on development and use of educational software. Probably, many guidelines find little or no use, and many new projects are initiated by developers who were not familiar with available guidelines. Moreover, too rigorous use of guidelines may limit the creativity of the developers. However, guidelines raise important questions at least for those involved in the process of developing them. Important guidelines include (8) and (9) at http://www.imbi. uni-freiburg.de/medinf/gmdsqc/e.htm. The World Federation for Medical Education, a non-governmental organization (NGO) with relation to the WHO, (http://www.sund.ku.dk/wfme/) has established a standing advisory committee for developing guidelines for medical educational software with participants from the USA, UK, Russia, Germany and Scandinavia. The first version of the guidelines was published in 1998 (10). The latest version (November 2001) is available at http://www.sund.ku.dk/wfme under activities. In the guideline development process it is striking that one key factor for international spread is that software should be open for adaptation to local needs. Teachers should be able to take ownership of the teaching materials.

Considering the very high quality of all four papers in this section of the yearbook, it should be worthwhile to consider use of the software outside the areas of origin. In many cases this requires portation of the software from stand-alone computers to the Internet. In this sense, let me make my last sentence a wish for the future. Let us hope that more top-quality medical educational software will be made available via the Internet under conditions that allow teachers to adapt it to their local needs and allows patients, physicians and students to globally benefit from it for free.

Reference

1. Daetwyler C, editor. Use of Computers in Medical Education Part I: Theoretical contributions. Innsbruck: StudienVerlag; 2001.
2. Daetwyler C, editor. Use of Computers in Medical Education Part II: Practical Examples. Innsbruck: StudienVerlag; 2001.
3. Christensen TD, Attermann J, Pilegaard HK, Andersen NT, Maegaard M, Hasenkam JM. Self-management of oral anticoagulant therapy for mechanical heart valve patients. Scand Cardiovasc J 2001; 35(2):107-13.
4. Fowler MSK. UML Distilled: A Brief Guide to the Standard Object Modeling Language. 2nd ed. Addison-Wesley; 1999.
5. Alexander S, McKenzie J. An evaluation of information technology projects for university learning. Canberra: CUTSD, Commonwealth of Australia; 1998.
6. Laurillard D. Effective teaching with multimedia methods. Rethinking University Teaching, A framework for the effective use of educational technology. London and New York: Routledge Falmer, 1993. p. 223-56.
7. Dørup J, Hansen MS, Geneser F. User-Centered Design of Medical Learning Software. In: Daetwyler C, editor. Use of Computers in Medical Education Part II: Practical Examples. Innsbruck: StudienVerlag; 2001.
8. Atkins MJOC. Evaluating Multimedia Applications for Medical Education. Association for Medical Education in Europe. AMEE Guide No 6; 1995.
9. Schulz S, Auhuber T, Schrader U, Klar R. Quality criteria for electronic publications in medicine. Stud Health Technol Inform 1998;51:217-26.
10. WFME advisory committee. World Federation for Medical Education (WFME) Guidelines for Using Computers in Medical Education. Med Educ 1998;32:205-8.

Address of the author:
Jens Dørup, MD PhD, Associate Professor
Section for Health Informatics
University of Aarhus,
Vennelyst Boulevard 6
8000 Aarhus C, Denmark.
E-mail: jd@hi.au.dk
URL: http://www.hi.au.dk/jd

Self-Study from Web-Based and Printed Guideline Materials

A Randomized, Controlled Trial among Resident Physicians

Douglas S. Bell, MD; Gregg C. Fonarow, MD; Ron D. Hays, PhD; and Carol M. Mangione, MD, MSPH

Background: On-line physician education is increasing, but its efficacy in comparison with existing self-study methods is unknown.

Objective: To compare knowledge, learning efficiency, and learner satisfaction produced by self-study of World Wide Web–based and print-based guidelines for care after acute myocardial infarction.

Design: Randomized, controlled trial.

Setting: 12 family medicine and internal medicine residency programs at four universities.

Participants: 162 residents.

Interventions: In proctored sessions, participants were randomly assigned to study from printed materials or from SAGE (Self-Study Acceleration with Graphic Evidence), a Web-based tutorial system. Both methods used identical self-assessment questions and answers and guideline text, but SAGE featured hyperlinks to specific guideline passages and graphic evidence animations.

Measurements: Scores on multiple-choice knowledge tests, score gain per unit of study time, and ratings on a learner satisfaction scale.

Results: Immediate post-test scores on a 20-point scale were similar in the SAGE and control groups (median score, 15.0 compared with 14.5; $P > 0.2$), but SAGE users spent less time studying (median, 27.0 compared with 38.5 minutes; $P < 0.001$) and therefore had greater learning efficiency (median score gain, 8.6 compared with 6.7 points per hour; $P = 0.04$). On a scale of 5 to 20, SAGE users were more satisfied with learning (median rating, 17.0 compared with 15.0; $P < 0.001$). After 4 to 6 months, knowledge had decreased to the same extent in the SAGE and control groups (median score, 12.0 compared with 11.0; $P = 0.12$).

Conclusions: On-line tutorials may produce greater learning efficiency and satisfaction than print materials do, but one self-study exposure may be insufficient for long-term knowledge retention. Further research is needed to identify instructional features that motivate greater final learning and retention.

Ann Intern Med. 2000;132:938-946.

For author affiliations, current addresses, and contributions, see end of text.

Many primary care physicians have not learned about key advances in caring for patients after acute myocardial infarction, including the use of β-blockers (1) and angiotensin-converting enzyme inhibitors (2). Although professional organizations have disseminated guidelines for the care of acute myocardial infarction (3, 4), important therapies continue to be underused (5). Physicians read guidelines to stay up-to-date (6), but reading without additional interaction is relatively ineffective for learning (7) and has little effect on practice (8). Physicians therefore need better methods for learning from guidelines. Self-assessment tests are often used to enhance self-study of printed materials (9, 10), but physicians can now choose from a growing number of World Wide Web sites that offer on-line self-study (11).

Since the 1960s, computer-assisted instruction has been explored as a method for medical education (12–15). In theory, computer-assisted instruction can enhance self-study by tailoring presentations to learners' individual needs and by including interactive simulations (16). Two previous studies comparing computer-assisted instruction systems with carefully constructed self-study controls found mixed results (17, 18). In both of these studies, the systems were developed for and tested among medical students before the advent of the Web. Therefore, physicians have little direct evidence to inform their choices among currently available self-study methods.

We conducted a randomized trial to compare the educational outcomes produced by a Web-based tutorial on myocardial infarction guidelines with those produced by self-assessment–based and study from print versions of the same guidelines. We hypothesized that print-based self-study would result in substantial learning but Web-based self-study would produce incrementally greater knowledge gains, retention, learning efficiency, and satisfaction. We conducted this trial among residents rather than community physicians because residents frequently use self-study materials and because we anticipated that they would be more feasible to recruit.

Methods

Design of Self-Study Alternatives

Guidelines and Learning Objectives

The American College of Cardiology (ACC), the American Heart Association (AHA), and the American College of Physicians–American Society of Internal Medicine (ACP–ASIM) allowed us to use their guidelines for this trial. We wrote 20 "cognitive" learning objectives (19), covering knowledge from one or both guidelines that would be important for physicians who provide primary care to patients after myocardial infarction. One of the authors, an expert in evidence-based cardiology, edited the objectives for content validity and importance. The final set of learning objectives is shown in the **Appendix Table**.

Knowledge Tests

We wrote multiple-choice questions that had one correct response demonstrating the knowledge in a single learning objective. Thirty attending physicians and fellows in internal medicine, family medicine, and cardiology critiqued the clarity and difficulty of prospective questions by using an electronic mail quiz system that tracked each question's average score (20). These data were used to assemble a 20-question pretest and a different 20-question posttest. The tests included one question per learning objective and were approximately equivalent in overall difficulty. Expected scores on the final pretest and post-test differed by less than 6%. For each question on the final test forms, participants could place a check mark next to the statement, "I would like to review available evidence or recommendations on this topic." We referred to this feature as the "review flag." For both of the self-study alternatives in this trial, learners initially completed the pretest on paper.

Web-Based Self-Study Materials

We constructed a Web-based learning system called SAGE (Self-Study Acceleration with Graphic Evidence). Participants who used SAGE copied their pretest answers into the system and were then taken to the "main tutorial page," which presents an overview of the user's pretest results for each learning objective. By clicking on hyperlinks, users could view a sequence of learning resources for each objective. The first resource for each objective was the relevant pretest answer. From there, users could click on hyperlinks to view the relevant guideline passages (highlighted segments of text in an on-line version of the complete guideline document). When guidelines referred to landmark clinical trials, users could click on a link to open a graphic evidence browser (**Figure 1**). Complete instructions for using SAGE were provided in the system. The program was intended to combine two strategies of computer-assisted instruction: a tutorial strategy, which focuses the learner on deficits in previous knowledge, and a simulation strategy, which reinforces knowledge through interaction with graphic models of

randomized trial evidence. We wrote software for SAGE in Server-side JavaScript, using the Netscape Enterprise Server (Mountain View, California) running on a Sun Ultrasparc2 workstation (Mountain View, California). For animated statistical graphics, we wrote a Java applet.

Printed Self-Study Materials

Printed materials for the control group included the same self-assessment test and guidelines as the Web-based materials. The printed materials included 1) a booklet showing the correct answer for each pretest question and the learning objective each question was intended to evaluate and 2) complete reprints of the ACP–ASIM and ACC/AHA guidelines. Learners were instructed to compare their pretest answers with the correct answers and look up the evidence or guideline recommendations for each learning objective that they may not have met by using the outline structure of the ACP–ASIM guidelines and the index of the ACC/AHA guidelines. Materials in the control group were intended to provide learning through self-assessment and study from the actual guideline documents as distributed by the specialty societies. The control materials contained the same pretest answers and guideline content as SAGE but lacked the hypermedia navigation features and the detailed, interactive, graphic presentations of landmark trial evidence. Of note, however, the guideline materials for both self-study groups contained all of the information that learners would need to meet each learning objective, including narrative descriptions of the key trial results that were available graphically in SAGE.

Study Sample

We recruited residency programs in family and internal medicine at four universities. Approval for research involving humans was obtained from each university's institutional review board. A total of 5 family medicine and 7 internal medicine programs agreed to participate. We recorded the name, sex, and training year of every resident across all 12 programs in a confidential recruitment database. Letters were placed in residents' mailboxes inviting them to attend a 1.25-hour learning session in which they would be randomly assigned to study from computer or printed materials on the care of myocardial infarction. An honorarium of $30 was offered for completing the trial. The trial was also announced at resident conferences. All residents who attended a session and gave consent became eligible participants.

Self-Study Sessions

Participants used the self-study materials in a single session that began with the pretest and ended

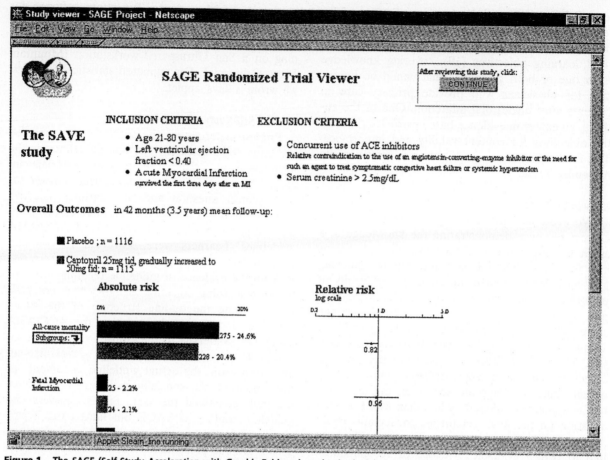

Figure 1. **The SAGE (Self-Study Acceleration with Graphic Evidence) randomized trial viewer.** When guidelines refer to landmark clinical trials, users can select an "evidence link" to open the randomized trial viewer, displaying a standard graphic view of the trial's results in terms of absolute risks and relative risks. If the trial reported subgroup results for an outcome, a "Subgroups" pop-up menu is shown below the outcome label. Selecting a subgroup variable, such as "Age," starts an animation sequence in which the absolute risk bar for each treatment splits into a separate risk bar for each subgroup. The bars then rearrange, ending with adjacent treatment and control bars and new relative risk estimates for each subgroup. ACE = angiotensin-converting enzyme; tid = three times per day.

with an immediate post-test. After completing the pretest, participants kept carbon copies of their answers, returned their originals, and received their randomly generated study group assignment. Those assigned to the control group were given the printed materials, and those assigned to SAGE went to an adjacent computer classroom, where they logged on and entered their pretest answers. Participants in both groups were asked to study until they felt that they had met the learning objectives, at which point the self-study materials were removed and they immediately took the post-test on paper. Each session was proctored to ensure that all learning was attributable to self-study from the assigned material without use of extraneous materials or discussion with colleagues. No irregularities occurred. Participants could not attend more than one session and were not allowed to keep the printed self-study materials or to access SAGE after completing their session.

Study Group Assignment

Individual participants were randomly assigned to study groups by a computer program that generated

blocked randomization stratified by the participants' sex and residency year. As each resident arrived at a session, he or she was registered on a laptop computer that contained coded records from the recruitment database. As the first participants finished the pretest, a randomization program run on the laptop generated a balanced pool of assignments for each sex–residency year category (using a block size of 2 [21]). For each registered participant, the program chose an assignment at random from the appropriate pool. As participants turned in their pretests, they and the investigators looked up their assignments on the laptop screen. Study group assignment was therefore simultaneously revealed to the participants and to the investigators.

Outcome Measures

Knowledge scores from multiple-choice tests were calculated by assigning 1 point per correct answer; unanswered items were considered incorrect. This created scores that could range from 0 to 20 points. The primary outcome of the trial was knowledge on the immediate post-test. The time

Table 1. Characteristics of Trial Participants Compared with Nonparticipants and the Control Group Compared with the Web-Based Self-Study Group*

Characteristic	Participants (n = 162)	Nonparticipants (n = 379)	P Value	Control Group (n = 76)	SAGE Group (n = 82)	P Value
Mean age ± SD, y	29.1 ± 2.7	NA		29.4 ± 2.9	28.8 ± 2.5	0.19
Male sex, %	58.6	50.9	0.1	57.9	61.0	>0.2
Specialty, %			>0.2			
Family medicine	30.9	28.8		29.0	29.3	
Internal medicine	69.1	71.2		71.0	70.7	>0.2
Residency training year, %			0.06			
First year	29.6	39.6		26.3	35.4	
Second year	38.3	29.8		42.1	32.9	
Third year	32.1	30.6		31.6	31.7	>0.2
University, %			0.001			
A	48.1	14.5		48.7	45.1	
B	24.1	16.9		25.0	25.6	
C	14.2	26.9		17.1	12.2	
D	13.6	41.7		9.2	17.1	>0.2
Previous World Wide Web experience, %						
Never used	3.1	NA		3.9	2.4	
Used <5 times ever	11.1			13.2	9.8	
Used >5 times but never weekly	38.9			42.1	35.4	
Used at least weekly at times	46.9			40.8	52.4	

* The chi-square test was used for categorical variables, and the t-test was used for the continuous variable (age). NA = not available; SAGE = Self-Study Acceleration with Graphic Evidence.

spent studying was measured by using a time-stamp machine for participants in the control group and the server log for participants in the SAGE group. Learning efficiency was calculated as the point gain from pretest to immediate post-test divided by the time spent studying. A follow-up test that included all items from the immediate post-test was used to measure knowledge retention after 4 to 6 months. Participants completed the follow-up test in the presence of a proctor.

Learner satisfaction was measured by using five items taken from an ACP–ASIM course evaluation survey for continuing medical education activities. An additional item from the survey was used to measure learners' evaluation of the pretest. Participants responded to each item by circling a number ranging from 1 to 4, with higher numbers representing more positive attitudes. A learner satisfaction scale was constructed by summing responses for the five satisfaction items, thereby creating a scale with possible scores ranging from 5 to 20 points. The SAGE program automatically recorded the use of individual learning resources.

Statistical Analysis

Using chi-square tests for categorical variables and t-tests for continuous variables, we compared the characteristics of participants with the available characteristics of residents who did not participate and the characteristics of the SAGE group with those of the control group. We used the Wilcoxon rank-sum test to compare outcomes between study groups because each outcome was non-normally distributed according to the Shapiro–Wilk test (22). Confidence intervals for medians were estimated by using the Conover method (23). Outcome comparisons included all available data, and participants

were grouped according to their study group assignment (intention-to-treat analysis). We used the Cronbach α coefficient (24) to estimate the internal consistency reliability of the learner satisfaction scale. We used stratified analysis (25) to estimate the effect of previous knowledge, as measured by the pretest, on SAGE users' odds of accessing individual learning resources. Adjustment for the effects of clustering by participant (26, 27) did not substantially change these odds ratios. All reported P values are two-tailed.

Assuming that a P value less than 0.05 was statistically significant, 144 participants (72 in each group) would provide a power of 0.85 to detect a difference of one-half standard deviation in post-test scores between groups (a medium effect). Because of resource limitations, the trial was not powered for subgroup analyses.

Results

Characteristics of Participants

A total of 162 residents (30% of the 541 residents in the 12 training programs) attended a session. Among nonparticipants, it was not logistically possible to differentiate those who truly declined to participate from those who were unable to participate because of vacations, "away" rotations, or immediate patient care responsibilities. **Table 1** compares the characteristics of participants with the known characteristics of nonparticipants. Women and interns tended to be underrepresented and second-year residents tended to be overrepresented, but these differences were not statistically significant. Participation varied significantly by university.

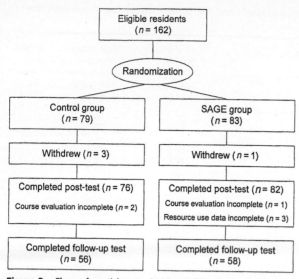

Figure 2. Flow of participants. SAGE = Self-Study Acceleration with Graphic Evidence.

Through randomization, 79 participants were assigned to the control group and 83 were assigned to the SAGE group (**Figure 2**). Because no participants used unassigned self-study materials, there was no crossover between groups. Three participants withdrew from the control group, and 1 withdrew from the SAGE group. Of these 4 participants, 1 withdrew because of post-call fatigue and 3 withdrew because of immediate patient care demands. Therefore, 76 participants in the control group and 82 participants in the SAGE group completed the immediate post-test. Data on learner satisfaction were incomplete for 3 participants (because some questions were left blank) and data on resource use were incomplete for 3 SAGE participants (because of anomalies in SAGE log-off) (**Figure 2**). The control group and the SAGE group did not differ significantly for any characteristics (**Table 1**). After 4 to 6 months, 114 of 158 participants took the follow-up test (overall follow-up rate, 72%) (**Figure 2**).

Knowledge, Learning Efficiency, and Satisfaction

Table 2 summarizes the effect of each self-study method on knowledge scores, time spent studying, and learning efficiency. Previous knowledge and knowledge immediately after the self-study program did not differ significantly between groups ($P > 0.2$ for both comparisons). The median time spent studying, however, was 30% less in the SAGE group ($P < 0.001$), which resulted in a 28% better learning efficiency for SAGE participants ($P = 0.04$). After 4 to 6 months, retention of post-test knowledge in each group decreased by 3.0 to 3.5 learning objectives; between-group differences were not statistically significant ($P = 0.12$).

The satisfaction scale had a Cronbach α coeffi-

cient of 0.88, indicating adequate internal consistency for between-group comparisons (28). The median satisfaction score was 15.0 in the control group and 17.0 in the SAGE group, a statistically significant difference ($P < 0.001$) (**Table 2**). When evaluating the course, SAGE users rated the self-study session higher on each question that assessed aspects of satisfaction with learning (P values, 0.02 to <0.001) but did not give higher scores to the pretest ($P = 0.17$).

Use of Individual Resources within the Web-Based Self-Study Program

Hyperlinks within SAGE allowed each user to access up to 20 answers to questions, 28 guideline passages, and graphic evidence from 12 clinical trials. On average, SAGE users accessed 86% of all available answers to questions, 43% of all available guideline passages, and 8% of all available graphic evidence animations. **Table 3** shows the use of these learning resources stratified by participants' previous knowledge and selection of the "review flag." Participants used resources more frequently when they had answered the relevant pretest question incorrectly; however, they accessed only 53% of the guideline passages that pertained to these unmet objectives. Participants also used more resources when they had chosen the review flag on the pretest. However, even when participants had answered incorrectly and had selected the review flag, they still accessed only 59% of the relevant guideline passages and 19% of the relevant graphic evidence animations.

Table 2. Knowledge Scores, Study Time, and Learning Efficiency according to Study Group Assignment*

Measure	Control Group ($n = 76$)	SAGE Group ($n = 82$)	P Value
Knowledge score†			
Pretest	9.0 (9.0–10.0)	10.0 (9.0–11.0)	>0.2
Immediate post-test	14.5 (14–15)	15.0 (14.0–15.0)	>0.2
Follow-up after 4–6 months‡	11.0 (10.0–12.0)	12.0 (11.0–13.0)	0.12
Study time, *min*§	38.5 (31–44)	27.0 (25.0–30.0)	<0.001
Learning efficiency, *points/h*‖	6.7 (5.9–8.1)	8.6 (7.1–11.7)	0.04
Learner satisfaction scale score¶	15.0 (15.0–16.0)	17.0 (16.0–18.0)	<0.001

* Values are expressed as the median (95% CI). The Wilcoxon rank-sum test was used for between-group comparisons, and 95% CIs were estimated by using the Conover method. SAGE = Self-Study Acceleration with Graphic Evidence.
† Number of questions answered correctly on a 20-item multiple-choice test. The pretest and immediate post-test contained different questions but assessed the same 20 learning objectives. The follow-up test contained the same 20 questions as the post-test.
‡ Fifty-six participants in the control group and 58 participants in the SAGE group completed the follow-up test (overall response rate, 72%).
§ No absolute limit; participants were asked to study until they felt that they had met the learning objectives.
‖ For each participant, learning efficiency = (post-test score – pretest score)/study time in hours.
¶ Scale range, 5–20.

Table 3. Use of Available Learning Resources in SAGE (Self-Study Acceleration with Graphic Evidence)*

Learning Objective	Use of Learning Resources		
	Answers to Questions ($n = 1580$)	Guideline Passages ($n = 2212$)	Graphic Evidence ($n = 984$)
Use according to previous knowledge†			
Resources used for unmet objectives, %	95	53	13
Resources used for met objectives, %	77	32	4
Unmet/met odds ratio (95% CI)	5.3 (3.7–7.4)	2.5 (2.1–2.9)	3.5 (2.1–5.7)
Use according to selection of "review flag"‡			
Resources used for unmet objectives			
With review flag selected, %	96	59	19
With review flag not selected, %	94	49	9
Flag/no flag odds ratio (95% CI)	1.6 (0.85–3.1)	1.5 (1.2–1.8)	2.4 (1.3–4.1)
Resources used for met objectives			
With review flag selected, %	95	50	9
With review flag not selected, %	70	24	3
Flag/no flag odds ratio (95% CI)	8.6 (4.4–17.0)	3.1 (2.3–4.8)	3.5 (1.5–8.1)

* Each SAGE user had the opportunity to access 20 answers to questions, 28 guideline passages, and graphic evidence from 12 clinical trials. Use data were incomplete for three participants.
† Each resource use opportunity was classified according to whether the user had answered the associated pretest question correctly or incorrectly, indicating a met or an unmet learning objective.
‡ Resource use opportunities were subclassified according to users' selection of a "review flag" on the pretest. Review flags were selected for 42% of unmet objectives and 27% of met objectives.

Discussion

All physicians are expected to perform self-assessment (29) and to spend time reading authoritative medical literature (30), but conscientious self-study can be arduous (31). We hypothesized that the efficiency, efficacy, and appeal of self-study could be improved by using two computer-based instructional features: hyperlinks from self-assessment results to authoritative guideline passages, and animated depictions of evidence from randomized trials. Our results show that using a Web site with these features improved residents' learning efficiency and satisfaction more than self-study from printed materials with the same learning objectives, self-assessment questions, and guideline content. Residents did not, however, achieve greater knowledge by using Web-based self-study features. Without additional reinforcement, residents who used either type of self-study could not recall most of their learning after 4 to 6 months.

Our findings are consistent with some of the results from two previous randomized trials among medical students, which compared computer-assisted instruction with content-equivalent printed materials. A system combining patient simulation and tutorial features did not improve the amount learned, but it did improve learning efficiency (17). In contrast, a multimedia textbook system did not significantly improve the amount learned or learning efficiency compared with printed materials (18). The latter trial also found that knowledge scores decreased significantly after 11 to 22 months (32). These findings of poor long-term retention are consistent with psychologists' observations that the odds of remembering a fact after a single exposure decrease as a function of time since the exposure (33).

The features of SAGE did not function entirely as intended. Hyperlinks were meant to improve the thoroughness as well as the speed of physicians' self-study. Instead of being more thorough, however, those in the SAGE group stopped working significantly sooner than those in the control group, leaving many resources unused even when their pretest results indicated a need for them. The "review flag" feature of the pretest seemed to stimulate additional study, but further research is necessary to identify more powerful motivators. Graphic evidence was intended to visually reinforce recommendations that were supported by landmark clinical trials, but this feature was rarely used. Clearly, SAGE users were drawn more strongly toward accessing the next learning objective than toward viewing evidence. Additional research is needed to investigate the reasons for this apparent lack of interest in understanding trial evidence.

Our study has several limitations. First, because participants knew the research hypotheses, a placebo-like bias was possible, especially on the satisfaction survey. However, participants in the SAGE and control groups expressed equal satisfaction for the pretest, which was identical in both groups. Second, participant attributes, such as stage of training, may have influenced the ability to benefit from SAGE. Our numbers did not provide sufficient power to support subgroup analyses, but our participants had a diverse range of previous training, pretest scores, and previous Web experience, which indicates that our observed effects apply to a relatively diverse population. Finally, results from "real-world" use of our materials could be somewhat different from those found in the setting of a controlled trial. Real-world results might be worse if participants in our study increased their effort simply because they were under observation. In contrast, real-world results might be better because users could revisit most Web- or print-based materials over time. This reinforcement would probably enhance long-term retention.

As the Internet continues its rapid growth (34), physicians are becoming increasingly interested in on-line education, primarily because of its convenience (35). A growing variety of providers are meeting this demand with products that include quiz-based tutorials (36, 37) and hypermedia patient simulations (38). Our findings directly show that on-line tutorials may provide more efficient and more appealing learning experiences than similar print-based exercises. Our results also show, however, that one pass through self-study materials may be insufficient to achieve long-term retention.

Further research is needed on Web-based instruction regarding guideline implementation. Features not present in SAGE, such as patient simulations and video presentations from experts, should

Appendix Table. SAGE (Self-Study Acceleration with Graphic Evidence) Resources Available for Each Learning Objective*

Category, Topic, and Learning Objective	Linked Learning Resources		
	ACP–ASIM Guideline Passage	ACC/AHA Guideline Passage	Evidence Animation
Testing			
Left ventricular function measurement			
Know the prognostic factor considered most important in guiding the selection of additional testing for patients who have survived the acute phase of a myocardial infarction	Yes	Yes	No
Know the options for quantitative assessment of left ventricular function and know their relative advantages	Yes	No	No
Know the clinical predictors of preserved left ventricular function in patients after myocardial infarction	Yes	No	No
Coronary angiography			
Recognize indications for post–myocardial infarction angiography in patients who did not undergo primary percutaneous transluminal coronary angioplasty	Yes	Yes	No
Noninvasive stress testing			
Know the recommended use of stress testing for stable, low-risk patients after myocardial infarction	Yes	Yes	No
Serum lipid profile			
Know when, after myocardial infarction, a serum cholesterol measurement should accurately reflect a patient's lipid status	Yes	Yes	No
Medications			
ACE inhibitors			
Identify the indications for and expected benefits of long-term ACE inhibition after myocardial infarction	No	Yes	SAVE study AIRE study SOLVD
Know the recommended course for ACE inhibitor therapy after acute myocardial infarction	No	Yes	ISIS-4
Identify contraindications to ACE inhibitors	No	Yes	No
Aspirin			
Identify the expected benefits of aspirin therapy for patients after myocardial infarction	No	Yes	ISIS-2
Lipid-lowering agents			
Know the strength of evidence for the effect of 3-hydroxy-3-methylglutaryl coenzyme A reductase inhibitors on important clinical end points	Yes	Yes	4S
Identify the recommended indications for starting and adjusting lipid-lowering drug therapy in patients with coronary artery disease	No	Yes	No
Recognize relative advantages and differing uses of medications available for lipid-lowering therapy	No	Yes	No
β-Adrenergic blockers			
Identify the benefits expected from treating patients with β-blockers after myocardial infarction	No	Yes	BHAT NMSTMI ISIS-1 MIAMI study
Calcium-channel blockers			
Know the patient subsets in which calcium-channel blockers should be avoided and know the strength of the evidence supporting this recommendation	No	Yes	MDPIT
Antiarrhythmic agents			
Know recommended and contraindicated uses of antiarrhythmic agents after myocardial infarction	Yes	Yes	CAST
Surgery			
Coronary artery bypass surgery			
Know the patient features that predict a mortality benefit from coronary artery bypass grafting	No	Yes	No
Special programs			
Smoking cessation counseling			
Identify expected benefits of smoking cessation after myocardial infarction	Yes	Yes	No
AHA step II diet			
Know the low-fat diet recommended for patients after myocardial infarction	No	Yes	No
Exercise rehabilitation			
Know the strength of the evidence supporting exercise rehabilitation programs for patients after myocardial infarction	Yes	Yes	No

* 4S = Scandinavian Simvastatin Survival Study; ACC = American College of Cardiology; ACE = angiotensin-converting enzyme; ACP–ASIM = American College of Physicians–American Society of Internal Medicine; AHA = American Heart Association; AIRE = Acute Infarction Ramipril Efficacy; BHAT = Beta Blocker Heart Attack Trial; CAST = Cardiac Arrhythmia Suppression Trial; ISIS = International Study of Infarct Survival; MDPIT = Multicenter Diltiazem Post Infarction Trial; MIAMI = Metoprolol in Acute Myocardial Infarction; NMSTMI = Norwegian Multicenter Study on Timolol after Myocardial Infarction; SAVE = Survival and Ventricular Enlargement; SOLVD = Studies of Left Ventricular Dysfunction.

be tested for their efficacy. Even without enhanced efficacy, on-line tutorials might improve guideline dissemination if they could attract increased physician participation or repeated use. However, these hypotheses also need to be tested. Power to detect interactions with previous training or learning styles might be achieved by conducting larger studies or by testing instruction on separate topics using a crossover design. As more knowledge is gained about Web-based self-study, its effects on physician practice will need to be measured. Future research should combine Web-based self-study with other types of guideline implementation, such as reminder systems and physician incentives. Until more research is conducted, however, health care organizations may find that investments in Web-based instruction do not yield predictable returns.

From University of California, Los Angeles, School of Medicine, Los Angeles, California.

Presented in part at the Society for General Internal Medicine Annual Meeting, 30 April–1 May 1999, San Francisco, California.

Acknowledgments: The authors thank the SAGE trial participants and the following chief residents, program directors, and administrators who were instrumental in their residents' participation: David Graham, MD, Oregon Health Sciences University, Portland, Oregon; Jodi Friedman, MD, and Roland Sakiyama, MD, University of California, Los Angeles, Los Angeles, California; Harry Hollander, MD, and Jill Thomas, University of California, San Francisco, San Francisco, California; Stephanie Silas, MD, H. James Williams, MD, Ita M. Killeen, MD, and Judi Weston, University of Utah, Salt Lake City, Utah. They also thank LuAnn Wilkerson, PhD, Anju Relan, PhD, and Martin Shapiro, MD, PhD, for insightful critical review of the instructional design and the trial design.

Grant Support: In part by a National Research Service Award (T32 PE19001-09) from the Health Resources and Services Administration of the U.S. Department of Health and Human Services. Additional project support was provided by the University of California, Los Angeles, Stein–Oppenheimer Fund and by the GTE Foundation through the University of California, Los Angeles, Center for Digital Innovation. Dr. Mangione was partially supported by the Robert Wood Johnson Foundation as a Generalist Faculty Scholar (award no. 029250).

Requests for Single Reprints: Douglas S. Bell, MD, University of California, Los Angeles, Division of General Internal Medicine and Health Services Research, 911 Broxton Plaza, Room 218, Los Angeles, CA 90095-1736; e-mail, sagequery@gim.med.ucla.edu.

Requests To Purchase Bulk Reprints (minimum, 100 copies): Barbara Hudson, Reprints Coordinator; phone, 215-351-2657; e-mail, bhudson@mail.acponline.org.

Current Author Addresses: Drs. Bell, Hays, and Mangione: Department of Medicine, Division of General Internal Medicine and Health Services Research, University of California, Los Angeles, 911 Broxton Plaza, Los Angeles, CA 90095-1736.
Dr. Fonarow: Department of Medicine, Division of Cardiology, University of California, Los Angeles, CHS 67-130A, Los Angeles, CA 90095-1679.

Author Contributions: Conception and design: D.S. Bell, G.C. Fonarow, R.D. Hays, C.M. Mangione.
Analysis and interpretation of the data: D.S. Bell, G.C. Fonarow, R.D. Hays, C.M. Mangione.

Drafting of the article: D.S. Bell, G.C. Fonarow, R.D. Hays, C.M. Mangione.
Critical revision of the article for important intellectual content: D.S. Bell, G.C. Fonarow, R.D. Hays, C.M. Mangione.
Final approval of the article: D.S. Bell, G.C. Fonarow, R.D. Hays, C.M. Mangione.
Provision of study materials or patients: D.S. Bell, G.C. Fonarow, C.M. Mangione.
Statistical expertise: D.S. Bell, R.D. Hays, C.M. Mangione.
Obtaining of funding: D.S. Bell, C.M. Mangione.
Administrative, technical, or logistic support: D.S. Bell, C.M. Mangione.
Collection and assembly of data: D.S. Bell.

References

1. **Ayanian JZ, Hauptman PJ, Guadagnoli E, Antman EM, Pashos CL, McNeil BJ.** Knowledge and practices of generalist and specialist physicians regarding drug therapy for acute myocardial infarction. N Engl J Med. 1994; 331:1136-42.
2. **Chin MH, Friedmann PD, Cassel CK, Lang RM.** Differences in generalist and specialist physicians' knowledge and use of angiotensin-converting enzyme inhibitors for congestive heart failure. J Gen Intern Med. 1997;12:523-30.
3. Guidelines for risk stratification after myocardial infarction. American College of Physicians. Ann Intern Med. 1997;126:556-60.
4. **Ryan TJ, Anderson JL, Antman EM, Braniff BA, Brooks NH, Califf RM, et al.** ACC/AHA guidelines for the management of patients with acute infarction. A report of the American College of Cardiology/American Heart Association Task Force on Practice Guidelines (Committee on Management of Acute Myocardial Infarction). J Am Coll Cardiol. 1996;28:1328-428.
5. **O'Connor GT, Quinton HB, Traven ND, Ramunno LD, Dodds TA, Marciniak TA, et al.** Geographic variation in the treatment of acute myocardial infarction: the Cooperative Cardiovascular Project. JAMA. 1999;281:627-33.
6. **Grol R, Zwaard A, Mokkink H, Dalhuijsen J, Casparie A.** Dissemination of guidelines: which sources do physicians use in order to be informed? Int J Qual Health Care. 1998;10:135-40.
7. **Gagne RM.** The Conditions of Learning and Theory of Instruction. 4th ed. Fort Worth, TX: Holt, Rinehart and Winston; 1985.
8. **Freemantle N, Harvey EL, Wolf F, Grimshaw JM, Grilli R, Bero LA.** Printed educational materials: effects on professional practice and health care outcomes (Cochrane Review). In: The Cochrane Library. Oxford: Update Software; 1999.
9. **Burg FD, Grosse ME, Kay CF.** A national self-assessment program in internal medicine. Ann Intern Med. 1979;90:100-7.
10. **Day SC, Grosso LJ, Norcini JJ.** Methods of preparing for the certifying examination in internal medicine and their efficacy. J Gen Intern Med. 1994; 9:167-9.
11. **Sikorski R, Peters R.** Tools for change: CME on the Internet. JAMA. 1998; 280:1013-4.
12. **Entwisle G, Entwisle DR.** The use of a digital computer as a teaching machine. J Med Educ. 1963;38:803-12.
13. **Harless WG, Lucas NC, Cutter JA, Duncan RC, White JM, Brandt E.** Computer-assisted instruction in continuing medical education. J Med Educ. 1969;44:670-4.
14. **Hoffer EP, Barnett GO, Farquhar BB, Prather PA.** Computer-aided instruction in medicine. Annu Rev Biophys Bioeng. 1975;4:103-18.
15. **Piemme TE.** Computer-assisted learning and evaluation in medicine. JAMA. 1988;260:367-72.
16. **Atkinson RC, Wilson HA.** Computer-assisted instruction. Science. 1968; 162:73-7.
17. **Lyon HC Jr, Healy JC, Bell JR, O'Donnell JF, Shultz EK, Moore-West M, et al.** PlanAlyzer, an interactive computer-assisted program to teach clinical problem solving in diagnosing anemia and coronary artery disease. Acad Med. 1992;67:821-8.
18. **Santer DM, Michaelsen VE, Erkonen WE, Winter RJ, Woodhead JC, Gilmer JS, et al.** A comparison of educational interventions. Multimedia textbook, standard lecture, and printed textbook. Arch Pediatr Adolesc Med. 1995;149:297-302.
19. **Kern DE, Thomas PA, Howard DM, Bass EB.** Goals and objectives. In: Curriculum Development for Medical Education: A Six-Step Approach. Baltimore: Johns Hopkins Univ Pr; 1998.
20. **Bell DS, Mangione CM.** A system for pilot testing clinical knowledge questions using pseudo-anonymous electronic mail [Abstract]. Proc AMIA Annu Fall Symp. 1998:971.
21. **Matts JP, Lachin JM.** Properties of permuted-block randomization in clinical trials. Control Clin Trials. 1988;9:327-44.
22. **Shapiro SS, Wilk MB.** An analysis of variance test for normality. Biometrika. 1965;52:591-611.
23. **Conover WJ.** Practical Nonparametric Statistics. 2d ed. New York: J Wiley; 1980.
24. **Cronbach LJ.** Coefficient alpha and the internal structure of tests. Psychometrika. 1951;16:297.
25. **Greenland S, Rothman KJ.** Introduction to stratified analysis. In: Rothman KJ, Greenland S. Modern Epidemiology. 2d ed. Philadelphia: Lippincott-Raven; 1998:253-79.

26. **Huber PJ.** The behavior of maximum likelihood estimates under non-standard conditions. Proceedings of the Fifth Berkeley Symposium on Mathematical Statistics and Probability. 1967;1:221-33.

27. **White H.** Maximum likelihood estimation of misspecified models. Econometrica. 1982;50:1-25.

28. **Nunnally JC, Bernstein IH.** Psychometric Theory. New York, McGraw-Hill; 1994:264-5.

29. American Medical Association. AMA Physician Recognition Award: category 2 activities. Available at http://www.ama-assn.org/med-sci/pra2/i-5cate.htm#Self-assessment activities. Accessed 16 Nov 1999.

30. American Medical Association. AMA Physician Recognition Award: basic requirements. Available at http://www.ama-assn.org/med-sci/pra2/i-3reqs.htm#Read. Accessed 16 Nov 1999.

31. **Burnum JF.** Trial by self-assessment. Ann Intern Med. 1997;126:84-5.

32. **D'Alessandro DM, Kreiter CD, Erkonen WE, Winter RJ, Knapp HR.** Longitudinal follow-up comparison of educational interventions: multimedia textbook, traditional lecture, and printed textbook. Acad Radiol. 1997;4:719-23.

33. **Healy AF, McNamara DS.** Verbal learning and memory: does the modal model still work? Annu Rev Psychol. 1996;47:143-72.

34. The Strategis Group. U.S. Internet breaks the 100 million mark. Available at http://www.strategisgroup.com/press/pubs/iut99.html. Accessed 16 Nov 1999.

35. **Richardson ML, Norris TE.** On-line delivery of continuing medical education over the World-Wide Web: an on-line needs assessment. AJR Am J Roentgenol. 1997;168:1161-4.

36. American Academy of Pediatrics. Pediatrics in review. Available at http://www.pedsinreview.org/cme/. Accessed 3 Nov 1999.

37. Medscape, Inc. Medscape CME Center. Available at http://cmecenter.medscape.com. Accessed 3 Nov 1999.

38. American College of Physicians. Clinical problem-solving cases. Available at http://cpsc.acponline.org/. Accessed 3 Nov 1999.

Computer-aided learning for the education of patients and family practice professionals in the personal care of diabetes

Emma-Jane Berridge [a],*, Abdul Roudsari [a], Sheila Taylor [b], Steve Carey [c]

[a] *Centre for Measurement and Information in Medicine, School of Informatics, City University, Northampton Square, London EC1V 0HB, UK*
[b] *Diabetes and Endocrinology Day Centre, St Thomas' Hospital, Lambeth Palace Road, London SE1 7EH, UK*
[c] *Department of Diabetes and Endocrinology, Division of Medicine, GKT Medical School, St Thomas' Hospital, Lambeth Palace Road, London SE1 7EH, UK*

Received 8 December 1998; received in revised form 26 August 1999; accepted 8 December 1999

Abstract

Diabetes Mellitus is approaching pandemic proportions across the globe. It is a disproportionately expensive condition, accounting for 5–9% of annual NHS expenditure. Family practices often play a huge role in the care of diabetic patients. Many GPs elect to play a larger role in diabetes care, but the increasing burden on the multidisciplinary secondary care team means that some of the burden has to fall to family practitioners. In order to provide a high standard of care, the practitioner requires access to continuing education regarding diabetes care. The value of patient education is undisputed. In light of this situation a computer-aided learning (CAL) system is being developed for the education of both patients and practitioners concerning diabetes and its care. The proposed system takes a two pronged approach, being aimed at both patient and practitioner. This interactive system employs multimedia technology to teach practical skills and promote and consolidate theoretical understanding. It is hoped this system will improve patient self-care, and in the long-term reduce the incidence of diabetic complications and their associated costs. © 2000 Elsevier Science Ireland Ltd. All rights reserved.

Keywords: Computer-aided learning; Diabetes mellitus; Primary care; Patient education

1. Introduction

Multimedia computer-aided learning (CAL) is established as a useful and cost-effective adjunct to conventional education, and its successful application in varied domains has been widely evident in recent years [1–5]. In the domain of diabetes, several CAL systems have been developed which, subject to user evaluation, have achieved encouraging results [6–8]. Several impressive examples have been developed for various aspects of diabetes patient education, but as yet, CAL has not been applied in professional continuing education for non-specialists involved in diabetes care. However, where CAL has been

* Corresponding author. Tel.: +44-20-74778371; fax: +44-20-74778364.

developed for professionals in various other areas of medical and paramedical education, promising results have been found [9–12].

The prevalence of diabetes is increasing dramatically [13] and the care of diabetic patients is increasingly devolved to primary care [14]. In this climate, the lack of continuing education for non-specialist nurses involved in diabetes care must be addressed. The care of this complex condition requires significant expertise. Patient education is a fundamental part of diabetes self-care [15,16], and therefore non-specialist professional education is vital for the effective communication of complex knowledge and myriad practical skills to the patient. The ability to disseminate theoretical knowledge and practical skills in an effective and cost-effective way is essential to a forward thinking but cost-restrained NHS. The development of computer-aided learning providing education for both patients and primary care professionals will provide a useful and cost-efficient solution to the current deficit of specialist continuing education to non-specialist professionals and will supplement nurse-led patient education.

A comprehensive diabetes CAL application with two specific branches for patients and for non-specialist healthcare professionals has therefore been designed and partially implemented. Despite the number of CAL products developed in recent years, there exist few explicit guidelines or concrete methodologies for the design, development and evaluation of CAL for patient or professional education. A methodology has therefore been developed for the design, development, implementation and evaluation of CAL applied to the broad and complex domain of diabetes, based on top-level requirements for the system. This paper describes the methodology and charts the progress of the project to date.

2. System design and development

The design and development of this dual-branched CAL system follows several distinct phases. An iterative approach has been adopted, with evaluation undertaken at various points and evaluation information fed back to the design and development process. Systematic evaluation of a representative sub-set at various stages helps ensure that design and development proceeds in a sensible way which satisfies potential users. This formative evaluation during development is supplemented with final evaluation by patients and practice nurses of the finished system. Fig. 1 depicts this evolutionary process and each step in the design, development and implementation of the system is described below.

2.1. Establish requirements

In order to establish top-level requirements for our system, two simple questionnaires were devised. These questionnaires sought information on a national and a local scale regarding the provision of specialist diabetes education for practice nurses. As such, one was sent to all 69 Health Authorities (HAs) in England, which requested details of diabetes education provision for primary care practitioners under each HA. Of the 38 respondents, all provide some kind of continuing education in diabetes. However, there is great regional variability in the depth and nature of this education, and only 47% of our responding Health Authorities use the English National Board of Nursing and Midwifery (ENB) diabetes management courses. The ENB course is a prerequisite for diabetes specialist nurses.

Our second simple, structured and locally focussed questionnaire was sent to all practices in the boroughs of Lambeth, Southwark and Lewisham, South London. This acted as a preliminary needs assessment. Responses to our questionnaire indicated that while the majority (83%) of our 54 respondents — those practice nurses responsible for diabetes care in their practice — have attended continuing diabetes education in the last 2 years, 41% of all respondents still feel they need additional support and education. Interest in the use of CAL for patient and nurse education was demonstrated through 54% of respondents willing to be involved with the project at a later date. The Health Authority contracted Diabetes Resource Team (DRT) in Lambeth, Southwark and Lewisham provides strong support (telephone support, resource packs, service outlines, training programmes) to practices in these boroughs, but a desktop reference guide and continuing education tool would provide immediate and ongoing educational support.

2.2. Identify objectives

Having established the need for a cost-effective educational tool, objectives for the project were identified. Through collaboration with members of the multidisciplinary secondary care team at St Thomas' Hospital, London and the DRT, a number of objectives were established.

Our learning tool should:

- Deliver interesting and high quality information on diabetes to motivate users to learn more and to inspire concordance with the self-care regimen
- Foster a deeper understanding of the lifestyle modifications necessary in diabetes self-care
- Promote familiarity with the practical skills necessary within diabetes care and self-care
- Contain up to date evidence-based information

- Be accessible both as a modular educational tool and as a quick reference guide to both patients and healthcare professionals
- Provide a directory of support services available to both patients and healthcare professionals

2.3. Identify design principles

An effective CAL system in the context of this project should therefore motivate patients to self-care, and should educate both patients and nurses about risk factors and warning signs in order to promote timely diagnosis and appropriate referral. With timely diagnosis, appropriate referral and improved patient self-care, an improvement in health outcomes can be achieved. A number of principles for the design of the system were identified in order to achieve the objectives of the system.

The system aims to deliver high quality diabetes education, relevant to user needs:

- With content based upon the most recent consensus guidelines from the World Health Or-

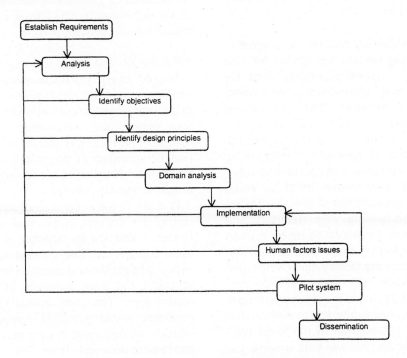

Fig. 1. The iterative design and development process.

ganisation, the International Diabetes Federation and the BDA, [17–19] structured into various modules

- With a simple user interface and easy to learn navigation procedure in order that content, rather than how to use the system is the primary focus
- Using multimedia, interactive tasks and self-assessment tests in order to motivate users and to help consolidate their knowledge and understanding of diabetes, its care and self-care
- With branching and hyperlinking between related parts of the system
- Taking an evidence-based approach — developed with current research in mind and containing a reference section of publications consulted in the development of the system and for further reading
- Including a searchable index, employing hypertext to allow quick and easy access to the preferred part of the system
- With text in the system linked to a glossary of terms, and with a searchable glossary readily accessible from the main window's menu bar.

2.4. Domain analysis

In order to establish the breadth and content of our domain, domain analysis was carried out with the assistance of a group of experts from the multidisciplinary team. The initial step was a brainstorming exercise, in which diabetes specialist nurses (DSNs) were asked to identify the various roles they play on a daily basis, and from there to brainstorm all the tasks involved and information to be conveyed to patients within each of these roles.

From this vast, unstructured list of the roles, tasks and education points identified by the DSNs, preliminary module headings were established, and related information keywords clustered around them. Where there were overlaps, with information relevant in more than one module, these were noted for later consideration in the context of hypertext/media and branching within the system. Our team of nurses was consulted at intervals to confirm that this rudimentary organisation of the various aspects of their different roles was both sensible and meaningful.

2.4.1. Development of concept maps

The result of the brainstorming exercise indicated the breadth of our domain, then, and with the addition of preliminary module headings, allowed us to see the beginning of some kind of structure. In order to add further structure to this vast list of concepts, the headings and keywords were mapped and expanded into hierarchical concept maps. This hierarchical tree structure of modules and sub-topics was developed using Microsoft Organisation Chart (Banner Blue Software, Fremont, California, 1995). Links to similar or related information points elsewhere in the structure were highlighted and cross-referenced within the maps. The structure and finer details of content were further refined though collaboration with the multidisciplinary team, and using guidelines from British and international bodies [17–20].

The resulting concept maps provide an exhaustive plan of the domain of diabetes. There are 26 maps in all, representing the breakdown of the system into 23 modules (14 on the patient branch and nine additional practice nurse-specific modules), each of which contains between three and 11 sub-topics. Fig. 2 illustrates the size and complexity of the domain with detail from the 'What is diabetes?' module concept map.

2.4.2. Verification of concept maps

In order to verify that the information contained was correct and the structure sensible, the concept maps were subject to evaluation by experts. During their development, verification of structure and content of the maps was obtained through consultation with members of the multidisciplinary team at St Thomas' Hospital, London, whose advice was sought at regular intervals.

In order to assess the overall structure and content of the concept maps, they were subject to further evaluation by another group of experts upon completion. The concept maps were sent with a straightforward questionnaire to a sample of DSNs and other members of the multidisciplinary team. The questionnaire requested scored responses to the perceived completeness of the information contained in each module map. These scores were on a scale from 1–6 — incomplete to complete. The aim of the evaluation exercise was

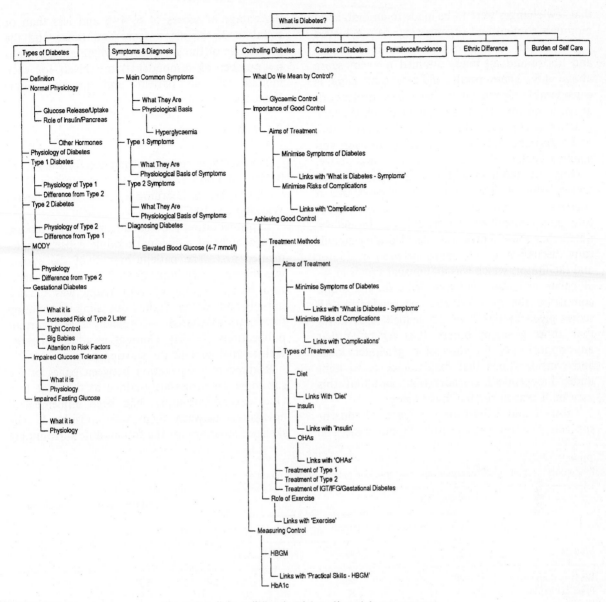

Fig. 2. Detail from 'What is Diabetes?' module concept map.

to establish to what degree experts agreed with the structure and content, and to elicit any further information deemed necessary for inclusion in an educational system for patients and non-specialist nurses. The ideal score for each map was therefore 6, indicating complete agreement with the map. The questionnaire allowed space for free text responses to the organisation, content and

structure of the information where the score for a map fell below 6. Where there was some degree of disagreement with content and structure, comments were taken into account and the concept maps modified accordingly.

Of the 14 modules in the patient branch of the system, 29% achieved a mean score of 5.5 and above. This high degree of consensus indicated that few changes were to be made to an individual module's content and organisation. 64% achieved a good degree of consensus — a mean score of 5 and above-and all maps attained a mean score above 4.5. These results indicate that there is considerable agreement by healthcare professionals with the completeness of the maps. Of the nine practice nurse maps, 44% achieved a mean score of 5.5 and above; 89%, a score of 5 and over, and again, all achieved a mean score of 4.5 and above.

Only two modules of the total of 23 obtained scores below 4. The score of 3 indicates that a substantial amount of work is necessary on structure and content of the module. It should be noted that these scores were decided after significant discussion of the maps between evaluator and facilitator, which was an unusual situation — all other evaluators had considered the maps and completed the questionnaire independently. All scores given by this evaluator tended to be lower than those given by others. It is suggested that any opportunity for discussion generates ideas and considerations that may not come to light under independent consideration, and that this may be a reason for the lower scores.

Tables 1 and 2 illustrate the degree of consensus achieved for each of our 23 modules. The percentage of scores of 6, 4–5 and less than or equal to 3, the mean score and range and the percentage of the ideal score (where ideal score is 6 × number of respondents) are given for each module of the patient and practice nurse branches, respectively.

2.5. Content creation

The system is being implemented for the PC (to be delivered on CD-ROM) using Asymetrix Toolbook (Asymetrix Learning Systems, Inc. Bellevue, Washington, 1997).

Implementation proceeded from the bottom up, with content of individual module subsets implemented first. The patient branch of the system was the first to be implemented. A skeleton structure based on our concept maps was created initially and content fleshed out using information from various sources — guidelines and various publications [21–24]. Content is added directly, with textual content the starting point.

Rudimentary navigation between pages of the sub-topic was necessarily added at this time too. Once several sub-topics had been implemented, navigation between them was considered. The skeleton structure for the full module surrounding

Table 1

Evaluators' responses to concept maps developed for patient branch modules

Module	Score (%) Complete agreement 6	Partial agreement 4–5	Little agreement ≤3	Mean	Range	% of ideal
What is diabetes?	40	60	–	5.2	4–6	87
Practical skills	20	60	20	4.6	3–6	77
Insulin	20	80	–	4.8	4–6	80
OHAs	60	40	–	5.6	5–6	93
Hypos	–	100	–	4.8	4–5	80
Intercurrent illness	–	100	–	4.8	4–5	80
Complications	60	40	–	5.6	5–6	93
Diet	50	50	–	5.25	4–6	87.5
Exercise	20	80	–	5	4–6	83
Drinking, smoking, drugs	40	60	–	5.4	5–6	90
Travel and holidays	20	80	–	5.2	5–6	87
Sex and pregnancy	20	60	20	4.6	3–6	77
Stress	75	25	–	5.5	4–6	92
Employment	80	20	–	5.8	5–6	97

Table 2
Evaluators' responses to concept maps developed for practice nurse branch modules

Module	Score (%) Complete agreement	Partial agreement	Little agreement	Mean	Range	% of ideal
	6	4–5	≤3			
What is diabetes?	75	25	–	5.75	5–6	96
Clinical tasks	25	75	–	5	4–6	83
Psychological/physical assessment	50	50	–	5.25	4–6	87.5
Social/lifestyle assessment	50	50	–	5.5	5–6	92
Medical history	75	25	–	5.75	5–6	96
Complications	67	33	–	5.67	5–6	94
Annual review	–	100	–	5	5	83
Quality of life	33	67	–	5	4–6	83
Education principles	–	100	–	4.75	4–5	79

these sub-topics was implemented next, and necessarily also navigation tools for the whole module. This generated the need to consider navigation for the full system, in terms of navigating around and between modules and their sub-topics. A strategy for navigating the system was therefore implemented. The skeleton structure for all modules and sub-topics of the patient branch were added, with top level (empty) pages created for content to be added and sub-topics expanded later.

The glossary of terms hyperlinked to textual content and a separate searchable and cross-referenced hypertext glossary have been added, and glossary content is expanded on an ad hoc basis as further module content is added. Other tools such as a searchable index and index of references will be implemented at the final stage. In order to assess the propriety and ease of use of our navigation method, evaluation was undertaken at this early stage. As full modules are completed, these, too, are evaluated by the multidisciplinary team.

The concept maps have been followed carefully but implementation, even in its early stages, illuminated minor problems with the organisation (e.g. unwieldy amounts of information clustered in one sub-topic which could be divided and branching extended). In light of such difficulties, the concept maps are provisionally amended where necessary. An iterative implementation process has evolved; the original maps have not been discarded, as they may later emerge to be more appropriate than the amended version. Clearly, this is a somewhat intuitive process.

2.5.1. Use of multimedia

As the module subsets are fleshed out, they are initially empty pages, simple to generate within Toolbook, which are filled with textual content according to the system maps. The generation of textual content on an ad lib basis inspires various other means of representing the information non-textually, and of consolidating this information through the use of tasks and games. In the first instance these are marked with placeholders to be developed later. A list of these media assets is created as appropriate positions for multimedia content are identified.

Alongside the textual content, then, are video, audio, still graphics and animation.

2.5.1.1. Video. Video clips are employed within the system to demonstrate practical procedures such as drawing up and injecting insulin — procedures more accurately explained using video than textual accounts. Video is also used to provide some variety in the means of delivering information. Also, clips of patients discussing certain aspects of diabetes care are included to reassure the user that other 'normal' people like themselves have diabetes and are also dealing with the challenge of self-care. Similarly, clips depicting members of the interdisciplinary team are used to reassure users of the validity and accuracy of the information provided.

2.5.1.2. Graphics. The system contains still graphics to illustrate textual content and to further consolidate certain points. Graphics are also used in the development of interactive tasks and games, as well as in self-assessment tests, for example, involving the user making food choices and examining feet.

2.5.1.3. Audio. Voiceovers are employed to provide variety in information delivery, and to provide authoritative instructions. Voiceovers, where included, have the option to be disabled.

2.5.1.4. Animation. Animation is also employed to illustrate various points. Animated clips depicting the body's reaction to glucose ingestion in both the diabetic and non-diabetic person, for example, provide a useful illustration of physiological processes, and may promote a greater understanding where dense text explaining the same processes is a chore to follow for all but the most motivated patients.

Table 3 provides an overview of criteria guiding the choice of media use.

2.5.2. Categories of content type

A number of specific categories of content type can be identified within the domain, to be represented in different ways using various media. In multimedia development, constraints exist regarding the quantity and types of multimedia assets employed in the system, where disk space and funds are often limited. The sheer vastness of the domain of diabetes necessarily impacts upon the quantity of multimedia resources employed in the current project with cost and disk space at a premium. Identifying different types of content and how they are best represented using certain media, then, allows us to begin to prioritise regarding multimedia asset use. Subtopics within the system are arranged into these categories and similar rules are adopted in the implementation of similar topics. The content types identified in the domain of diabetes can be seen in Table 4.

2.5.3. Content evaluation

As implementation proceeds, modules are subject to rigorous evaluation both by users and by technical experts. An evolutionary approach to prototyping has been adopted, and this formative evaluation highlights any necessary modifications, which can be incorporated before development proceeds further.

An assessment of the value and accuracy of the content within the system, including assessment of glossary content, is to be undertaken by members of the multidisciplinary team. As complete modules are implemented, evaluation proceeds by asking a sample of specialists to systematically browse module content and complete a structured questionnaire regarding completeness, accuracy and structure of content. As well as assessing accuracy and clarity of content and propriety of information representation, this multidisciplinary evaluation will also concentrate on usefulness and ease-of-use of the system. The results of these evaluations will feed back into the design and development process. In this way, evaluation informs and shapes the development process. Evaluation will run concurrently with implementation of further modules.

2.6. Human factors issues

It is of some concern that computers may be found to be confusing, threatening, or difficult to use. In a learning tool it is essential that the educational material is the focus of attention, and so 'the interface should facilitate the user's tasks rather than calling attention to itself' [25]. The interface must therefore be simple and input devices should require minimal training to use [26].

The interface of the current system is therefore, in accordance with our design principles, designed to be easy to understand and use even for those with little or no experience of using a PC. In order that the system is easy to learn, the interface and navigational tools are consistent throughout.

Given the importance of the information conveyed by the system, it is essential that it is easy to see and is engaging.

Table 3
Criteria guiding multimedia choice

Medium	Advantages	Disadvantages	Use	Example
Text	Cheap to produce Easy to produce Facilitates hypertext and branching Resource-light	Care with readability level User literacy? Dense = off-putting?	Bullet lists FAQs Introductions Step by step with graphics	FAQ sections Basic explanations Step by step drawing up Insulin + still pictures
Still graphics	Add variety Aid abstraction Illustration/clarity can be easy to produce Easier to remember than text and numbers	Specialist software to produce Specialist hardware may be required Some expertise required	With step by step instructions Illustrating points Presenting data Icons and bullets Tests and tasks	Injection sites Syringe sizes Prevalence graphs Lipohypertrophy /footcare illustrations
Animation	Promotes interest Clear practical demonstrations can add humour	Expensive to produce Specialist software Expertise required Resource-hog Over use can be distracting	Where video can't be created Animated bullets Screen transitions Animated charts	Physiological processes Cartoon explanations Animated prevalence graphs
Video	Adds variety Promotes interest Clear practical demonstrations Compression improving	Expensive to produce — specialist hard & software Expertise required Resource-hog	Talking heads Practical demonstrations Storytelling	Injection technique Home monitoring techniques Patient experience talking heads Authoritative advice (nurse)
Voice over	Effective and natural communication Adds soothing tone Influential/persuasive Improves retention	Relatively expensive Relative resource hog Over use can be distracting	Authoritative instructions Soothing tone Adding info to graphics	Navigation instructions Complication prevention (authoritative) Unpleasantness of complications (soothing)
Music and sound effects	Adds atmosphere Adds emotion Enlivens presentation Reinforces visuals	Can be hard to obtain Expertise required to create Equipment expensive	In interactive tasks Reinforce graphical messages Variety/humour	Verbal instructions with still images for insulin storage

Table 4
Categories of content type identified in the domain of diabetes and examples of their representation using multimedia

Content type	Examples	Media employed
Theoretical	Physiology of diabetes; glucose metabolism	Animation of process; interactive 'What happens if...' drag and drop games
Practical	Injection technique; blood glucose monitoring	Video demonstration; textual step-by-step with still graphics
Strategic	The 'sick day rules'; planning to go abroad	Textual/graphical/pop-up hit list of points

2.6.1. Text

Text is easy to read — large enough and clear on the background — in order to hold user attention. Each page of textual content looks the same, and hypertext 'contents' pages within each sub-topic are consistent. Text is 12 point and the font consistent within context. The size of text boxes is limited and scrolling fields omitted to promote ease of use. Where textual content exceeds the size of a text field, the user can choose to view more content with a hypertext link to another page.

2.6.2. Colour

The use of colour in the interface helps highlight important information and can be used to guide users to important information [27]. As such, hypertext links to related information are indicated with coloured text, and glossary entries are also coloured. Colouring glossary entries not only highlights these as important keywords, but also allows the possibility of looking up these terms as necessary.

The use of colour can also be distracting, however, so in accordance with our principle that content should be the focus of user attention, textual content is black on a white background for clarity.

2.6.3. Video

Video is centrally placed on an uncluttered screen and the user interface consistent throughout. Where video and animated clips are available, the clip always occupies the same location in the workspace, and the clip control panel is always consistent.

2.6.4. Menu bar and control panel

Navigation needs to be easy to use/learn, and consistent in order to facilitate ease of use for new and returning users. Windows conventions are followed regarding the design and layout of the menu bar through which users can select modules, open other resources such as the glossary and references and quit the program. A navigation control panel containing a list box for sub-topic selection and other tools for navigation is present on every page.

2.6.5. Interface evaluation

A number of different interface options were subject to peer review within the Centre for Measurement and Information in Medicine as part of the evolutionary prototyping process. These were subject to simple, informal tests by a small number of participants, which involved users browsing through content from the entry-level menu to content items several levels deep. On the basis of users' experiences and comments regarding clarity and user-friendliness of the interface, a final user interface design was chosen which can be seen in Fig. 3.

2.6.6. Navigation issues

Navigation must be simple for users to understand and easy to learn. Further, navigation must be carefully planned to prevent the user from getting lost in deep menu structures and hyperlinks.

Users navigate the system by selecting a module from a menu on the main window's menu bar. This generates a list of sub-topics in a single-select list box within the 'control panel' (also containing other navigation buttons) at the side of the workspace and navigates to the module introduction page. The user selects a sub-topic from the list and an introduction page for that sub-topic is opened in the workspace. From this introduction page the user has a choice of destinations, which can be reached from a hypertext list.

2.6.7. Navigation evaluation

Evaluation of the navigation methodology employed was undertaken by a sample of 17 practice nurses. Practice nurses already involved in diabetes care were chosen as evaluators as they represent a portion of the target audience and because a cross-section of computer literacy was expected. Participants were asked to complete a short set of tasks in which they were required to navigate from one specific point in the system to another. The tasks attempted to take users deep into the structure in order to ascertain whether they felt comfortable and well oriented even at a relatively deep level. A certain amount of diabetes specific knowledge was pre-supposed in order that users could be given simple cues about where to navi-

gate to rather than step-by-step instructions on how to navigate there. Although they clearly represent a substantial part of our target audience and must therefore have an opportunity to comment on the system, patients were omitted from evaluation at this stage, due to the amount of diabetes knowledge pre-supposed in the written task.

The majority of respondents found the system easy to navigate (94%), and found themselves well oriented most of the time (94%). The method of choosing modules from a menu bar item and selecting sub-topics from a single select list box were found to be sensible by all users, and the use of internal navigation instructions (e.g. Return to..., Jump to..., etc.) deemed useful alongside the sub-topic single select list box (82%). Although our informal observation of users indicated that several had initial difficulty in selecting modules from a menu bar item, this was not expressed in the results. This indicated that the navigation was easy to learn, if not easy to use initially. In light of this, it would have been useful to have video-

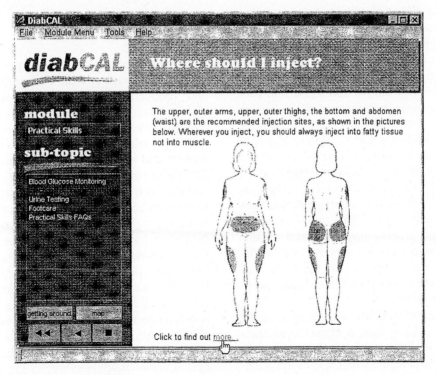

Fig. 3. DiabCAL screen shot, illustrating the user interface.

taped users navigating the system to identify exactly where they had problems, and to reflect these in our evaluation results. The project's resources were not sufficient to provide for this, however subsequent evaluations will include more formal observation of users in order that evaluation results more accurately reflect the experiences of our user group.

Overall, responses to the navigation method were encouraging. However, several users expressed a wish for the navigation instructions page to be accessible from the help menu at all times as well as available on entry to the system (88%). Also, some evaluators felt a map would be a useful addition, allowing users to orientate themselves relative to the whole system (47%). These results have been taken into account and the system modified accordingly. In order to ensure that our modifications satisfy users, navigation issues will be examined again as part of the overall system evaluation.

2.7. Piloting system

A number of different methods for the evaluation of computer-aided learning can be identified [28] and the present project relies upon two of these. As part of the design and development process, formative evaluation [29] is systematically employed, helping to inform and shape that process. Formative evaluation involves the collection of information during design and development, which informs decisions and ultimately improves the product. The evaluations involved in the creation of our concept maps, the evaluation of navigation and verification of content, as well as the peer reviews involved in interface design have all impacted upon and fed back into the design and development process, improving and refining design at each stage. The involvement of potential users and of experts ensures that the system satisfies both and improves the chances of success of the completed system.

A second type of evaluation to be used in the development of the system is impact evaluation [30], in which the impact of our full product on user learning and understanding is assessed. Piloting the system will therefore involve a structured

quantitative analysis of the usefulness of the system for patient and practice nurse learning. Ethical approval for the involvement of patients in the study is currently being sought. Pre- and post-use tests will establish how much users have learnt using the CAL system, and ease-of-use of the final product will also be examined.

Technical evaluation will also be undertaken at the latter stage of system development, in which experts will assess the structure and navigation of the system. The results of these final evaluations will be presented upon completion.

2.8. Dissemination

Subject to satisfactory findings from the piloting of the system, the full system will be packaged for distribution on CD-ROM for the stand-alone PC. The system will be available for use in general practice (for both practice nurse, patient and for use by the two in patient education sessions) and, it is hoped, might also be distributed for use in libraries and community centres.

3. Status report

Domain analysis, the mapping of the domain into concept maps and the evaluation of structure and verification of knowledge have been completed. Several full modules have been implemented on a basic level: textual content has been added, placeholders for multimedia content implemented and an asset list of multimedia resources for those modules created, with media clips sketched out for creation at a later stage. Test video clips have been created and run. Navigation has been implemented and evaluated to the satisfaction of our user group, and skeleton structure for the whole system is in place. Glossaries have been developed, and further glossary content will be added alongside the addition of content of further modules. The content of the full modules is subject to review by members of the multidisciplinary team, in which related glossary content will also be assessed for validity and completeness. Further module subtopics are under development, and these will be subject to equivalent review by the multidisciplinary team upon completion. The system's other resources (the resources directory, index of references, help files) will be implemented at the final stage, and evaluated for completeness, usefulness, and ease of use, again by members of the multidisciplinary team.

4. Summary

Current epidemiological research projects a rapid increase in the prevalence of diabetes in the next 10 years. The pressure on healthcare professionals to provide optimal care for existing and newly diagnosed patients in order to reduce the risks and costs associated with diabetes and its complications is therefore enormous, and increasing. As pressure increases on the specialist secondary care team, the responsibility for diabetes care in primary practice necessarily increases. The lack of standardised specialist training available to non-specialists in primary care, akin to that of the diabetes specialist nurse, reveals a need for self-paced continuing training which can be addressed by computer aided learning. The value of patient education in the improvement of self-care and reduction of risk is undisputed. An effective and cost-effective tool to supplement nurse-led patient education will help to reduce the pressure on practice nurses and will provide motivating and relevant educational material to patients.

The design and development of this computer-aided learning system for the education for patients and practice nurses has been partially implemented. Formative evaluation has been undertaken at various stages to ensure that the system satisfies diabetes experts and potential users. The iterative development process will continue until the final piloting of the finished system by our target community. The results of these final evaluations will be presented upon completion.

Acknowledgements

Emma-Jane Berridge was supported by a grant from the Economic and Social Research Council, UK.

References

[1] C.C. Jaffe, P.J. Lynch, Computer assisted instruction in radiology: opportunities for more effective learning, Am. J. Roentgenol. 164 (1995) 463–467.

[2] R.M. Rippey, D. Bill, M. Abeles, et al., Computer-based patient education for older persons with osteoarthritis, Arthritis Rheum. 30 (1987) 932–935.

[3] H. Birn, M. Horsted, A. Aarslev, L. Bjerregaard, Simple and time-saving computer programs for chairside assistants, J. Dent. Educ. 53 (1989) 577–580.

[4] E.C. Besa, L.Z. Nieman, R.R. Joseph, Interactive computer-based programs for a cancer learning center, J. Cancer Educ. 10 (1995) 137–140.

[5] J.K. Chambers, A.K. Frisby, Computer-based learning for end-stage renal disease (ESRD) patient education: current status and future directions, Adv. Renal Replace. Ther. 2 (1995) 234–245.

[6] R. Lo, B. Lo, E. Wells, M. Chard, J. Hathaway, The development and evaluation of a computer-aided diabetes education program, Aust. J. Adv. Nurs. 13 (1996) 19–27.

[7] J.L. Day, G. Rayman, L. Hall, P. Davies, Learning diabetes: a multimedia learning package for patients, carers and professionals to improve chronic disease management, Med. Inform. 22 (1997) 91–104.

[8] L.A. Wheeler, M.L. Wheeler, P. Ours, C. Swider, Evaluation of computer based diet education in persons with diabetes mellitus and limited educational background, Diabet. Care 8 (1985) 537–544.

[9] K. Premkumar, Development and evaluation of an evaluation tool for multimedia resources in health education, Int. J. Med. Inform. 50 (1998) 243–250.

[10] J. Cheek, Use with care: possibilities and constraints offered by computers in nursing clinical education, Int. J. Med. Inform. 50 (1998) 111–115.

[11] M.H. Khadra, A.I. Guinea, D.A. Hill, The acceptance of computer assisted learning by medical students, Aust. New Z. J. Surg. 65 (1995) 610–612.

[12] A. Demirjian, B. David, Learning medical and dental sciences through interactive multimedia, Med. Inform. 8 (1995) 1705.

[13] A.F. Amos, D.J. McCarty, P. Zimmet, The rising global burden of diabetes and its complications: estimates and projections to 2010, Diabet. Med. 14 (Suppl 5) (1997) S1–S85.

[14] B. Leese, The costs of diabetes and its complications, Soc. Sci. Med. 35 (1992) 1303–1310.

[15] S. Farrant, D. Dowlatshahi, M. Ellwood-Russell, P.H. Wise, Computer-based learning and assessment for diabetic patients, Diabet. Med. 1 (1984) 309–315.

[16] E.D. Lehmann, The diabetes control and complications trial (DCCT): a role for computers in patient education?, Diabet. Nutrit. Metab. 7 (1994) 308–316.

[17] H. King, W. Gruber, T. Lander (Eds.), Implementing National Diabetes Programmes: report of a World Health Organisation meeting, WHO, 1995.

[18] International Diabetes Federation Consultative Section on Diabetes Education, International Consensus Standards of Practice for Diabetes Education, Class, London, 1997.

[19] British Diabetic Association, Recommendations for the Management of Diabetes in General Practice, BDA, London, 1997.

[20] Royal College of Nursing, Diabetes Clinical Guidelines for Practice Nurses, RCN, London, 1994.

[21] P.H. Sönksen, C. Fox, S. Judd, Diabetes at your fingertips, Class, London, 1998.

[22] M. MacKinnon, Providing diabetes care in general practice, Class, London, 1998.

[23] Nutrition Subcommittee of the British Diabetic Association's Professional Advisory Committee, Dietary recommendations for people with diabetes; an update for the 1990s, Diabet. Med. 9 (1992) 189–202.

[24] British Diabetic Association, Recommendations for the management of diabetes in general practice, BDA, London, 1997.

[25] Microsoft Corporation, The windows interface: an application design guide, Microsoft, Redmond, Washington DC, 1992.

[26] B. Richards, A.W. Colman, R.A. Hollingsworth, The current and future role of the Internet in patient education, Int. J. Med. Inform. 50 (1998) 279–285.

[27] A.G. Sutcliffe, Human-Computer Interface Design, MacMillan, London, 1995.

[28] J.B. Krygier, C. Reeves, D. DiBiase, J. Cupp, Design, implementation and evaluation of multimedia resources for geography and earth science education, J. Geog. High. Educ. 21 (1997) 17–38.

[29] T. Reeves, Evaluating schools infused with technology, Educ. Urban Soc. 24 (1992) 519–534.

[30] R. Reiser, H. Kegelmann, Evaluating instructional software: a review and critique of current methods, Educ. Technol. Res. Dev. 42 (1994) 63–69.

A Virtual-Reality-Based Telerehabilitation System with Force Feedback

Viorel G. Popescu, *Student Member, IEEE*, Grigore C. Burdea, *Senior Member, IEEE*, Mourad Bouzit, *Member, IEEE*, and Vincent R. Hentz

Abstract—A PC-based orthopedic rehabilitation system was developed for use at home, while allowing remote monitoring from the clinic. The home rehabilitation station has a Pentium II PC with graphics accelerator, a Polhemus tracker, and a multipurpose haptic control interface. This novel interface is used to sample a patient's hand positions and to provide resistive forces using the Rutgers Master II (RMII) glove. A library of virtual rehabilitation routines was developed using WorldToolKit software. At the present time, it consists of three physical therapy exercises (DigiKey, ball, and power putty) and two functional rehabilitation exercises (peg board and ball game). These virtual reality exercises allow automatic and transparent patient data collection into an Oracle database. A remote Pentium II PC is connected with the home-based PC over the Internet and an additional video conferencing connection. The remote computer is running an Oracle server to maintain the patient database, monitor progress, and change the exercise level of difficulty. This allows for patient progress monitoring and repeat evaluations over time. The telerehabilitation system is in clinical trails at Stanford Medical School (CA), with progress being monitored from Rutgers University (NJ). Other haptic interfaces currently under development include devices for elbow and knee rehabilitation connected to the same system.

Index Terms—Client-server system, haptic feedback, orthopedic rehabilitation, telerehabilitation, virtual reality.

I. INTRODUCTION

THE RESEARCH planning report of the National Center for Medical Rehabilitation Research indicates that in 1993 there were approximately 40 million disabled Americans [14]. This staggering number includes people with restricted mobility, with reduced sensorial capacity, or with communication and intellectual deficits. The aging of the American population, coupled with the negative impact age has on disabilities (including recurrence of previously controlled conditions) has increased the number of disabled in recent years. Societal cost has similarly increased to $300 billion, according to a report of the Institute of Medicine [2]. The above cost does not account for the psychological impact on the disabled, their family, and the environment. While the number of patients needing rehabilitation (including long-term therapy) has increased, the resources available to them have unfortunately diminished, in part due to restrictions in managed healthcare agreements.

The reduction in the covered duration of therapy thus has a negative impact on the patient's condition and on the recovery process. The duration of the rehabilitation therapy is important, as is timeliness of treatment. Indeed, assessment and therapy have to occur early on, or else the same therapy duration will have diminished results. Timeliness and duration of rehabilitative therapy are problematic for those in remote rural locations or living in depressed urban areas. In such instances, generally there are no clinics in the vicinity of the patient's home. Avoiding travel to the clinic altogether would mean that adequate therapeutic intervention can be done at home, after an initial assessment at the clinic. However, therapists may not be able to travel to the patient's remote home or may be unwilling to do so.

The leading cause of activity limitations for Americans is orthopedic impairments. Such patients typically follow a regimen of combined clinic and home rehabilitation exercises. Home exercises are done on simple mechanical systems that are loaned to the patient or constructed for them. Since these mechanical devices are not networked, there is no way a therapist can either monitor a patient's progress or change exercise difficulty levels remotely. There is also no way to verify that the patient has actually done the prescribed home rehabilitation exercises. Therefore, there is a need for a home telerehabilitation system that will record data from a patient's rehabilitation routines and will allow the therapist to remotely monitor the patient's progress.

Historically, computer-based biomechanical evaluation tools were first used for monitoring the rehabilitation process. Greenleaf Medical developed "Eval" and "Orca" systems for orthopedic evaluation [9], [8]. The systems offer easy data collection and storage and tools for analyzing the patient information stored in the database. Other companies (Lafayette Instrument Company[1] and Electronic Healthcare Systems Inc.[2]) are offering software for patient monitoring and evaluation. Data is stored in custom databases and patient reports can be displayed. The systems described above were designed to be used in the clinic so that they do not include either a networking or a rehabilitation component. No forces are applied to the patient by these devices.

Prototype systems that do provide forces for manual therapy have been developed by Hogan at MIT [10], Luecke at Iowa State University [12], Takeda and Tsutsul at Nagasaki Institute Applied Science [24], and, more recently, Rovetta at the Milano Politechnic Institute [22]. All of these prototypes have certain advantages versus the clinical practice. For example, the MIT

Manuscript received July 7, 1999; revised September 8, 1999. This work was supported by the National Science Foundation under Grant BES-9708020 and by Rutgers University (CAIP Center Grant, and Special Research Opportunity Award).

V. G. Popescu, G. C. Burdea, and M. Bouzit are with the CAIP Center, Rutgers University, Piscataway, NJ 08854 USA.

V. R Hentz is with the Division of Hand Surgery, Department of Functional Restoration, Stanford Medical School, Stanford, CA 94304 USA.

Publisher Item Identifier S 1089-7771(00)02131-2.

[1][Online]. Available: http://www.licmef.com/assessme1.htm

[2][Online]. Available: http://dm3host.com/websites2/ehs/charttrad.html

system showed faster upper limb motor rehabilitation for stroke patients who exercised with a robot. The Iowa State system allowed independent force control for each finger, while the Nagasaki system was extremely light and powerful through the use of pneumatic "muscle" actuators. The Milano Politechnic system is portable (uses a laptop) and is intended for patients that need neuromotor rehabilitation (such as those with Parkinson's disease). However, all the systems cited above also have drawbacks, due mainly to their complexity (for example, the use of robot manipulators), making them difficult for use at home. In the case of the Milano Politechnic system, forces to only one finger are measured, and only one virtual finger is shown. Furthermore, there is no networking component in either of these systems, so that at-home monitored rehabilitation is not possible.

A virtual-reality(VR)-based system for hand rehabilitation was also developed by Burdea and colleagues [5], [6]. The system differs from the other prototypes mentioned above as it includes a diagnosis module (with standard diagnosis instruments), a rehabilitation module using VR simulations, and the Rutgers Master I haptic glove [3]. Proof of concept trials done with a small group of patients were promising, especially in regard to the subjective evaluation of the system by the patients. Problems remained due to the DataGlove technology used at the time for hand readings, as well as the slow graphics workstation used (Sun 10-Zx). This system, like the ones before, was not networked, as it was intended for clinic rather than at-home use.

An example of a system for computer-based patient monitoring and remote evaluation is the "electric house call" (EHC) [18] developed by researchers at the Georgia Institute of Technology in collaboration with the Medical College of Georgia and the Eisenhower Army Medical Center. Six at-home patient measurements were demonstrated, with data stored at the clinic using a client/server database architecture. In the area of home rehabilitation, Ward and Bullinger recently patented a system where a remote clinician can monitor and set the range of motion of body joints through a "dual-plane joint monitor" [26]. There is no VR component to their proposed system and no forces are measured or applied by the patented apparatus.

This paper describes another client/server telemedicine application in orthopedic rehabilitation. This telerehabilitation system contains a PC workstation, a novel multipurpose haptic control interface, the Rutgers Master II (RMII) force feedback glove, a microphone array for hands-free voice input, and videoconferencing hardware. The system is in clinical trials at Stanford Medical School (client site), with rehabilitation progress being monitored from Rutgers University (server site). Section II describes the telerehabilitation system hardware. Section III presents the VR rehabilitation library of exercises. The deformation and haptic rendering models are detailed in Section IV. Section V describes the patient database, the client/server architecture, and the network system setup. Concluding remarks are given in Section VI.

II. TELEREHABILITATION SYSTEM HARDWARE

The prototype of the home orthopedic rehabilitation system is shown in Fig. 1(a) [20]. It consists of a Powerdigm Pentium II PC equipped with an InsideTrack 3-D tracker [19], a FireGL

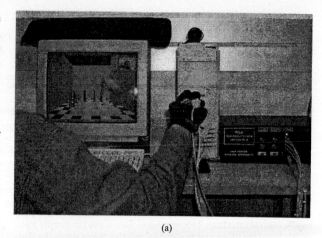

(a)

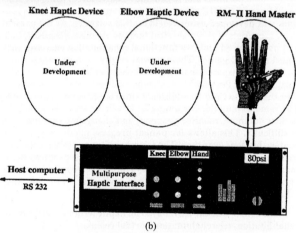

(b)

Fig. 1. Telerehabilitation workstation. (a) Experimental prototype. (b) The RMII connected to the MHCI [20].

4000 graphics accelerator, a custom microphone array, and a net camera. The Pentium PC is connected to a novel multipurpose haptic control interface (MHCI) which can drive several rehabilitation haptic interfaces (for the hand, elbow, and knee). The MHCI is a redesigned version of the RM-II Smart Controller Interface, with a new haptic control loop, an upgraded imbedded PC, and multiplexing capabilities. It can switch between the hand, elbow, and knee haptic devices seamlessly, as required by the VR exercise routine to be executed. The system is self-configurable, depending on the patient's needs, without any hardware changes (connect, disconnect, etc.).

Currently the system is used with the RM-II haptic glove while the elbow and knee units are under development. As shown in Fig. 1(b), the RM-II glove is an exoskeletal structure that provides forces at the patient's fingertips and contains its own noncontact position sensors [7]. Thus, the system is simplified (no need for a separate sensing glove) and light (about 100 g). The feedback actuators have glass/graphite structures with very low static friction. The combination of high, sustained feedback forces (16 N at each fingertip) and low friction provides high dynamic range (300). This makes the RM-II capable of high sensitivity and resolution in the feedback forces it can produce. The pistons have protective metallic

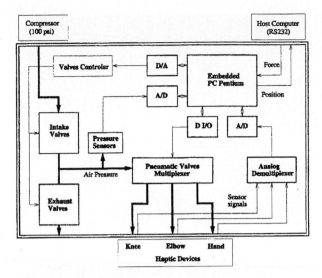

Fig. 2.   The multipurpose haptic control interface.

caps at the top to prevent overextending patients' fingers. The patient–RM-II device interaction benefits from air compliance which augments patient's safety. Additional safety features are included in the software exercises, allowing patients to shut off the system in case of emergency. The InsideTrak measures the patient's wrist position 60 times/s, while the RM-II provides 187 finger position updates/s.

The internal view of the prototype multipurpose haptic control interface is shown in Fig. 2. It consists of high-bandwidth pneumatic valves, a pneumatic multiplexer, an embedded Pentium board, several other electronic boards, and a power supply. The pneumatic valves were carefully selected for their response time and air flow in order to maximize the haptic device bandwidth. The solenoid valves operate at a frequency of 500 Hz with a flow of 200 Nl/min and an opening (or closing) response time of less than 2 ms. The MHCI pressure regulator was built with two of these fast valves, one each for exhaust and intake. The embedded Pentium (100 MHz) controls the valves using pulsewidth modulation (PWM) based on feedback from pressure sensors installed on the valve output pipes. Experimental results showed that the resulting closed-loop control assures a precise and stable output pressure control with a mechanical feedback bandwidth of 10–20 Hz [17]. This is approximately four times larger than the corresponding bandwidth of the off-the-shelf Buzmatics controller used in the previous RM-II electronics interfaces. Additionally, the real-time software running on the embedded Pentium reads and filters data from the RM-II sensors through an analog demultiplexer and A/D board and transforms it into the patient's joint angles. The transformation needs user calibration data transferred during the initial calibration stage of the rehabilitation routines.

The communication between the MHCI and the host is through a standard RS232 serial port, which brings total hardware independence (the system was tested on a SGI Infinite Reality, on a Sun Ultra 60, and on several Pentium PC's). Data sent to the host contain joint angles, measured forces, or device state, while received data from the host include commands or forces to be displayed to the patient. At a rate of 57 500 bit/s,

the RS232 line can transmit up to 187 RM-II position data sets/s or 166 data sets that contain both position and finger force readings every second.

A microphone array [11] provides hands-free voice input by focusing on the patient's head siting approximately 3 ft in front of the monitor. Additionally, a net color camera connected to the PC parallel port is used for teleconferencing with the clinic. It can provide up to 15 fps QCIF images when running on a local machine.

III. The Virtual Reality Exercise Library

The high-level software used by the telerehabilitation system has three components: the VR exercises routines, the database of patients' files, and the networking component. The rehabilitation exercises were developed using the commercial World-ToolKit graphics library [23], with a simple virtual environment in order to keep the patient focused. All exercises contain a high-resolution virtual hand from Viewpoint DataLabs [25] and several objects (DigiKey, peg board, rubber ball, power putty) created with AutoCAD [1] or WTK Modeler.

Several hand gestures allow patients to interact with the virtual objects: whole-hand grasping, two-finger grasping (lateral pinch), selecting (pointing), and releasing. Contact detection between hand segments and the objects triggers a grasping gesture. Objects stay "attached" to the virtual hand until a release gesture is executed by the patient. The "select" gesture is executed with the index finger touching a virtual object. This gesture is used only at the beginning of each exercise to interactively set the rehabilitation routine level of difficulty and object stiffness.

The rehabilitation routines are broadly classified into two categories: physical therapy (PT) and functional rehabilitation. PT exercises use force feedback to improve the patient's motor skills (exercise muscles and joints). Functional rehabilitation is done to regain lost skills (such as those needed in activities of daily living or job-related skills). Functional rehabilitation exercises, therefore, have much greater diversity and their output depends on each exercise design. The essential feature of these exercises is the patient's interactivity with the VE. Each therapy exercise has several levels of difficulty corresponding to the maximum force that can be applied, the time allowed, and other parameters.

The first PT exercise models a rubber ball squeezing routine, as illustrated in Fig. 3(a). The ball stiffness is color-coded and can be selected by the patient at the beginning of the exercise. Ball dynamics simulate gravity and Newtonian laws. Once it is grasped, the ball deforms in contact with the virtual hand while force feedback is displayed to the patient and recorded in the database. The exercise terminates when either the patient presses an exit key or the allowed time was exhausted. The second PT exercise implements a virtual version of the DigiKey [15], which is an individual finger exerciser, illustrated in Fig. 3(b), [5]. The model was modified to include the thumb instead of the pinky due to the RM-II kinematics configuration. The DigiKey maximum force levels were color-coded to match the commercially available set. After grasping the selected DigiKey, contact detection is checked between fingers and the corresponding cylinder ends; while in contact, the virtual cylinders are driven by the patient's finger movements. Forces proportional to the displacement of

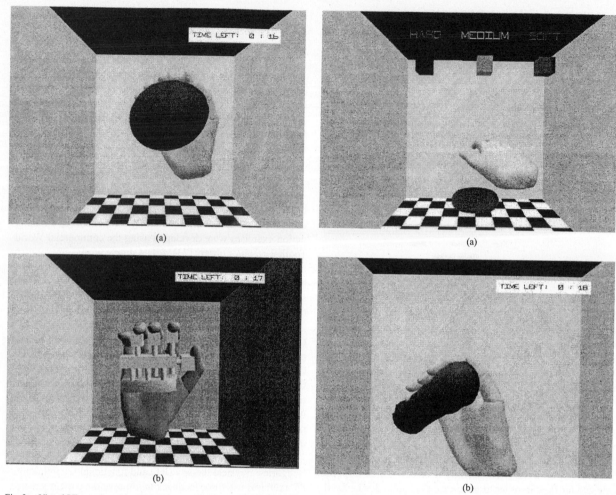

Fig. 3. Virtual PT exercises: (a) rubber ball squeezing and (b) DigiKey model (adapted from [5]).

Fig. 4. Virtual power putty molding PT exercise. (a) Putty selection. (b) Full grip. [21] © IEEE.

the DigiKey cylinders are fed back to the patient and stored transparently and simultaneously in the database.

The third PT exercise is a molding of virtual "power putty," as illustrated in Fig. 4(a) and (b). The patient selects either an ellipsoid or sphere unmolded putty shape, each with three selectable hardness levels. The ellipsoidal premolded putty is used for full grip, fingers only, thumb press only, or wrist rotation exercises. The spherical premolded putty is used for finger pinch, where the putty is squeezed between the thumb and fingers. A "reshape" button allows the patient to reset the putty to its premolded shape before repeating the exercise.

The first functional rehabilitation exercise is a peg board insertion task, illustrated in Fig. 5(a) [5]. The simulation uses a virtual peg board with nine holes and a corresponding number of pegs. The exercise has three levels of difficulty: "novice," "intermediate," and "expert," each with a different clearance between the peg and hole (smallest for the "expert" level). The amount of time allowed to complete the exercise is set by the therapist. Visual and auditory cues increase the simulation realism and help the patient overcome visual distortions. Pegs are grasped with a lateral pinch gesture and change color when in a correct insertion position. Exercise results are stored in the form of number

of holes filled, time spent to perform the exercise, and number of errors made (missed hole or an attempt to put two pegs in one hole). The second functional rehabilitation exercise is the ball game shown in Fig. 5(b). The patient has to throw the ball so that it hits the target wall above a marked area. When the ball bounces back, the patient has to catch it after at most one bounce off the ground. The ball speed parameter ("fast" or "slow" ball) is selected at the beginning of the exercise. Any correct catch increases the patient "catch" counter, while a miss will increase the "miss" counter. The ball deforms when caught by the patient and loses energy while bouncing. This exercise is useful to train feedforward ballistic-type movements and hand–eye coordination. Throwing and catching movements help improve accuracy and speed control.

IV. DEFORMATION AND HAPTIC RENDERING MODELS

Virtual objects which correspond to real rehabilitation devices deform when grasped by the patient, as described above. The deformation model uses the displacement vector of the mesh points (see [4] for a review of physical deformation methods). The method is simple, can be executed in real time, and fits well

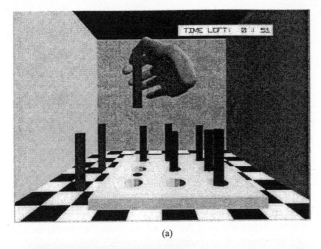

(a)

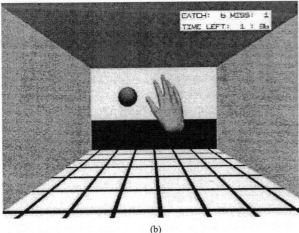

(b)

Fig. 5. Functional rehabilitation exercises. (a) Peg board (adapted from [5]). (b) Ball game. [21] © IEEE.

with the haptic rendering approach described below. The model allows for both elastic as well as plastic deformations. The elastic deformation model uses a nondeformed reference object, while the plastic deformation model updates the reference object after each simulation frame. The elastic deformation is modeled as a superposition of a global and a local deformation. The global deformation model uses a morphing technique. The position, normal, and color of all object vertices are interpolated linearly between a normal state (corresponding to an opened hand) and a maximum deformation state (corresponding to fully closed hand). The interpolation parameter α is the normalized mean of finger joint angles

$$\alpha = \sum_{i=0}^{\text{joints \#}} \theta_i \Big/ \sum_{i=0}^{\text{joints \#}} \theta_{i\,\text{max}}. \quad (1)$$

The local deformation model is controlled by a 3×3 mesh of points placed on the surface of the fingertip. Contact distances are calculated between these points and the closest vertices of the intersecting object surface within a certain radius of influence. The radius of influence is typically the size of the largest dimension of the fingertip bounding box. The penetration distance relative to the reference object is weighted with a second

degree polynomial

$$D = k * u$$
$$\cdot \left(\langle \vec{P}_{\text{surface point}} - \vec{P}_{\text{fingertip}}, \vec{N}_{\text{surface point}} \rangle \right),$$

where

$$k = 1 - (d/\text{radius of influence})^2 ,$$
$$d = \left\| \vec{P}_{\text{fingertip}} - \vec{P}_{\text{surface point}} \right\| \quad (2)$$

and $u(\ )$ is the unity step function (deformations are calculated only for positive penetration distances). The deformations from different points of the haptic interaction mesh are not summed up but a maximum value is calculated to obtain vertex displacement.

The haptic control loop in the MHCI runs at a much higher rate (500 Hz) than the graphics refresh rate (currently set at 20 fps in this application). Two models were used to implement the haptic control loop. In the first case used for DigiKey, peg board, and ball game exercises, the haptic rendering loop runs entirely on the MHCI, and the host PC only commands the beginning and the end of haptic feedback. Haptic interaction parameters (spring, friction, and dumping constants + intervals where the model applies) are transmitted by the host when the force feedback loop is activated. Forces are calculated locally on the MHCI using Hooke's deformation law. More complex deformation models can be implemented using dumping and friction parameters. This local model works well for grasping objects with a simple shape.

In the second case for ball and power putty exercises, the haptic rendering model resides entirely on the PC workstation. Here the PC host calculates and sends 20 force targets per second (synchronized with the graphics loop) to be displayed by the MHCI to patient fingers. The forces are based on the displacement vector calculated for the deformation model. The force vector is determined by the formula

$$\mathbf{F} = k_{\text{stiffness}} * u$$
$$\cdot \left(\langle \vec{P}_{\text{surface point}} - \vec{P}_{\text{fingertip}}, \vec{N}_{\text{surface point}} \rangle \right). \quad (3)$$

V. The Clinical Database and Client/Server Architecture

Patient data is stored during the therapeutic exercises and organized in several tables: patient table (personal data), index table (exercise index, type and date), and exercise tables. The database Graphical User Interface (GUI) was designed using Oracle Forms, Reports, and Graphics [16]. The patient entry form provides the graphical interface to input data, query, update, browse, or delete records. The exercise form displays a listing of sessions of specified type performed by the patient.

"Raw data" corresponding to the forces exerted by the patient's fingers are displayed when pressing the "show" button. Fig. 6(a) is a sample graph for the thumb forces during a DigiKey exercise [20]. Finger forces "raw data" is, however, of little use to the clinician. These data are therefore processed in order to extract meaningful information for patient remote assessment. The finger force mean, standard deviation, and effort (force integral) for each session are computed and displayed. A time history of these parameters over several rehabilitation sessions is subsequently created, as shown in Fig. 6(b). The graph shows a target (goal) parameter, which is set by the therapist. The patient

THUMB

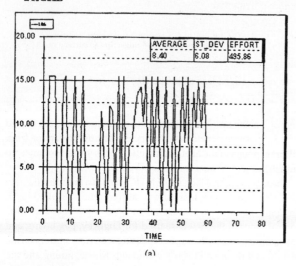

(a)

THUMB

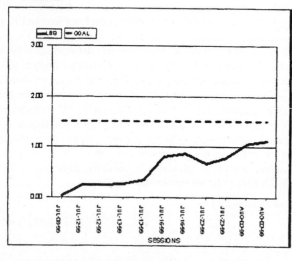

(b)

Fig. 6. Clinical database. (a) Graph containing "raw data" for a given session. (b) A patient's progress history versus the set goal [20].

has to achieve this goal over a specified number of sessions, if the rehabilitation therapy is effective when implemented at home. This goal can be remotely modified by the clinician after assessing patient progress in order to fine tune the treatment to a particular patient's speed of recovery.

The above database is stored at the server side (clinic), as illustrated in Fig. 7 [20]. The therapist has remote access to the patient's exercise routines without having to travel to the patient's home. After looking at the graphs, the therapist can also judge whether the routine was performed in a satisfactory fashion or not. A client server networking component has a menu style GUI developed on a WinNT platform. The database update module written using ProC transfers data from VR rehabilitation exercises into the clinic database. The asynchronous transfer uses a TCP/IP connection and transfers local files stored subsequent to each exercise routine. The data file transferred contains exercise type, patient ID, execution time, and exercise raw data.

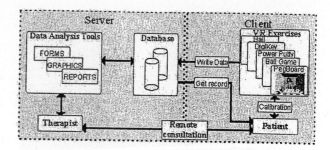

Fig. 7. Telerehabilitation system software architecture [20].

The client site (the patient's home) is running the real-time VR exercises previously described. While wearing the rehabilitation haptic devices, the patient controls the system using voice commands. The speech interface uses a Microsoft speech recognition engine [13], with a small grammar implemented for our application. Care has to be taken when programming all software components to share a single processor machine. The VR exercises thus run with higher priority to allow a maximum graphics frame rate. Videoconferencing tools installed at the server and client sites use CuSeeMe videoconferencing software [27]. The graphical interface thus allows a patient to start VR exercises and open a video channel for consultation with the therapist; it also includes documentation in the form of help and mpeg tutorial movies for correct execution of the rehabilitation routines. During several teleconferencing system trials, we obtained uneven performances, in some cases with only 2–3 frames/s. Internet2 became available for the project in late 1999 and allowed about 10 frames/s.

The quality of network services is very important for the system reliability and performance. Several parameters affect the network services: data file size, time to transfer, and failure rate. The amount of data collected from the exercise depends on its type and duration. For physical therapy exercises, we are recording forces applied by the patient at a sampling rate of five reads/s. For a 1-min exercise, that means about 10 kbit of data. Functional rehabilitation exercises need only tens of bytes to be transferred to the database. Transfer time and failure rates need to be measured experimentally. A recovering procedure was designed to prevent patient data loss. Failures are recorded in a log and transfer is reinitiated for each failure. The client server communication was tested in a LAN before the actual start of clinical trials. The average time for data transfer and failure rate were measured in an experiment with 1000 database updates over the LAN. It took an average of 2.01 s for a DigiKey exercise to be stored in the remote database. There were no failures over these 1000 database updates. Networking data collected so far from the experiment involving Stanford University and Rutgers University sites showed an average transfer time of 30 s for the DigiKey exercise and 4 s for PegBoard.

VI. CONCLUSION AND FUTURE RESEARCH

A PC-based telerehabilitation system using virtual reality and force feedback interfaces was developed for home use. The haptic hardware used to apply forces on the patient's body includes a novel multipurpose haptic control interface and the RM-II glove.

A library of VR exercises was modeled after standard rehabilitation routines. This simulation library contains both physical therapy and functional rehabilitation routines. Data collected during the exercises is stored remotely at the server site (clinic) using the Internet. Here the therapist can analyze it, evaluate the patient's progress, and modify VR exercise parameters or rehabilitation goals over the network. Remote consultation is supported using a videoconferencing system.

Developing new haptic devices for rehabilitation is an ongoing research effort in our laboratory. Elbow, knee, and ankle interfaces are currently being designed and built for control by the same multipurpose haptic control interface hardware. Elbow and knee units are one-degree-of-freedom systems using symmetrically mounted pneumatic actuators to oppose flexion extension motion. The Rutgers ankle interface uses a Stewart platform with six double acting pneumatic actuators. Clinical trials with the telerehabilitation system described here are underway at Stanford Medical School.

The system is currently being extended to include several client sites (patient homes with rehabilitation workstations) and a central server clinic. This configuration, called multiplexed telerehabilitation, should allow the testing of the full potential of telerehabilitation technology. Additional issues of patient identification, data security, and remote consultation multiplexing have to be addressed. A new web-based distributed architecture for the multiplexed telerehabilitation system is under development. This innovative design assumes fast speed networks (Internet2) and takes advantage of newly developed Internet technologies (Java3D) to create a distributed system (database, multimedia, VR exercises) which resides entirely on the web.

REFERENCES

[1] *AutoCAD User's Manual*, Sausalito, CA, 1994.
[2] E. Brandt and A. Pope, Eds., *Enabling America*. Washington, DC: National Academy Press, 1997.
[3] G. Burdea, N. Langrana, E. Roskos, D. Silver, and J. Zhuang, "A portable dextrous master with force feedback," *Presence*, vol. 1, no. 1, pp. 18–28, 1992.
[4] G. Burdea, *Force and Touch Feedback for Virtual Reality*. New York, NY: Wiley, 1996.
[5] G. Burdea, S. Deshpande, V. Popescu, N. Langrana, D. Gomez, D. DiPaolo, and M. Kanter, "Computerized hand diagnostic/rehabilitation system using a force feedback glove," in *Proc. MMVR 5*, 1997, pp. 141–150.
[6] G. Burdea, S. Deshpande, B. Liu, N. Langrana, and D. Gomez, "A Virtual reality-based system for hand diagnosis and rehabilitation," *Presence*, vol. 6, no. 2, pp. 229–240, 1997.
[7] D. Gomez, G. Burdea, and N. Langrana, "Integration of the Rutgers Master II in a Virtual Reality Simulation," in *Proc. VRAIS'95*, 1995, pp. 198–202.
[8] Greenleaf Medical Systems, Business Overview. (1997), Palo Alto, CA. [Online]http://www.greenleafmed.com/Products/pointofcare.html
[9] S. Fox, "EVAL-revolutionizing hand exams," *ADVANCE for Occupational Therapists*, vol. 7, no. 3, pp. 7–7, 1991.
[10] H. Krebs, N. Hogan, M. Aisen, and B. Volpe, "Application of robotics and automation technology in neuro-rehabilitation," in *Japan-USA Symposium on Flexible Automation*, vol. 1, NY, 1996, pp. 269–275.
[11] Q. Lin, C.-W. Che, D.-S. Yuk, and J. Flanagan, "Robust distant talking speech recognition," in *Proc. ICASSP'96*, Atlanta, GA, 1996, pp. 21–24.
[12] G. Luecke, Y. Chai, J. Winkler, and J. Edwards, "An exoskeleton manipulator for application of electro-magnetic virtual forces," in *Proc. ASME WAM*, vol. DSC-58, 1996, pp. 489–494.
[13] Microsoft Corp, "Whisper Speech Recognizer,", http://research.microsoft.com/msrinfo/demodwnf.htm, 1998.
[14] National Center for Medical Rehabilitation Research, "Research plan for the national center for medical rehabilitation research,", NIH Publication no. 93-3509, 1993.
[15] North Coast Medical Inc., "Digi-Key,", San Jose, CA, 1994.
[16] *Oracle User's Manual*, Redwood City, CA, 1995.
[17] G. Patounakis, M. Bouzit, and G. Burdea, "Study of the electromechanical bandwidth of the rutgers master," Rutgers University, Tech. Rep. CAIP-TR-225, May 22, 1998.
[18] J. Peifer, A. Hooper, and B. Sudduth, "A patient-centric approach to telemedicine database development," in *Proc. MMVR 6*. Amsterdam: IOS Press, 1998, pp. 67–73.
[19] *Fastrak User's Manual*, McDonnell Douglas Electronics Co., Colchester, VT, 1993.
[20] V. Popescu, G. Burdea, M. Bouzit, M. Girone, and V. Hentz, "PC-based telerehabilitation system with force feedback," in *Proc. MMVR 7*. Amsterdam, 1999, pp. 261–267.
[21] V. Popescu, G. Burdea, and M. Bouzit, "Virtual reality modeling for a haptic glove," in *Proc. Computer Animation '99*, Geneva, Switzerland, 1999, pp. 195–200.
[22] A. Rovetta, F. Lorini, and M. Canina, "A new project for rehabilitation and psychomotor disease analysis with virtual reality support," in *Proc. MMVR 6*. Amsterdam, 1998, pp. 180–185.
[23] *WorldToolKit User's Manual*, Sausalito, CA, 1994.
[24] T. Takeda and Y. Tsutsul, "Development of a virtual training environment," in *Advances in Robotics, Mechatronics, and Haptic Interfaces, Proc. ASME WAM*, vol. DSC-49, 1993, pp. 1–10.
[25] *Viewpoint Catalog*, 3rd ed., Orem, UT, 1994.
[26] F. Ward and M. Bullinger, "Joint monitor," U.S. Patent 5 754 121, May 19, 1998.
[27] *CuSeeMe User Guide*, Nashua, NH, 1997.

Viorel G. Popescu (S'93) received the B.S. and M.S. degrees from the University "Politechnica" of Bucarest in 1993. He is currently working toward the Ph.D. degree at the Electrical and Computer Engineering Department, Rutgers University, New Brunswick, NJ.

His research involves haptic display systems and medical application of virtual reality.

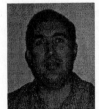

Grigore C. Burdea (S'87–M'87–SM'90) received the Ph.D. degree from New York University, New York, NY, in 1987.

He is presently an Associate Professor of Computer Engineering at Rutgers University, New Brunswick, NJ. He has authored the books *Virtual Reality Technology* (New York: Wiley, 1994) and *Force and Touch Feedback for Virtual Reality* (New York: Wiley, 1996) and co-edited the book *Computer-Aided Surgery* (Cambridge, MA: MIT Press, 1996).

Dr. Burdea will chair the upcoming IEEE Virtual Reality 2000 Conference.

Mourad Bouzit (M'99) received the Ph.D. degree in robotics and computer science from the University of Paris VI, Paris, France, in 1996.

He is presently a Post-Doctoral Fellow at the Center for Advanced Information Processing, Rutgers University, Piscataway, NJ. His research topics include teleoperation, dextrous telemanipulation, artificial hand and force feedback systems for virtual reality applications. He prototyped the LRP Master, the first French force feedback data glove for virtual reality.

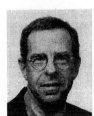

Vincent R. Hentz received the M.D. degree from the University of Florida, Gainesville, in 1968.

He is presently Professor of Functional Restoration at Stanford University School of Medicine, Stanford, CA. He has authored four books and 25 book chaptersl

Dr. Hentz is currently President of the American Society for Surgery of the Hand.

Impact of a Computer-assisted Education Program on Factors Related to Asthma Self-management Behavior

Ross Shegog, PhD, L. Kay Bartholomew, EdD, MPH, Guy S. Parcel, PhD,
Marianna M. Sockrider, MD, DrPH, Louise Mâsse, PhD,
Stuart L. Abramson, MD, PhD

Abstract **Objective**: To evaluate *Watch, Discover, Think and Act* (WDTA), a theory-based application of CD-ROM educational technology for pediatric asthma self-management education.

Design: A prospective pretest posttest randomized intervention trial was used to assess the motivational appeal of the computer-assisted instructional program and evaluate the impact of the program in eliciting change in knowledge, self-efficacy, and attributions of children with asthma. Subjects were recruited from large urban asthma clinics, community clinics, and schools. Seventy-six children 9 to 13 years old were recruited for the evaluation.

Results: Repeated-measures analysis of covariance showed that knowledge scores increased significantly for both groups, but no between-group differences were found ($P = 0.55$); children using the program scored significantly higher ($P < 0.01$) on questions about steps of self-regulation, prevention strategies, and treatment strategies. These children also demonstrated greater self-efficacy ($P < 0.05$) and more efficacy building attribution classification of asthma self-management behaviors ($P < 0.05$) than those children who did not use the program.

Conclusion: The WDTA is an intrinsically motivating educational program that has the ability to effect determinants of asthma self-management behavior in 9- to 13-year-old children with asthma. This, coupled with its reported effectiveness in enhancing patient outcomes in clinical settings, indicates that this program has application in pediatric asthma education.

■ **J Am Med Inform Assoc.** 2001;8:49–61.

Affiliations of the authors: Baylor College of Medicine (RS, MMS, SLA) and University of Texas-Houston Health Science Center (LKB, GSP, LM), Houston, Texas.

This work was supported in part by National Institutes of Health contract N01 H039220 from the National Heart, Lung, and Blood Institute and by the Texas Children's Hospital, Children's Asthma Center.

Correspondence and reprints: Ross Shegog, PhD, Allergy and Immunology, Abercrombie Suite 380, Texas Children's Hospital, 6621 Fannin Street, MC 1-3291, Houston, TX 77030-2399; e-mail: <rshegog@sph.uth.tmc.edu>.

Received for publication: 12/6/99; accepted for publication: 8/30/00.

Background

This paper describes an evaluation of the impact of *Watch, Discover, Think and Act* (WDTA), a computer-based educational program designed to teach asthma self-management skills to urban, minority children.[1–3] The impact evaluation assesses the program's immediate effect on knowledge, self-efficacy, and attributions, which are variables related to the target behavior of self-management. It also examines the motivational aspects of the program on children who use it.

Asthma Self-management

Asthma is among the most common chronic diseases in the United States, and its medical and social consequences are more severe in inner-city populations.[4] Asthma is characterized by chronic inflammation of the airways that leads to episodes of bronchospasm and excess mucus production. It has a high prevalence (about 5 percent of children under 18 years old) and contributes significantly to school absenteeism.[5–7] Asthma morbidity and mortality rates have increased substantially among children since 1980, and the asthma death rate among children 5 to 14 years old rose from 1.7 to 3.2 per million between 1980 and 1993.[8] Asthma morbidity, mortality, and hospitalization rates have been disproportionately high among the poor and medically underserved. African American and Hispanic children in the inner cities have been reported to be more likely to have asthma than white children. The annual prevalence of asthma among children living in inner cities is 1.5 to 2 times higher than that of the U.S. population as a whole.[9–12]

Asthma requires constant self-management by the patient to maintain control of symptoms, prevent exacerbations, attain normal lung function, and maintain normal activity levels. Self-management refers to the behaviors that people with asthma and their family members perform to lessen the impact of this chronic illness (Table 1). Self-management includes adherence to medical regimens as well as the complex cognitive-behavioral tasks of self-monitoring, decision making, and communicating about both symptoms and treatment regimens.[13–15] Determinants of asthma self-management behavior include a person's behavioral capability for management behaviors[16–18] and degree of self-efficacy in performing those behaviors.[13,17–19] Attribution has also been implicated in children's self-management behaviors and in control of asthma and other diseases.[20–22]

Computer-based Patient Education

Computers have diverse uses in health promotion and disease prevention—for example, as tools for education on AIDS and responsible sexuality and as adjuncts to medical therapy for alcohol rehabilitation and rheumatoid arthritis.[23–26] The use of virtual fantasy worlds, such as the Starbright Pediatric Network for pediatric inpatients, has been shown to reduce dependence on medications and to enhance pain management.[27] The Health Touch database system has been shown to facilitate physician–patient interaction in primary care practice.[28] Furthermore, empirical research has identified the value of using computers to provide behavior-change messages tailored to client belief characteristics, such as stage of change and health beliefs, and to demographic characteristics, such as gender and ethnicity.[29]

Several computer-based applications have been developed to assist in asthma management and education. For adult asthma patients, computer-assisted instruc-

Table 1 ■

Asthma Self-management

Monitor:

- Monitor symptoms of asthma "directly" and compare with personal standard. Use object measures (e.g, peak flow meter) to monitor and compare symptoms with personal standard.

- Monitor for personal environmental triggers

- Monitor asthma self-management efforts and compare with personal standard

Identify problems:

- Using monitoring (as described above), identify when a problem exists.

Implement solutions:

- Keep regular appointments with health care providers.

- Refer to asthma action plan.

- Maintain medication for chronic condition as prescribed.

- Maintain "normal" exercise levels.

- On the basis of symptoms or the environment, make medication adjustments, including administration of rescue medication, as prescribed.

- Avoid or remove asthma triggers.

- Call health care professional in an acute situation.

- Communicate with family members and with health care providers.

Evaluate:

- Evaluate success of actions and return to monitoring.

tion (CAI) has been used to help them monitor and avoid house dust-mite allergen.[30] Several CAI programs have been developed for children with asthma. These include Clubhouse Asthma,[31] Bronkie the Bronchiasaurus,[32] Wee Willie Wheezie,[33] Air Academy: The Quest for Airtopia,[34] and Asthma Command.[35] Bronkie the Bronchiasaurus has been shown to positively affect knowledge, self-efficacy, and communication about asthma in children who use it.[36] Airtopia has been shown to positively affect asthma knowledge in children when used in the context of a general health curriculum.[34] Asthma Command has been evaluated in clinic settings where children who used the program showed increases in knowledge and in self-reported asthma management, compared with children in the control group.[35] There were no demonstrated differences in visits to physicians, emergency rooms, or hospitals.

Although these trends are encouraging, there remains a need for programs that can be tailored to the asthma characteristics of the individual child and that can help patient and families learn self-management skills. We describe here such a program, WDTA, a second-generation asthma CAI program that has been rigorously evaluated.[3]

Watch, Discover, Think and Act Computer-assisted Instruction

The WDTA computer-based education program has taken a motivational approach to teaching asthma self-management skills to urban, minority children.[1-3] The program is a multimedia application that uses three types of computer-based instructional strategies—a simulation of real-world activities in which the child can learn and practice self-regulatory processes; tutorials with which the child can learn and practice asthma-specific skills; and a game treatment to enhance motivation. The broad objectives of the program are to provide asthma self-management skills training as an adjunct to medical care and enhance clinical care provided for the asthma patient by supplying information to health care providers and parents regarding the child's asthma self-management capabilities and progress.

The program specifically targets change in factors that may be determinants of this self-management. The program was developed using social cognitive theory change methods to improve the child's knowledge, self-efficacy, and attributions.[37] These methods include verbal reinforcement, guided practice with feedback, persuasion, goal setting, incentives, and symbolic modeling. The program addresses the need

to individualize asthma education and to teach self-regulatory skills, components of what Creer et al.[38] refer to as a second generation of asthma self-management programs.[38]

Overview of the Game Procedure and Graphical User Interface

Watch, Discover, Think and Act is an interactive multimedia computer program for providing intensive, tailored self-management education to inner-city children, of upper elementary and middle school ages, who have asthma. Designed for use in primary care clinics and physician's offices, it gives these children the opportunity—in a safe, non-threatening, even fun, computer environment—to learn how to manage their asthma .

Originally developed on CD-ROM for the Apple platform, using MacroMind Director 5.0 authoring software,[39] WDTA makes use of text, graphics, animation, sound, and video clips.

The program comprises four stages—data input, introduction, game scenarios, and data output. The first use of the program occurs after the encounter with the physician. A clinic staff member helps the child with data input, using the keyboard and mouse to provide information about the child's physician and about the child, such as name, age, and duration of asthma. Information on personal asthma symptoms and environmental triggers, medications, and peak flow make up the child's asthma profile.

Once this information has been entered, the child self-navigates through the program using the mouse. During the introduction stage, the child chooses a character and a coach. The character represents a child approximately 12 years old who has asthma. The child can choose whether the character and coach are male or female and can choose between African American and Hispanic ethnicity. The coach is a teenager, slightly older than the target population for the game, who has learned to manage asthma.

The child is given an overview of the game, which involves a mission to rescue plans for anti-pollution technology from the castle of Dr. Foulair. The goal of the game is to move the character through three real-life scenarios with multiple scenes (home, school, and neighborhood) and then to Dr. Foulair's castle. To progress from one scenario to the next, the child must successfully manage the character's asthma by following the four self-regulation steps of watching (monitoring symptoms and environmental triggers, taking maintenance or preventive medication, and keeping

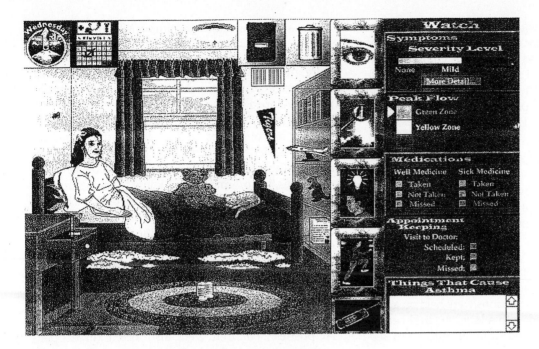

Figure 1 Watch, Discover, Think and Act computer game screen.

appointments), discovering (deciding whether an asthma problem exists and what its probable cause is), thinking (deciding on a list of possible actions), and acting (choosing an action such as taking rescue or symptom relief medicine, removing or avoiding triggers, getting help). The child must also collect mission handbook pages to complete tutorials on asthma and click and drag tools to be used in the castle.

The game scenarios include 18 real-world and 4 castle situations that present the problems that inner-city children with asthma must deal with successfully to manage their disease. The game screen shown in Figure 1 shows one of the scenario scenes containing environmental asthma triggers (dust, fur, and feathers), tools (the peak flow meter in the table drawer), and mission handbook tutorial pages (on the bookshelf). Tutorial components contain information developed de novo as well as components drawn from National Institutes of Health source material.[40,41] In the tutorials, video segments depicting medicine-taking procedures were obtained by permission to use pre-existing educational materials.[42]

In Figure 1, four self-regulatory icons for WDTA are vertically aligned to the right of the scene, near the center of the screen. Below these, a fifth icon represents a cellular phone with which to contact the coach. The health status boxes on the far right of the screen show the character's symptoms, peak flow, medication taking, appointment scheduling, and personal triggers; they appear during the "watch" step of the asthma self-management process. The WDTA pro-

gram tracks each child's progress so that children can resume the game where they left off on a previous visit.

The data output stage provides information for the child, the parents, and the health care provider. Players receive constant feedback from the game as to their progress, and at the end of each session children receive a certificate that congratulates them on the progress made and reiterates the four steps of self-regulation. To guide further asthma education, the parents and physician receive a progress report that indicates the scenario the child reached, the child's use of the self-regulation steps, and tutorial scores.

METHODS

Design and Sample

A prospective pretest posttest trial with randomly assigned intervention and comparison subjects was used for the study. The WDTA program was evaluated in terms of its effect on cognitive impact variables of knowledge, self-efficacy, and attribution; factors associated with successful asthma management. The hypothesis was that children using the intervention would experience improvement in these cognitive variables. A sample of 76 children was recruited from six clinics and seven schools in a large urban area.

Five subjects were lost to posttesting because of lack of availability for follow-up ($n = 4$) and refusal to participate further ($n = 1$). The resulting study sample comprised 71 children who were 8 to 13 years old and had been diagnosed as having asthma by their health care providers. The mean age of subjects in the study was 10.7 years. Forty-six boys and 25 girls completed the posttest. Based on subject self-report, the study sample was primarily white non-Hispanic (47.9 percent) and African American (40.8 percent). The remaining five children were Hispanic (11.3 percent).

Intervention and Data Collection Protocol

Children were recruited over ten months and assigned to intervention or comparison groups after parents gave written consent and children signed assent forms. The children in the intervention group received intervention in the form of playing WDTA, and those in the comparison group received no intervention. Data for each subject were collected in three sessions over a three-week period. Sessions were held on a university campus affiliated with a large medical center. Baseline data were collected from all children in session one. Measures included paper-and-pencil assessments of knowledge, self-efficacy, and attributions regarding asthma self-management.

Session two for each subject occurred one week after session one. In session two, children in the intervention group independently used WDTA. Following children's completion of the program instructions, the investigator assessed each learner's comprehension and provided further orientation to ensure understanding of how to use the program correctly. The children progressed through the first three levels of the program. At the end of the third level, the investigator asked the children whether they wanted to continue to the fourth level or to stop using the program. Process data of achievement and time on task was collected in this session. Children in the comparison group received no intervention in the second session and were not required to spend time at the study site. Session three occurred one week later. In this session, posttest data were collected from each child. In addition to the measures previously listed, these data included attitudes toward computer-assisted instruction.

Measurement

For data collection, a pencil-and-paper format was used and questionnaires were given to each subject or parent (depending on the instrument) to complete without assistance. However, the investigator observed children completing example items of each questionnaire to ensure that they understood the instructions before they proceeded.

Child Knowledge of Asthma Management

Knowledge was assessed in two ways—by a questionnaire and by three open-ended questions. The Child Knowledge of Asthma Management Questionnaire was developed to assess change in knowledge in children between 7 and 12 years old and was based on the educational objectives of the design document for WDTA. Each item provided the child with a statement about asthma self-management and possible responses of "yes," "no," and "don't know." The instrument was pilot-tested on a study sample of 101 children who had diagnoses of asthma. In the pilot sample, the Cronbach coefficient alpha for the 30-item questionnaire was 0.86 for children 7 to 13 years of age, and scores ranged from 5 to 30. The mean was 20.4 (±6.1), and skewness was −0.99 (SE skew, 0.26). In a clinical study involving 171 urban children with asthma who were 7 to 16 years of age, the alpha was 0.73.[2]

At posttest, children were also asked three open-ended questions about strategies for asthma self-management, and their answers were matched to a set of possible correct responses. The questions (and ranges of accurate responses) were as follows: What are the four steps that you should follow to manage your asthma? (0–4) What can you do to stop a problem before it starts? (0–10) What can you do to stop an asthma problem after it starts? (0–16)

Child Self-efficacy for Asthma Self-management

Self-efficacy is the belief that one has the skill and ability necessary to perform a behavior in a variety of circumstances and in the face of various obstacles.[37] Self-efficacy was assessed using a 23-item questionnaire developed to determine change in confidence in performing self-regulatory and asthma-specific behaviors in children 7 to 12 years old. The questionnaire included confidence in monitoring symptoms, environment, medicine taking, and health care use; confidence in deciding whether there is an asthma problem; and confidence in determining appropriate solutions and acting on them. Pilot testing on 101 children with asthma revealed an internal consistency using a Cronbach coefficient alpha of 0.88. In the intervention trial of 171 urban-dwelling children with asthma who were 7 to 16 years old, the Cronbach coefficient alpha was 0.77, indicating acceptable internal consistence.[2]

Causal Attributions

Attributions relate to the belief that self-management behavior is controllable and is subject to personal effort.[43] Attributions were assessed using a 22-item questionnaire developed for this study to determine change in causal attribution along the dimensions of locus and stability in children 7 to 12 years old. The item format was modeled on that used in the Children's Attributional Style Questionnaire, also known as the KASTAN-R[44] (N. Kaslow, personal communication, 1994). For each item in the questionnaire, the child is provided with a positive or negative self-management outcome. The subject is asked to imagine experiencing the outcome presented. An example of a positive outcome is "you go camping and have no asthma problems the whole time." An example of a negative self-management outcome is "you always have breathing problems when you swim." Two stems accompany each outcome. The child is asked to choose the stem that gives the best reason why the event would happen to him or her. For each item, one attribution dimension (i.e., locus or stability) is varied while the other dimension is kept constant. Pilot-testing of this questionnaire determined coefficient alphas for the locus subscales, which were 0.54 (success), 0.53 (failure), and 0.64 (combined). Coefficient alphas for the stability subscales were 0.70 (success), 0.67 (failure), and 0.74 (combined). The locus and stability subscales were not significantly correlated ($r = 0.14$, $P = 0.31$).

Attribution Classification

Children were asked to classify the four principal self-management behaviors (taking care of asthma, avoiding triggers, watching for symptoms, and taking medicine) in terms of the attributional dimensions of locus, stability, and controllability. Children were provided with a self-management behavior (e.g., taking medicine) and asked to check boxes on a semantic differential scale. This instrument uses a format based on Russell's causal dimension scale, which was developed to assess causal attribution dimensions in adults.[45] Scale items assessing perceptions of locus were "something other people do for you or get you to do" vs. "something you do yourself." Scale items assessing perception of control were "something you cannot control" vs. "something you can control." Scale items assessing perception of stability were "something you sometimes do" vs. "something you always do." The coefficient alpha for the 12-item scale is 0.75, based on baseline data from the 71 children in the current study.

Demographic and Health Information

Demographic information was obtained from primary caregivers, who were asked about their child's medicines, personal best peak flow, asthma triggers, and symptoms. Information on the use of emergency and hospital services, school grades, and absenteeism was also obtained. Parents also completed a six-item severity scale, developed by Rosier et al.,[46] which classified severity as low, moderate, mild, or high. The scale assesses number of episodes, coughing or wheezing, and curtailment of activities. An item reliability of 0.89 has been reported by the developers of the scale.[46] In the intervention trial of 171 inner-city children with asthma, the coefficient alpha for the scale was 0.77.[2]

Computer Experience

Children were also asked three questions about their computer experience. Responses to a question about how often they used computers ranged from "not at all" to "a few times a day." To find out what they used computers for, the children were asked to check all that applied from a list of eight common applications, such as word processing, games, and graphics or art and to list other uses. The children indicated where they used computers by checking all that applied from home, school, and friend's home and by listing other locations.

Motivation

The motivational impact of the WDTA (referred to as intrinsic motivation) was assessed using methodology similar to that described by Parker and Lepper.[47] In that study, children were given a choice of computer treatments that they could use. In the current study, motivational value of the program was assessed by determining the number of children continuing to the end of the program (level four) after being given the option to stop using the program at level three. Children were also asked to indicate on a four-point Likert scale how much they liked the computer game, liked to work with it, and liked the story that went with it. Possible responses ranged from "I didn't like it" to "I liked it very much." In addition, the children were asked to compare WDTA with their favorite board game, computer game, and school subject and with other asthma education they had had, using a three-point Likert scale with categories of "less fun," "as much fun," and "more fun." The children were interviewed about the game and asked what they would tell their best friend and other children with asthma about the game.

Attitude toward Computer-assisted Learning

Attitude toward computer-assisted instruction was assessed with the Attitude toward Computer-assisted Learning scale by Askar et al.[48] The scale consists of ten items, scored on a three-point response scale—

yes (3), sometimes (2), and no (1); the negatively worded items are reversed to a positive direction for scoring purposes. Askar et al. report the alpha reliability estimate of the total score to be 0.81.[48]

Process of Computer Use

Four characteristics of the child's computer use were collected—fidelity, time on task, tutorial score, and levels completed. The fidelity of program use was observed by the investigator, who rated children on seven categories using a five-point scale (never, rarely, sometimes, usually, always). The categories were as follows: needing assistance; understanding the program directions; following the WDTA self-regulatory sequence; making appropriate decisions in the game scenarios; engaging with the game scenarios; and attending to the tutorial segments.

Data Analysis

Sample Size Estimates

Data from the pilot test of the Child Knowledge of Asthma Management and the Child Self-efficacy for Asthma Self-management questionnaires with 101 children 7 to 13 years of age with asthma were used to calculate sample size requirements. On the basis of these data and predetermined estimates of alpha at 0.05 and power at 0.80, a sample of 80 subjects was calculated to be adequate to determine a difference 0.4 SD between groups using an analysis of covariance (ANCOVA) procedure.[49]

Statistical Analysis

The study sought to answer two questions: Is the computer program intrinsically motivating for children who use it? Do those children exposed to the computer program experience significantly greater change in knowledge, self-efficacy, and attributions than children who are not exposed?

To answer the first question, an 80 percent threshold for wanting to continue playing the game beyond the third level was set to indicate that the program was intrinsically motivating. To answer the second question, separate 2 × 2 repeated-measures analyses of variance were conducted to determine whether a significant change in knowledge, self-efficacy, and attribution had occurred in the intervention group compared with the comparison group. Analysis of covariance was conducted on the open-ended knowledge questions, which were collected only at posttest. Pretest scores from the Child Self-management Knowledge Questionnaire were used as covariates for this analysis.

RESULTS

Asthma Severity, Computer Use, and Demographic Variables

Forty-six percent of the study population was classified as having moderate-to-severe asthma. Most of the children in the study were reported by their parents as receiving above-average grades at school, with 73 percent reporting typical grades of As and Bs. Another 23.9 percent of children's parents reported their child's typical grades to be Bs and Cs. The children in the study were also experienced with computers. One third of the children in the study sample reported using computers a few times a day, and 90 percent of them reported using computers a few times a month. Computers were used principally in the school (81.7 percent of the children) and the home (61.9 percent). Computers were used for a variety of purposes, including school projects (70.4 percent), games (63.4 percent), and word processing (56.3 percent). In the study sample, 97.2 percent of caregivers had completed high school or had some college or a higher degree, and most study subjects came from two-parent households (68.6 percent). Most primary caregivers reported being employed full-time (67.1 percent), and 4.3 percent were employed half-time. Only 9.9 percent of the study sample were Medicaid recipients.

Differences between Groups at Baseline

There were no statistically significant differences between the two groups in any of the variables that might have affected performance on the CAI program (Table 2). The groups were also compared on mean impact variables at baseline. The mean score for the knowledge pretest was found to be significantly greater in the intervention group ($P = 0.027$). No difference was found for the other variables.

Motivational Value of *Watch, Discover, Think and Act*

With respect to the intrinsic motivation of the program, all the children in the intervention group who had time to do so (32 of 38) continued to use the program when told they could stop. This represents 84.2 percent of the sample and exceeds the 80 percent a priori criteria set for the study. The six children who did not proceed to the fourth level did not complete the entire game because of time constraints but indicated that they would have continued to play if time had permitted.

Table 2 ∎

Demographic and Severity Variables, by
Number (%), for the Total Sample,
Intervention, and Control Groups

Variable	Total Study Population, $N = 71$	Intervention Subjects, $n = 38$	Comparison Subjects, $n = 33$	Signifi-. cance
Sex:				
Male	46 (64.8)	25 (65.8)	21 (63.9)	0.24[b]
Female	25 (35.2)	13 (34.2)	12 (36.4)	
Ethnicity:				
Hispanic	5 (7.0)	2 (5.3)	3 (9.1)	
Asian	1 (2.6)	1 (2.6)	—	
Black	29 (40.8)	16 (42.1)	13 (39.4)	0.53[b]
White	34 (47.9)	17 (44.7)	17 (51.5)	
Other	2 (2.8)	2 (5.3)	—	
Asthma severity:				
Low	11 (15.5)	5 (13.2)	6 (18.2)	
Mild	27 (38.0)	13 (34.2)	14 (42.4)	0.32[b]
Moderate	25 (35.2)	17 (44.7)	8 (24.2)	
Severe	8 (11.3)	3 (7.9)	5 (15.2)	
School grades:				
As & Bs	52 (73.2)	25 (65.8)	27 (81.8)	
Bs & Cs	17 (23.9)	12 (31.6)	5 (15.2)	0.27[b]
Cs & Ds	2 (2.8)	1 (2.6)	1 (3.0)	
Computer experience:				
None at all	—	—	—	
Few times/yr	7 (9.9)	3 (7.9)	4 (12.1)	
Few times/mo	17 (23.9)	11 (28.9)	6 (18.2)	0.73[b]
Few times/wk	24 (33.8)	12 (31.6)	12 (36.4)	
Few times/day	23 (32.4)	12 (31.6)	11 (33.3)	

NOTE: Mean ages, in years (SD), were as follows: total study population, 10.69 (±1.14); intervention subjects, 10.92 (±1.17); comparison subjects, 10.42 (±1.06); signficance, 0.067a.
[a] Two-tailed *t*-test.
[b] Chi-square test.

No significant pretest-posttest difference was found between the groups regarding attitude about using computers as a learning medium. The children in the intervention group showed increased positive attitudes toward computers following the intervention, but this was not significant ($P = 0.327$). The children indicated that they liked the game (91.1 percent) and liked working with the computer (86.3 percent). They also liked the story that went with the program (72.3 percent). The children indicated that the WDTA program was as much or more fun than their favorite board game (88.9 percent), computer game (72.2 percent), subject in school (91.6 percent), and other asthma education (91.7 percent).

Program Effectiveness

With respect to the effectiveness of the program, Table 3 presents pretest and posttest mean scores for the impact variables. Knowledge posttest scores were significantly higher than pretest scores for the study sample ($F_1 = 37.87$, $P = 0.00$). However, repeated-measures analysis of variance revealed no between-group differences in knowledge ($F_1 = 0.35$, $P = 0.55$). A posttest-only analysis was found to be significant between the groups for the open-ended questions about the four-step self-regulation process ($F_1 = 189.18$, $P = 0.00$), prevention strategies ($F_1 = 12.33$, $P = 0.00$), and treatment strategies ($F_1 = 17.48$, $P = 0.00$). Because of the difference in baseline knowledge between the groups, an ANCOVA analysis was conducted using pretest knowledge scores as the covariate. Children in the intervention group had significantly greater scores on the open-ended knowledge questions than children in the comparison group when we controlled for knowledge pretest scores (all $P < 0.01$).

Assessment of the self-efficacy change scores revealed the existence of an influential data point greater than three SD from the mean. Using the criteria provided by Stevens,[50] this case represents an outlier. Subsequent analysis of the self-efficacy data was conducted with and without the outlier in the study sample. When the outlier was included ($n = 71$), repeated-measures analysis revealed no difference between the groups ($F_1 = 2.33$, $P = 0.13$) with an observed power of 0.325. When the outlier was omitted, a significant improvement in self-efficacy was apparent ($F_1 = 4.45$, $P = 0.04$), with an observed power of 0.547. The influential case did not differ significantly from other cases on the other variables tested.

Analysis of the total score and subscale scores of the Asthma Self-management Attribution Questionnaire revealed no difference between the intervention and comparison groups. However, the total score for attribution classification revealed a significant difference between the intervention and comparison groups; children in the intervention group exhibited significantly more positive attributions with respect to asthma self-management ($F_1 = 4.45$, $P = 0.04$). Observed power for this analysis was 0.548.

Process Variables

Observations of the children's progress on the computer program revealed that most did not require assistance with the program (69.4 percent). This is probably because standard help was provided to all children at the beginning of the first scenario. Most children (80.6 percent) followed the program directions. However, they tended to stray from the watch-discover-think-act self-regulatory sequence. Sixty-six

Table 3 ■

Pretest and Posttest Means for Impact Variables of Knowledge, Self-Efficacy, and Attribution

Variable	Group	n	Pretest Mean (SD)	Posttest Mean (SD)
Knowledge questionnaire	Intervention	38	18.6 (±5.1)	21.1 (±5.4)
	Control	33	15.7 (±5.8)	17.8 (±6.3)
Knowledge:				
Self-regulation	Intervention	38	—	3.3 (±1.3)
	Control	32	—	0.06 (±0.3)
Prevention	Intervention	38	—	2.7 (±1.1)
	Control	33	—	1.8 (±1.0)
Treatment	Intervention	38	—	2.7 (±1.4)
	Control	33	—	1.5 (±0.8)
Self-efficacy*	Intervention	38	53.4 (±9.7)	56.5 (±9.8)
	Control	32	51.6 (±9.7)	51.5 (±10.7)
Attribution:				
Locus (+)	Intervention	35	2.6 (±1.0)	2.9 (±0.9)
	Control	32	2.9 (±0.9)	3.0 (±0.9)
Locus (−)	Intervention	37	3.2 (±1.1)	3.5 (±0.8)
	Control	32	3.3 (±0.7)	3.6 (±0.7)
Locus (Total)	Intervention	35	5.6 (±1.8)	6.4 (±1.6)
	Control	32	6.3 (±1.3)	6.6 (±1.2)
Stability (+)	Intervention	37	4.3 (±1.8)	4.8 (±1.8)
	Control	33	4.2 (±1.8)	4.5 (±1.7)
Stability (-)	Intervention	36	4.8 (±1.7)	5.0 (±1.7)
	Control	32	4.6 (±1.8)	5.3 (±1.7)
Stability (Total)	Intervention	36	9.0 (±2.8)	9.9 (±2.7)
	Control	32	8.8 (±2.3)	5.3 (±1.7)
Attribution classification	Intervention	37	36.1 (±7.1)	39.5 (±6.4)
	Control	33	35.3 (±7.9)	36.5 (±6.7)

* Outlier removed.

percent of the children were observed to use the process only sometimes, rarely, or never. Most children (64.6 percent) usually or always made appropriate game decisions in the scenarios, such as choosing appropriate triggers and solutions to an asthma problem or taking appropriate actions for an asthma problem. Furthermore, most (91.7 percent) usually or always understood and attended to the tutorials. The children were observed to be always or usually engaged in the game activities (97.2 percent). Most (94.4 percent) were observed to usually answer the tutorial questions correctly. This is reflected by the children's high achievement scores on the tutorial questions; the mean scores for all tutorials were greater than 87 percent.

DISCUSSION

Attention, Motivation and Appeal

A fundamental tenet of social cognitive theory is that if learning is to occur, the learner must attend to what is learned.[37] This program's ability to attract children's attention and to keep them engaged in the learning activity is encouraging. All the children in the study wanted to continue to the end of the game, and they remained fully engaged in using the program, even after periods as long as 2.5 hours. This is even more compelling when we consider that the children in the study were sophisticated computer users. They compared the WDTA computer application favorably with other games and education programs they had used. Krendl and Lieberman's research in computer-based education[51] suggested that effects on motivation might be simply effects of the novelty of the medium. Given that the computer was not new to the children in this study, we could not attribute the program's success to novelty alone. Children in both groups had very positive views of using computers to learn.

Snyder and Palmer[52] noted the potential for instructional designers to create intricate, involving, and illustrated contexts into which educational activities can be embedded. Proponents have noted the potential motivational advantages of such procedures,[47,52–54] whereas opponents have viewed such developments as "sugarcoated" instruction that is likely to produce less lasting and less efficient learning.[54] While the debate over "edutainment" continues, it must be acknowledged that although an education program may maintain the attention of the learner, it is only a first step in engendering change in the educational variables the program is designed to affect.

Enhancement of Knowledge, Self-Efficacy and Attribution

Children who used WDTA were able to provide a more extensive array of behavioral strategies for asthma management. They were able to reiterate the components of a four-step problem-solving framework, describe behavioral strategies to prevent asthma episodes, and describe behavioral strategies to treat asthma symptoms to a significantly greater extent than those in the comparison group. The potential of the WDTA computer program to positively influence asthma self-management behavioral capability is further demonstrated by the between-group difference in self-efficacy. Enhanced self-efficacy theoretically leads to greater likelihood of the child attempting asthma self-management at home and to greater persistence in the endeavor.[37] Confidence to carry out self-management behaviors was not altered in the comparison group but improved significantly in the intervention group. The simulated experience of successfully negotiating a series of asthma self-management situations and performing simulated self-regulatory actions could change a child's self-perceived ability to perform these behaviors. The application provides a number of methods to elicit self-efficacy change in learners, including persuasion related to self-management actions, guided practice with corrective feedback, and social and symptom reinforcement for self-management success.[3]

The application is also designed to elicit change in attributions regarding asthma self-management behavior. To engender a move to more internal attributions, the learner is provided with direct control over the asthma self-management of a chosen character and is accompanied by an older peer coach who persuades the character that asthma self-management is largely in his or her own hands. The coach also demonstrates that self-management is based largely on effort and is not subject to external authority figures or to circumstances that cannot be changed. Repeated self-management experiences and situations reiterate the message that self-management failure is due to unstable (changeable) causes, such as lack of effort or modifiable environmental circumstances that can be managed in the future.

A significant group difference was apparent in how children classified asthma self-management behaviors. Children who had used the computer program classified the behaviors as more internal ("something I do myself"), more controllable ("something I can control"), and more stable ("something I always do"). This movement in perceived attributions indicates a move to feelings of greater autonomy in the children using the computer program. This change in attribution is theoretically related to enhanced self-efficacy and is important if these children are to be active asthma self-managers.[55,56]

Taken together, these results suggest that the program can influence factors related to asthma self-management. The strength of these findings should be considered in light of the relatively small sample size of 71 children.

Study Limitations

The study was limited because of the small sample size and some measurement problems. The significant change in knowledge scores in both groups points to the measurement instrument being a potential intervention in itself. This was a group of children with above-average school grades and, perhaps, above-average motivation. We might, therefore, predict some learning from noticing what they didn't know on pretest and seeking to find the answers. Parallel forms of the Asthma Knowledge Questionnaire might have provided a more stringent test. Although WDTA was effective in affecting behavioral determinants in a laboratory setting with children of moderate socioeconomic status, the effectiveness of the program in changing outcomes in a clinical setting of low-socioeconomic-status, predominantly minority children was unknown. The efficacy of the program in a laboratory setting indicated that a broader clinical-based study was warranted.

Effects on Self-management and Behavioral Outcomes: Use in Clinical Settings

A subsequent prospective pretest-posttest clinical trial with randomly assigned intervention and comparison subjects in four inner-city pediatric asthma clinics provided information on how the program might affect asthma self-management behavior.[2] The clinic sites served an inner city, primarily Medicaid-recipient (government-funded) population. Two sites were affiliated with large teaching hospitals headed by respiratory specialists with staffs of rotating fellows. The other two clinics were inner-city community sites staffed by pediatricians. Inclusion in the study was voluntary. No sites refused participation.

The computers were mounted on trolleys for ease of transportation. Clinic rooms or offices provided for the children to play the game were isolated from the distractions of clinic activity. Patients who met the inclusion criteria—age (6 to 17 years), moderate-to-severe asthma (as defined by their physicians), English speaking (parents could be Spanish speaking), and no chronic disease other than asthma—were invited by the research coordinator to participate. Patient participation was voluntary.

On the first visit the patient would see the physician and then be introduced to the computer by research staff for data entry and orientation. The first session with the computer comprised data entry, orientation, and play through at least one scenario game screen. This session lasted approximately 40 minutes. The intention was for the child to use the program unassisted; however, research assistants were available if the child needed help. On subsequent visits to the clinic, the children played the computer game for approximately 30 minutes before seeing the physicians. The computer's record keeping allowed the children to continue the program from where they left off. After each play session, the child and the physician received printouts with reinforcing messages, a reminder of the self-regulatory process taught, and the scores in the game. Research assistants completed the self-management sections of the plan, and physicians completed the sections on medications and treatment for episodes. Children in the comparison group continued to have regularly scheduled clinic appointments.

Results of the outcome study in the clinical sites indicated that children who were older and those who scored higher at pretest improved their knowledge of how to manage asthma. Self-management improved for intervention children who had a more conservative estimate of their self-efficacy at pretest and for children with higher pretest scores. Children in the intervention group had a lower rate of hospitalization, and there were differences in functional status that suggest improvement for children in the intervention group. Use of the self-management program was associated with a decrease in symptoms for those children whose symptoms were milder.

Feasibility for Clinic Use

Support for asthma self-management must include the participation of health care providers so that education can be individualized to the child's treatment regimen; getting this participation can prove challenging.[57] Health care providers work under growing time constraints, and in the two evaluation studies, enlisting their participation was difficult. The WDTA program is by no means a substitute for an National Asthma Education Program–recommended asthma action plan. Rather, the two work in concert.

The information from the child's asthma action plan is incorporated into the game parameters of WDTA, and the program gives the child simulated experience in managing asthma according to his or her plan. Optimally, the health care provider collaborates with the family in creating an action plan and helps them identify the child's triggers. In our experience, physicians usually fail to provide the action plan. Wide dissemination of the program will require support, such as an implementation manual and training to enable the health care team to incorporate the use of the action plan and help the child use the computer game. An additional challenge is managing the system. Although self-contained and easily maintained, the computer still requires staff to troubleshoot, enter data, and introduce the patient to the program. The WDTA program was subsequently withdrawn from the clinics pending ongoing evaluation of the system based on program modifications.

Program Modifications

The results of these two evaluation studies allowed us to plan a second iteration of WDTA. Three major modifications were planned and executed. They were development of a version for younger children, increase in the amount of guidance and feedback for the older children regarding their use of the self-regulatory processes, and development of Spanish-language versions.

Development of the Program for Younger Children

We found that the instructions were not adequate to allow the learners to go through the program on their own. Another problem with the program was the amount of detailed information offered in the tutorial segments. Although the 9- to 13-year-olds in the impact study remained engaged in these tutorials, younger learners in the clinic-based study found the information presented overwhelming. Furthermore, the indicators of health status were too complex for the younger children (ages 7 to 8 years). Therefore, a new version was developed that incorporated a smaller amount of tutorial information into the simulations, simplified the health status feedback, and provided more coaching throughout.

More Guidance Regarding the Self-regulatory Process

The observations that many children could not explain the self-regulatory buttons and that some of the children in the two evaluation studies tended to not follow the four-step self-regulatory sequence in order prompted the development of increased program guidance, reinforcement, and control. In the new version the children are guided to use watch, discover, think, then act in that order, and they receive more obvious score accrual for doing so.

Spanish Version

The WDTA program was developed for urban, low-income children and was evaluated in the southwestern United States, where many children have Spanish as a first language. Therefore, the second iteration included a Spanish translation that was made using both focus group methods to test possible translations of asthma-related words as well as the back-translation method that has become the accepted standard in health education.[58] Currently, all versions of the program are being used and evaluated as a part of a multi-component health-education and health services program and evaluation study in 60 elementary schools in grades one through five.

Future Research

The primary recommendation, and next logical step, for future research related to this and other technologically based programs is to conduct a diffusion study to determine the best way to achieve dissemination, adoption, implementation, and maintenance in clinics. Additional research issues involve examining the effect of parental asthma education on child behavior, conducting an evaluation of the program outside clinics, examining the effects of providing further tailoring in the program, evaluating the effectiveness of versions designed for younger children and for Spanish speakers, examining the effect of the program on patient–physician interaction, and adapting and evaluating the program for other diseases.

References ■

1. Watch, Discover, Think, and Act [computer program],version 1.02. Claverton, Md: Macro International Inc., 1995.
2. Bartholomew LK, Gold RS, Parcel GS, et al. Watch, Discover, Think and Act: evaluation of computer-assisted instruction to improve asthma self-management in inner-city children. Patient Educ Couns. 2000;39:269–80.
3. Bartholomew LK, Shegog R, Parcel GS, et al. Watch, Discover, Think, and Act: a model for patient education program development. Patient Educ Couns. 2000;39:253–68.
4. Halfon N, Newacheck PW. Childhood asthma and poverty: differential impacts and utilization of health services. Pediatrics. 1993;91(1):56–61.
5. Taylor WR, Newacheck PW. Impact of asthma on health. Pediatrics. 1992;90:657–62.
6. Crain EF, Weiss KB, Bijur PE, Hersh M, Westbrook L, Stein RE. An estimate of the prevalence of asthma and wheezing among inner-city children. Pediatrics. 1994;94:356–62.
7. Weiss KB, Gergen PJ, Wagener DK. Breathing better or worse? The changing epidemiology of asthma morbidity and mortality. Annu Rev Public Health. 1993;14:491–531.
8. Centers for Disease Control. Asthma mortality and hospitalization among children and young adults: United States, 1980–1993. MMWR Morb Mortal Wkly Rep. 1996;45(17):350–3.
9. Carr W, Zeitel L, Weiss K. Variations in deaths in New York City. Am J Public Health. 1992;82:59–65.
10. Marder D, Targonski O, Orris P, Persky V, Addington W. The effect of racial and socioeconomic factors on asthma mortality in Chicago. Chest. 1992;101:426s–9s.
11. Targonski PV, Persky VW, Orris O, Addington W. Trends in asthma mortality among African Americans and whites in Chicago, 1968 through 1991. Am J Public Health. 1994;84:1830–3.
12. Weitzman M, Gortmaker S, Sobol A. Racial, social, and environmental risks for childhood asthma. Am J Dis Child. 1990;144:1189–94.
13. Clark NM, Zimmerman BJ. A social cognitive view of self-regulated learning about health. Health Educ Res. 1990;5:371–9.
14. Bailey WC, Clark NM, Gotsch AR, Lemen RJ, O'Connor GT, Rosenstock IM. Asthma prevention. Chest. 1992;102(3):216s–31s.
15. Thorensen CE, Kirmil-Gray K. Self-management psychology and the treatment of childhood asthma. J Allergy Clin Immunol. 1983;72(5):596–610.
16. Clark NM, Rosenstock IM, Hassan H, Evan D, Wasilewski Y, Feldman C, Mellins B. The effect of health beliefs and feelings of self-efficacy on self-management behavior of children with chronic disease. Patient Educ Couns. 1988;11:131–9.
17. Tobin DL, Wigal JK, Winder JA, Holroyd KA, Creer TL. The "Asthma Self-Efficacy Scale." Ann Allergy. 1987;59:273–7.
18. Wigal JK, Stout C, Brandon M, Winder JA, Creer TL, Kotses H. The Knowledge, Attitude, and Self-efficacy Asthma Questionnaire. Chest. 1993;104:1144–8.
19. Parcel GS, Meyer MP. Development of an instrument to measure children's health locus of control. Health Educ Monogr. 1978;6:149–59.
20. Seligman MEP, Peterson C, Kaslow NJ, Tanenbaum RL, Alloy LB, Abramson LY. Attributional style and depressive symptoms among children. J Abnorm Psychol. 1984;93(2):235–8.
21. Kuttner MJ, Delamater AM, Santiago JV. Learned helplessness in diabetic youths. J Pediatr Psychol. 1990;15(5):595–604.
22. Weiner B. An attributional theory of achievement motivation and emotion. Psychol Rev. 1985;92(4):548–73.
23. Paperny DM, Starn JR. Adolescent pregnancy prevention by health education computer games: computer-assisted instruction knowledge and attitudes. Pediatrics. 1989;183:742–52.
24. Kann LK. Effects of computer-assisted instruction on selected interaction skills related to responsible sexuality. J School Health. 1987;57:282–7.
25. Meier ST, Sampson JP. Use of computer-assisted instruction in the prevention of alcohol abuse. J Drug Educ. 1989;9:245–56.
26. Wetstone SL, Sheehan TJ, Votaw RG, Peterson MG, Rothfield N. Evaluation of a computer-based education lesson for patients with rheumatoid arthritis. J Rheumatol. 1985;12:907–12.
27. Starbright Foundation Web site. Available at:

http://www.starbright.org/projects/sbw/index.html, 1999.

28. Williams RB, Boyles M, Johnson RE. Patient use of a computer for prevention in primary care practice. Patient Educ Couns. 1995;25:283–92.

29. De Vries H, Brug J. Computer-tailored interventions motivating people to adopt health promoting behaviors: introduction to a new approach. Patient Educ Couns. 1999;36:99–105.

30. Huss K, Salerno M, Huss RW. Computer-assisted reinforcement of instruction: effects on adherence in adult atopic asthmatics. Res Nurs Health. 1991;14:259–67.

31. Clubhouse Asthma [software]. Raleigh, NC: MindJourney Software, 1999. Clubhouse Asthma Web site. Available at: http://www.clubhouseasthma.com.

32. Wave Quest Inc. Bronkie the Bronchiasaurus [video game]. Mountain View, Calif: Raya Systems Inc., 1992–1995. Licensed by Nintendo, 1991.

33. The Wee Willie Wheezie asthma computer game [online]. Formerly available at GSF (National Research Center for Environment and Health, Germany) Web site, at: http://www.gsf.de/wjst/gamepage.htm, 1997.

34. Yawn BP, Algatt-Bergstrom PJ, Yawn RA, et al. An in-school CD-ROM asthma education program. J School Health. 2000;70(4):153–9.

35. Rubin DH, Hecht AR, Marinangeli PC, Erenberg FG. Asthma Command. Am J Asthma Allergy. 1989;2(2):108–12.

36. Lieberman DA. Interactive video games for health promotion: effects on knowledge, self-efficacy, social support, and health. In: RL Street, WR Gold, T Manning (eds). Health Promotion and Interactive Technology. Mahwah, NJ: Lawrence Erlbaum, 1997.

37. Bandura A. Social Foundations of Thought and Action: A Social Cognitive Theory. Englewood Cliffs, NJ: Prentice Hall, 1986.

38. Creer TL, Kotses H, Wigal JK. A second-generation model of asthma self-management. Pediatr Allergy Immunol. 1992;6:143–65.

39. Macromedia Inc. Macromind Director 5.0. Available at: http://www.macromedia.com/software/director/.

40. National Asthma Education Program. Expert Panel Report 2: Guidelines for the Diagnosis and Management of Asthma. Bethesda, Md: NAEP, National Heart, Lung and Blood Institute, 1997. Public Health Service report 97-4051.

41. National Asthma Education Program. Teach Your Patients About Asthma: A Clinician's Guide. Bethesda, Md: NAEP, National Heart, Lung and Blood Institute, 1992. Public Health Service report 92-2737.

42. Glaxo Wellcome, Inc. Managing Your Asthma: Understanding Proper Inhaler and Peak Flow Technique.

Research Triangle Park, NC: Glaxo Wellcome, Inc. Publication GVL335R0.

43. Weiner B. An attributional theory of achievement motivation and emotion. Psychol Rev. 1985;92(4):548–73.

44. Seligman MEP, Peterson C, Kaslow NJ, Tanenbaum RL, Alloy LB, Abramson LY. Attributional style and depressive symptoms among children. J Abnorm Psychol. 1984;93(2):235–8.

45. Russell D. The causal dimension scale: a measure of how individuals perceive causes. J Pers Soc Psychol. 1982;42:1137–45.

46. Rosier M, Bishop J, Nolan T, Robertson CF, Carlin JB, Phelan PD. Measurement of functional severity of asthma in children. Am J Respir Crit Care Med. 1994;149:1434–441.

47. Parker LE, Lepper MR. Effects of fantasy contexts on children's learning and motivation: making learning more fun. J Pers Soc Psychol. 1992;62(4):625–33.

48. Askar P, Yavuz H, Koksal M. Student's perceptions of computer assisted instruction environment and their attitudes towards computer-assisted learning. Educ Res. 1992; 34:133–9.

49. Cohen J. Statistical Power Analysis for the Behavioral Sciences. 2nd ed. Hillsdale, NJ: Lawrence Erlbaum, 1988.

50. Stevens J. Applied Multivariate Statistics for the Social Sciences. 2nd ed. Hillsdale, NJ: Lawrence Erlbaum, 1988.

51. Krendl KA, Lieberman DA. Computers and learning: a review of recent research. J Educ Comput Res. 1988;4(4): 367–89.

52. Snyder T, Palmer J. In Search of the Most Amazing Thing: Children, Education and Computers. Menlo Park, Calif: Addison-Wesley, 1986.

53. Loftus GR, Loftus ER. Mind at Play. New York: Basic Books, 1983.

54. Bowers CA. The Cultural Dimensions of Educational Computing: Understanding the Non-Neutrality of Technology. New York: Teachers College Press, 1988.

55. Bandura A. Self-efficacy: The Exercise of Control. New York: WH Freeman, 1997.

56. Skinner CS, Kreuter MW. Using theories in planning interactive computer programs. In: Street RL, Gold WR, Manning T (eds). Health Promotion and Interactive Technology: Theoretical Applications and Future Directions. Mahwah, NJ: Lawrence Erlbaum, 1997.

57. Developing and implementing educational strategies and interventions for controlling asthma in inner city and high risk populations: final report. Claverton, Md: Macro International Inc., 1994. National Heart, Lung and Blood Institute contract N01-H0-39220.

58. Marin G, Marin BV. Research with Hispanic Populations. Newbury Park, Calif: Sage, 1991.

Section 7:

Reprinted by kind permission of:
American Medical Informatics
Association (602)
Lippincott Williams & Wilkins (592)
Oxford University Press (584, 610, 620)

R. Hofestädt

Synopsis

Bielefeld University, Faculty of Technology
Bioinformatics Department
Bielefeld, Germany

Bioinformatics

The papers selected for this section describe important topics of Bioinformatics. Methods of Molecular Biology are important for the future of Medicine. Therefore, methods of computer science, e.g. database systems, information systems and analysis tools, have to be developed and implemented. In Germany, the Ministry of Science recently started new programs to build Bioinformatic Centres at five universities and five research centres. The main reason to support this new research topic is the fact that the exponential growth of molecular data can only be handled using methods of computer science. The selected five papers in this section of the Yearbook 2002 demonstrate the current situation of the electronical infrastructure of Molecular Biology. The paper by Berman et al. describes the Protein Data Bank (PDB). Today more than 300 molecular databases are available via the Internet and PDB represents the knowledge of analysed proteins. Database systems that represent information about genes, gene regulation processes, metabolic reactions, enzymes, signal pathways etc. also exist. Beyond molecular database systems, different information systems are available that also allow information fusion to solve specific questions and problems. In this sense, the paper by Kolaskar and Naik shows an information system for identifying viruses. All these database systems only represent molecular data selected from published experimental results. For future aspects, modelling and simulation must be integrated and will help analyse the molecular mechanisms. Data modelling is one important aspect addressed by Paton et al.. Their paper presents a collection of data models

for genomic data. However, to understand the metabolic behaviour of cell simulation, tools for metabolic processes have to be implemented. Rzhetsky et al. present a new model for the analysis of gene controlled metabolic networks. Modelling and simulation is the backbone for the implementation of the virtual cell. We are far from implementing the first version of this vision today. However, one important application of Bioinformatics is Medicine. The last paper, by Miller, represents a current discussion of the future of Bioinformatics in the field of Health Informatics. This paper is based on a presentation made to the Symposium of the American College of Medical Informatics in 2000.

Bioinformatics

Based on the Human Genome Project, the new interdisciplinary subject of Bioinformatics has become an important research topic during the last decade. Methods of Molecular Biology allow automatic sequencing and synthesis of nucleic and amino acids. Based on this technology robots able to sequence small genomes in one month's time are developed. The automatic assembly and annotation of the sequence data can only be done using methods of computer science. This is one of the main reasons for the success of this new research topic. Today, beside the genome and protein sequence data, a new domain of data is arising–the so-called proteomic project, which allows the identification of protein profiles. The molecular data is stored in database systems available via the Inter-

net. Based on that data, different questions can be solved by implementing specific analysis tools. Regarding the DNA sequence, we are looking for tools that will predict DNA-functional units. Today, we call this topic "From the Sequence to the Function" or "Post Genomics". The main application area of this new research topic is Molecular Medicine. Therefore, Bioinformatics has also become an important topic of Medical Informatics. Regarding current definitions of Bioinformatics, we can see two different views: The German definition of Bioinformatics is a global definition. On the one hand, the application of the methods and concepts of computer science in biology represent the main focus. This is also the common definition. On the other hand, looking onto the history of computer science, we can identify important innovations coming from the analysis of molecular mechanisms. Regarding this aspect, we can distinguish between direct and indirect innovations. The implementation of neuronal networks, genetic algorithms or DNA Computing methods try to solve severe problems using molecular mechanisms. We can call this research topic the biological paradigm of computing. Moreover, the definition of formal systems, like the cellular automaton (J. v. Neumann), the finite state automaton (H. Kleene) or L-systems (A. Lindenmayer), is based on the idea of the implementation of analysis tools for modelling neural networks.

The common definition of Bioinformatics addresses the application of methods and concepts of computer science in the field of biology. Bioinformatics currently stresses three main topics. The first major topic is sequence analysis or genome informatics. Its basic tasks are: assembling sequence fragments, automatic annotation, and implementation of database systems, like EMBL, TRANSFAC, PIR, GENBANK, KEGG etc.. The sequence alignment problem still represents the kernel of sequence analysis tools. Their development and implementation represents the second aspect of sequence analysis. Nevertheless, sequence analysis is not a new topic. It was, and still is, a topic of Theoretical Biology or Computational Biology. Protein Design is the second current major research topic of Bioinformatics. The first task is to implement specific database systems that represent knowledge about the proteins. Today many different systems, like PIR or SWISSPROT, are available. The main idea of this topic still is to develop and implement a model, that will allow the automatic calculation of the 3D structure, including the prediction of the molecular behaviour of this protein. Until now, molecular modelling has been unsuccessful. Protein design is also not a new research topic. Its roots can be found in Biophysics, Pharmaco Kinetics and Theoretical Biology. The third current major Bioinformatics topic is Metabolic Engineering, which was defined by J. Bailey. Its goal is to analyze and synthesize metabolic processes. The basic molecular information of metabolic pathways is stored in database systems, like KEGG, WIT, etc.. Models and specific algorithms, based on the molecular knowledge represented by these database and information systems, allow the implementation of analysis tools.

Prospects for the future - Virtual Cell

The idea of Metabolic Engineering represents the basic idea of the Virtual Cell. Using molecular data and molecular knowledge, the implementation of specific models allows the implementation of simulation tools. Behind the algorithmic analysis of molecular data, modelling and simulation methods and concepts allow the analysis and synthesis of complex gene controlled metabolic networks. The current and available knowledge and data of Molecular Biology is still rudimentary. Furthermore, the experimental data available in molecular databases have a high error rate, while biological knowledge has a high rate of uncertainty. Therefore, only modelling and simulation methods will suffice to discuss arising important questions. Such formal descriptions can be used to specify of a simulation environment. Therefore, modelling and simulation can be interpreted as the basic step for implementing virtual worlds that allow virtual experiments.

The papers of this section show parts of the electronic infrastructure of Molecular Biology and the application of molecular data to model and simulate metabolic processes. The concepts available in literature are based on specific questions, such as the gene regulation process phenomena, or the biochemical process control. To solve current questions, we must implement integrative models which can be used to implement the virtual cell. If we take a look at the Internet, we can see that only online representations of cellular illustrations, taken directly from books, are available today (http://www.life.uiuc.edu/plantbio/cell/). The state of the art methods and concepts for the implementation of a virtual cell have been documented by the seminars organized at Dagstuhl, including a summer school focusing on: Modelling and Simulation of Gene Regulation and Metabolic Pathways

· http://www-bm.cs.uni-magdeburg. de/iti_bm/ibss/
· http://www-bm.cs.uni-magdeburg. de/iti_bm/dagstuhl/
· http://www-bm.cs.uni-magdeburg. de/iti_bm/dagstuhl2001/

Based on these events, MIT Press will publish a book by the end of 2001. One chapter of this book will include a description of M. Tomita's E-Cell system, which represents the first implementation of the virtual cell. His work represents a specific software solution and cannot be used globally (www.e-cell.org). Many new virtual cell projects are following the E-Cell project. However, it will take much time to implement a useful and powerful virtual cell. Rudimentary knowledge is one problem confronting the implementation of such systems. Furthermore, data and information are still missing. We are not yet able to understand the quantitative behaviour of simple metabolic processes.

Benefits

Bioinformatics will present the electronical infrastructure of Molecular Biology and will support drug design, molecular diagnosis and gene therapy. Based on molecular methods, modelling tools will be implemented that allow computer-supported design of new drugs. Information systems, in combination with methods of artificial intelligence, will support molecular diseases detection. Therefore, first information and expert systems for the detection of metabolic diseases as well as tools for the analysis of genotype/phenotype correlations have already been implemented. Diagnosis and therapy of metabolic diseases will be supported by database systems, knowledge based systems and molecular expert systems. Therefore, it is important to integrate Bioinformatics into the Medical Informatics curriculum. Thus, the future of Molecular Medicine is correlated with the future of Molecular Biology. Gene therapy is only one example, that demonstrates that methods of Bioinformatics are important. On the one hand, the analysis of all genes is supported by Bioinformatics methods. On the other hand, gene therapy is based on the idea of gene transfer methods. The molecular effect of the transfer of one or more genes into another organism must be tested and simulated using Bioinformatics methods, which allow the implementation of hypothetical worlds. The first task is to understand the gene regulatory mechanism, while the second task is to control the molecular effect of the gene product. The later can be discussed using the molecular information stored in the molecular database systems. Identification of negative side effects can only occur with help of available molecular data from different database systems, used in combination with modelling and simulation methods. Beside this scientific approach, simple methods of information fusion of molecular data can be used and implemented in modern health care systems today. These tools will support expert systems or simple information systems, that are able to monitor patient data, for example a specific drug therapy.

Barriers

Bioinformatics methods in use are database systems, information systems, analysis tools, modelling, and simulation. Evaluation processes of molecular database systems show that most database systems represent much incorrect and/or junk data. The mistakes are caused by false experimental and/or published data. Moreover, the copy process from the selected papers to the database entry, which is done by humans, also shows a high error rate. However, there are many scientists saying that most of the molecular database systems represent junk data. Although some tests have shown that the error rate is very high, it will not be easy to solve this problem in the future. Until now no efforts to implement software tools, that will reduce this error rate can be seen in the area of Bioinformatics. Another problem is that we are not able to implement analysis tools for many of the open questions. We need clear definitions and specifications to develop analysis tools. This is not the case in the field of Biology. For example the fundamental term „homology of sequences" has hundreds of definitions. For this reason, so many different alignment algorithms exist. The other reason is the high complexity of time and space of most of these problems. Complexity is the main argument against the implementation of the virtual cell within the next decades. Finally, the main barriers come directly from Molecular Biology.

Today, it seems as though we will never understand basic molecular mechanisms, such as the fundamental process of gene regulation.

Prospects for the near future

Information systems for scientists, patients and doctors, to represent the basic knowledge of Molecular Biology are available already. Moreover, their data is growing exponentially. Today, molecular data is available via the Internet and can be used to support therapy, diagnosis and drug design. The molecular diagnosis of metabolic diseases is a current research topic. Thousands of metabolic diseases are known and about 500 relevant inborn errors are discussed in the literature. Based on medical data of inborn errors, the German Human Genome Project initiated a project, to discuss the actual benefits of molecular information fusion in combination with modelling and simulation methods. Databases such as METAGENE, KEGG, TRANSFAC and MDCave will be integrated into this project. Using gene regulation and metabolic processes modelling, the analysis process will be supported. This running project shows that genotype/phenotype correlations can be identified using current molecular data and knowledge.

References:

1. Attwood TK, Parry-Smith DJ. Introduction to Bioinformatics. Prentice-Hall, Hempstead; 1999
2. Bailey J. Toward a Science of Metabolic Engineering. Science 1991;252:1668-74.
3. Collado-Vides J, Hofestädt R. Gene Regulation and Metabolism. MIT Press. In press 2001
4. Frenkel K. The Human Genome Project and Informatics. Commun ACM 1991; 11:41-51.
5. Goldberg DE. Genetic Algorithms in Search, Optimization and Machine Learning. Amsterdam Bonn Singapore: Addison-Wesley; 1989.
6. Heijne G v. Sequence Analysis in Molecular Biology. San Diego New York London Toronto: Academic Press; 1987.
7. Hofestädt R, Collado-Vides J, Löffler M, Mavrovouniotis M. Modelling and Simulation of Metabolic Pathways, Gene Regulation and

Cell Differentiation. Bioessays 1996;18:333-5.
8. Hofestädt R. Computer Science and Biology. Biosystems 1997;43:69-71.
9. Hofestädt R, Lengauer T, Löffler M, Schomburg D, editors. Bioinformatics. Heidelberg: Springer; 1997.
10. Hofestädt R, Scholz U. Information Processing for the Analysis of Metabolic Pathways and Inborn Errors. Biosystems 1998;47:91-102.
11. Kanehisa M. Post-Genome Informatics. Oxford: Oxford University Press; 2000.
12. Pevzner P. Computational Molecular Biology: An Algorithmic Approach. Cambridge: MIT Press; 2000.
13. Setubal J, Meidanis J. Introduction to Computational Molecular Biology. Boston: PWS Publishing Company; 1997
14. Waterman M. Introduction to Computational Biology. Boston: Chapman Hall; 1992.

www-glossary

EMBL – Gene sequences
http://www.ebi.ac.uk/ebi_docs/embl_db/ebi/topembl.html
GEPASI – Biochemical simulation
http://gepasi.dbs.aber.ac.uk/softw/gepasi.html
KEGG – Metabolic pathways
http://genome.ad.jp
GENBANK – Gene sequences
http://www.ncbi.nlm.nih.gov/Web/Genbank/index.html
HGMD – Human Gene Mutation Database
http://archive.uwcm.ac.uk/uwcm/mg/hgmd0.html
MatInspector – Promoter detection
http://genomatix.gsf.de
MDCave – Molecular data of inborn errors
http://mdcave.genophen.de
METAGENE – Medical data of inborn errors
http://www.metagene.de
OMIM – Online Mendelian Inheritance in Man
http://www.ncbi.nlm.nih.gov/Omim/
PIR – Protein information
http://pir.georgetown.edu/
PDB – Protein Data Bank
http://www.rcsb.org/pdb/
SRS – Database integration
http://srs6.ebi.ac.uk
SWISSPROT – Protein information
http://www.expasy.ch/sprot/
TRANSFAC – Gene regulation
http://transfac.gbf.de/
WIT – Metabolic pathways
http://wit.mcs.anl.gov/WIT2/

Address of the author:
Ralf Hofestädt
Bielefeld University, Faculty of Technology
Bioinformatics Department
P.O. Box 100 131
D-33501 Bielefeld, Germany
E-Mail: hofestae@techfak.uni-bielefeld.de

The Protein Data Bank

Helen M. Berman[1,2,*], John Westbrook[1,2], Zukang Feng[1,2], Gary Gilliland[1,3], T. N. Bhat[1,3], Helge Weissig[1,4], Ilya N. Shindyalov[4] and Philip E. Bourne[1,4,5,6]

[1]Research Collaboratory for Structural Bioinformatics (RCSB), [2]Department of Chemistry, Rutgers University, 610 Taylor Road, Piscataway, NJ 08854-8087, USA, [3]National Institute of Standards and Technology, Route 270, Quince Orchard Road, Gaithersburg, MD 20899, USA, [4]San Diego Supercomputer Center, University of California, San Diego, 9500 Gilman Drive, La Jolla, CA 92093-0505, USA, [5]Department of Pharmacology, University of California, San Diego, 9500 Gilman Drive, La Jolla, CA 92093-0500, USA and [6]The Burnham Institute, 10901 North Torrey Pines Road, La Jolla, CA 92037, USA

Received September 20, 1999; Revised and Accepted October 17, 1999

ABSTRACT

The Protein Data Bank (PDB; http://www.rcsb.org/pdb/) is the single worldwide archive of structural data of biological macromolecules. This paper describes the goals of the PDB, the systems in place for data deposition and access, how to obtain further information, and near-term plans for the future development of the resource.

INTRODUCTION

The Protein Data Bank (PDB) was established at Brookhaven National Laboratories (BNL) (1) in 1971 as an archive for biological macromolecular crystal structures. In the beginning the archive held seven structures, and with each year a handful more were deposited. In the 1980s the number of deposited structures began to increase dramatically. This was due to the improved technology for all aspects of the crystallographic process, the addition of structures determined by nuclear magnetic resonance (NMR) methods, and changes in the community views about data sharing. By the early 1990s the majority of journals required a PDB accession code and at least one funding agency (National Institute of General Medical Sciences) adopted the guidelines published by the International Union of Crystallography (IUCr) requiring data deposition for all structures.

The mode of access to PDB data has changed over the years as a result of improved technology, notably the availability of the WWW replacing distribution solely via magnetic media. Further, the need to analyze diverse data sets required the development of modern data management systems.

Initial use of the PDB had been limited to a small group of experts involved in structural research. Today depositors to the PDB have varying expertise in the techniques of X-ray crystal structure determination, NMR, cryoelectron microscopy and theoretical modeling. Users are a very diverse group of researchers in biology, chemistry and computer scientists, educators, and students at all levels. The tremendous influx of data soon to be fueled by the structural genomics initiative, and the increased recognition of the value of the data toward understanding biological function, demand new ways to collect, organize and distribute the data.

In October 1998, the management of the PDB became the responsibility of the Research Collaboratory for Structural Bioinformatics (RCSB). In general terms, the vision of the RCSB is to create a resource based on the most modern technology that facilitates the use and analysis of structural data and thus creates an enabling resource for biological research. Specifically in this paper, we describe the current procedures for data deposition, data processing and data distribution of PDB data by the RCSB. In addition, we address the issues of data uniformity. We conclude with some current developments of the PDB.

DATA ACQUISITION AND PROCESSING

A key component of creating the public archive of information is the efficient capture and curation of the data—data processing. Data processing consists of data deposition, annotation and validation. These steps are part of the fully documented and integrated data processing system shown in Figure 1.

In the present system (Fig. 2), data (atomic coordinates, structure factors and NMR restraints) may be submitted via email or via the AutoDep Input Tool (ADIT; http://pdb.rutgers.edu/adit/) developed by the RCSB. ADIT, which is also used to process the entries, is built on top of the mmCIF dictionary which is an ontology of 1700 terms that define the macromolecular structure and the crystallographic experiment (2,3), and a data processing program called MAXIT (MAcromolecular EXchange Input Tool). This integrated system helps to ensure that the data submitted are consistent with the mmCIF dictionary which defines data types, enumerates ranges of allowable values where possible and describes allowable relationships between data values.

After a structure has been deposited using ADIT, a PDB identifier is sent to the author automatically and immediately (Fig. 1, Step 1). This is the first stage in which information about the structure is loaded into the internal core database (see section on the PDB Database Resource). The entry is then annotated as described in the validation section below. This process involves using ADIT to help diagnose errors or

*To whom correspondence should be addressed at: Department of Chemistry, Rutgers University, 610 Taylor Road, Piscataway, NJ 08854-8087, USA. Tel: +1 732 445 4667; Fax: +1 732 445 4320; Email: berman@rcsb.rutgers.edu

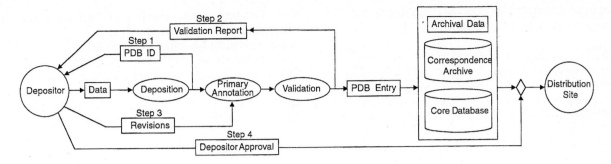

Figure 1. The steps in PDB data processing. Ellipses represent actions and rectangles define content.

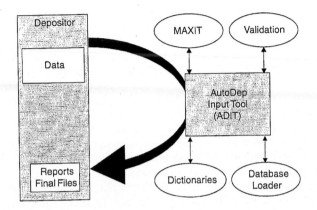

Figure 2. The integrated tools of the PDB data processing system.

inconsistencies in the files. The completely annotated entry as it will appear in the PDB resource, together with the validation information, is sent back to the depositor (Step 2). After reviewing the processed file, the author sends any revisions (Step 3). Depending on the nature of these revisions, Steps 2 and 3 may be repeated. Once approval is received from the author (Step 4), the entry and the tables in the internal core database are ready for distribution. The schema of this core database is a subset of the conceptual schema specified by the mmCIF dictionary.

All aspects of data processing, including communications with the author, are recorded and stored in the correspondence archive. This makes it possible for the PDB staff to retrieve information about any aspect of the deposition process and to closely monitor the efficiency of PDB operations.

Current status information, comprised of a list of authors, title and release category, is stored for each entry in the core database and is made accessible for query via the WWW interface (http://www.rcsb.org/pdb/status.html). Entries before release are categorized as 'in processing' (PROC), 'in depositor review' (WAIT), 'to be held until publication' (HPUB) or 'on hold until a depositor-specified date' (HOLD).

Content of the data collected by the PDB

All the data collected from depositors by the PDB are considered primary data. Primary data contain, in addition to the coordinates, general information required for all deposited structures and information specific to the method of structure determination.

Table 1 contains the general information that the PDB collects for all structures as well as the additional information collected for those structures determined by X-ray methods. The additional items listed for the NMR structures are derived from the International Union of Pure and Applied Chemistry recommendations (IUPAC) (4) and will be implemented in the near future.

Table 1. Content of data in the PDB

Content of all depositions (X-ray and NMR)
Source – specifications such as genus, species, strain, or variant of gene (cloned or synthetic); expression vector and host, or description of method of chemical synthesis
Sequence – Full sequence of all macromolecular components
Chemical structure of cofactors and prosthetic groups
Names of all components in structure
Qualitative description of characteristics of structure
Literature citations for the structure submitted
Three-dimensional coordinates
Additional items for X-ray structure determinations
Temperature factors and occupancies assigned to each atom
Crystallization conditions, including pH, temperature, solvents, salts, methods
Crystal data, including the unit cell dimensions and space group
Presence of non-crystallographic symmetry
Data collection information describing the methods used to collect the diffraction data including instrument, wavelength, temperature, and processing programs
Data collection statistics including data coverage, R_{sym}, data above 1, 2, 3 sigma levels and resolution limits
Refinement information including R factor, resolution limits, number of reflections, method of refinement, sigma cutoff, geometry rmsd, sigma
Structure factors – h, k, l, Fobs, σ Fobs
Additional items for NMR structure determinations
Model number for each coordinate set that is deposited and an indication if one should be designated as a representative, or an energy minimized average model provided
Data collection information describing the types of methods used, instrumentation, magnetic field strength, console, probe head, sample tube
Sample conditions, including solvent, macromolecule concentration ranges, concentration ranges of buffers, salts, antibacterial agents, other components, isotopic composition
Experimental conditions, including temperature, pH, pressure, and oxidation state of structure determination and estimates of uncertainties in these values
Non-covalent heterogeneity of sample, including self-aggregation, partial isotope exchange, conformational heterogeneity resulting in slow chemical exchange
Chemical heterogeneity of the sample (e.g., evidence for deamidation or minor covalent species)
A list of NMR experiments used to determine the structure including those used to determine resonance assignments, NOE/ROE data, dynamical data, scalar coupling constants, and those used to infer hydrogen bonds and bound ligands. The relationship of these experiments to the constraint files are given explicitly
Constraint files used to derive the structure as described in Task Force recommendations

The information content of data submitted by the depositor is likely to change as new methods for data collection, structure determination and refinement evolve and advance. In addition, the ways in which these data are captured are likely to change as the software for structure determination and refinement produce the necessary data items as part of their output. ADIT, the data input system for the PDB, has been designed so as to easily incorporate these likely changes.

Validation

Validation refers to the procedure for assessing the quality of deposited atomic models (structure validation) and for assessing how well these models fit the experimental data (experimental validation). The PDB validates structures using accepted community standards as part of ADIT's integrated data processing system. The following checks are run and are summarized in a letter that is communicated directly to the depositor:

Covalent bond distances and angles. Proteins are compared against standard values from Engh and Huber (5); nucleic acid bases are compared against standard values from Clowney *et al.* (6); sugar and phosphates are compared against standard values from Gelbin *et al.* (7).

Stereochemical validation. All chiral centers of proteins and nucleic acids are checked for correct stereochemistry.

Atom nomenclature. The nomenclature of all atoms is checked for compliance with IUPAC standards (8) and is adjusted if necessary.

Close contacts. The distances between all atoms within the asymmetric unit of crystal structures and the unique molecule of NMR structures are calculated. For crystal structures, contacts between symmetry-related molecules are checked as well.

Ligand and atom nomenclature. Residue and atom nomenclature is compared against the PDB dictionary (ftp://ftp.rcsb.org/pub/pdb/data/monomers/het_dictionary.txt) for all ligands as well as standard residues and bases. Unrecognized ligand groups are flagged and any discrepancies in known ligands are listed as extra or missing atoms.

Sequence comparison. The sequence given in the PDB SEQRES records is compared against the sequence derived from the coordinate records. This information is displayed in a table where any differences or missing residues are marked. During structure processing, the sequence database references given by DBREF and SEQADV are checked for accuracy. If no reference is given, a BLAST (9) search is used to find the best match. Any conflict between the PDB SEQRES records and the sequence derived from the coordinate records is resolved by comparison with various sequence databases.

Distant waters. The distances between all water oxygen atoms and all polar atoms (oxygen and nitrogen) of the macromolecules, ligands and solvent in the asymmetric unit are calculated. Distant solvent atoms are repositioned using crystallographic symmetry such that they fall within the solvation sphere of the macromolecule.

In almost all cases, serious errors detected by these checks are corrected through annotation and correspondence with the authors.

It is also possible to run these validation checks against structures before they are deposited. A validation server (http://pdb.rutgers.edu/validate/) has been made available for this purpose. In addition to the summary report letter, the server also provides output from PROCHECK (10), NUCheck (Rutgers University, 1998) and SFCHECK (11). A summary atlas page and molecular graphics are also produced.

The PDB will continually review the checking methods used and will integrate new procedures as they are developed by the PDB and members of the scientific community.

Other data deposition centers

The PDB is working with other groups to set up deposition centers. This enables people at other sites to more easily deposit their data via the Internet. Because it is critical that the final archive is kept uniform, the content and format of the final files as well as the methods used to check them must be the same. At present, the European Bioinformatics Institute (EBI) processes data that are submitted to them via AutoDep (http://autodep.ebi.ac.uk/). Once these data are are sent to the RCSB in PDB format for inclusion in the central archive. Before this system was put in place it was tested to ensure consistency among entries in the PDB archive. In the future, the data will be exchanged in mmCIF format using a common exchange dictionary, which along with standardized annotation procedures will ensure a high degree of uniformity in the archival data. Structures deposited and processed at the EBI represent ~20% of all data deposited.

Data deposition will also soon be available from an ADIT Web site at The Institute for Protein Research at Osaka University in Japan. At first, structures deposited at this site will be processed by the PDB staff. In time, the staff at Osaka will complete the data processing for these entries and send the files to the PDB for release.

NMR data

The PDB staff recognizes that NMR data needs a special development effort. Historically these data have been retrofitted into a PDB format defined around crystallographic information. As a first step towards improving this situation, the PDB did an extensive assessment of the current NMR holdings and presented their findings to a Task Force consisting of a cross section of NMR researchers. The PDB is working with this group, the BioMagResBank (BMRB) (12), as well as other members of the NMR community, to develop an NMR data dictionary along with deposition and validation tools specific for NMR structures. This dictionary contains among other items descriptions of the solution components, the experimental conditions, enumerated lists of the instruments used, as well as information about structure refinement.

Data processing statistics

Production processing of PDB entries by the RCSB began on January 27, 1999. The median time from deposition to the completion of data processing including author interactions is less than 10 days. The number of structures with a HOLD release status remains at ~22% of all submissions; 28% are held until publication; and 50% are released immediately after processing.

When the RCSB became fully responsible there were about 900 structures that had not been completely processed. These included so called Layer 1 structures that had been processed by computer software but had not been fully annotated. All of

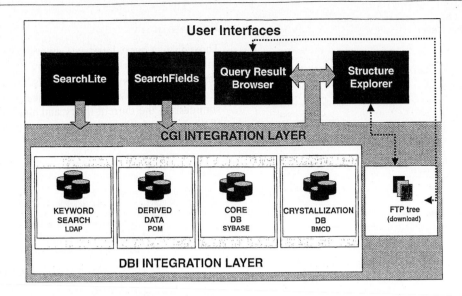

Figure 3. The integrated query interface to the PDB.

these structures have now been processed and are being released after author review.

The breakdown of the types of structures in the PDB is shown in Table 2. As of September 14, 1999, the PDB contained 10 714 publicly accessible structures with another 1169 entries on hold. Of these, 8789 (82%) were determined by X-ray methods, 1692 (16%) were determined by NMR and 233 (2%) were theoretical models. Overall, 35% of the entries have deposited experimental data.

Table 2. Demographics of data in the PDB

Experimental Technique	Molecule Type				
	Proteins, Peptides, and Viruses	Protein-Nucleic Acid Complexes	Nucleic Acids	Carbohydrates and Other	Total
X-ray Diffraction and Other	7946	390	439	14	8789
NMR	1365	53	270	4	1692
Theoretical Modeling	202	16	15	0	233
Total	9513	459	724	18	10714

Data uniformity

A key goal of the PDB is to make the archive as consistent and error-free as possible. All current depositions are reviewed carefully by the staff before release. Tables of features are generated from the internal data processing database and checked. Errors found subsequent to release by authors and PDB users are addressed as rapidly as possible. Corrections and updates to entries should be sent to deposit@rcsb.rutgers.edu for the changes to be implemented and re-released into the PDB archive.

One of the most difficult problems that the PDB now faces is that the legacy files are not uniform. Historically, existing data ('legacy data') comply with several different PDB formats and variation exists in how the same features are described for different structures within each format. The introduction of the

advanced querying capabilities of the PDB makes it critical to accelerate the data uniformity process for these data. We are now at a stage where the query capabilities surpass the quality of the underlying data. The data uniformity project is being approached in two ways. Families of individual structures are being reprocessed using ADIT. The strategy of processing data files as groups of similar structures facilitates the application of biological knowledge by the annotators. In addition, we are examining particular records across all entries in the archive. As an example, we have recently completed examining and correcting the chemical descriptions of all of the ligands in the PDB. These corrections are being entered in the database. The practical consequence of this is that soon it will be possible to accurately find all the structures in the PDB bound to a particular ligand or ligand type. In addition to the efforts of the PDB to remediate the older entries, the EBI has also corrected many of the records in the PDB as part of their 'clean-up' project. The task of integrating all of these corrections done at both sites is very large and it is essential that there is a well-defined exchange format to do this; mmCIF will be used for this purpose.

THE PDB DATABASE RESOURCE

The database architecture

In recognition of the fact that no single architecture can fully express and efficiently make available the information content of the PDB, an integrated system of heterogeneous databases has been created that store and organize the structural data. At present there are five major components (Fig. 3):

- The core relational database managed by Sybase (Sybase SQL server release 11.0, Emeryville, CA) provides the central physical storage for the primary experimental and coordinate data described in Table 1. The core PDB relational database contains all deposited information in a tabular form that can be accessed across any number of structures.

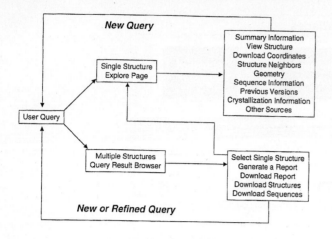

Figure 4. The various query options that are available for the PDB.

- The final curated data files (in PDB and mmCIF formats) and data dictionaries are the archival data and are present as ASCII files in the ftp archive.
- The POM (Property Object Model)-based databases, which consist of indexed objects containing native (e.g., atomic coordinates) and derived properties (e.g., calculated secondary structure assignments and property profiles). Some properties require no derivation, for example, B factors; others must be derived, for example, exposure of each amino acid residue (13) or Cα contact maps. Properties requiring significant computation time, such as structure neighbors (14), are pre-calculated when the database is incremented to save considerable user access time.
- The Biological Macromolecule Crystallization Database (BMCD; 15) is organized as a relational database within Sybase and contains three general categories of literature derived information: macromolecular, crystal and summary data.
- The Netscape LDAP server is used to index the textual content of the PDB in a structured format and provides support for keyword searches.

It is critical that the intricacies of the underlying physical databases be transparent to the user. In the current implementation, communication among databases has been accomplished using the Common Gateway Interface (CGI). An integrated Web interface dispatches a query to the appropriate database(s), which then execute the query. Each database returns the PDB identifiers that satisfy the query, and the CGI program integrates the results. Complex queries are performed by repeating the process and having the interface program perform the appropriate Boolean operation(s) on the collection of query results. A variety of output options are then available for use with the final list of selected structures.

The CGI approach [and in the future a CORBA (Common Object Request Broker Architecture)-based approach] will permit other databases to be integrated into this system, for example extended data on different protein families. The same approach could also be applied to include NMR data found in the BMRB or data found in other community databases.

Database query

Three distinct query interfaces are available for the query of data within PDB: Status Query (http://www.rcsb.org/pdb/status.html), SearchLite (http://www.rcsb.org/pdb/searchlite.html) and Search-Fields (http://www.rscb.org/pdb/queryForm.cgi). Table 3 summarizes the current query and analysis capabilities of the PDB. Figure 4 illustrates how the various query options are organized.

Table 3. Current query capabilities of the PDB

Query Options	
SearchLite	Any word or combination of words in the PDB
SearchFields	*General information*: PDB identifier, citation author, chain type (protein, DNA etc.), PDB HEADER, experimental technique, deposition/release date, citation, compound information, EC number, text search
	Sequence and secondary structure: chain length, FASTA search, short sequence pattern, secondary structure content
	Crystallographic experimental information: resolution, space group, unit cell dimensions, parameters
Status	PDB identifier, deposition author, title, holding status, deposition date, release date
Result Analysis	
Single Structure: Structure Explorer	
Summary	Compound name, authors, experimental method, classification, source, primary citation, deposition date, release date, resolution, R-value, space group, unit cell parameters, polymer chain identifiers, number of residues, HET groups, number of atoms
View Structure	VRML, RasMol, QuickPDB (Java Applet), Chime, still images
Download/Display file	HTML and text formats for display; PDB and mmCIF formats with different compression options for download
Structural Neighbors	List of sites for finding structural homologues
Geometry	Unusual dihedral angles, bond angles and bond lengths
Other Sources	Links to other sources of information (Table 4)
Sequence Details	Chain Ids, number of residues per chain, molecular weight, chain type, secondary structure assignment; download sequence only in FASTA format
Crystallization Information	Conditions under which the crystals were obtained
Previous versions	Versions of the structure replaced by the current version if applicable
Nucleic Acid Database Atlas Entry	Detailed information from the Nucleic Acid Database (NDB) if applicable
Quick Report	Nucleic acid geometry if applicable
Structure Factors	Experimental data if available
Multiple Structure: Results Browser	
Summary List	Deposition date, resolution, experimental method, classification, compound name
Download Structures or Sequences	mmCIF and PDB compressed files (gzip, tar, compressed); sequences in FASTA format
Query Refinement	Iterative query over result set using OR, AND or NOT Boolean logic
Tabular Report	Cell dimensions, primary citation, structure identifiers, sequence, experimental details, refinement details
Query Review	Summary of queries submitted thus far with the option to return

SearchLite, which provides a single form field for keyword searches, was introduced in February 1999. All textual information within the PDB files as well as dates and some experimental data are accessible via simple or structured queries. Search-Fields, accessible since May 1999, is a customizable query form that allows searching over many different data items including compound, citation authors, sequence (via a FASTA search; 16) and release or deposition dates.

Two user interfaces provide extensive information for result sets from SearchLite or SearchFields queries. The 'Query Result Browser' interface allows for access to some general information, more detailed information in tabular format, and the possibility to download whole sets of data files for result sets consisting of multiple PDB entries. The 'Structure Explorer' interface provides information about individual structures as well as cross-links to many external resources for macromolecular structure data (Table 4). Both interfaces are accessible to other data resources through the simple CGI application programmer interface (API) described at http://www.rcsb.org/pdb/linking.html

Table 4. Static cross-links to other data resources currently provided by the PDB

Resource	Information Content
3dee (21)	Structural domain definitions
BMCD (15)	Crystallization information about biomacromolecules
CATH (22)	Protein fold classification
CE (14)	Complete PDB and representative structure comparison and alignments
DSSP (23)	Secondary structure classification
Enzyme Structures Database (http://www.biochem.ucl.ac.uk/bsm/enzymes/)	Enzyme classifications and nomenclature
FSSP (24)	Structurally similar families
GRASS (25)	Graphical representation and analysis
HSSP (26)	Homology derived secondary structures
Image (27)	Image library of biological macromolecules
MMDB (28)	Database of three dimensional structures
Medline (http://www.nlm.nih.gov/databases/medline.html)	Direct access to Medline at NCBI
NDB (29)	Database of three dimensional nucleic acid structures
PDBObs (30)	Obsolete structures database
PDBSum (31)	Summary information about protein structures
SCOP (32)	Structure classifications
STING (33)	Simultaneous display of structural and sequence information
Tops (34)	Protein structure motif comparisons topological diagrams
VAST (35)	Vector Alignment Search Tool (NCBI)
Whatcheck (36)	Protein structure checks

The website usage has climbed dramatically since the system was first introduced in February 1999 (Table 5). As of November 1, 1999, the main PDB site receives, on average, greater than one hit per second and greater than one query per minute.

Table 5. Web query statistics for the primary RCSB site (http://www.rcsb.org)

Month	Daily Avg		Monthly Totals			
	Hits	Files	Sites	Kbytes	Files	Hits
August 99	63768	47675	34928	31781561	1477927	1976818
July 99	75693	54427	38698	35652864	1687265	2346495
June 99	33256	27054	11586	11164410	622264	764894
May 99	26890	22085	12405	12463441	684650	833597
April 99	21140	17099	12261	9925351	512990	634224
March 99	8406	6911	6292	3560629	214255	260610
February 99	2944	2433	2246	844536	68133	82453
January 99	1563	1353	1153	92014	35202	40641

DATA DISTRIBUTION

The PDB distributes coordinate data, structure factor files and NMR constraint files. In addition it provides documentation and derived data. The coordinate data are distributed in PDB and mmCIF formats. Currently, the PDB file is created as the final product of data annotation; the program pdb2cif (17) is used to generate the mmCIF data. This program is used to accommodate the legacy data. In the future, both the mmCIF and PDB format files created during data annotation will be distributed.

Data are distributed to the community in the following ways:
- From primary PDB Web and ftp sites at UCSD, Rutgers and NIST that are updated weekly.
- From complete Web-based mirror sites that contain all databases, data files, documentation and query interfaces updated weekly.
- From ftp-only mirror sites that contain a complete or subset copy of data files, updated at intervals defined by the mirror site. The steps necessary to create an ftp-only mirror site are described in http://www.rcsb.org/pdb/ftpproc.final.html
- Quarterly CD-ROM.

Data are distributed once per week. New data officially become available at 1 a.m. PST each Wednesday. This follows the tradition developed by BNL and has minimized the impact of the transition on existing mirror sites. Since May 1999, two ftp archives have been provided: ftp://ftp.rcsb.org , a reorganized and more logical organization of all PDB data, software, and documentation; and ftp://bnlarchive.rcsb.org , a near-identical copy of the original BNL archive which is maintained for purposes of backward compatibility. RCSB-style PDB mirrors have been established in Japan (Osaka University), Singapore (National University Hospital) and in UK (the Cambridge Crystallographic Data Centre). Plans call for operating mirrors in Brazil, Australia, Canada, Germany, and possibly India.

The first PDB CD-ROM distribution by the RCSB contained the coordinate files, experimental data, software and documentation as found in the PDB on June 30, 1999. Data are currently distributed as compressed files using the compression utility program gzip. Refer to http://www.rcsb.org/pdb/cdrom.html for details of how to order CD-ROM sets. There is presently no charge for this service.

DATA ARCHIVING

The PDB is establishing a central Master Archiving facility. The Master Archive plan is based on five goals: reconstruction of the current archive in case of a major disaster; duplication of the contents of the PDB as it existed on a specific date; preservation of software, derived data, ancillary data and all other computerized and printed information; automatic archiving of all depositions and the PDB production resource; and maintenance of the PDB correspondence archive that documents all aspects of deposition. During the transition period, all physical materials including electronic media and hard copy materials were inventoried and stored, and are being catalogued.

MAINTENANCE OF THE LEGACY BNL SYSTEM

One of the goals of the PDB has been to provide a smooth transition from the system at BNL to the new system. Accordingly, AutoDep, which was developed by BNL (18) for data deposition, has been ported to the RCSB site and enables depositors to complete in-progress depositions as well as to make new depositions. In addition, the EBI accepts data using AutoDep. Similarly, the programs developed at BNL for data query and distribution (PDBLite, 3DBbrowser, etc.) are being maintained by the remaining BNL-style mirrors. The RCSB provides data in a form usable by these mirrors. Finally the style and format of the BNL ftp archive is being maintained at ftp://bnlarchive.rcsb.org

A multitude of resources and programs depend upon their links to the PDB. To eliminate the risk of interruption to these services, links to the PDB at BNL were automatically redirected to the RCSB after BNL closed operations on June 30, 1999 using

Table 6. PDB information sources

Source	Information Content
http://www.rcsb.org/pdb/	Main PDB Web site
http://rutgers.rcsb.edu/pdb/ (Rutgers) http://nist.rcsb.org/pdb/ (NIST)	RCSB member institution PDB Web sites
http://rutgers.rcsb.org/pdb/mirrors.html	List of all RCSB PDB Mirrors
http://pdb.rutgers.edu/adit/	ADIT Web site
http://pdb.rutgers.edu/validate/	ADIT Validation Server
http://www.rcsb.org/pdb/newsletter/index.html	RCSB PDB Newsletter
http://www.rcsb.org/pdb/linking.html	Enzyme classifications and nomenclature
http://www.rcsb.org/pdb/ftpproc.final.html	FTP mirroring information
http://www.rcsb.org/pdb/cdrom.html	CD-ROM ordering information
info@rcsb.org	General help desk
deposit@rcsb.rutgers.edu	Data processing correspondence

a network redirect implemented jointly by RCSB and BNL staff. While this redirect will be maintained, external resources linking to the PDB are advised to change any URLs from http://www.pdb.bnl.gov/ to http://www.rcsb.org/

CURRENT DEVELOPMENTS

In the coming months, the PDB plans to continue to improve and develop all aspects of data processing. Deposition will be made easier, and annotation will be more automated. In addition, software for data deposition and validation will be made available for in-laboratory use.

The PDB will also continue to develop ways of exchanging information between databases. The PDB is leading the Object Management Group Life Sciences Initiative's efforts to define a CORBA interface definition for the representation of macromolecular structure data. This is a standard developed under a strict procedure to ensure maximum input by members of various academic and industrial research communities. At this stage, proposals for the interface definition, including a working prototype that uses the standard, are being accepted. For further details refer to http://www.omg.org/cgi-bin/doc?lifesci/ 99-08-15 . The finalized standard interface will facilitate the query and exchange of structural information not just at the level of complete structures, but at finer levels of detail. The standard being proposed by the PDB will conform closely to the mmCIF standard. It is recognized that other forms of data representation are desirable, for example using eXtensible Markup Language (XML). The PDB will continue to work with mmCIF as the underlying standard from which CORBA and XML representations can be generated as dictated by the needs of the community.

The PDB will also develop the means and methods of communications with the broad PDB user community via the Web. To date we have developed prototype protein documentaries (19) that explore this new medium in describing structure–function relationships in proteins. It is also possible to develop educational materials that will run using a recent Web browser (20).

Finally it is recognized that structures exist both in the public and private domains. To this end we are planning on providing a subset of database tools for local use. Users will be able to load both public and proprietary data and use the same search and exploratory tools used at PDB resources.

The PDB does not exist in isolation, rather each structure represents a point in a spectrum of information that runs from the recognition of an open reading frame to a fully understood role of the single or multiple biological functions of that molecule. The available information that exists on this spectrum changes over time. Recognizing this, the PDB has developed a scheme for the dynamic update of a variety of links on each structure to whatever else can be automatically located on the Internet. This information is itself stored in a database and can be queried. This feature will appear in the coming months to supplement the existing list of static links to a small number of the more well known related Internet resources.

PDB ADVISORY BOARDS

The PDB has several advisory boards. Each member institution of the RCSB has its own local PDB Advisory Committee. Each institution is responsible for implementing the recommendations of those committees, as well as the recommendations of an International Advisory Board. Initially, the RCSB presented a report to the Advisory Board previously convened by BNL. At their recommendation, a new Board has been approached which contains previous members and new members. The goal was to have the Board accurately reflect the depositor and user communities and thus include experts from many disciplines.

Serious issues of policy are referred to the major scientific societies, notably the IUCr. The goal is to make decisions based on input from a broad international community of experts. The IUCr maintains the mmCIF dictionary as the data standard upon which the PDB is built.

FOR FURTHER INFORMATION

The PDB seeks to keep the community informed of new developments via weekly news updates to the Web site, quarterly newsletters, and a soon to be initiated annual report. Users can request information at any time by sending mail to info@rcsb. org . Finally, the pdb-l@rcsb.org listserver provides a community forum for the discussion of PDB-related issues. Changes to PDB operations that may affect the community, for example, data format changes, are posted here and users have 60 days to discuss the issue before changes are made according to major consensus. Table 6 indicates how to access these resources.

CONCLUSION

These are exciting and challenging times to be responsible for the collection, curation and distribution of macromolecular structure data. Since the RCSB assumed responsibility for data deposition in February 1999, the number of depositions has averaged approximately 50 per week. However, with the advent of a number of structure genomics initiatives worldwide this number is likely to increase. We estimate that the PDB, which at this writing contains approximately 10 500 structures, could triple or quadruple in size over the next 5 years. This presents a challenge to timely distribution while maintaining high quality. The PDB's approach of using modern data management practices should permit us to scale to accommodate a large data influx.

The maintenance and further development of the PDB are community efforts. The willingness of others to share ideas, software and data provides a depth to the resource not obtainable otherwise. Some of these efforts are acknowledged below. New input is constantly being sought and the PDB invites you to make comments at any time by sending electronic mail to info@rcsb.org

ACKNOWLEDGEMENTS

Research Collaboratory for Structural Bioinformatics (RCSB) is a consortium consisting of three institutions: Rutgers University, San Diego Supercomputer Center at University of California, San Diego, and the National Institute of Standards and Technology. The current RCSB PDB staff include the authors indicated and Kyle Burkhardt, Anke Gelbin, Michael Huang, Shri Jain, Rachel Kramer, Nate Macapagal, Victoria Colflesh, Bohdan Schneider, Kata Schneider, Christine Zardecki (Rutgers); Phoebe Fagan, Diane Hancock, Narmada Thanki, Michael Tung, Greg Vasquez (NIST); Peter Arzberger, John Badger, Douglas S. Greer, Michael Gribskov, John Kowalski, Glen Otero, Shawn Strande, Lynn F. Ten Eyck, Kenneth Yoshimoto (UCSD). The continuing support of Ken Breslauer (Rutgers), John Rumble (NIST) and Sid Karin (SDSC) is gratefully acknowledged. Current collaborators contributing to the future development of the PDB are the BioMagResBank, the Cambridge Crystallographic Data Centre, the HIV Protease Database Group, The Institute for Protein Research, Osaka University, National Center for Biotechnology Information, the ReLiBase developers, and the Swiss Institute for Bioinformatics/Glaxo. We are especially grateful to Kim Henrick of the EBI and Steve Bryant at NCBI who have reviewed our files and sent back constructive criticisms. This has helped the PDB to continuously improve its procedures for producing entries. The cooperation of the BNL PDB staff is gratefully acknowledged. Portions of this article will appear in Volume F of the International Tables of Crystallography. This work is supported by grants from the National Science Foundation, the Office of Biology and Environmental Research at the Department of Energy, and two units of the National Institutes of Health: the National Institute of General Medical Sciences and the National Institute of Medicine.

REFERENCES

1. Bernstein,F.C., Koetzle,T.F., Williams,G.J., Meyer,E.E., Brice,M.D., Rodgers,J.R., Kennard,O., Shimanouchi,T. and Tasumi,M. (1977) *J. Mol. Biol.*, **112**, 535–542.
2. Bourne,P., Berman,H.M., Watenpaugh,K., Westbrook,J.D. and Fitzgerald,P.M.D. (1997) *Methods Enzymol.*, **277**, 571–590.
3. Westbrook,J. and Bourne,P.E. (2000) *Bioinformatics*, in press.
4. Markley,J.L., Bax,A., Arata,Y., Hilbers,C.W., Kaptein,R., Sykes,B.D., Wright,P.E. and Wüthrich,K. (1998) *J. Biomol. NMR*, **12**, 1–23.
5. Engh,R.A. and Huber,R. (1991) *Acta Crystallogr.*, **A47**, 392–400.
6. Clowney,L., Jain,S.C., Srinivasan,A.R., Westbrook,J., Olson,W.K. and Berman,H.M. (1996) *J. Am. Chem. Soc.*, **118**, 509–518.
7. Gelbin,A., Schneider,B., Clowney,L., Hsieh,S.-H., Olson,W.K. and Berman,H.M. (1996) *J. Am. Chem. Soc.*, **118**, 519–528.
8. IUPAC–IUB Joint Commission on Biochemical Nomenclature (1983) *Eur. J. Biochem.*, **131**, 9–15.
9. Zhang,J., Cousens,L.S., Barr,P.J. and Sprang,S.R. (1991) *Proc. Natl Acad. Sci. USA*, **88**, 3346–3450.
10. Laskowski,R.A., McArthur,M.W., Moss,D.S. and Thornton,J.M. (1993) *J. Appl. Crystallogr.*, **26**, 283–291.
11. Vaguine,A.A., Richelle,J. and Wodak,S.J. (1999) *Acta Crystallogr.*, **D55**, 191–205.
12. Ulrich,E.L., Markley,J.L and Kyogoku,Y. (1989) *Protein Seq. Data Anal.*, **2**, 23–37.
13. Lee,B. and Richards,F.M. (1971) *J. Mol. Biol.*, **55**, 379–400.
14. Shindyalov,I.N. and Bourne,P.E. (1998) *Protein Eng.*, **11**, 739–747.
15. Gilliland,G.L. (1988) *J. Cryst. Growth*, **90**, 51–59.
16. Pearson,W.R. and Lipman,D.J. (1988) *Proc. Natl Acad. Sci. USA*, **24**, 2444–2448.
17. Bernstein,H.J., Bernstein,F.C. and Bourne,P.E. (1998) *J. Appl. Crystallogr.*, **31**, 282–295.
18. Laboratory,B.N. (1998) AutoDep, version 2.1. Upton, NY.
19. Quinn,G., Taylor,A., Wang,H.-P. and Bourne,P.E. (1999) *Trends Biochem. Sci.*, **24**, 321–324.
20. Quinn,G., Wang,H.-P., Martinez,D. and Bourne,P.E. (1999) *Pacific Symp. Biocomput.*, 380–391.
21. Siddiqui,A. and Barton,G. (1996) Perspectives on Protein Engineering 1996, 2, (CD-ROM edition; Geisow,M.J. ed.) BIODIGM Ltd (UK). ISBN 0-9529015-0-1.
22. Orengo,C.A., Michie,A.D., Jones,S., Jones,D.T., Swindels,M.B. and Thornton,J.M. (1997) *Structure*, **5**, 1093–1108.
23. Kabsch,W. and Sander,C. (1983) *Biopolymers*, **22**, 2277–2637.
24. Holm,L. and Sander,C. (1998) *Nucleic Acids Res.*, **26**, 316–319.
25. Nayal,M., Hitz,B.C. and Honig,B. (1999) *Protein Sci.*, **8**, 676–679.
26. Dodge,C., Schneider,R. and Sander,C. (1998) *Nucleic Acids Res.*, **26**, 313–315.
27. Suhnel,J. (1996) *Comput. Appl. Biosci.*, **12**, 227–229.
28. Hogue,C., Ohkawa,H. and Bryant,S. (1996) *Trends Biochem. Sci.*, **21**, 226–229.
29. Berman,H.M., Olson,W.K., Beveridge,D.L., Westbrook,J., Gelbin,A., Demeny,T., Hsieh,S.H., Srinivasan,A.R. and Schneider,B. (1992) *Biophys. J.*, **63**, 751–759.
30. Weissig,H., Shindyalov,I.N. and Bourne,P.E. (1998) *Acta Crystallogr.*, **D54**, 1085–1094.
31. Laskowski,R.A., Hutchinson,E.G., Michie,A.D., Wallace,A.C., Jones,M.L. and Thornton,J.M. (1997) *Trends Biochem. Sci.*, **22**, 488–490.
32. Murzin,A.G., Brenner,S.E., Hubbard,T. and Chothia,C. (1995) *J. Mol. Biol.*, **247**, 536–540.
33. Neshich,G., Togawa,R., Vilella,W. and Honig,B. (1998) Protein Data Bank Quarterly Newsletter, 84.
34. Westhead,D., Slidel,T., Flores,T. and Thornton,J. (1998) *Protein Sci.*, **8**, 897–904.
35. Gibrat,J.-F., Madej,T. and Bryant,S.H. (1996) *Curr. Opin. Struct. Biol.*, **6**, 377–385.
36. Hooft,R.W.W., Sander,C. and Vriend,G. (1996) *J. Appl. Crystallogr.*, **29**, 714–716.

Online identification of viruses

A.S. Kolaskar[1,2], P.S. Naik[1]

[1]Bioinformatics Centre, University of Pune, Pune, India; and [2]Bioinformatics, American Type Culture Collection, Manassas, USA

Received: May 4, 1999 Revised: February 17, 2000 Accepted: February 24, 2000

A computerized animal virus information system is developed in the Sequence Retrieval System (SRS) format. This database is available on the Word Wide Web (WWW) at the site http://bioinfo.ernet.in/www/avis/avis.html. The database has been used to generate large number of identification matrices for each family. The software is developed in C.Unix shell scripts and Hypertext Marked-up Language (HTML) to assign the family to an unknown virus deterministically and to identify the virus probabilistically. It has been shown that such web based virus identification approach provides results with high confidence in those cases where identification matrix uses large number of independent characters. Protein sequence data for animal viruses have been analyzed and oligopeptides specific to each virus family and also specific to each virus species are identified for several viruses. These peptides thus could be used to identify the virus and to assign the virus family with high confidence showing the usefulness of sequence data in virus identification.

Key words: Virus identification, web based

In the microbial world, viruses the obligate parasites have established themselves as very important biological species. Viruses require hosts for their growth and reproduction, which could be bacteria, plants and animals. Thus, the nature and characteristics of viruses differ. Based on the hosts, viruses are categorized as animal viruses, plant viruses and phages. Further, the distinctive features among the macro characters as well as differences at molecular level have helped the taxonomists to classify known viruses into 184 genera and 54 families [1]. Most of the classification of viruses is carried out at the species level and macro character values are generally used for their classification. In very rare cases, molecular properties, particularly the sequences of oligopeptides/oligonucleotides are used for classification and identification [2]. One of the main reasons for such a lacuna is nonavailability of comprehensive data on viruses at one place that the experts can use to formulate rules of classification.

Identification and classification of viruses is of paramount importance not only because of its esoteric nature, but because these viruses cause serious damage to crops, animal and human health as well as environment. Design of control strategy is possible only if the identification is done at an early stage. Though

viruses have played an important role in early development of molecular biology, the role/function of several viruses is still unknown. For example, Herpesvirus 6 is present in most Indian population in an inactivated form and causes no damage. Activated Herpesvirus 6 in an human immunodeficiency virus (HIV) positive mother seems to help in transmitting HIV. The coexistence of more than one virus and thus the function of these viruses in the presence of each other are still not understood and studied.

In the light of the above mentioned facts a computerized database on animal viruses called the Animal Virus Information System (AVIS) was created at our center in the University of Pune, India and is available at the web site: http://bioinfo.ernet.in/www/avis/avis.html [3]. This database was used to develop a computerized method to identify the virus on the World Wide Web (WWW). This approach is discussed in succeeding sections.

Materials and Methods

AVIS database

The information on viruses in AVIS is at two main levels: alphanumeric information and pictorial information. Pictorial information contains mostly high-resolution electron micrographic pictures of the viruses. The alphanumeric information is broadly divided into 17 different categories as given in table 1. The experts

Corresponding author: Dr. A.S. Kolaskar, Bioinformatics Centre, University of Pune, Pune 411007, India.

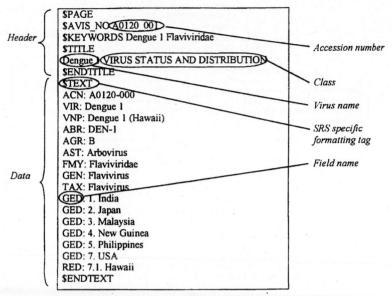

Fig. 1. Record of AVIS formatted for SRS. The example for the VIRUS STATUS AND DISTRIBUTION record of the Dengue 1 virus.

verify the data and thus the correctness of the data is maintained. Data is updated regularly by searching the literature using keywords in an automatic fashion.

The information on about 1700 animal viruses is organized in the Sequence Retrieval System (SRS) format and implemented on the web using the SRS search engine. SRS was developed at the European Bioinformatics Institute, UK [4]. SRS is considered as one of the standard formats to access biological databases on the web and several databases including the nucleic acid and protein sequence databases are available in this format. SRS uses the "Icarus" scripting language to parse flat file databases. SRS produces almost all of the query reports dynamically for the web. SRS also allows linking of other databases loaded on the computer system. The SRS formatted database file of AVIS was indexed with the indexing programs available with the SRS package and was loaded on the computer. The record structure of the AVIS database in the SRS format is given in figure 1.

The AVIS also contains two subdatabases: (i) Database containing all viral nucleic acids sequences. This information is extracted from Genbank and European Molecular Biology Laboratory (EMBL) databases of nucleic acids sequences. The data is organized in the Genbank format. (ii) Database consists of virus protein sequences. These sequences are extracted from NBRF-PIR and Swiss-Prot and organized in the NBRF-PIR format. The protein sequence information is organized under the virus family. Conversion of sequence data into the NBRF-PIR format allows the data analysis to be carried out using PSQ and NAQ software that is available in the public domain, and also available along with the ATLAS CDs from PIR International [5]. In order to use these software along with the virus sequence data in the web environment, necessary utilities were written using the Unix shell script language.

Virus identification

The software has been developed to identify viruses online through the web. The software developed for virus identification uses the schema given in figure 2. As can be seen from figure 2, the process of

Table 1. Classes created for the virus database

No.	Classes
1	Virus status and distribution
2	Original source of the virus
3	Method of isolation and validity
4	Physicochemical properties
5	Stability of infectivity and virulence
6	Virion morphology
7	Morphogenesis
8	Hemagglutination
9	Antigenic relationship
10	Susceptibility of cell systems
11	Natural Host range
12	Experimental viremia
13	Histopathology
14	Human disease
15	Links with other data banks
16	Pictorial information
17	References

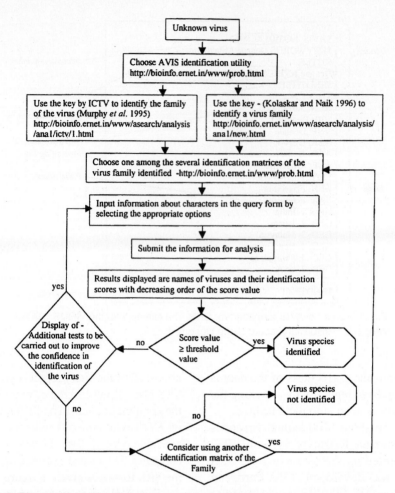

Fig. 2. Diagram illustrating the computer aided identification of viruses on the WWW.

identification has been divided into two parts: (i) assignment of the family uses a deterministic approach and (ii) identification of a virus species using a probabilistic approach.

The software consists of two main modules, input module and the compute module. The input module consists of three components: (i) input for identification of a virus family, (ii) input of character values to create identification matrix and (iii) direct input of identification matrix developed by the user. In each of these cases, a predesigned screen allows an user to feed in the data, by clicking one of the possible alternatives. These pop-up screens are user-friendly. The programs are written in HTML and Unix Shell scripts. The compute module is divided into three parts: (i) assignment of the virus family, (ii) creation of the identification matrix, and (iii) identification of the virus species and display of results. The programs for the compute module are written in Unix shell scripts and C.

The assignment of the family to the unknown virus is carried out deterministically using the key given in

figure 3. The character-based keys using neg-entropy as a measure were developed. Use of such characters showed that only 12 characters are necessary and sufficient to identify one of the 25 animal virus families [6] (Table 2). The International Committee on Taxonomy of Viruses (ICTV) has also developed the keys giving higher importance to (i) nature of viral genome, (ii) the strandedness of the viral genome and (iii) the replication strategy of the virus [7]. These ICTV keys can also be used to assign the family. The software developed allows choice of any one of the above methods.

Only after virus family is assigned, the process of virus identification is continued. To carry out virus identification, the first step is to create identification matrices for each family using the characters those provide high resolution and thus have different values for different viruses. Development of such matrices is described in detail in our earlier communication [8], but the brief outline of the method used with an example is given in figure 4.

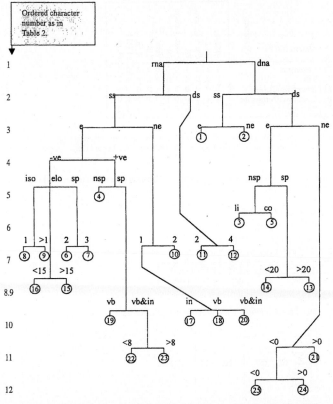

Fig. 3. A tree drawn using 12 ordered characters as given in table 2. The short-form given here are explained in table 2. The Families identified are represented as encircled numbers and correspond to the superscripts in table 2. Note that the tree has 22 nodes and a maximum of 7 steps to identify any family.

Assignment of virus family using sequence data

For viruses belonging to each family, a study has been carried out to find out which protein is sequenced for most of the members of the family. For each family, multiple alignment was carried out for available protein sequences using CLUSTALW [9]. The bias and penalty

Table 2. Hierarchically ordered characters used to form identification key

SL No.	Ordered characters	Families identified	
		Number	Name
1	RNA/DNA (rna/dna)	0	
2	Double/Single stranded (ds/ss)	0	
3	Enveloped/Nonenveloped (e/ne)	2	*Polydnaviridae*[1], *Parvoviridae*[2]
4	RNA -ve sense/+ve sense (-ve/+ve)	0	
5	Virion shape isometric/ elongated/nonspherical/spherical (iso/elo/nsp/sp)	2	*Herpesviridae*[3], *Coronaviridae*[4]
6	Genome linear/coiled (li/co)	1	*Baculoviridae*[5]
7	No. of genome segments (1/> 1/2/3/4)	7	*Arenaviridae*[6], *Bunyaviridae*[7], *Paramyxoviridae*[8], *Orthomyxoviridae*[9], *Nodaviridae*[10], *Birnaviridae*[11], *Reoviridae*[12]
8	DNA size in kb (< 20/> 20)	2	*Poxviridae*[13], *Hepednaviridae*[14]
9	RNA size in kb (< 15/> 15)	2	*Filoviridae*[15], *Rhabdoviridae*[16]
10	Host type vertebrate/insect/ vertebrate + insect (in/vb/vb & in)	4	*Tetraviridae*[17], *Caliciviridae*[18], *Retroviridae*[19], *Picornaviridae*[20]
11	Percentage Carbohydrate content (< 0/> 0 & < 8/> 8)	3	*Adenoviridae*[21], *Togaviridae*[22], *Flaviviridae*[23]
12	Percentage Lipid content (< 0/> 0)	2	*Iridoviridae*[24], *Papovaviridae*[25]

Note: The animal virus family identified using these ordered keys is also given.

Viruses (OTUs)	Characters	BHK-21	BS-C1	Chick embryo	PK	Mouse embryo	PS	Vero	KB	SPIK	MA111	PK15
P1	Uukuniemi	1	1	1	1	0	0	0	0	0	0	0
P2	Sabo	1	0	0	0	1	0	0	0	0	0	0
P3	Jamestown Canyon	1	0	0	0	0	1	1	0	0	0	0
P4	California Encephalitis	0	1	1	0	0	1	0	1	1	0	0
P5	Buttonwillow	1	0	0	0	0	1	1	0	1	1	1

The data is represented as follows : The cytopathic effects observed on these cell lines by the five chosen viruses are represented as : 1 for yes, 0 for no and unknown. Number of OTUS = n = 5

The distances dP_k dP_1 is obtained by calculating the Euclidean distances of the viruses by using the Jaccard's coefficent is :

dP_1	0.00				
dP_2	0.89	0.00			
dP_3	0.91	0.86	0.00		
dP_4	0.84	1.00	0.92	0.00	
dP_5	0.94	0.92	0.70	0.88	0.00
	dP_1	dP_2	dP_3	dP_4	dP_5

The average distance for the P_kth row with respect to other OTUs is :

$$W_k = \left[\left[\sum_{\substack{l=1 \\ k \neq l}}^{n} dP_k\, dP_1 \right] / (n-1) \right] \cdot 100$$

Where dP_k dP_1 is the euclidean distance between $OTUP_k$ and $OTUP_1$

The resulting weight matrix obtained is as follows :

P1	89	89	89	89	01	01	01	01	01	01	01
P2	91	01	01	01	91	01	01	01	01	01	01
P3	84	01	01	01	01	84	84	01	01	01	01
P4	01	91	91	01	01	91	01	91	91	01	01
P5	86	01	01	01	01	86	86	01	86	86	86

Fig. 4. Procedure used to develop the Virus Identification Matrix in Probabilistic identification. An example of a few viruses of the *Bunyaviridae* family.

values are varied so as to get the best multiple alignment results [10]. Peptides, common in every virus of a given family or genus having a length greater than or equal to six was picked up. Such peptides are called "putative signature peptides" of the virus family or genus under study. Presence of each of these peptides in the whole database was studied through a program called MATCH. If the putative signature peptides were found to be present only in the viruses of the family/genus under study but absent in every other sequence in the whole data base even with three mismatches, then that peptide is called the signature peptide of the family/ genus. Unique peptides are obtained for 16 families by analyzing protein sequence data. These peptides are given in table 3. Such unique peptides thus can be used

to assign the family of the unknown virus.

Identification using signature peptides

Identification of a member virus of a particular family is possible with the use of signature sequences. This procedure can be used to confirm identification. Signature peptides were obtained for the members of the *Flavivirus* genus. The sequences of the envelope glycoprotein (Egp) of 19 *Flaviviruses* extracted from sequence databases were studied. In the multiple alignment program, a single linkage cluster is developed which brings two sequentially most similar proteins close together. Amino acid sequences of such most homologous protein pairs were aligned. By examining the alignment, an oligopeptide having at least 10 amino

Table 3. Unique peptide sequences for animal virus families obtained from analysis of virus protein sequence data

Family	Genus	Protein	Unique peptide
Togaviridae	*Alphavirus*	Structural polyprotein	AYEHXXV/TXPN
Filoviridae	*Filovirus*	Nucleocapsid protein	PQLSAIALGVAT AHGSTLAGVNV GEQYQQLREAA
Iridoviridae	*Lymphocystivirus* *Iridovirus*	Capsid protein	TSXFIDXAT IEKXXYGG
Papovaviridae	*Papillomavirus*	L1 protein	CKYPDF/Y GHPLF/YNKV/L
	Polyomavirus	Coat protein VP1	PDPXXNEN GVGPLCK QVEEVR
		Coat protein VP2	WXLPLXLGLYG
Arenaviridae	*Arenavirus*	Surface glycoprotein	MLXKEYXXRQXXTP PTHXHIXGXXCPXPHR LXLXGRSC
Flaviviridae	*Flavivirus*	Nonstructural protein 1 Envelope glycoprotein	CWYXMEIRP DRGWGNXCGXFGKG
Adenoviridae		Hexon protein	FKPYSGTA GVLAGQ PNYCFPL NPFNHHRN
Caliciviridae	*Calicivirus*	Coat protein	LXPXXNPYLXH SGSGVFGGKLAA MLQYPHVLFDARQ HGSIPSDLIP VFQXNRHFDF TXGWSTP PDGWPDTTI
Paramyxoviridae	*Paramyxovirus* *Morbillivirus*	Hemagglutinin neuraminidase Hemagglutinin	NRKSCS DVLTPLFKIIGDE
Picornaviridae	*Enterovirus* *Rhinovirus* *Hepatovirus* *Cardiovirus* *Apthovirus*	Genome polyprotein	DGYXXQXXXXXDD
Nodaviridae	*Nodavirus*	Coat protein precursor	FLKCAFA DPGKGIPD FRYASM
Parvoviridae	*Parvovirus* *Dependovirus*	Coat protein VP1	TPWXXXXXNXXXXXFXP
Orthomyxoviridae	Influenza-A Influenza-B Dhori	Nucleoprotein	GQIXXXPXFXXXR
	Influenza-C	Nucleoprotein	TQIXXXAXFXXXR
Hepadnaviridae	*Orthohepadnavirus*	Core antigen	EYLVSFGVWI
Herpesviridae	*Rhadinovirus* Major *Lymphocryptovirus*	Capsid protein	PXXYXXXXXXXXNXVTA GNXPXXLXPXXF
	Simplexvirus *Varicellavirus* *Betaherpesvirinae* *Cytomegalovirus*		HPGXXXTXVRXD
Birnaviridae	*Birnavirus*	Structural protein VP2	GPASIPD

Note: Single letter amino acid code is used x represent any amino acid.

Table 4. Identification matrices created for different virus families

Family	Type of identification matrices	No. of OTUs/ viruses in the matrix	No. of characters considered
Bunyaviridae	Cytopathic effects observed on cell lines	63	43
	Natural host range — mosquitoes	95	120
Rhabdoviridae	Natural host range	46	150
Togaviridae	Natural host	28	218
	Experimental viremia	28	21
	Cytopathic effects observed on cell lines	22	18
Reoviridae	Natural host range	62	124
Flaviviridae	Natural host range	62	278
	Experimental viremia	58	53
	Amino acid composition of envelope protein	14	20
	Amino acid composition of nucleocapsid protein	13	20
	Antigenic relationship	48	48
	Cytopathic effects observed on cell lines	52	18
	Human disease	28	27
Coronaviridae	Amino acid composition of nucleocapsid protein	10	20
Parvoviridae	Amino acid composition of coat protein VP1	8	20
Poxviridae	Amino acid composition of fusion protein	8	20

acid residues out of which at least four amino acids are different in two proteins were picked up. These unique peptides in the Egp of the virus are termed as candidate signature peptides. Using the program such as MATCH, a search was carried out to confirm its uniqueness, by allowing three mismatches. The initial search was carried out on related proteins, namely Egp of *Flaviviridae* family. Only after the uniqueness with three mismatches was established at this level, a search on the full database of protein sequences was carried out again by allowing three mismatches. If no other matching peptide was observed, then the peptide was termed as signature peptide.

Results

It has been observed that the software developed to identify a virus on the WWW can identify an unknown virus with a high degree of confidence [8]. Character based identification matrices have been prepared using AVIS to identify viruses belonging to different families. The list of identification matrices created for *Bunyaviridae, Rhabdoviridae, Togaviridae, Flaviviridae, Coronaviridae, Parvoviridae* and *Poxviridae* are listed in table 4. It can be seen from table 4 that seven different identification matrices are generated for *Flaviviridae* family. A combined matrix was also developed. Accuracy of identification of virus species in this family was almost 99%. This is because of our interest in development of vaccines against flaviviruses. The

usefulness of such matrix approach in identification of viruses was checked. Our results have shown that one can identify the virus with 99% accuracy provided the matrix is sufficiently large and prepared using independent character values. Additional matrices for various other families will soon be added to make the web based identification more useful to virologists. The users are requested to visit the web site http://bioinfo.ernet.in/www/prob.html at regular intervals to find out the new matrices.

Sequence information of viruses is increasing at a rapid rate. Peptides specific to each of the 16 animal virus families are identified from our analysis of protein sequence alignment approach. These virus family specific peptides are listed in the table 3. The proteins used to obtain the virus family specific peptides are also listed in this table. It can be seen from table 3 that wherever possible an attempt has been made to identify the genus specific peptide. For example the peptide NRKSCS from hemagglutinin neuraminidase is specific to genus *Paramyxovirus*. The peptide DVLTPLFKIIGDE from hemagglutinin is specific to genus *Morbillivirus*. Both these genus belong to virus family *Paramyxoviridae*. The peptides listed in the last column of table 3 are present only in the protein from the virus family under consideration and in no other protein present in the protein sequence data bank. Note that MATCH was run with zero mismatches. In most cases, more than one peptide are found to be unique

Table 5. Unique peptides for members of the family *Flaviviridae*

Virus	Unique peptide	Unique up to number of mismatches
St. Louis encephalitis virus	VNPFISTGGAN	3
	EGRPAT	0
Murray valley encephalitis virus	VTANPYVASSTA	3
Japanese encephalitis virus	LDVRMINIEA[S/V]Q	3
West Nile virus	TTKATGWIIQK	3
Kunjin virus	STKATGRTILKE	3
Langat virus	DGAEAWNEAGR	3
	FTCEDKK	0
	VGFSGTRP	0
Yellow fever virus	MRVTKDTN[D/G][N/S]NL	3
Powassan virus	KDNQDWNSVE	3
Dengue type 1 virus	GTVLVQV	0
Dengue type 2 virus	GTIVIRV	0
Dengue type 3 virus	TEATQL	0
	GTILIKV	0
Dengue type 4 virus	TTAKEVA	0
	GTTVVKV	0
Tick borne encephalitis virus	GFLTSVGKA	0
Louping ill virus	NPHWNNVER	0

Note: Peptides if unique up to 3 number of mismatches, they are termed as signature peptides. The peptides are from the envelope glycoproteins from the respective viruses.

and thus the presence of all these peptides in the proteins of the virus mentioned in this table helps to assign the virus family with high degree of confidence. Table 3 shows that one can use these unique peptides to assign the family of the virus for 16 virus families.

From the database Egp sequences of 19 *Flaviviruses* were extracted. In figure 5, conserved amino acids from all 19 Egps of the *Flaviviruses* are given. Figure 5 shows that the peptide [98]DRGWGNXCGXFGKG[111] is conserved (X represents any amino acid). As can be seen in figure 5, at position 104 though X is used to represent occurrence of any amino acid, only two amino acids occur namely glycine frequently and histidine rarely. In a similar fashion at position 107, leucine is highly preferred and in rare cases phenylalanine occurs though it is represented by X (Fig. 5). Occurrence of DRGWGNXCGXFGKG, in any other protein sequences in the PIR and Swiss-Prot databank was studied. Even with the allowance of three mismatches, the oligopeptide DRGWGNXCGXFGKG did not occur in any other protein except in Egps of *Flaviviruses*. This suggests that the above peptide can be used as a

signature of the genus *Flavivirus*.

Discussion

The animal virus information system AVIS has been analyzed and character values are grouped to form the identification matrix, an approach used by microbiologists for bacterial identification. It has been showed that this approach is equally useful in virus identification. As the quality and quantity of data on viruses increases and it gets captured in the structured computerized database the automatic generation of identification matrices with high resolution becomes easy. The method described here can be extended. The results of *Flaviviridae* family described support the statement that the probabilistic identification with high accuracy can be achieved. Molecular sequence data, from proteins and nucleic acids, that is rapidly accumulating has the potential to substantially improve the identification and taxonomy of viruses. The attempt described in this manuscript of analysis of protein sequences suggests that the method developed is useful and also sufficiently general. The results suggest that

```
  1234567890  1234567890  1234567890  1234567890

    G     D                                    T
--C-_---R-_  ---G--G---  ----LE---C  -T-----KP-_     40
    H     A                                    S

                                               E
-D--------  -------R--C  ----------  ---CP--G-_-     80
                                               P

  L E E                  G   L                K
-_-_-_-KR-----  -C-----DRG  WGN-_-CG-_-FGK  G----C-_--   120
  N                      H   F                M

         G          L     V             N
C-------_-  ------_-Y-  _----H----  -----_----    160
         L          I     I             N

                                Y
----------  ----------  -----_-G---  -C--------    200
                                F

                     W      HR   E D    L
----------  --------_-  V-_-W-_-_-L-  _-PW-------   240
                     F      DK   A N    Y

    W       V     P              E    G        A   G
---_----  -_-F--_-HA--  -----L--Q-_  _-----_-L-_-   280
    L       M     A              T    A        S   E

                        L            M L
----------  ------GH-_-  C---_-_--  --G--Y--C-     320
                        V            L V

               TQ G                         K P
----------  --_-_-_-T---  ---------P  C-_-_--     360
               SG D                         R A

             T N                       L       DS
----------  -_-_-P-----  -------_-E-  --P--_-I-     400
             S T                       V       EN

V        L                L                G       G
_-G-----_--  -W---GS-_-G  -----T--_  -R----_--A     440
I        I                I                R       R

   F                 K       F    Y    FG       W
WD-_-S-GG--  -S-G-_-----  _-G--_--_-S  G--_------    480
   L                 R       L    F              F

                 R S S                 L        V
G------G--  -_-_-_---  ---G-----_  ---_--      520
                 K T A                 M        C
```

Fig. 5. Conserved amino acids in the envelope glycoproteins of the 19 *Flaviviruses**. "Hyphen mark" indicates nonconserved position with more than 2 types of amino acid residues occurring at each of these positions. The results were obtained after multiple alignment of sequences of envelope glycoproteins. "Highlight" indicates amino acids which occur more than 80% in the alignment.

*Viruses considered: Dengue 1, Dengue 2, Dengue 3, Dengue 4, Japanese encephalitis, Kunjin, Murray Valley encephalitis, St. Louis encephalitis, Louping ill, Tick borne encephalitis, Langat, West Nile, Yellow fever, Negishi, Omsk hemorrhagic fever, Tyuleniy, Saumarez Reef, Kysanur forest disease and Powassan.

the confidence of assigning virus family using the oligopeptide sequence is high compared to identification of virus species using such an approach. The level of confidence in virus family assignment using family specific peptide goes higher when proteins from number of viruses belonging to a particular family. For example 116 protein sequences of 14 members of *Picornaviridae* family belonging to five genera were studied and the family specific peptide DGYXXQXXXXXDD was obtained. A virus polyprotein having this peptide has more than 95% chance to belong to *Picornaviridae*.

However, such a high level of confidence can not be assigned to few other families as protein sequences for few species of those families are available in the sequence databank. As the sequence data on virus increases the above approach becomes powerful and accurate.

The method to identify a virus using the virus species specific peptide is an extension of above approach. In this study one extract a peptide that is present only in that virus and does not exit in any other protein sequence. Unique or virus specific peptides obtained for members of the *Flaviviridae* family are given in table 5. It may be mentioned that one finds very high identity in the sequences of the Egp for the viruses, which are closely related. For example there is only 6% difference between the Egp of the viruses Tick borne encephalitis and Louping ill and thus it is difficult to pick-up virus specific oligopeptides.

Such oligopeptides could not be obtained for five out of the 19 viruses studied. Virus specific oligopeptides can be used as polymerase chain reaction probes to identify viruses as is described in earlier studies [11]. The procedure used here to identify signature peptides of a particular virus is sufficiently general in nature. False negative results can occur if one has chosen the peptide corresponding to hot spots or if only a few protein sequences from a particular virus family/genus have been selected to obtain unique signature. Available sequence data of strains indicate that the number of mutations in such short regions is smaller than the number of mismatches allowed. Such submolecular markers thus can be used in association with identification matrices to identify unknown virus.

References

1. Mayo MA, Pringle CR. Virus taxonomy — 1997. J Gen Virol 1998;79:649-57.
2. Koonin EV, Dolja VV. Evolution and taxonomy of positive strand RNA viruses: implications of comparative analysis of amino acid sequences. Crit Rev Biochem Mol Biol 1993;28: 375-430.
3. Kolaskar AS, Naik PS. Computerization of virus data and its usefulness in virus classification. Intervirology 1992;34:133-41.
4. Etzold T, Ulyanov A, Argos P. SRS: Information retrieval system for molecular biology data banks. Methods Enzymol 1996;266:114-28.
5. Barker WC, Garavelli JS, Haft DH, Hunt LT, Marzec CR, Orcutt BC, Srinivasarao GY, Yeh LSL, Ledley RS, Mewes HW, Pfeiffer F, Tsugita A. The PIR international protein sequence database. Nucleic Acids Res 1998;26:27-32.
6. Kolaskar AS, Naik PS. Concerted use of multiple database for taxonomic insights. In: Dubois JE, Ghershon N, eds. The Information Revolution: Impact of Science and Technology. Berlin: Springer 1996:236-70.
7. Murphy FA, Fauquet CM, Bishop DHL, Ghabrial SA, Jarvis AW, Martelli GP, Mayo MA, Summers MD. Virus taxonomy. Classification and nomenclature of viruses, sixth Report of the International Committee on Taxonomy of Viruses. Arch Virol 1995;(Suppl 10):S1-586.
8. Kolaskar AS, Naik PS. Computer-aided virus identification on the world wide web. Arch Virol 1998;143:1513-21.
9. Thompson J D, Higins DG, Gibson TJ. CLUSTALW: improving the sensitivity of progressive multiple alignment through sequence weighting, positions-specific gap penalties and weight matrix choice. Nucleic Acids Res 1994;22:4673-80.
10. Date S, Kulkarni R, Kulkarni B, Kulkarni-Kale U, Kolaskar AS. Multiple alignment of sequences on parallel computers. Comput Appl Biosci 1993;9:397-402.
11. Leary TP, Muerhoff AS, Simons JN, Pilot-Matias TJ, Erker JC, Chalmers ML, Schlauder GG, Dawson GJ, Desai SM, Mushahwar IK. Consensus oligonucleotide primers for the detection of GB virus C in human cryptogenic hepatitis. J Virol Methods 1996;56:119-21.

Opportunities at the Intersection of Bioinformatics and Health Informatics:

A Case Study

PERRY L. MILLER, MD, PHD

Abstract   This paper provides a "viewpoint discussion" based on a presentation made to the 2000 Symposium of the American College of Medical Informatics. It discusses potential opportunities for researchers in health informatics to become involved in the rapidly growing field of bioinformatics, using the activities of the Yale Center for Medical Informatics as a case study. One set of opportunities occurs where bioinformatics research itself intersects with the clinical world. Examples include the correlations between individual genetic variation with clinical risk factors, disease presentation, and differential response to treatment; and the implications of including genetic test results in the patient record, which raises clinical decision support issues as well as legal and ethical issues. A second set of opportunities occurs where bioinformatics research can benefit from the technologic expertise and approaches that informaticians have used extensively in the clinical arena. Examples include database organization and knowledge representation, data mining, and modeling and simulation. Microarray technology is discussed as a specific potential area for collaboration. Related questions concern how best to establish collaborations with bioscientists so that the interests and needs of both sets of researchers can be met in a synergistic fashion, and the most appropriate home for bioinformatics in an academic medical center.

■ **J Am Med Inform Assoc. 2000;7:431–438.**

This paper provides a "viewpoint discussion" based on a presentation made to the American College of Medical Informatics (ACMI) Symposium, which was held in

Affiliation of the author: Yale University, New Haven, Connecticut.

This work was supported in part by NIH grant G08-LM05583 from the National Library of Medicine.

Correspondence and reprints: Perry L. Miller, MD, PhD, Center for Medical Informatics, Yale University School of Medicine, P.O. Box 208009, New Haven, CT 06520-8009; e-mail: perry.miller@yale.edu.

Received for publication: 2/16/00; accepted for publication: 5/4/00.

February 2000 at San Marco Island, Florida. The activities of one day of that three-day symposium centered on the intersection of bioinformatics[1] and health informatics. The implicit theme was to help identify opportunities for researchers in health informatics to become involved in the rapidly growing field of bioinformatics. In general, there are two types of such opportunities. One set of opportunities occurs where bioinformatics research itself intersects with the clinical world. The second set of opportunities occurs where bioinformatics research can benefit from the technologic expertise, techniques, and approaches that health informaticians have used extensively in the clinical arena.

Several related questions were also addressed. One question concerned how best to establish collaborations with bioscientists so that the interests and needs of both sets of researchers can be met in a synergistic fashion. A second question concerned the appropriate home for bioinformatics in an academic medical center.

Since these questions are very broad and complex, they can be difficult to discuss in abstract terms. This paper uses the experience of the Yale Center for Medical Informatics (YCMI) as a case study to structure a discussion of these issues.

What is Bioinformatics?

The term "bioinformatics" has been used with different scopes and meanings by different groups of researchers. The term could refer to a range of activities:

- *Informatics involving genomics.* A number of researchers in the field of genomics have used the term "bioinformatics" to refer to the applications of informatics within their discipline. In the early 1990s, this work tended to focus on chromosome mapping and sequencing. Now that a number of smaller genomes have been fully sequenced and many genes in the human genome have been at least partially identified, genomic informatics has expanded into exploring the function of these genes, giving rise to fields such as functional genomics and structural genomics. As these trends continue, the distinction between genomic informatics and informatics in support of bioscience as a whole will become less distinct.

- *Informatics involving the biosciences.* Beyond genomics, computers are being used in a wide range of ways to support the biosciences. For example, the national Human Brain Project has coined the term "neuroinformatics" to describe the storage, analysis, and integration of experimental neuroscience data at many levels of bioscience research. If one defines "bioinformatics" as involving the biosciences as a whole, then one question concerns its relationship to the field of computational biology, whose scope is also evolving.

- *Informatics involving bioscience and clinical research.* Since genomic data will increasingly become the subject of a wide range of clinical research, one could define bioinformatics to include this work as well.

- *All biomedical and health informatics.* At the most general level, "bioinformatics" might be defined to

include all medical and health informatics in addition to the biosciences. There will certainly be an increasing number of intersections between work in these areas.

In this paper, "bioinformatics" is loosely defined to include the first two areas discussed above—informatics involving the biosciences, including genomics.

The Spectrum of Biomedical Informatics at the Yale Center

Table 1 outlines the spectrum of biomedical informatics activities at the YCMI. The three areas of research are increasingly likely to intersect in the near future.

Genomic Informatics

Over the past decade, the YCMI has been involved in a number of projects in support of genomics and genetics. An early project explored the use of parallel computation in biological sequence analysis and genetic linkage analysis, in collaboration with faculty in the Department of Computer Science.[2] Another project provided Internet-based informatics support for the collaborative Genome Center, involving the Albert Einstein College of Medicine and Yale, to map human chromosome 12.[3]

Table 1 ■

The Spectrum of Biomedical Informatics at the Yale Center for Medical Informatics

Areas of Research	Purpose
Genomic informatics: Yeast Genome Analysis Center Human genome diversity Microarray projects	Working up from the genetic blueprint
Neuroinformatics: Informatics in support of olfactory research, including molecular modeling and neuronal modeling	Storing, integrating, and modeling experimental data at many biological levels in the most complex organ system
Clinical informatics: Informatics support for clinical research Computer-based clinical decision support Network-based clinical information access Electronic patient record system research and development	Working with the fuzziness of clinical data and disease

Current YCMI activities in genomic informatics focus on three areas. One long-standing collaboration, with the laboratory of Prof. Kenneth Kidd (Genetics),[4] centers on human genome diversity. A second major collaboration is with Prof. Michael Snyder, director of Yale's Yeast Genome Analysis Center.[5] A recent and rapidly growing set of collaborations involve the support of microarray technology, as discussed further below. All these collaborations have involved the development of databases and informatics tools for internal use at Yale and also for providing public access to the data via the Web.

With regard to integrating genomic informatics with clinical practice, now that many genes and gene fragments have been identified, there are tremendous opportunities to work up from the genetic blueprint to explore gene expression, functional genomics, and structural genomics on a massive scale, including their implications for human disease.

Clinical Informatics

Clinical informatics and genomic informatics are at far ends of the spectrum shown in Table 1. Here the field of medical and health informatics has long been confronting the development of informatics techniques that deal with the fuzziness of clinical data and disease. At the YCMI, we have been working on many different projects:

- Informatics support for clinical research. One rapidly growing YCMI project involves the development and use of Trial/DB,[6] a Web-accessible database designed to collect data for clinical trials and clinical research. In addition to its use at Yale, Trial/DB is being supported by the National Cancer Institute to serve as the "special studies database" for its national Cancer Genetics Network (CGN). The CGN by definition focuses specifically on clinical studies that have a genetic component.

- Computer-based clinical decision support. Faculty at the YCMI have a long-standing research interest in computer-based clinical decision support, including implementing clinical practice guidelines and providing access to network-based reference information in the context of care for particular patients. We are also working with our medical center to move incrementally toward the electronic patient record. As more and more genetic tests become available, test results will become an important part of the patient record, and there will be many opportunities to use this information to provide clinical decision support.

Thus, we anticipate increasing interplay between the genomic and clinical levels, which will have a major impact on our informatics activities.

Neuroinformatics

In Table 1, neuroinformatics sits between genomic informatics and clinical informatics and is really a placeholder for informatics activities involving many different tissues and organ systems. Once the genetic blueprint is known, the next step is to determine what it means in a range of different tissues and organ systems, including the kidney, the liver, the gastrointestinal tract, the heart, and the endocrine system, among others. Neuroinformatics focuses on the central nervous system, which is clearly the most complex organ system.

The goal of the field of neuroinformatics is to provide enabling informatics technology that supports neuroscience research at many different levels[7,8] (Table 2). These include the genetic level, the cellular level, the physiologic and pharmacologic levels, and, eventually, the level of behavioral research. The research includes experimental microanatomic studies (e.g., imaging cells) and macroanatomic studies (e.g., imaging brains). Each type of experiment uses different experimental techniques and generates different types of experimental data. Historically, different laboratories have tended to focus on one or two of these levels.

At each of these levels, large amounts of experimental data are being generated in a form that can be stored and analyzed online. To fully understand a neuroscience phenomenon, however, it is ultimately important to gather data at many different levels and analyze all those data in an integrated fashion.

In summary, neuroinformatics in a sense "connects" genomic informatics and clinical informatics in the areas of neuroscience research. As such, it is representative of many other bioscience disciplines that are addressing similar issues in other tissues and organ systems. The three levels shown in Table 1 represent a spectrum of informatics activities that will become increasingly integrated in many different ways.

Bioinformatics and Health Informatics: Selected Areas of Intersection

Health informaticians have many potential opportunities to become involved in collaborations involving bioinformatics. One set of opportunities occurs where bioinformatics research intersects the clinical world:

- *Clinical correlation of genetic variation.* Genetic variation might be caused by different mutations of a

Table 2 ∎

Examples of Experimental Neuroscience Data at Different Levels of Brain Function

Levels of Brain Function	Types of Data
Behavior	Performance quantification, video monitoring, drug testing
Distributed systems	2-D and 3-D axon tracing between regions, electrophysiologic recordings (spike timing), brain imaging, and 3-D brain maps
Specific regions	2-D and 3-D cytoarchitectonics of layers and functional columns, transmitter-receptor localization, anatomic, physiologic, and metabolic maps
Nerve cells	3-D cell morphology, 3-D functional imaging, electrophysiologic recordings of action-potential firing patterns and membrane currents
Neuronal components	3-D imaging of axon terminals, growth cones, dendrites, dendritic spines, 3-D localization of organelles and synaptic microcircuits
Microcircuits	3-D fine structure and imaging of synaptic patterns, synaptic pharmacology, action-potential firing patterns and synaptic currents, and potentials
Organelles	2-D and 3-D fine structure and molecular composition of synapses, mitochondria, microtubules, etc.; recordings of synaptic currents and potentials
Molecules	3-D molecular models of receptors, channels, enzymes and structural proteins, molecular physiology, and pharmacology of transmitters, modulators, hormones, guidance molecules, growth factors and gene-transcription factors
Genes	DNA and protein sequences

SOURCE: Shepherd et al.[9] Used with permission.

single gene or by mutations of different genes that are related, for example, because they code for different enzymes in a single metabolic pathway.

- Genetic variation may be correlated with different levels of severity of a disease or different presentations of signs and symptoms.[10]

- Patients with different genetic makeups may have different responses to treatment. The new field of pharmacogenetics is exploring the possibility of tailoring treatment of disease to a patient's underlying genetic makeup.

- A patient's genetic makeup may make the patient more susceptible, or relatively resistant, to risk factors associated with a disease.

- A patient's prognosis might differ depending on underlying genetic factors.

∎ *Comparison of gene expression in normal and disease states.* Microarray technology is a potentially productive area for collaborations, as discussed in a later section. This technology will be used both in the biosciences and in clinically oriented projects.

∎ *Genetic test results as part of the patient record.* We have already mentioned the potential inclusion of genetic test results in a patient medical record and

their use in computer-based clinical decision support. Legal and ethical issues that arise from inclusion of this information in the electronic patient record will also need to be addressed.

A second set of opportunities occurs where bioinformatics research can benefit from techniques and approaches that informaticians have used extensively in the clinical arena:

∎ *Data mining.* As large and diverse databases of biological data are developed, there will be opportunities to explore many different approaches to data mining, to understand the complex interactions and implications of the data.

∎ *Database organization and knowledge representation.* There will also be many opportunities to explore research issues in database design and interoperability; in data querying; in representing knowledge derived from data, which guides the analysis of the data; and in inferencing based on the knowledge. The creation, use, and maintenance of standardized biomedical vocabularies will also be needed. Such vocabularies will include not only standardized sets of terms but also standardized sets of relationships between those terms and standardized sets of attributes describing those terms.

■ *Computer modeling of normal and disease processes at many levels.* Modeling is already being used at many different levels to understand biological phenomena. As more and more data become available, there will be opportunities to create computer models, of many different types, that are closely tied to the data. Ideally, experimental data should refine a model, and analysis using the model should suggest further laboratory experiments, in an iterative, cyclic fashion.

Storing and Analyzing Microarray Data: A Case Study

The microarray, a recently developed technology, offers a wide range of informatics opportunities.[11–14] Yale is currently installing two microarray analyzers, one in the School of Medicine and one on Yale's main campus. These use a technology whereby "DNA chips" measure whether and to what degree different genes are expressed in experimental tissue samples. Each DNA chip can analyze the presence or absence and the approximate level of expression of tens of thousands of genes.

For example, one group of Yale researchers will use this technology to study hematologic disease involving white blood cells (WBCs). They will take WBCs at different stages of cell differentiation and in a single experiment see which of roughly 10,000 genes are expressed in two samples that have been combined (e.g., a normal sample and a cancerous sample at the same stage of differentiation). The test for each gene (really a small DNA fragment that is part of a gene) is seen on the microarray as a single spot in a massive array of spots. The two samples (from normal and abnormal WBCs) will be tagged with fluorescent markers of different colors (red and green), so that each gene can be tested in both samples in a single microarray experiment.

Each experiment will generate 10,000 data points. Each point will have several associated values, reflecting the actual intensity and relative intensity of both fluorescent markers at each of the 10,000 spots. The researchers estimate they will ultimately perform up to five such experiments a day.

In addition, other laboratories will be using the same machine to generate similar numbers of data for many different experiments. It takes roughly 10 minutes to perform each microarray analysis. Slides can be loaded to allow the machine to perform analyses automatically 24 hours a day.

As a result, we see microarray experiments as an ex-

citing opportunity to expand our activities in genomic informatics:

■ Huge amounts of data will be generated. In the near future, microarrays will probably be able to analyze all 60,000 to 100,000 human genes in a single experiment.

■ These experiments will have major needs for bioinformatics, far beyond the need previously experienced by our bioscience collaborators.

■ There are extensive opportunities to explore many different approaches to data mining and analysis.

■ There is also a need for people who understand database design issues. For example, as an increasing number of different microarray experiments are performed, it will useful if entity-attribute-value (EAV) technology can be used so that new database tables do not need to be programmed for each experiment.

■ The data need to be robustly and flexibly linked to many external databases and software analytic tools, so that their meaning and implications can be fully explored.

■ Supercomputer capabilities, including parallel computation, are clearly needed for the performance of all the required analyses.

■ Microarray research will be performed both by bioscientists and by clinically oriented researchers.

As a result, a broad, stable infrastructure of informatics staff and faculty will be required to support the high volume of microarray experiments that will soon be performed.

Establishing Collaboration with Bioscientists: Informatics Support vs. Informatics Research

If health informaticians are to become centrally involved in bioinformatics, they need to establish robust collaborations with bioscientists. In the forging of such collaborations, it is important to understand that informaticians can play two general types of informatics roles—specifically, providing informatics support for bioscience research and performing informatics research that uses the bioscience domain as a context for addressing basic informatics research issues.

In this regard, it is important to point out that bioscientists typically have motivations that are very different from those of the clinician collaborators with whom many health informaticians have worked in the past. Clinician collaborators are, typically, primarily involved in clinical practice and are looking for additional interesting research projects in which they can become involved. For such collaborators, embarking on a clinical informatics research project allows them to provide their clinical expertise and participate in sophisticated research that relates to their field. If this research results in additional visibility and publications, they have reason to be happy.

Bioscientist collaborators may have a very different motivation. They are already doing research. They are looking to informaticians to provide tools to help them perform their research more effectively. They are, typically, not looking for additional areas for research peripheral to their field, nor do they want to devote their time to such projects. They have more than enough research in their own field to keep them busy, and their time is precious. As a result, they will not be satisfied with the clinical informatics model of serving as domain experts in informatics research projects, even if the projects are in their field. They want help solving their immediate research problems.

As a result, bioscientists typically want informaticians to provide them with informatics support. Conversely, academic informaticians want at some level to be performing informatics research, although they are certainly willing to provide informatics support if this leads to interesting research opportunities.

The YCMI's neuroinformatics experience in the national Human Brain Project (HBP) provides, as a case study, a chance to discuss these issues more concretely. The YCMI's HBP work involves the integration of multidisciplinary sensory data, using the olfactory system as a model system. This HBP work involves both neuroinformatics support and neuroinformatics research.

Neuroinformatics Support

Our neuroinformatics support activities involve building a variety of databases and tools. In general, we have attempted to build databases that can serve the needs of our collaborating laboratories and also serve as pilot resources for the field as a whole. These databases include ORDB, containing information about olfactory receptors[15]; OdorDB, containing information about odor molecules; NeuronDB, containing information about neuronal cell properties[16]; and ModelDB, containing neuronal models that can be searched, examined, downloaded via the Web, and run locally.

The development of these databases involved a great deal of practical work with our collaborators to fine-tune their design, functionality, and interface so that they can be readily useful to, and usable by, neuroscientists. It is important to emphasize, however, that "just" performing good neuroinformatics support requires that informatics faculty work closely with the neuroscientists to understand the biological problems, to appreciate the needs of the neuroscience researchers, and to develop well-structured solutions to enable neuroscience research.

Neuroinformatics Research

In developing these tools, we have been able to define interesting neuroinformatics research projects. As discussed in more detail below, however, this did not happen immediately. Our current neuroinformatics research includes:

- *The EAV/CR data model.* The entity-attribute-value (EAV) model has been used in a number of clinical information systems to store clinical data. This data model has the advantage, over strictly relational databases, that a large number of clinical data items can be accommodated without massive numbers of tables and that new data items can be included without restructuring and reprogramming the database. We have extended the EAV data model to include complex data items (classes) as values and to allow relationships between data items to be explicitly represented in the database. We call the resulting data model EAV/CR (entity-attribute-value with classes and relationships) and believe that it is well suited to handling heterogeneous bioscience data.[17] We have implemented an EAV/CR database framework and have migrated the operational versions of all four of our HBP databases (ORDB, OdorDB, NeuronDB, and ModelDB) to the EAV/CR model.[18]

- *Tools to support the iterative modeling process.* Another area of neuroinformatics research that we are currently exploring involves developing database approaches and related tools to support the iterative process of neuronal modeling. These tools will maintain an organized record of the different versions of the model, the input data used to test each version, and the results of running the model with those data.

The Problem and the Solution

In a neuroscience collaboration, one would like to strike a balance between neuroinformatics support and neuroinformatics research, so that both can be pursued in a synergistic fashion. The problem that we encountered in our HBP work was essentially that of "the chicken and the egg." At the start of our HBP activities, in particular, there was no critical mass of neuroinformatics support activities to provide a context for neuroinformatics research. In addition, our neuroinformatics support activities were applied and pragmatic, reflecting the real-world needs of our neuroscience collaborators. It was therefore difficult (in retrospect, impossible) to perform neuroinformatics research that was directly tied to our collaborators' immediate research needs.

The problem was that we had not achieved a robust level (a critical mass) of neuroinformatics support activities to provide a context for neuroinformatics research. Once we had achieved a sufficiently robust level of neuroinformatics support (which took about five years), we could then embark on neuroinformatics research that was built on our support and therefore directly tied to our collaborators' research needs. This, in turn, meant that the results of our neuroinformatics research could be folded back to enhance our neuroinformatics support, in a fully synergistic fashion.

For example, as described above, we were able to integrate the operational versions of all four of our HBP databases into our EAV/CR data model. We believe that this provides a strong pilot proof of concept for the EAV/CR model and also provides a robust, flexible database environment for the further development of these and future HBP databases at Yale.

Finding an Academic Home for Bioinformatics

An important question concerns the most appropriate home for bioinformatics in an academic medical center. One possible academic home is in a bioscience department. To the extent that a particular computational technique is unique to a department, then that department may well be a logical home for researchers who focus on that technique. This would be particularly true if such faculty members need to be fully trained in that department's discipline.

To the extent that bioinformatics faculty members require broad training in informatics issues and have skills that are applicable across many bioscience fields, however, there is logic to basing those faculty members in a broader academic unit containing colleagues who share this informatics background. Two general types of such a unit are:

- An academic bioscience informatics unit comprising faculty trained in informatics focused on the biosciences

- An academic biomedical informatics unit comprising faculty trained in bioscience informatics and faculty trained in clinical and health informatics

A unit of the later type would promote—among all faculty, staff, and students—work at the intersection of clinical and bioscience informatics as well as a broader appreciation of biomedical informatics as a whole. As the current trends in bioinformatics continue, the latter model is likely to become an increasingly logical solution. It is clear, however, that many historical, political, and practical considerations will influence how any individual academic medical center approaches this issue.

References ■

1. Altman RB. Bioinformatics. In: Shortliffe EH, Perreault LE, Wiederhold G, Fagan LM (eds). Medical Informatics: Computer Applications in Health Care and Biomedicine. New York: Springer-Verlag, in press.
2. Sittig DF, Shifman MA, Nadkarni P, Miller PL. Parallel computation for medicine and biology: experience with Linda at Yale University. Int J Supercomput Appl. 1992;6:147–63.
3. Miller PL, Nadkarni PM, Kidd KK, et al. Internet-based support for biomedical research: a collaborative genome center for human chromosome 12. J Am Med Inform Assoc. 1995; 2:351–64.
4. Cheung KH, Osier MV, Kidd JR, Pakstis AJ, Miller PL, Kidd KK. Alfred: an allele frequency database for diverse populations and DNA polymorphisms. Nucleic Acids Res. 2000; 28:361–3.
5. Kumar A, Cheung KH, Ross-Macdonald P, Coelho PSR, Miller P, Snyder M. Triples: a database of transposon mutagenesis in S cervisiae. Nucleic Acids Res. 2000;28:81–4.
6. Nadkarni PM, Brandt C, Frawley S, et al. ACT/DB: a client–server database for managing entity-attribute-value clinical trials data. J Am Med Inform Assoc. 1998;5:139–51.
7. Martin JB, Pechura CM (eds). Mapping the Brain and Its Functions: Integrating Enabling Technologies into Neuroscience Research. Washington, DC: National Academy Press, 1991.
8. Koslow SH, Huerta MF (eds). Neuroinformatics: An Overview of the Human Brain Project. Mahwah, NJ: Lawrence Erlbaum Associates, 1997.
9. Shepherd GM, Mirsky JS, Healy MD, et al. The Human Brain Project: neuroinformatics tools for integrating, searching, and modeling multidisciplinary neuroscience data. Trends Neurosci. 1998;21:460–8.
10. Nadkarni PM, Reeders ST, Zhou J. CECIL: a database for storing and retrieving clinical and molecular information on patients with Alport syndrome. Proc 17th Symp Comput Appl Medl Care. 1993:649–53.
11. Bassett DE, Eisen MB, Boguski MS. Gene expression informatics: it's all in your mine. Nature Genetics. 1998(suppl 21):51–5.
12. National Human Genome Research Institute, Division of Intramural Research. Microarray project Web site. Available at: http://www.nhgri.nih.gov/DIR/LCG/15K/HTML. Accessed Jun 28, 2000.

13. Stanford University Department of Biochemistry. Patrick O. Brown Laboratory homepage. Available at: http://cmgm.stanford.edu/pbrown. Accessed Jun 28, 2000.

14. Albert Einstein College of Medicine (AECOM). Functional Genomics Project Web site. Available at: http://sequence.aecom.yu.edu/bioinf/funcgenomic.html. Accessed Jun 28, 2000.

15. Skoufos E, Healy MD, Singer MS, Nadkarni PM, Miller PL, Shepherd GM. Olfactory Receptor Database: a database of the largest eukaryotic gene family. Nucleic Acids Res. 1999; 27:343–5.

16. Mirsky JS, Nadkarni PM, Healy MD, Miller PL, Shepherd GM. Database tools for integrating neuronal data to facilitate construction of neuronal models. J Neurosci Methods. 1998;82:105–21.

17. Nadkarni P, Marenco L, Chen R, Skoufos E, Shepherd G, Miller P. Organization of heterogeneous scientific data using the EAV/CR representation. J Am Med Inform Assoc. 1999; 6:478–93.

18. Marenco L, Nadkarni P, Skoufos E, Shepherd G, Miller P. Neuronal database integration: the Senselab EAV data model. AMIA Annu Symp. 1999:102–6.

Conceptual modelling of genomic information

Norman W. Paton[1], Shakeel A. Khan[2], Andrew Hayes[2], Fouzia Moussouni[1], Andy Brass[2], Karen Eilbeck[2], Carole A. Goble[1], Simon J. Hubbard[3] and Stephen G. Oliver[2]

[1]*Department of Computer Science, University of Manchester, Oxford Road, Manchester M13 9PL, UK,* [2]*School of Biological Sciences, University of Manchester, Oxford Road, Manchester M13 9PL, UK and* [3]*Department of Biomolecular Sciences, UMIST, PO Box 88, Manchester, UK*

Received on November 12, 1999; revised and accepted on February 3, 2000

Abstract

Motivation: Genome sequencing projects are making available complete records of the genetic make-up of organisms. These core data sets are themselves complex, and present challenges to those who seek to store, analyse and present the information. However, in addition to the sequence data, high throughput experiments are making available distinctive new data sets on protein interactions, the phenotypic consequences of gene deletions, and on the transcriptome, proteome, and metabolome. The effective description and management of such data is of considerable importance to bioinformatics in the post-genomic era. The provision of clear and intuitive models of complex information is surprisingly challenging, and this paper presents conceptual models for a range of important emerging information resources in bioinformatics. It is hoped that these can be of benefit to bioinformaticians as they attempt to integrate genetic and phenotypic data with that from genomic sequences, in order to both assign gene functions and elucidate the different pathways of gene action and interaction.
Results: This paper presents a collection of conceptual (i.e. implementation-independent) data models for genomic data. These conceptual models are amenable to (more or less direct) implementation on different computing platforms.
Availability: Most of the information models presented here have been implemented by the authors using an object database. The implementation of a public interface to this database is in progress. We hope to have a public release in the autumn of 2000, available from http://img. cs.man.ac.uk/gims.
Contact: norm@cs.man.ac.uk

Introduction

The recent availability of complete genome sequences provides biologists with new opportunities for identi-fying and understanding properties of the genome that have hitherto been out of reach, and for conducting comparisons of genomes. The exploitation of this new information resource is, however, dependent upon the provision of effective tools for the management, integra-tion and presentation of genome sequences and related information.

The storage, sharing, and analysis of genomic data sets is made more challenging still by the emergence of new information resources for which there are few established bioinformatics techniques, such as transcriptome data from hybridization-array analyses. The fact that many insights are likely to emerge from the combined use of core genome sequence data with the data on functional analyses, in turn implies that consistent and integrated representations of genomic data are likely to be important to post-genomic bioinformatics.

This paper provides conceptual models that describe eukaryotic genome sequence data and genome organi-sation, plus a number of important functional data sets, namely protein interaction data, transcription data, and results from gene deletions. The information models presented have been developed in the context of a project that is focusing initially on the management of *Sac-charomyces cerevisiae* data, but where the models are biased towards *S.cerevisiae*, we seek to make this explicit. The models are described using Unified Modelling Lan-guage (UML) (Booch *et al.*, 1999), the emerging standard object-modelling language.

The work described in this paper is by no means unique in providing object-oriented models of biological data. One of the authors was involved in an early project on the use of object databases with protein structure data (Gray *et al.*, 1990). However, more recent work presents conceptual or object-based models for biological data. For example, Okayama *et al.* (1998) describes the conceptual schema of a DNA database using an extended entity-relationship model. Chen and Markowitz (1995) have

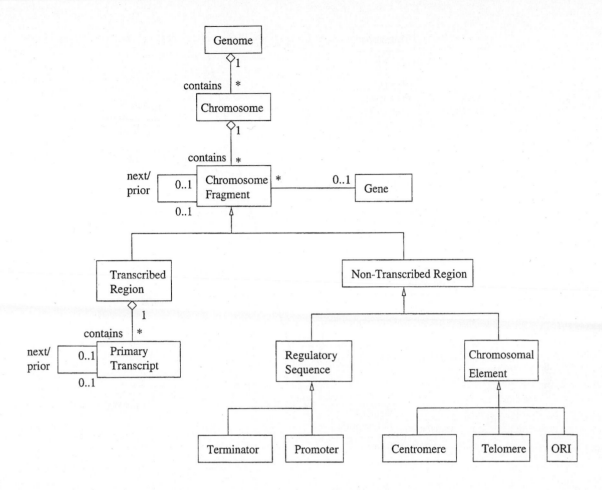

Fig. 1. Basic schema diagram for genomic data.

indicated how an extended object data model can be used to capture the properties of scientific experiments, and Medigue *et al.* (1999) include models for representing genomic sequence data.

A number of researchers have also explored the use of object-oriented implementation technologies for biological data. For example, Ellis *et al.* (1998) describes how a metabolic pathway database has been developed using Java and a commercial secondary storage manager. The ooTFD transcription factors database is outlined in Ghosh (1999). In the genomic setting, Hu *et al.* (1998) indicates how the object-oriented middleware CORBA has been used to provide distributed access to a genome mapping database, and Jungfer and Rodriguez-Tome (1998) describes how CORBA was employed in the construction of a map viewer. Most closely related to the current work is that described in Eilbeck *et al.* (1999), which describes the implementation of a protein interaction database that uses one of the conceptual models presented in this paper. In Maltchenko (1998), a proposal is made for some generic object classes for use in a distributed computing

environment; this seems less suitable to the authors than a carefully defined collection of less generic classes.

It is probably also important to differentiate this work from the earlier work of some of the authors on an ontology for biological data in the TAMBIS project (Baker *et al.*, 1999). The purpose of an ontology is not so much to provide a conceptual representation of structures for storing data, but rather to provide a description of the terminology used in a domain. As a result, for example, it would not be obvious how to derive a database schema from the TAMBIS ontology. In addition, a further distinction between the TAMBIS ontology and the models presented in this paper is that the latter focus on genomic data sets, which are outside the scope of the TAMBIS ontology.

The purpose of this paper is to provide clear conceptual models for genomic data that can be used to direct subsequent implementation activities. By separating the information models from a description of a system, it is hoped that important issues relating to the way in which data can be described will be made explicit, to the benefit of developers of future information systems for genomic data.

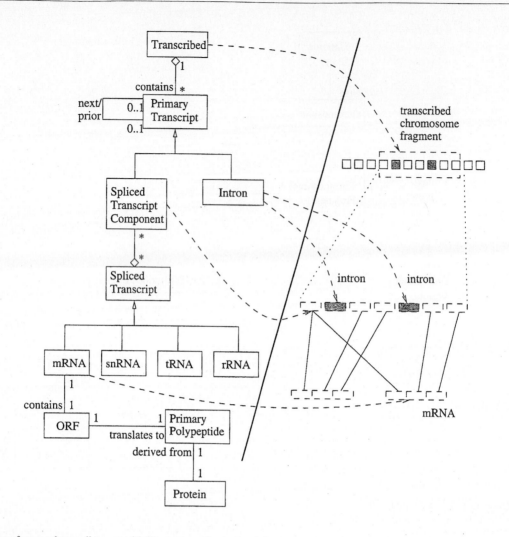

Fig. 2. Fragment of core schema diagram with illustration of associated data.

Systems and methods

This section presents the information models using the class diagram notation of UML (Booch *et al.*, 1999).

In UML class diagrams, such as that in Figure 1, classes are drawn in rectangles, with the name of the class at the top, and optionally with the attributes and operations of the class shown below. In this paper, we list the attributes of the class only when these are felt to be important to the understanding of the model as a whole—listing all the reasonable attributes of all the classes would consume a prohibitive amount of space. Generalization relationships (e.g. *Terminator* and *Promoter* are both kinds of *Regulatory Sequence*) are drawn using a line with an arrowhead at the most general class. Relationships between classes are represented by lines connecting the classes, with the name of the role that the class plays in the relationship written beside the line, along with the multiplicity, which indicates the number of objects that may participate in the relationship. Where the relationship

represents a part/whole relationship, the line depicting the relationship is adorned with an open diamond at the whole end of the relationship. For example, a *Genome* contains *many* (denoted by *) *Chromosome*s, each of which is part of *one* Genome.

Genome sequence model

Here we describe the basic information that must be stored to describe a fully sequenced genome. The focus is on the fully sequenced genome, rather than on the information from which the final sequence is derived. The schema diagram for the core data set is presented in Figure 1.

The model in Figure 1 describes the basic components of a genome. The complete *Genome* consists of a collection of chromosomes. Each *Chromosome* can be considered to be a long sequence of DNA, which in turn consists of a sequence of (potentially overlapping) *Chromosome Fragment*s. These fragments are either *Transcribed* regions of DNA or *Non-Transcribed* regions

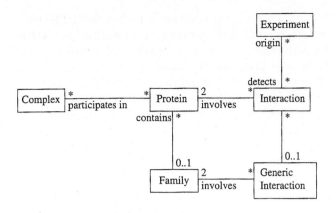

Fig. 3. Class diagram for protein interaction data.

(i.e. both *Transcribed* and *Non-Transcribed* regions are kinds of *Chromosome Fragment*).

Different approaches to the modelling of genomic information may place different interpretations on some biological terms, even for familiar notions such as *Gene* and *ORF*. In the model in Figure 1, a *Gene* is a segment of the chromosome that is transcribed into RNA. Its flanking non-transcribed sequences/regions (the *Regulators*) are included as parts of the *Gene*. There is a possibility that two adjacent genes may overlap, where a part of the coding sequence, of the preceding one, acts as the promoter for the following one. This can be handled in the model because *Chromosome Fragments* may overlap. Thus, within the model (as in genetics), 'gene' is defined in functional terms and no artificial constraints are placed on that portion of the DNA sequence that represents a 'gene'.

The *Non-Transcribed* regions are either *Regulators*, which control the expression of genes, or *Chromosomal Elements*, which include the *Centromere*, the *Telomeres* and the Origins of Replication (*ORI*).

The *Transcribed* chromosome fragments are illustrated more fully in Figure 2. Each *Transcribed* region contains a collection of *Primary Transcripts*. Each of the primary transcripts is either an *Intron* or a *Spliced Transcript Component*. In the model, there is no direct relationship between *Intron* and *Regulator*, and information on the regulatory function of an *Intron* would be captured using attributes of *Intron*. In addition, the model in its present form deals only with the simplest form of alternate splicing. While adequate for *S.cerevisiae*, this part of the model will have to be extended if it is to be applied to more complex eukaryotes.

The *Spliced Transcript Components* are assembled (with the *Introns* removed) to form *Spliced Transcripts*. Each *Spliced Transcript* is categorized as being some kind of RNA. An additional complicating factor is that a single

Spliced Transcript Component can be used in the synthesis of more than one *Spliced Transcript*. For example, Figure 2 illustrates two different *Spliced Transcripts* that share common *Spliced Transcript Components*.

Every *mRNA* contains an open reading frame (*ORF*), which consists of a series of triplets (codons) that specify the amino-acid sequence of the *Primary Polypeptide* that a gene encodes. The ORFs begin with an initiation (start) codon, usually ATG, and end with a termination codon, either TAA, TAG or TGA. The *Primary Polypeptide* undergoes certain post-translational modifications to become a functional *Protein*.

As the emphasis in the paper is on fully sequenced genomes, no models are provided for mapping data. An example of a model for mapping data can be found in Barrilot *et al.* (1999).

There is a question as to where information on experiments or on the literature should be provided in class diagrams such as those provided in Figures 1 and 2. As there could be interest in providing such information at many different points in the diagram, it might be appropriate to provide an abstract superclass that allows literature or experimental details to be provided for all classes in these diagrams.

Protein–protein interaction data

Here and in the following subsections we describe information models that are related to the core genome sequence. The models provided have been selected because they can be used to describe experimental results that are becoming available as a result of systematic functional analyses.

Protein–protein interactions are essential to most cellular processes such as signal transduction, DNA replication, and metabolism. Experimental techniques, particularly the yeast two-hybrid system, are being used to provide comprehensive analyses of interactions. For example, the protein–protein interactions of bacteriophage T7 were mapped using yeast two-hybrid to reveal 22 interactions between 53 proteins (Bartels *et al.*, 1996). Since then, attempts have been made to systematically map the interactions between the 6000 or so expressed proteins in yeast (Fromont-Racine *et al.*, 1997).

A class diagram for protein-protein interaction data is provided in Figure 3. This intersects with Figure 2 at the class *Protein*. In this model, every *Interaction* involves two proteins, which allows the model to capture the details about each interface. Each *Interaction* can in turn be validated by many *Experiments*. As the different experimental methods for protein interaction detection can produce results of differing quality, information on the experimental techniques used gives an indication of the confidence that can be held in the interaction. For example, an interaction detected by yeast two-hybrid *and* affinity

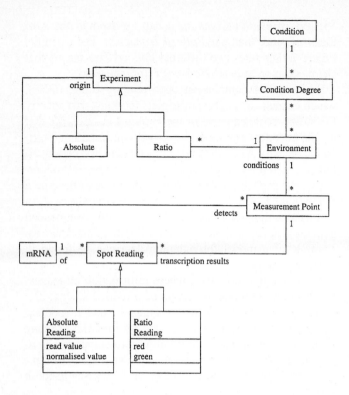

Fig. 4. Schema diagram for transcriptome data.

chromatography would be considered to be more likely than one detected by yeast two-hybrid alone.

The class *Complex* contains information about proteins interacting in groups of more than two. One source of complexes used to populate this section of the database is MIPS (Mewes *et al.*, 1998), in which there are 230 multi-protein complexes at the time of writing.

The class *Generic Interaction* is used to describe categories of interaction that are apparent in many species. This generality is captured by relating individual *Interaction*s with the *Generic Interaction* of which they are an example. Generic interactions are in turn described in terms of the gene families that participate in them. An example of a *Generic Interaction* is that the families *MAPKKK* and *MAPKK* interact in the pheromone signalling pathway. A specific example of this is that in *S.cerevisiae* the protein *Ste11* (a member of the family *MAPKKK*) interacts with *Ste7* (a member of the family *MAPKK*).

Transcriptome data

Gene expression data provide important clues as to the function of novel genes identified during genome sequencing (Planta *et al.*, 1999), and also provide insights on the behaviour of cells in different conditions (Spellman *et al.*, 1998). The recent development of experimental techniques that allow transcript levels to be measured

for every gene in an organism simultaneously (the transcriptome) will make available a substantial information resource that will, in turn, require novel bioinformatic techniques in the area of functional analysis. The focus of this section is on the modelling of transcriptome data.

Transcriptome data can be generated using different experimental techniques applied to DNA arrays that yield different kinds of data. A DNA array is generally prepared (a) by crosslinking a PCR product on a solid support like a glass slide or a nylon membrane, or (b) by synthesizing oligonucleotides on a gene-chip.

There are now a number of transcriptome studies on *S.cerevisiae* for which the data are publicly available. For instance, protein-encoding genes whose expression is phased in the yeast cell cycle have been identified by two groups (Spellman *et al.*, 1998). In this work, the relative abundance of each transcript in the test sample (from each time point of a yeast culture where the cells undergo division in a synchronous manner) is compared with the reference (time-zero) sample, by measuring as the ratio of red to green fluorescence. The greater relative abundance of a particular transcript (mRNA) in the test sample results in a higher ratio of red-labelled to green-labelled copies of the corresponding cDNA. From a modelling perspective, the key feature of the results is that a *relative* expression level, at different times in the cell cycle, is obtained on a *per-gene* basis.

In an alternative approach, by EUROFAN, the regulation of expression of all protein-encoding genes in yeast was investigated under carbon and nitrogen limitation conditions. Following normalization, the abundance of each transcript is expressed as its fractional contribution to the total level of transcription. To identify genes under carbon or nitrogen control, levels of expression of individual ORFs are compared between the two conditions. From a modelling perspective, the key feature of the results of this experiment is that each data item is a normalized *absolute* expression level for each gene.

A fragment of data from an absolute-value expression experiment is provided in Figure 5. This figure shows two filters that have been hybridized with radiolabelled cDNAs prepared from mRNA extracts taken from steady-state carbon-limited and nitrogen-limited cultures. Each 'spot' represents an ORF that is expressed under each condition. The intensity (or darkness) of the spot is proportional to the level of expression of the particular gene. The spots that have been highlighted with arrows show major differences between the two conditions. The context (e.g. growth condition) in which a particular gene is expressed provides clues as to its function.

The class diagram for transcriptome data is given in Figure 4. The *mRNA* class is common to this schema diagram and to that in Figure 2. Arrays employed in yeast transcriptome analysis currently comprise oligonucleotides or PCR

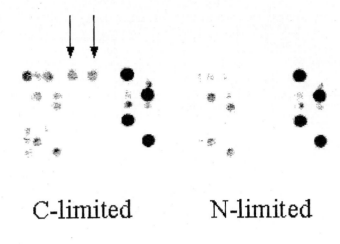

C-limited   N-limited

Fig. 5. Example expression data results.

products containing sequences exclusively derived from ORFs. The current model does not deal with the fact that, because of genetic redundancy, more than one spot in the array may be hybridized by a single mRNA class (Delneri *et al.*, 1999).

There are two kinds of *Experiment*, *Absolute* experiments and *Ratio* experiments[†] reflecting whether the technique used in the experiment measures the absolute quantity of mRNA expressed or the amount of mRNA expressed relative to some baseline (in practice, whether the two-colour fluorescence technique or radioisotopic labelling was used). Each *Experiment* has a collection of *Measurement Point*s, each of which is at some time from the start of the experiment. The *Environment* of a *Measurement Point* is a description of the conditions that prevail at the time of the measurement. In particular, an *Environment* records the extent (i.e. *Condition Degree*) to which some property (i.e. *Condition*) holds when a measurement is taken.

The relationship between *Ratio* and *Environment* captures the environment of the baseline. Thus in a *Ratio* experiment in which there are *n* *Measurement Point*s, there will be *n* + 1 *Environment*s, one for each *Measurement Point* and one for the baseline.

Each *Measurement Point* associates the description of the *Environment* with a collection of *Spot Reading*s. Each *Spot Reading* is either an *Absolute Reading* or a *Ratio Reading*, depending on the type of *Experiment* being carried out. An *Absolute Reading* captures the quantity of a particular gene expressed at the time of the measurement, plus some normalized value (such as the percentage of the total mRNA present in the cell that this reading represents).

[†] Although in ratio experiments the ratios are computed from absolute expression levels, the absolute values are not normally made public.

To relate the model with the experimental values in Figure 5: each *mRNA* species represents a position in the array; the *read value* of each *Absolute Reading* represents the intensity of the 'spot' at a specific position; there is a separate image of the array for each *Measurement Point*, and the *Condition* and *Condition Degree* classes represent the labels on the images of the arrays, such as *C-limited* and *N-limited*. In the case of *C-limited*, the *Condition* is carbon limitation, and the degree of the condition is the dilution rate (e.g. 0.1 h^{-1}).

The rapidly increasing production of transcriptome data sets has led to a number of proposals for modelling such data. For example Brazma *et al.* (1999) presents a design for a repository of array data. The models for transcriptome data presented in this paper focus principally on the information that is derived from the array experiments, whereas the models in Brazma *et al.* (1999) seek to capture as much detail as possible on the techniques used and the images obtained. We consider that the wider scope of the models in Brazma *et al.* (1999) is appropriate in the context of a repository, and that the emphasis in the models presented in this paper is appropriate for an information resource that focuses on the integration of different kinds of information for analysis purposes.

Genome modifications

Genome sequencing projects reveal the presence of many genes with unknown functions. Knowing the function of all the genes in the genome is important to the long-term value of the genome data, and systematic approaches can be taken that seek to assign functions to novel genes. For example, upon completion of the yeast genome sequence, an international, integrated effort was initiated to determine the possible functions of as many novel genes as possible (Oliver, 1996). In order to achieve this, ORFs with unknown functions were deleted by a PCR-mediated gene replacement method (Baudin *et al.*, 1993; Wach *et al.*, 1994).

The modelling of experiments relating to naturally occurring or induced modifications to a genome involves describing the modification that has taken place, the ploidy of the strain, and the consequences of the modification for the organism.

The schema for describing genome modifications is given in Figure 6. A *Strain* is described as a collection of modifications to *Gene*s in a *Genome*. A *Strain* is associated with a collection of variations in the phenotype of the organism. In experiments involving yeast, the *effect*s of a *Variation* that are recorded include the viability and rate of growth of the strain. This is straightforward to describe, but modelling phenotypic behaviour in other organisms is likely to present a significant challenge for controlled vocabularies or ontologies, and is beyond the scope of this paper.

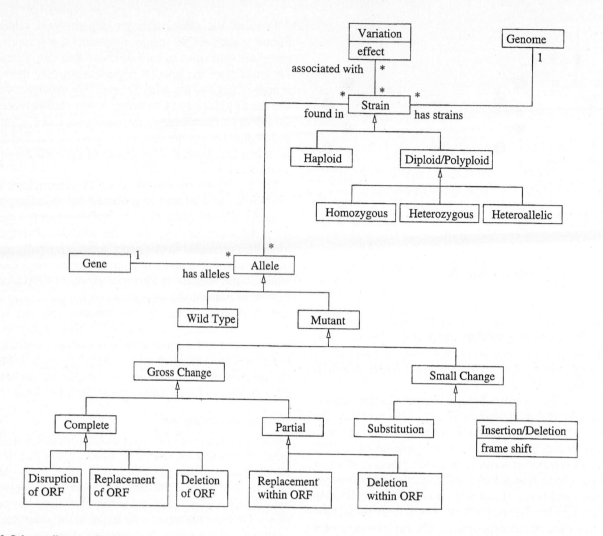

Fig. 6. Schema diagram alleles.

The interpretation of the significance of a variation in phenotype depends on the ploidy of the strain. For example, if an essential novel gene is deleted from a diploid strain, the strain may still show viability, whereas a haploid strain is sure to be non-viable. In the model in Figure 6, a *Strain* may be *Haploid* or *Diploid/Polyploid*, reflecting the number of copies of the chromosomes in the organism.

Each of the modifications to a *Gene* in a *Strain* is represented as an *Allele*. *Allele*s are classified as either *Wild Type*s or *Mutant*s. The model for describing *Mutant*s is much richer than that for *Wild Type*s, as the nature of the genetic change in any marker genes may not be known.

The modifications within a *Mutant* allele are classified according to their size. This is by no means the only possible dimension that could be used for classification—for example, the hierarchy could have been based on the type of the modification (e.g. insertion, replacement). During

modelling, a range of alternative classifications were explored, and that based on the size of the modification seemed the most natural for use with the data sets to which we had access. This, however, is the only model in the paper that has not yet been implemented and used with real data sets, and thus the model has yet to be validated in practice. Whatever dimension is chosen for the classification of the modifications is likely to seem somewhat arbitrary.

A *Small Change* is a modification involving not more than three nucleotides, and may be either a *Substitution*, an *Insertion* or a *Deletion*.

A *Gross Change* is any larger modification to a gene. A *Complete* change involves either the *Disruption* of the gene (i.e. inserting a sequence into the gene that prevents the expression of a functional product), the *Replacement* of the gene with another gene that can be expressed, or the *Deletion* of the entire gene. A *Partial* change in the gene involves either *Replacement* or *Deletion* of a length of sequence within the gene.

An example of an experiment that yields data that can be captured using the model in Figure 6 is described in El-Moghazy *et al.* (1999). In that experiment, one of the two copies of YLL035w, that encodes a hypothetical protein in yeast, was replaced with the KanMx marker gene in a heterozygous diploid strain of *S.cerevisiae* (FY1679). This can be represented in the model as a *Diploid* strain, where the strain has two *Allele*s for the *Gene* YLL035w, one of which is a *Wild Type*, and the other a *Mutant*. The *Mutant* is an example of a *Partial Replacement*. The subsequent popping out of the marker gene by homologous recombination resulted in a partial deletion of YLL035w. Sporulation resulted in four haploid spores (two with the same wild-type allele and two with the same partially deleted allele). Spores with the wild-type allele did not show any change in phenotype, while the effect of deletion on the haploid was the loss of its viability. This latter case is represented in the model as two *Haploid* strains. One of these strains has one *Wild Type* allele, and the other has one *Mutant* allele. The *Mutant* allele is a *Partial Deletion*.

A database of human mutations, including a description of a relational data model, is given in Attimonelli *et al.* (1999).

Implementation

This section presents an overview of the implementation context for the previous models under development in the Genome Information Management System (GIMS) project, which can be seen as a scientific data warehouse. A data warehouse is a repository for data that is also available elsewhere, where the data is replicated to allow complex analyses over that data. In Widom (1995), it is stated that the warehousing approach is appropriate in applications in which:

- clients require specific, predictable portions of the available information;

- clients require high performance;

- native applications at the information sources require high performance;

- clients want access to private copies of the information so that it can be modified, annotated and summarized.

All of these points are applicable to genome information management. However, there are a number of ways in which genome information management differs from classical business data warehousing applications (Anahory and Murray, 1997).

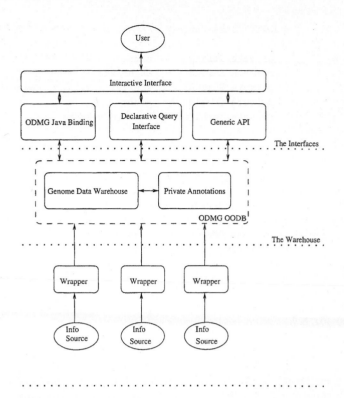

Fig. 7. Architecture of GIMS system.

- The core data set is much more complex (i.e. the core data set is that of the genome, rather than, for example, a collection of sales transactions).

- The data sets that 'surround' the core data set in *star schemas* are themselves likely to be complex, containing experimental results (e.g. expression data, protein-protein interaction data), rather than more straightforward product or supplier information.

- The role of aggregation in analyses is currently seen as less central to genome information management. Instead, the complexities in the analysis of genomic data often come from the substantial number of data types that may be visited during a single task, as analyses often involve navigation through a wide range of objects.

The architecture of the GIMS system is outlined in Figure 7. The core warehouse is an ODMG compliant object database (Cattell *et al.*, 1997), in our case POET. POET was chosen largely because it conforms with the ODMG standard, as we were keen not to develop a highly vendor-specific implementation. The database is accessed by the user interface through the standard ODMG Java binding, the declarative query language OQL, and a generic application programming interface. The latter is

```
public class Genome
{
  private String      name;
  private String      organism;
  private String      source;
  private double      size;
  private SetOfObject hasChromosomes;
  ...
}

public class Chromosome
{
  private String       number;
  private int          size;
  private Genome       hasGenome;
  private ListOfObject hasFragments;
  ...
}
```

Fig. 8. Java definitions for *Genome* and *Chromosome*.

necessary because some features of the user interface require access to the database in a manner that is data-type independent. For example, the classes used to implement forms in the browser are generic in the sense that their implementation contains no domain-specific code—the same user interface classes could be used to browse instances from any database.

At present, the core warehouse is populated principally using data from MIPS (Mewes *et al.*, 1997), and associated information is generally drawn via wrappers from remote sites. The principal way of accessing data within GIMS is expected to exploit *canned queries*—a canned query is a parameterized request for the result of a query or an analysis which has been anticipated by the developers of the database and coded as part of the interface. An early activity in the GIMS project was a requirements analysis which identified over 50 analysis tasks that potential users indicated they might be interested to ask over a genome information management system. These tasks will form the starting point for a canned query interface in a public version of GIMS in due course.

To give a flavour of the implementation, Figure 8 contains parts of the definitions of *Genome* and *Chromosome* in the syntax of the POET Java binding. Classes from Figure 1 are represented by database classes, and relationships are represented by attributes of these classes. For example, the fact that a *Chromosome* is associated with a single *Genome* is represented by the attribute *hasGenome* of *Chromosome*, and the fact that a *Chromosome* contains an ordered collection of *Chromosome Fragments* is represented by the *hasFragments* attribute of *Chromosome*. Inverses are stored for all relationships, so that they can

be explored in either direction. As well as the information provided by the Java class definitions, POET also provides a configuration file for describing indexes, extents, etc.

Discussion and conclusions

This paper has presented conceptual models for describing both genome sequences and related functional data sets. Although conceptual models can seem quite straightforward with hindsight, they are often difficult to develop; construction of the models presented in this paper was a lengthy and iterative process. The models produced have served as the starting point for an implementation activity in which the UML class diagrams are mapped to an object database schema. However, as conceptual representations of the data sets, these models could equally be mapped to different implementation platforms, such as alternative data models, or to object models for handling distributed data (e.g. CORBA) or transient data (e.g. Java).

The biological focus of the paper is, however, the key motivation for this work. Genome sequencing and functional genomics projects are making available new information resources that will motivate the development of a new generation of genome-level bioinformatics. However, it is clear that the information storage and analysis challenges of genomics are extremely great. Effective analysis of genomes will require high performance access to a diverse collection of complex information resources, which are typically developed at a range of sites. These information resources are made available in a wide range of formats, and generally in a form that allows the data to be browsed or downloaded, but not necessarily analysed effectively in conjunction with other information sources.

A number of researchers have investigated tools for distributed querying of biological sequence information sources (e.g. Buneman *et al.*, 1995; Chen *et al.*, 1997; Baker *et al.*, 1998). While some of us are involved in one such activity, we believe that the warehousing approach will be at least as relevant in the genomic area. The key difference in genomics is that typical analyses are likely to be much more complex than in non-genomic bioinformatics. In genomics, value is added through the close association of specific data resources, so that genomes can be compared with each other, and information from high throughput experiments, such as those relating to gene expression and protein-protein interactions, can be easily associated and displayed.

This paper seeks to provide one building block that is important to post-genomic bioinformatics—information models for a range of important, genome-level data sets. To be of practical use such models must be implemented, and search, analysis or visualization techniques developed for use with the models. However, all of these tasks will be made significantly more straightforward if the underlying data sets are described in a consistent and coherent manner. In providing high-level models of important data sets, we hope to provide a worthwhile foundation on which others can build.

Acknowledgements

We are pleased to acknowledge the support of the *BB-SRC/EPSRC* Bioinformatics Programme. Our understanding of transcriptome bioinformatics has benefited from interactions with Mike Cornell, Norman Morrison and Magnus Rattray. Karen Eilbeck was supported by a BBSRC CASE award with GlaxoWellcome.

References

Anahory,S. and Murray,D. (eds) (1997) *Data Warehousing in the Real World*. Addison-Wesley.

Attimonelli,M. *et al.* (1999) Update of the Human MitBASE database. *Nucleic Acids Res.*, **27**, 143–146.

Baker,P., Brass,A., Bechhofer,S., Goble,C., Paton,N. and Stevens,R. (1998) TAMBIS—transparent access to multiple biological information sources. In *Proceedings of the International Conference on Intelligent Systems for Molecular Biology*. AAAI Press, pp. 25–34.

Baker,P., Goble,C., Bechhofer,S., Paton,N., Stevens,R. and Brass,A. (1999) An ontology for bioinformatics applications. *Bioinformatics*, **15**, 510–520.

Barrilot,E. *et al.* (1999) A proposal for a standard CORBA interface for genome maps. *Bioinformatics*, **15**, 157–169.

Bartels,P., Bucher,P. and Hofmann,K. (1996) A protein linkage map of Escherichia coli bacteriophage—T7. *Nature Gen.*, **12**, 72–77.

Baudin,A., Ozier,K., Dennoul,A., Lacroute,F. and Cullin,C. (1993) A simple and efficient method for direct gene deletion in *S.cerevisiae*. *Nucleic Acid Res.*, **21**, 3329–3330.

Booch,G., Rumbaugh,J. and Jacobson,I. (eds) (1999) *The Unified Modelling Language User Guide*. Addison-Wesley.

Brazma,A., Robinson,A., Vilo,J., Vingron,M., Hoheisel,J., Fellenberg,K. and Muilu,J. (1999) Establishing a public repository for DNA array-based gene expression data. *EBI Technical Report* http://www.ebi.ac.uk/microarray/.

Buneman,P., Davidson,S., Hart,K., Overton,C. and Wong,L. (1995) A data transformation system for biological data sources. In *Proceedings of the 21st VLDB* Morgan Kaufmann, pp. 158–169.

Cattell,R. *et al.* (1997) *The Object Database Standard: ODMG 2.0*. Morgan Kaufmann.

Chen,I.-M.A., Kosky,A., Markowitz,V. and Szeto,E. (1997) Constructing and maintaining scientific database views in the framework of the Object Protocol Model. In *Proceedings of the SSDBM*. IEEE Press.

Chen,I.-M.A. and Markowitz,V. (1995) Modeling scientific experiments with an object data model. In *Proceedings of Data Engineering*. IEEE Press, pp. 391–400.

Delneri,D., Gardner,D. and Oliver,S. (1999) Analysis of the seven-member AAD gene set demonstrates that genetic redundancy in

yeast may bemore apparent than real. *Genetics*, 1591–1600.

Eilbeck,K., Brass,A., Paton,N. and Hodgman,C. (1999) INTER-ACT: an object oriented protein-protein interaction database. In*Proceedings of Intelligent Systems in Molecular Biology (ISMB)*. AAAI Press, pp. 87–94.

El-Moghazy,A., Zhang,N., Ismail,T., Wu,J., Butt,A., Khan,S., Merlotti,C., Woodwark,K., Gardner,D. and Oliver,S. (1999) Functional analysis of six ORFs on the left arm of chromosome XII in Saccharomyces cerevisiae reveals two essential genes, one of which is under cell-cycle control. *Yeast*, in press.

Ellis,L., Speedie,S. and McLeish,R. (1998) Representing metabolic pathway information: an object-oriented approach. *Bioinformatics*, **14**, 803–806.

Fromont-Racine,M., Rain,J. and Legrain,P. (1997) Toward a functional analysis of the yeast genome through exhaustive two-hybrid screens. *Nature Genetics*, **16**, 277–282.

Ghosh,D. (1999) Object oriented Transcription Factors Database (ooTFD). *Nucleic Acids Res.*, **27**, 315–317.

Gray,P., Paton,N., Kemp,G. and Fothergill,J. (1990) An Object-oriented database for protein structure analysis. *Protein Engineering*, **4**, 235–243.

Hu,J., Mungall,C., Nicholson,D. and Archibald,A. (1998) Design and implementation of a CORBA-based genome mapping system prototype. *Bioinformatics*, **14**, 112–120.

Jungfer,K. and Rodriguez-Tome,P. (1998) Mapplet: a CORBA-based genome map viewer. *Bioinformatics*, **14**, 734–738.

Maltchenko,S. (1998) The Bio-objects project. Part 1: The Object Data Model core elements. *Bioinformatics*, **14**, 479–485.

Medigue,C., Rechenmann,F., Danchin,A. and Viari,A. (1999) Imagene: an integrated computer environment for sequence annotation and analysis. *Bioinformatics*, **15**, 2–15.

Mewes,H., Albermann,K., Heumann,K., Liebl,S. and Pfeiffer,F. (1997) MIPS: a database for protein sequences, homology data and yeast genome information. *Nucleic Acids Res.*, **25**, 28–30.

Mewes,H., Hani,J., Pfeiffer,F. and Frishman,D. (1998) MIPS: a database for protein sequences and complete genomes. *Nucleic Acids Res.*, **26**, 33–37.

Okayama,T., Tamura,T., Gojobori,T., Tateno,Y., Ikeo,K., Miyazaki,S., Fukami-Kobayashi,K. and Sugawara,H. (1998) Formal design and implementation of an improved DDBJ DNA database with a new schema and object-oriented library. *Bioinformatics*, **14**, 472–478.

Oliver,S. (1996) From DNA sequence to biological function. *Nature*, **379**, 597–600.

Planta,R. *et al.* (1999) Transcript analysis of 250 novel yeast genes from chromosome XIV. *Yeast*, **15**, 329–350.

Spellman,P. *et al.* (1998) Comprehensive identification of cell cycle-regulated genes of the yeast *Saccharomyces cerivisiae* by microarray hybridization. *Mol. Biol. Cell*, **9**, 3273–3297.

Wach,A., Bracht,A., Pohlmann,R. and Philippsen,P. (1994) PCR synthesis of marker cassettes with long flanking homology regions for gene disruption in *S.cerevisiae*. *Yeast*, **10**, 1793–1808.

Widom,J. (1995) Research problems in data warehousing. In *Proceedings of the 4th International Conference on Information and Knowledge Management*, pp. 25–30.

A knowledge model for analysis and simulation of regulatory networks

Andrey Rzhetsky [1, 2,*], *Tomohiro Koike* [1, 3], *Sergey Kalachikov* [1], *Shawn M. Gomez* [1], *Michael Krauthammer* [2], *Sabina H. Kaplan* [1], *Pauline Kra* [2, 4], *James J. Russo* [1] *and Carol Friedman* [2, 5]

[1] *Columbia Genome Center, Columbia University,* [2] *Department of Medical Informatics, Columbia University,* [3] *Hitachi Software Engineering Co. Ltd,* [4] *Department of French, Yeshiva University and* [5] *Department of Computer Science, Queens College of the City University of New York*

Received on October 7, 1999; revised on April 24, 2000; accepted on July 20, 2000

Abstract

Motivation: In order to aid in hypothesis-driven experimental gene discovery, we are designing a computer application for the automatic retrieval of signal transduction data from electronic versions of scientific publications using natural language processing (NLP) techniques, as well as for visualizing and editing representations of regulatory systems. These systems describe both signal transduction and biochemical pathways within complex multicellular organisms, yeast, and bacteria. This computer application in turn requires the development of a domain-specific ontology, or knowledge model.

Results: We introduce an ontological model for the representation of biological knowledge related to regulatory networks in vertebrates. We outline a taxonomy of the concepts, define their 'whole-to-part' relationships, describe the properties of major concepts, and outline a set of the most important axioms. The ontology is partially realized in a computer system designed to aid researchers in biology and medicine in visualizing and editing a representation of a signal transduction system.

Availability: The knowledge model can be reviewed at http://genome6.cpmc.columbia.edu/tkoike/ontology/

Contact: ar345@columbia.edu

Introduction

A large body of knowledge that has become available recently through the internet consists of electronic versions of articles published in scientific journals, such as *Science* or *Cell*. This creates new opportunities for automated knowledge acquisition: if information contained in these articles can be extracted and organized, it could then be stored in a knowledge base and used in computational analyses such as data mining. While there is a prototype

---

*To whom correspondence should be addressed.

computer system for extracting medical knowledge from research articles in medicine (e.g. Hahn *et al.* (1996)), to our knowledge there is no equivalent system within the fields of Genomics and Molecular Biology. We aim to fill this gap by designing a system for the automatic extraction of functional information describing regulatory relationships between genes and proteins from online versions of research articles. Below, we provide the rationale for developing such a system.

The natural sciences proximal to molecular biology and medicine currently enjoy exponential growth. Individual researchers often find themselves unable to keep pace with the rate of information accumulating in multiple fields just outside their focus. Virtually every field of modern biology is likely to profit from the methodological advances that help scientists cope with information overflow. This is especially true for signal transduction-related research, where numerous investigators would benefit from systematic compilation, integration, and synthesis of thousands of disparate pieces of information scattered among individual research articles. For example, at the time that this paper was being revised, a search through the PubMed system using the keywords 'cell cycle' and 'apoptosis' produced lists of 169 293 and 29 961 articles, respectively (see http://www3.ncbi.nlm.nih.gov/Entrez/medline.html to access PubMed). It would be difficult and extremely time-consuming to navigate each of these articles manually. The biological community at large clearly needs specialized computer applications for the analysis of complex regulatory schemes; Such a program would facilitate the automatic retrieval of regulatory data from electronic versions of scientific publications using *natural language processing* (NLP) techniques (e.g. see literature on MedLEE, Friedman *et al.*, 1994), visualization and editing of representations of regulatory systems, and computer analysis and simulation of regulatory networks.

Each of these tasks requires the development of a domain-specific *ontology* tailored to the specific task of analyzing complex regulatory pathways in a particular organism. In this article we introduce such an ontology and describe properties that distinguish it from the already existing ontologies.

Background

Ontology

An ontology, conceptualization or *domain model* for a specialized field of science is usually defined as a collection of concepts representing domain-specific entities, concept definitions, a set of relationships among concepts ('semantic network'), properties of each concept, the range of allowed values for each property, and, in some cases, a set of explicit axioms defined on these concepts (Gruber, 1993).

Regulatory pathways

Regulation of tissue and organ development, as well as cell cycling and differentiation, is governed by a complex series of interactions between proteins and genes, in which one protein can 'switch off' or 'switch on' another protein, which in turn may stop or start its action on other proteins or genes. When a regulatory protein A is known to *increase* expression of gene B, biologists often say that 'A upregulates gene B,' while they say that 'A downregulates gene B' if protein A causes a *decrease* in the expression of gene B. While the actual regulation process is continuous and gradual, it is convenient to represent a regulatory network as a network of logical switches that can be turned on and off by other switches within the same network. For example, a process illustrating the regulation of long-term potentiation in human neurons is shown in Figure 1. In this figure, glutamate (here defined as a small molecule) binds and activates metabotropic receptor (a protein). Metabotropic receptor, in conjunction with G-protein activates another protein, PLC/PIC, and so on. Biologists may describe this as 'glutamate acts *upstream* of PLC/PIC,' and that 'PLC/PIC acts *downstream* of metabotropic receptor.'

In graph theory, a regulatory pathway is usually represented as an oriented graph with vertices corresponding to substances and edges corresponding to interactions (*Actions* in our ontology). So long as any oriented graph is completely defined by two sets, a set of vertices and a set of edges, any complex pathway can be fully encoded with a list of substances (vertices) and a list of interactions (edges) between them.

It is common practice in biology to represent large segments of regulatory networks with non-uniquely defined 'fuzzy' names. For example, in the sentence '*activation of MKK3 kinase triggers cell death*,' 'cell death' is a process including actions and substances that are not specified in the sentence, and '*MKK3 kinase*' is a substance (protein). Depending on the context, the term 'cell death' can represent one or a few different pathways leading to apoptosis, or it may correspond to just a fragment of the most downstream portion of a particular apoptotic pathway. Furthermore, the level of details showed in descriptions of the same regulatory pathway, usually considerably varies among journal papers. For example, the oriented graph shown in Figure 1 is commonly referred to in research articles as 'long-term potentiation' even though the number of proteins and genes included into a particular regulatory scheme can vary tenfold.

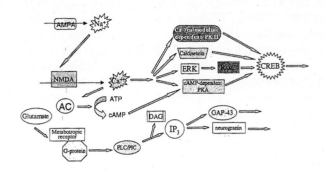

Fig. 1. Example of representation of a regulatory pathway (long-term potentiation in human neurons).

Natural language processing (NLP) techniques aimed at extracting information from electronic texts

In medicine, text reports of patient visits to their physicians are a vast source of clinical information, but such information in this 'raw' textual form is not useful for automated clinical applications (there may be numerous representations of the same piece of information) and although electronically available, this information remains locked within the text. Text is difficult to access because it is extremely diverse and meanings of words vary depending on their context. In spite of these underlying difficulties, NLP in the medical domain has begun to show promising results. For example, there are two NLP systems (Friedman *et al.*, 1994; Haug *et al.*, 1990; Hripcsak *et al.*, 1995) which are currently integrated into operational clinical information systems. Evaluating these systems clearly demonstrated that automated applications using NLP perform as well as or almost as well as medical experts in identifying abnormal conditions (Friedman *et al.*, 1994; Haug *et al.*, 1990; Hripcsak *et al.*, 1995).

Existing related systems

The molecular biology community possesses a number of online databases related to genomics research (Burks, 1999). GenBank (Benson *et al.*, 1998) contains nucleic acid sequence information, GDB (Fasman *et al.*, 1997) specializes in the location of genes on chromosomes, and PDB (Abola *et al.*, 1997) offers three-dimensional protein structures. Two databases targeted to the clinical community are OMIM (Pearson *et al.*, 1994), a database that maintains clinical phenotypes and their links to human genes, and Helix (Tarczy-Hornoch *et al.*, 1998), a database containing information about diseases, genetic testing, and laboratories in the United States that perform this testing.

Work in representing complex information has been done with a domain *independent* knowledge-based system called OWEB (Hon *et al.*, 1998), which was developed specifically for building and supporting shareable online scientific data resources. OWEB models complex information by using a knowledge base that contains meta-information about the data resources. This meta-information consists of a hierarchical taxonomy of concepts, specifications of relations between these concepts, as well as real-world objects, which are instances of concepts and relations. One application of this system resulted in the development of MHCWeb (Hon *et al.*, 1998), an online immunological knowledge base that contains information about peptide molecules and the set of major histocompatibility complex (MHC) molecules to which they bind, along with experimental and publication information.

Another complex modeling tool is the Oncology Thinking Cap (OncoTCAP) Ramakrishnan *et al.* (1998), which was developed to support learning and provide a means by which medical students, clinicians, and researchers can develop research and treatment strategies through simulation. OncoTCAP provides a simulation-modeling tool for expressing the complex concepts and explicit relationships associated with cancer research, treatment, apoptotic and mutational mechanisms, cell repair processes, treatment scheduling, and genetic characteristics.

Our research is similar to MHCWeb and OncoTCAP in that it models complex information and makes explicit relationships between informational concepts. Our work differs from the two systems in that our aim is to automatically acquire functional genomics knowledge through the extraction of relevant information from published articles using natural language processing methods.

For the construction of our ontology it was useful to include concepts from the UMLS (Unified Medical Language System of the National Library of Medicine in Washington, DC, McCray *et al.*, 1993), a comprehensive source of biomedical knowledge. The UMLS integrates biomedical terminology and organizes concepts into a hierarchy of classes. Some parts of UMLS, such as the Methathesaurus which incorporates classifications of diseases like ICD9, are immediately relevant to our ontology; other aspects of UMLS are either unrelated to our task or lack specifics essential for the computer representation and modeling of regulatory pathways. A detailed analysis of UMLS regarding the genomics domain is provided by Yu *et al.* (1999).

Other existing biological ontologies such as EcoCyc (Karp, 1991), Molecular Biology Ontology (Schulze-Kremer, 1997; Schulze-Kremer and King, 1992) and several other ontologies (Hafner *et al.*, 1994; Hafner and Fridman, 1996; Karp, 1998; Karp and Riley, 1993; Schulze-Kremer, 1998) are useful for our study as points of reference, but insufficient for our goal because they were developed for different applications.

EcoCyc (Karp, 1998) is a carefully designed ontology aimed at representing, modeling and visualizing *biochemical pathways in bacteria* (Karp *et al.*, 1999). Many features are relevant to our application: EcoCyc can both represent a range of complex biochemical reactions and allow for qualitative as well as quantitative modeling of each reaction. However, since this system targets only the representation of bacterial pathways, it does not reflect the multiplicity of cell types, tissues, organs, and developmental stages of multicellular organisms. Moreover, it deals mostly with linear or simple cyclic pathways typical of bacteria, rather than more complex graphs corresponding to regulatory networks in multicellular species. The design of EcoCyc was designed for input of data to be done by human experts and consequently does not consider issues arising when information is automatically extracted from literature using NLP techniques, such as conflicts between statements. Finally, EcoCyc is a proprietary commercially implemented ontology, not readily available in its complete form to the general public.

MBO, a Molecular Biology Ontology (Schulze-Kremer, 1997; Schulze-Kremer and King, 1992), is a *general* ontology for molecular biology which aims to collect 'all relevant concepts that are required to describe biological objects, experimental procedures and computational aspects of molecular biology.' As a general ontology, MBO contains large amounts of information that are important to their application whereas our model has a different focus. Our intention is to describe signal transduction as well as biochemical pathways in both complex and simple organisms through visualization and simulation.

Methods

In order to design the ontology, we manually collected more than 300 online journal articles from *Science, Nature, Proceedings of the National Academy of Sciences of the USA, Cell*, and *Current Biology*, which addressed regulation of 'programmed cell death' in animals. We then manually analyzed these articles with the aim of reconstructing a moderately complete regulatory network for this system. The selection of papers for this analysis was done through an iterative keyword search against an online reference database (MEDLINE, see http://www3.ncbi.nlm.nih.gov/Entrez/medline.html), followed by downloading relevant papers from Internet sites of the mentioned journals and manual review. The keywords used for the initial search were 'apoptosis' and the name of the publication, e.g. *Science*. We used the reconstructed network to iteratively and manually design a parsimonious representation capturing much of the information that a biologist might consider important when analyzing a regulatory network. While designing ontology we followed recommendations aimed at facilitating future 'graceful evolution' of the ontology (Cimino, 1998). Each iteration of the development process included a fine-tuning of the knowledge model followed by model verification through description of a part of the apoptotic network with the currently available tools of the ontology. Altogether four iterations of this kind were carried out.

Further, we downloaded twenty review articles from *Current Biology* and *Trends in Genetics*, all of which contained descriptions of relatively large regulatory pathways. We then manually analyzed descriptions of pathways in these articles attempting to use our knowledge model for the representation of information contained in each of these articles with the aim of verifying our ontology. Because the last verification required little fine-tuning of the model, we concluded that the model is sufficiently mature for current purposes. However, in the future it may be necessary to amend concepts and concept properties as the system moves toward novel computational problems and new aspects of the complex biological reality. Note that the current evaluation of the knowledge model is not a rigorous one because it was performed by the model developers rather than by a group of impartial experts.

Results and discussion

It is convenient to describe our ontology by considering its three main aspects: *taxonomy* of the concepts, *relations* between them, *properties* of the concepts, and axioms defined in the ontology; below we will follow this scheme.

Taxonomy of terms

The 'IS-A' relationships between concepts (relationships between a general concept and more concrete concepts, representing instances of the general concept) are often represented as trees (taxonomies) in which each edge represents one binary relation of this kind and each node is

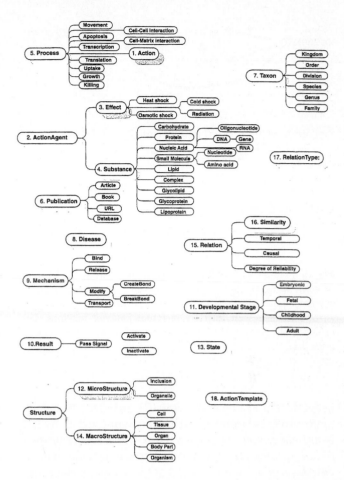

Fig. 2. Top-level taxonomy ('IS-A' relationships, indicated with continuous lines, and 'is associated with' relationships, indicated with dashed lines) of concepts. *Substances* and *Actions* are the central concepts in this ontology; *Taxon, Structure, Publication,* and *Disease* are required to specify the living organism, the structure within the organism, the source of the information and the malady associated with each individual *Action* and *Substance*. *Stimulus* and *Process* are categories associated with the external triggers of the regulatory cascades in a living organism, and the macroevents within an organism that involve multiple regulatory steps, correspondingly. Finally, *Relation* is a separate concept permitting the ordering of *Actions* and *Processes* in three different ways (cf. Figure 4).

occupied by a concept (see Figure 2). Each of the basic concepts, depicted in this figure serves as a root for a separate tree: *Action, ActionAgent, Process, Publication, Taxon, Disease, Mechanism, Result, Developmental Stage, MicroStructure, State, MacroStructure, Relation, Similarity, RelationType,* and *ActionTemplate*. The most important among these concepts are *ActionAgent* and *Action*. The former most frequently corresponds to a *Substance* (a protein, a gene or other molecule) and the latter to an *interaction* between two or more molecules in a regulatory

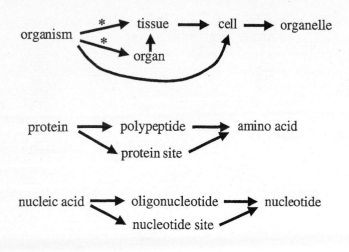

Fig. 3. Example of 'PART-TO-WHOLE' relationships ('HAS-A') between some of the categories shown in Figure 1. Each arrow corresponds to a single 'HAS-A' relationship between two concepts. Arrows marked with asterisks represent *optional* relations. For example, not every organism has organs and tissues because many organisms are unicellular. Note that, unlike the taxonomies of categories, these graphs are not trees.

network. For example, proteins IP3 and GAP-43 belong to the group *substances*, and activation of GAP-43 by IP3 is an *interaction* (see Figure 1). A less frequent type of *ActionAgent* is *Effect*, introduced here to reflect inputs or outcomes of an action that can not be correctly characterized within *Substances*. Among the most common examples of input *Effect* found in the biological literature are heat shock, cold shock, osmotic shock, radiation, electrical stimulation, tension, and starvation. Mechanisms of *Action* in our model are limited to their 'normal' repertoire in animal signal transduction systems. One can think of 'abnormal' actions that we are not including into our ontology at this stage.

Next in rank by importance are *Process* and *Relation*. In our ontology, *Process* represents a set of several *Substances*, at least some of which are linked by *Actions* or *Relations*. *Process* also represents a set of other *Processes* or a mixture of *Actions* and *Processes*. Finally, *Publication, Taxon, Structure, Developmental Stage, and Disease* encapsulate pieces of auxiliary information about *ActionAgents, Processes* and *Actions*. These concepts indicate the source of knowledge (e.g. a book), taxonomic position of the organism (e.g. *Homo sapiens*), anatomical structure (which can be a macro-structure, such as an organ or a tissue, or a micro-structure, such as a mitochondrion), a stage in ontogenesis (e.g. fetal), and a malady (e.g. cancer), respectively. The concept *Disease* corresponds to a large list of specific maladies and syndromes, which are taken from UMLS (data not shown).

Note, that although the current 'IS-A' graph is a strict

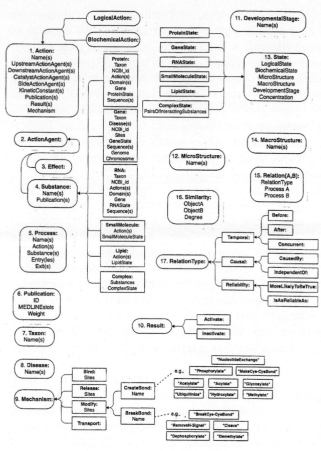

Fig. 4. Properties of major concepts. The frame *Publication* contains a slot called 'MEDLINE slots' referring to types of information ('fields') used in the MEDLINE reference database (http://www3.ncbi.nlm.nih.gov/Entrez/). These fields include: title of publication, names of the authors, year, journal volume, journal number, page numbers, abstract, keywords and some others. The frame *Actions* has a slot called *KineticConstants,* which refers to constants characterizing kinetics of the interaction between two or more molecules. The slots *MicroStructure* and *MacroStructure* in the frame *State* must refer to the location of the corresponding substance within the organism at several structural levels: organ, tissue, cell type, and organelle (see Figure 7).

taxonomy (tree), the future evolution of the knowledge model may require addition of edges representing relation of multiple inheritance between concepts. In this case the oriented graph will cease to be a tree but it will always remain acyclic.

Relations between concepts

To bring our ontology closer to the language used by biologists, we defined a network of 'HAS-A' relations (= 'part-whole' relations between concepts). A part of this network is shown in Figure 3. This network explicitly specifies 'part–whole' relations between concepts and the possibility that terms may have several different meanings, common in the language of experimental biology and medicine, where the same word, e.g. *cell*, may refer to distinct entities with very different properties (e.g. cells in Eukaryotes, Eubacteria and Archaea), and can correspond to either a part of an organism, or the whole organism.

Properties of concepts, slots and admissible values

The properties of the above concepts can be conveniently described using *frame* representation (Gruber, 1993).

In this representation, each concept is described with a 'frame' having a *name* (e.g. *Substance*) unique for the given domain and *slots* which can be filled by values of a specified type and range (see Figure 4). For example, following an expert's advise (Cimino, 1998) that a well-designed ontology needs to 'have the unique identifiers for the concepts which are free of hierarchical or other implicit meaning (i.e. nonsemantic concept identifiers),' we provided each concept with a slot 'ConceptID,' which should hold a unique numeric value for each concept. The slot *Name(s)* may contain a single string or a set of strings representing alternative names of the same substance, and the slot *Publication(s)* must refer to a concept object defined with the frame named *Publication*. Figure 4 depicts the current knowledge model, which utilizes these features and illustrates the concepts first introduced in Figure 2.

Similarities and differences with EcoCyc

We adopted a number of important features from the EcoCyc (Karp, 1998) ontology. Most importantly, the structure of the concept *Action* in our ontology is based on the concepts *reaction* and *enzymatic reaction* in EcoCyc. Following EcoCyc, we explicitly specify *sideAction-Agents* and *mainActionAgents*, a *CatalystActionAgent*. Likewise, our concepts *UpstreamActionAgents and DownstreamActionAgents* are not unlike the EcoCyc concepts reaction left side and reaction right side, respectively. In the Biochemical Representation A phosphorylates B in Figure 6, The *sideActionAgent* is ATP, the *mainActionAgent* is B, and the *CatalystActionAgent* is A. Meanwhile, the logical representation of the same action, the *UpstreamActionAgent* is A and the *DownstreamActionAgent* is B.

Also analogous to EcoCyc's *isozyme-sequence-similarity* is our concept *Similarity*. Our definition describes both primary sequences and three-dimensional protein structures, where similarity at the sequence level is not required (see Murzin and Bateman, 1997).

The concept *ActionAgent* is somewhat parallel to the *compound* concept of EcoCyc. In addition, it includes *Effect*, which is not a substance. For example, in the statement 'ultraviolet light can induce expression of the p53 gene,' 'ultraviolet light' is an *effect* and p53 gene is a *substance* (gene) activated via an unspecified mechanism.

EcoCyc (Karp, 1998) is very well designed for representing metabolic pathways of bacteria, and therefore it includes details of cell morphology of prokaryotic species (e.g. *cytoplasm, membrane, inner-membrane, outer-membrane, membrane-spanning, periplasm*). Because our model seeks to describe signal transduction and biochemical pathways in eukaryotes as well as bacterial, it includes the additional concepts of tissues, body parts, organs, developmental stages, and cellular organelles that distinguish multicellular eukaryotes from prokaryotes (see Figure 4).

Signal transduction pathways are currently described as a mixture of two representations, logical and biochemical

Analyzing the language of current biological literature reveals a curious mixture of two different representations of regulatory pathways, which we will denote here as *logical* and *biochemical* (see Figure 6). The 'logical' representation handles changes in 'logical states' of the proteins and genes, while the 'biochemical' representation defines the chemical or physical mechanism leading to a change in the logical state of a substance. A single logical description 'A activates B' can correspond to a multiplicity of biochemical descriptions. Regulatory diagrams in present-day research articles often blend both logical and biochemical descriptions in the same figure. Moreover, situations where only the logical description of an action may be inferred from experimental data are common. The availability of only a biochemical action description is a dominant feature in the portrayal of *metabolic pathways*, such as synthesis of fatty acids; in contrast, actions with only well-defined logical descriptions are foremost in the portrayal of *signal transduction pathways*, such as cell cycle regulation. Similar to the described duality of *Action*, we define two properties of *State* for each substance: *LogicalState* and *BiochemicalState*. Without contextual information, a property cannot be directly inferred from the other. For example, a protein that is phosphorylated (*BiochemicalState*) can be in either active or inactive *LogicalState*.

In signal transduction literature it is possible to observe both logical and biochemical representations of an action combined within a single sentence of a research article. For example, in the following sentence taken from an actual research article (Boussiotis *et al.*, 1997)

'Activated Raf-1 phosphorylates and activates MEK-1...'

one can clearly distinguish the logical action between proteins Raf-1 and MEK-1 ('activate') and the biochemical mechanism of the action ('phosphorylate').

Because signal transduction pathways use a rather limited repertoire of biochemical reactions, such as *phospho-*

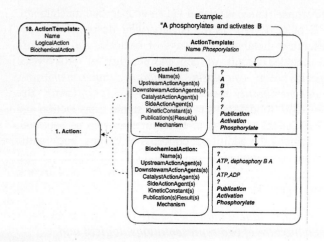

Fig. 5. An additional concept of *ActionTemplate* is designed to store rules of conversion of *LogicalAction* to corresponding *BiochemicalAction* and *vice versa*.

rylation, dephosphorylation, cleavage, etc. (see Figure 6), a logical description can often be converted to its corresponding biochemical description (or vice versa) automatically. For this purpose we introduce the *ActionTemplate* concept, which defines rules of converting of a logical action representation into the corresponding biochemical representation, or the other way around, assuming that the required information is present (see Figure 5).

Consensus-level conceptualization vs observation-level conceptualization

Most of the existing knowledge models, including EcoCyc (Karp, 1998), are oriented toward *consensus-level* conceptualization. This means that data inconsistencies are removed or resolved by domain experts before the data is represented with a knowledge model. This is impractical in the case of automatic extraction of data from original research articles: the 'raw' data obtained in this way are bound to contain inconsistencies and even mutually exclusive statements. Therefore, in our application we adopt an *observation-level* conceptualization rather than a consensus-level conceptualization. Each statement in our knowledge base will be given a 'weight,' a real number measuring the 'credibility' of the statement and computed as described below.

We reason that as controversies and occasional errors are unavoidable realities of a productive research process, Natural Language Processing analysis is destined to produce some contradictory and incorrect statements. Observation-level conceptualization would potentially allow the retention of original natural language passages containing primary information, thus enabling an individual researcher accessing our system to make independent

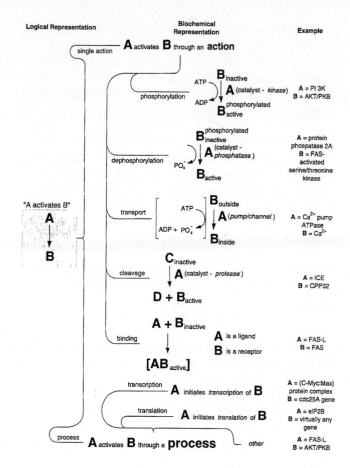

Fig. 6. Multiple biochemical representations corresponding to a single logical representation. A similar figure corresponds to the logical representation 'A inhibits B.'

decisions on the quality of different pieces of information. In order to determine the 'credibility' of a statement, we introduce a set of weights that take into account the reliability of an individual journal, the publication year, particular authors, and the section within an article (e.g. 'Discussion') in which particular statements appeared. (Similarly, if a statement in a research article is a citation of the previous work, it may be given lower weight than that of an original experimental observation.) This should provide a flexible mechanism for re-defining the regulatory model along with an accumulation of knowledge about previous errors. It would be desirable, for example, to exclude from analysis a statement that appeared in a retracted article, in an article with an erratum published later, or derived from an experiment that was not successfully reproduced. (A hypothetical example: one may decide to exclude all papers published before 1990 because of an unreliable, older experimental technique that was replaced in 1990.)

A weight for each binary action (statement) can be

possibility that terms may have several different meanings, common in the language of experimental biology and medicine, where the same word, e.g. *cell*, may refer to distinct entities with very different properties (e.g. cells in Eukaryotes, Eubacteria and Archaea), and can correspond to either a part of an organism, or the whole organism.

Properties of concepts, slots and admissible values

The properties of the above concepts can be conveniently described using *frame* representation (Gruber, 1993).

In this representation, each concept is described with a 'frame' having a *name* (e.g. *Substance*) unique for the given domain and *slots* which can be filled by values of a specified type and range (see Figure 4). For example, following an expert's advise (Cimino, 1998) that a well-designed ontology needs to 'have the unique identifiers for the concepts which are free of hierarchical or other implicit meaning (i.e. nonsemantic concept identifiers),' we provided each concept with a slot 'ConceptID,' which should hold a unique numeric value for each concept. The slot *Name(s)* may contain a single string or a set of strings representing alternative names of the same substance, and the slot *Publication(s)* must refer to a concept object defined with the frame named *Publication*. Figure 4 depicts the current knowledge model, which utilizes these features and illustrates the concepts first introduced in Figure 2.

Similarities and differences with EcoCyc

We adopted a number of important features from the EcoCyc (Karp, 1998) ontology. Most importantly, the structure of the concept *Action* in our ontology is based on the concepts *reaction* and *enzymatic reaction* in EcoCyc. Following EcoCyc, we explicitly specify *sideAction-Agents* and *mainActionAgents*, a *CatalystActionAgent*. Likewise, our concepts *UpstreamActionAgents and DownstreamActionAgents* are not unlike the EcoCyc concepts reaction left side and reaction right side, respectively. In the Biochemical Representation A phosphorylates B in Figure 6, The *sideActionAgent* is ATP, the *mainActionAgent* is B, and the *CatalystActionAgent* is A. Meanwhile, the logical representation of the same action, the *UpstreamActionAgent* is A and the *DownstreamActionAgent* is B.

Also analogous to EcoCyc's *isozyme-sequence-similarity* is our concept *Similarity*. Our definition describes both primary sequences and three-dimensional protein structures, where similarity at the sequence level is not required (see Murzin and Bateman, 1997).

The concept *ActionAgent* is somewhat parallel to the *compound* concept of EcoCyc. In addition, it includes *Effect*, which is not a substance. For example, in the statement 'ultraviolet light can induce expression of the p53 gene,' 'ultraviolet light' is an *effect* and p53 gene is a *substance* (gene) activated via an unspecified mechanism.

EcoCyc (Karp, 1998) is very well designed for representing metabolic pathways of bacteria, and therefore it includes details of cell morphology of prokaryotic species (e.g. *cytoplasm, membrane, inner-membrane, outer-membrane, membrane-spanning, periplasm*). Because our model seeks to describe signal transduction and biochemical pathways in eukaryotes as well as bacterial, it includes the additional concepts of tissues, body parts, organs, developmental stages, and cellular organelles that distinguish multicellular eukaryotes from prokaryotes (see Figure 4).

Signal transduction pathways are currently described as a mixture of two representations, logical and biochemical

Analyzing the language of current biological literature reveals a curious mixture of two different representations of regulatory pathways, which we will denote here as *logical* and *biochemical* (see Figure 6). The 'logical' representation handles changes in 'logical states' of the proteins and genes, while the 'biochemical' representation defines the chemical or physical mechanism leading to a change in the logical state of a substance. A single logical description 'A activates B' can correspond to a multiplicity of biochemical descriptions. Regulatory diagrams in present-day research articles often blend both logical and biochemical descriptions in the same figure. Moreover, situations where only the logical description of an action may be inferred from experimental data are common. The availability of only a biochemical action description is a dominant feature in the portrayal of *metabolic pathways*, such as synthesis of fatty acids; in contrast, actions with only well-defined logical descriptions are foremost in the portrayal of *signal transduction pathways*, such as cell cycle regulation. Similar to the described duality of *Action*, we define two properties of *State* for each substance: *LogicalState* and *BiochemicalState*. Without contextual information, a property cannot be directly inferred from the other. For example, a protein that is phosphorylated (*BiochemicalState*) can be in either active or inactive *LogicalState*.

In signal transduction literature it is possible to observe both logical and biochemical representations of an action combined within a single sentence of a research article. For example, in the following sentence taken from an actual research article (Boussiotis *et al.*, 1997)

'Activated Raf-1 phosphorylates and activates MEK-1…'

one can clearly distinguish the logical action between proteins Raf-1 and MEK-1 ('activate') and the biochemical mechanism of the action ('phosphorylate').

Because signal transduction pathways use a rather limited repertoire of biochemical reactions, such as *phospho-*

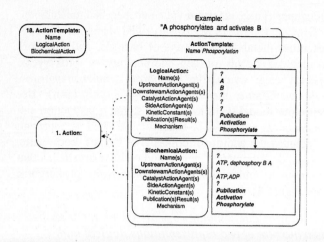

Fig. 5. An additional concept of *ActionTemplate* is designed to store rules of conversion of *LogicalAction* to corresponding *BiochemicalAction* and *vice versa*.

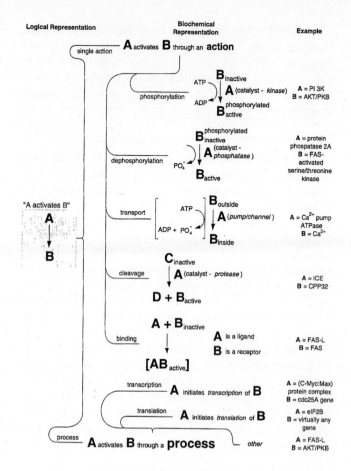

Fig. 6. Multiple biochemical representations corresponding to a single logical representation. A similar figure corresponds to the logical representation 'A inhibits B.'

rylation, dephosphorylation, cleavage, etc. (see Figure 6), a logical description can often be converted to its corresponding biochemical description (or vice versa) automatically. For this purpose we introduce the *ActionTemplate* concept, which defines rules of converting of a logical action representation into the corresponding biochemical representation, or the other way around, assuming that the required information is present (see Figure 5).

Consensus-level conceptualization vs observation-level conceptualization

Most of the existing knowledge models, including EcoCyc (Karp, 1998), are oriented toward *consensus-level* conceptualization. This means that data inconsistencies are removed or resolved by domain experts before the data is represented with a knowledge model. This is impractical in the case of automatic extraction of data from original research articles: the 'raw' data obtained in this way are bound to contain inconsistencies and even mutually exclusive statements. Therefore, in our application we adopt an *observation-level* conceptualization rather than a consensus-level conceptualization. Each statement in our knowledge base will be given a 'weight,' a real number measuring the 'credibility' of the statement and computed as described below.

We reason that as controversies and occasional errors are unavoidable realities of a productive research process, Natural Language Processing analysis is destined to produce some contradictory and incorrect statements. Observation-level conceptualization would potentially allow the retention of original natural language passages containing primary information, thus enabling an individual researcher accessing our system to make independent decisions on the quality of different pieces of information. In order to determine the 'credibility' of a statement, we introduce a set of weights that take into account the reliability of an individual journal, the publication year, particular authors, and the section within an article (e.g. 'Discussion') in which particular statements appeared. (Similarly, if a statement in a research article is a citation of the previous work, it may be given lower weight than that of an original experimental observation.) This should provide a flexible mechanism for re-defining the regulatory model along with an accumulation of knowledge about previous errors. It would be desirable, for example, to exclude from analysis a statement that appeared in a retracted article, in an article with an erratum published later, or derived from an experiment that was not successfully reproduced. (A hypothetical example: one may decide to exclude all papers published before 1990 because of an unreliable, older experimental technique that was replaced in 1990.)

A weight for each binary action (statement) can be

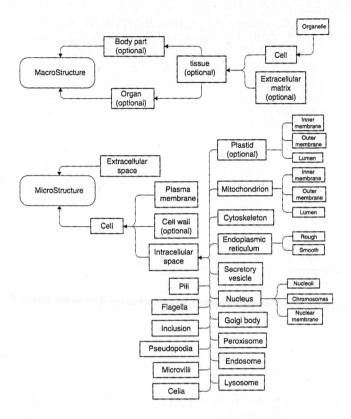

Fig. 7. Models corresponding to concepts *MicroStructure* and *MacroStructure*.

computed according to the following 'equations' where *W(x)* is defined as 'the weight of *x*.'

W(a statement) = A weighted sum of W(all sentences related to this statement)

W(a sentence related to the statement) = W(journal, year, authors, article, etc.).

The sum of the first 'formula' is weighted in order to allow for downweighting multiple identical statements from the same paper and from different papers of the same authors. In the simplest scheme, the weight of a sentence would be defined as a product of the individual weights of journal, year, author, etc. Once all the weights are explicitly defined, it is trivial to compute a weight for each statement and for each statement's negation. For each set of conflicting statements, only the statement with the largest weight would be selected for visualization and simulation. The goal of this is to create a scenario in which a researcher can easily trace individual statements and corresponding sentences, remove erroneous data, and downweight equivocal statements. We intend to implement an 'iterative editing' regime, where a researcher can begin to visualize or simulate a pathway, then 'descend'

to statements and sentences (each sentence highlighted within the text of the corresponding article or shown independently) related to a particular part of the pathway, redefine weights, and again 'ascend' to a modified visual representation and dynamic model of the same pathway, repeating this cycle as often as desired. This weight scheme may potentially accommodate fluctuations in the dominant scientific paradigm: different paradigms would correspond to different sets of weights for the same collection of statements.

Axioms

The area of molecular biology describing signal transduction incorporates a set of axioms that are implicit for biologists, but should be specified explicitly within a knowledge model. The fundamental axiom of molecular biology can be formulated in the following way; 'For every protein there is a unique mRNA, and for every mRNA there is a unique gene or a unique set of genes.' Among other important axioms are the following three:

1. If *ActionAgent* A is upstream to *ActionAgent* B in an action, and the action *Result* is defined, the *ActionAgent* A is active.

2. If *ActionAgent* A is situated downstream in an action and the action *Result* is *Activate*, the *ActionAgent* A is active.

3. If *ActionAgent* A is situated downstream in an action and the action result is *Inactivate*, the ActionAgent A is *inactive*.

A few other axioms used in logical and biochemical representation of actions are shown in Figure 8.

Conclusion

With the goal of developing computational tools for the analysis of signal transduction pathways, we have introduced ontology suitable for the description and modeling of regulatory pathways in multicellular and unicellular species. This ontology has a number of common features with EcoCyc and several other existing ontologies, but differs significantly from them in a number of features, most important of which is that it allows for modeling both Boolean ('logical') and biochemical pathways, multiple cells, tissues, and organ types, as well as representing partial and/or conflicting information.

Acknowledgements

This study was partially supported by grants from the Center for Advanced Technology, New York State, and from Hitachi Software Engineering Co. Ltd.

Logical result-related axioms

1. Transitivity. If A activates B and B activates C, it is valid to state that A activates C.

2. Additivity. A logical result of a pathway can be calculated as a sum of results of separate actions along the pathway.

Biochemical mechanism-related axioms (in the form **mechanism**[subject substance, object substance])

1. **Transcribe**[gene]

2. **Translate**[mRNA]

3. **Phosphorylate**[protein (kinase), protein]

4. **Dephosphorylate**[protein (phosphatase), protein]

5. **Methylate**[protein (methylase), gene OR protein OR lipid]

6. **Demethylate**[protein (demethylase), protein OR lipid]

7. **Cleave**[protein, gene OR protein OR lipid OR RNA OR
　　　　　　　　small molecule OR carbohydrate]
  Cleave[RNA, RNA]
  Cleave[small molecule, protein OR gene OR lipid OR RNA OR
　　　　　　　　small molecule OR carbohydrate]

8. **Bind**[protein, protein OR RNA OR gene]
  Bind[RNA, RNA OR gene]
  Bind[small molecule, protein OR gene OR lipid OR RNA OR small
　　　　　　　　molecule]

9. **Transport**[protein, protein OR gene OR lipid OR RNA OR small molecule]
  Transport[RNA, small molecule]

Fig. 8. Major axioms of the knowledge model described in this paper. A more complete set of axioms will be made available through the Internet in near future.

References

Abola,E.E., Sussman,J.L., Prilusky,J. and Manning,N.O. (1997) Protein Data Bank archives of three-dimensional macromolecular structures. *Meth. Enzymol.*, **277**, 556–571.

Benson,D.A., Boguski,M.S., Lipman,D.J., Ostell,J. and Ouellette,B.F. (1998) GenBank. *Nucleic Acids Res.*, **26**, 1–7.

Boussiotis,V.A., Freeman,G.J., Berezovskaya,A., Barber,D.L. and Nadler,L.M. (1997) Maintenance of human T cell anergy: blocking of IL-2 gene transcription by activated Rap1. *Science*, **278**, 124–128.

Burks,C. (1999) Molecular biology database list. *Nucleic Acids Res.*, **27**, 1–9.

Cimino,J.J. (1998) Desiderata for controlled medical vocabularies in the twenty-first century. *Meth. Infect. Med.*, **37**, 394–403.

Fasman,K.H., Letovsky,S.I., Li,P., Cottingham,R.W. and Kingsbury,D.T. (1997) The GDB Human Genome Database Anno 1997. *Nucleic Acids Res.*, **25**, 72–81.

Friedman,C., Alderson,P.O., Austin,J.H., Cimino,J.J. and Johnson,S.B. (1994) A general natural-language text processor for clinical radiology. *J. Am. Med. Inform. Assoc.*, **1**, 161–174.

Gruber,T.R. (1993) *Towards Principles for the Design of Ontologies Used for Knowledge Sharing: Knowledge Systems Laboratory.* Stanford University.

Hafner,C.D., Baclawski,K., Futrelle,R.P., Fridman,N. and Sampath,S. (1994) Creating a knowledge base of biological research papers. *Ismb*, **2**, 147–155.

Hafner,C.D. and Fridman,N. (1996) Ontological foundations for biology knowledge models. *Ismb*, **4**, 78–87.

Haug,P.J., Ranum,D.L. and Frederick,P.R. (1990) Computerized extraction of coded findings from free-text radiologic reports. Work in progress. *Radiology*, **174**, 543–548.

Hon,L., Abernethy,N.F., Brusic,V., Chai,J. and Altman,R.B. (1998) MHCWeb: converting a WWW database into a knowledge-based collaborative environment. *Proc. AMIA Symp.*, 947–951.

Hripcsak,G., Friedman,C., Alderson,P.O., DuMouchel,W., Johnson,S.B. and Clayton,P.D. (1995) Unlocking clinical data from narrative reports: a study of natural language processing. *Ann. Int. Med.*, **122**, 681–688.

Karp,P.D. (1991) Artificial intelligence methods for theory representation and hypothesis formation. *Comput. Appl. Biosci.*, **7**, 301–308.

Karp,P.D. (1998) Metabolic databases. *Trends Biochem. Sci.*, **23**, 114–116.

Karp,P.D. and Riley,M. (1993) Representations of metabolic knowledge. *Ismb*, **1**, 207–215.

Karp,P.D., Riley,M., Paley,S.M., Pellegrini-Toole,A. and Krummenacker,M. (1999) Eco Cyc: Encyclopedia of *Escherichia coli* genes and metabolism. *Nucleic Acids Res.*, **27**, 55–58.

McCray,A.T., Aronson,A.R., Browne,A.C., Rindflesch,T.C., Razi,A. and Srinivasan,S. (1993) UMLS knowledge for biomedical language processing. *Bull. Med. Libr. Assoc.*, **81**, 184–194.

Murzin,A.G. and Bateman,A. (1997) Distant homology recognition using structural classification of proteins. *Proteins*, (Suppl 1), 105–112.

Pearson,P., Francomano,C., Foster,P., Bocchini,C., Li,P. and McKusick,V. (1994) The status of online Mendelian inheritance in man (OMIM) medio 1994. *Nucleic Acids Res.*, **22**, 3470–3473.

Schulze-Kremer,S. (1997) Adding semantics to genome databases: towards an ontology for molecular biology. *Ismb*, **5**, 272–275.

Schulze-Kremer,S. (1998) Ontologies for molecular biology. *Pacific Symp. Biocomput.*, 695–706.

Schulze-Kremer,S. and King,R.D. (1992) IPSA-inductive protein structure analysis. *Protein Eng*, **5**, 377–390.

Tarczy-Hornoch,P., Covington,M.L., Edwards,J., Shannon,P., Fuller,S. and Pagon,R.A. (1998) Creation and maintenance of helix, a web based database of medical genetics laboratories, to serve the needs of the genetics community. *Proc. AMIA Symp.*, 341–345.

Yu,H., Friedman,C., Rzhetsky,A. and Kra,P. (1999) Representing genomic knowledge in the UMLS semantic network. *AMIA 1999 Fall Annual Symposium*.

Authors' Index of Selected Articles

MeSH Index of Selected Articles

MeSH Index of Selected Articles (continued)